Inflammatory Bowel Disease

Inflammatory Bowel Disease

Edited by

JOSEPH B. KIRSNER, M.D., Ph.D.

Louis Block Distinguished Service Professor of Medicine
Formerly Chief of Staff and Deputy Dean for Medical Affairs
University of Chicago
Department of Medicine
Chicago, Illinois

ROY G. SHORTER, M.D.

Consultant, Departments of Pathology and Medicine,
Mayo Clinic and Mayo Foundation
Professor of Medicine and Pathology, Mayo Medical School
Rochester, Minnesota

THIRD EDITION

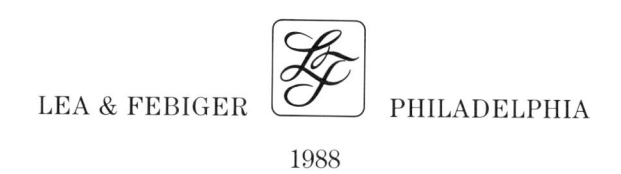

LEA & FEBIGER   PHILADELPHIA

1988

LEA & FEBIGER
600 Washington Square
Philadelphia, Pa. 19106
(215) 922-1330

Library of Congress Cataloging-in-Publication Data

Inflammatory bowel disease.

Includes bibliographies and index.

1. Ulcerative colitis. 2. Enteritis, Regional.
I. Kirsner, Joseph B., 1909-   . II. Shorter, Roy G. (Roy Gerrard), 1925-   . [DNLM: 1. Colitis, Ulcerative. 2. Crohn Disease. WI 522 I43]
RC862.C63I54 1988   616.3′447   87-2966
ISBN 0-8121-1092-7

Copyright © 1988 by Lea & Febiger. Copyright under the International Copyright Union. All Rights Reserved. This book is protected by copyright. No part of it may be reproduced in any manner or by any means without written permission of the publisher.

PRINTED IN THE UNITED STATES OF AMERICA

Print No.   3   2   1

to Minnie and Rhiannon

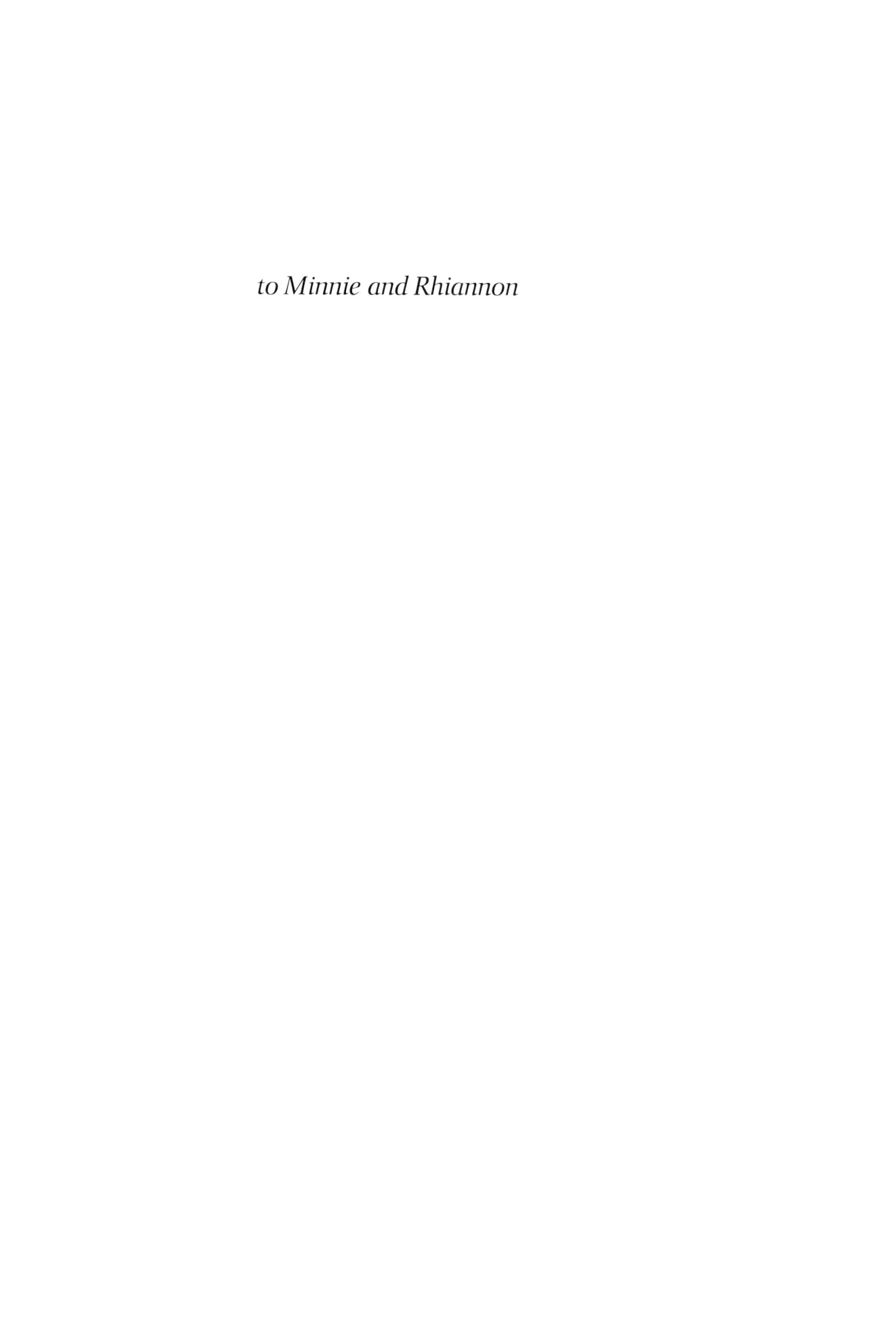

Preface

Idiopathic inflammatory bowel disease (IBD: ulcerative colitis, and Crohn's disease) is a major medical and surgical problem in the western world that has challenged and fascinated many physicians and an ever-increasing number of investigators in various disciplines. As a result, knowledge concerning inflammatory bowel disease has advanced since the first two editions of *Inflammatory Bowel Disease* were published. While the cause or causes of chronic ulcerative colitis (CUC) and Crohn's disease (CD) remain elusive, more has been learned about their clinical manifestations, courses, complications, and treatments. Research into IBD has yielded important information on many aspects of gastrointestinal function, including mechanisms of intestinal inflammation as well as the immunologic capabilities of the gut. This research has also indicated new directions for future study.

In order to review and correlate these advances, this third edition of *Inflammatory Bowel Disease* has virtually been rewritten. Of the 43 contributing authors, each an active investigator of IBD, 32 are new to this edition. Preceded by a completely revised chapter on epidemiology, the section on etiopathogenesis includes reviews of experimental IBD, the intestinal microflora, intestinal defense mechanisms, the membranous epithelial M cell, and the immunologic and genetic features of IBD. The second section includes the clinical and laboratory findings in CUC and CD, both in adults and in children; the pathophysiology of these diseases; the differential diagnosis; and their gastrointestinal and extraintestinal complications, including the risks of gastrointestinal malignancy. The effects of IBD on fertility, and the problems introduced by the coexistence of pregnancy and CUC or CD, are also considered. In the fourth and fifth sections, other authors deal with the pathology, and the endoscopic and radiologic findings in IBD, respectively. The first part of the section on therapy details the medical treatment of CUC and CD in adults and children, including the nutritional consequences and their management in IBD. Then the opinions of a gastroenterologist on the indications for surgical therapy are presented, followed by the opinions of a surgeon. Other contributors deal with the complications of surgical intervention, the conventional ileostomy, the newer operations for ulcerative colitis and Crohn's disease, and the physiologic consequences of surgical treatment. The book concludes with a chapter on prognosis, documenting the improved outlook for those with CUC or Crohn's disease, and a chapter on the fallibility of activity indices in Crohn's disease.

In such a volume, it is necessary that there be some areas of repetition, these are intended to be convenient for the reader; in addition, it is inevitable that some disagreements emerge. Indeed, if the latter did not exist, our understanding of IBD would be so complete that a book on the topic would no longer be appropriate.

The theme of this third edition of *Inflammatory Bowel Disease* is expressed by the words of Louis Pasteur: "In the field of observation, chance only favors the prepared mind." This book "prepares" clinicians and investigators with the information on IBD that has been accumulated up to now, and thus increases the possibility that soon there will be significant advances toward finding the causes and cure.

Chicago, Illinois JOSEPH B. KIRSNER
Rochester, Minnesota ROY G. SHORTER

Acknowledgment

The editors thank their secretaries Ms. Jean Dornseif and Ms. Sandy Groth for their invaluable help in the preparation of this book.

Contributors

THEODORE M. BAYLESS, M.D.
Professor of Medicine
The Johns Hopkins School of Medicine
Director, Meyerhoff Digestive Disease-Inflammatory
Bowel Disease Center
Johns Hopkins Hospital
Baltimore, MD

W.L. BEEKEN, M.D.
Professor of Medicine
University of Vermont
Burlington, Vermont

GEORGE E. BLOCK, M.D., F.A.C.S.
Thomas D. Jones Professor of Surgery
University of Chicago Medical Center
Department of Surgery
Chicago, IL

BEVERLY M. CALKINS, M.S., M.P.H., D.H.Sc.
Assistant Professor
Department of Epidemiology and Biostatistics
School of Medicine
Case Western Reserve University
Cleveland, OH

HARLEY C. CARLSON, M.D., PH. D.
Consultant, Department of Diagnostic Radiology
Mayo Clinic and Mayo Foundation
Professor of Radiology
Mayo Medical School
Rochester, MN

ROGER R. DOZOIS, M.D., M.S., F.A.C.S.
Associate Professor of Surgery,
Mayo Medical School
Consultant in Colon and Rectal Surgery
Mayo Clinic
Rochester, MN

DOUGLAS A. DROSSMAN, M.D.
Associate Professor of Medicine and Psychiatry
Division of Digestive Diseases
University of North Carolina School of Medicine
Chapel Hill, NC

DAVID L. EARNEST, M.D.
Professor of Medicine
Chief of Gastroenterology
The University of Arizona
Health Sciences Center
Tucson, AZ

CHARLES O. ELSON, M.D.
Professor of Medicine
Director, Division of Gastroenterology
University of Alabama at Birmingham
Birmingham, AL

RICHARD G. FARMER, M.D., F.A.C.P.
Chairman, Division of Medicine
The Cleveland Clinic Foundation
Cleveland, OH

DONALD J. GLOTZER, M.D.
Associate Professor of Surgery
Harvard Medical School
Surgeon, Beth Israel Hospital
Boston, MA

SHERWOOD L. GORBACH, M.D.
Chief, Infectious Disease Section
New England Medical Center Hospital
Professor of Medicine and Microbiology
Tufts University School of Medicine
Boston, MA

RICHARD J. GRAND, M.D.
Chief, Division of Pediatric Nutrition and
Gastroenterology
New England Medical Center
Tufts University School of Medicine
Boston, MA

NORTON J. GREENBERGER, M.D.
Peter T. Bohan Professor & Chairman
Department of Medicine
Director, Division of Gastroenterology
University of Kansas School of Medicine
Kansas City, KS

STEPHEN B. HANAUER, M.D.
Assistant Professor of Medicine
University of Chicago Medical Center
Chicago, IL

KENNETH A. HUIZENGA, M.D.
Professor of Medicine
Mayo Medical School
Senior Consultant Gastroenterology and Internal Medicine
Mayo Clinic and Mayo Foundation
Rochester, MN

DAVID G. JAGELMAN, M.S. (LONDON), F.R.C.S. (ENGLAND), F.A.C.S.
Staff Surgeon, Department of Colorectal Surgery
Cleveland Clinic Foundation
Cleveland, OH

HENRY D. JANOWITZ, M.D.
Consultant in Gastroenterology
Clinical Professor of Medicine, Emeritus
Mt. Sinai School of Medicine
New York, NY

KURSHEED N. JEEJEEBHOY, M.D.
Professor of Medicine,
Department of Medicine
University of Toronto
Head of Division of Gastroenterology
Toronto General Hospital
Toronto, Ontario, Canada

KEITH A. KELLY, M.D., M.S.
Roberts Professor of Surgery, and Chairman,
Department of Surgery
Mayo Clinic and Mayo Medical School
Rochester, MN

BARBARA S. KIRSCHNER, M.D.
Associate Professor of Pediatrics
Pritzker School of Medicine, University of Chicago
Co-Director, Section of Pediatric Gastroenterology
Wyler Children's Hospital
Chicago, IL

JOSEPH B. KIRSNER, M.D., PH.D.
Louis Block Distinguished Service
Professor of Medicine
The Division of the Biological Sciences and the Pritzker School of Medicine
The University of Chicago Hospitals and Clinics
Chicago, IL

PETER F. KOLACK, M.D.
Department of Gastroenterology
Lahey Clinic Medical Center
Burlington, MA

BURTON I. KORELITZ, M.D.
Chief, Section of Gastroenterology
Department of Medicine
Lenox Hill Hospital
Clinical Professor of Medicine
New York Medical College
New York, NY

CHARLES J. LIGHTDALE, M.D.
Director, Diagnostic Gastrointestinal Unit
Memorial Sloan-Kettering Cancer Center
Associate Professor Clinical Medicine
Cornell University Medical College
New York, NY

LLOYD MAYER, M.D.
Chief, Division of Clinical Immunology
Associate Professor of Medicine
Mount Sinai School of Medicine
New York, NY

RICHARD B. MCCONNELL, M.D., F.R.C.P.
Emeritus Consultant Physician
Royal Liverpool and Broadgreen Hospitals
Liverpool, England

ALBERT I. MENDELOFF, M.D., M.P.H., F.A.C.P.
Professor of Medicine
Johns Hopkins University School of Medicine
Senior Associate in Epidemiology
Johns Hopkins University School of Hygiene
Baltimore, MD

SAMUEL MEYERS, M.D.
Associate Clinical Professor of Medicine
Mount Sinai School of Medicine
City University of New York
New York, NY

KATHLEEN J. MOTIL, M.D., PH.D.
Assistant Professor
USDA/ARS Children's Nutrition Research Center
Department of Pediatrics
Section of Nutrition and Gastroenterology
Baylor College of Medicine
Texas Children's Hospital
Houston, TX

F. WARREN NUGENT, M.D.
Senior Consultant in Gastroenterology
Lahey Clinic Medical Center
Burlington, MA

MICHAEL J. OSTRO, M.D.
Assistant Professor of Medicine
Department of Medicine
Toronto Western Hospital
Division of Gastroenterology
Toronto, Ontario, Canada

SIDNEY F. PHILLIPS M.D., F.R.A.C.P., F.A.C.P.
Director, Gastroenterology Unit
Mayo Clinic
Professor of Medicine
Mayo Medical School
Rochester, MN

ROBERT RIDDELL, M.D.
Professor of Pathology
Chief of Service, Anatomical Pathology
McMaster University
Hamilton, Ontario, Canada

DAVID B. SACHAR, M.D.
Professor of Clinical Medicine
Mount Sinai School of Medicine
City University of New York
Director, Division of Gastroenterology
The Mount Sinai Hospital
New York, NY

WOLFGANG H. SCHRAUT, M.D., PH.D., F.A.C.S.
Associate Professor
Department of Surgery
University of Chicago Medical Center
Chicago, IL

KENNETH W. SCHROEDER,
Assistant Professor of Medicine
Mayo Medical School
Consultant, Gastroenterology and Internal Medicine
Mayo Clinic and Mayo Foundation
Rochester, MN

ERNEST SEIDMAN, M.D., F.R.C.P.(C)
Assistant Professor of Pediatrics
Faculty of Medicine
University of Montreal
Attending Physician
Division of Gastroenterology
Hôpital Sainte-Justine
Montréal, Québec, Canada

PAUL SHERLOCK, M.D. (DECEASED)
Former Chairman, Department of Medicine
Memorial Sloan-Kettering Cancer Center
Professor of Medicine
Cornell University
New York, NY

ROY G. SHORTER, M.D., F.R.C.P., F.A.C.P., F.R.C.PATH.
Professor of Medicine and Pathology
Mayo Medical School
Rochester, MN

JOHN W. SINGLETON, M.D.
Professor of Medicine
University of Colorado School of Medicine
Denver, Co

W. ALLAN WALKER, M.D.
Professor of Pediatrics
Harvard Medical School
Chief, Combined Program in Gastroenterology and Nutrition
Children's Hospital and Massachusetts General Hospital
Boston, MA

JEROME D. WAYE, M.D.
Clinical Professor of Medicine
Mount Sinai School of Medicine
City University of New York
Chief, Gastrointestinal Endoscopy Units
Mount Sinai Hospital and Lenox Hill Hospital
New York, NY

JACQUELINE L. WOLF, M.D.
Assistant Professor of Medicine
Harvard Medical School
Associate Physician
Brigham and Women's Hospital
Gastroenterology Division, Departments of Medicine
Brigham and Women's Hospital, Harvard Medical School, and Harvard Digestive Diseases Center
Boston, MA

Contents

Section 1. Epidemiology   1

1. The Epidemiology of Idiopathic Inflammatory Bowel Disease   3
   A.I. MENDELOFF AND B.M. CALKINS

Section 2. Etiology and Pathogenesis   35

2. Experimental Inflammatory Bowel Disease   37
   W.L. BEEKEN

3. Intestinal Microflora in Inflammatory Bowel Disease– Implications for Etiology   51
   S.L. GORBACH

4. Intestinal Defenses   65
   E. SEIDMAN AND W.A. WALKER

5. The Membranous Epithelial (M) Cell: A Portal of Antigen Entry   75
   J.L. WOLF

6. Genetic Aspects of Idiopathic Inflammatory Bowel Disease   87
   R.B. MCCONNELL

7. The Immunology of Inflammatory Bowel Disease   97
   C.O. ELSON

Section 3. Clinical Aspects   165

8. Clinical Features, Course, and Laboratory Findings in Ulcerative Colitis   167
   J.W. SINGLETON

9. Clinical Features, Laboratory Findings, and Course of Crohn's Disease   175
   R.G. FARMER

10. Differential Diagnosis of Chronic Ulcerative Colitis and Crohn's Disease of the Colon   185
    F.W. NUGENT AND P.F. KOLACK

11. Psychosocial Aspects of Ulcerative Colitis and Crohn's Disease   209
    D.A. DROSSMAN

12. Ulcerative Colitis and Crohn's Disease in Children   227
    K.J. MOTIL AND R.J. GRAND

13. Pathophysiology of Symptoms and Clinical Features of Inflammatory Bowel Disease   239
    S.F. PHILLIPS

14. Gastrointestinal Complications of Ulcerative Colitis and Crohn's Disease   257
    K.A. HUIZENGA AND K.W. SCHROEDER

15. Neoplasia and Gastrointestinal Malignancy in Inflammatory Bowel Disease   281
    C.J. LIGHTDALE AND P. SHERLOCK

16. Extraintestinal Complications of Inflammatory Bowel Disease   299
    L. MAYER AND H. JANOWITZ

17. Fertility and Pregnancy in Inflammatory Bowel Disease 319
B.I. KORELITZ

Section 4. Pathology 327

18. Pathology of Idiopathic Inflammatory Bowel Disease 329
R.H. RIDDELL

Section 5. Endoscopy and Radiology 351

19. Endoscopy in Idiopathic Inflammatory Bowel Disease 353
J.D. WAYE

20. Radiology of Inflammatory Bowel Disease 377
H.C. CARLSON

Section 6. Therapy 429

21. Medical Therapy in Ulcerative Colitis 431
S.B. HANAUER AND J.B. KIRSNER

22. Medical Therapy of Crohn's Disease 477
S. MEYERS AND D.B. SACHAR

23. Medical Management of Inflammatory Bowel Disease in Children 503
B.S. KIRSCHNER

24. Nutritional Consequences and Therapy in Inflammatory Bowel Disease 513
K.N. JEEJEEBHOY AND M.J. OSTRO

25. Indications for Surgery in Inflammatory Bowel Disease: A Gastroenterologist's Opinion 529
N.J. GREENBERGER

26. Indications for Surgery in Inflammatory Bowel Disease—A Surgeon's Opinion 549
D.J. GLOTZER

27. The Surgical Management of Idiopathic Inflammatory Bowel Disease 585
D.J. GLOTZER

28. The Conventional Ileostomy 645
D.G. JAGELMAN

29. Newer Operations for Ulcerative Colitis and Crohn's Disease 655
R.R. DOZOIS AND K.A. KELLY

30. Complications of the Surgical Treatment of Ulcerative Colitis and Crohn's Disease 685
G.E. BLOCK AND W.H. SCHRAUT

31. Physiologic Consequences of Surgical Treatment in Inflammatory Bowel Disease 715
D.L. EARNEST

Section 7. Prognosis 745

32. Prognosis of Idiopathic Inflammatory Bowel Disease 747
T.M. BAYLESS

33. The Fallibility of Activity Indices in Crohn's Disease (CD) 765
R.G. SHORTER

Index 767

Section 1 · *Epidemiology*

1 · The Epidemiology of Idiopathic Inflammatory Bowel Disease

A. I. MENDELOFF, M.D., M.P.H., F.A.C.P. AND BEVERLY M. CALKINS, M.S., M.P.H., D.H.Sc.

The first studies of the epidemiology of inflammatory bowel disease were published in the late 1950's and early 1960's. Some of the forms of idiopathic inflammatory bowel disease considered in this book have existed for centuries, but without historic data the epidemiologist must look at their occurrence in various populations as if they are newly discovered entities. Thus, the development of epidemiologic data on inflammatory bowel disease is relatively recent. This chapter will ask questions about the distribution of these disorders in human populations throughout the world to identify possible avenues of investigation that need further study.

Problems in Epidemiologic Approaches to Inflammatory Bowel Disease

Although cases of ulcerative colitis and Crohn's disease have been recorded from all over the world, this chapter will concentrate on those studies based on populations with defined demographic characteristics. A number of these studies have not only measured incidence and prevalence, but also compared the characteristics of the patients with various control populations. It is rather remarkable that, during the three and a half decades during which such studies have been carried out in the United States, Scandinavia, Great Britain, and other parts of Europe, different investigators have reached agreement on some fundamental characteristics of cases.

The term "clinical" refers to the bedside, and "clinical data" refer to manifestations of disease in people who are ill. "Epidemiologic data" refer to the total population, both well and sick; "epidemiologic techniques" predict or identify certain features that are associated with ill rather than healthy members of the population. Subjects with disease move from the "normal" population into the category of patients carrying a definite "diagnosis." These patients form the background for the development of clinical data that can then be given an appropriate epidemiologic and statistical treatment.

Diagnosis

The onset of inflammatory bowel disease is characterized by a gradual, insidious development of chronic complaints such as episodic diarrhea, colicky abdominal pain, weight loss, melena, blood, and/or mucus in the stool. Some ulcerative colitis patients may present with abrupt, explosive diarrhea. The first symptoms of Crohn's disease may be gastrointestinal complications such as obstruction, perforation, abscess, hemorrhage, or peritonitis. A significant amount of time may elapse between first symptoms and the definitive diagnosis. Iversen et al. tabulated the number of cases definitely diagnosed as ulcerative colitis per year against the number of years of symptoms preceding the diagnosis (Table 1-1).[1] Only about 40% of patients were diagnosed within the first year of their symptoms, and even 30 years after the onset of symptoms, patients were being diagnosed for the first time. Recent data from an Oakland, California health maintenance organization confirm that only about 30 to 40% of ulcerative colitis and Crohn's disease patients are hospitalized within the first year of diagnosis.[2] In Sweden, the onset-to-diagnosis interval for ulcerative colitis has been studied for sequential five-year time periods and for the location of the lesions. No changes have been shown for 1955 to 1979 for the symptom-onset-to-diagnosis interval or for the location of lesions in the bowel (total, left-sided, or proctitis only). The symptom-onset-to-diagnosis interval in this report was 2.1 to 2.4 years.[3] Other data from Rochester, Minnesota have shown a median onset-to-diagnosis interval of four months for Crohn's disease patients.[4] Studies of series of children with Crohn's disease have found that the onset-to-diagnosis interval is about 18 months.[5] Thus, because of the somewhat insidious onset of inflammatory bowel disease, bringing patients to prompt medical attention is difficult, as is studying truly incident cases.

The technology and training of medical professionals needed to distinguish ulcerative colitis from Crohn's disease, and from other etiologically specific inflammations of the gut, are not currently uniformly distributed around the world. A lack of pathologic specimens at various stages of their progression has also limited development of knowledge about the natural history of inflammatory bowel disease. Unfortunately, in most parts of the world where diarrheal diseases are still prevalent, a dearth of information about the frequency and natural history of chronic inflammations of the gut is a problem. Complicating the diagnostic process is the fact that experience with amebiasis, shigellosis, and lymphopathia venereum indicates that each can produce inflammatory reactions that persist for some time after the initial inciting pathogen can no longer be isolated.[6] Thus, at some point in this sequence of events it is possible to confuse the clinical, radiologic, proctoscopic, and perhaps even the histologic appearance of the bowel with the types of responses usually associated with ulcerative colitis or Crohn's disease. Not long ago it was thought by some authoritative investigators that ulcerative colitis was a form of chronic bacillary dysentery, and Crohn's disease was some atypical variant of intestinal tuberculosis. Furthermore, because a correct diagnosis is a prerequisite for classifying patients, any lack of agreement on diagnostic criteria is a serious obstacle for those who study the disease in various parts of the world. Diagnostic guidelines have been suggested and validated by the Organisation Mondiale de Gastroenterologie.[7] Investigators who conduct epidemiologic studies must recognize that changes in diagnostic criteria and/or in the nomenclature of a disease may introduce errors in classification that can seriously mislead and confuse.

TABLE 1-1. *Distribution of one thousand hypothetical cases of ulcerative proctitis and colitis Copenhagen County, Denmark.*

Duration of Symptoms (Years)	Remaining Patients	Number Diagnosed	Number of Deaths	Proportion of All Patients Diagnosed
0	1,000			
1	600	387	13	0.39
2	482	109	9	0.18
3	400	75	7	0.16
4	347	47	6	0.12
5	303	39	5	0.11
10	105	89	19	0.07
15	116	67	12	0.08
20	73	35	8	0.07
25	46	22	5	0.07
30	24	19	3	0.10
		21	3	
Total		910	90	

*Reproduced with permission from Iversen, E., et al.: Scand. J. Gastroenterol., *3*:593, 1968.

Another diagnostic problem is the lack of accurate diagnostic tools in some centers, particularly those used for bacterial cultures of stools, parasitologic identification, sigmoidoscopy, biopsy, interpretation of findings, and radiologic investigations. Most physicians depend on endoscopy to diagnose ulcerative colitis, whereas they rely on radiology, at least in part, for the diagnostic study of Crohn's disease. Thus, the epidemiologist tends to have more confidence in those studies carried out in sophisticated medical centers. The obvious problem of developing studies in such a setting is that the patient population is likely to be biased. A balance must be struck between the best clinical data and the most reliable population data in order to understand all the epidemiologic features of these two disorders. In this discussion, it is assumed that a majority of the clinical cases reported represent clear-cut instances of either ulcerative colitis or of Crohn's disease, although in any large series, misclassification may be up to 20%.

Case Ascertainment

The process of collecting a group of cases for study must rely on two key points: first, a patient who is aware that a problem needing care exists; and second, a physician with sufficient training, awareness, and access to diagnostic techniques to make a correct diagnosis or referral. Increased physician interest may produce more cases that might otherwise go unrecognized. For example, case ascertainment of communicable diseases, required by law to be reported to public health authorities, is more thorough during epidemic periods than during endemic periods. Thus, increased awareness can produce more cases without an actual increase in the prevalence of the disease in a population.

Changes in the distribution, quality, and access to medical care also influence case ascertainment. As more sophisticated diagnostic techniques and more trained personnel become available in rural and underdeveloped areas, incidence rates may show an artificial increase. As programs of care are developed for poor populations (which, in the United States, usually means minority groups), more cases may be recognized in these groups. Thus, reports of incidence in areas or groups that have previously reported none should be regarded as baseline estimates and used as comparisons with other populations and with follow-up determinations of incidence.

Investigators must also be aware of the referral pattern for inflammatory bowel disease in a locality of a study. If a large diagnostic and treatment facility is located near but outside of the proposed area of a study, many cases may be lost through referral, possibly introducing a bias when studying only those cases left behind.

Another problem with case ascertainment is the process of assigning patients' hospitalization diagnoses to diagnosis-related groups based on the primary International Classification of Disease codes. Because diagnosis-related groups are used in the United States for hospitalization payments, the assignment of primary International Classification of Disease codes may be influenced by economic considerations rather than strictly by the medical data. Whether patients can be readily and correctly identified for research purposes by this new process is still unclear. Certainly, the potential for misclassification seems greater, but this issue has not yet been assessed. Finally, the effect of record retrieval on case ascertainment must be considered. This problem is an increasingly important one, with the emphasis on medical record confidentiality and the bureaucratic mechanisms that are used to control access to medical records. The many factors impinging on case ascertainment have made research on inflammatory bowel disease complicated and expensive. Perhaps the most immediate solution would be a multi-center collaborative effort.

Size and Location of Population

The ecology of many of the geographic areas of the world has changed rapidly in recent decades. These changes include migrations of populations in response to wars or industrial and agricultural development that force them into changing environments. It is difficult to observe all these variables while studying changes in the occurrence of diseases. Data presented by both Acheson and Goligher suggest that it is possible to find cases of ulcerative colitis and Crohn's disease in many locations,[8,9] but the varying degrees of frequency reported have not been correlated with geographic features such as climate, sunlight, rainfall, soil characteristics, or altitude.

The size of a population is a key element to the success of a study of inflammatory bowel disease. Because it does not occur at high rates, compared to colon cancer, for example, much larger base populations are needed so enough cases can be accrued to study. The large populations needed complicate the logistics and increase the expense of studies. The density of proposed study populations is also a consideration. More time and manpower are necessary to contact dispersed individuals. The degree to which the base population is characterized demographically is an important component. Areas that have undercounted segments of some portions of the age distribution or of certain racial groups cannot serve as sources of satisfactory statistical analysis. Thus, three basic factors of the base population must be present for a study to be logistically feasible: adequate size, characterization, and geographic definition. With regard to population size, a minimum for inflammatory bowel disease studies is about one million persons for a single year study.

Reliability of Published Data on Incidence

One of the most disturbing features of the investigations reported is the imprecision of the data relating to the population under age 15. This group of children, which makes up from 20 to 25 percent of the total United States population (1980 census) and an even greater proportion of the population of less industrialized societies, is poorly studied. Physicians are naturally reluctant to submit children to radiologic, endoscopic, and biopsy procedures unless they are obviously ill; and they are not likely to investigate the asymptomatic siblings of patients with these diseases for data relating to familial occurrence. Consequently, in the total childhood population, those children with minimal symptoms will probably never be seen by a physician, and thus will never be counted in any tabulation. Children who are seen in the hospital probably are those with severe disease, especially in the countries where health insurance for medical care does not exist. It is likely that only well-educated or reasonably affluent parents would insist on follow-up studies of an affected child or of siblings with mild symptoms. The mobility of populations may make the diagnosis of patients difficult to record completely, because patients may often move to different areas and physicians. Thus, the morbidity and mortality rates for these diseases will probably reflect the fate of those patients who are severely ill, especially in rural or underdeveloped areas.

Determining Characteristics Antedating Diagnosis

Because of the low occurrence of inflammatory bowel disease cases in populations, the most effective research design is the case-control study. The nature of this design requires cases and controls to recall factors antecedent to a particular time or event. The foibles of the human memory are an important concern with respect to the validity of the data obtained in this way. During the months between the onset of symptoms and the diagnosis of inflammatory bowel disease, many changes can occur in the lives of patients that can dim the memory regarding medical history, medication usage, and psychologic, dietary, and other lifestyle factors. Given the inherent recall bias that may affect the accuracy of data obtained on newly diagnosed (incident) cases, using prevalent cases to determine antecedent factors associated with the onset of the disease may compound the problem of recall bias. Thus, the use of incident cases is preferable whenever possible. In addition, measurement of many physiologic features, such as immune mechanisms, serum levels of hormones and other factors, and the flora of the gut, as well as dietary, lifestyle, and psychologic factors, may be changed by the disease process or its treatment. Even certain demographic variables may be changed, such as divorces, lost or changed occupations, reduced incomes, and delayed or terminated educational programs because of the interference that inflammatory bowel disease brings into the lives of its victims.

With such problems facing the investigator, the question might be asked if good studies of inflammatory bowel disease are possible. The answer is yes, perhaps more so in areas where record linkage has been established; but in the United States, carefully planned studies have also made significant contributions to the understanding of the population at risk of inflammatory bowel disease. Understanding the limitations of different research designs, analyses, or data resources can assist greatly in the careful interpretation of findings.

Separating Genetic and Environmental Factors

As Susser has stated, theoretically no trait can be exclusively genetic or environmental in origin,[10] but determining what factors are stronger determinants of disease requires an attempt to separate genetic from environmental inferences. The purpose for doing this is practical. An understanding of the mechanisms involving environmental factors is important because these factors may be highly susceptible to intervention and prevention strategies. Although not currently alterable, an understanding of the mechanisms involving genetic factors is important for genetic counseling. Therefore, a clear understanding both of genetic and environmental mechanisms can improve diagnosis and treatment.

The process of determining genetic or environmental factors begins with establishing the presence or absence of familial aggregation, that is the clustering of cases in family units. Because family members share genes and environment, familial aggregation of a disease only raises the *suspicion* of investigators that genetic factors may be involved. Thus, both environmental and genetic hypotheses must be given serious consideration.

In the presence of familial aggregation, the first question usually posed is whether the familial distribution pattern fits any mendelian model for single genes. The distribution of genetic traits within the family unit can be analyzed by using expected values derived from the mendelian assumption that genes are either dominant or recessive, or either autosomal or sex-linked. Another analytic approach is to explore the possibility of a linkage between a genetic trait and a disease. Finding such a linkage would virtually confirm the genetic transmission of a disease. Finally, measuring heritability can be useful in estimating the genetic or environmental components of a disease.

Environmental factors in the presence of familial aggregation generally can be characterized in three ways: nonmendelian clustering, cohabitational effects, and maternal transmission. Nonmendelian clustering is similar to the pattern observed for acute contagious disease, particularly time of onset and sex clusters. Cohabitation effects are those manifestations of disease in genetically unrelated persons who live together, such as spouses. Finally, maternal transmission involves both intrauterine and postnatal factors.

If familial aggregation cannot be established, genetic factors may still be involved. To determine this, biologic markers and endogamous groups must be examined. Biologic markers include blood type and HLA patterns. Endogamous groups result from the expression of a recessive gene in a homozygous pair. This occurs when the gene pool is limited, such as in consanguineous marriages or in geographically or socially isolated groups. Environmental factors in the absence of familial aggregation are examined by the epidemiologic approaches of characterizing cases by person, place, and time. Research design strategies to separate genetic and environmental factors include twin studies, clusters of cases characterized by the closeness of relations, and comparisons of relatives raised separately. This last design is perhaps the strongest indicator of a genetic or an environmental basis for a disease.

Morbidity and Mortality

Incidence

In Tables 1-2 and 1-3, selected reports of the average annual incidence and prevalence of ulcerative colitis and Crohn's disease are compiled from selected areas.[2,4,14,11-58] It is of considerable interest that these investigations, conducted over two and a half decades and in a variety of western populations, are in general agreement. The annual incidence is, for the sum of both disorders, 5 to 15 new cases per 100,000 population. The data for incidence, taking into account the many uncertainties on which they are based, indicate that ulcerative colitis is a disease that seems to be more frequent in English stock (United Kingdom, New Zealand, and Australia), the United States, and northern Europe; less frequent in central Europe and the Middle East; and infrequent in South America, Asia, and Africa. Crohn's disease has its highest incidence in the United States, the United Kingdom, and Scandinavia; is less frequent in central Europe, and is infrequent in African, Asian, and South American populations.

Perhaps differences between regions could be explained by the inclusion of milder cases in the numerator, particularly ulcerative proctitis. Danish data would suggest that at least 60% of the total ulcerative colitis population has ulcerative proctitis;[16] a survey conducted in Baltimore has indicated that less than 10% of the proctitis population is ever hospitalized.[59] Thus, most of the variation in the reported series of ulcerative colitis incidence probably is determined by whether or not ulcerative proctitis is recognized by the diagnostic facilities doing the reporting.

TABLE 1-2. *Incidence and prevalence rates (per 100,000 population) of ulcerative colitis, by area reporting.* *

Area	Time Period	Incidence	Prevalence
North America:			
Baltimore, MD[11,12]	1960–1963	3.0	
	1973	3.8	
	1977–1979	2.2	
Rochester, MN[13,14]	1935–1944	2.0	
	1945–1954	3.2	
	1955–1964	4.0	39
	1960–1969	16.1	
	1970–1979	14.3	
Oakland, CA[2]	1971–1982	6.3[a]	
		4.35[b]	
		1.33[c]	
15 United States areas[15]	1973	3.5	
Scandinavia:			
Copenhagen, Denmark[16,17]	1962–1978	8.1	117
	1961–1967	7.3	44.1
Sweden[3,+]	1955–1959	1.7	
	1960–1964	3.2	
	1965–1969	4.5	
	1970–1974	4.7	
	1975–1979	4.3	
Norway[18–20]	1946–1950	0.9	
	1951–1955	1.5	
	1956–1960	2.1	
	1964–1969	3.3	
Great Britain:			
Cardiff, Wales[21]	1968–1977	7.2	
Oxford, England[22]	1951–1960	5.2	65.7
North Tees, Scotland[23]	1971–1977	15.1	99.0
Europe:			
Czechoslovakia[24]	1961–1965	1.4	
South Pacific:			
New Zealand Maori[25]	1965–1958	5–6	
Africa, Asia, South America[56–58]		rarely found	

*United States data is based on hospital incidence; other data are population-based.
+Rates estimated from graph from Gollup, J. H., Phillips, S. F., Melton, L. J., and Zinsmeister, A. R.: Unpublished data, 1986.
[a]Total incidence rate
[b]First hospitalization incidence rate
[c]Hospitalization within one year of diagnosis

This is not to disparage the ability of the physicians in such facilities, but merely to point out that physicians can only diagnose conditions in patients they see. For example, in some sections of any country large numbers of proctitis patients may never be diagnosed simply because they never see a physician or because the patients may seek care from centers which do not submit their records to those collecting data. Thus, the ratio of proctitis to colitis may be crucial to the total incidence of ulcerative colitis. Particularly in children, the observation of proctitis by a pediatrician or general practitioner may not prompt other diagnostic tests which could establish the existence of more extensive colitis. The studies from Scandinavia,[18,60] and from Olmsted County (Minnesota),[13,14] do permit us to estimate that about half of the ulcerative colitis cases have disease limited to the rectum.

The situation regarding Crohn's disease is somewhat different. The symptoms of this disorder are generally more insidious in the chronic form, making accurate recognition of the disease difficult. On the other hand, acute ileitis, a rather rare and dramatic clinical entity

TABLE 1-3 *Incidence and prevalence rates (per 100,000 population) of Crohn's disease, by area reporting.**

Area	Time Period	Incidence	Prevalence
North America:			
Baltimore, MD[11,12]	1960–1963	1.2	
	1973	2.2	
	1977–1979	3.1	
15 United States areas[15]	1973	2.4	
Oakland, CA[2]	1971–1982	5.5[a]	
		4.8[b]	
		1.89[c]	
Olmsted County, MN[4,26]	1935–1954	8.4	
	1955–1964	12.0	
	1965–1975	13.5	28.0
	1973–1977	4.1	
	1978–1982	3.9	
	1982		60.6
Rochester, MN[4,26]	1935–1964	6.6	106.0
	1973–1977	8.2	
	1978–1982	4.6	
	1982		108.1
Sherbrooke, Ontario, Canada[27]	1969–1971	0.7	6.3
Scandinavia:			
Copenhagen, Denmark[28]	1961–1967	7.3	44.1
Copenhagen County, Denmark[17]	1961–1969	1.3	
	1970–1978	2.7	34.0
Turku, Finland[29]	1950–1970	0.3	
Norway[18,30]	1956–1963	2.6	
	1964–1969	1.0	
Central Sweden[31–32]	1956–1959	1.4	
	1960–1964	2.6	
	1965–1969	4.0	
	1970–1973	5.1	
Gothenburg, Sweden[34]	1951–1955	1.2	
	1956–1960	1.6	
	1961–1965	6.3	
	1966–1970	6.3	
Stockholm, Sweden[5]	1955–1959	1.5	
	1960–1964	2.2	
	1965–1969	3.6	
	1970–1974	4.5	
	1975–1979	4.1	
Malmo, Sweden[35]	1958–1973	4.8	75.2
Great Britain:			
Cardiff, Wales[36,37]	1934–1976	4.8	56.0
Aberdeen, Scotland[38,39]	1955–1957	1.2	
	1958–1960	1.9	
	1961–1963	2.8	
	1964–1966	3.3	
	1967–1969	4.5	
	1970–1972	4.3	
	1973–1975	2.6	
Clydesdale, Scotland[40]	1961–1970	1.5	
North Tees, Scotland[23]	1971–1977	5.3	35.0
Northern Ireland[41]	1966–1973	1.3	
Belfast, North Ireland[41]	1966–1973	3.5	
County Down, North Ireland[41]	1966–1973	0.3	
Gloucester, England[42]	1966–1970	1.5	
Blackpool, England[43]	1971–1975	3.3	
	1976–1980	6.1	

TABLE 1-3 *Continued*

Area	Time Period	Incidence	Prevalence
London, England[44]			13.0
Nottingham, England[45]	1958–1973	3.6	26.5
Oxford, England[22]	1951–1960	0.8	9.0
Europe:			
Northern Bohemia[46]	1972–1979	1.6-2.0	12.0
Bologna, Italy[47]	1972–1973	0.8	
Galicia, Spain[48]	1976–1983	0.14	1.22
Madrid, Spain[49]		0.7	
Basel, Switzerland[50]	1960–1966	1.1	
	1967–1969	2.6	
Middle East:			
Israel[51,52]	1961–1970		14.0
	1971–1975	0.5	14.0
Beersheva, Israel[53,54]	1976–1980	1.8	14.0
Tel Aviv, Israel[55]	1970–1976	1.28	12.3
Africa, Asia, South America[56–58]		rarely found	

*United States data are based on hospital incidence; other data are population-based.
[a]Total incidence rate
[b]First hospitalization incidence rate
[c]Hospitalization within one year of diagnosis

symptomatically similar to acute appendicitis and usually requiring hospitalization, is easily tabulated, but is probably not importantly related to chronic Crohn's disease. Thus, only approximately half or less of the reported cases of acute ileitis that may be tabulated as Crohn's disease should be regarded as valid cases of that disorder.[34]

Annual incidence rates presume that accurate dating of the onset of these diseases can be determined from a clinical history. As previously mentioned, in the studies by Iversen and associates, however, only about 40% of all ulcerative colitis patients are diagnosed within the first year of symptoms (Table 1-1).[1] Thus, an accurate date of onset can probably only be established for the most seriously ill patients. For the majority of patients, it is difficult to determine the exact time of onset of the first episode of colitis. With Crohn's disease, a less acute disorder, the accurate dating of onset is equally unreliable. Thus, the available figures on incidence represent a reasonable but not precise estimate.

In the United States, data on incidence have been obtained from the Mayo Clinic in Rochester, Minnesota, the hospitals of the greater Baltimore area and the Permanente Medical Group, Inc. in Oakland, California (a health maintenance organization). The Oakland and Rochester data have the advantage of record linkage of inpatient and outpatient records. The findings from these two areas are important, because the only other data from the United States are derived hospital incidence rates from the Baltimore Standard Metropolitan Statistical Areas (SMSA). Clearly, the development of data using only hospitalized cases has an inherent bias; it cannot be known what proportion of all incident cases are hospitalized for diagnosis. Study of this question in the Oakland health maintenance organization, however, has shown that about 45% of Crohn's disease patients and six percent of ulcerative colitis patients are hospitalized at or within one year of diagnosis.[2]

Trends in Incidence

The trend of incidence rates for ulcerative colitis among whites in Baltimore[12] and in Stockholm appears to be downward.[3] For the same time period, it appears that in most other reporting areas, such as England and Wales,[45] Denmark,[16,17] Israel,[52,53] Finland,[61] and New Zealand,[62] the rates are stabilizing. In Norway and North Tees (Scotland)[18-20,23] however, recent reports indicate increasing rates. Increases in hospitalizations have also been reported in Japan,[63] and among immigrants to Great Britain.[64] Changes in the availability of medical care and attention given to these problems in these populations, however, may account for the observed changes.

The Crohn's disease rates in Aberdeen (Scotland)[39] have increased sharply during the 1950s and early 1960s, stabilized in the late 1960s, and declined in the early 1970s. North Tees (Scotland),[23] Cardiff (Wales),[36,37] Oakland (California),[2] and Baltimore (Maryland),[12] report either stabilizing or declining rates in the past decade.* Olmsted county (Minnesota),[13] Clydesdale (Scotland),[40] Denmark,[17,28] Finland,[29] Norway,[18,30] Switzerland,[50] Israel,[51-55] England and Wales,[65] and South Africa,[66,67] all report large increases in rates. Hospital admissions for Crohn's disease in Japan have increased since newly diagnosed cases were first reported in the mid-1960s.[63] Rates for ulcerative colitis and Crohn's disease reported for nonwhite populations are quite low, making trends difficult to detect.[12,68] Information on rates for ulcerative colitis and Crohn's disease in nonindustrialized nations is also too limited for comment.

Comparing secular changes in rates of disease over time within and between several areas is of interest because the clues provided can suggest directions for further etiologic studies. Such comparisons are subject to certain limitations, however. The availability and delivery of medical care varies from area to area, which affects case ascertainment. The availability and delivery of care, however, will be more consistent within than between areas. Thus, although comparison of rates between areas may not be useful because of differences in the medical care system, analysis of trends within an area is of value. Comparisons between areas could also be affected by varying diagnostic criteria, diagnostic trends, and/or improvements in diagnostic technology, modalities that are less likely to vary within an area. To examine the possibility that ulcerative colitis cases diagnosed by criteria of a past time period might be classified as Crohn's disease cases now, reviews of older cases have been made to determine the possible crossover resulting from changing criteria. Miller determined in his study that only 6% of formerly diagnosed ulcerative colitis cases would be classified as Crohn's disease by current criteria.[45] A similar study was made in the Oakland series; 2% of Crohn's disease cases and 10% of ulcerative colitis cases had been misclassified. The misclassification was not related to the age of the patient at diagnosis but to the sex; men were misclassified more than women.[2] Thus, the importance of changing diagnostic practices cannot be ignored.

*Editor's note: See also Rose, J. D. R., et al.: Gut (abstract), 27:1275, 1986.

The difference in the trends of rates for ulcerative colitis and Crohn's disease, with the hospitalization rate of Crohn's disease now exceeding that of ulcerative colitis, could imply increased recognition of Crohn's disease as a separate disease entity. Although improvement in diagnosis and recognition of Crohn's disease as an entity that differs from ulcerative colitis has become more widespread, this does not explain the observed increase. The differences in trends for these diseases probably are real, and they suggest that the causal agent(s) or factor(s) for these diseases may not be the same.

Prevalence

Because a study of the prevalence of these disorders would require an intensive clinical, endoscopic, and radiologic study of every member of a sample of a population, the prevalence is generally based on conclusions from the data on incidence. But the actual mechanics of this inferential process are not clearly established. It is assumed that once a patient has an inflammatory bowel disease he or she will have it until the organ is removed, as in ulcerative colitis, or until death. The same assumption is made for the prevalence of duodenal ulcer and cholelithiasis, despite the occasional radiographic disappearance of ulcers and gallstones over a lifetime in some patients; the patient is thought to have the disease no matter how inactive it may be. The implications of this thought process are disquieting with respect to data collection, particularly for proctitis. For patients with clearly diagnosed ulcerative colitis or Crohn's disease some follow-up data do exist supporting the idea that the disease remains active enough to warrant the concept of a large pool of individuals with these disorders existing in the population.[9,60] Attempts to define the course of inflammatory bowel disease by tabulating the number of patient years of follow-up, during which symptoms of the disease persist, have been recorded and reported by a number of workers. Although Jalan and associates found relapses among about 25% of the patient years tabulated,[60] Goligher's data suggest that patients with these diseases will usually experience a clinical relapse for half the patient years investigated.[9] Data from Rochester have indicated that only about 10% of Crohn's disease patients recede into a prolonged asymptomatic state of 10 years or more.[4] These data provide little evidence that ulcerative colitis tends to recede into a prolonged asymptomatic state while supporting the concept that every patient diagnosed should be regarded as affected with the disease until the colon is resected. Some serious methodologic questions about patient year techniques have been raised by Sheps, however.[69] Because the time necessary to study inflammatory bowel disease by this approach is prolonged, there may not be constant risk for all members of a sample during the study period.

In 1958, Houghton and Naish published a study of the admission rate to Bristol hospitals of patients with inflammatory bowel disease.[70] They estimated that during a twelve year period every patient with ulcerative colitis would be admitted for treatment once; by this, they assumed that for each patient for the first time there were 12 patients in the population at large with the same disease. The actual rates for prevalence as shown in Tables 1-2 and 1-3 are astonishingly close to those predicted by Houghton and Naish, on the average about ten times the annual incidence figures for both diseases. For countries with highly heterogeneous populations, such as the United States, it is probably impossible to estimate national prevalence data based on the extrapolations of the incidence in one area multiplied by a single numerical factor. Without a record linkage system, it cannot be definitely known that the same patients are not counted more than once; given the mobility of the United States population and its freedom of access to various centers, there is no doubt that this does occur.

It should be mentioned that the data from the United States are derived almost entirely from studies involving one metropolitan area on the east coast (the greater Baltimore area) and one rural area (Olmsted County, Minnesota). The data from the United Kingdom and Scandinavia are derived from well characterized populations to which fairly uniform diagnostic criteria have been applied. Few reports from underdeveloped countries exist. The wide range of prevalence indicated in Tables 1-2 and 1-3 is probably a result of differences in case ascertainment and availability of medical care for the areas represented. In 1985, inflammatory bowel disease in the United States probably affected 440,000 to 540,000 persons. This number was compiled by using as an estimate of "true" population risk, an annual incidence of 15/100,000 for an estimated United States population of 240 million persons, and multiplying the resulting annual incident cases by factors 12 to 15 to determine the probable range of prevalent cases.

Mortality

Deaths coded as a result of inflammatory bowel disease (Ninth Revision of the International Classification of Diseases, codes 555, 556) represent postoperative deaths, acute complications of peritonitis, hemorrhage, or sepsis. It is likely that these deaths are correctly coded and truly represent the actual mortality. Death certificates recording mortality from less common complications of the disease, such as amyloidosis, biliary tract disease, or pancreatitis, usually indicate inflammatory bowel disease as the underlying cause of death. The mortality caused by ulcerative colitis and Crohn's disease is not large, about 0.05 percent of all United States deaths. Because of the small numbers involved, the death rates from ulcerative colitis and Crohn's disease (Table 1-4) were combined into one set of values to provide more meaningful data for race. In spite of this effort, the age group categories for "other" races contain many empty cells in the numerators. Despite this limitation, annual average mortality rates for the United States for 1970 to 71 and 1982 are shown in Table 1-4 (age-adjusted to the 1970 United States census population).[71-75] In the past, ulcerative colitis cases made up nearly 90% of the deaths. More recently the proportion of ulcerative colitis and Crohn's disease deaths is about equal. The mortality rates for whites are about 1 per 100,000 for ages 20 to 29, 3 to 4 per 100,000 for ages 50 to 59, and continue to rise with age (data not shown.) Age-adjusted rates for white females are higher than white males, following the pattern for the incidence rates noted earlier; age-specific rates are higher for white females than white males at most ages (data not shown.) For each sex, the age-adjusted rates for whites are somewhat above those for blacks and "other" races, with

TABLE 1-4. *Mortality rates for inflammatory bowel disease in the United States.*

Race and Sex	Rates* 1970–1971	1982
Males:		
White	5.88	2.68
Blacks	3.72	1.17
Other	1.39	3.40
Females:		
White	7.24	3.48
Blacks	2.87	0.71
Other	3.13	1.96

*Rates are per 1,000,000 population and age-adjusted to the 1970 United States census population for US rates.

the exception of "other" males. A decline in death rates is indicated for all race and sex groups except for "other" males. No strikingly unusual pattern for these mortality rates is suggested by the data. Given these facts, a review of mortality rates for various sex, age, or racial groups is more likely to suggest treatment-related factors than disease-onset-related factors. The decline in the death rates for most race and sex groups probably reflects improvements in medical care.

Demographic Characteristics

Populations can be characterized by the epidemiologic method into groupings that have special susceptibility or resistance to the occurrence of a disease. Systematic exploration using this approach with respect to the occurrence of inflammatory bowel disease has barely begun, but already some features of significance have been identified.

Sex

Women appear to be at about 30% increased risk of developing ulcerative colitis or Crohn's disease (Table 1-5) when population groups of predominantly English or Northern European origin are considered. In almost all other countries with mixed racial stock, the female preponderance of ulcerative colitis is reduced, and is not found in Crohn's disease. In recent studies from Europe and England, there appears to be an increased incidence of Crohn's colitis among older women.[40] In all series, mortality rates follow the incidence rates, but it is not clear what implications the sex differences have on the etiology or the determining features of either disease.

Age

In all extensive series of these disorders, the incidence of ulcerative colitis in patients under the age of six far exceeds that of Crohn's disease for patients of the same age. For investigative purposes, the under-six population might be regarded as resistant to the development of Crohn's disease, and thus worthy of special study. For ages six to ten, ulcerative colitis occurs with increasing frequency, whereas Crohn's disease remains infrequent. At age ten both diseases begin to show greatly increased frequencies. Therefore, the mode for incidence of both diseases, for both sexes, is between the ages of 15 and 25 years. For the ages 20 to 50 the two diseases are almost identical with respect to annual incidence.

TABLE 1-5. *Sex-specific incidence rates (per 100,000) of Crohn's disease and ulcerative colitis by area.*

Area	Time Period	Ulcerative Colitis Male	Ulcerative Colitis Female	Crohn's disease Male	Crohn's disease Female
North America:					
Olmsted County, MN[26]					
	1935–1975			4.2	4.4
Baltimore, MD[11,12]	1960–1963	2.49	3.54	1.65	0.66
	1973	2.72	4.82	1.97	2.49
	1977–1979	2.11	2.35	2.34	3.81
Scandinavia:					
Central Sweden[31–33]	1956–1967			2.6	2.4
	1968–1973			4.3	5.7
Stockholm, Sweden[5]	1955–1974			2.8	3.1
Copenhagen, Denmark[16,17,28]					
	1961–1966	6.7	7.6		
Norway[18–20,30]	1946–1955	1.05	1.30		
	1956–1960	2.04	2.07		
	1956–1963			2.6	2.5
Great Britain:					
Oxford, England[22]	1951–1960	4.5	5.9	0.8	0.8
North Tees, Scotland[23]	1970–1977	9.4	11.4	4.6	5.8
Northeast Scotland[38,39]	1955–1961			1.4	1.9
	1962–1968			1.6	3.0
Clydesdale, Scotland[40]	1961–1965			1.0	1.4
	1966–1970			1.6	2.2

A special and fascinating issue is the occurrence of what appears to be a second mode at ages 55 to 60 in most but not all series of cases. Figures 1-1 and 1-2 illustrate four age distributions: two for Crohn's disease, both with the secondary rise; Figures 1-3 and 1-4 illustrate age distributions for ulcerative colitis, one with and one without the secondary rise. The first mode occurs consistently in the third decade of life, but the second mode is more variable, in the fifth to seventh decades. Bimodality has also been noted for aplastic anemia,[76] multiple sclerosis,[77-82] and Hodgkin's disease,[83] with different etiologic factors suggested for the different ages. The United States data for Baltimore for ulcerative colitis and Crohn's disease,[12] and Oakland, for Crohn's disease only,[2] show bimodality more frequently than do the European series. However, the possibility that this observation is artifactual cannot be discounted because the smaller series tend to show bimodality while the larger series do not. Most of the data showing bimodality were obtained prior to 1970; the most recent series from Baltimore, Central Sweden, Norway, and Copenhagen show less prominent bimodality.

If a more definite bimodal pattern for Crohn's disease and a less definite one for ulcerative colitis exist, together with a different pattern in secular trends, this would reinforce the concept that these diseases are separate entities with different etiologic factors.[12,43] Perhaps ulcerative colitis and Crohn's disease themselves are each heterogeneous disease entities, each with different etiologic factors or host factors that act at different periods of life. The suggestion by Rogers and co-workers that mesenteric vascular disease may account for this secondary rise has many attractive features;[84] the pathologic findings in these cases do not support this thesis, however. This is unfortunate, because ischemic changes would provide a way to reconcile the variability of the size of the secondary rise in the distribution of rates in different series studied, would make the rather difficult clinical courses noted in older patients more understandable, and would explain their more frequently segmental or strictured responses of the colon. An entirely different interpretation of the bimodal incidence curve has been offered by Burch and associates.[85] It is their contention that the best way to explain a new susceptibility to ulcerative colitis is to postulate an immunologic change, such as a clonal response. The large series of cases reported by Jalan and co-workers, however, while demonstrating an expectedly higher

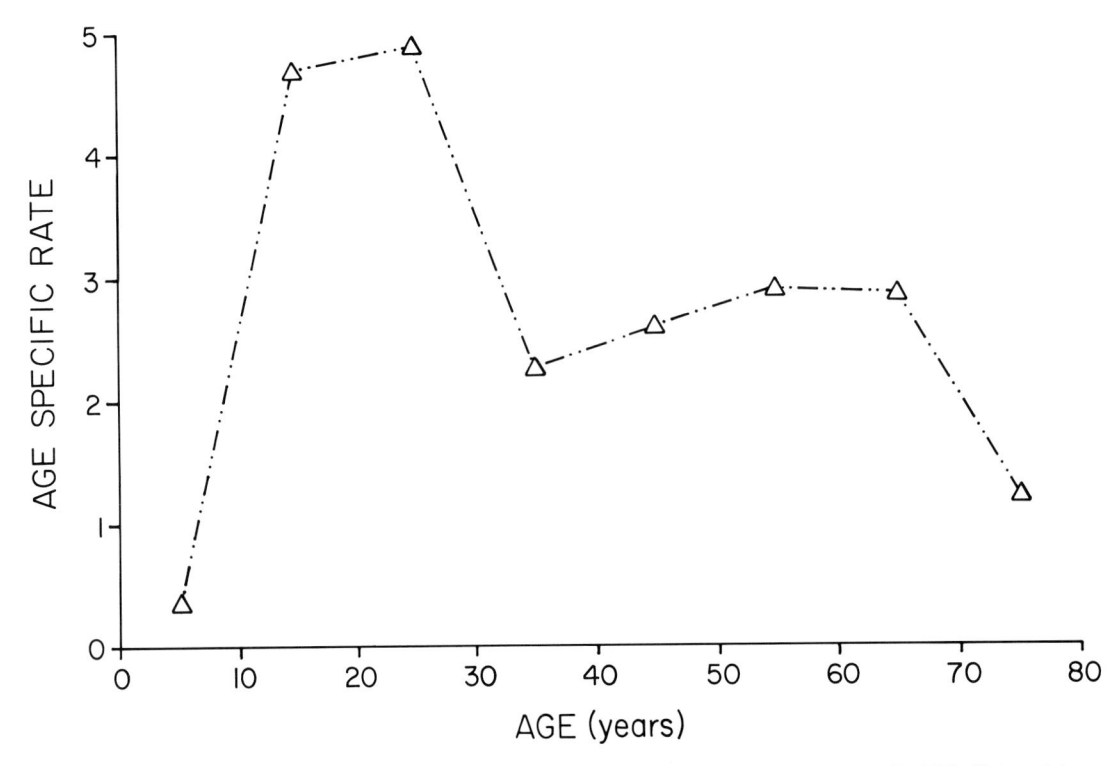

Fig. 1-1. Age-specific incidence rates (per 100,000 population) for Crohn's disease in Baltimore, 1960–1979. (Adapted from Calkins, B. M., Lilienfeld, A. M., Garland, C. F., and Mendeloff, A. I.: Dig. Dis. Sci., 29: 913, 1984.)

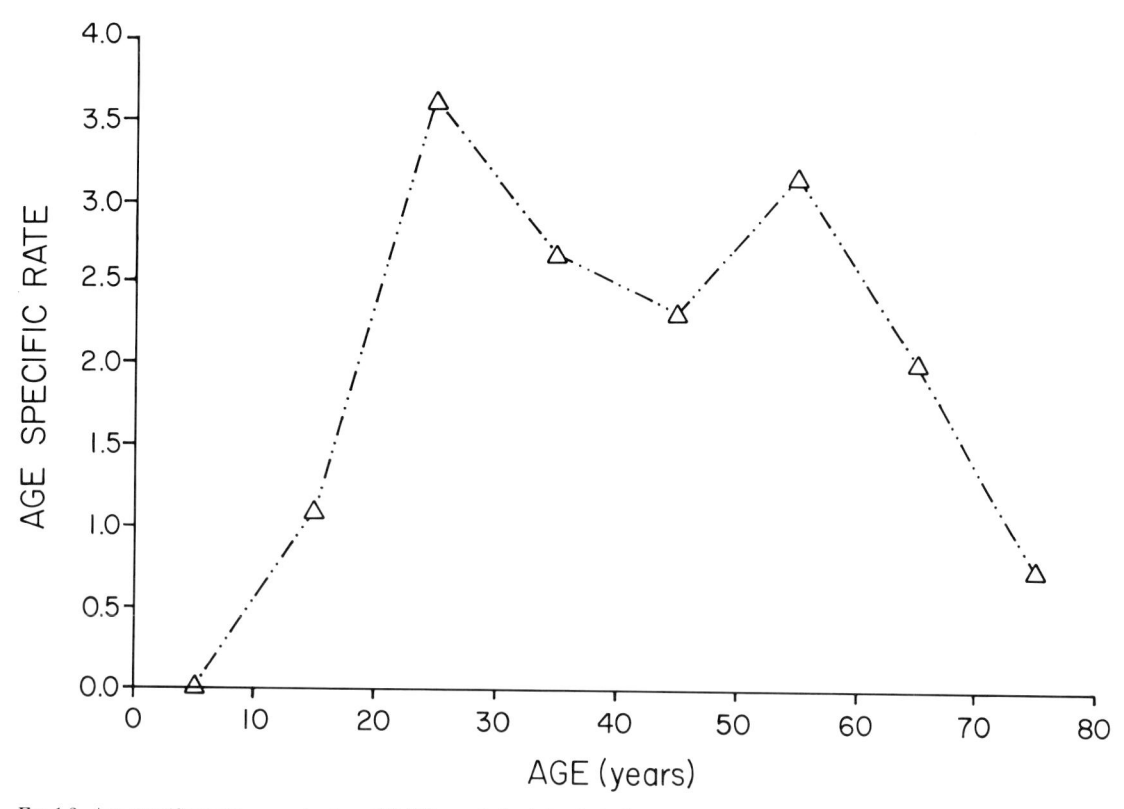

FIG. 1-2. Age-specific incidence rates (per 100,000 population) for Crohn's disease in Norway, 1956–1969. (Adapted from Myren, I., et al.: Scand. J. Gastroenterol., 6: 511, 1971; and Gjone, E., Orning, O. M., and Myren, J.: Gut, 7: 372, 1966.)

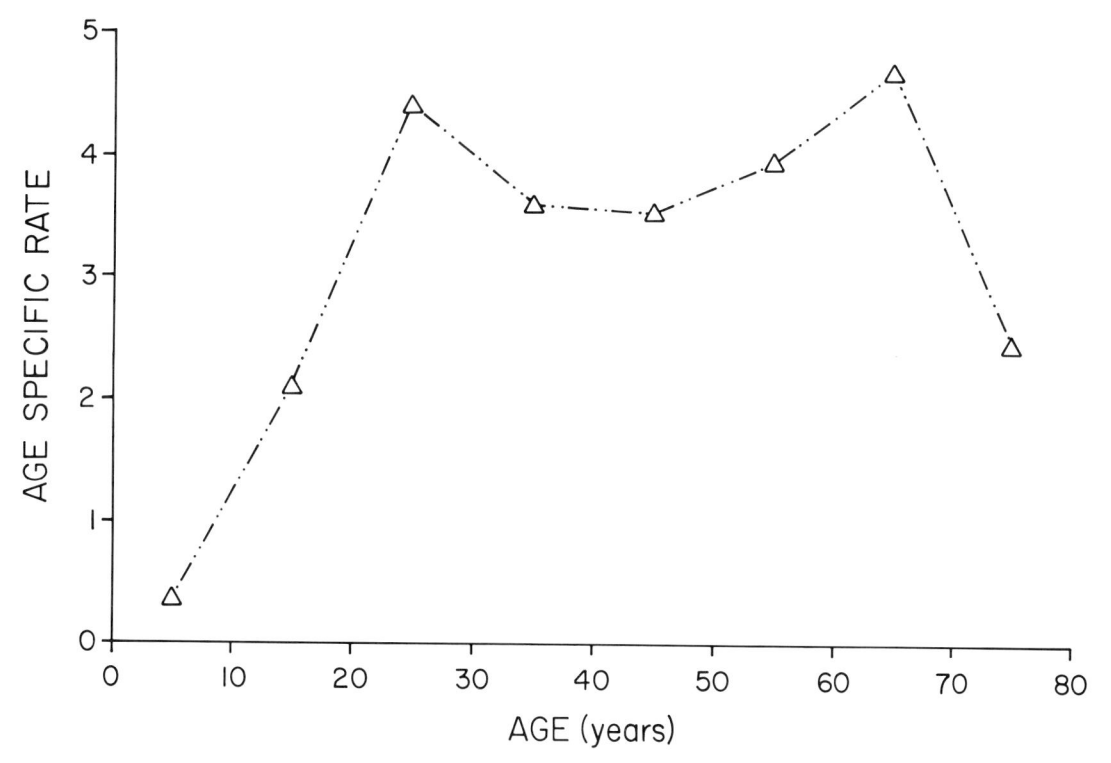

FIG. 1-3. Age-specific incidence rates (per 100,000 population) for ulcerative colitis in Baltimore, 1960–1979. (Adapted from Calkins, B. M., Lilienfeld, A. M., Garland, C. F., and Mendeloff, A. I.: Dig. Dis. Sci., 29: 913, 1984.)

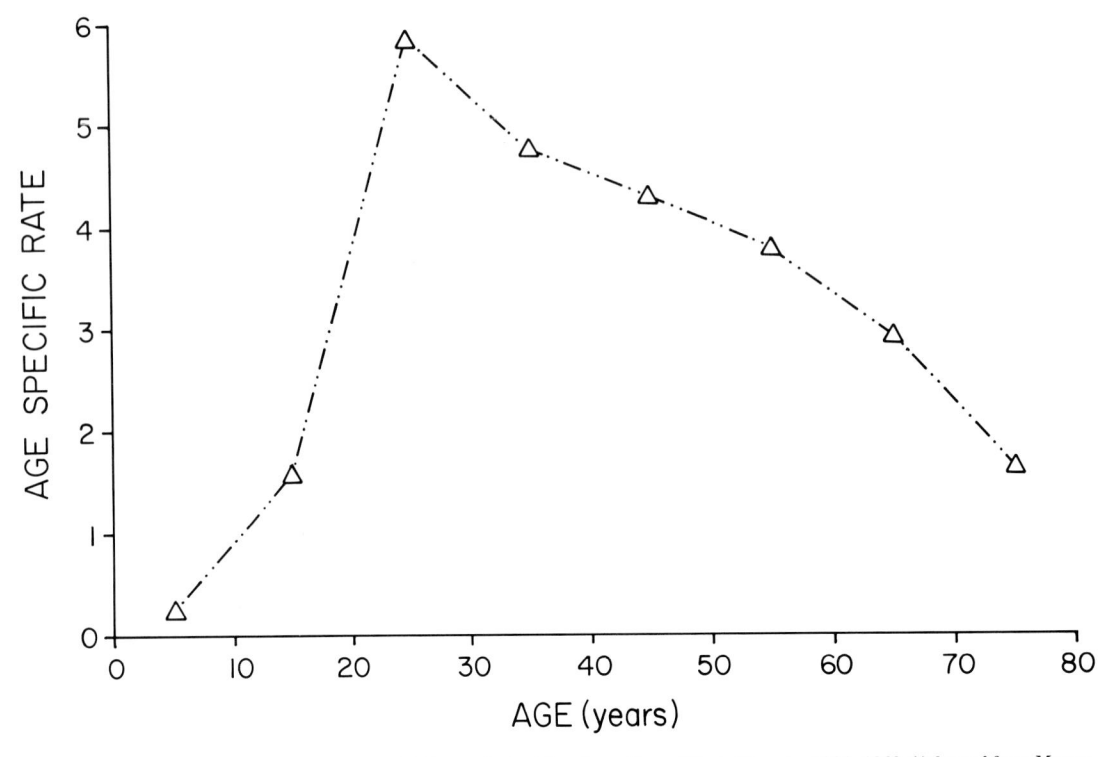

FIG. 1-4. Age-specific incidence rates (per 100,000 population) for ulcerative colitis in Norway, 1964–1969. (Adapted from Myren, et al.: Scand. J. Gastroenterol., 6: 511, 1971.)

mortality for those first manifesting ulcerative colitis after the age of 50, shows that the relapses of the disease may be less frequent and severe in this group and that more of the deaths are caused by diseases related to aging than to colitis itself.[60] If members of the older group develop colitis at a later age because of clonal change, the behavior of the disease should be at least as severe as it is among the young. A thorough discussion of possible ways of explaining the secondary rise can be found in the article by Evans and Acheson.[22]

Race

The incidence of inflammatory bowel disease among the peoples of South America, Asia, and Africa cannot be analyzed in statistically meaningful terms. There is no doubt that such disease has been described in these populations. Mortality data would suggest that from 1960 to 1980, American black and American Indian populations were at low risk for both of these diseases.[86] The greater Baltimore area has good incidence data for the urban nonwhite population (Table 1-6).[12] In early surveys, the nonwhite population of both sexes appeared to be one-third as likely to develop ulcerative colitis and one-fifth as likely to have Crohn's disease as the white population, but the difference between the races appears to be closing with time. The Crohn's disease rate for nonwhites of both sexes has increased in Baltimore, more sharply for nonwhite females than males. In contrast, the ulcerative colitis rate has increased for nonwhite males and decreased for nonwhite females, but the rate for nonwhite females still exceeds the rate for nonwhite males. The increase in rates among the nonwhite population

TABLE 1-6. *Incidence rates (per 100,000) by race for Baltimore.*

Time Period and Race	Ulcerative Colitis	Crohn's Disease
1960–1963:		
Whites	8.24	4.07
Nonwhites	2.49	0.63
1973:		
Whites	5.12	3.76
Nonwhites	2.41	0.69
1977-79:		
Whites	2.85	3.46
Nonwhites	2.08	2.68

could represent an increasing availability of medical care, but some real increase in risk is also likely. In New Zealand, the Maoris were reported as suffering an incidence of ulcerative colitis one-twentieth that of their English-descended white neighbors.[25] In Japan the incidence of ulcerative colitis, low in former decades, is now thought to be increasing steadily, although it is still much less than that reported in the western white population.[87]

Ethnicity

Ethnicity is a term used in research to indicate a certain homogeneity of population groups within racial groups. The homogeneity observed is of different orders of purity, of course, and represents many common cultural, religious, lifestyle, dietary, and/or health practices.

The Jewish population has been shown to be at higher risk of developing inflammatory bowel disease (Table 1-7). In a comparison of the proportion of Jewish patients with ulcerative colitis in two London hospitals in 1950, Paulley first described a twofold increase of the incidence of this disease compared with the proportion of total Jewish patients discharged from the two hospitals.[88] In the United States from 1953 to 1957, Acheson found that, among 2,320 male veterans discharged from Veterans Administration hospitals with a diagnosis of either ulcerative colitis or Crohn's disease, there were four times as many Jews as occurred in a 12.5% sample of all patients discharged in October 1956 from these same hospitals.[89] This predominance of Jews in the inflammatory bowel disease group occurred regardless of place of birth, United States or foreign. A study of Crohn's disease among active United States soldiers by Rappaport also noted a fourfold increase among Jews in the population at risk.[90] In Malmo, Sweden, Crohn's disease occurred five times more frequently in Jews than the expected rate,[35] and in Hellers' study in Sweden a similar Jewish predominance was noted.[5] In groups of patients seen at large United States referral clinics, the preponderance of Jewish persons has been noted for many years.[91,92]

In the only large-scale study of this problem in the United States, Monk and associates, using 1960 census tract data in Baltimore, interviewed patients with ulcerative colitis, Crohn's disease, irritable bowel syndrome, diverticulitis of the colon, or cancer of the colon appearing in Baltimore hospitals from 1960 to 1963.[93] Case characteristics were compared to those of the general populations, selected by census tracts, and matched for sex, age, ethnic group, and socioeconomic status. The frequency of ulcerative colitis among Jews proved to be about 3.5 times the rate among non-Jews. For Crohn's disease, the rate was 6 times higher for Jewish males and 3 times higher for Jewish females than the rates for the corresponding non-Jews. In fact, when

TABLE 1-7. *Inflammatory Bowel Disease incidence rates* among Jewish and non-Jewish persons.*

Area	Time Period	Rates* Jewish	Non-Jewish
North America:			
Baltimore, MD:[11,12]			
All inflammatory bowel disease	1960–1963	8.4	2.7
	1977–1979+	25.0	14.6
Ulcerative colitis	1960–1963	13.1	3.8
	1977–1979	9.8	5.8
Crohn's disease	1960–1963	3.6	1.7
	1977–1979	15.2	8.9
New York, NY[91]		12.6†	5.4
Scandinavia:			
Malmo, Sweden[35]	1965–1973	24.0†	6.0
Stockholm, Sweden[5]	1960–1974	10.0	3.0
Middle East:			
Tel Aviv, Israel[51]	1970–1976	1.3	
Beersheva, Israel[52]	1976–1980	1.8	
Africa:			
Cape Town, South Africa[66,67]		7.2	1.2

*Rates per 100,000 population
+Unpublished data from Calkins and Mendeloff.
†As estimated in Krawiec, J., et al.: Isr. J. Med. Sci., *20:* 16, 1984.

Jewish patients with Crohn's disease were subtracted from patients with the disease, the rates for the remaining white Baltimore population were identical to those found by Evans and Acheson in their study of the area around Oxford, England. Table 1-7 shows that the trend in the Baltimore area for Jewish and non-Jewish persons is toward higher rates in 1977 to 1979 than in 1960 to 1963, but the ratio of difference between the rates appears to be smaller in 1977 to 1979 than previously observed.

Of the characteristics studied in patients with ulcerative colitis and Crohn's disease in the Baltimore area, Jewish ethnicity was the single most distinctive feature. The higher prevalence in Jews might be accounted for by religious, social, or genetic factors, but in the Baltimore study neither the degree of orthodoxy nor intermarriage played any role in incidence. Social and educational factors were no more discriminatory in Jewish cases and controls than in non-Jewish cases and controls. Further discussion of these points with regard to irritable bowel syndrome and ulcerative colitis in this same population is found in an article by Mendeloff and associates.[94] The familial incidence of ulcerative colitis does seem to be markedly increased for Jewish patients seen in the United States, but has not proved to be so preponderant in English and northern European studies. The predominance of Jewish patients in the North American series of inflammatory bowel disease and the less striking incidence among Jews in other parts of the world, particularly the unexceptional incidence of ulcerative colitis and Crohn's disease in Israel, must contain important implications for etiology.

Marital Status

Studies have presented conflicting information on the association of marital status to inflammatory bowel disease. Some have found single status to be more common among patients,[93,95] but others have found no clear pattern.[65] It is important to keep in mind that the symptoms of the disease, such as pain, diarrhea, and growth retardation, and its treatment, steroid-induced changes in appearance, and ileostomy, may affect the possibility of getting married. Therefore, any noted association may be a result of therapy and not related to disease etiology.

Urban and Rural Distribution

Urban and rural differences in the incidence and prevalence of Crohn's disease and ulcerative colitis may provide valuable clues to their etiology and history. An early study of ulcerative colitis in the United States Army, by Acheson and Nefzger, suggested a preponderance of cases among urban-dwellers.[96] The differences, however, were largely because of differences in the distribution of persons of Jewish descent. Monk and colleagues reported that ulcerative colitis and Crohn's disease cases identified in Baltimore were less likely than controls to be from a rural background.[93] A study of Crohn's disease in Olmsted County, Minnesota between 1945 and 1975, showed a higher urban incidence in both sexes over the entire study period.[26] Epidemiologic studies of ulcerative colitis and Crohn's disease completed in Scandinavia,[5,31,32] and also Great Britain,[22] usually have shown no urban and rural differences. An exception is the study of Crohn's disease in northeastern Scotland completed by Kyle.[38] He reported the incidence of Crohn's disease between 1955 and 1969 to be much lower among rural residents, especially males. Finally, Wigley and MacLaurin found ulcerative colitis to be less common in rural populations of New Zealand.[25] More recent reports from many countries are somewhat unclear because of the difficulty of keeping the urban and rural dwelling status separate from occupational factors. Both diseases exist in rural populations and may be increasing there, according to documentation in a number of reports.

Socioeconomic Factors

Socioeconomic factors are used to describe a collection of demographic, educational, income, and occupational factors, which have all been shown to be important etiologically in many diseases. Ulcerative colitis and Crohn's disease have also been associated with socioeconomic status. In a study of ulcerative colitis cases and controls in the United States Army in 1944, a higher proportion of cases than controls had come from professional, managerial, or proprietary-level employment prior to entering active service.[96] A Copenhagen study of ulcerative colitis cases also showed a higher percentage were at a senior salaried level than the proportion of employees in the general population.[97] The 1960 to 1963 hospital incidence survey in Baltimore showed a higher proportion of male, non-Jewish ulcerative colitis cases from professional and managerial levels of employment than was found in a population sample.[93] By contrast, the husbands of female ulcerative colitis cases were more likely to be blue collar level employees. A study of Crohn's disease in England has shown results similar to those for ulcerative colitis with a higher proportion of white collar occupations among cases than in the comparison groups,[65] but a study in Scotland found the opposite.[38]

The educational level of ulcerative colitis cases was not found to be different from the comparison population in the Baltimore survey,[93] but higher educational levels were found to be characteristic of ulcerative colitis in the Copenhagen study.[97] For Crohn's disease, neither male cases nor husbands of female cases differed significantly in occupation from a comparison population in the Baltimore survey, but both male and female cases had more years of schooling than the comparison population.[93]

The farming occupation may favor a low risk of inflammatory bowel disease. This was the only occupational group significantly underrepresented in Kyle's series of Crohn's disease in Scotland.[38,39] In the Baltimore and in the Olmsted County data, however, no significantly low risk for people brought up on farms could be established.[26,93] In the United States, recent and rapid changes in the number of farmers, their educational level, and the managerial practices of farming have made a determination of what factors can be implicated in the 1980's more difficult when describing farmers as an occupation.

Genetic and Environmental Hypotheses

Familial Aggregation

The study of disease occurrence in families is useful to begin the process of separating genetic and environmental factors that may have a part in the development of a disease. A condition that occurs at a rate within families more often than in the general population is familially aggregated. The increased frequency of inflammatory bowel disease in families of patients with the disease has been documented in many countries. A typical finding is that in Cardiff,[98] where the prevalence of Crohn's disease in the siblings of 139 patients was 1602 per 100,000, as compared to the community-wide prevalence of 56. This 30-fold increase agrees with other reports in the literature of non-population-based studies of Crohn's disease. For ulcerative colitis the best data have come from specialized clinics, which have shown that from 10 to 40% of cases have first degree relatives with inflammatory bowel disease.[95] An important observation is that in the total family membership investigated there is a mixture of Crohn's disease and ulcerative colitis. A thoroughgoing review of the roles of heredity and environment in these two disorders comes from McConnell's laboratory, which has reported that the incidence of a second family member developing inflammatory bowel disease is probably two to three times the expected rate in the general population (see Table 1-8). In specialized tertiary care centers, rates for familial occurrence range from 15 to 30%, with even higher rates for the relatives of Jewish probands.[95]

The greatest risk for inflammatory bowel disease seems to occur in those who share the most genes with the propositus. Parent-child and sibling-sibling occurrences are found more frequently than those in less close relatives (Table 1-8).[99] The possibility that such occurrences are because of chance is unlikely. Distinguishing between genetic and shared environmental influences is difficult, however, because there are few attractive environmental hypotheses and testing these is not easily accomplished. These diseases have been described in siblings living geographically apart for many years. Unrelated spouses and children have been reported to develop Crohn's disease within a short time span, but these are rare and could have occurred by chance.[99,100-102] When a family is identified in which either disease is the sole disorder in more than one member, the condition is likely to be Crohn's disease.

Because ascertainment of inflammatory bowel disease cases in relatives of index cases is a function of physician interest and of family cooperation in submitting to expensive and unpleasant tests documenting diagnosis, studies are often plagued by low response rates and are limited to anamnestic diagnoses. Thus, the literature on the familial incidence of these disorders may represent an underestimation. Conversely, acceptance of unvalidated reports of cases among family members may represent an overestimation of familial occurrence. The incidence rates for Crohn's disease have increased in the Western world since 1960, suggesting an emergence of new environmental factors; the proportion of familial cases has paralleled this increase.[98] For ulcerative colitis, there has been no such rapid rise in incidence rates, but familial cases, including Crohn's disease in relatives, continue to be identified in proportions similar to those reported 20 years ago.[98] Consequently, while the trend in incidence rates for these two diseases appears to be different, familial patterns of the two diseases appear to be similar. In spite of the many problems and uncertainties in current studies of familial aggregation, investi-

TABLE 1-8. *Rate of occurrences of inflammatory bowel disease in affected siblings and parents.**

	Index Patients	Affected Sibs/ Total Sibs+ Rate (%)	Affected Parents Total Parents Rate (%)
Ulcerative colitis:			
Group I: 1955–1959	52	1/120(1)	5/104(5)
Group II: 1960–1964	50	2/117(2)	9/100(9)
Group III: 1965–1969	60	5/121(4)	6/120(5)
Group IV: 1970–1974	75	11/153(7)	11/150(8)
Total	237	19/511(4)	31/564(6)
Crohn's disease:			
Group I: 1955–1959	25	2/59(7)	4/50(8)
Group II: 1960–1964	48	8/79(10)	9/96(9)
Group III: 1965–1969	96	15/224(7)	18/192(3)
Group IV: 1970–1974	152	14/322(4)	17/304(3)
Total	321	39/684(6)	48/642(8)

*Adapted from Farmer, R. G., Michever, W. M., and Mortimer, E. A.: Clin. Gastroenterol., 9: 271, 1980.
+No inflammatory bowel disease occurred in 94 half-siblings.

gators and clinicians believe that these diseases have *some* familial association, whether genetic or environmental in origin. Further studies of mendelian and nonmendelian clusters, twins, maternal transmission, cohabitation effects, biological markers, and the usual person, place, and time characteristics of disease patterns are needed to further clarify the role of genetic and environmental factors.

Genetic Features

There is no simple mendelian genetic mechanism at work in the transmission of inflammatory bowel disorders. Aggregate studies of familial occurrence invariably include families in which both ulcerative colitis and Crohn's disease occur. It is unusual for the two diseases to occur together in the same sibship, but more common for a parent to have one disorder and one child or more to have the other. No genetic markers of either disease have yet been validated, either for mucosal immune responses or for those postulated to control physiologic functions of the gut, as, for example, those noted in peptic ulcer heterogeneity—blood groups, serum pepsinogens I and II, HLA haplotypes, immunoglobulins, and T-cell and B-cell populations. Associations of inflammatory bowel disease with rare genetic syndromes, suggesting a recessive inheritance pattern, are sparse; Crohn's disease in Turner's syndrome and in the Hermansky-Pudlak syndrome have been reported in individual cases.[103–105] In inflammatory bowel disease, many studies of the HLA system have been made in affected and in unaffected family members; identical patterns are more often found in the affected siblings than in unaffected siblings, but from family to family the HLA type is highly variable.[106–108] Thus, if any genetic hypothesis can be generated from a review of studies, it is that the gene locus, more than the HLA type, may be associated with the development of inflammatory bowel disease, and particularly with Crohn's disease. The emergence of ankylosing spondylitis, a well-studied disease highly associated (80%) with HLA-B27, as an important association of inflammatory bowel disease, has produced a number of reports attempting to define a genetic link in inflammatory bowel disease patients to the HLA-B27 marker. The results have been confusing, and appear to indicate that when ankylosing spondylitis or sacroiliitis appear in patients with inflammatory bowel disease, about half the patients do not possess the HLA-B27 haplotype.[109] The issue is further complicated by uncertainties in defining the clinical syndrome of ankylosing spondylitis. Viewed from the other end of the spectrum, there may be as yet undefined *deficiencies* of markers that exert either higher relative risk for, or more protection against the development of inflammatory bowel disease. In any case, markers are desperately needed if any progress in defining the heterogeneity of these diseases is to be made.

As has been demonstrated for most chronic disorders, genetic heterogeneity plays an important role in accounting for the diversity of subgroups encompassed by the phenotypes. It is likely that the results of therapy in inflammatory bowel disease, so unpredictable, are directly related to the inevitable diversity of the persons being treated. Approaches to the development of various markers and unusual syndromes to demarcate subgroups at higher or lower risk for developing these diseases, and for responding to various therapeutic manipulations, are needed. Markers for control of gut physiology, as far as they are currently known and understood, have not been identified as yet in inflammatory bowel disease patients; the diseases predominantly represent inflammatory responses, and the markers for diverse aspects of these responses have largely been confined to mucosal immunologic characteristics.[110,111] It is fair to assume that more precision in identifying both these immune mechanisms and the heterogeneity of response to inflammation mediators will be achieved in the near future, but at present little is known. Epidemiologic evidence that either ulcerative colitis or Crohn's disease result from perturbations of normal mucosal immune responses to some agent, transmissible or otherwise, is currently weak. A lymphocytotoxic antibody was described more commonly among household contacts of patients with inflammatory bowel disease than in similarly related family members who live separately.[112] This is an indication of a familial cohabitation effect. Biochemical markers are perhaps more promising, although they are just beginning to be developed. A glycoprotein deficiency in ulcerative colitis has been reported by Podolsky,[113] fattyacid (butyrate) oxidation deficiency has been claimed in ulcerative colitis by Roediger,[114] and a variety of lysosomal enzyme deficiencies has been noted by O'Morain.[111] Such studies need to be applied to family members at risk for inflammatory bowel disease, and some description of their persistence obtained from patients throughout their course.

For the present, the McConnell synthesis is that "from a *genetic* point of view both ulcerative colitis and Crohn's disease should be lumped together as one disease, inflammatory bowel disease. Consideration of their epidemiology indicated that they may also have a shared environmental etiology" (emphasis supplied).[115] The data available at present indicate that genes at several loci subserve the predisposition to inflammatory bowel disease; to paraphrase McConnell: if a few relevant genes are present, the clinical picture is that of ulcerative colitis; a more complete genotype leads to the development of Crohn's disease (see Chap. 6) This position is not universally accepted, but there are no other genetic data that challenge it.

Twin Studies

A study of twins is a more direct method than familial aggregation of examining genetic versus environmental factors that may be involved in a disease. Monozygotic twins (identical) share identical genes and a similar environment. Dizygotic twins (nonidentical) share no more genes than do other full siblings born in singleton births. Dizygotic twins, however, share a more similar environment than other full siblings by virtue of having developed in utero at the same time and shared nearly the same environment pre- and postnatally. Thus, if monozygotic twins are concordant for a disease more often than dizygotic twins, genetic rather than environmental factors are implicated. Epidemiologic studies of inflammatory bowel disease in twins have not been previously reported, which is understandable because both the event of twinning and the occurrence of ulcerative colitis and Crohn's disease are not common. A review of cases of Crohn's disease among twins reported in the literature has shown that seven of eight pairs are concordant for Crohn's disease, and all are monozygous (Table 1-9).[116-122] For, ulcerative colitis, the concordance within twins appears to be much lower, from the literature surveyed.[123-134] Five of 22 pairs of twins were concordant for ulcerative colitis, but all concordant twins were monozygous. Six of the 17 discordant twins were monozygous. It has been shown, however, that twins who are concordant for a disease are more likely to be ascertained and reported, because the fact that the patients are twins and both have the same disease is of interest.[135] All these reports are uncontrolled and based on reports of a single or a small number of twin pairs from clinical series, but these reports do not indicate whether the proportion of twins in clinical series is higher than expected. These reports do suggest that an examination of inflammatory bowel disease among twins would be helpful in clarifying the genetic and environmental basis of inflammatory bowel disease.

Association with Other Diseases

The systemic conditions—aphthous stomatitis, erythema nodosum, uveitis, and pyodermata—that have been noted for many years in ulcerative colitis have now been found to characterize the course of patients with Crohn's disease as well. In addition, liver enlargement and various inflammatory responses in the liver are found in patients suffering from each of these dis-

TABLE 1-9. *Clinical reports of ulcerative colitis and Crohn's disease in twins.*[*]

Study	Number of Twin Pairs	Twinning[+]	Sex[**]	Number Involved One Twin	Number Involved Both Twins
		Crohn's Disease			
Edwards[116]	1	Mz	F		X
Freysz et al.[117]	1	Mz	F		X
Neiderle[118]	1	Mz	F		X
Hislop and Grant[119]	1	Mz	F		X
Crismer et al.[120]	1	Mz	M		X
Janowitz[121]	1	Mz	M		X
Lennard-Jones, 1972[§]	1	Mz	M		X[ǀ]
Anfanger[122]	1	Mz	M	X	
Concordance rate by pooling reports:					
Mz	7/8(88%)				
		Ulcerative Colitis			
Lyons and Postlethwaite[123]	1	Mz	M		X
Webb[124]	1	Mz	M		X
Sleight et al.[125]	1	Mz	F		X
Sanford[126]	1	Mz	M		X
Fausa et al.[127]	1	Mz	F		X
Gregg and Baggenstoss[128]	1	Mz	M	X	
Marie and Ledoux-Lebard[129]	1	Mz	F	X	
Qazi et al.[130]	1	Mz	F	X	
Bacon[131]	1	Dz	M,F	X	
Tidrick, 1962[§]	1	Dz	F	X	
Finch and Hess[132]	1	Dz	Not specified	X	
Binder, 1973[§]	3	Mz	2F,1M	X	
Binder et al.[133]	7	Dz	3F,4M	X	
Kirsner[134]	1	Dz	Not specified	X	
Concordance rate by pooling reports:					
Mz	5/11(45%)				
Dz	0/11(0%)				

[*]Adapted from Kirsner, J. B., and Shorter, R. G.: N. Engl. J. Med., *306*: 775, 1982.
[+]Mz = monozygotic; Dz = dizygotic.
[**]M = male; F = female.
[§]Personal communication to Kirsner.
[ǀ]Crohn's disease of the colon only.

eases.[136] It is probable that patients with Crohn's disease more often have granulomatous lesions in the liver than do those with ulcerative colitis, and that "pericholangitis," chronic active hepatitis, and various forms of cirrhosis are more commonly seen in patients with pancolitis of the ulcerative type, but not much can be made of these differences in frequency of complicating reactions in such patients. It is unlikely that the differences are of fundamental importance in casting light on the etiology of these diseases; they may merely reflect the differing interests and persistence of physicians taking care of large numbers of patients in medical centers at various times. The relationship of sacroiliitis to spondylitis is not always clear, and many of the reports have relied on the appearance of the sacroiliac joints in x-ray films made during performance of barium enemas, films that are not designed to provide the best views of these joints. It may be concluded that the population groups that are susceptible to the underlying bowel inflammation are also likely to respond in other body systems. Indeed, it seems that little can be gained by deciding that one or the other of these reactions is more or less common in one disease or the other. A family in which the classical form of ankylosing spondylitis disease is associated with Crohn's disease is illustrated in Figure 1-5.

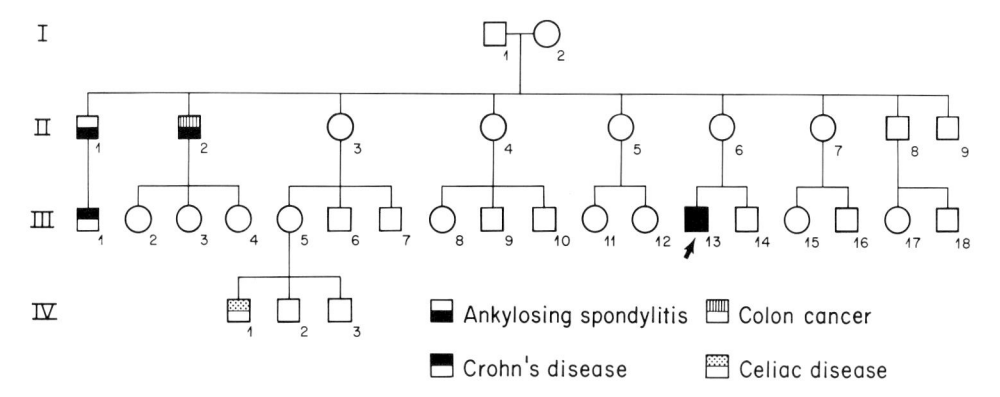

FIG. 1-5. A family in which both ankylosing spondylitis and Crohn's disease occurred in the proband; two uncles had ankylosing spondylitis and one cousin had Crohn's disease.

Infectious Agents and Transmission[*]

An infectious hypothesis is a natural one for inflammatory bowel disease because of the large number of bacterial, viral, and other organisms that are closely associated with the gastrointestinal tract; the large number of other inflammatory conditions of the bowel associated with infectious agents; the intensive infiltration of lymphocytes and polymorphonuclear leukocytes, as well as granuloma formation (in Crohn's disease), which is similar to other infectious processes; the familial association of patients suggesting a common source contamination; and, finally, anecdotal reports of beneficial responses to various antibiotics. An infectious hypothesis, while a viable possibility for Crohn's disease and ulcerative colitis, has not been well addressed from an epidemiologic viewpoint. With respect to ulcerative colitis, a cytomegalovirus has been suggested to have a role in etiology,[137] but this has been disputed.[138] Investigators believe that the nature of the inflammatory response in Crohn's disease makes it more likely to have an infectious etiology. Cave et al. attempted to pass disease from Crohn's disease tissue to animals.[139-141] A granulomatous development was found in rabbit foot pads and in the gastrointestinal tract, but this work has not been replicated.[142] A cell-wall deficient pseudomonas bacterium has been cultured from Crohn's disease tissue, and antibodies to this organism in Crohn's disease patients' serum have been found.[143] This work has been partially confirmed by Yoshimura et al. but it has not been demonstrated whether this organism is etiologically related to Crohn's disease or just an opportunist in the inflamed bowel.[144] A lymphoma-like lesion has been induced in immunologically supressed mice injected with Crohn's disease tissue filtrates.[145] This would suggest a small viral particle, but this work has not been replicated. Another candidate currently receiving attention is a cell-wall defective mycobacterial agent in Crohn's disease tissue. Burnham et al. cultured Mycobacterium kansasii from Crohn's disease lymph nodes and other uncharacterized cell-wall defective agents from 22 of 27 Crohn's disease patients.[146] More recently, investigators have isolated a new form called Mycobacterium linda, felt to be related to Mycobacterium paratuberculosis, and cell-wall defective spheroplasts from Crohn's disease patients.[147-154] They also have reported transmitting an ileal inflammatory disease to goats using the culture material. This is of interest because goats are known to develop granulomatous bowel disease. While this work is interesting, it remains controversial because the results have been only partially confirmed; similar organisms have been found in noninflammatory bowel disease intestinal tissues, and no serologic studies have confirmed the specificity of the findings.[*] The problems of identifying an infectious agent in inflammatory bowel disease patients are that the relationship of such agents to disease onset is problematic. Because of the protracted time involved in establishing a diagnosis, it is not easily determined whether an agent is causally related. Some agents identified in patients may be simply opportunists. Other agents may have

[*]See also Chaps. 2 and 3

[*]Editor's note: See also Sang-nae Cho, et al.: Gut, 27:1353, 1986; and Graham, D. Y., et al.: Gastroenterology, 92:436, 1987.

a role in exacerbations but not in the onset process. Further studies of Crohn's disease patient populations are needed to demonstrate that any particular organism is consistently found among them and is not a contaminant of cultures.

If an organism is isolated, its infectivity and transmissibility should be studied carefully. Transmission of an organism involved in the etiology of ulcerative colitis or Crohn's disease should demonstrate that the new cases are related by time or space parameters in a geographic area. Several such studies have been carried out, but have failed to show time or space clustering of cases.[155, 156] As previously mentioned, however, the early detection of Crohn's disease is usually difficult to document, and thus the latent period between a possible exposure event and the first symptoms or the first diagnosis is not well established. Consequently, the amount of time necessary for a postulated transmission of the causative agent or an adjustment of geographic variables that may play a role need further investigation. Over the years, a number of case reports of inflammatory bowel disease occurring in multiple members of families have accumulated, including members who are not blood relatives. A typical report is that of Hershfield who reported that both parents and a son developed Crohn's disease within an 18-month period.[157] Several other reports of parent-child "transmission" are found in the literature.[158–160] Husband-wife "transmission" is quite rare.[161] Given the established incidence rates, these events are likely to have occurred by chance. The likelihood that blood relatives are at increased risk, however, is supported by increasingly sophisticated literature on the familial features of these diseases. Within the limitations of present understanding, it must be concluded that no *epidemiologic* data other than familial aggregation currently supports the "transmissible agent hypothesis."

Psychologic Factors

In general, clinicians believe that most diseases, once they become established, recur and remit in relation to interpersonal conflicts and the anxieties of daily life. The reliability of epidemiologic data on these points in large numbers of the population is often questionable, particularly when using the case-control design in which psychological evaluation is made after diagnosis among cases. Attempts to characterize large groups by questioning individuals to establish the facts of their life histories—place of birth, level of education, social and economic expectations for lifestyle, marital status and family composition, life events and stresses, and geographic and social mobility—have not met with general acceptance by groups of behavioral scientists, sociologists, or clinical psychiatrists. The principal objection is that those persons suffering most severely may neither communicate freely about such matters nor be able to convey to the questioner the depth of their reactions and the meaning of events and situations in their lives.

In the Baltimore study, such data were meticulously sought and analyzed in patients and in various control groups; a special control group was selected from patients with irritable bowel syndrome, closely matched on age, sex, and ethnic origins to the patients with inflammatory bowel disease.[93,94] Analyses of these data showed that inflammatory bowel disease patients did not have unusual health histories and that inflammatory bowel disease patients did not have significantly more life stress factors as identified by sociologists. The patients with irritable bowel syndrome did show considerably higher "stress indices" than did the patients with ulcerative colitis who, in this respect, were indistinguishable from the other control populations.

A recently reported study of ulcerative colitis and psychiatric disorders found no greater frequency of diagnosable psychiatric disorders among ulcerative colitis patients than among controls. The patients with both ulcerative colitis and a psychiatric disorder did not appear to have more serious gastrointestinal involvement, nor did the more serious ulcerative colitis cases have more serious or frequently occurring psychiatric disorders. Personality profiles and "life events" patterns were also similar for cases and controls.[162]

As noted earlier, psychiatrists would probably have anticipated such results, because many believe that a "hopeless, helpless" response, which they believe underlies the psychological makeup of inflammatory bowel disease patients, cannot be identified by superficial questioning and the establishment of certain historic data in large numbers of people. Recent studies have emphasized depression and anxiety as more characteristic of patients with Crohn's disease than those with ulcerative colitis.

Diet

Because dietary intake is the single most important environmental exposure factor of the digestive system, it is natural to suspect that diet may play some role in inflammatory bowel disease. Dietary studies are somewhat problematic in that the relevant dietary exposure may have occurred many years prior to diagnosis, and even if this were not the case, the prolonged onset-to-diagnosis interval may alter dietary practices. Refinements of dietary intake methodology need to be made. It is probably not surprising then that few studies have been carried out on the preillness diet of inflammatory bowel disease patients. Black African populations, Chinese, East Indians, and Japanese suffer low incidence rates of inflammatory bowel disorders, as is the case with colon polyps, diverticular disease, and colon cancer. Whether their dietary fiber intake is an important feature of this low incidence rate has not yet been studied. The Japanese diet has recently been shown to be no different in fiber content than that of the West,[163] but there is some evidence that Japanese inflammatory bowel disease rates are rising from their previously low levels.[63] Most studies of fiber intakes of westernized subjects has been conducted on prevalent cases, with considerable uncertainty as to the exact characteristics of their diet antecedent to the onset of inflammatory bowel disease. Several studies have shown that Crohn's disease patients were eating diets somewhat lower (15%) in total dietary fiber than controls at the time that their illness was first identified; whether this is a biologically significant difference is questionable.[164] For patients with established inflammatory bowel disease, diets totally lacking in fiber have been shown to be useful in establishing remissions,[165] but diets high in total dietary fiber have also been shown to be helpful in reducing relapses.[166] The overall conclusion at this time would be that dietary fiber intake is most likely not an important determinant of the onset of inflammatory bowel disease.

A study has been made of the intake of dietary refined sugars with respect to inflammatory bowel disease. Thornton and others have reported a higher preillness intake of refined sugars and a deficit of raw fruit and vegetables among Crohn's disease cases.[165,167–170] The amount of difference in the intake of refined sugar was shown by these reports to be about double among cases when compared to controls.[171] A small number of patients (6) who were interviewed within six months of diagnosis in this study were not shown to have higher preillness consumption of refined sugar. Thus, the findings of a higher intake of refined sugar among Crohn's disease cases could simply represent dietary changes made after diagnosis and a memory bias of the preillness diet highly influenced by these changes. No differences in fat or protein intake among these studies have been reported. In an early study, milk consumption was suggested as a causal factor in ulcerative colitis development, but subsequent studies have not supported this hypothesis for either ulcerative colitis or Crohn's disease.[172–175] In a case control study one author found inflammatory bowel disease cases were less likely to take breakfast than controls, and were more likely to consume corn based cereal products.[176] These findings also have not been supported by other research.[177]

The postnatal diet has also received some attention as a possible determinant of later inflammatory bowel disease occurrence. Two reports of case-control studies of ulcerative colitis and Crohn's disease have shown an association of formula feeding with later disease development.[180,181] The importance of a longer duration of breast feeding as a protection against later development of Crohn's disease has also been demonstrated.[181] An absence of an association of breast feeding with Crohn's disease has also been reported, however.[182] Several factors noted previously tend to support a role for infant dietary exposures; first, the higher occurrence of ulcerative colitis and Crohn's disease among persons of Jewish descent in the United States and low occurrence of breast feeding in this same group;[183] second, the downward and then upward trend in the occurrence of breast feeding in the population, and the upward and now apparently stabilizing (or perhaps declining) trend in the incidence of these diseases.[12,43,184] If breast feeding is an important factor for protecting against later development of ulcerative colitis or Crohn's disease, then the incidence trend in the younger age groups should be shown to be the most responsive, with first an increase and then a stabilization (or a decline). The rates of increase for the population under thirty years of age appear to be the highest, but the numbers in any incidence series reported are not large enough to draw reliable conclusions about trends for specific age categories.[12] However, even if both an increasing occurrence of breast feeding and a decreasing incidence of ulcerative colitis and Crohn's disease could be established, the inferences that could be drawn from these trends alone would be limited at best.

The development of an adult chronic intestinal/bowel disorder as a result of exposure in infancy to elements in the diet is not without an existing accepted model and is biologically plausible. It has long been postulated that celiac disease is the result of childhood exposure to the gluten fraction in cereal proteins.[185] Although genetic and other etiologic factors that set the stage for gluten sensitive enteropathy are unknown, gluten exposure in childhood is a necessary component to the activation of the disease. In spite of the large number of persons exposed to formula feeding during the past four to five decades, the relatively small proportion of these persons who develop inflammatory bowel disease suggests that the influence of formula feeding on risk may not be large. Certainly, formula feeding by itself is probably not either a necessary or a sufficient causal factor.

Smoking

Several recent reports have indicated that a larger percentage of ulcerative colitis patients are persons who never smoked or former smokers more often than comparison groups (Table 1-10).[170,186–191] In contrast, patients with Crohn's disease have been found to have the same or higher frequencies of cigarette smoking than a control group.[170,190–192] In assessing these results, it should be noted that several of these studies used prevalent rather than incident

TABLE 1-10. *The relative risk of developing ulcerative colitis and Crohn's disease for various categories of smoking status.*

	Number of Cases	Number of Controls	Relative Risk (95% Confidence Interval)
Ulcerative colitis:			
Harries et al.:[187]			
Never smoked	110	83	1.0
Ex-smokers	102	46	1.67 (1.07-2.62)
Current smokers	18	101	0.13 (0.08-0.23)
Logan et al.:[189]			
Never smoked	52	76	1.0
Ex-smokers	46	24	2.80 (1.54-5.10)
Current smokers	22	99*	0.32 (0.18-0.57)
Calkins et al.:[190]			
(Cases compared with hospital controls)			
Never smoked	45	29	1.0
Ex-smokers	24	18	0.86 (0.37-1.99)
Current smokers	16	33	0.31 (0.14-0.71)
(Cases compared with neighborhood controls)			
Never smoked	45	40	1.0
Ex-smokers	24	20	1.07 (0.48-2.36)
Current smokers	16	23	0.62 (0.28-1.42)
Crohn's disease:			
Somerville et al.:[192]			
Never smoked	59	64	4.0 (1.9-8.1)
Current smokers	45	35	3.50 (1.80-6.60)
Smoking at onset	52	41	4.8 (2.4-9.7)
Calkins et al.:[190]			
(Cases compared with hospital controls)			
Never smoked	49	53	1.0
Ex-smokers	17	26	0.71 (0.32-1.55)
Current smokers	66	51	1.40 (0.79-2.47)
(Cases compared with neighborhood controls)			
Never smoked	49	68	1.0
Ex-smokers	17	28	0.84 (0.39-1.81)
Current smokers	66	44	1.08 (1.18-3.66)

*For two controls, smoking status was uncertain.

cases of ulcerative colitis and Crohn's disease. Such a practice, while advantageous for producing a large enough sample of cases, may introduce biases of unknown direction and magnitude. All of the studies to date have suffered from one or more design problems: low statistical power, inappropriate control groups, lack of adjustment or matching for confounding variables, inadequate smoking history and dose-response information, and a dearth of information relating to smoking behavior and symptoms. It should be noted that the excess risk appears to be limited to former smokers in some reports,[193,194] but not all.[191] A prevalence survey of Mormons, who are generally nonsmokers, in Great Britain has shown ulcerative colitis to be five times more common in this predominantly nonsmoking population than in the general population, but no excess prevalence of Crohn's disease was found.[195] A significant deficit of smoking-related mortality experiences (cardiovascular disease and lung cancer deaths) has also been noted among ulcerative colitis cases,[196,197] which indirectly confirms the smaller number of smokers among ulcerative colitis cases to explain these lower cardiovascular disease and lung cancer mortality rates.[198]

In addition to these studies, two case histories have been published of patients with ulcerative colitis who achieved remission of symptoms while smoking and an exacerbation of symptoms at the cessation of smoking.[199,200] On the other hand, a study of a larger case series (8 smokers and 94 nonsmokers) of ulcerative colitis patients has shown more relapses and a greater severity of pain during relapse (neither being statistically significant) among ulcerative colitis smokers when compared to ulcerative colitis nonsmokers.[201] In the same study, Crohn's disease smokers were reported to experience statistically significantly more relapses, hospital admissions, surgery, pain, diarrhea, and changes in white cell count than Crohn's disease nonsmokers, suggesting an aggravating role for smoking in the disease. The case histories in the literature are interesting because they raise the suggestion of a possible etiologic or therapeutic role for cigarette smoking in ulcerative colitis. If smoking is therapeutic or possibly preventive, that would indeed be astonishing after the decades of study and multiplicity of publications linking smoking with many other chronic diseases.

The consistency of the nonsmoking feature of ulcerative colitis cases and the difference of the smoking association between ulcerative colitis and Crohn's disease suggests that the associations are real and not artifactual. Perhaps the most important implication of the reported case histories is that a study of the mechanism by which nicotine or other tobacco ingredients may act to control symptoms would be of great value. An understanding of this mechanism, if operative, would be helpful in developing a similar, nonaddictive product that could be used therapeutically.

Oral Contraceptives

The worldwide adoption of oral contraceptive drugs began in 1965, reached a peak of usage in 1978, and has remained stable since.[202] This pattern is similar to that for the incidence rates of Crohn's disease in females of childbearing age; one important study identified ulcerative colitis and Crohn's disease as diseases more prevalent among oral contraceptive users than among nonusers.[203] In addition, remission of symptoms after discontinuing the use of oral contraceptives has been reported by a number of investigators.[204–211] A larger proportion of Crohn's disease cases have been reported by Rhodes to be users of oral contraceptives.[212] The odds ratio for oral contraceptive use among Crohn's disease patients was determined by Lesko to be 1:9.[213] If confirmed, these findings could explain the excess risk among women noted earlier. But in the Baltimore area, the confidence intervals for the odds ratios for all inflammatory bowel disease patients and ulcerative colitis and Crohn's disease patients separately all include unity.[214] As with the studies on smoking, these studies suffer from design problems. The Rhodes et al. study did not use an especially selected control group, but compared oral contraceptive use among patients with that of the general population.[212] The Lesko findings could be explained if women with established Crohn's disease used oral contraceptives to avoid pregnancy believing that pregnancy and child rearing would further complicate their lives.[213] The Baltimore data were not collected in such a way as to distinguish estrogenic and nonestrogenic hormones, or the reason for hormone use.[214] It has also been suggested that estrogens may produce symptoms and clinical findings in some patients that mimic Crohn's disease because any manifestation of the disease disappears with the cessation of use.[211] This issue has just begun to be explored and warrants further study; however, even if confirmed, these findings could perhaps explain only the excess risk among women noted earlier.

Summary

This chapter has reviewed the methods currently used in the investigation of the epidemiology of inflammatory bowel disease for which frequency and mortality are low and genetic and environmental determinants may be multiple. During the two and a half decades during which such studies have been carried out in both hemispheres, different investigators have reached agreement on some fundamental characteristics of cases. These characteristics and the current findings on various hypotheses that have been studied are summarized in Table 1-11.

For the future, if the distribution of features in the population at risk is to provide more insight into the etiology and course of these diseases, it will be necessary to develop better fundamental means of acquisition and recording of data, especially methods of identifying cases diagnosed and treated as out-patients exclusively. Many of these requisites have been discussed by authorities in the field; the WHO expert Committee on Health Statistics has published a number of technical reports on the subject, and the 1967 report is especially recommended.[215,216] Emphasis has been made in this review on the possible benefits to be derived from more intensive studies of families; again, the WHO technical report of 1971 (254) goes into considerable detail on the proper methodology for such studies. A record linkage program for all citizens is probably a prerequisite for proper interpretation of trends in incidence and prevalence. This system, well described by Acheson, starts with birth certificates and moves then into a family master file.[217] Such record linkages are worked out for the United Kingdom and should be started in the United States if any reasonable understanding of the relation of genetic to environmental factors in chronic disease is to be achieved. Emphasis has been made in this chapter on the possible benefits to be derived from more intensive studies of families; again, the WHO technical report of 1971 goes into considerable detail on the proper methodology for such studies. Further clarification of the diagnostic characteristics of early disease is important to ascertain cases before many changes in antecedent characteristics have occurred. Increased public awareness of all of the symptoms of gastrointestinal dysfunction that should be brought to the attention of qualified gastroenterologists would likely result in earlier ascertainment and diagnosis of inflammatory bowel disease, as well as other problems. Finally, the impact of diagnosis-related groups on the classification of inflammatory bowel disease cases needs evaluation.

Whatever new methodologic approaches are developed, many areas of investigation remain open for study. The verification of the incidence

TABLE 1-11. *General characteristics of inflammatory bowel disease cases and findings on selected hypotheses.*

	Ulcerative Colitis	*Crohn's Disease*
Risk groups:		
Sex	Females—30% higher risk	Females—30% higher risk
Age groups (years)	15–35	15–35
		?60–70
Race	Whites	Whites
Ethnicity	Jews	Jews
Urban-rural dwellers	?Urban	?Urban
Occupation	White collar	White collar
Education	Higher levels	Higher levels
Hypotheses:		
Family/genetics	Few shared genes	Many shared genes
Infectious agents	?	?Mycobacterium
Transmissibility	doubtful	doubtful
Psychiatric factors	?No	?No
Diet:		
fiber	?	?
refined sugar	?	?Yes
postnatal	?Formula feeding	?Formula feeding
Smoking	?Protective	?Risk
Oral contraceptives	?Yes	?Yes

trends in various populations is important; investigators must be sure that the primary classifications have been consistent over past decades in order to determine whether trends in incidence or mortality have occurred. Diseases that change incidence over a few decades, as has been suggested for Crohn's disease, are likely affected by environmental causes. Study of the trends in incidence in age-specific categories and in birth cohorts would be useful. For example, if incidence is shown to be higher in a particular birth cohort over time, this suggests that some common environmental exposure may be involved in etiology. Confirming the risk at specific ages is important to establish or refute the observation of bimodality. Further study of racial, religious, ethnic, and social characteristics are needed. For example, studies of Hispanic and Asian groups within the United States, and of Amish, Mormon, and Seventh-day Adventist religious groups would help to identify groups with differential risk. Further study of Jewish groups in the United States, Europe, and Israel are needed to determine why United States Jews are at higher risk. Studies in nonwesternized countries are needed. Studies of employees involved in particular occupations would also be useful.

The establishment of familial aggregation epidemiologically has been attempted without success to date. The logistics of confirming diagnoses of anamnestic reports among family members are formidable, but further studies of familial aggregation are needed. As a minimal effort, registries of families in which multiple cases of inflammatory bowel disease occur should be developed. These families should be intensively studied by genetic, nutritional, psychologic, and metabolic techniques; family members thought to be unaffected should be closely followed at intervals for possible development of early disease. In such registries, the relationship of disease occurrence to identifiable changes in the environment, defined chemically, physically, or psychologically can be examined. In families with inflammatory bowel disease, the population under the age of 15 presents a unique opportunity for longitudinal studies. Because this age group is highly susceptible and probably experiences the most complete range of clinical manifestations, special means should be developed for classifying children as early in life as possible. The potential for malignancies in children with either disease is serious, therefore the requisite follow up of these children can provide an opportunity for a detailed exploration of the genetic susceptibility to cancer in families; attention should be paid to possible carcinogens being produced in these patients, or perhaps to their failure to detoxify known carcinogens or oncongenic viruses. Studies in twin and adoption registries would be useful to clarify the contribution of genetics to risk. Carefully planned studies of Asian migrants to Hawaii and California would be useful. Finally, the association with other diseases must be better defined with a parallel appraisal of peculiarities in drug metabolism, enterohepatic circulation, or immunologic reactivity.

Further studies of possible bacterial or viral agents involved in inflammatory bowel disease pathogenesis are needed. Biologic markers related to risk need to be defined. While psychologic factors do not appear to be a fruitful area for etiologic search, these factors may contribute to the establishment of the disease and its pattern of remissions and exacerbations. Psychologic factors might be reconsidered causally if improved instruments for measuring these factors prior to the onset of the disease are developed. Carefully planned studies of dietary factors antecedent to disease onset are needed. Postnatal feeding factors, breast-formula feeding, age at weaning, first foods introduced, may be a particularly fruitful area for study of disease in the young. Study of the effect of these postnatal factors on developmental patterns of the digestive and immune system should be made. The relationship of smoking and/or the constituents of tobacco to risk and/or therapy should be explored. Studies of oral contraceptive users and nonusers should also be made to determine the effect on the risk of acquiring inflammatory bowel disease. Because few solid leads have been established, new ideas for exposure factors are needed.

References

1. Iversen, E., et al.: An epidemiological model of ulcerative colitis. Scand. J. Gastroenterol., *3*:593, 1968.
2. Hiatt, R. A.: Unpublished data, 1987.
3. Nordenvall, B., et al.: Incidence of ulcerative colitis in Stockholm County, 1955–1979. Scand. J. Gastroenterol., *20*:783, 1985.
4. Gollup, J. H., Phillips, S. F., Melton, L. J., and Zinsmeister, A. R.: Epidemiologic aspects of Crohn's disease: A population-based study in Olmsted County, Minnesota, 1943–82. Unpublished data, 1986.
5. Hellers, G.: Crohn's Disease in Stockholm County, 1955–74. A study of epidemiology, results of surgical treatment and long term prognosis. Acta Chir. Scand. (Suppl.) *490*:1, 1979.

6. Sanderson, I. R., and Walker-Smith, J. A.: Indigenous amoebiasis: an important differential diagnosis of chronic inflammatory bowel disease. Br. Med. J., *289*:823, 1984.
7. Myren, J., et al.: The O.M.G.E. Multinational Inflammatory Bowel Disease Survey 1976–1982. Scand. J. Gastroenterol., *19*(Suppl 95):1, 1984.
8. Acheson, E. D.: Epidemiology of ulcerative colitis and regional enteritis. *In* Recent Advances in Gastroenterology. Edited by J. Badenoch, and B. N. Brooke. Boston, Little, Brown and Co., 1965.
9. Goligher, J. C.: Ulcerative Colitis. Baltimore, Williams & Wilkins, 1968.
10. Susser, M.: Separating heredity and environment. Am. J. Prev. Med., *1*:5, 1985.
11. Monk, M., Mendeloff, A. I., Siegel, C. I., and Lilienfeld, A.: An epidemiological study of ulcerative colitis and regional enteritis among adults in Baltimore. I. Hospital incidence and prevalence, 1960–1963. Gastroenterology, *53*:198, 1967.
12. Calkins, B. M., Lilienfeld, A. M., Garland, C. F., and Mendeloff, A. I.: Trends in the incidence rates of ulcerative colitis and Crohn's disease. Dig. Dis. Sci., *29*:913, 1984.
13. Sedlack, R. E., Nobrega, F. R., Kurland, L. T., and Sauer, W. G.: Inflammatory colon disease in Rochester, Minnesota, 1935–1964. Gastroenterology, *62*:935, 1972.
14. Stonnington, C. M., Phillips, S. F., Melton, L. J., and Zinsmeister, A. R.: Chronic ulcerative colitis: incidence and prevalence in a community. GUT *28*:402, 1987.
15. Garland, C. F., et al.: Incidence rates of ulcerative colitis and Crohn's disease in fifteen areas of the United States. Gastroenterology, *81*:1115, 1981.
16. Bonnevie, O., Riis, P., and Anthonisen, P.: An epidemiological study of ulcerative colitis in Copenhagen County. Scand. J. Gastroenterol., *3*:432, 1968.
17. Binder, V., et al.: Incidence and prevalence of ulcerative colitis and Crohn's disease in the county of Copenhagen, 1962 to 1978. Gastroenterology, *83*:563, 1982.
18. Myren, I., et al.: Epidemiology of ulcerative colitis and regional enterocolitis (Crohn's disease) in Norway. Scand. J. Gastroenterol., *6*:511, 1971.
19. Ustvedt, J. H.: Ulcerative colitis: A study of all cases discharged from Norwegian hospitals in the ten-year period 1946–1955. *In* Recent Studies in Epidemiology. Edited by J. Pemberton. Springfield, Il., Charles C Thomas, 1958.
20. Gjone, E., and Myren, J.: Colitis ulcerosa i Norge. Nord. Med., *71*:143, 1964.
21. Morris, T., and Rhodes, J.: Incidence of ulcerative colitis in the Cardiff region, 1968–1977. Gut, *25*:846, 1984.
22. Evans, J. G., and Acheson, D. E.: An epidemiological study of ulcerative colitis and regional enteritis in the Oxford area. Gut, *6*:311, 1965.
23. Devlin, H. B., Datta, D., and Dellipiani, A. W.: The incidence and prevalence of inflammatory bowel disease in North Tees health district. World J. Surg., *4*:183, 1980.
24. Nedbal, J., and Maratka, Z.: Ulcerative proctocolitis in Czechoslovakia. Am. J. Proctol., *19*:106, 1968.
25. Wigley, R. D., and MacLaurin, B. P.: A study of ulcerative colitis in New Zealand, showing a low incidence in Maoris. Br. Med. J., *2*:228, 1962.
26. Sedlack, R. E., Whisnant, J., Elveback, L. R., and Kurland, L. R.: Incidence of Crohn's disease in Olmsted County, Minnesota, 1945–1975. Am. J. Epidemiol., *112*:759, 1980.
27. Gelpi, A.: Inflammatory bowel disease among college students. West. J. Med., *129*:369, 1978.
28. Hoj, L., Brix-Jensin, P., Bonnevie, O., and Riis, P.: An epidemiological study of regional enteritis and acute ileitis in Copenhagen County. Scand. J. Gastroenterol., *8*:381, 1973.
29. Havia, T., and Thomasson, G.: Crohn's disease. followup study. Acta Chir. Scand., *138*:844, 1972.
30. Gjone, E., Orning, O. M., and Myren, J.: Crohn's disease in Norway, 1956–1963. Gut, *7*:372, 1966.
31. Bergman, L., and Krause, U.: The incidence of Crohn's Disease in Central Sweden. Scand. J. Gastroenterol., *10*:725, 1975.
32. Norlen, B. J., Krause, U., and Bergman, L.: An epidemiological study of Crohn's disease. Scand. J. Gastroenterol., *5*:385, 1970.
33. Krause, U.: Epidemiology in Sweden. *In* Regional Enteritis (Crohn's Disease). Edited by A. Engel, and T. Larson. Stockholm, Nordiska Bokhandelns Forlan, Scandia International Symposia, 1971.
34. Kewenter J., Hulten, L., and Kock, N. G.: The relationship and epidemiology of acute terminal ileitis and Crohn's disease. Gut, *15*:801, 1974.
35. Brahme, F., Lindstrom, C., and Wenckert, A.: Crohn's disease in a defined population. Gastroenterology, *69*:342, 1975.
36. Harries, A. D., Baird, A., Rhodes, J., and Mayberry, F. F.: Has the rising incidence of Crohn's disease reached a plateau? Br. Med. J., *284*:235, 1982.
37. Mayberry, J., Rhodes, J., and Hughes, L. E.: Incidence of Crohn's disease in Cardiff between 1934 and 1977. Gut, *20*:602, 1979.
38. Kyle, J.: An epidemiological study of Crohn's disease in northeast Scotland. Gastroenterology, *61*:826, 1971.
39. Kyle, J., and Stark, G.: Fall in the incidence of Crohn's disease. Gut, *21*:340, 1980.
40. Smith, I. S., et al.: Epidemiological aspects of Crohn's disease in Clydesdale, 1961–1979. Gut, *16*:62, 1975.
41. Humphreys, W. G., and Park, T. G.: Crohn's disease in Northern Ireland—a retrospective study of 159 cases. Ir. J. Med. Sci., *144*:437, 1975.
42. Tresadern, J. C., Gear, M. W. L., and Nicol, A.: An epidemiological study of regional enteritis in the Gloucester area. Br. J. Surg., *60*:366, 1973.
43. Lee, F. I., and Costello, F. T.: Crohn's disease in Blackpool—incidence and prevalence, 1968–80. Gut, *26*:274, 1985.
44. Wright, J. T.: The prevalence of Crohn's disease in an East London borough. 4th World Congress of Gastroenterology. Advance Abstracts, *389*:1970.
45. Miller, D. S., Keighley, A. C., and Langman, M. J. S.: Changing patterns in epidemiology of Crohn's disease. Lancet, *2*:691, 1974.
46. Bitter, J., and Zuvocova, J.: Crohnova choroba v severoceskem kraji. Cesk. Gastroenterol. Vyz., *35*:137, 1981.
47. Lanfranchi, G. A., et al.: Uno studio epidemiologico sulle malattie infiammatorie intestinali nella provincia de Bologna. G. Clin. Med., *57*:235, 1976.
48. Ochoa, R.: Epidemiologia. *In* Simposio Sobre La Enfermedad de Crohn en Galicia. Edited by M. Fiol, R. Ochoa, and P. Perez. Rev. Esp. Enferm. Apar. Dig., *50*:469, 1977.
49. Paredes, J. G., and Garcia, J. M. P.: Crohn's disease in the central area of Spain. *In* Developments in Gastroenterology. I. Recent Advances in Crohn's Disease. Edited by A. S. Peña, I. T. Weterman, and C. C. Booth. The Hague, Martinus Nijhoff, 1981.
50. Farhlandr, H., and Baerlocher, C.: Clinical features and epidemiological data on Crohn's disease in Basle area. Scand. J. Gastroenterol., *6*:657, 1971.

51. Gilat, T., et al.: Ulcerative colitis in the Jewish population of Tel Aviv-Yafo. I. Epidemiology. Gastroenterology, 66:335, 1974.
52. Gilat, T., and Rozen, P.: Epidemiology of Crohn's disease and ulcerative colitis: etiologic implications. Isr. J. Med. Sci., 15:305, 1979.
53. Krawiec, J., et al.: Aspects of the epidemiology of Crohn's disease in the Jewish population in Beer Sheva, Israel. Isr. J. Med. Sci., 20:16, 1984.
54. Odes, H. S., Krawiec, J., and Weitzman, S.: Prevalence of Crohn's disease in Israel. N. Engl. J. Med., 306:750, 1982.
55. Rozen, P., Zonis, J., Yekutiel, P., and Gilat, T.: Crohn's disease in the Jewish population of Tel Aviv-Yafo: epidemiologic and clinical aspects. Gastroenterology, 76:25, 1979.
56. Hutt, M. S. R.: Epidemiology of chronic intestinal disease in middle Africa. Isr. J. Med. Sci., 15:314, 1979.
57. Rolon, P. A.: Gastrointestinal pathology in South America. Isr. J. Med. Sci., 15:318, 1979.
58. Falla-Alvarez, L., and Albacete, R.: Further experience with chronic regional enteritis in Cuba. South Med. J., 51:1556, 1958.
59. Mendoloff, A. I.: Unpublished data, 1975.
60. Jalan, K. N., et al.: An experience of ulcerative colitis. III. Long-term outcome. Gastroenterology, 59:598, 1970.
61. Moller, C., and Linden, F.: Ulcerative colitis in Finland. I. Cases treated at central hospitals, 1956–1967. Dis. Colon Rectum, 14:259, 1971.
62. Eason, R. J., Lee, S. P., and Tasman-Jones, C.: Inflammatory bowel disease in Auckland, New Zealand. Aust. NZ. J. Med., 12:125, 1982.
63. Ishikawa, M., et al.: Crohn's disease, non-specific ulcers of the small intestine, and idiopathic proctocolitis in a Japanese university hospital from 1954 to 1974. Tohoku J. Exp. Med., 118:97, 1976.
64. Das, S. K., and Montgomery, R. D.: Chronic inflammatory bowel disease in Asian immigrants. Practitioner, 221:747, 1978.
65. Keighley, A., Miller, D. S., Hughes, A. O., and Langman, M. J. S.: The demographic and social characteristics of patients with Crohn's disease in the Nottingham area. Scand. J. Gastroenterol., 11:293, 1976.
66. Brom, B., et al.: Crohn's disease in the Cape: A follow-up study of 24 cases and a review of the diagnosis and management. S. Afr. Med. J., 42:1099, 1968.
67. Novis, B. H., Marks, I. N., Bank, S., and Louw, J. H.: Incidence of Crohn's diseasest at Groote Schuur Hospital during 1970–1974. S. Afr. Med. J., 49:693, 1975.
68. Segal, I., Tim, L. O., Hamilton, D. G., and Walker, A. R. P.: The rarity of ulcerative colitis in South African blacks. Am. J. Gastroenterol., 74:332, 1980.
69. Sheps, M. C.: On the person-years concept in epidemiology and demography. Milbank Mem. Fund Q., 44:68, 1966.
70. Houghton, E. A. W., and Naish, J. M.: Familial ulcerative colitis and regional ileitis. Gastroenterologia (Basel), 89:65, 1958.
71. 1970 Census of Population. United States Department of Commerce, Washington, DC, 1973.
72. 1980 Census of Population. United States Department of Commerce, Washington, DC, 1983.
73. National Center for Health Statistics, Vital Statistics of the United States, 1970. United States Department of Health, Education, and Welfare, Public Health Service, Rockville, MD, 1974.
74. National Center for Health Statistics, Vital Statistics of the United States, 1971. United States Department of Health, Education, and Welfare, Public Health Service, Rockville, MD, 1974.
75. National Center for Health Statistics, Vital Statistics of the United States, 1982. United States Department of Health and Human Services, Public Health Service, Hyattsville, MD, unpublished.
76. Szklo, M., et al.: Incidence of aplastic anemia in metropolitan Baltimore: a population-based study. Blood, 66:115, 1985.
77. Dean, G., and Kurtzke, J. F.: On the risk of multiple sclerosis according to age at immigration to South Africa. Br. Med. J., 3:725, 1971.
78. Poskanzer, D. C., Schapira, K., and Miller, H.: Epidemiology of multiple sclerosis in the counties of Northumberland and Durham. J. Neurol. Neurosurg. Psychiatry, 26:368, 1963.
79. Poskanzer, D. C., Schapira, K., and Miller, H.: Multiple sclerosis and poliomyelitis. Lancet, 2:917, 1963.
80. Morariu, M. A., and Linden, M.: Multiple sclerosis in American blacks. Acta Neurol. Scand., 62:180, 1980.
81. Alter, M.: Multiple sclerosis in the negro. Arch. Neurol., 7:83, 1962.
82. Fischman, H. R.: Multiple sclerosis: A new perspective on epidemiological patterns. Neurology., 32:864, 1982.
83. Paffenbarger, R. S., Wing, A. L., and Hyde, R. T.: Brief communication: characteristics in youth indicative of adult-onset Hodgkin's disease. J. Natl. Cancer Inst., 58:1489, 1977.
84. Roger, B. H. G., Clark, L. M., and Kirsner, J. B.: The epidemiologic and demographic characteristics of inflammatory bowel disease: an analysis of a computerized file of 1400 patients. J. Chronic Dis., 24:743, 1971.
85. Burch, P. R. J., de Dombal, F. T., and Watkinson, G.: Aetiology of ulcerative colitis. II. A new hypothesis. Gut, 10:277, 1969.
86. Mendeloff, A. I., and Dunn, J. P.: Digestive Diseases. American Public Health Association Vital and Health Statistics Monograph. Cambridge, Harvard University Press, 1971.
87. Matsunaga, F.: Clinical studies of ulcerative colitis and its related diseases in Japan. *In* Proceedings World Congress Gastroenterology. Baltimore, Williams & Wilkins, 1958.
88. Paulley, J. W.: Ulcerative colitis: A study of 173 cases. Gastroenterology, 16:566, 1950.
89. Acheson, E. C.: The distribution of ulcerative colitis and regional enteritis in United States veterans with particular reference to the Jewish religion. Gut, 1:291, 1960.
90. Rappaport, H., Burgoyne, F. H., and Smetana, H. F.: The pathology of regional enteritis. Milit. Surg., 109:463, 1951.
91. Korelitz, B. I.: From Crohn to Crohn's disease: 1979. An epidemiologic study in New York City. Mt. Sinai J. Med. (NY), 46:533, 1979.
92. Wright, J. P., et al.: The Cape Town experience of Crohn's disease. *In* Crohn's Workshop: A Global Assessment of Crohn's Disease. Edited by E. C. G. Lee. London, H M & M Heyden, 1981.
93. Monk, M., Mendeloff, A. I., Siegel, C. I., and Lilienfeld, A.M.: An epidemiological study of ulcerative colitis and regional enteritis among adults in Baltimore, II. Social and demographic factors. Gastroenterology, 56:847, 1969.
94. Mendeloff, A. I., et al.: Illness experience and life stresses in patients with irritable colon and with ulcerative colitis. N. Engl. J. Med., 282:14, 1970.
95. Singer, H. C., Anderson, J. G. O., Fischer, H., and Kirsner,

J. B.: Familial aspects of inflammatory bowel disease. Gastroenterology, *61*:423, 1971.
96. Acheson, E. D., and Nefzger, M. D.: Ulcerative colitis in the United States Army in 1944. Gastroenterology, *44*:7, 1963.
97. Bonnevie, O.: A socio-economic study of patients with ulcerative colitis. Scand. J. Gastroenterol., *2*:129, 1967.
98. Mayberry, J. F., Rhodes, J., and Newcombe, R. G.: Familial prevalence of inflammatory bowel disease in relatives of patients with Crohn's disease. Br. Med. J., *280*:84, 1980.
99. Farmer, R. G., Michever, W. M., and Mortimer, E. A.: Studies of family history among patients with inflammatory bowel disease. Clin. Gastroenterol., *9*:271, 1980.
100. Whorwell, P. H., et al.: Crohn's disease in a husband and wife. Lancet, *2*:186, 1978.
101. Craxi, A., Olive, L., and Distefauo, G.: Ulcerative colitis in a married couple. Ital. J. Gastroenterol., *11*:184, 1979.
102. Zetsel, L.: Crohn's disease in a husband and wife. Lancet, *2*:583, 1978.
103. Price, W. H.: A high incidence of chronic inflammatory bowel disease in patients with Turner's syndrome. J. Med. Genet., *16*:263, 1979.
104. Schinella, R. A., et al.: Hermansky-Pudlak syndrome with granulomatous colitis. Ann. Intern. Med., *92*: 20, 1980.
105. Nishimura, H., Kino, M., Kubo, S., and Kawamura, K.: Hashimoto's thyroiditis and ulcerative colitis in a patient with Turner's syndrome. JAMA, *254*:357, 1985.
106. Smolen, J. S., et al.: HLA antigens in inflammatory bowel disease. Gastroenterology, *82*:34, 1982.
107. Peña, A. S., et al.: HLA antigen distribution and HLA haplotype segregation in Crohn's disease. Tissue Antigens, *16*:56, 1980.
108. Eade, O. E., et al.: Discordant HLA haplotype segregation in familial Crohn's disease. Gastroenterology, *79*:271, 1980.
109. Van den Berg-Loonen, E. M., et al.: Histocompatibility antigens and other genetic markers in ankylosing spondylitis and inflammatory bowel disease. J. Immunogenet., *4*:167, 1977.
110. O'Morain, C., Smethurst, P., Levi, A. J., and Peter, T. J.: Biochemical analysis of enzymic markers of inflammation in rectal biopsies from patients with ulcerative colitis and Crohn's disease. J. Clin. Pathol., *36*:1312, 1983.
111. O'Morain, C., Smethurst, P., Levi, A. J., and Peter, T. J.: Organelle pathology in ulcerative and Crohn's colitis with special reference to the lysosomal alterations. Gut, *25*:455, 1984.
112. Krosmeyer, S. J., Williams, R. C., Wilson, I. D., and Strickland, R. G.: Lymphocytotoxic antibody in inflammatory bowel disease. N. Engl. J. Med. *293*:1117, 1975.
113. Podolsky, D. K., and Isselbacher, K. J.: Glycoprotein composition of colonic mucosa. Specific alteration in ulcerative colitis. Gastroenterology, *87*:991, 1984.
114. Roediger, W. E. W.: The colonic epithelium in ulcerative colitis: an energy-deficiency disease. Lancet, *2*:712, 1980.
115. McConnell, R. B.: Inflammatory bowel disease: newer views of genetic influences. *In* Developments in Digestive Disease. Vol 3. Edited by J. E. Berk. Philadelphia, Lea & Febiger, 1980.
116. Edwards, H. C.: Crohn's Disease. Recent Advances In Surgery. 4th Ed. London, Churchill, 1954.
117. Freysz, H., Haemmerli, A., and Dartagener, M.: Ileitis regionalis bei einem weiblichen zwillinspaar. Gastroenterologia (Basel), *89*:75, 1958.
118. Niederle, M. B.: Regional ileitis in monozygotic female twins. Arch. Mal. l'Appar. Dig. Mal. Nutr., 50:1245, 1961.
119. Hislop, I. G., and Grant, A. K.: Genetic tendency in Crohn's disease. Gut, *10*:994, 1969.
120. Crismer, R., Dreze, C., and Donival, P.: Ileite de Crohn chez des jemeaux univitellins. Acta Genet. Med. Gemellol. (Roma), *12*:358, 1963.
121. Janowitz, H. D.: Cited by Sherlock, P., et al.: Familial occurrence of regional enteritis and ulcerative colitis. Gastroenterology, *45*:413, 1963.
122. Anfanger, H.: Regional ileitis in children. J. Mt. Sinai Hosp., *22*:187, 1955.
123. Lyons, D. K., and Postlethwaite, R. W.: Chronic ulcerative colitis in twins. Gastroenterology, *10*:545, 1948.
124. Webb, L. R.: The occurrence of chronic ulcerative colitis in two males. Gastroenterology, *15*:523, 1950.
125. Sleight, D. R., Galpin, G. E., and Condon, R. E. : Ulcerative colitis in monozygotic twins and a female sibling. Gastroenterology, *61*:507, 1971.
126. Sanford, F. E.: Genetic implications in ulcerative colitis. Am. J. Surg., *37*:512, 1971.
127. Fausa, O., et al.: Ulcerative colitis in monozygotic twins. Scand. J. Gastroenterol., (Suppl.), *7*(16):38, 1972.
128. Gregg, J. A., and Baggenstoss, A. H.: Discordance for ulcerative colitis in identical twins concordant for cholestatic liver disease, report of two cases. Am. J. Dig. Dis., *15*:667, 1970.
129. Marie, J., and Ledoux-Lebard, G.: Rectocolitis: hemorragiques chez un enfant. Caractere familial de l'affection. Arch. Mal. l'Appar. Dig. Mal. Nutr., *31*:76, 1942.
130. Qazi, Q. H., Pikin, E., and Fierst, S.: Discordant occurrence of ulcerative colitis in identical twins. Gastroenterology, *65*:134, 1973.
131. Bacon, H. D.: Ulcerative Colitis. Philadelphia, J. B. Lipincott, 1958.
132. Finch, S. M., and Hess, J. H.: Ulcerative colitis in children. Am. J. Psychiatry, *9*:819, 1962.
133. Binder, V., Weeks, E., Olson, J. H., Anthonisen, P., and Riis, P.: A genetic study of ulcerative colitis. Scand. J. Gastroenterol., *1*:49, 1966.
134. Kirsner, J. B.: Unpublished data, 1972.
135. Tattersall, R. B., and Pyke, D. A.: Diabetes in identical twins. Lancet, *2*:1120, 1972.
136. Schrumpf, E., et al.: HLA antigens and immunoregulatory T-cells in ulcerative colitis associated with hepatobiliary disease. Scand. J. Gastroenterol., *17*:187, 1982.
137. Farmer, G. W., et al.: Viral investigations in ulcerative colitis and regional enteritis. Gastroenterology, *65*:8, 1973.
138. Collins, J., et al.: No evidence of cytomegalovirus in ulcerative colitis tissue evaluated by culture, nucleic acid hybridization and monoclonal antibody. Gastroenterology, *88*:1353, 1985 (abstract).
139. Cave, D. R., et al.: Further animal evidence of a transmissible agent in Crohn's disease. Lancet, *2*:1120, 1973.
140. Cave, D. R., Mitchell, D. N., and Brooke, B. N.: Observations on the transmissibility of Crohn's disease and ulcerative colitis. Gut, *16*:401, 1975 (abstract).
141. Orr, M. M., et al.: Chronic lesions of rabbit bowel due to contact with antiseptic skin preparation. Gut, *16*:401, 1975 (abstract).
142. Bolton, P. M., et al.: Negative findings in laboratory animals for a transmissible agent in Crohn's disease. Lancet, *2*:1122, 1973.
143. Parent, K., and Mitchell, P.: Cell wall-defective variants of Pseudomonas-like (Group Va) bacteria in Crohn's disease. Gastroenterology, *75*:368, 1978.
144. Yoshimura, H. H., Markensich, D. C., and Graham, D. Y.: Mycobacteria isolated from patients with Crohn's disease. Gastroenterology, *88*:1639, 1985 (abstract).

145. Peña, A. S., et al.: Reproducibility of a potential serodiagnostic system in Crohn's disease using primed nude mouse lymph nodes and the difference with lymphocytotoxic antibodies. Gastroenterology, 88:1536, 1985 (abstract).
146. Burnham, W. R., et al.: Mycobacteria as a possible cause of inflammatory bowel disease. Lancet, 2:693, 1978.
147. Chiodini, R., et al.: Characteristics of an unclassified Mycobacterium species isolated from patients with Crohn's disease. J. Clin. Microbiol., 20:966, 1984.
148. Chiodini, R., et al.: In vitro antimicrobial susceptibility of a Mycobacterium species isolated from patients with Crohn's disease. Antimicrob. Agents Chemother., 26:930, 1984.
149. Chiodini, R., et al.: Possible role of mycobacteria in inflammatory bowel disease I. An unclassified Mycobacterium species isolated from patients with Crohn's disease. Dig. Dis. Sci., 29:1073, 1984.
150. Thayer, W. R., et al.: Possible role of mycobacteria in inflammatory bowel disease II. Mycobacterial antibodies in Crohn's disease. Dig. Dis. Sci., 29:1080, 1984.
151. Chiodini, R. J., et al.: Mycobacterial spheroplasts isolated from patients with Crohn's disease. Gastroenterology, 88:1348, 1985 (abstract).
152. Cho, W., et al.: Mycobacterial etiology of Crohn's disease: serologic study using common mycobacterial antigens and the species-specific glycolipid antigen from M. paratuberculosis. Gastroenterology, 88:1348, 1985 (abstract).
153. Van Kruiningen, et al.: Experimental disease in goats induced by a Mycobacterium from a patient with Crohn's disease. Gastroenterology, 88:1623, 1985 (abstract).
154. Gitnick, G., et al.: Mycobacteria in Crohn's disease. Gastroenterology, 88:1348, 1985 (abstract).
155. Miller, D. S., et al.: Crohn's disease in Nottingham: a search for time-space clustering. Gut, 16:454, 1975.
156. Miller, D. S., et al.: A case control method for seeking evidence of contagion in Crohn's disease. Gastroenterology, 71:385, 1976.
157. Hershfield, N. B.: Crohn's disease in a mother, father and son. Can. Med. Assoc. J., 131:1190, 1984.
158. Kirsner, J. B., and Shorter, R. G.: Recent developments in "nonspecific" inflammatory bowel disease (first of two parts). N. Engl. J. Med., 306:775, 1982.
159. Rosenberg, J. L., Kraft, F. C., and Kirsner, J. B.: Inflammatory bowel disease in all three members of one family. Gastroenterology, 70:759, 1976.
160. Achord, J. L., Gunn, C. H., and Jackson, J. F.: Regional enteritis and HLC concordance in multiple siblings. Dig. Dis. Sci., 27:330, 1982.
161. Kirsner, J. B.: Genetic aspects of inflammatory bowel disease. Clin. Gastroenterol., 2:557, 1973.
162. Helzer, J. E., et al: A controlled study of the association between ulcerative colitis and psychiatric diagnoses. Dig. Dis. Sci., 27:513, 1982.
163. Minowa, M., Bingham, S., and Cummings, J. H.: Dietary fibre intake in Japan. Hum. Nutr. Appl. Nutr., 32A:113, 1983.
164. Thornton, J. R., Emmett, P. M., and Heaton, K. W.: Diet and Crohn's disease: characteristics of the pre-illness diet. Br. Med. J., 2:762, 1979.
165. O'Morain, C., Segal, A. W., and Levi, A. J.: Elemental diet as primary treatment of acute Crohn's disease: a controlled trial. Br. Med. J., 288:1859, 1984.
166. Heaton, K. W., Thornton, J. R., and Emmett, P. M.: Treatment of Crohn's disease with an unrefined-carbohydrate, fibre-rich diet. Br. Med. J., 2:764, 1979.
167. Miller, B., Fervers, F., Rohbeck, R., and Strohmeyer, G: Zuckerkonsum bie Patienten mit Morbus Crohn. Vehrh. Dtsch. Ges. Inn. Med., 82:922, 1976.
168. Martini, G. A., and Brandes, J. W.: Increased consumption of refined carbohydrates in patients with Crohn's disease. Klin. Wochenschr., 54:367, 1976.
169. Kasper, H., and Sommer, H.: Dietary fiber and nutrient intake in Crohn's disease. Am. J. Clin. Nutr., 32:1898, 1979.
170. Thornton, J. R., Emmett, P. M., and Heaton, K. W.: Smoking, sugar, and inflammatory bowel disease. Br. Med. J., 290:1786, 1985.
171. Jarnerot, G., Jarnmark, I., and Nilsson, D.: Consumption of refined sugar by patients with Crohn's disease, ulcerative colitis, or irritable bowel syndrome. Scand. J. Gastroenterol., 18:999, 1983.
172. Truelove, S. C.: Ulcerative colitis provoked by milk. Br. Med. J., 1:154, 1961.
173. Taylor, D. B., and Truelove, S. C.: Circulating antibodies to milk proteins in ulcerative colitis. Br. Med. J., 2:924, 1961.
174. Dudek, B., Spiro, H. M., and Thayer, W. R.: A study of ulcerative colitis and circulating antibodies to milk proteins. Gastroenterology, 49:544, 1965.
175. Jewell, D. P., and Truelove, S. C.: Reaginic hypersensitivity in ulcerative colitis. Gut, 13:903, 1972.
176. James, A. H.: Breakfast and Crohn's disease. Br. Med. J., 1:943, 1977.
177. Rawcliffe, P. M., and Truelove, S. C.: Breakfast and Crohn's disease—I. Br. Med. J., 2:539, 1978.
178. Archer, L. N. J., and Harvey, R. F.: Breakfast and Crohn's disease-II. Br. Med. J., 2:540, 1978.
179. Mayberry, J. F., Rhodes, H., and Newcombe, R. G.: Breakfast and dietary aspects of Crohn's disease. Br. Med. J., 2:1401, 1978.
180. Acheson, E. D., and Truelove, S. C.: Early weaning in the aetiology of ulcerative colitis—a study of feeding in infancy in cases and controls. Br. Med. J., 2:929, 1961.
181. Hellers, G.: Some epidemiological aspects of Crohn's disease in Stockholm county, 1955–1979. In Recent Advances in Crohn's Disease. Edited by A. S. Peña, I. T. Weterman, C. C. Booth, and W. Strober. The Hague, Martinus Nijhoff, 1981.
182. Whorwell, P. J., et al.: Bottle feeding, early gastroenteritis, and inflammatory bowel disease. Br. Med. J., 1:382, 1979.
183. Hirschman, C., and Sweet, J. A.: Social background and breast feeding among American mothers. Soc. Biol., 21:39, 1974.
184. Martinez, G. A., and Nelezienski, J. P.: The recent trend in breast feeding. Pediatrics, 64:686, 1979.
185. Zamcheck, N., and Broitman, S. A.: Nutrition in diseases of the intestines. In Modern Nutrition in Health and Disease. Edited by R. S. Goodhart, and M. E. Shils. Philadelphia, Lea & Febiger, 1973.
186. Bures, J., Fixa, B., Komarkova, O., and Fingerland, A.: Letter. Br. Med. J., 285:440, 1982.
187. Harries, A. D., Baird, A., and Rhodes, J.: Non-smoking. A feature of ulcerative colitis. Br. Med. J., 284:706, 1982.
188. Jick, H., and Walker, A. M.: Cigarette smoking and ulcerative colitis. N. Engl. J. Med., 308:261, 1983.
189. Logan, R. F. A., Edmond, M., Somerville, K. W., and Langman, M. J. S.: Smoking and ulcerative colitis. Br. Med. J., 288:751, 1984.
190. Calkins, B., et al.: Smoking factors in ulcerative colitis and Crohn's disease in Baltimore. Am. J. Epidemiol., 120:498, 1984.

191. Benoni, C., and Nilsson, A.: Smoking habits in patients with inflammatory bowel disease. Scand. J. Gastroenterol., *19*:824, 1984.
192. Somerville, K. W., Loban, R. F. A., Edmond, M., and Langman, M. J. S.: Smoking and Crohn's disease. Br. Med. J., *289*:954, 1984.
193. Amery, K. V.: Smoking and ulcerative colitis. Letter. Br. Med. J., *288*:1307, 1984.
194. Logan, R. F. A. L., and Langmann, M. J. S.: Smoking and ulcerative colitis. Letter. Br. Med. J., *288*:1307, 1984.
195. Penny, W. J., Penny, E., Mayberry, J. F., and Rhodes, J.: Mormons, smoking and ulcerative colitis. Lancet, *2*:1315, 1983.
196. Gyde, S., et al.: Mortality in ulcerative colitis. Gastroenterology, *83*:36, 1982.
197. Gyde, S. N., Prior, P., Taylor, K., and Allan, R. N.: Cigarette smoking, blood pressure, and ulcerative colitis. Gut, *24*:A998, 1983.
198. Gyde, S. N., et al.: Ulcerative colitis: Why is the mortality from cardiovascular disease reduced? Q. J. Med., *77*:351, 1984.
199. Roberts, C. J., and Diggle, R.: Letter. Br. Med. J., *285*:440,1982.
200. de Castella, J.: Letter. Br. Med. J., *284*:1706, 1982.
201. Holdstock, G., Savage, D., Harman, M., and Wright T.: Should patients with inflammatory bowel disease smoke? Br. Med. J., *288*:362, 1984.
202. Kols, A., et al.: OCs—Update on Usage, Safety, and Side Effects. Popul. Rep., *A5*:A189, 1982.
203. Royal College of General Practitioners: Oral Contraceptives and Health. London, Pitman Medical, 1974.
204. Morowitz, D. A., and Epstein, B. H.: Spectrum of bowel disease associated with use of oral contraceptives. Med. Annals of the District of Columbia, *42*:6, 1973.
205. Bernardino, M. E., and Lawson, T. L.: Discrete colonic ulcers associated with oral contraceptives. Dig. Dis. Sci., *21*:503, 1976.
206. Simon, L., and Figus, I. A.: Akut Colitis ulcerosa-spontan regressioval. A hormondis anticonceptio ujabb mellekhatasa? Orv. Hetil., *117*:2987, 1976.
207. Bonfils, S., et al.: Acute spontaneously recovering ulcerating colitis. Dig. Dis. Sci., *22*:429, 1977.
208. Favier, D.: Colite erosive chez des malades prenant des contraceptifs oraux. Nouv. Presse. Med., *6*:2074, 1977.
209. Conri, C., et al.: Maladie de Crohn colique et contraception orale. Sem. Hop. Paris, *55*:1735, 1979.
210. Camilleri, M., et al.: Periportal sinusoidal dilatation, inflammatory bowel disease, and the contraceptive pill. Gastroenterology, *80*:810, 1981.
211. Tedesco, F. J., Volpicelli, N. A., and More, F. S.: Estrogen- and progesterone-associated colitis: a disorder with clinical and endoscopic features mimicking Crohn's colitis. Gastrointest. Endosc., *28*:247, 1982.
212. Rhodes, J. M., Cockel, R., Allan, R. N., and Hawker, P. C.: Colonic Crohn's disease and use of oral contraception. Br. Med. J., *288*:595, 1984.
213. Lesko, S., et al.: Oral contraceptive use and Crohn's disease. Am. J. Epidemiol., *120*:466, 1984.
214. Calkins, B. M., Mendeloff, A. I., and Garland, C. F.: Unpublished data, 1987.
215. Epidemiological methods in the study of chronic disease. Eleventh report of the WHO expert committee on health statistics. WHO Tech. Rep. Ser., *365*:1, 1967.
216. Methodology for family studies of genetic factors. WHO Tech. Rep. Ser., *46*:5, 1971.
217. Acheson, E. D.: Medical record linkage—the method and its application. R. Soc. Health J., *86*:216, 1966.

Section 2 · *Etiology and Pathogenesis*

2 · Experimental Inflammatory Bowel Disease

WARREN L. BEEKEN, M.D.

The obscure etiology of ulcerative colitis and Crohn's disease has resulted in many attempts to develop experimental models of these disorders. An animal model that accurately reflected human inflammatory bowel disease would greatly aid the study of the epidemiology, various etiologic agents, immune mechanisms, the biochemistry of mucosal and transmural inflammation, various forms of treatment, and the evolution of cancer in chronic inflammation.

The classification of experimental models is difficult and somewhat artificial, because most examples of intestinal inflammation in experimental animals exhibit overlapping biochemical, microbiologic, or immunologic aspects. Several excellent reviews of experimental inflammatory bowel disease are available that describe the earlier models.[1-5] These are included for completeness, but this chapter will also review newer immunologic models of ileitis and colitis, animal transmission studies, and recently described spontaneous animal models. A number of models described in abstract form are included to present the broad spectrum of techniques used to induce experimental intestinal inflammation. This chapter is designed to provide an up-to-date catalogue of animal models that might be of interest to students and investigators of human inflammatory bowel disease.

Production of Intestinal Inflammation in Animals

Indirect Manipulation

Forceful intrarectal injection of water during a water ski spill has been known to cause acute colitis,[6] but trauma is generally not thought to cause inflammatory bowel disease as usually seen in humans. Indirect manipulations of lymphatic, vascular, or neurologic systems have resulted in some interesting experimental lesions, however.

LYMPHATIC OBSTRUCTION

Reichert and Mathes produced lymphangitis and intestinal muscular hypertrophy in dogs by injecting mesenteric lymphatics with 26% oxychloride,[7] a potent sclerosant. Mucosal ulcerations and granulomas were not demonstrable. Oral administration of silica to experimental animals induces lymphoid hyperplasia, thickening of the terminal ileum, occasional foreign body granulomas but minimal mucosal abnormalities.[8] Occlusion of the mesenteric lymphatics of dogs by cauterization causes lymphedema, lymphocytic infiltration of the bowel wall, submucosal fibrosis, and shortened villi, lasting more than one year.[9] Kalima and colleagues produced obstruction of the mesenteric lymphatics of pigs by injection of formalin and induced ulcerations, intra-abdominal lesions, fistula, granuloma, and hyperplastic lymphoid tissue.[10] Animals also demonstrated growth retardation for periods of up to 14 weeks. It is generally accepted that none of these models reproduces the lesions of ulcerative colitis or Crohn's disease, however.

VASCULAR CHANGES

Several investigators have developed models for ischemic bowel disease in dogs by arterial occlusion.[11-13] Lesions vary from mucosal congestion to extensive necrotic ulceration, but these are not characteristic of inflammatory bowel disease. Histamine administration has been reported to produce a transient colitis, resulting from enhanced vascular permeability.[14] Although increased vascularity has been documented by angiography in both the transmural lesions of Crohn's disease and the mucosal abnormalities of ulcerative colitis,[15] it is currently believed that vascular alterations are not of primary importance in either disorder.

NEUROGENIC MANIPULATION

Moeller and Kirsner described colonic inflammation in dogs secondary to cholinergically mediated hypermotility,[16] and Berger and Lium invoked abdominal postganglionic sympathectomy as a technique for production of colitis.[17] Because the role of stress in inflammatory bowel disease remains so controversial, studies of the effect of stress-induced neurogenic stimulation on intestinal function at the cellular level would be of interest.

Topical Application of Irritant Chemicals

ACETIC ACID

Macpherson and Pfeiffer produced colitis in rats using mucosal or serosal application of acetic acid in concentrations between 10 and 50%.[18] Mucosal application resulted in acute colitis and weight loss over periods of up to 2 months, whereas serosal application resulted in fistulas and abdominal adhesions. The histology of these lesions included neutrophil infiltration, decreased mucus, denuded epithelium, deep ulcers, and pseudopolyps. Other investigators have administered 10% acetic acid to rats by enema, documented colitis by endoscopic and histologic examination, and demonstrated that prostaglandin (PGE_2) levels were increased.[19] Administration of indomethacin inhibited the endoscopic, histologic, and biochemical changes. A preliminary report documents an increase in the lipoxygenase products leukotriene B4 and 5-12- and 15-hydroxy-icosatetranoic acid in acetic acid-treated animals.[20] Indomethacin administration did not diminish lipoxygenase products, but another compound, nordihydroguaiaretic acid, inhibited both lipo- and cyclo-oxygenase metabolism in this model. Preliminary evidence suggests that oral administration of 5-aminosalicylic acid and metaclopromide together prevents acetic acid-induced colitis.[21]

TRINITROBENZENOSULFONIC ACID (TNB)

Intrarectal infusion of 20 mg of TNB in 0.25 ml of 35% ethanol has been reported to produce chronic granulomatous inflammation.[22] In this interesting model, TNB acted as a hapten and ethanol permitted its subepithelial penetration. Additional preliminary data indicate that in TNB colitis, lipoxygenase and cyclo-oxygenase products increase transiently and normalize by one week, but myeloperoxidase reaches a peak between 24 and 72 hours and remains elevated.[23] The mechanism of granuloma formation in this model is unclear, and further confirmatory studies are needed.

DIFLUOROMETHYL ORNITHINE (DFMO)

Another interesting preliminary report describes delayed maturation of intestinal cells, mucosal injury, and diarrhea in rats treated with DFMO, a compound that inhibits synthesis of polyamines that stimulate growth of the rat intestine.[24] Cellular DNA and disaccharide levels were diminished by DFMO, and effects were greater in weaning animals than in adults.

PEPSIN INHIBITORS

Marcus and Watt administered the pepsin inhibitors sodium lignosulfate and sulfated amylopectin to rabbits and guinea pigs, demonstrating that these compounds resulted in diarrhea, growth retardation, and intestinal bleeding.[25] Histologic examination showed multiple stellate ulcers in the cecum and proximal colon with neutrophilic and mononuclear phagocyte infiltration. The left colon and rectum were unaffected.

CARRAGEENAN

Carrageenan is a sulfated polygalactose widely used in the food industry and deemed safe for human consumption in molecular weights above 100,000.[26] Most reports indicate that native, undegraded forms of carrageenan used as food additives do not induce inflammatory bowel disease in laboratory animals.[27-29] Engster and Abraham reported, however, that native iota-carrageenan, having an average molecular weight of 107,000, caused cecal thinning and slight erosion of the epithelium, with macrophage infiltration of the lamina propria, crypt abscesses, and cellular infiltration when fed to the guinea pig.[30] Degraded forms of carrageenan with molecular weights of 20,000 to 40,000 are considered to be the most potent in producing cecal and colonic ulceration. When administered in drinking water, degraded carrageenan produces an ulcerative colitis in as little as two weeks.[28,30,31] The colitis is heralded by decreased mucin and sialic acid prior to the appearance of ulceration.[32] Macrophages become laden with degraded carrageenan,[33] and phagocytosis is suppressed.[34] Sulfate-depleted iota-carrageenan is toxic to monocytes in vitro, but does not induce proliferative responses in autologous or allogeneic mixed leukocyte reactions. Toxicity to monocytes and lymphocytes is induced by 6 days of culture in 100 μg carrageenan per ml.[35] Other investigators report that concentrations as low as 5 μg per ml are toxic to peripheral blood monocytes in vitro, and that it increases lectin-dependent cellular cytotoxicity for human epipharyngeal carcinoma targets (HEP-2) at levels of 25 μg per ml.[36] It also enhances Concanavalin A (ConA) induced proliferation of peripheral blood mononuclear cells in vitro, and after oral administration of carrageenan there is a dose-dependent suppression of lymphocyte responsiveness to in vitro stimulation by phytohemagglutinin.[37] Carrageenan-treated guinea pigs have normal delayed hypersensitivity reactions, but Ig synthesis is depressed.[38] Macrophage functions and antibody synthesis appeared to be more sensitive to carrageenan than those involved in the induction of cell-mediated immunity. Nicklen et al. found that 0.5% food grade carrageenan given in water over 90 days to adult rats did not alter biliary and systemic antibody responses to gut bacteria or oral immunization by sheep red blood cells, but hemagglutination reactions to parenterally administered sheep erythrocyte cells were diminished.[39]

Vanderwaaij, Cohen, and Anver reported that elimination of anaerobic gram-negative intestinal bacteria using trimethoprim-sulfamethoxazole prevented the development of carrageenan-induced colitis in guinea pigs.[40] They concluded that Enterobacteriaceae were responsible, presuming that these organisms stimulated an immune response after penetration of the mucosa. Onderdonk and Bartlett subsequently found that B. vulgatus is required for carrageenan-induced colitis,[41] and that immunization with B. vulgatus prior to carrageenan administration increased the severity of the inflammation;[42] they also found that spleen cells from a strain-specific B. vulgatus immunized guinea pig could adoptatively transfer this enhancement to other animals.[43]

A preliminary report documents the development of severe focal glandular atypism in rabbits with carrageenan colitis of 28 months' duration, suggesting an important link between chronic inflammation and epithelial cell dysplasia.[44] Rats fed carrageenan at levels of 1 to 10% in the diet develop colorectal adenomas, squamous cell carcinomas, or adenocarcinomas.[45] Although the carrageenan model is not an exact replica of human inflammatory bowel disease, it has many facets of the disease in man and continues to be one of the more important experimental models.

LECTINS

Another potentially important model of inflammatory bowel disease is that induced in rats fed a diet high in lectin-rich beans.[46,47] Animals developed duodenitis and jejunitis characterized by an increase in epithelial and lamina proprial lymphocytes and eosinophils with disruption of the microvilli, and many adherent E. coli. Feeding purified albumin or globulin lectin also has resulted in duodenitis, but association with bacteria was not observed. The role of transmigration of bacteria or bacterial toxins after epithelial damage through contact with lectins is not fully known, and the role of the ubiquitous lectins in stimulating subepithelial immune responses to invasive bacteria is a matter for future research.

OTHER TOXIC CHEMICALS

Ethanol, formalin, detergents, a variety of hypertonic mineral salts, and even nonsteroidal anti-inflammatory reagents are capable of injuring the human intestinal mucosa. These agents currently offer little in the study of inflammatory bowel disease, but do provide models of inflammation that may have general relevance to human enteritis.

Immunologic Methods

TOPICAL CHEMOTACTIC PEPTIDES

N-formylated peptides, synthetic analogs of chemotactic bacterial products, when administered rectally to mice have been found by Chester and colleagues to produce neutrophil infiltration, ulceration, and necrosis proportional to the duration of contact and the concentration.[48] Formylmethionyl-leucyl phenylalanine and formylnorleucyl phenylalanine are more potent than formylmethionine that, interestingly, is not chemotactic in vitro. The mechanism of injury is speculative, but may be related to neutrophil degranulation rather than to chemotaxis alone. This model should have relevance to any form of acute colitis regardless of its etiology.

DINITROCHLOROBENZENE (DNCB)

Dinitrochlorobenzene, another irritant hapten, produces a chronic delayed hypersensitivity reaction in the guinea pig colon if skin sensitization is followed by rectal instillation.[49] Intraperitoneal administration of spleen and lymph node cells from DNCB sensitized animals transferred susceptibility to production of colitis by rectal DNCB alone.[50] Azathioprine partially inhibits the development of this colitis. Rabin and Rogers used the skin-rectal DNCB model in rabbits with similar results.[51] The colitis was characterized by depletion of goblet cell mucus, lymphocyte and neutrophil infiltration, crypt abscesses, and mucosal ulceration apparent at 3 and 14 days post-treatment, followed by regeneration by 35 days. This process involved only the colon and rectum, with no lesions being found in the small intestine, liver, or kidney. Repeated rectal application of DNCB results in accumulation of lymphoid cells in hepatic portal tracts and a positive skin test to autologous colon extracts, however.

SENSITIZATION TO E. COLI

Halpern and colleagues reported that the inoculation of E. coli into rat foot pads produced diarrhea, bleeding, and chronic colitis.[52] They also documented colitis in rats immunized with canine colonic mucosa. Subsequent work demonstrated that E. coli-induced colitis could be prevented by oral administration of E. coli.[53]

Bicks and Walker observed that when rabbit antiserum to homogenate of dog colon was infused into dogs pretreated with a formalin enema, vascular congestion, polymorphonuclear leukocyte infiltration of colonic crypts, ulceration, and necrosis occurred.[54] Somewhat later, Mitscheke and Kracht described a chronic ulcerating cecitis in rats immunized with homologous colonic mucosa.[55] In similar studies, Leveen et al. demonstrated that duck or rabbit antiserum to dog colon antigen, when infused into dogs, produced chronic colitis characterized by remissions and exacerbations.[56] Rabin and Rogers subsequently immunized guinea pigs with saline extract of rabbit colon in Freund's adjuvant and transfused sensitized lymphocytes into guinea pigs.[57] Nineteen percent of animals treated by immunization alone developed histologic changes, whereas 40% of the lymphocyte recipients developed colitis. The lesions consisted of depletion of mucus, mononuclear cell infiltration, edema, dilated lymphatics, and infiltration by mast cells. No changes were observed with inoculation of normal control lymphocytes, dead lymphocytes, or lymphocytes from guinea pigs immunized with egg albumin. It was postulated that immunization occurred because a bacterial antigen was inoculated with the colon extract.

IMMUNE COMPLEX MODEL

Goldgraber and Kirsner studied the Arthus phenomenon induced in the colon of rabbits by systemic immunization to egg albumin followed by subserosal injection of the protein in the proximal and distal colon.[58] They described hyperemia and edema with polymorphonuclear leukocyte infiltration within 24 hours, followed sequentially by lymphocyte infiltration, intramuscular vasculitis, the development of giant cells, and hemorrhage by 144 hours. They also described the Shwartzman-Sanarelli phenomenon in rabbits using colonic injection of Serratia marcescens lysate as the initial inoculum, followed one day later by intravenous administration of the antigen.[59] Autopsies at intervals over four weeks showed edema, inflammation, hemorrhage, necrosis, and vascular thrombi within several days, followed by ulceration, fibroblast proliferation, and finally the development of foreign body granulomas.

Kraft, Fitch, and Kirsner investigated Auer colitis induced by systemic sensitization to egg albumin, rectal instillation of 0.4% formalin, and a final challenge with intravenous egg albumin.[60] The local immune complex reaction was characterized by rapid development of hyperemia, hemorrhage, ulcers, and a thickened bowel wall, with microscopic findings of infiltration of neutrophils, macrophages, eosinophils, lymphocytes, and plasma cells. Antigen-antibody complexes were identified in the regions of inflammation. Later, Hodgson et al. administered preformed immune complexes (human serum albumin-rabbit immunoglobulin) intravenously to rabbits pretreated by intrarectal administration of 1% formalin.[61] Animals treated with formalin alone developed transient congestion that cleared by 48 hours. Animals given immune complexes developed acute inflammatory changes that evolved over a 6 week period to minimal lymphocyte infiltration. Within 3 months, the mucosa was normal except for architectural distortion of crypts. They also demonstrated in the Auer model that preimmunization of rabbits with Kunin enterobacterial common antigen resulted in a colitis that lasted for up to 6 months.[62] In a more recent report, Brown and Zipser demonstrated that the acute blood flow changes accompanying immune complex colitis were inhibited by indomethacin and ibuprofen, but not by the thromboxane inhibitor, dazoxiben. They postulated that the increased vascularity was prostaglandin-mediated.[63]

GRAFT-VERSUS-HOST DISEASE

Dogs rendered immunologically unresponsive by chemotherapy or irradiation develop the intestinal lesions of graft-versus-host reaction.[64] The greatest changes occur in the distal ileum where a spectrum of pathologic changes is seen consisting of flattening of the epithelium, crypt distortion, leukocyte infiltration, and necrosis. This is a fascinating immunologic model of enteritis, requiring further study as clinical transplantation increases. At present, the implications for aiding our understanding of idiopathic ileitis and colitis are obscure.

Animal Transmission Studies

Attempts to induce ulcerative colitis or Crohn's disease in animals by inoculation of preparations derived from inflammatory bowel disease tissue are legion. Since the earliest report of granulomatous enteritis by Dalzeil,[65] and the subsequent description by Crohn and colleagues,[66] the suspicion of an infectious agent has persisted. In 1970, the work of Mitchell and Rees, who adapted the mouse foot-pad model of leprosy to the study of Crohn's disease, added great renewed impetus to the search for transmissible agents.[67] Unfortunately, their work could not be confirmed, but the search continues. Over the past 15 years, however, no study has provided reproducible evidence that transmissible infectious agents are responsible for ulcerative colitis or Crohn's disease (see Tables 2-1 and 2-2). The types of inocula employed for these studies have varied widely, and the animal recipients have been similarly diverse. Fecal filtrates, crude tissue homogenates, filtrates, tissue culture harvests, and various other preparations have all been administered. In the mid-1970's, reports by Aronson et al. and Gitnick

TABLE 2-1. *Summary of Animal Transmission Studies of Ulcerative Colitis.*

Year	Investigator	Recipient	Inoculum	Route	Results
1950	Victor[68]	Monkey	Fecal filtrate	Rectal	Negative
		Dog		Rectal	Negative
		Mice		IP	Negative
		Mice	Colonic homogenate	Cerebral	Negative
1962	Schneierson[69]	Guinea pig	Tissue culture harvest	Intestinal	Negative
1964	Hardin[70]	Rabbit	Colonic filtrate	IP	Negative
1974	Taub[71]	Mice	Lymph node homogenate	Foot pad	Negative
1976	Cave[72]	Mice	Colonic filtrate	Foot Pad	Positive
				IP	Positive
1976	Taub[73]	Mice	Colonic filtrate	Foot pad	Positive
1977	Simonowitz[74]	Rabbit	Colonic filtrate	Intestinal	Positive
1979	Beeken[75]	Rabbit	Colonic filtrate	IV	Negative
1980	Cohen[76]	Rabbit	Colonic filtrate	Intestinal	Negative
1980	Cave[77]	Rabbit	Colonic homogenate	Intestinal	Negative
1984	Yoshimura[78]	Rabbit	Colonic filtrate	IV	Negative

TABLE 2-2. *Summary of Animal Transmission Studies of Crohn's Disease.*

Year	Investigator	Recipient	Inoculation	Route	Result
1962	Schneierson[69]	Guinea Pig	Tissue culture harvest	Intestinal	Negative
1970-76	Mitchell[67,79]	Mice	Intestinal homogenate	Foot pad	Positive
			Lymph node homogenate	Foot pad	Positive
1972-74	Taub[80]	Mice	Homogenate	Ear/Foot pad	Positive*
1973	Bolton[81]	Guinea Pig	Intestinal homogenate	Foot pad	Negative
		Rat		Ear	
		Mice		Groin	
1973-75	Cave[82,83]	Rabbit	Intestinal homogenate	Intestinal	Positive
1975	Orr[84]	Rabbit	Streptococcal L forms	Intestinal	Positive
1975	Heatley[85]	Rabbit	Homogenate	Intestinal	Negative
		Rat	Homogenate	Foot pad	
		Mice		Oral	
1976	Taub[73]	Mice	Homogenate	Ear/Foot pad	Positive*
1977	Simonowitz[74]	Rabbit	Homogenate	Colonic	Positive*
1977	Donnelly[86]	Rabbit	Homogenate	Intestinal	Positive*+
1978	Ahlberg[87]	Piglets	Homogenate	Intestinal	Negative
		Rats		SC	
1979	Parent[88]	Rabbit	Pseudomonas L forms	Colonic	Positive**
1979	Beeken[75]	Rabbit	Intestinal filtrates	IV	Negative
			Tissue culture harvest		
1980-83	Das[89,90]	Mice	Lymph node filtrates	IP	Lymphoma
1980	Cave[77]	Rabbit	Homogenates	Intestinal	Negative
1984	Yoshimura[78]	Rabbit	Intestinal filtrate	IV	Negative
1985	Sartor[91]	Rat	Streptococcal cell wall	Intestinal	Positive

* Control tissue also positive
+ Lesions at 6 months–none at 12
** Foreign body granuloma

and colleagues stimulated the hope that viral agents might be etiologically related to inflammatory bowel disease.[92-94] However, subsequent work provided evidence that the agents in question were actually nonreplicating cytoplasmic cytotoxins.[78,95-97] Parent and Mitchell cultured a cell wall-defective Pseudomonas bacterium from Crohn's disease tissue but this work could not be consistently confirmed and lies dormant at the moment. Among these many studies, several remain as viable possibilities. Das and colleagues have inoculated filtrates of mesenteric lymph nodes or intestinal mucosa from patients with Crohn's disease into BALB/c nude mice and produced lymphoma or lymphoid hyperplasia in a significant percentage of animals.[89,90] Inoculation of ulcerative colitis filtrates or those from normal colon produced no changes. In addition, 22 to 80% of sera from patients with Crohn's disease reacted with the induced lymphoma according to the severity of symptoms. Electron microscopy has disclosed c-type viral particles in five lymphomas induced by Crohn's disease filtrates and in one control lymphoma. While these studies continue to command interest, so far their relevance to the etiology of inflammatory bowel disease remains speculative.

In another interesting model, Sartor and colleagues found chronic granulomatous inflammation in the rat after intramural inoculation of a peptidoglycan-polysaccharide complex derived by enzymatic digestion and chloroform-methanol extraction of group A or Group D streptococci cell walls.[91] Approximately 45% of inoculated animals showed lesions, compared to 20% of control animals inoculated with albumin. None of the animals developed symptoms of bowel disease, but at necropsy, thickening of the intestinal cell wall, adhesions, and mesenteric contraction were evident at all intervals of study. The immediate reaction was characterized by neutrophil, eosinophil, and macrophage infiltration, accompanied by edema, hemorrhage, and focal necrosis at the injection sites. After 2 weeks, this was largely replaced by a chronic inflammatory response characterized by periodic acid-Schiff (PAS) positive macrophages surrounded by lymphocytes, plasma cells, and eosinophils. Changes persisted for up to 6 months in the group A inoculated animals and for 3 months in the group D recipients. Classic granulomas were observed, and immunofluorescent studies showed peptidoglycan-polysaccharide antigen to be localized in the majority of these. This model provides a provocative new avenue of investigation in the experimental animal and emphasizes once more the potentially important role of bacterial antigens in the genesis of inflammatory bowel disease.

A new infectious animal model has been reported by James and colleagues, who induced colitis in Macaque monkeys by rectal instillation of lymphogranuloma venereum.[99] Sequential study documented functional changes of mucosal natural killer cell activity in rectum, colon, spleen, and peripheral blood. The numbers of peripheral blood, rectal NK cells, and the lysis of K562 target cells all were reduced after infection. These studies may have more relevance to sexually transmitted disorders than ulcerative colitis and Crohn's disease, but they use an important approach for sequential evaluation of immunologic events during development of the inflammatory response to an infectious agent.

Other evidence for an infectious transmissible agent in inflammatory bowel disease was reported in 1984 by Chiodini and colleagues.[100] They identified an unclassified Mycobacterium from three patients with Crohn's disease. The organisms were unusually fastidious and mycobactin-dependent, and required up to 18 months of incubation for isolation. Careful biochemical analysis indicated that the organism may be a subspecies of M. paratuberculosis or a new species.[101] Tests of in vitro antimicrobial susceptibility indicated that the organism was sensitive to streptomycin, rifampin, kanamycin, viomycin sulfate, clofazimine, and cefazolin, and resistant to isoniazid, p-aminosalicylic acid, cycloserine, 2-thiophenecarboxylic acid hydrazide, trimethoprim, diaminodiphenyl sulfone, sulfamethoxazole, sulfadimethoxine, polymyxin B, metronidazole, neomycin, and carbenicillen.[100,102] Oral administration of one of these organisims has induced ileitis in infant goats.[103] Animals were autopsied at 3, 5, 6, and 10 months, and each had granulomas and ulceration in the Peyer's patches of the ileum. The mycobacterium was cultured from all 4 animals, and it was seen in histologic sections of 2 animals. In addition to isolating the organism from 4 patients, they identified spheroplasts in specimens from 12 additional patients with Crohn's disease. Culture of 9 resections from patients with ulcerative colitis and 14 with noninflammatory bowel disease were negative. Dalziel's 1913 description of Crohn's disease suggested that the disorder might be a result of M. paratuberculosis,[65] an organism known to cause granulomatous ileitis (Johne's disease) in goats and other domestic animals. This organism closely resembles the unclassified mycobacterium described by Chiodini's group. Unfortunately, any enthusiasm for assigning this new organism an etiologic role is tempered by the likelihood that it is an intestinal resident unrelated to the etiology of Crohn's disease, as recent work suggests,* and by the observation that treatment trials with antimycobacterial therapy have not resulted in improvement.[104]

Spontaneous Animal Models of Ileitis and Colitis

Spontaneous Infections

The histologic findings of epithelial cell destruction, microulceration, granulocyte and mononuclear cell infiltration, and crypt abscesses so frequently seen in ulcerative colitis also occur in bacterial enteritis. Moreover, the presence of lymphocytes, macrophages, and granulomas in Crohn's disease resemble the changes seen in tuberculosis, other mycobacterial infections, and chlamydial disease in experimental animals. These similarities have stimulated numerous investigations of animal models of infectious enteritis. Unfortunately, most of the infectious models are self-limited and do not truly resemble ulcerative colitis or Crohn's disease in man. Nonetheless, they provide important models by which the immunologic and biochemical changes that accompany the development of mucosal inflammation and transmural disease may be investigated. Table 2-3, modified from a tabulation by Mayberry, Rhodes, and Heatley,[2] lists examples of naturally occurring animal models of intestinal inflammation which may have indirect relevance to human inflammatory bowel disease. The reader is referred to their article for further descriptions of these entities.[2] These infections may confound the investigator if they occur sporadically during studies of other models of inflammatory bowel disease, or they may provide unique opportunities to elucidate particular phenomena of intestinal inflammation.

---

*Editor's note: See also Sang-nae Cho, et al.: Gut, 27:1353, 1986; and Graham, D. Y., et al.: Gastroenterology, 92:436, 1987.

TABLE 2-3. *Spontaneous Animal Models of Inflammatory Bowel Disease Resulting from Infectious Agents.*

Year	Investigator	Species	Disease	Organism
1917	Tyzzer[105]	Mice	Colitis	Bacillus pyliformis
1918	McFadyean[106]	Cattle	Ileitis	M. paratuberculosis
		Sheep		
		Goats		
		Swine		
		Horses		
		Monkeys		
1931	Beister[107]	Swine	Ileitis	C. sputorum
1945	Hjarre[108]	Chickens	Ileocolitis	E. coli
1967	Van Kruiningen[109]	Boxer dogs		Chlamydia; LGV-like
1967	Boothe[110]	Hamster	Ileitis	Rod-shaped bacillus
1968	Tomita[111]	Hamster	Ileitis	DNA virus
1972	Gribble[112]	Nonhuman primates		M. avium
1974	Berkhoff[113]	Quail	Ileocolitis	Gram + anaerobes
1974	Doughri[114]	Cattle	Ileitis	Chlamydia CW613
1974	Widmer[115]	Fox hound	Ileitis	Trichuris
1975	Tolin[116]	Turkey	Enteritis	Adeno-like virus
1978	Reid[117]	Chicken/Turkey	Ileocolitis	Coccidiosis
1980	Tyrrell[118]	Mouse	"Enteritis"	Coronavirus
		Turkey		
		Pig		
		Cattle		
		Dog		
		Cat		

Spontaneous Idiopathic Disorders

Because the etiologies of ulcerative colitis and Crohn's disease in man remain so elusive, spontaneous models of idiopathic colitis and ileitis in experimental animals are of particular interest. Spontaneous disease has been described in rats, dogs, pigs, sheep, and horses as listed in Table 2-4. The general consensus is that most of these disorders do not closely resemble human inflammatory bowel disease with the notable exception of the colitis described in primates. The report in 1969, by Stout and colleagues,[124] of colitis in gibbons was soon followed by the description of ileitis in gorillas and orangutans by Scott in 1974.[126] In 1981 Chalifoux and Bronson described ulcerative colitis in the marmoset, which has attracted a great deal of attention both as a potential model for human gastrointestinal disease and because the disease seriously threatens the species.[129] In April of 1984 the National Institutes of Health and Oakridge Associated Universities sponsored a workshop entitled "Is the Marmoset an Experimental Model for the Study of Gastrointestinal Disease?" The proceedings of this workshop are summarized thus. Fifty to 70% of marmosets in captivity have been demonstrated to have colitis either at autopsy or by sigmoidoscopic examination during life. The disease is characterized by crypt abscesses and mononuclear cell and neutrophil infiltration. No granulomas are found. The onset of colitis may be as early as 18 days of age. Sixty percent of animals survive for one year and their life span may be up to 18 years. After 4 years of colitis most animals develop adenocarcinoma of the colon. The disease improves with sulfasalazine and forced tube feeding, but it recurs within 6 to 8 weeks of stopping treatment. Unlike human ulcerative colitis, inflammation also occurs in the jejunum and ileum, the disease involves predominantly the ascending colon, and toxic megacolon has not been described. Some investigators have also documented less hemorrhage, less ulceration, and less dysplasia in the marmoset disease. Death may be a result of sepsis, colitis, or colon cancer.

The Yale primate colony was apparently free of colitis between 1973 and 1982 and no carcinomas were documented. However, 3 months after moving this colony to the New England Regional Primate Center in Southboro, Massachusetts, ulcerative colitis began to appear and carcinoma was identified. Accordingly, an intensive search for infectious agents was undertaken. No Shigella, Yersinia, or Salmonella were identified but

TABLE 2-4. *Spontaneous Animal Models of Idiopathic Inflammatory Bowel Disease.*

Year	Investigator	Species	Disease
1941	Stewart[119]	Rats	Cecum
1951	Emsbo[120]	Swine	
1954	Strande[121]	Cocker Spaniel Dogs	Ileum-colon
1961	Geil[122]	Rats	Cecum
1962	Wensvoort[123]	Sheep	Ileitis
1969	Stout[124]	Gibbons	Colitis
1972	Van Kruiningen[125]	Dogs-different varieties	Ileum-colon
1974	Scott[126]	Gorillas	Colitis
1974	Cimprich[127]	Horses	Small bowel
1976	Merritt[128]	Horses	Ileum-colon
1981	Chalifoux[129]	Marmoset	Colitis

Campylobacters were cultured in 21% (15 out of 71). A search for viral agents was also undertaken and 18 out of 68 animals were found to have corona virus. All of these animals had diarrhea and most were adults. Corona viruses are fastidious, pleomorphic, RNA viruses, 80 to 120 nanometers in diameter, which infect human respiratory and intestinal epithelial cells. They are found in normal subjects,[130] in those with gastroenteritis,[131] and have been implicated in necrotizing enteritis.[132] Specific antibodies are common in human sera, but the agent has not been implicated in human ulcerative colitis.[133] Coronaviruses cause enteritis in the mouse, turkey, pig, calf, dog, and cat,[118] and they also occur in many primates.[134] The finding of corona virus in marmosets raises the possibility that it may play an etiologic role in their colitis. However, the agent may be an opportunistic organism of no significance, or be a secondary invader that perpetuates an immune response initiated by another agent. Studies are in progress to define the role of corona virus in marmoset colitis.

Other aspects are also being investigated. Boland et al. reported that peanut-binding lectin identified oncodevelopmental mucins in 90% in S. oedipus with severe acute inflammation and tumor, but it was present in less than 40 percent of animals with milder inflammation and no cancer.[135] These data suggest that severe inflammatory changes might predispose to epithelial dysplasia and the development of neoplasm in this species.

This animal model of an ulcerative colitis and colonic carcinoma deserves careful study. Major questions of immediate concern are: what is the incidence of colitis in the wild; is colitis present in newborns in captivity; can the model be subjected to serial study; and, what are the criteria for a normal mucosa in this species?

So far there are no exact experimental replicas of human inflammatory bowel disease, and no exact replicas occur spontaneously in other animal species. Nonetheless, investigation of animal models of enteritis can provide important insights into various aspects of the inflammatory response that have relevance to the idiopathic human disorders. It could be argued that any experimental means of producing enteritis in animals may increase our understanding of mechanisms of intestinal inflammation, but some techniques are less artificial than others, and these logically deserve emphasis in future investigations. Certainly, further studies of primate colitis, especially in the cotton topped marmoset, will be of great importance because of the potential relationship to human ulcerative colitis. Similarly, the finding of granulomatous ileitis in infant goats fed mycobacteria isolated from human Crohn's disease tissue requires further investigation to determine its significance. Could the mycobacterium be the cause of Crohn's disease or, perhaps more likely, is it a contaminant or opportunistic passenger that causes Johne's disease in goats but has no relevance to human disease? A number of other investigations emphasize the induction of inflammation by other bacterial antigens, and additional research is required to place this growing body of information in its proper perspective. Finally, the induction of intestinal inflammation by oral administration of lectins and carrageenan suggests that the ingestion of other nonmicrobial immunogenic compounds deserves consideration in searching for mediators of inflammatory bowel disease. Experimental animal models are aiding our understanding of intestinal inflammation; in the future, animal models are likely to play an important role in unravelling the etiologies of human inflammatory bowel disease.

References

1. MacPherson, B., and Pfeiffer, C. J.: Experimental colitis. Digestion, *14*:424, 1976.
2. Mayberry, J. F., Rhodes, J., and Heatley, R. V.: Infections which cause ileocolic disease in animals: Are they relevant to Crohn's disease? Gastroenterology, *78*:1080, 1980.
3. Schacter, H., and Kirsner, J. B.: Crohn's Disease of the Gastrointestinal Tract. New York, John Wiley and Sons, 1980.
4. Melnyk, C. S.: Experimental enteritis and colitis. *In* Inflammatory Bowel Disease. J. B. Kirsner and R. G. Shorter. Philadelphia, Lea & Febiger, 1980.
5. Cave, D. R.: Etiology: Transmissible agents in inflammatory bowel disease. *In* Inflammatory Bowel Disease. Edited by R. N. Allen, M. R. B. Keighley, J. Alexander, and C. Hawkins. New York, Churchill Livingston, 1983.
6. Bundgaard, A., and Jarnum, S.: Water ski spill and ulcerative colitis. Lancet, *2*:1157, 1984.
7. Reichert, F. L., and Mathes, M. W.: Experimental lymphedemia of the intestinal tract and its relation to regional cicatrizing enteritis. Ann. Surg. *104*:601, 1936.
8. Chess, S., et al.: Production of chronic enteritis and other systemic lesions by ingestion of finely divided foreign materials. Surgery, *27*:221, 1950.
9. Jesseph, J. E.: Morphologic changes in the ileum secondary to experimental chronic mesenteric lymphatic occlusion. Gastroenterology, *42*:777, 1962.
10. Kalima, T. V., Saloniemi, H., and Rahko, T.: Experimental regional enteritis in pigs. Scand. J. Gastroenterol., *11*:353, 1976.
11. Schwartz, S., Lash, J., Sternhill, V., and Boley, S. J.: Reversible vascular occlusion of the colon. Surg. Gynecol. Obstet., *116*:53, 1963.
12. Boley, S. J., et al.: Experimental aspects of peripheral vascular occlusion of the intestine. Surg. Gynecol. Obstet., *121*:789, 1965.
13. Marsten, A., Marcuson, R. W., Chapman, M., and Arthur, J. F.: Experimental study of devascularization of the colon. Gut, *10*:121, 1969.
14. Kirsner, J. B.: Experimental "colitis" with particular reference to hypersensitivity reactions in the colon. Gastroenterology, *40*:307, 1961.
15. Brahme, F., and Lindstrom, C.: A comparative radiographic and pathological study of intestinal vaso-architecture in Crohn's disease and ulcerative colitis. Gut, *11*:928, 1970.
16. Moeller, H. C., and Kirsner, J. B.: The effect of drug-induced hypermotility on the gastrointestinal tract of dogs. Gastroenterology, *26*:303, 1954.
17. Berger, R. L., and Lium, R.: Abdominal postganglionic sympathectomy: A method for the production of an ulcerative colitis-like state in dogs. Ann. Surg., *152*:266, 1960.
18. MacPherson, B. R., and Pfeiffer, C. J.: Experimental production of diffuse colitis in rats. Digestion, *17*:135, 1978.
19. Mann, N. S., and Demers, L. M.: Experimental colitis studied by colonoscopy in the rat: Effect of indomethacin. Gastrointest. Endosc., *29*:77, 1983.
20. Phyall, W. B., Rush, J. A., and Fondacaro, J. D.: Identification of lipooxygenase products in an animal model of gut inflammation. Gastroenterology, *88*:1541, 1985 (abstract).
21. Mangala, J. C., and Aanda, K. K.: Ulcerative colitis animal model-role of metaclopromide (M) in the fast delivery of oral 5-aminosalicylic acid (5-ASA) to colon. Clin. Res., *33*:323A, 1985.
22. Morris, G. P., et al.: An animal model for chronic granulomatous inflammation of the stomach and colon. Gastroenterology, *86*:1188, 1984 (abstract).
23. Boughton-Smith, N. K., Wallace, J. L., and Whittle, B. J. R.: Temporal relationship between arachadonic acid metabolism and myeloperoxidase activity in a rat model of Crohn's disease. Gastroenterology, *88*:1332, 1985 (abstract).
24. Alarcon, P. A., Lee, P. C., and Lebenthal, E.: Induction of mucosal injury and diarrhea in weanling rats by difluoromethyl ornithine (DFMO). Gastroenterology, *88*:1302, 1985.
25. Marcus, R., and Watt, J.: Ulcerative disease of the colon in laboratory animals induced by pepsin inhibitors. Gastroenterology, *67*:473, 1974.
26. Carrageenan, salts of carrageenan and chondrus extract: Withdrawal of proposal and termination of rulemaking proceeding. Fed. Reg., *44*(133):40343, 1979.
27. Abraham, R., and Coulston, F.: Ulcerative lesions due to carrageenan. Z. Gastroenterol., *17*(suppl.):154, 1979.
28. Benitz, K. F., Goldberg, L., and Coulston, F.: Intestinal effects of carrageenans in the Rhesus monkey (Macaca mulatta). Food Cosmet. Toxicol., *11*:565, 1973.
29. Poulson, E.: Short-term peroral toxicity of undergraded carrageenan in pigs. Food Cosmet. Toxicol., *11*:219, 1973.
30. Engster, M., Abraham, R. Cecal response to different molecular weights and types of carrageenan in the guinea pig. Toxicol. Appl. Pharmacol., *38*:265, 1976.
31. Abraham, R., Fabian, R. J., Goldberg, M. B., and Coulston, F.: Role of lysosomes in carrageenan-induced cecal ulceration. Gastroenterology, *67*:1169, 1979.
32. Al Suhail, et al.: Studies of the degraded carrageenan induced colitis of rabbits. II. Changes in epithelial glycoprotein O-acetylated sialic acids associated with the induction and healing phases. Histochem. J., *16*:555, 1984.
33. Grasso, P., Sharratt, M., Carpanini, F. M. B., and Gangolli, S. D.: Studies on carrageenan and large bowel ulceration in mammals. Food Cosmet. Toxicol., *11*:555, 1973.
34. Rumjanek, V. M., Watson, S. R., and Sljivic, H.: A re-evaluation of the role of macrophages in carrageenan-induced immunosuppression. Immunology, *33*:423, 1977.
35. Sugawara, I., and Ishizaka, S.: Desulfated carrageenan and cytotoxicity of human monocytes. Agents Actions, *13*:354, 1983.
36. Perl, A., Gonzalez-Rabello, R., and Gergely, P.: Stimulation of lectin dependent cell mediated toxicity against adherent HEP 2 cells by carrageenan. Clin. Exp. Immunol., *54*:567, 1983.
37. Bash, J. A., and Vago, J. R.: Carrageenan-induced suppression of T lymphocyte proliferation in the rat: In vivo suppression induced by oral administration. J. Reticuloendothel. Soc., *28*:213, 1980.
38. Neveu, P. J., and Thierry, D.: Effects of carrageenan, a macrophage toxic agent, on antibody synthesis and delayed hypersensitivity in the guinea pig. Int. J. Immunopharmacol., *4*:175, 1982.
39. Nicklin, S., and Miller, K.: Effect of orally administered food grade carrageenans on antibody mediated and cell mediated immunity in the inbred rat. Food Cosmet. Toxicol., *22*:615, 1984.
40. Van Der Waaij, D., Cohen, B. J., and Anver, M. R.: Mitigation of experimental inflammatory bowel disease in guinea pigs by selective elimination of the aerobic gram-negative intestinal microflora. Gastroenterology, *67*:460, 1974.
41. Onderdonk, A. B., and Bartlett, J. G.: Bacteriological studies of experimental ulcerative colitis. Am. J. Clin. Nutr., *32*:258, 1979.

42. Onderdonk, A. B., Cisneros, R. L., and Bronson, R. T.: Enhancement of experimental ulcerative colitis by immunization with Bacteriodes vulgatus. Infect. Immun., *42*:783, 1983.
43. Onderdonk, A. B., Steeves, R. M., Cisnaros, R. L., and Bronson, R. T.: Adoptive transfer of immune enhancement of experimental ulcerative colitis. Infect. Immun., *46*:64, 1984.
44. Kitano, A., and Kobayashi, K.: Epithelial dysplasia induced by carrageenan in rabbit colon. Gastroenterology, *88*:1447, 1985.
45. Oohashi, Y., Ishioka, T., Wakabayashi, K., and Kuwabara, N.: A study on carcinogenesis induced by degraded carrageenan arising from squamous metaplasia of the rat colorectum. Cancer Lett., *14*:267, 1981.
46. King, T. P., Pusztai, A., and Clarke, M. W.: Kidney bean (phaseolus vulgaris) lectin-induced lesions in rat small intestine: 1. Light microscope studies. J. Comp. Pathol., *90*:585, 1984.
47. Wilson, A. B., King, T. P., Clarke, E. M. W., and Posztai, A.: Kidney bean (phaseolus vulgaris) lectin-induced lesions in rat small intestine: 2 microbiological studies. J. Comp. Pathol., *80*:597, 1980.
48. Chester, J. F., Ross, J. S., Malt, R. A., and Weitzman, S. A.: Acute colitis produced by chemotactic peptides in the mouse. Gastroenterology, *88*:1348, 1985.
49. Bicks, R. O., and Rosenberg, E. W.: A chronic delayed hypersensitivity reaction in the guinea pig colon. Gastroenterology, *46*:543, 1964.
50. Bicks, R. O., et al.: Delayed hypersensitivity reactions in the intestinal tract. 1. Studies of 2-4 dinitrochlorobenzine-caused guinea pig and swine colon lesions. Gastroenterology, *53*:422, 1967.
51. Rabin, B. S., and Rogers, S. J.: A cell mediated immune model of inflammatory bowel disease in the rabbit. Gastroenterology, *75*:29, 1978.
52. Halpern, B., Zweibam, B., Oriol Palow, R., and Morard, J. C.: Experimental immune ulcerative colitis. *In* Immunopathology 5th International Symposium Mechanisms of Inflammation Induced by Immune Reactions. Edited by P. A. Miescher, and P. Grabar. New York, Grune and Stratton, 1967.
53. Zweibaum, A., Morard, J. C., and Halpern, B.: Realization d'une colite ulcero-hemorrhagique experimentale par immunisation bacterienne. Path. Biol. (Paris), *16*:813, 1968.
54. Bicks, R. O., and Walker, R. H.: Immunologic "colitis" in dogs. Am. J. Dig. Dis., *7*:574, 1962.
55. Mitschke, H., and Kracht, J.: Experimental investigations on immunopathology of colon. Beitr. Path. Anat., *136*:261, 1968.
56. Leveen, H. H., Falk, G., and Schotman, B.: Experimental ulcerative colitis produced by anticolon sera. Ann. Surg. *154*:275, 1961.
57. Rabin, E., and Rogers, S.J.: Transfer of colon inflammatory disease from immune to normal guinea pigs by lymphocytes. Int. Arch. Allergy Appl. Immunol., *63*:201, 1980.
58. Goldgraber, M.B., and Kirsner, J.B.: The arthus phenomenon in the colon of rabbits: A serial histological study. Arch. Pathol., *67*:556, 1959.
59. Goldgraber, M.B., and Kirsner, J.B.: The Schwartzman phenomenon in the colon of rabbits: A serial histological study. Arch. Pathol., *68*:539, 1959.
60. Kraft, S.C., Fitch, F.W., and Kirsner, J.B.: Histological and immunohistochemical features of the Auer colitis in rabbits. Am. J. Pathol., *43*:913, 1963.
61. Hodgson, H.J.F., Potter, B.J., Skinner, J., and Jewell, D.P.: Immune complex mediated colitis in rabbits. Gut, *19*:225, 1978.
62. Mee, A.S., McLaughlin, J.E., Hodgson, H.J.F., and Jewell, D.P.: Chronic immune colitis in rabbits. Gut, *20*:1, 1979.
63. Brown, J.A., and Zipser, R.D.: Regulation of colonic blood flow in experimental colitis: Role of prostaglandins. (abstract) Gastroenterology, *88*:1336, 1985.
64. Kolb, H., et al.: Pathology of acute graft-versus-host disease in the dog. Am. J. Pathol., *96*:581, 1979.
65. Dalzeil, T.K.: Chronic interstitial enteritis. Brit. Med. J. *11*:1068, 1913.
66. Crohn, B.B., Ginzburg, L., and Oppenheimer, G.D.: Regional ileitis. A pathological and clinical entity. J. Amer. Med. Assoc., *99*:1323, 1932.
67. Mitchell, D.N., and Rees, R.J.W.: Agent transmissible from Crohn's disease. Lancet, *2*:168, 1970.
68. Victor, R.G., Kirsner, J.B., and Palmer, W.L.: Failure to induce ulcerative colitis experimentally with filtrates of feces and rectal mucosa. A preliminary report. Gastroenterology, *14*:398, 1950.
69. Schneierson, S.S., et al.: Studies on the viral etiology of regional enteritis and ulcerative colitis: A negative report. Am. J. Dig. Dis., *7*:839, 1962.
70. Hardin, C.A., Vancil, M.E., Weder, A.A., and Schmidt, C.: Observations on human colonic cellular suspensions and filtrates as etiologic agents in ulcerative colitis. Am. J. Dig. Dis., *8*:531, 1964.
71. Taub, R.N., Sachar, D.B., and Siltzbach, L.E.: Transmission of ileitis and sarcoid granulomas to mice. Trans. Assoc. Am. Physicians, *87*:219, 1974.
72. Cave, D.R., Mitchell, D.N., and Brooke, B.N.: Evidence of an agent transmissible from ulcerative colitis tissue. Lancet, *1*:1311, 1976.
73. Taub, R.N., Sachar, D., Janowitz, H., and Siltzbach, L.E.: Induction of granulomas in mice by inoculation of tissue homogenates from patients with inflammatory bowel disease and sarcoidosis. Ann. N. Y. Acad. Sci., *278*:560, 1976.
74. Simonowitz, D., et al.: The production of an unusual tissue reaction in rabbit bowel injected with Crohn's disease homogenates. Surgery, *82*:211, 1977.
75. Beeken, W.L.: Infectious agents in inflammatory bowel disease. *In* Developments in Digestive Diseases. Edited by J. Edward Berk. Philadelphia, Lea & Febiger, 1979.
76. Cohen, Z., Jirsch, D., Archibald, S., and Leung, M.K.: The production of granulomas in rabbit bowel. Gastroenterology, *78*:1152, 1980 (abstract).
77. Cave, D., et al.: Infectious agents in inflammatory bowel disease (IBD). A status report. Gastroenterology, *78*:1185, 1980 (abstract).
78. Yoshimura, H.H., Estes, M.K., and Graham, D.Y.: Search for evidence of a viral aetiology for inflammatory bowel disease. Gut, *25*:347, 1984.
79. Mitchell, D.N., and Rees, R.J.W.: Further observations on the transmissibility of Crohn's disease. Ann. N. Y. Acad. Sci., *278*:546, 1976.
80. Taub, R.N., and Siltzbach, L.E.: Induction of granulomas in mice by injection of human sarcoid and ileitis homogenates. *In* Proceedings of VI International Conference on Sarcoidosis. Baltimore, University Press, 1972.
81. Bolton, P.M., et al.: Negative finding in laboratory animals for a transmissible agent in Crohn's disease. Lancet, *2*:1122, 1973.
82. Cave, D.R., Mitchell, D.N., and Brooke, B.N.: Further evidence of a transmissible agent in Crohn's disease. Lancet, *2*:1120, 1973.

83. Cave, D.R., Mitchell, D.N., and Brooke, B.N.: Experimental animal studies of the etiology and pathogenesis of Crohn's disease. Gastroenterology, 69:619, 1975.
84. Orr, M.M.: Experimental intestinal granulomas. Proc. Roy. Soc. Med., 68:34, 1975.
85. Heatley, R.V., et al.: A search for a transmissible agent in Crohn's disease. Gut, 16:523, 1975.
86. Donnelly, B.J., Delaney, P.V., and Healy, T.M.: Evidence for a transmissible factor in Crohn's disease. Gut, 18:360, 1977.
87. Ahlberg, J., et al.: Negative findings in search for a transmissible agent in Crohn's disease. Acta. Chir. Scand. (Suppl.), 482:45, 1978.
88. Mitchell, P.D., and Parent, K.: Cell wall-defective pseudomonas-like bacteria: Their possible significance in the etiology of Crohn's disease. Z. Gastroenterol. (Verh.), 17:109, 1979.
89. Das, K.M., Valenzuela, J., and Morecki, R.: Crohn's disease lymph node homogenates produce murine lymphoma in athymic mice. Proc. Natl. Acad. Sci. U. S. A., 77:588, 1980.
90. Das, K.M., et al.: Studies of the etiology of Crohn's disease using athymic nude mice. Gastroenterology, 84:364, 1983.
91. Sartor, R.B., Cromartie, W.J., Powell, D.W., and Schwab, J.H.: Granulomatous enterocolitis induced by purified bacterial cell wall fragments. Gastroenterology, 89:587, 1985.
92. Aronson, M.D., Phillips, C.A., Beeken, W.L., and Forsyth, B.R.: Isolation and characterization of a viral agent from intestinal tissue of patients with Crohn's disease and other intestinal disorders. Progr. Med. Virol., 21:165, 1975.
93. Gitnick, G.L., Arthur, M.H., and Shibata, I.: Cultivation of viral agents in Crohn's disease. Lancet, 2:215, 1976.
94. Gitnick, G.L., Rosen, V.J., Arthur, M.H., and Hertweck, S.A.: Evidence for the isolation of a new virus from ulcerative colitis patients. Comparison with virus derived from Crohn's disease. Dig. Dis. Sci., 24:609, 1979.
95. Phillpotts, R.J., Herman Taylor, J., and Brooke, B.N.: Virus isolation studies in Crohn's disease: A negative report. Gut, 20:1057, 1979.
96. O'Morain, C., et al.: Cytopathic effects in cultures inoculated with material from Crohn's disease. Gut, 22:823, 1981.
97. McLaren, L.C., and Gitnick, G.: Ulcerative colitis and Crohn's disease tissue cytotoxins. Gastroenterology, 82:1381, 1982.
98. Parent, K., and Mitchell, P.: Cell wall defective variants of Pseudomonaslike (Group Va) bacteria in Crohn's disease. Gastroenterology, 75:368, 1978.
99. James, S.P., Graeff, A.S., Quinn, T.C., and Strober, W.: Natural Killer (NK) cell activity is decreased in lamina propria lymphocytes (LPL) isolated from non-human primates with colitis due to lymphogranuloma venereum (LGV). Gastroenterology 88:1430. 1985.
100. Chiodini, R.J., et al.: Possible role of Mycobacteria in inflammatory bowel disease. I. An unclassified mycobacterium species isolated from patients with Crohn's disease. Dig. Dis. Sci., 29:1073, 1984.
101. Chiodini, R.J., Van Kruiningen, H.J., Merkal, R.S., and Thayer, W.R.: Characteristics of an unclassified Mycobacterium species isolated from patients with Crohn's disease. J. Clin. Microbiol., 20:966, 1984.
102. Chiodini, R.J., et al.: In vitro antimicrobial susceptability of a Mycobacterium species isolated from patients with Crohn's disease. Antimicrob. Agents Chemother., 26:930, 1984.
103. Van Kruiningen H.J., et al.: Experimental disease in infant goats induced by a Mycobacterium isolated from a patient with Crohn's disease. Dig. Dis. Sci., 31:1351, 1986.
104. Shaffer, J.L., et al.: Controlled trial of rifampicin and ethambutol in Crohn's disease. Gut, 25:203. 1984
105. Tyzzer, E.: A fatal disease of the Japanese waltzing mouse characterized by a spore boring bacillus. J. Med. Res., 37:307, 1917.
106. McFadyean, J.: The histology of the lesions of Johne's disease. J. Comp. Pathol. Therap., 31:73, 1918.
107. Beister, H.E., and Schwartz, L.H.: Intestinal adenoma in swine. Am. J. Pathol., 7:175, 1931.
108. Hjarre, A., and Wramby, G.: Under sokningar over en med specitika granulom forlopando honssjukdom orsakad av mukioda koli bacterier (Kili granulom). Skan. Veterinaerfidskr., 35:449, 1945.
109. Van Kruiningen, H.J.: Granulomatous colitis of boxer dogs: Comparative aspects. Gastroenterology, 53:114, 1967.
110. Boothe, A.D., and Cheville, N.F.: The pathology of proliferative ileitis in the Golden Syrian hamster. Pathol. Vet. (Basel), 4:31, 1967.
111. Tomita, Y., and Jonas, A.M.: Two viral agents isolated from hamsters with a form of regional enteritis: A preliminary report. Am. J. Vet. Res., 29:445, 1968.
112. Gribble, D.H.: Granulomatous enteritis and intestinal amyloidosis in nonhuman primates. Vet. Pathol., 9:81, 1972.
113. Berkhoff, A.G., and Campbell, S.G.: Etiology and pathogenesis of ulcerative enteritis (Quail disease). The experimental disease. Avian Dis., 18:205, 1974.
114. Doughri, A.M., Young, S., and Storz, J.: Pathologic changes in intestinal Chlamydial infection of newborn calves. Am. J. Vet. Res., 37:939, 1974.
115. Widmer, W.R., and Van Kruiningen, H.J.: Trichuris induced transmural ileocolitis in a dog: An entity mimicking regional enteritis. J. Am. Animal Hosp. Assoc., 10:581, 1974.
116. Tolin, S.A., and Domermuth, C.H.: Hemorrhagic enteritis of turkeys: Electron microscopy of the causal virus. Avian. Dis., 19:118, 1975.
117. Reid, W.M.: Coccidiosis in Diseases of Poultry. Edited by M.S. Hofstad, B.W. Calnek, C.F. Hembolett, W.M. Reid, and H.W. Yoder. Ames, Iowa State University Press, 1978.
118. Tyrrell, D.A.J.: Biology of coronaviruses 1980. In Biochemistry and Biology of Coronaviruses. Edited by V. ter Meulen, S. Siddell, and H. Wege. Adv. Exp. Med. Biol., 142:419, 1981.
119. Stewart, H.L., and Jones, B.F.: Pathologic anatomy of chronic ulcerative colitis: A spontaneous disease of the rat. Arch. Pathol., 31:37, 1941.
120. Emsbo, P.: Terminal or regional ileitis in swine. Nord. Vet. Med., 3:1, 1951.
121. Strande, A., Sommers, S.C., and Petrak, M.: Regional enterocolitis in Cocker Spaniel dogs. Arch. Pathol., 51:357, 1954.
122. Geil, R.G., Lavis, C.L., and Thompson, S.W.: Spontaneous ileitis in rats. Am. J. Vet. Res., 22:932, 1961.
123. Wensvoort, P.: Rekkers of strekkers een aandoening by lammeren. Tijdschr. Diergeneeskd., 87:841, 1962.
124. Stout, C., Snyder, R.L.: Ulcerative colitis-like lesion in Siamang gibbons. Gastroenterology, 57:256, 1969.
125. Van Kruiningen, H.J.: Canine colitis comparable to regional enteritis and mucosal colitis of man. Gastroenterology, 62:1128, 1972.
126. Scott, G.B.D., and Keymer, I.F.: Ulcerative colitis in apes:

A comparison with the human disease. J. Pathol., *115*:241, 1975.
127. Cimprich, R.E.: Equine granulomatous enteritis. Vet. Pathol., *11*:535, 1974.
128. Merritt, A.M., Cimprich, R.E., and Beech, J.: Granulomatous enteritis in nine horses. J. Am. Vet. Med. Assoc., *169*:603, 1976.
129. Chalifoux, L.V., and Bronson, R.T.: Colonic adenocarcinoma associated with chronic ulcerative colitis in cotton topped marmosets (Sanguinus oedipus). Gastroenterology, *80*:942, 1981.
130. Clarke, S.K.R., Caul, E.O., and Egglestone, S.I.: The human enteric coronaviruses. Postgrad. Med. J., *55*:135, 1979.
131. Marshall, J.A., et al.: Coronavirus-like particles and other agents in the feces of children in Efate, Vanuatu. J. Trop. Med. Hyg., *85*:213, 1982.
132. Chany, C., Moscovici, O., Lebon, P., and Rousset, S.: Association of coronavirus infection with neonatal necrotizing enterocolitis. Pediatrics, *69*:209, 1982.
133. Storz, J., Kaluza, G., Niemann, H., and Rott, R.: An enteropathogenic bovine coronavirus. *In* Biochemistry and Biology of Coronoviruses. Edited by V. ter Meulen, S. Siddell, and H. Wege. Adv. Exp. Med. Biol., *142*:171, 1981.
134. Smith, G.C., Lester, T.L., Heberling, R.L., and Kalter, S.S.: Coronavirus-like particles in nonhuman primate feces. Arch. Virol., *72*:105, 1982.
135. Boland, C.R., and Clapp, N.K.: Oncodevelopmental mucins in the colons of new world monkeys with ulcerative colitis and cancer. Gastroenterology, *88*:1330, 1985.

3 · Intestinal Microflora in Inflammatory Bowel Disease—Implications for Etiology

SHERWOOD L. GORBACH, M.D.

The intestinal epithelium is an important barrier to invasion by the intraluminal microbial populations of the bowel. This relationship between the host and its microflora is disturbed in idiopathic inflammatory bowel disease (IBD) in man. Arguments have been raging for many years over the possible role of indigenous microbes in initiating the chain of events leading to this group of disorders. This chapter will review our current knowledge of human intestinal microbiology with particular reference to etiologic factors in idiopathic inflammatory bowel disease.

Normal Flora

The intestinal microflora has specific longitudinal and cross-sectional distributions that are remarkably stable.[1-5] The upper gastrointestinal tract, encompassing the stomach, duodenum, jejunum, and upper ileum, harbors a sparse microflora composed largely of facultative and anaerobic species derived from the oropharynx. The concentration of microorganisms in the upper bowel is generally less than 10^5/ml. These organisms are relatively inert metabolically, and this property, in addition to their low numbers, permits normal absorption of dietary foodstuffs.

The lower ileum shows an increase in microbial elements. It occupies a transitional zone between the sparse flora of the upper bowel and the luxuriant populations of the colon. The major change in the ileum is the appearance of gram-negative, enteric bacilli (coliforms) and small numbers of obligate anaerobes. The total concentration of bacteria in the ileum is generally 10^4 to 10^7/gm, although there is considerable variation among normal subjects.

The colon is a complex ecosystem with high concentrations of microorganisms (10^{11}/gm) and a wide variety of species. Early studies had noted a 1– to 2–log discrepancy between direct microscopic counts of bacteria in feces and the viable counts of cultivable strains. It was thus assumed that many of the organisms seen on direct smear were dead. More recently, however, investigators have been using rigorous anaerobic techniques developed for rumen microbiology.[6,7] With these methods, it is possible to grow virtually all microorganisms that are observed under the microscope. The "dead" forms are, in reality, fastidious anaerobes. Indeed, these techniques have shown that obligate anaerobes predominate over coliforms by approximately 1000:1. The major species are Bacteroides, anaerobic streptococci (peptostreptococci), clostridia, and bifidobacteria.

The cecum and large bowel are characterized by stasis and decreased transit time. These features provide a physiochemical environment of low oxidation-reduction potential (Eh), a situation well suited for growth of fastidious anaerobic microorganisms. The low Eh does not arise de novo, but is a complex interaction between the indigenous flora and its niche within the large bowel. For example, the ceca of germ-free mice have an Eh of -49 ± 50 mv, whereas conventional mice with a normal microflora maintain a markedly reduced atmosphere of -236 ± 17 mv.[8]

Control Mechanisms

Several control mechanisms are important in maintaining the normal relationships between microorganisms and their preferred sites in the gut. At the portal of entry, gastric acid destroys most unwelcome intruders from the outside environment. The upper small bowel uses propulsive motility to rid itself of organisms that manage to escape the acid barrier. Motility may be impaired by surgery (blind loops), radiation therapy, autonomic neuropathy (diabetes), infiltrating diseases (scleroderma), or drugs; in each instance, bacterial overgrowth is a natural sequel.

The ileum is protected to some degree from the colonic flora by the ileocecal valve. Surgical removal of the valve, or its incompetence caused by local disease, leads to proximal spread of microorganisms normally restricted to the terminal ileum and large bowel. This situation often pertains in Crohn's disease.

Microbial regulation in the large bowel is provided by metabolic products of the indigenous flora itself.[8-10] Such mechanisms act to maintain stable population levels and to prevent implantation by pathogens. The resident microbes produce short-chain fatty acids such as acetic, butyric, and propionic. These substances act in synergism with the reduced oxidation-reduction potential and the pH to maintain the normal ecology. Under such conditions, strains of Shigella and Salmonella are unable to implant. Treatment with antibiotics abolishes this protective mechanism and facilitates incursion by these pathogens.

Bacterial-mucosal Relationships

In addition to the longitudinal arrangement of the normal flora, there is also a cross-sectional distribution. Biopsies of the small intestine in man have revealed small numbers of bacteria embedded in the mucous layer overlying the epithelial cells.[11] Cultures of these bacteria have yielded the same strains that are present in the lumen, that is, lactobacilli, streptococci, and occasional obligate anaerobes. Penetration of the intestinal epithelium by bacteria is a pathologic finding; mucosal invasion is characteristic of infectious diarrhea caused by Salmonella, Shigella, and certain strains of Escherichia coli. Bacterial penetration without inflammation is seen in Whipple's disease. Microorganisms are also associated with ulcerating lesions in IBD.

More comprehensive studies of bacteria-mucosa interrelationships have been performed in experimental animals.[12] The distal ileum and the colon of rodents contain microorganisms in intimate association with the epithelial cells. Specially stained histologic sections reveal spiral-shaped bacteria with varying oxygen tolerances, and fusiform-shaped obligate anaerobes. These organisms are densely packed over the epithelial cells in concentrations of 10^{10} to 10^{11}/gm. Their ends are fixed in the mucus overlying the intestinal cells, but there is no evidence of penetration. Because of the stability and reproducibility of these mucosa-associated bacterial forms, they have been labeled "autochthonous flora." Whether such a flora exists in the distal bowel of man is still speculative, because the appropriate studies have not been performed.

Endogenous Microflora in Ulcerative Colitis

Bacterial elements of the normal flora have been implicated in the pathogenesis of chronic ulcerative colitis (CUC) by several investigators. While these were fashionable for several decades, none has stood the test of time and critical reexamination.[13,14] Bargen suggested that a "diplostreptococcus" was prevalent in the feces of colitis patients.[15] He claimed that intravenous challenge with these organisms in rabbits reproduced ulcerating disease of the large bowel. However, Bargen noted that similar bacteria from healthy controls also produced the disease in rabbits. The theory began to fall apart when other investigators found the organism in stools from patients with a variety of other diseases. Moreover, the biochemical characteristics were highly variable, suggesting that Bargen was isolating many species of fecal streptococci and giving them all his appellation "diplostreptococcus."

An anaerobic bacterium known as Bacteroides necrophorum was implicated by Dack, Dragstedt, Heniz, and Kirsner in the pathogenesis of CUC.[16] This organism was cultured from colons that had been surgically removed from patients undergoing diverting ileostomies. In such circumstances, the colon was found to undergo a transformation of microflora with decreased number of aerobic bacteria and a preponderance of the anaerobic, gram-negative rods. B. necrophorum was also found in the feces of patients with chronic ulcerative colitis during periods of exacerbation, but not during periods of quiescence. Finally, many patients with chronic ulcerative colitis had serum agglutinin titers for this organism while normal individuals did not.

Several objections have been raised to these studies. In the first place, the exact identification of Bacteroides necrophorum has not been settled. This organism is probably similar to strains that were known previously as Bacteroides funduliformis and Sphaerophorus necrophorus. The most recent taxonomy places such strains in the species Fusobacterium necrophorum. There is a large variety of anaerobic gram-negative rods in the gastrointestinal tract. Currently the only reliable methods for differentiating these are by biochemical tests, growth in bile salts, susceptibility to antibiotics, and, most importantly, analysis of volatile acid fermentation products by gas-liquid chromatography.[7] These techniques were not available to earlier workers so that there is no assurance that the strains of Bacteroides necrophorum isolated by Dack et al. belonged to a single taxonomic group.[16]

Another problem with this work is that it is now recognized that B. necrophorum is part of the normal flora of the bowel and oropharynx; its presence is ubiquitous in healthy individuals. It can also be shown that these strains are capable of producing ulcers when injected into the skin or mucous membranes of experimental animals. It should be pointed out however, that Dack et al. never fulfilled Koch's postulates by causing intestinal lesions in previously healthy animals with this organism.[16]

The cultures of colonic contents reported by Dack et al. revealed a mixed assortment of morphotypes, according to their own illustrations;[16] B. necrophorum was not isolated in pure culture. Further problems arose when other workers could not duplicate their findings. Meleney noted that he could recover the specific strains of B. necrophorum from only 3 of 40 colitis cases,[17] but he did find the organism in unrelated infections of the throat, bone, liver, and chest. It would appear in retrospect that Bacteroides necrophorum may have been increased under certain conditions such as severe diarrhea or in an isolated colon. The changes in microflora were probably secondary to the disease process itself, however, rather than being of etiologic significance.

Another attractive concept is that an imbalance or "dysbiosis" of the intestinal microflora might lead to mucosal invasion and colitis. Seneca and Henderson presented evidence that the total aerobic flora of the colon increased in patients with chronic ulcerative colitis.[18] Their techniques were unconventional, so it has been difficult to confirm this work. Other investigators found no change in the fecal flora of mild to moderately ill patients with CUC.[19, 20] Severely ill patients showed modest increases in intestinal flora, especially in the coliform elements. Treatment with corticosteroids lowered these counts if there was associated clinical improvement.[19]

Among the normal flora components, coliforms are increased in the fecal effluent of patients with CUC, especially during periods of relapse.[20] The anaerobic flora is generally unchanged in patients with IBD.

It has been claimed that certain E. coli strains in the stools of CUC patients produce necrotoxins, hemolysins, or enterotoxins.[21] In another study, the adhesive properties of coliforms from fecal flora of CUC patients and normal controls were compared.[22] In general, CUC patients tended to have one serotype of coliforms that dominated the fecal flora, while normal controls had a variety of serotypes. The CUC patients had at least one type of adhesive or invasive fecal coliform more frequently (35% in active cases and 27% in inactive cases) than did patients with other types of colitis (5%) or the normal controls (5%).

Diarrhea may cause changes in the microflora, regardless of the primary etiology.[3] For example, alterations have been reported in infectious diarrheas caused by Shigella, E. coli or V. cholerae, in "nonspecific" diarrhea, in hypolactasic subjects fed lactose, and in diarrhea induced by purging the bowel with isotonic fluid. These changes fall into three major categories:

1. Increase in certain coliform species that are uncommon in the normal flora, such as Enterobacter, Proteus, Klebsiella, and Pseudomonas. Such strains may gain prevalence while the usual flora of E. coli is suppressed. This can result in a net increase in a total coliform count.

2. Decline in obligate anaerobes. The anaerobic strains that ordinarily are predominant in the fecal flora may actually decline below the coliform count. In particularly brisk diarrhea, such as cholera, obligate anaerobes may fall to low, even undetectable, concentrations.
3. Retrograde contamination of the upper small bowel by elements of the fecal flora. Colonization of the jejunum by pathogens has important implications in enterotoxin-associated diarrhea. The abnormal flora may persist for several weeks following an acute episode. This abnormality can also be seen in diarrhea induced by saline perfusion of the lower intestine.

From the available data there is no justification for ascribing etiologic significance to alterations in the balance of the normal flora in chronic ulcerative colitis. The changes that have been described may be secondary to rapid transit through the large bowel, effectively bypassing the normal control mechanisms described above. It is hazardous to assign a primary role to changes in flora on the basis of simple bacteriologic surveys of fecal microbial populations.

Chronic Ulcerative Colitis and Bacillary Dysentery

The pathologic changes caused by virulent Shigella closely mimic those of "idiopathic chronic ulcerative colitis" in the acute period. Because of this similarity and the occasional case of chronic shigellosis, several investigators have attempted to portray CUC as chronic bacillary dysentery in which the infecting Shigella can no longer be cultured.[23-25]

The pathogenesis of bacillary dysentery has been elucidated by using various mutant strains of Shigella.[26] The first step is attachment of the pathogenic organism to the surface of the colonic epithelial cell, a phenomenon that can be identified by fluorescent microscopy. While the ability to attach is an absolute requirement for a pathogenic strain, the disease cannot be produced unless the organism also possesses the capacity to penetrate the epithelium. Following attachment and penetration, the Shigella strain can be seen in the lamina propria, leaving in its wake mucosal ulcerations and an intense inflammatory response.

The precise mechanism of tissue destruction by Shigella has not been explained. An exotoxin was originally demonstrated in S. dysenteriae by Shiga,[27] and more recently in other species of Shigella as well.[28] A controversy exists, however, as to whether this toxin is important in the pathogenesis of acute colitis in the natural host, man.[29,30]

The advocates of Shigella as an important cause of CUC lost credibility in recent years when the decline in bacillary dysentery in the United States and Europe failed to influence the incidence of idiopathic chronic ulcerative colitis. Furthermore, careful bacteriologic studies of patients with acute CUC have failed to recover Shigella in most cases. With the availability of selective media and enrichment techniques, these organisms should not be overlooked by careful observers.

The point can always be raised that the initial event is bacillary dysentery caused by a microorganism that cannot be cultured by current methodology. This "What if. . . . " approach to scientific criticism has been strengthened in the case of colitis by the recent recognition of E. coli strains that penetrate the large bowel mucosa, causing bacillary dysentery.[31] The acute onset and rapid recovery of this disease are in marked contrast to chronic ulcerative colitis. However, this condition does cause us to wonder if there are other microorganisms presently unrecognized that can cause a more indolent disease.

Entamoeba histolytica has "entered the ring" as a possible contender for the pathologic agent in chronic ulcerative colitis.[32] This agent no doubt causes acute colitis that may lapse into a chronic stage if not adequately treated. The pathology of amebiasis is different from that seen in most cases of CUC, however. The lesion in amebiasis is characterized by tissue liquefaction and undermining necrosis with a relative paucity of acute inflammatory cells. This produces the typical "collar-button" appearance on proctoscopic examination. Furthermore, amebae usually can be seen in microscopic sections when examined by experienced observers. It is also apparent that broad-spectrum antibiotics usually provide rapid relief for the acute symptoms of intestinal amebiasis, although the cyst stage of the parasite may persist. The salutary effects of tetracycline in acute amebiasis has not been reproduced in treating acute chronic ulcerative colitis. Invoking E. histolytica as a causative agent is reminiscent of Elsdon-Dew's classic remark that "Amebiasis is the refuge of the diagnostically destitute."

After reviewing the several microorganisms that have been implicated as "the pathogen" in CUC, it is obvious that none has satisfied Koch's postulates of: (1) isolation from all cases, (2) growth in some in vitro culture system, and (3) passage to an appropriate animal model. It is still intriguing that chronic ulcerative colitis primarily affects the colon, an area that is in intimate contact with luxuriant microbial populations. Furthermore, the microscopic appearance of mucosal ulcerations, crypt abscesses, and abundant inflammatory cells is also seen in colitis caused by certain infectious agents, such as Shigella and E. coli. The conundrum of chronic ulcerative colitis is its self-perpetuating nature, its episodic relapse, and its disappointing response to a variety of antimicrobial agents.

Bacterial Flora in Crohn's Disease

Studies of the microflora in Crohn's disease (CD) have been hampered by our lack of understanding of the ileal flora in health. Because the area of the intestine commonly involved is relatively inaccessible, investigators have been forced to rely on capsules for sampling the lower reaches of the ileum. More recently, a long plastic tube has been employed. Some patients have also been studied during surgical procedures, but the interpretation of data thus obtained is influenced by preoperative medications and the period of fasting.

Based on available evidence, it would appear that the ileal flora in healthy individuals is highly variable. Some subjects have a minimal flora comprised of organisms derived from the oropharynx. Others have relatively high concentrations of bacteria (10^5 to 10^7/ml) that include coliforms and obligate anaerobes derived from the colon. In all subjects, however, there is a striking difference across the ileocecal valve.[33, 34] Five centimeters proximal to this structure the microflora may be relatively sparse, but just across the valve there is a sharp increase by several logs. The flora of the cecum is predominantly anaerobic, and reflects the bacterial populations throughout the large intestine.

Abnormalities of small intestinal flora in patients with Crohn's disease depend on the anatomic features of the small intestine. Patients with stricture or resection of the ileum have shown an abnormal flora in the proximal small bowel. Krone et al. demonstrated that coliforms, enterococci, clostridia, and Bacteroides were present in jejunal aspirates of patients with structural abnormalities of the ileum.[35] In the study by Gorbach and Tabaqchali,[36] facultative microorganisms such as coliforms could be found in the upper small bowel of patients with CD. Obligate anaerobes were restricted to areas of stasis associated with stricture formation. Loss of the ileocecal valve had the effect of contaminating the upper intestine with colonic bacteria. Prizoni et al. could demonstrate an abnormal flora in 2 of 6 patients with CD.[37] The study by Vince et al. showed that 4 of 13 patients with Crohn's disease had an abnormal flora in the jejunum and midgut.[38] The increase in bacterial counts in the upper intestine was observed *only* in patients with obvious stasis or with fistula formation. Subjects with normal motility or with relatively localized disease in the distal ileum had an upper intestinal flora similar to normal subjects.

Two groups of investigators studied the fecal microflora in Crohn's disease patients, before and after treatment with metronidazole and sulfonamide compounds (either trimethoprim/sulfamethoxazole, or salazopyrin).[39, 49] As expected, obligate anaerobes, such as Bacteroides, decreased in patients receiving metronidazole, but there were no reproducible changes in patients treated with a sulfonamide. In their analysis of results, Hudson et al. could find no correlation between clinical improvement and changes in the microflora associated with the antimicrobial therapy.[40] Other workers have found increased numbers and varieties of streptococci, especially enterococci.[41, 42] It has been suggested by van de Merwe and Mol that Eubacterium and Peptostreptococcus species, both elements of the normal microflora, are greatly increased in patients with Crohn's disease.[43]

Some investigators have cultured tissues of Crohn's disease patients, obtained by endoscopic biopsy or at surgery. Hudson et al. found the same types of organisms associated with the rectal mucosa in Crohn's disease patients as in their fecal flora.[40] The study by Ambrose et al. used samples of ileal serosa and mesenteric lymph nodes harvested at surgery.[44] They found potentially pathogenic bacteria in serosal tissues of 27% of Crohn's disease patients, compared with 15% of controls, and in the mesenteric lymph nodes of 33% Crohn's disease patients, compared to 5% of controls. The types of organisms generally were those expected in the normal flora, such as E. coli, Proteus, Bacteroides, and streptococci. They postulated that these organisms "leaked" from the bowel in Crohn's disease patients because of the damaged mucosa.

Many individuals with Crohn's disease have malabsorption of fat and vitamin B_{12}. The pathophysiologic events suggest that there may be an element of the "stagnant-loop syndrome" in such patients, that is, the bacterial flora is directly interfering with absorptive function. Krone et al. noted that some Crohn's disease patients with steatorrhea had deconjugated bile acids in the upper intestine.[35] These findings were ascribed to bacterial overgrowth. Vince et al. also found deconjugation of bile salts with steatorrhea in Crohn's disease patients but, in this series, bacterial overgrowth could not be implicated.[38] Some patients had these findings without overgrowth, while others had overgrowth without steatorrhea. Rutgeers et al.,[45] using the ^{14}C-glycocholate breath test along with fecal analysis, found evidence of bacterial overgrowth and abnormal ileal dysfunction in 26 of 61 patients (44%).

In summary, one-third of patients with Crohn's disease have been found to have an abnormal microflora in the upper small bowel. Bacterial overgrowth is more common when there has been surgical removal of the ileocecal valve. A smaller number of patients have obligate anaerobes in the upper intestine, and this finding is usually associated with stricture or stasis. Even when an abnormal intestinal flora is demonstrated, this is not necessarily the cause of malabsorption. Because the ileal mucosa is directly involved with the disease process, there may be malabsorption of fat and vitamin B_{12} that can simulate the stagnant loop syndrome. Careful studies of bile salt deconjugation and micellar concentrations, along with judicious therapeutic trials with antibiotics, are required in these complex cases.

Antibodies Against Normal Flora Bacteria

The damaged intestinal mucosa in IBD patients provides greater contact between the host's antibody-forming mechanisms and the intestinal flora. Consequently, several investigators have found high circulating serum antibodies against normal flora bacteria in IBD patients. Among the aerobic/facultative bacteria, antibodies to specific serotypes of Escherichia coli and Streptococcus faecalis were found to be elevated.[46-49] High levels of circulating antibody against anaerobic bacteria have also been encountered. For example, antibodies against anaerobic gram-positive cocci and rods, such as Peptostreptococcus and Eubacterium, have been found in inflammatory bowel disease patients, particularly those with Crohn's disease.[50-52] Circulating antibodies against Bacteroides have also been demonstrated in inflammatory bowel disease patients.[48,49] Of interest, Gump et al. found that antibodies against a specific species of Bacteroides, namely Bacteroides vulgatus, were elevated in CD patients;[53] this is the same species of Bacteroides identified by Onderdonk et al. to provide immune enhancement of experimentally-induced disease in a guinea pig model of IBD.

It is important when reviewing studies of the normal flora in inflammatory bowel disease to distinguish between a primary etiologic event and a secondary role in complications. On the basis of current data, it is impossible to ascribe a primary etiologic role to components of the normal intestinal microflora in IBD. On the other hand, intestinal bacteria may be involved in complications of IBD. Thus, increased antibody formation, anticolon antibodies, and immune complexes could be related to the normal flora components.[55]

Antibodies Against Microbial Pathogens

Blaser et al. conducted a comprehensive study of Crohn's disease patients and healthy age- and sex-matched controls, measuring their serum antibodies to a variety of bacterial pathogens.[56] The antigens used in their complement-fixation assays included Campylobacter, Yersinia, Listeria, Brucella, and Mycobacterium. These organisms were selected because they are transmitted by the oral route, they may produce a granulomatous disease in the intestine, and they are not generally found in the normal intestinal flora. The serum from CD patients had enhanced antibody activity to all seven of these antigens when compared to controls. Interestingly, there was no difference between CD patients and the controls for a common mycobacterial antigen known as arabinomannan. Patients with widespread mycobacterial disease, such as lepromatous leprosy or cavitary tuberculosis, generally have high serum reactivity to this antigen. Lack of reactivity to this antigen may be seen in patients with relatively low numbers of organisms in their tissues, however, such as those with scrofula or tuberculoid leprosy. Furthermore, Grange et al. found elevated titers of IgA and IgM in CD patients, using a sonicate of BCG mycobacteria.[57] Blaser et al. concluded that the elevated titers in Crohn's disease to several bacterial antigens represented "increased bowel wall permeability", rather than any primary pathogenic mechanism.[56]

As new microbial pathogens are described,

they are tested in those diseases that remain undiagnosed in our nosology. Yersinia enterocolytica has been "hoisted" in inflammatory bowel disease, and then "lowered" when a negative report appeared in the literature.[58] Chlamydia, another fashionable microorganism, was initially associated with elevated serologic titers in Crohn's disease but subsequently it lost credibility because of several reports showing no association.[58–61]

Experimental Colitis[*]

An experimental model of chronic ulcerative colitis, using a red seaweed extract, carrageenan, in guinea pigs, has shown the relationship of the intestinal microflora to the pathologic events. Animals fed carrageenan develop ulcerations in the cecum and colon, similar to those seen in chronic ulcerative colitis. The disease develops in animals with a conventional microflora, but *not* in germ-free animals.[62] A similar effect could be demonstrated by treating the conventional animals with antimicrobial drugs. Metronidazole and clindamycin each prevented the cecal ulcerations associated with carrageenan, but no effect was seen with gentamicin, trimethoprim/sulfamethoxazole, and vancomycin.[63] Salazopyrin gave 50% reduction in cecal ulcerations. These results indicate that the anaerobic flora, that is, the component suppressed by metronidazole or clindamycin, was acting in a synergistic manner with carrageenan to produce these cecal ulcerations. Subsequent studies by Onderdonk and co-workers showed that the major promoting organism in the microflora was Bacteroides vulgatus.[54] When this organism was administered with the carrageenan, it seemed to enhance the cecal pathology. The organism must come from an IBD patient, because a similar strain from a normal individual gave no augmentation. In addition, prior immunization with Bacteroides vulgatus, or using adoptive transfer of spleen cells from immunized animals, also caused enhancement of pathology when the immunized animals were fed carrageenan, compared to nonimmunized controls.

These studies indicate the seminal role of the microflora, particularly the anaerobic component and Bacteroides vulgatus, in the development of this experimental disease. Whether these findings relate to the human disease is speculative. It is interesting that Gump et al. found elevated titers of serum antibodies to Bacteroides vulgatus in CD patients, when compared to matched controls.[53]

Clostridium Difficile and Inflammatory Bowel Disease

The agent of pseudomembranous colitis and certain forms of antibiotic-associated diarrhea (without colitis) has been conclusively identified as Clostridium difficile, a gram-positive, spore-forming, anaerobic rod.[64,65] This organism is found only rarely in the fecal flora of healthy adults, although it can be isolated from stools of neonates. C. difficile was originally isolated from the stools of patients with clindamycin-associated pseudomembranous colitis. The disease is now known to be associated with virtually all antibiotics used in clinical practice. The most common drugs, reflecting the pattern of usage, are cephalosporins and penicillins. Among the drugs implicated in this condition are salazopyrin and metronidazole, two agents widely used in inflammatory bowel disease. This disease has been reproduced in a hamster model, either by injecting the organism or a cell-broth filtrate containing the necrotizing toxin into the cecum.

Trinka and Lamont reported the presence of C. difficile toxin in the feces of patients with chronic ulcerative colitis or Crohn's disease,[66] despite earlier reports to the contrary.[64] Toxin-positive stools were found with equal frequency in CUC and CD patients, although there was an apparent increase in the isolation rate from more severe cases. Nine of their patients were treated with vancomycin, and they reported a satisfactory, although somewhat dilatory, improvement with this specific therapy. They specifically mentioned that only 3 of 11 patients with toxin-positive stools had received antibiotics in the two months prior to testing their stool. In the same issue of Gastroenterology, a contradictory article written by Meyers et al. appeared.[67] Performing a similar study, they identified the C. difficile toxin in 4 of 44 patients with CUC or CD. In each of the toxin-positive cases, however, both among IBD patients and "diarrhea controls," of which there were five, *all* had received antibiotics sometime in the preceding six months. These authors concluded that previous antibiotic usage had predisposed these patients to colonization by C. difficile, and they were unable to associate the clinical status of the patient with the presence of this organism. Other authors have been unable to correlate the

[*]See also Chap. 2.

presence of C. difficile or its toxins with inflammatory bowel disease. Wright et al. studied multiple stool specimens from ten patients with mild to severe Crohn's disease.[68] None of the samples was positive for C. difficile cytotoxin. The study by Dorman et al. examined stool specimens from 50 CD patients.[69] Most had inactive disease, although a few had relapses during the course of investigation. The organism was recovered from only 8% of patients, and none had positive cytotoxin tests. Similarly, Rolny et al., in a study of 53 IBD "inpatients," found only 5% with a positive cytotoxin test.[70]

Further clarification of the relationship between C. difficile and inflammatory bowel disease has come from the excellent study by Greenfield et al.[48] Using either a positive culture or the presence of cytotoxin as the indicator, they found a positive result in 13% of CD patients, 14% of CUC patients, 12% of a control group of "inpatients" with other forms of diarrhea, and 1% of healthy controls. Of their 109 inflammatory bowel disease patients, 28% had either a positive culture or toxin titer on at least one occasion during the one-year study. A higher incidence of positive tests was seen in IBD patients taking either antibiotics (31%) or salazopyrin (13%), when compared to IBD patients taking no antimicrobial drugs (6%). The incidence of positive tests in IBD patients was not related to their clinical condition, but it correlated significantly with hospital admissions. The finding of increased positive tests in the control patients with diarrhea because of other causes has been reported by other investigators.[72,73]

The issue of C. difficile in inflammatory bowel disease raises several important concerns, both on a practical level for the "treating physician" and on a theoretical level for the investigating scientist. It seems clear that this organism has no primary role in the causation of inflammatory bowel disease. It may, however, be related to clinical relapse, although this would appear to be a relatively rare cause of deterioration in the clinical picture. The diagnosis should be based on a positive cytotoxin assay, with necessary controls as described by Chang et al.[74] A positive fecal culture for the organism is adjunctive information. It should be recognized that a carrier state exists in which the organism may be found in the feces for a period of up to nine months after acquisition, usually related to antibiotic exposure.[75] Such carriers generally have a negative cytotoxin assay. It is preferable, then, to have a positive toxin assay when ascribing clinical symptoms to this organism, because it is toxin that produces the disease, not the organism itself. Epidemiologic features should also be considered in IBD patients. As noted by Greenfield et al., hospital admission is correlated with acquisition of C. difficile.[17] This association may be related to the presence of the organism in the hospital environment and the tendency of hospitalized patients to acquire it. Another important issue, however, is that antimicrobial drugs are widely used in IBD patients, especially salazopyrin and metronidazole. Colonization by C. difficile has been associated with a wide variety of antimicrobial agents, including clindamycin, ampicillin, cephalosporins, erythromycin, tetracycline, metronidazole, as well as the sulfonamide found in salazopyrin. Once the organism is acquired it may remain in the fecal flora, with its toxins, for up to nine months after the antibiotic exposure. In some patients this produces relapsing diarrheal episodes, but most people live in symbiosis with the organism, without experiencing symptoms.

Only a small percentage of patients with inflammatory bowel disease harbor C. difficile or its toxins, generally related to prior antibiotic use or hospitalization. When exacerbation of clinical symptoms is present along with a positive cytotoxin assay, it would be justified to treat such a patient with either vancomycin, metronidazole (presuming that this drug has not been used earlier), or bacitracin. It should be pointed out that the response to these antibiotics should be prompt, at least within five days. Failure to respond within this time frame would indicate that this organism is playing no role in the clinical condition.

Novel Pathogens in Inflammatory Bowel Disease

Employing hypertonic culture medium, Parent and Mitchell have reported the isolation of cell-wall defective bacteria, known as L-forms, in homogenized tissue obtained at surgery from CD patients.[76] These organisms were isolated from all eight CD patients using small bowel or lymph node tissue, but in none of nine CUC patients or twenty "control" patients with other illnesses. Cell-wall defective organisms should revert to the parent bacterial strain when subcultured on conventional medium. These variants behaved in this manner, reverting to conventional organisms, subsequently identified as Pseudomonas-like Group Va (taxonomy according to the Center for Disease Control, U. S. A.).[77] In a subsequent abstract, these investigators were unable to reproduce disease when the organisms were injected into rabbits.[78] It should be noted that all patients in these studies had received preoperative antibiotic bowel preps, and this may be an important point because L-forms can be induced by the use of antibiotics.

In the study by Belsheim et al. a variety of L-form bacteria were isolated from patients with inflammatory bowel disease.[79] However, none of the Pseudomonas strains isolated by Parent and Mitchell was recovered by these workers. Instead, their major isolates were E. coli (57%), enterococci (26%), Pseudomonas aeruginosa (9%), and several other fecal-type bacteria. These cell-wall defective enteric bacteria were isolated from 27 of 71 CD patients, 51 of 121 CUC patients, and 2 of 140 controls.

Other investigators have looked for traces of these organisms in intestinal tissue by various immunologic and genetic techniques. Graham et al. constructed DNA probes from Parent and Mitchell's reverted cell-wall defective Pseudomonas strains.[80] With these labeled probes, they examined intestinal tissue and found DNA homology in 3 of 23 CD patients, 2 of 10 CUC patients, and 0 of 15 controls. These workers also attempted to culture cell-wall defective organisms from these tissues, using hypertonic culture media. They were unable to isolate any of these cell-wall defective organisms from these same tissues. They did detect, however, pleomorphic, unclassified organisms in the hypertonic cultures of 14 or 53 CD patients, 0 of 16 CUC patients, and 0 of 11 controls. These organisms did not revert, remaining as L-forms: thus, they were unable to classify the organisms any further. A similar type of study was reported by Whorwell et al., who used indirect immunofluorescence for the antigens of Pseudomonas maltophilia.[81] None of the tissues from CD patients was positive in this study.

Studies of circulating antibodies against the revertant forms of cell-wall deficient bacteria have yielded conflicting results in CD patients. Shafii et al. used indirect immunofluorescence for antibody against two strains of the Pseudomonas cell-wall defective variants described by Parent and Mitchell.[82] Serum samples from 22 or 25 CD patients were positive, whereas 0 of 23 CUC patients and 0 of 15 control patients gave positive results. In a similar study, Gump et al. found antibody against the Pseudomonas-like variant in 51% of CD patients, compared to 25% of age- and sex-matched controls.[53]

To date, there is no evidence that the cell-wall deficient forms of Pseudomonas are primary pathogens in inflammatory bowel disease. It may be that these organisms are trapped by, or penetrate, a more permeable intestinal wall in Crohn's disease. Hence, positive cultures of various types of L-forms can be obtained, some of which revert to recognizable enteric bacteria, while others remain in the L-form state. Yet the relative infrequency of isolation, the lack of consistency from laboratory to laboratory, and the failure to reproduce the disease in an animal model, all militate against the significance (in an etiologic sense) of these cell-wall deficient bacterial forms.

Mycobacteria

Early Studies

Several histologic features of Crohn's disease suggest that a mycobacterium or a related agent might be involved. The granulomatous tissue reaction together with the abnormalities of delayed hypersensitivity share features with tuberculosis and leprosy.

Mitchell and Rees pursued the possible relation of CD to leprosy, using an animal model that has proven successful with M. leprae.[83] The footpad of a mouse is injected with infected material from leprosy patients. The low temperature in this part of the body apparently favors growth of the leprosy bacillus and, after several weeks, swelling and an inflammatory reaction can be demonstrated. Biopsy of the footpad reveals abundant mycobacteria and typical histologic features. Following this protocol, Mitchell and Rees injected mouse footpads with cell-free extracts of affected ileum from patients with active Crohn's disease. They used normal mice and immunologically deficient animals (thymectomy and whole body X-irradiation), because the immunologically deficient animal gives an earlier and more active response to infection with M. leprae. The results with Crohn's disease were interesting, but not definitive. At 46 days, 5 of 8 animals injected with CD tissue showed positive histologic findings of a granulomatous reaction. At 169 days, 8 of 48 animals were positive. In addition, 2 mice had ileal granulomas. Positive Kveim tests were noted in 6 animals, all of which had positive footpad biopsies.

These results were confirmed by Taub et al., who induced similar granulomas with ileal tissue from Crohn's disease and also with lymph nodes from patients with sarcoid.[84] No disease, however, was noted with tissue from patients with chronic ulcerative colitis. The passage of granulomas was inhibited by phenol treatment or by the freezing and thawing of the material prior to its injection. In addition, transfer could be accomplished from animal to animal, following the initial induction of disease. Subsequent studies by Cave et al. reproduced the disease in mice and caused a similar lesion in rabbits.[85, 86] The animals had a long latent period, usually 2 to 9 months, maintained their disease for up to 6 months, and could pass the disease to other animals. The putative agent was killed by autoclaving, phenol treatment, and slow freezing. It was successfully passaged 3 to 4 times in animals and went through a 0.2-micron filter.

The studies by Cave et al. showed that tissue from patients with Crohn's disease and chronic ulcerative colitis could induce granulomatous disease in mice.[85, 86] In rabbits, however, the CD tissue produced granulomas, while the CUC material caused a round cell infiltrate in the intestinal mucosa.

The results of these experiments were not unanimously acclaimed by all scientists, however, because Bolten et al. and Heatley et al. were unable to confirm the findings using similar protocols in mice.[88, 89] Nevertheless, the negative studies used bovine albumin and a shorter observation time, and it has been suggested that these factors may have explained the divergence of findings.

In addition to the conflicting results, however, there have been problems with interpretation of these investigations. Granulomatous lesions in the intestinal wall can be induced by injection of equine serum into previously sensitized rabbits.[90] Similar lesions have been caused by injecting the bowel wall with E. coli.[91] Thus, the granulomatous reaction is nonspecific and can be produced by a number of immunologic challenges that may have nothing to do with IBD. It is also disturbing that the same type of reactions reported with CD and CUC tissue were induced by tissue from patients with unrelated bowel disorders, colonic interposition, familial polyposis, cancer of the rectum, and occasionally by normal tissue.[84]

Culture Isolation Studies

Taking a somewhat different "tack," Burnham, Stanford, and co-workers cultivated mesenteric lymph nodes in Lowenstein Jensen medium at various temperatures for periods up to nine months (this medium is used for culturing mycobacteria such as M. tuberculosis and atypical mycobacteria). Positive cultures were noted to have a "fine surface growth of organisms which are irregular in shape and stained acid-fast by the Ziehl-Neelsen method." Such positives were found in 33 of 50 CD patients, 11 of 20 with CUC, and 2 of 26 controls. However, they were unable to cause reversion of these cell-wall defective organisms, apparently mycobacteria, to orthodox strains.[92] A single exception was from one of their original patients with Crohn's disease from whom they isolated Mycobacterium kansasii. On electronmicroscopy they also saw organisms from the original culture that resembled Mycoplasma, although these strains could not be subcultured.

Subsequent studies by Stanford reported cultivation of acid-fast and gram-positive "masses" from lymph nodes from Crohn's disease patients, chronic ulcerative colitis patients, and occasionally from patients with other diseases.[93] In a collateral study by White, this acid-fast material from Crohn's disease patients was felt to represent mycolic acids;[94] however, others, using antigens from Mycobacterium kansasii, were unable to demonstrate immunofluorescence in tissue of Crohn's disease patients, indicating the absence of the organism, at least in substantial numbers.[95] Serum antibodies to M. kansasii were found in 9 or 11 Crohn's disease patients, but in none of 22 controls.

Another group added some evidence suggesting a possible role for a Mycobacterium species in Crohn's disease patients, using prolonged incubation in enriched culture medium. Chiodini et al. isolated a previously unrecognized Mycobacterium in two Crohn's disease patients.[96] These strains most likely resembled M. paratuberculosis, and they were tentatively placed in Runyon Group III. In another publication, this group claimed to have isolated a Mycobacterium strain in 3 of 22 Crohn's disease patients.[97] In an accompanying paper by Thayer et al. serum antibody was tested in Crohn's disease patients, using an antigen from M. paratuberculosis with an ELISA technique.[98] Twenty-three percent of Crohn's disease patients were positive for serum antibody against this organism, and this was significantly higher than chronic ulcerative colitis patients or controls. However, healthy controls with a PPD-positive skin test had serum antibodies to this organism in titers similar to those found in Crohn's disease patients. A recent study by Graham's group failed to find consistent antibody responses in the serum to Mycobacterium paratuberculosis in CD. Furthermore, in another report from the same group of a cultural study of gut specimens obtained from patients with CD, CUC, or nonimflammatory bowel diseases, no consistent relationship could be found between the presence or species of Mycobacterium and Crohn's disease.

Van Kruiningen et al. also have carried out animal challenge studies with their Mycobacterium isolate. Goats developed granulomatous disease of the distal small intestine, along with humoral and cell-mediated immunity, when challenged by the oral route with this organism.[96,97] This Mycobacterium was subsequently isolated from the duodenum, jejunum, colon, and mesenteric lymph nodes of the diseased goat, as early as three months after oral challenge.

We would love to believe that the etiologic agent of Crohn's disease has at last been discovered. Certainly, it is tempting to accept the Mycobacterium connection, especially the organism reported by Chiodini et al.[96] The pathology, with its granuloma formation and altered cell-mediated immunity, resembles that caused by the Mycobacterium group of organisms. For example, there is a remarkable counterpart in ruminants, known as Johne's disease, which is caused by a Mycobacterium. The problems with these reports, however, are legion; in fact, the organism has been isolated from only 3 of 22 Crohn's disease patients, according to one of the more recent reports.[97] There is no mention of isolation attempts from controls. The inoculation studies in animals, while encouraging, are not entirely convincing, because it is known that such granulomatous reactions can be induced in experimental animals by inoculation with any of a variety of foreign antigens, both living and dead. Again, there were no controls using other protein inoculations or other species of Mycobacterium in the goats. The antibody studies, reported by Thayer et al., also lack some credibility.[98] The antigen was *not* the same organism isolated in the Crohn's disease patients, but a strain of M. paratuberculosis. Only 23% of Crohn's disease patients had significant antibody to this organism. Similar results, however, were observed in PPD-positive controls. These findings suggest that contact with Mycobacterium is found in at least some Crohn's disease patients. The question is whether this organism is a true pathogen or whether it is an idle bystander in the intestinal microflora. The intestinal mucosa of Crohn's disease patients is abnormal, and there seems to be increased sampling of antigens within the intestinal lumen. It is apparent from other studies that Crohn's disease patients have higher antibody levels to a variety of intestinal bacteria and viruses, some of which are pathogens, and others merely members of the microflora.

The findings of Graham's group raise doubt as to the suggested significance of any Mycobacterium studied to date to the etiology of CD.[99,100] On the basis of these investigations, and extrapolating from observations on known mycobacterial diseases, it is possible to make some speculations on a possible pathogen in Crohn's disease. It is likely to be a highly fastidious organism, requiring enriched culture media and prolonged incubation, such fastidiousness being a feature of certain mycobacteria pathogenic to humans, especially the leprosy bacillus. The organism is likely to be rare in tissues, or it would have been seen in the multiple histologic studies in CD carried out by many investigators. There may even be "burnt-out" cases that have cured themselves, leaving no viable organisms in tissues. Low numbers of mycobacteria are common in human intestinal tuberculosis and in tuberculoid leprosy. The putative pathogen might have strong host specificity, so inoculation in other animals would prove extremely difficult. Again, this is a trait of several mycobacterial species known to infect humans. The organism should cause infection by an oral challenge, because this is the most likely route of transmission in CD. The immune mechanisms probably would be mostly cell-mediated, with relatively little or no circulating antibody response. This type of immunity is found in human tuberculosis and other mycobacterial diseases as well. Unfortunately, if such an organism is operating in CD, the fact that it is so fastidious and host-specific not only would render it difficult to identify, but also make it even more difficult to satisfy Koch's postulates to prove its pathogenicity. The latter remain the ultimate arbiters of claims for infection by any specific microorganism as significant in the etiology of CUC or CD.

Currently, for those who favor a specific infectious etiology, the axiom is: "back to the drawing board."

References

1. Donaldson, R. M. Jr.: Normal bacterial population of the intestine and their relation to intestinal function. N. Engl. J. Med., *270*:938, 1984.
2. Floch, M. H., Gorbach, S. L., and Luckey, T. D.: Symposium: The intestinal microflora. Am. J. Clin. Nutr., *23*:1425, 1970.
3. Gorbach, S. L.: Intestinal microflora. Gastroenterology, *60*:1110, 1971.

4. Hentges, D. J.: Human Intestinal Microflora in Health and Disease. New York, Academic Press, 1983.
5. Simon, G. L., and Gorbach, S. L.: Intestinal flora in health and disease: A review. Gastroenterology, 86:174, 1984.
6. Moore, W. E. C., Cato, E. P., and Holderman, L. V.: Anaerobic bacteria of the gastrointestinal flora and their occurrence in clinical infections. J. Infect. Dis., 120: 641, 1969.
7. Virginia Polytechnic Institute Anaerobic Laboratory: Outline of Clinical Methods in Anaerobic Bacteriology. Blackburg, Virginia Polytechnic Institute, 1972.
8. Maier, B. R., et al.: Shigella, indigenous flora interactions in mice. Am. J. Clin. Nutr., 25:1433, 1972.
9. Meynell, G. G.: Antibacterial mechanisms of the mouse gut. II. The role of Eh and volatile fatty acids in the normal gut. Br. J. Exp. Pathol., 44:209, 1963.
10. Hentges, D. J.: Inhibition of Shigella flexneri by the normal intestinal flora. II. Mechanisms of inhibition by coliform organisms. J. Bacteriol., 97:513, 1969.
11. Plaut, A. G., et al.: Studies in intestinal microflora. III. The microbial flora of human small bowel intestinal mucosa and fluids. Gastroenterology, 53:868, 1967.
12. Savage, D. C.: Associations and physiological interactions of indigenous microorganisms and gastrointestinal epithelia. Am. J. Clin. Nutr., 25:1372, 1972.
13. Weinstein, G.: Bacteriological aspects of ulcerative colitis. Gastroenterology, 40:323, 1961.
14. deDombal, F. T., Burch, P. R. J., and Watkinson, G.: Aetiology of ulcerative colitis. I. A review of past and present hypotheses. Gut, 10:270, 1969.
15. Bargen, J. A.: Experimental studies on etiology of chronic ulcerative colitis. J. Am. Med. Assoc., 83:332, 1924.
16. Dragsteadt, L. R., Dack, G. M., and Kirsner, J. B.: Chronic ulcerative colitis: A summary of evidence implicating Bacterium necrophorum as an etiologic agent. Ann. Surg., 114:653, 1941.
17. Meleney, F.: Discussion. Ann. Surg., 114:661, 1941.
18. Seneca, H., and Henderson, E.: Normal intestinal bacteria in ulcerative colitis. Gastroenterology, 15:34, 1950.
19. Gorbach, S. L., et al.: Studies of intestinal microflora: V. Fecal microbial ecology in ulcerative colitis and regional enteritis; relationship to severity of disease and chemotherapy. Gastroenterology, 54:575, 1968.
20. Gorbach, S. L., et al.: Studies of intestinal microflora: V. Fecal microbial ecology in ulcerative colitis and regional enteritis; relationship to severity of disease and chemotherapy. Gastroenterology, 54:575, 1968.
21. Cooke, E. M.: Properties of strains of Escherichia coli isolated from the faeces of patients with ulcerative colitis, patients with acute diarrhoea and normal persons. J. Pathol. Bacteriol., 95:101, 1968.
22. Dickinson, R. J., Varian, S. A., Axon, A. T. and Cooke, E. N.: Increased incidence of fecal coliforms with in vitro adhesive and invasive properties in patients with ulcerative colitis. Gut, 21:787, 1980.
23. Hurst, A. F.: Ulcerative colitis. Guy's Hosp. Rep., 71:26, 1921.
24. Macie, T. T.: Ulcerative colitis due to chronic infection with Flexner-bacillus. J. Am. Med. Assoc., 98:1706, 1932.
25. Felsen, J., and Wolarsky, W.: Acute and chronic bacillary dysentery and chronic ulcerative colitis. J. Am. Med. Assoc., 153:1069, 1953.
26. Formal, S. B., LaBrec, E. H., and Schneider, H.: Pathogenesis of bacillary dysentery in laboratory animals. Fed. Proc., 23:29, 1965.
27. Keusch, G. T., et al.: Pathogenesis of Shigella diarrhea. I. Enterotoxin production by Shigella dysenteriae 1. J. Clin. Invest., 51:1212, 1972.
28. Keusch, G. T., and Jacewicz, M.: The pathogenesis of Shigella diarrhea. VI. Toxin and antitoxin in Shigella flexneri and Shigella sonnei infections in humans. J. Infect. Dis., 135:552, 1977.
29. Gemski, P. Jr., et al.: Shigellosis due to Shigella dysenteriae I: Relative importance of mucosal invasion versus toxin production in pathogenesis. J. Infect. Dis., 126:523, 1972.
30. Keusch, G. T., et al.: Pathogenesis of Shigella diarrhea. Serum anticytotoxin antibody response produced by toxigenic and nontoxigenic Shigella dysenteriae I. J. Clin. Invest., 57:194, 1971.
31. Dupont, H. L., Formal, S. B., and Hornick, R. B.: Pathogenesis of Escherichia coli diarrhea. N. Engl. J. Med., 285:1, 1971.
32. Fradkin, W. Z.: Ulcerative colitis. Bacteriological aspects. NY J. Med., 37:249, 1937.
33. Gorbach, S. L., et al.: Studies of intestinal microflora. II. Microorganisms of the small intestine and their relations to oral and fecal flora. Gastroenterology, 53:856, 1967.
34. Bentley, D. W., et al.: The microflora of the human ileum and intra-abdominal colon: Results of direct needle aspiration at surgery and evaluation of the technique. J. Lab. Clin. Med., 79:421, 1972.
35. Krone, C. L., Theodore, F., and Sleisenger, M. H.: Studies on the pathogenesis of malabsorption, lipid hydrolysis and micelle formation in the intestinal lumen. Medicine, 47:89, 1968.
36. Gorbach, S. L., and Tabaqchali, S.: Bacteria, bile and the small bowel. Gut, 10:963, 1969.
37. Donaldson, R. M., McConnell, C., and Deffner, N.: Bacteriological studies in clinical and experimental blind loop syndromes. Gastroenterology, 52:1082, 1967.
38. Vince, A., et al.: Bacteriological studies in Crohn's disease. J. Med. Microbiol., 5:219, 1972.
39. Danielsson, D., Kjellander, J., and Jarnerot, G.: The effect of metronidazole and sulfasalazine on the fecal flora in patients with Crohn's disease. Scand. J. Gastroenterol., 16:2:183, 1981.
40. Hudson, M. J., et al.: The microbial flora of the rectal mucosa and faeces of patients with Crohn's disease before and during antimicrobial chemotherapy. J. Med. Microbiol., 18:335, 1984.
41. Cooke, E. M.: A quantitative comparison of the fecal flora of patients with ulcerative colitis and that of normal persons. J. Pathol. Bacteriol., 91:439, 1967.
42. Van der Wiel-Korstangie, J. A., and Winkler, K. C.: The fecal flora in ulcerative colitis. J. Med. Microbiol., 8: 491, 1975.
43. Van der Merwe, M., and Mol, G. J. J.: A possible role of Eubacterium and Peptostreptococcus species in the etiology of Crohn's disease. Antonie Van Leeuwenhock, 46:597, 1980.
44. Ambrose, N. S., Johnson, M., Burdon, D. W., and Keighly, M. R. B.: Incidence of pathogenic bacteria from mesenteric lymph nodes and ileal serosa during Crohn's disease. Br. J. Surg., 71:623, 1984.
45. Rutgeerts, P., Ghoos, Y., Vantrappen, G., and Eyssen, H.: Ileal dysfunction and bacterial overgrowth in patients with Crohn's disease. Eur. J. Clin. Invest., 11:199, 1981.
46. Brown, W. E., and Lee, E.: Radioimmunological measurements of naturally occurring bacterial antibodies. 1. Human serum antibodies reactive with Escherichia coli in gastrointestinal and immunologic disorders. J. Lab. Clin. Med., 82:125, 1973.
47. Tabaqchali, S., O'Donoghue, D. P., and Bettelheim, K. A.: Escherichia coli antibodies in patients with inflammatory bowel disease. Gut, 19:108, 1978.

48. Persson, S., and Danielsson, D.: On the occurrence of serum antibodies to Bacteroides fragilis and serogroups of E. coli in patients with Crohn's disease. Scan. J. Infect. Dis. (Suppl.), *19*:61, 1979.
49. Brown, W. R., and Lee, E.: Radioimmunological measurements of bacterial antibodies. Human serum antibodies reactive with Bacteroides fragilis and enterococcus in gastrointestinal and immunological disorders. Gastroenterology, *66*:1145, 1974.
50. Mathews, N., et al.: Agglutinins to bacteria in Crohn's disease. Gut, *21*:376, 1980.
51. Auer, I. O., et al.: Selected bacterial antibodies in Crohn's disease and ulcerative colitis. Scand. J. Gastroenterol., *18*:217, 1983.
52. Weinsinck, F., van de Merwe, J. P., and Mayberry, J. F.: An international study of agglutinins to Eubacterium, Pepostreptococcus and Coprococcus species in Crohn's disease, ulcerative colitis and control subjects. Digestion, *27*:63, 1983.
53. Gump, D., et al.: Lymphocytotoxic and microbial antibodies in Crohn's disease and matched controls. Antonie Van Leeuwenhock, *46*:597, 1981.
54. Onderdonk, A. B., Steeves, R. M., Cisneros, R. L., and Bronson, R. T.: Adoptive transfer of immune enhancement of experimental ulcerative colitis. Infect. Immun., *46*:64, 1984.
55. Kirsner, J. B., and Shorter, R. G.: Recent developments in "nonspecific" inflammatory disease. N. Engl. J. Med., *306*:775, 837, 1982.
56. Blaser, M. J., Miller, F. A., Lacher, J., and Singleton, J. W.: Patients with active Crohn's disease have elevated serum antibodies to antigens of seven enteric bacterial pathogens. Gastroenterology, *87*:888, 1984.
57. Grange, J. M., Gibson, J., Nassau, E., and Kardjito, T.: Enzyme-linked immunosorbent assay (ELISA): a study of antibodies to Mycobacterium tuberculosis in the IgG, IgA and IgM classes in tuberculosis, sarcoidosis, and Crohn's disease. Tubercle, *61*:145, 1980.
58. Swabrick, F. P., et al.: Chlamydia, cytomegalovirus and Yersinia in inflammatory bowel disease. Lancet, *2*:11, 1979.
59. Taylor-Robinson, D., O'Morain, C. A., and Thomas, B. J.: Low frequency of chlamydial antibodies in patients with Crohn's disease and ulcerative colitis. Lancet, *2*:1162, 1979.
60. Munro, J., et al.: Chlamydia and Crohn's disease. Lancet, *2*:45, 1979.
61. Mardh, P. A., Ursing, B., and Sandrgen, E.: Lack of evidence for an association between infection by microimmunofluorescence antibody test. Acta Pathol. Microbiol. Scand., (B) *88*:57, 1980.
62. Onderdonk, A. B., Franklin, M. L., and Cisneros, R. L.: Production of experimental ulcerative colitis in gnotobiotic guinea pigs with simplified microflora. Infect. Immun., *32*:225, 1981.
63. Onderdonk, A. B., and Bartlett, J. G.: Bacteriological studies of experimental colitis. Am. J. Clin. Nutr., *32*:258, 1979.
64. Bartlett, J. G., et al.: Antibiotic-associated pseudomembranous colitis due to toxin producing clostridia. N. Engl. J. Med., *298*:531, 1978.
65. Bartlett, J. G., and Chang, T. W.: Colitis induced by clostridium difficile. The Rev. Infect. Dis., *1*:370, 1979
66. Trinka, F., et al.: Oral vancomycin for antibiotic association pseudomembranous colitis. Lancet, *1*:97, 1978.
67. Meyers, S., et al.: Occurrence of clostridium difficile toxin during the course of inflammatory bowel disease. Gastroenterology, *80*:697, 1981.
68. Wright, J. M., Adams, S. P., Gribble, M. J., and Bowie, W. R.: Clostridium difficile in Crohn's disease. Can. J. Surg., *27*:435, 1984.
69. Dorman, S. A., Liggorioa, E., Winn, W. C. Jr., and Beeken, W. L.: Isolation of Clostridium difficile from patients with inactive Crohn's disease. Gastroenterology, *82*:1348, 1982.
70. Rolny, P., Jarnerot, G., and Mollby, R.: Occurrence of Clostridium toxin in inflammatory bowel disease. Scand. J. Gastroenterol., *18*:61, 1983.
71. Greenfield, C., et al.: Clostridium difficile and inflammatory bowel disease. Gut, *24*:713, 1983.
72. Falsen, E., et al.: Clostridium difficile in relation to enteric bacterial pathogens. J. Clin. Microbiol., *12*:297, 1980.
73. Gilligan, P. H., McCarthy, L. R., and Genta, V. W.: Relative frequency of Clostridium difficile in patients with diarrheal disease. J. Clin. Microbiol., *14*:26, 1981.
74. Chang, T. W., Laureman, M., and Bartlett, J. G.: Cytotoxicity assay in antibiotic-associated colitis. J. Infect. Dis., *140*:756, 1979.
75. Bartlett, J. G.: Clostridium difficile and inflammatory bowel disease (editorial). Gastroenterology, *80*:863, 1981.
76. Parent, K., and Mitchell, P.: Bacterial variants: etiologic agent in Crohn's disease? Gastroenterology, *71*:365, 1976.
77. Parent, K., and Mitchell, P.: Cell wall defective variants of Pseudomonas-like (Group Va) bacteria in Crohn's disease. Gastroenterology, *75*:368, 1978.
78. Parent, K., Mitchell, P., and Baltaos, E.: Pilot animal pathogenicity studies with cell wall defective Pseudomonas-like bacteria isolated from Crohn's disease patients. Gastroenterology *78*:1233, 1980.
79. Belsheim, M. R., Darwich, R. Z., Watson, W. C., and Schieven, B.: Bacterial L-form isolation from inflammatory bowel disease patients. Gastroenterology, *85*:364, 1983.
80. Graham, D. Y., Yoshimura, H. H., and Estes, M. K.: DNA hybridization studies of the association of Pseudomonas maltophilia with inflammatory bowel disease. J. Lab. Clin. Med., *101*:940, 1983.
81. Whorwell, P. J., Davidson, I. W., Beeken, W. L., and Wright, R.: Search by immunofluorescence for antigens of Rotavirus, Pseudomonas maltophilia, and Mycobacterium kansasii in Crohn's disease. Lancet, *2*:697, 1978.
82. Shafii, A., Sohper, S., Lev, M., and Das, K. M.: An antibody against revertant forms of cell-wall deficient bacterial variant in sera from patients with Crohn's disease. Lancet, *2*:332, 1981.
83. Mitchell, D. N., and Rees, R. J. W.: Agent transmissible from Crohn's disease tissue. Lancet, *2*:168, 1970.
84. Taub, R. N., et al.: Transmission of ileitis and sarcoid granulomas to mice. Trans. Assoc. Am. Physicians, *87*:219, 1974.
85. Cave, D. R., Mitchell, D. N., and Brooke, B. N.: Evidence of an agent transmissible from ulcerative colitis tissue. Lancet, *1*:1311, 1976.
86. Cave, D. R., et al.: Further animal evidence of a transmissible agent in Crohn's disease. Lancet, *2*:1120, 1973.
87. Cave, D. R., Mitchell, D. N., and Brooke, B. N.: Experimental animal studies of the etiology and pathogenesis of Crohn's disease. Gastroenterology, *69*:618, 1975.
88. Bolton, P. M., et al.: Negative findings in laboratory animals for a transmissible agent in Crohn's disease. Lancet, *2*:1122, 1973.
89. Heatley, R. V., et al.: A search for a transmissible agent in Crohn's disease. Gut, *16*:523, 1975.
90. Slaney, G.: Hypersensitivity granulomata and the alimentary tract. Ann. R. Coll. Surg. Engl., *31*:249, 1962.

91. Kane, S. P.: Experimental pathology of Crohn's disease. Clin. Gastroenterol., *1*:295, 1972.
92. Burnham, W. R., et al.: Mycobacteria as a possible cause of inflammatory bowel disease. Lancet, *2*:693, 1978.
93. Stanford, J. L.: Acid fast organisms in Crohn's disease and ulcerative colitis. *In* Recent Advances in Crohn's Disease. Edited by A. S. Peña, I. T. Weterman, C. C. Booth, and W. Strober. The Hague, Martinus Nijhoff Publishers, 1981.
94. White, S. A.: Investigation into the density of acid fast organisms located from Crohn's disease. *In* Recent Advances in Crohn's Disease. Edited by A. S. Peña, I. T. Weterman, C. C. Booth, and W. Strober. The Hague, Martinus Nijhoff Publishers, 1981.
95. Whits, S., Nassau, E., Gurnham, W., Stanford, J., and Lennard-Jones, E.: Further evidence for a mycobacterial aetiology of Crohn's disease. Gut, *19*:A443, 1978.
96. Chiodini, R. J., Van Kruiningen, H. J., Thayer, W. R., Merkal, R., and Coutu, J. A.: Possible role of mycobacteria in inflammatory bowel disease. I. An unclassified mycobacterium species isolated from patients with Crohn's disease. Dig. Dis. Sci., *29*:1073, 1984.
97. Van Kruiningen, H. J., et al.: Experimental disease in goats induced by mycobacterium from a patient with Crohn's disease. Gastroenterology, *88*:1623, 1985.
98. Thayer, W. R., et al.: Possible role of mycobacteria in inflammatory bowel disease. II. Mycobacteria antibodies in Crohn's disease. Dig. Dis. Sci., *29*:1080, 1984.
99. Sang-nae Cho, et al.: Mycobacterial aetiology of Crohn's disease: Serologic study using common mycobacterial antigens and a species-specific glycolipid antigen from Mycobacterium paratuberculosis. Gut, *27*:1353, 1986.
100. Graham, D. Y., Markesich, D. C., and Yoshimura, H. H.: Mycobacteria and inflammatory bowel disease. Results of culture. Gastroenterology, *92*:435, 1987.

4 · Intestinal Defenses

ERNEST SEIDMAN, M.D., F.R.C.P. (C) AND W. ALLAN WALKER, M.D.

The digestion and absorption of ingested nutrients have traditionally been considered the primary functions of the gastrointestinal tract. Recently, increased attention has been devoted to the immune functions of the gut and its physiologic role as an immune barrier.[1] The intestinal tract is perhaps second only to the lungs in terms of area of contact between the external environment and the internal milieu. Therefore, the intestinal tract represents a potential site for the uptake of harmful luminal antigens, toxins, enzymes, and pathogens.[2] In spite of this barrier function, there is increasing experimental and clinical evidence to suggest that antigenically intact macromolecules can escape complete digestion and penetrate the intestinal epithelial surface in quantities of immunologic importance.[3-5]

This chapter will focus on enteric antigen uptake and barrier mechanisms of the gastrointestinal tract to underscore the potential importance of this phenomenon in the pathogenesis of a number of immunologically mediated disorders, including idiopathic inflammatory bowel disease.[6]

Macromolecular Transport Mechanisms

Macromolecular uptake is believed to occur by one of four transport mechanisms across the intact epithelial cell membrane barrier:

1. Receptor-mediated endocytosis
2. Nonselective endocytosis
3. Direct penetration of cell membranes
4. Passage through intercellular junctions

Receptor-mediated Endocytosis

Receptor-mediated endocytosis refers to the process initiated by the extracellular macromolecule (ligand) binding to a specific receptor on the enterocyte plasma membrane (Fig. 4-1A). This binding stimulates the clustering of additional receptors in a coated pit area of the cell. Invagination and internalization of the coated pit follows, forming a coated vesicle. This uptake process is energy-dependent, because invagination is blocked by metabolic inhibitors of both glycolysis and oxidative phosphorylation. After invagination, macromolecules migrate within the membrane-bound vesicle (phagosome) to the supranuclear region of the cell. The vesicles then coalesce with lysosomes to form phagolysosomes, within which intracellular degradation normally occurs. The persistent attachment of the ligand to the surface receptor, or, in the case of IgA, to the secretory component, may prevent its intracellular degradation. The contents of the coated vesicle may then be discharged into the intercellular space by exocytosis.

Nonselective Endocytosis

A second mechanism of macromolecular transport occurs when extracellular proteins are nonselectively trapped and internalized through invaginations of noncoated regions of the cell (Fig. 4-1B). This type of uptake may be an important function of the specialized M cells that overlie Peyer's patch areas of the small bowel (Fig. 4-2). Electron microscopy has revealed that these cells have a paucity of microvilli, a poorly developed glycocalyx and an absence of lyso-

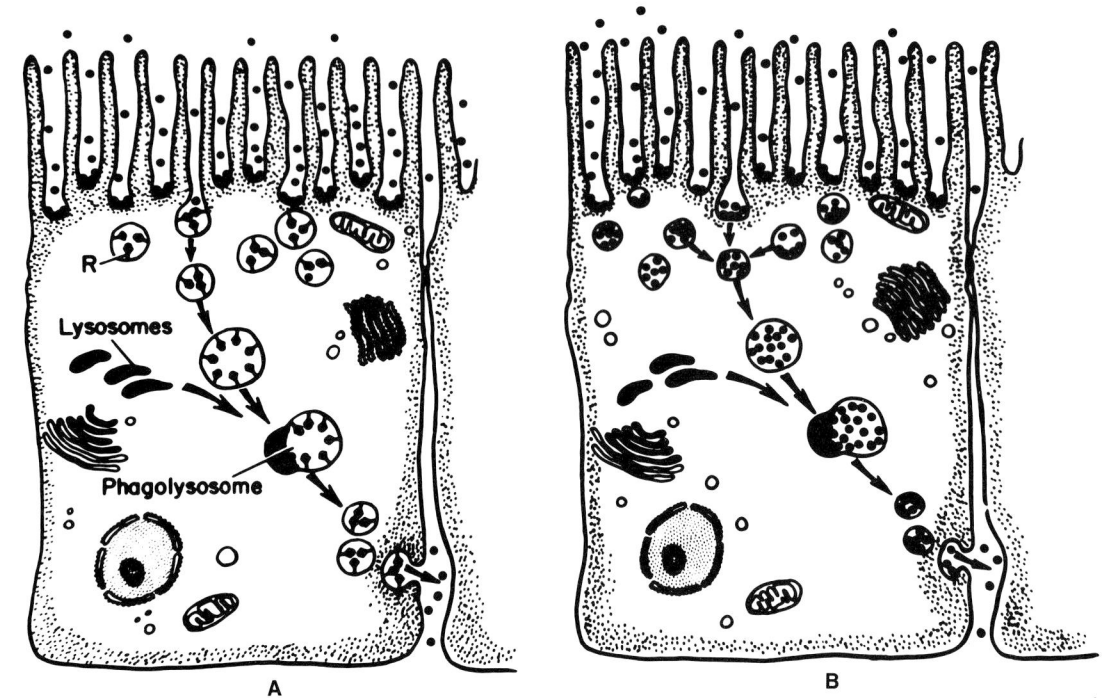

FIG. 4-1 A and B. Mechanisms of macromolecular absorption in the neonatal mammalian intestine. A. Selective transport of antigens occurs in the small intestine of the newborn via a specific receptor site (R), present on the microvillus membrane. Antigens thus transported may be protected from intracellular lysomal digestion because of attachment to the receptor site, and are transported in increased quantities out of the cell. B. A nonselective uptake and transport of other macromolecules occurs throughout the small intestine of most neonatal animals. Immature intestinal absorptive cells engulf large quantities of macromolecules. After intracellular digestion in phagolysosomes, small quantities are deposited in the intercellular space. (Reprinted with permission, from Walker, W. A., and Isselbacher, K. J.: Gastroenterology, 67:531, 1974.)

somal organelles.[7] This absorptive route represents an important mechanism by which luminal antigens reach the gut-associated lymphoid tissue, thereby affecting the local and systemic immune systems, as discussed in detail below.

Direct Penetration of Cell Membranes

A third potential portal of entry is by direct penetration through the cell membrane. This mechanism has been demonstrated to be an important entry route for certain bacterial and plant toxins, as well as for viruses. The direct penetration by macromolecular hormones and proteins has not been established.[8]

Passage Through Intercellular Junctions

Finally, the entry of macromolecules through the intercellular junctions may be an important mechanism, although conclusive data regarding this are lacking.

Factors Affecting Macromolecular Transport

Determinants controlling macromolecular uptake across the human intestinal epithelium may be divided into two major categories: immunologic and nonimmunologic factors (Table 4-1). Studies in many species, including man, have conclusively demonstrated that the immature gut is significantly more permeable to macromolecules prior to physiologic "closure."[9] This increased permeability of the gastrointestinal tract in the immature host (premature and newborn child) is a result of relative deficiencies in several of the factors discussed below.

Nonimmunologic factors

Gastric acid secretion and gastrointestinal proteolysis are important luminal defense mechanisms.[10] These functions are both significantly decreased in the neonatal period, potentially permitting higher intraluminal concentrations of bacteria and antigenically intact macromole-

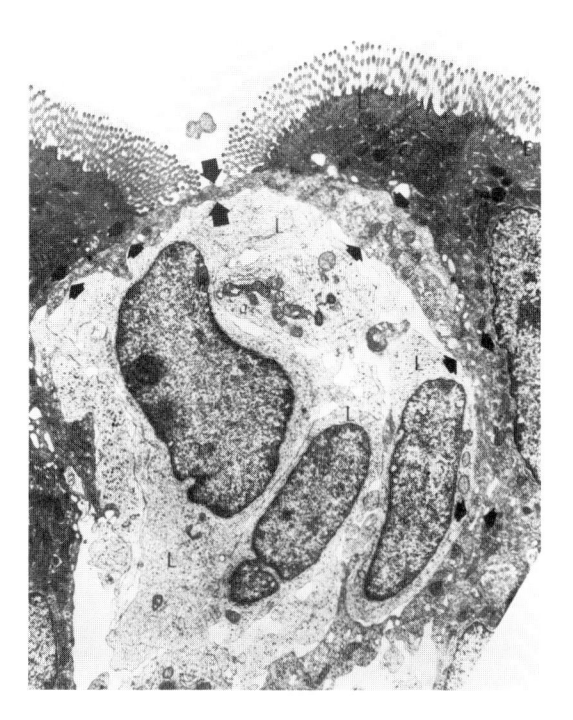

FIG. 4-2. Transmission electron micrograph from the noncolumnar region of the Peyer's patch epithelium, showing a cross-sectional view of the apex of an M cell, associated microvillus-covered epithelial cells, and at least three lymphoid cells (L). Note the attenuated cytoplasm of the M cells (between arrows) that bridges the surface between microvillus-covered cells, forming tight junctions with them and producing a barrier between the lympoid cells and the intestinal lumen. (Reprinted with permission, from Owen, R. L.: Gastroenterology, 72:440, 1977.)

cules. Furthermore, because bile acids offer some protection against microbes, the decreased bile acid secretion as well as the immaturity of the enterohepatic circulation in the newborn may adversely affect mucosal barrier function early in life.

Breast milk is known to contain various immunologic properties that may passively protect the neonatal gut.[11] In addition, natural feeding accelerates intestinal mucosal maturation, probably mediated by hormones (epidermal growth factor, thyroxin, and cortisol) present in breast milk.[12] In view of these factors, it comes as no surprise that breast feeding is associated with significantly lower antigen uptake in newborns.[9]

The normal gut flora is considered to be important in protecting the host against microbial pathogens.[10] The neonatal gut becomes colonized by the third day of life, but the nature of the flora depends on the type of feeding (breast vs. formula). Animal studies have revealed differences in microvillous membrane composition and mucous glycoproteins between developing and mature animals.[13,14] These factors are important in the increased susceptibility to enteric pathogens, the enhanced macromolecular transport, and potentially selective sensitization to particular microbial (enterobacterial) antigens seen in the immature, artificially fed host.

Immunologic Factors

Crabbe and Heremans demonstrated that plasma cells present in the intestinal lamina propria were primarily IgA-producing rather than IgG-producing cells, as seen in other peripheral lymphoid tissues.[15] Local secretory antibodies can inhibit the uptake of soluble protein antigens.[16,17] Therefore, the physiologic, transient deficiency of intestinal secretory antibodies during the newborn period may also play a role in the excessive intestinal permeability of the newborn,[18-20] as well as the increased incidence of food intolerance and atopy.[21]

Nature provides many factors in breast milk that may compensate for those lacking in the functionally immature gastrointestinal tract of the neonate. The enteromammary immune system (Fig. 4-3) is an important pathway by which immunocytes migrate from the gut to other mucosal surfaces, such as the mammary glands in

TABLE 4-1. *Factors controlling macromolecular uptake.*

I. Luminal
Gastric Acidity
Intestinal proteolysis
Bile Acids
Intestinal Flora
Peristalsis
Enteral Nutrition
Breast milk
Formula milk
II. Mucosal
Secretory IgA
Humoral Immunity
Cell-mediated Immunity
Epithelial Cell Membrane
Mucous Glycoproteins
III. Passive Defense
Transplacental IgG
Breast Milk Factors
Immune
Hormonal
IV. Hepatic
Reticuloendothelial Cells
Immune Complex (IgA) Clearance
Immune Modulation

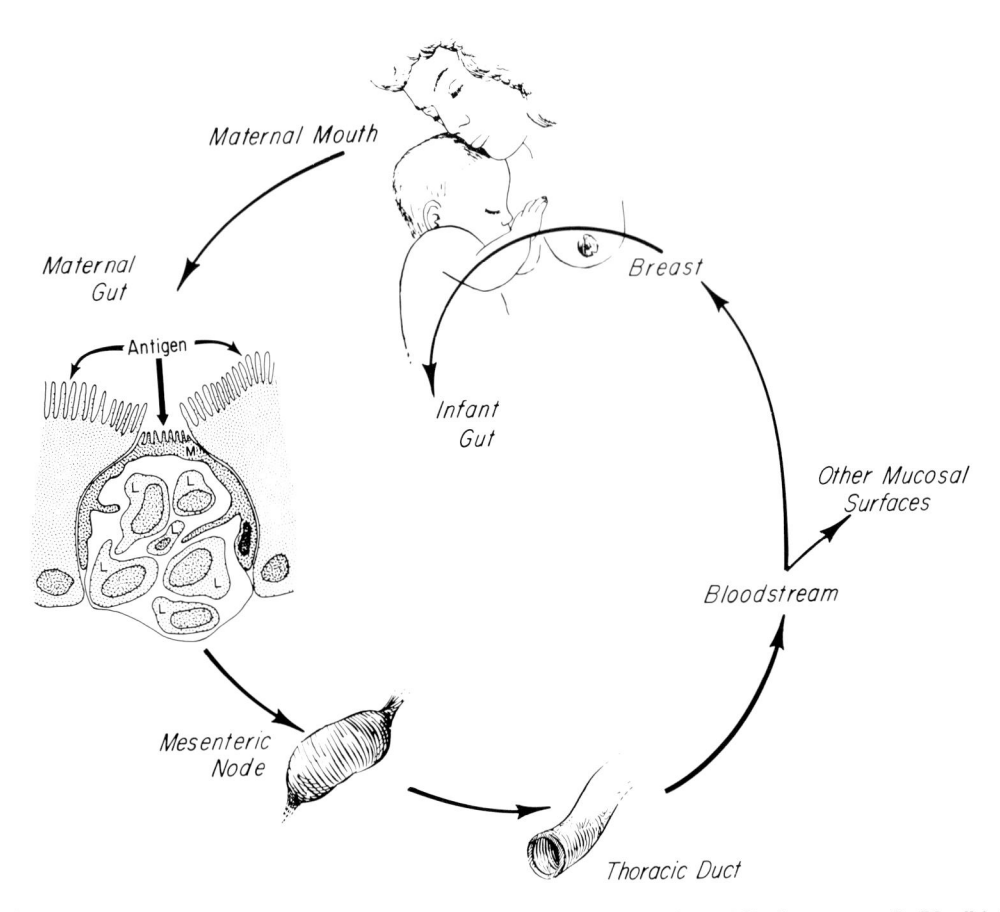

FIG. 4-3. Dietary antigen entering the maternal gut reaches lymphoid follicles through specialized transport cells (M cells). This antigen commits the lymphoblasts to specific IgA production, which then migrate via mesenteric nodes and the thoracic duct into the systemic circulation. During the periods of hormonal stimulation, such cells populate the breast and secrete sIgA, which then is ingested by and functions in the infant. T-cells, B-cells, and macrophages are also extruded into the breast milk and are immunologically active. (Reprinted with permission, from Kleinman, R. E., and Walker, W. A.: Dig. Dis. Sci., 24:876, 1979.)

lactating animals.[22] In this way, plasma cells in breast tissue release IgA antibodies directed against microbial and dietary antigens present in the maternal intestine of the neonate.[23] In the newborn animal, there are specific sites in the proximal small intestine where maternal sIgA binds to the glycocalyx of epithelial cells, serving much the same function as locally produced sIgA does in the mature animal.[24]

Food and other antigens from the maternal intestine can also reach the suckling newborn through breast milk. These antigens have occasionally been shown to produce an allergic colitis in newborns.[25] We have recently shown that maternal antibody can efficiently block the transfer of antigen into breast milk,[26] much as transplacentally-derived IgG diminishes intestinal macromolecular uptake.[27] The human neonate is primarily protected by the transfer of maternal IgG transplacentally. Although the postnatal acquisition of maternal immunoglobulins via receptor-mediated uptake from breast milk has been thought of as a murine system, evidence has been presented suggesting that maternal IgA may be absorbed by human neonates.[28,29]

Finally, T-lymphocytes present in colostrum appear to be preferentially activated by enteric-associated antigens rather than by systemic stimulation.[11,30] These cells also encounter favorable conditions for their survival in the neonatal intestine, where gastric acidity is buffered following the ingestion of colostrum.

Hepatic factors

The liver, which receives the major component of the mesenteric venous filtrate from the gastrointestinal tract, has an enormous capacity to phagocytose noxious substances present in the portal circulation. The liver is thus considered a

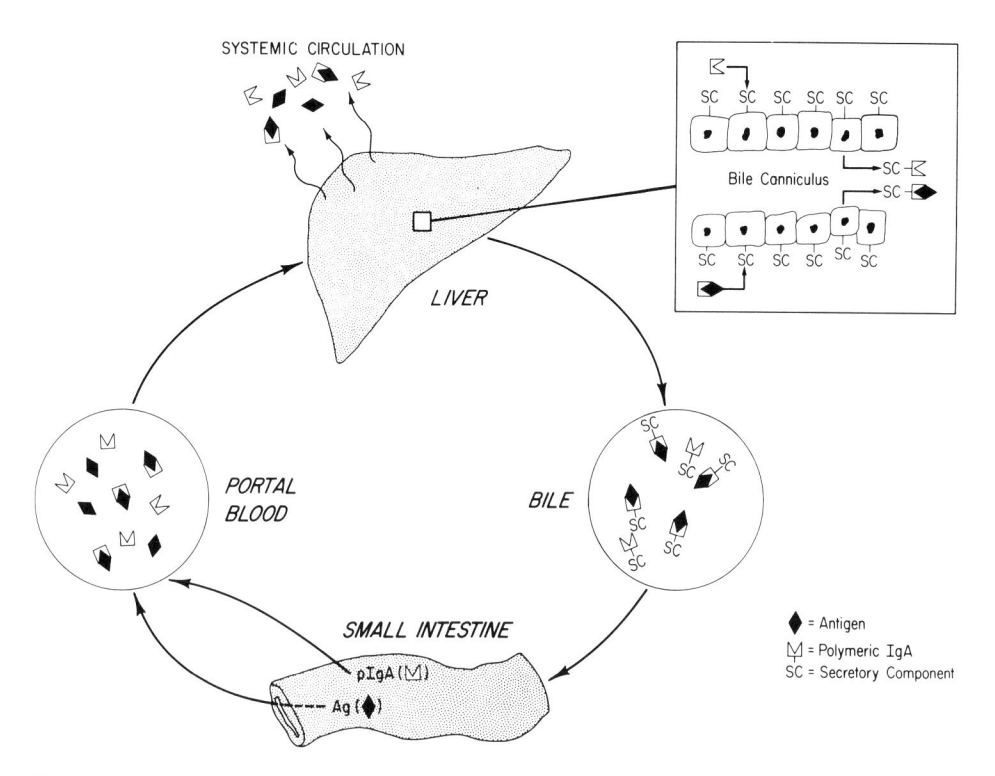

FIG. 4-4. Hepatobiliary transport of IgA and SC-IgA-antigen complexes. Enteric antigen that escapes digestion may complex with IgA in the lamina propria or in the portal circulation, be transported into biliary secretions, and return to the intestinal lumen. With compromise of hepatic circulation or obstruction of the extrahepatic bile ducts, IgA, antigen, or complexes of pIgA and antigen may return to the systemic circulation. (Reprinted with permission, from Kleinmen R. E., et al.: Hepatology, 2:379, 1982.)

second line of defense against biologically active substances absorbed from the external environment of the gut. Hepatic Kupffer's cells act as a filter, phagocytosing noxious substances and preventing their access to the systemic circulation. Aside from reducing enteric antigen access to the systemic circulation, the immune responses generated by antigen presentation into portal versus systemic circulation have been shown to differ.[31] These differing immune responses may reflect the capacity of macrophages to sequester antigens and modify the immunologic response.

It is now established that the liver can selectively transport dimeric IgA into bile, and subsequently into the intestinal lumen.[32] Human hepatobiliary transport of IgA is less efficient than in murine species, and therefore does not contribute as much IgA to the total intestinal pool of secretory IgA.[33] An important function of the serum-to-bile transport system of IgA (Fig. 4-4) may be to eliminate absorbed enteric antigens by returning them to the intestine as IgA-antigen complexes.[34-36]

These findings support the concept of the liver as an important second line of defense against the egress of enteric antigens into the systemic circulation. When the reticuloendothelial system malfunctions, as in destructive liver diseases, this filter system is defective and absorbed endotoxins and antigens may cause symptoms of clinical disease.[37]

In summary, the mature gut retains the capacity to absorb macromolecules from the intestinal lumen. The control of macromolecular uptake depends on a number of factors within the gut lumen and on its mucosal surface (see Table 4-1). Immediately postpartum, the human neonate must cope with bacterial products, pathogens, proteolytic enzymes, and food antigens.

The immature mucosal barrier of the newborn is deficient in a number of factors that normally regulate macromolecular uptake. The increased permeability of the immature, malnourished, or damaged gut is potentially capable of causing local intestinal or systemic disease states (Fig. 4-5). The second part of this chapter focuses on pathophysiologic uptake (Fig. 4-6), with particular reference to inflammatory bowel disease (IBD).

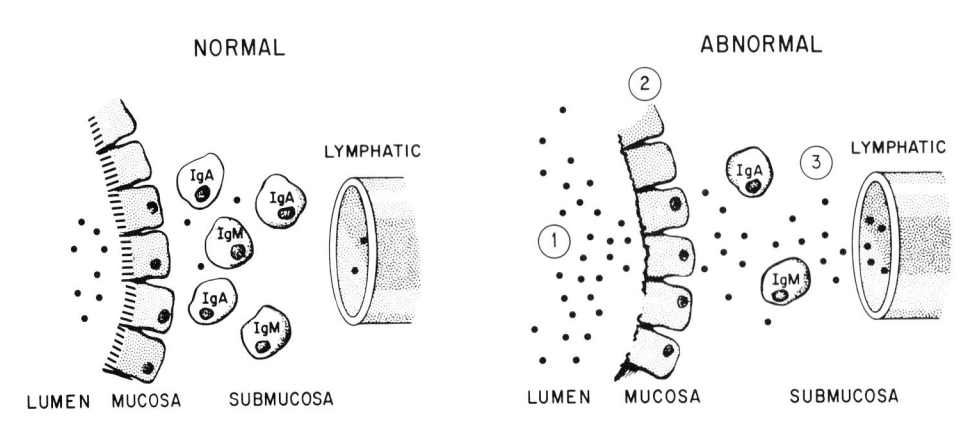

FIG. 4-5. Physiologic and pathologic uptake of antigens across the intestinal mucosal barrier into the systemic circulation. *Left.* Under normal conditions, factors within the intestinal lumen, on the surface of the epithelial cells, and within the lamina propria combine to limit the access of antigens to the systemic circulation. *Right.* When the barrier defenses are disrupted, excessive quantities of antigenic material may enter the circulation and contribute to clinical diseases. Factors contributing to pathologic absorption of antigens include decreased intraluminal digestion, disrupted mucosal barrier, and decrease in IgA-producing plasma cells in the lamina propria. (Reprinted with permission, from Walker, W. A.: Ped. Clin. North Am., 22:731, 1975.)

Clinical Conditions Associated with Pathologic Antigen Transport

Excessive transport of antigens across the intestine may predispose to immunologic or toxic reactions, leading to a number of gastrointestinal and systemic diseases (Fig. 4-6). Necrotizing enterocolitis (NEC) is an acute fulminating disease of neonates associated with focal or diffuse ulceration of the distal small intestine and colon.[38] The most common acquired gastrointestinal emergency in the newborn, NEC, appears to be the pathologic response of the immature intestine ensuing from multiple injurious factors. Epidemiologic data have invoked immaturity of the gastrointestinal immune barrier, perinatal gastrointestinal ischemia, microbial organisms or their toxins, and enteral alimentation in the development of NEC.

One of the most striking associations between gastrointestinal antigen handling and clinical disease is exemplified by gastrointestinal allergy. Several clinical patterns of food allergy and intolerance have been described that relate specifically to the ingestion of certain foods.[39] These conditions may be localized to

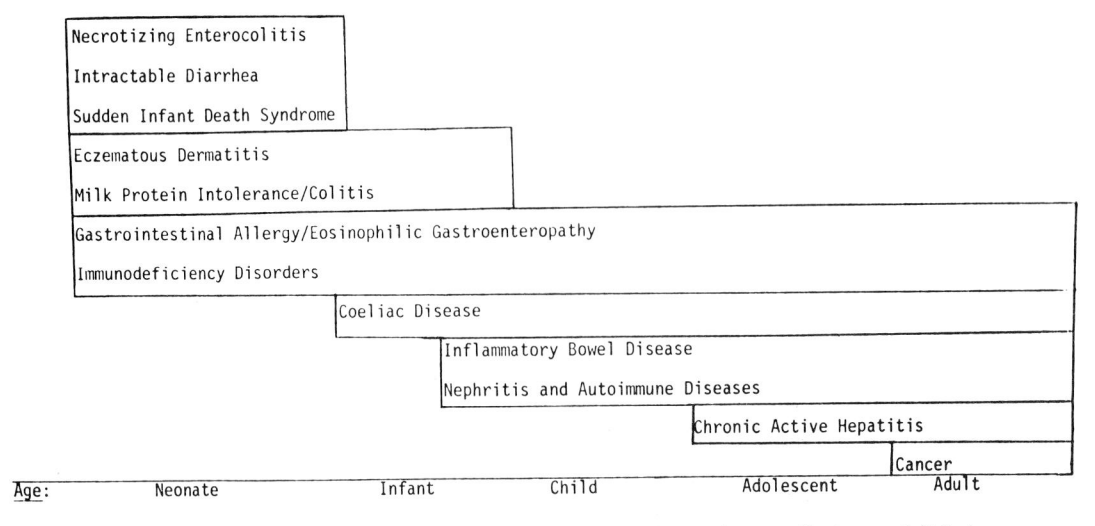

FIG. 4-6. Clinical disorders possibly associated with pathologic macromolecular uptake according to age of clinical occurrence. (Reprinted with permission, from Seidman, E. G., and Walker, W. A.: Gastrointestinal and hepatic disorders. *In* Immunologic Disorders in Infants and Children. Edited by E. R. Stiehm. Philadelphia, W. B. Saunders Co., 1986.)

the gut and present with diarrhea, gastrointestinal bleeding, or protein-losing enteropathy. They may, alternatively, be represented by systemic manifestations of allergy ranging from exanthema to anaphylaxis. Although the mechanisms underlying gastrointestinal food intolerance are not clear, it would appear that intestinal uptake of antigens is a necessary initial step in the pathogenesis. During the neonatal period, when increased antigen permeability exists, susceptible infants may become sensitized to specific ingested protein antigens.[40] Enteric antigen presentation may induce a mucosal immune response, or result in a state of systemic tolerance to that antigen.[22,41] Tolerance is readily induced in neonatal animals when an antigen is given via routes other than the gut.[42] However, feeding of a protein antigen (ovalbumin) to neonatal mice results in priming of both humoral and cell-mediated immune responses.[43,44] These factors, although incompletely understood, help explain the increased incidence of food allergy in childhood, as well as the fact that food allergy is the leading cause of colitis in infancy.[45]

Immunodeficiency states, whether congenital or acquired, are naturally-occuring models for the study of the pathologic basis for transport of macromolecules across the intestinal tract. Gastrointestinal symptoms constitute a major clinical component to both defects of humoral or cell-mediated immunity.[46] Although not clearly established, it is possible that pathologic transport of macromolecules may play a role in the pathogenesis of the intestinal manifestations in the immunodeficient host.

Immune Mechanisms in Idiopathic Inflammatory Bowel Disease

Role of Neonatal Sensitization to a Microbial/Mammalian Cross-Reacting Antigen

The etiology and pathogenesis of IBD remain unknown, despite several decades of intensive research.[47] Among the many hypotheses developed, there is a common theme involving the interaction of three factors: external agents, perhaps microbial; immunologic responses in the host; and genetic factors influencing such responses.[48]

In 1972, Shorter et al. developed a hypothesis for the etiology and pathogenesis of IBD centered on an intestinal cell-mediated immune reaction to a bacterial antigen, cross-reacting with antigens on colonic mucosal cells.[49] In this model, local immune sensitization of the gut-associated lymphoid tissue (GALT) to antigens absorbed occurs early in life because of immaturity of the newborn mucosal barrier (Fig. 4-7). The transport of macromolecules across the small intestinal mucosa into the systemic circulation has been shown to be significantly greater in neonatal animals than in adult animals of several species.[5,6] Macromolecular uptake across the colonic epithelium, although not of nutritional importance,[50] is an essential component of mucosal immunity.[1] Although the mature colonic epithelium is capable of absorbing macromolecules,[51] little knowledge is available concerning the effect of immaturity on colonic mucosal immune function.[52] Our recent observations support the concept of an increased colonic permeability to macromolecules in the immature host.[53]

According to Shorter's hypothesis,[49] a secondary, nonspecific colonic injury results in renewed augmented antigen exposure to the GALT (Fig. 4-7), as suggested by studies in rabbits with immune complex-mediated colitis.[54] A local hypersensitivity, cell-mediated immune response may theoretically ensue, perpetuated by the continued absorption of the cross-reacting microbial/colonic epithelial antigen (Fig. 4-7), resulting in "auto-immune" chronic inflammation.[49] Numerous cross-reactions exist between mammalian tissues and microbial antigens.[55,56] Rheumatic fever is a notable example of an autoimmune disease involving an abnormal humoral and cellular immune response to a shared microbial-mammalian antigen.[57]

An important finding was made by Kunin et al. when they detected a shared surface antigen present on almost all enterobacteriaceae,[58] known as the enterobacterial common antigen (ECA). E. coli strains rich in content of the ECA have been found in stool of healthy newborns as well as in the stool of patients recently having nonspecific gastroenteritis.[59,60] The opportunity thus exists for potential sensitization of the GALT to the ECA, and therefore to cross-reacting colonic epithelial antigens as originally proposed by Shorter and co-workers.[49]

It is thus of great interest that sera from patients with IBD contain high titers of antibodies reactive with the ECA that react in vitro with antigens of mucous-secreting colonic epithelial cells.[61,63] The lower incidence of elevated anticolon and anti-ECA antibodies in infectious dysenteries, as well as in nonhuman primates with chronic colitis,[64,65] suggest that this may not represent an epiphenomenon in IBD.

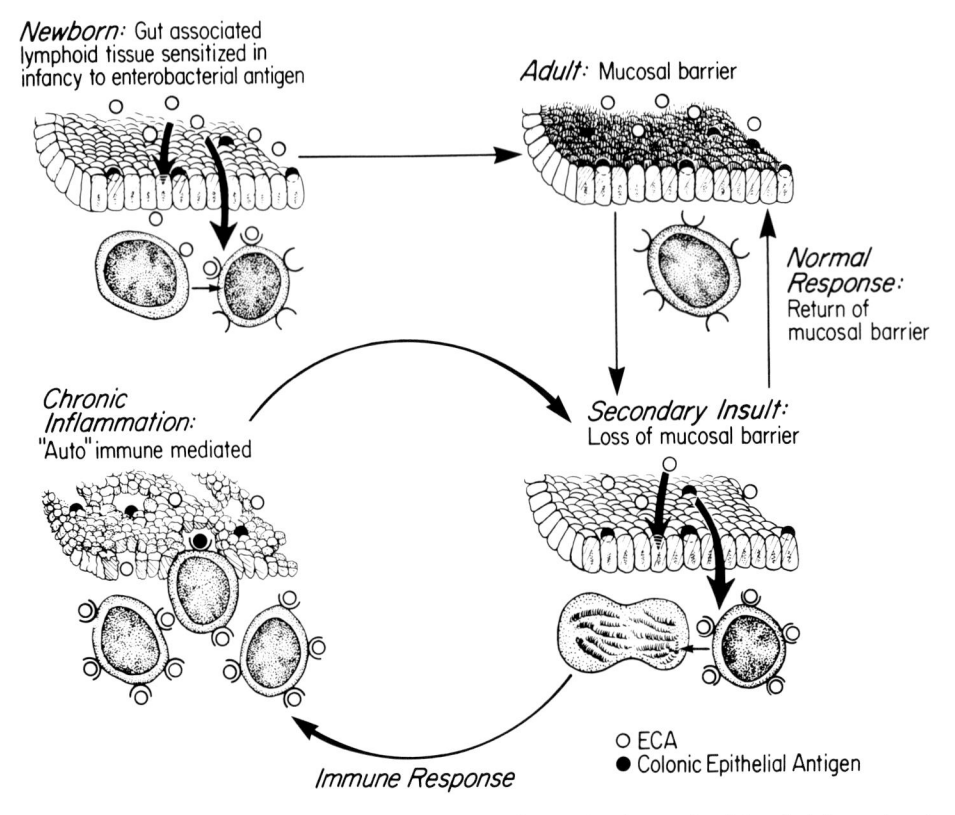

FIG. 4-7. Diagrammatic representation of an hypothesis for the etiology and pathogenesis of chronic inflammatory bowel disease, based on neonatal sensitization of gut-associated lymphoid tissue to a unique cross-reacting microbial (ECA)/mammalian (colonic epithelial) antigen. (Adapted from Shorter, R. G., Huizenga, K. A., and Spencer, R. J. Am. J. Dig. Dis., *17*:1024, 1972.)

From the standpoint of cellular immunity, peripheral and intestinal lymphocytes of ulcerative colitis patients manifest augmented cell-mediated immune responses to ECA and germ free colon antigens in vitro.[66-68] Furthermore, sera from IBD patients can induce normal lymphocytes to become cytotoxic for human colonic epithelial cells, and ECA can induce cytotoxicity against colon targets.[69,71] Subsequently, Stobo et al. concluded that the effector cells required for lysis of colonic target cells in vitro did not separate with the bulk of T-lymphocytes or B-lymphocytes, and that they possessed surface receptors for the Fc portion of IgG.[72] This implies that antibody-dependent cell-mediated cytotoxicity may be responsible for the effector arm of this response. Further support for this concept was provided by Shorter's report that macrophage-depleted isolates of mononuclear cells from colonic mucosa of IBD patients are cytotoxic in vitro for autologous colonic epithelial cells, and that the effectors possess receptors for the Fc portion of IgG.

In summary, this working hypothesis proposes that microbial antigens (ECA) cross-reacting with host colonic antigens may be responsible for the autoimmune features of IBD.[49] This hypothesis is based on the concept that initial enteric exposure of GALT to this agent occurs early in life, before the intestinal mucosal immune defenses mature. It is thus somewhat fitting that absence of, or early weaning from, breast feeding, which would generally delay "gut closure," is found in a higher proportion of patients with IBD.[74,75]

These studies suggest that ECA from intestinal flora might trigger an immunologic reaction, possibly an antibody-dependent cell-mediated cytotoxicity (ADCC), resulting in chronic intestinal (colonic) inflammation. It is critical to note, however, that studies to date have investigated these immune responses in IBD patients *after* the onset of the disease. Further studies are required to improve our understanding of the relationship between the increased mucosal permeability in newborns, host flora, the ontogeny of mucosal immune responses, and chronic inflammatory bowel disease.

References

1. Dobbins, W. O.: Gut immunophysiology: A gastroenterologist's view with emphasis on pathophysiology. Am. J. Physiol., *242*:G1, 1982.
2. Galant, S. P.: Biological and clinical significance of the gut as a barrier to penetration of macromolecules. Clin. Pediatr., *15*:731, 1976.
3. LeFevre, M. E., and Joel, D. D.: Intestinal absorption of particulate matter. Life Sci., *21*:1403, 1977.
4. Walker W. A.: Host defense mechanisms in the gastrointestinal tract. Pediatrics, *57*:901, 1976.
5. Udall, J. N., and Walker, W. A.: The physiologic and pathologic basis for transport of macromolecules across the intestinal tract. J. Pediatr. Gastroenterol. Nutr., *1*:295, 1982.
6. Walker, W. A., and Isselbacher, K. J.: Uptake and transport of macromolecules by the intestine: Possible role in clinical disorders. Gastroenterology, *67*:531, 1974.
7. Owen, R. L., and Jones, A. L.: Epithelial cell specialization within human Peyer's patches: An ultrastructural study of intestinal lymphoid follicles. Gastroenterology, *66*:189, 1974.
8. Goldstein, J. L., Anderson, R. G. W., and Brown, M. S.: Coated pits, coated vesicles and receptor-mediated endocytosis. Nature, *279*:679, 1979.
9. Udal, J. N., and Walker, W. A.: The physiologic and pathologic basis for transport of macromolecules across the intestinal tract. J. Pediatr. Gastroenterol. Nutr., *1*:295, 1982.
10. Ecknauer, R.: The barrier function of the gastrointestinal tract. Z. Gastroenterol., *20*:150, 1982.
11. Ogra, S. S., and Ogra, P. L.: Immunologic aspects of human colostrum and milk. J. Pediatr., *92*:550, 1978.
12. Widdowson, E. M., Colombo, V. E., and Artavans, C. A.: Changes in the organs of pigs in response to feeding for the first 24 hours after birth. II. The digestive tract. Biol. Neonate, *28*:272, 1976.
13. Pang, K. Y., Bresson, J. L., and Walker, W. A.: Development of the gastrointestinal barrier. Evidence for structural differences in microvillus membranes from newborn and adult rabbits. Biochem. Biophys. Acta, *727*:201, 1983.
14. Shub, M. D., Pang, K. Y., Swann, D. A., and Walker, W. A.: Age related changes in chemical composition and physical properties of mucus glycoproteins from rat small intestine. Biochem. J., *215*:405, 1983.
15. Crabbe, P. A., and Heremans, J. F.: The distribution of immunoglobulin containing cells along the human gastrointestinal tract. Gastroenterology, *51*:305, 1966.
16. Walker, W. A., Isselbacher, K. J., and Bloch, K. J.: Intestinal uptake of macromolecules. Effect of oral immunization. Science, *177*:608, 1970.
17. Walker, W. A., Wu, M., Isselbacher, K. J., and Bloch, K. J.: Intestinal uptake of macromolecules. III. Studies on the mechanism by which immunization interferes with antigen uptake. J. Immunol., *115*:854, 1975.
18. Rothberg, R. M.: Immunoglobulin and specific antibody synthesis during the first weeks of life of premature infants. J. Pediatr., *75*:391, 1969.
19. Robertson, D. M., Paganelli, R., Dinwiddie, R., and Levinsky, R. J.: Milk antigen absorption in the preterm and term neonate. Arch. Dis. Child., *57*:369, 1982.
20. Weaver, I. T., Laker, M,F., and Nelson, R.: Intestinal permeability in the newborn. Arch. Dis. Child., *59*:236, 1984.
21. Eastham, E. J., Lichauco, T., Grady, M. I., and Walker, W. A.: Antigenicity of infant formulas: Role of immature intestine in protein permeability. J. Pediatr., *93*:561, 1978.
22. Bienenstock, J.: The local immune response. Am. J. Vet. Res., *36*:488, 1975.
23. Kleinman, R. E., and Walker, W. A.: The enteromammary immune system: an important new concept in breast milk host defense. Dig. Dis. Sci., *24*:876, 1979.
24. Nagura, H., Nakane, P., and Brown, W. R.: Breast milk IgA binds to jejunal epithelium in suckling rats. J. Immunol., *120*:1333, 1978.
25. Lake, A. M., Whitington, P. F., and Hamilton, S. R.: Dietary protein-induced colitis in breast-fed infants. J. Pediatr., *101*:906, 1982.
26. Harmatz, P. R., et al.: Influence of circulating maternal antibody on the transfer of dietary antigen to neonatal mice via milk. Immunology, *57*:43, 1986.
27. Kleinman, R. E., et al.: Passive transplacental immunization: influence on the detection of enteric antigen in the systemic circulation. Pediatr. Res., *17*:449, 1983.
28. Ogra, S. S., Weintraub, D., and Ogra, P. L.: Immunologic aspects of human colostrum and milk. III. Fate and absorption of cellular and soluble components in the gastrointestinal tract of the newborn. J. Immunol., *119*:245, 1977.
29. Warren, R. J., Lepow, M. L., Bartsch, G. E., and Robbins, F. C.: The relationship of maternal antibody, breast and age to the susceptibility of newborn infants to infection with attenuated plioviruses. Pediatrics, *34*:4, 1964.
30. Parmely, M. J., Reath, D. B., and Beer, A. E.: Cellular immune responses of human milk T-lymphocytes to certain environmental antigens. Transplant. Proc., *9*:1477, 1977.
31. Triger, D. R., Cynamon, M. H., and Wright, R.: Studies on hepatic uptake of antigen. I. Comparison of inferior vena cava and portal routes of immunization. Immunology, *25*:941, 1973.
32. Kleinman, R. E., Harmatz, P. R., and Walker, W. A.: The liver: An integral part of the enteric mucosal immune system. Hepatology, *2*:379, 1982.
33. Delacroix, D. L. et al.: Changes in size, subclass, and metabolic properties of serum IgA in liver diseases and other diseases with high serum IgA. J. Clin. Invest., *71*:358, 1983.
34. Peppard, J., Orlans, E., Payne, A. W., and Andrew, E.: The elimination of circulating complexes containing polymeric IgA by excretion in the bile. Immunology, *42*:83, 1981.
35. Harmatz, P. R., et al.: Hepatobiliary clearance of IgA immune complexes formed in the circulation. Hepatology, *2*:328, 1982.
36. Bienenstock, J., and Befus, A. D.: Some thoughts on the biologic role of immunoglobulin A. Gastroenterology, *84*:178, 1983.
37. Popper, H., and Schaffner, F.: Progress in liver diseases. New York, Grune and Stratton, 1972.
38. Kliegman, R. M., and Fanaroff, A. A.: necrotizing enterocolitis. N. Engl. J. Med., *310*:1093, 1984.
39. Stern, M., and Walker, W. A.: Food allergy and intolerance. Pediatr. Clin. North Am., *32*:471, 1985.
40. Walker, W. A.: Mechanisms of antigen handling by the gut. Clin. Immunol. Allergy., *2*:15, 1982.
41. Bloch, K. J., Bloch, D. B., Stearns, M., and Walker, W. A.: Intestinal uptake of macromolecules. VI. Uptake of protein antigen in vivo in normal rats and in rats infected with Nippostrongylus brasiliensis or subjected to mild systemic anaphylaxis. Gastroenterology, *77*:1039, 1979.
42. Etlinger, H. H., and Chiller, J. M.: Maturation of the lymphoid system. I. Induction of tolerance in neonates with a T-dependent antigen that is an obligate immunogen in adults. J. Immunol., *122*:2558, 1979.

43. Hanson, D.: Ontogeny of orally induced tolerance to soluble proteins in mice. I. Priming and tolerance in newborns. J. Immunol., 127:1518, 1981.
44. Strobel, S., Ferguson, A.: Immune responses to fed protein antigens in mice. III. Systemic tolerance or priming is related to age at which antigen is first encountered. Pediatr. Res., 18:588, 1984.
45. Jenkins, H. R., et al.: Food allergy: The major cause of infantile colitis. Arch. Dis. Child., 59:326, 1984.
46. Seidman, E. G., and Walker, W. A.: Gastrointestinal manifestations of primary and secondary immunodeficiency states. Front. Gastrointest. Res., 1987 (in press).
47. Kirsner, J. B., and Shorter, R. G.: Recent developments in nonspecific inflammatory bowel disease. N. Engl. J. Med., 306:837, 1982.
48. Shorter, R. G., and Kirsner, J. B.: Immunology of idiopathic inflammatory bowel disease. *In* Gastrointestinal Immunity for the Clinician, Orlando, Grune and Stratton, 1985.
49. Shorter, R. G., Huizenga, K. A., and Spencer, R. J.: A working hypothesis for the etiology and pathogenesis of nonspecific inflammatory bowel disease. Am. J. Dig. Dis., 17:1024, 1972.
50. Potter, G. D., and Lester, R.: The developing colon and nutrition. J. Pediatr. Gastroenterol. Nutr., 3:485, 1984.
51. Kabacoff, B. L., Wohlman A., and Umhey, M.: Absorption of chymotrypsin by the intestinal tract. Nature, 199:815, 1963.
52. Ono, K.: Absorption of horseradish peroxidase by the principal cells of the large intestine of postnatal developing rats. Anat. Embryol., 151:53, 1977.
53. Seidman, E. G., et al.: Macromolecular uptake from colon: effects of age on permeability in rabbits. Gastroenterology, 88:1579, 1985.
54. Seidman, E. G., Hanson, D. G., and Walker, W. A.: Increased permeability to polyethylene glycol 4000 in rabbits with experimental colitis. Gastroenterology, 90:120, 1986.
55. Zabriskie, J. B.: Microbial-mammalian tissue cross-reactivities exemplified by group A streptococci. Recomb. DNA Tech. Bull., 4:117, 1981.
56. Springer, G. F., Wang, E. T., and Nichols, J. H.: Relations between bacterial lipopolysaccharide structures and those of human cells. Ann. NY Acad. Sci., 133:566, 1966.
57. Kaplan, M. H.: Autoantibodies to heart and rheumatic fever: The induction of autoimmunity to heart by streptococcal antigen cross-reactive with heart. Ann. NY Acad. Sci., 124:904, 1965.
58. Kunin, C. M.: Separation, characterization and biological significance of a common antigen in enterobacteriaceae. J. Exp. Med., 118:565, 1963.
59. Carrillo, J., Hashimoto, B., and Kumate, J.: Content of heterogenetic antigen in Escherichia coli and its relationship to diarrhea in newborn infants. J. Infect. Dis., 116:285, 1966.
60. Neter, E. O., et al.: Demonstration of antibodies against enteropathogenic E. coli in sera of children of various ages. Pediatrics, 16:801, 1955.
61. Broberger, O., and Perlmann, P.: Autoantibodies in human ulcerative colitis. J. Exp. Med., 110:657, 1959.
62. Langercrantz, R., et al.: Immunological studies in ulcerative colitis. III. Incidence of antibodies to colon-antigen in ulcerative colitis and other gastro-intestinal diseases. Clin. Exp. Immunol., 1:263, 1966.
63. Bartnik, W., and Shorter, R. G.: Inflammatory bowel disease: Immunologic developments. *In* Developments in Digestive Diseases. Edited by J. E. Berk. Philadelphia, Lea & Febiger, 1980.
64. Seidman, E. G., et al.: Antibodies to enterobacterial common antigen in humans and tamarins with chronic inflammatory bowel disease. Gastroenterology, 90:1625, 1986.
65. Thayer, W. R., et al.: Escherichia coli 0:14 and colon hemagglutinating antibodies in inflammatory bowel disease. 57:311, 1969.
66. Eckhardt, R., Heinisch, M., and Meyer zum Büschenfelde, K. H.: Cellular immune reactions against common antigen, small intestine, and colon antigen in patients with Crohn's disease, ulcerative colitis, and cirrhosis of the liver. Scand. J. Gastroenterol., 11:49, 1976.
67. Bull, D. M., and Ignaczak, T. F.: Enterobacterial common antigen-induced reactivity in inflammatory bowel disease. Gastroenterology, 64:43, 1973.
68. Bartnik, W., Remine, S. G., and Shorter, R. G.: Leukocyte migration inhibitory factor (LMIF) release by human colonic lymphocytes. Arch. Immunol. Ther. Exp., 29:397, 1981.
69. Shorter, R. G., Spencer, R. J., Huizenga, K. A., and Hallenbeck, G. A.: Inhibition of in vitro cytotoxicity of lymphocytes from patients with ulcerative colitis and granulomatous colitis for allogeneic colonic epithelial cells using horse anti-human thymus serum. Gastroenterology, 54:227, 1968.
70. Shorter, R. G., Cardoza, M. R., Spencer, R. J., and Huizenga, K. A.: Further studies of in vitro cytotoxicity of lymphocytes from patients with ulcerative and granulomatous colitis for allogeneic colonic epithelial cells, including the effects of colectomy. Gastroenterology, 56:304, 1969.
71. Shorter, R. G., et al.: Modification of in vitro cytotoxicity of lymphocytes from patients with chronic ulcerative colitis or granulomatous colitis for allogeneic colonic epithelial cells. Gastroenterology, 58:692, 1970.
72. Stobo, J. D., et al.: In vitro studies of inflammatory bowel disease: surface receptors of the mononuclear cell required to lyse allogeneic colonic epithelial cells. Gastroenterology, 70:171, 1976.
73. Shorter, R. G., McGill, D. B., and Bahn, R. C.: Cytotoxicity of mononuclear cells (MC) for autologous colonic epithelial cells (ACEC) in colonic diseases. Gastroenterology, 86:13, 1984.
74. Acheson, E. D., and Truelove, S. C.: Early weaning in the etiology of ulcerative colitis. Br. Med. J., 2:929, 1961.
75. Hellers, G.: Some epidemiological aspects of Crohn's disease in Stockholm County 1955-1979. *In* Recent Advances in Disease. Edited by A. J. Peña, I. T. Weterman, and C. C. Booth. Boston, Martinus Nijhoff Publishers, 1981.

# 5 · The Membranous Epithelial (M) Cell: A Portal of Antigen Entry*

JACQUELINE L. WOLF, M.D.

The etiology of idiopathic inflammatory bowel disease is unknown, even though investigators have devoted many years to trying to discover its elusive cause(s). Infectious agents such as mycobacteria,[1,2] cell-wall deficient bacteria,[3,4] and viruses have all been proposed,[5,7] but none has been shown to produce inflammatory bowel disease (see Chapter 3). Immunologic abnormalities found in patients could be primary abnormalities,[8-12] or, more likely, secondary phenomena seen in association with the disease (see Chapter 7). Immunologic abnormalities can occur in infectious diseases, as exemplified by the acquired immunodeficiency syndrome caused by the human T-cell leukemia virus III/lymphadenopathy-associated virus,[13,14] in which T_4 helper cells are destroyed,[15] and a variety of immunologic abnormalities occur.[16]

If inflammatory bowel disease is caused by an infectious organism, that organism must first penetrate the mucosal barrier of the host and then localize to a specific area in the small or large intestine where disease occurs. This breach of the epithelium could occur by direct passage across uninjured, healthy epithelium, or possibly across an epithelial surface that has been damaged either by the organism or by another cause. An important area through which antigen penetration of intact mucosa in adult animals occurs is the epithelium overlying the subepithelial follicles in the gastrointestinal tract (Peyer's patches and tonsils) and the respiratory tract.

Peyer's patches are located on the antimesenteric wall of the small bowel. In humans, Peyer's patches are more common in the ileum than the jejunum,[17] but in mice they are uniformly distributed throughout the small bowel.[18] The number of follicles associated with each Peyer's patch varies. In man, there are from 5 to more than 900 follicles per patch.[17] In the respiratory tract, the nodular aggregated lymphoid tissue occurs at bifurcations of bronchi and bronchioles.[19] Interspersed among the epithelial cells that overlie this aggregated lymphoid tissue in the gastrointestinal and respiratory tracts are the membranous epithelial (M) cells. M cells are specialized epithelial cells that transport antigens, including viruses and bacteria, from the lumen to the extracellular space, allowing their access to many cells, such as lymphocytes, macrophages, and plasma cells.

That Peyer's patches are important sites for antigen penetration has been known for many years. As early as 1922, Kumagai showed that rabbit appendix and/or Peyer's patches took up ink, Carmine dye, powdered erythrocytes, and living or dead mycobacteria.[20] Following oral inoculation of chimpanzees with poliovirus, it

---

*This work was supported in part by a grant from the National Foundation for Ileitis and Colitis.

was localized in the tonsils, cervical lymph nodes, and ileal Peyer's patches prior to hematogenous dissemination.[21] Similarly, following inoculation of chimpanzees and mice with Salmonella typhi,[22,23] and of mice with Salmonella enteritidis 5694,[24,25] which causes a typhoid fever-like illness, the initial infection occurs in ileal and cecal Peyer's patches and in the mesenteric nodes draining these areas. That the uptake of these macromolecules and infectious organisms occurs across an intact epithelium, that the M cell plays an important role in the uptake, and that the uptake may be part of the normal functioning of the epithelium in order for the host to mount an immunologic defense against these antigens have only been suggested in the last twenty years.

Membranous Epithelial (M) Cell

The term "M cells" has been used synonymously with "lymphoepithelial cells" and "follicle-associated epithelial cells." They were first identified by Schmedtje in 1965 and 1966 in the epithelium overlying the lymphoid follicles in rabbit appendix.[26,27] The apical surfaces stained poorly for alkaline phosphatase, but richly for neutral esterase. Lymphocytes were found within large cytoplasmic vacuoles of these cells. In 1967, Shimizu and Andrew showed that not only did the epithelial cells of rabbit appendix surround lymphocytes, but they also surrounded some endocytosed bacteria.[28] Similar cells were found by Oláh to overlie the tonsils of rabbits,[29] by Bockman and Cooper to overlie the bursa of Fabricius in chicks, the Peyer's patches of mice, and the appendix in rabbits,[30] and by Owen and Jones to overlie human Peyer's patches.[31] M cells were later shown to overlie the lymphoid collections in the human appendix,[32] and the human tonsils.[18] M cells have also been identified in pigs,[31,34] calves,[34-37] monkeys,[18] hamsters,[18] dogs,[18] rats,[18] and guinea pigs.[38]

Morphology of M Cells

The epithelium overlying the lymphoid follicles consists of absorptive cells, somewhat shortened in height compared to those of the villi, a paucity of goblet cells,[18] and cells that in 1 μm sections of resin embedded tissue have attenuated brush borders and separate lymphoid cells from the lumen by a small distance. These latter cells are putative M cells,[39] but their definitive identification depends upon examination of thin sections by scanning or transmission electron microscopy, or of freeze fracture replicas by transmission electron microscopy.

Scanning electron microscopy distinguishes many M cells in Peyer's patches from surrounding absorptive cells.[18,31,40] By this technique, a regular carpet of microvilli characterizes the absorptive cell apical surface, whereas the M cell apical surface has some microvilli and irregular ridges, with or without central concavities. The ridges are produced by microfolds that converge, branch, double-back and, occasionally, end abruptly.[31]

The morphologic appearances of sections of intestinal M cells examined by transmission electron microscopy show some variation from cell to cell,[18,40-42] which was thought to be caused by the relative maturity of the M cell.[41-42] A typical mature M cell is illustrated in Figure 5-1. The M cell shares tight junctions and desmosomes with adjacent epithelial cells, but not with the lymphoid cells that are enveloped by the M cell's cytoplasm. The apical surface of the intestinal M cell differs appreciably from that of the adjacent intestinal absorptive cells. Whereas the apical surface of the absorptive cell is characterized by regularly tall, thin, closely-packed microvilli (like a "picket fence"), the M cell's apical surface is characterized by microfolds and short, irregular, and often wider microvilli that are fewer in number than those of the absorptive cell. Compared to the absorptive cell, the M cell has fewer well-defined rootlets of actin filaments extending from the microvillus core into the terminal web. In the M cell, organelles, such as mitochondria, often are present just beneath the apical membrane. In the absorptive cell, however, the terminal-web area below the microvilli is devoid of organelles. Vesicles are abundant in the apical cytoplasm of the M cell. These vesicles endocytose and transport macromolecules[30,39,43-45] and microorganisms[37,46,50] through the M cell, releasing them into the extracellular space below the cell. The other organelles in M cells are similar in type and number to those in surrounding absorptive cells, with the exception of lysosomes, which are fewer in number in M cells.[51]

The mature M cell has a thin bridge of apical cytoplasm and a basally-located nucleus (Fig. 5-1). Its cytoplasm surrounds one or more intrusive cells, which are usually lymphocytes,[39,43] lymphoblasts,[52] or macrophages,[48,49,53,54] but occasionally are plasma cells,[52,54] or, rarely, pol-

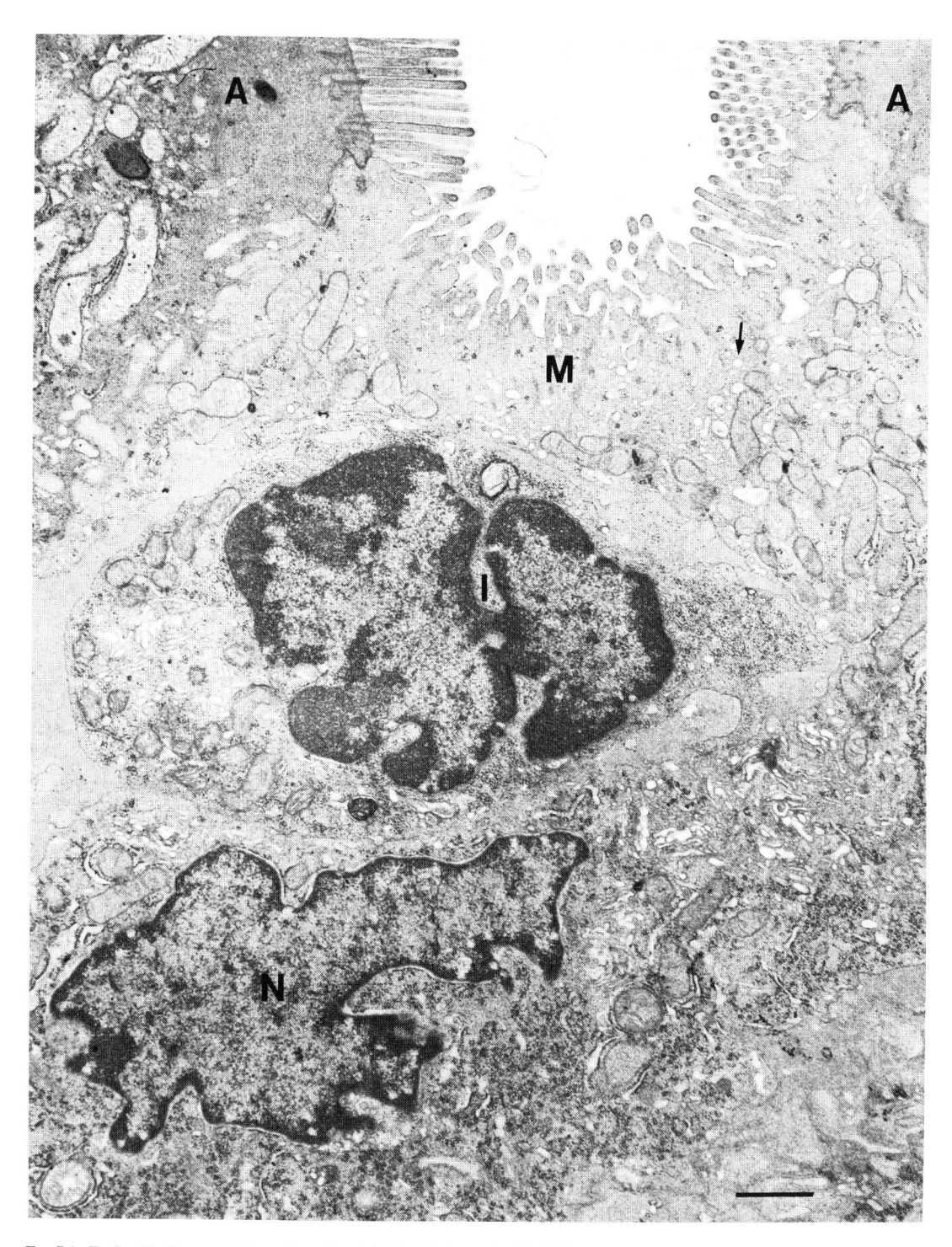

FIG. 5-1. Ileal epithelium overlying a Peyer's patch of an eight-week-old C3H/HeJ mouse. The M cell (M) has short, fat, irregular microvilli, a thin bridge of apical cytoplasm with many vesicles (arrow), and a basally oriented nucleus (N). Its cytoplasm envelops a mononuclear cell (I). The adjacent absorptive cells (A) have tall, thin microvilli. Bar equals 1 μm. (Reprinted with permission from Wolf, J. L., and Bye, W. A.: The membranous epithelial (M) cell and the mucosal immune system. Ann. Rev. Med., 35:98, Copyright © 1984 by Annual Reviews Inc.)

ymorphonuclear leukocytes.[55] These cells are not within the M cell cytoplasm, but are in the intercellular space that indents the M cell cytoplasm, forming a "central hollow."[56,57]

Immature M cells not only have more abundant and regular microvilli than do mature M cells, but also have sparser, shorter, and wider microvilli than the absorptive cells. There are more free ribosomes in immature M cells than in mature ones. Most immature M cells lack the mononuclear cell-containing central hollow, and, hence, are columnar in shape. Like mature M cells, immature cells have many apical vesicles and lack a well-defined terminal web.[38,41,42] Many cells having morphologic appearances halfway between mature and immature M cells occur in the epithelium overlying the Peyer's patches.[42]

Studies of the M Cell-Apical Membrane

Comparisons have been made of the apical membranes of M cells and absorptive cells to uncover differences that would account for their varied functions. Histochemical studies of the follicle-associated epithelium showed that the apical membrane of intestinal M cells has less alkaline phosphatase,[26,58,59] and more esterase,[58,59] than that of absorptive cells. In rabbit intestinal follicular epithelium, Ricinus communis agglutinins I and II and wheat germ agglutinin bind to the apical surfaces both of M cells and absorptive cells in fixed and unfixed tissue.[60] No dramatic difference is evident between binding of any of the three lectins to the microvilli and microfolds of M cells as compared with the binding to the microvilli of absorptive cells either in prefixed or unfixed tissue, suggesting no differences in their apical membrane terminal D-galactose, N-acetyl-D-galactosamine, sialic acid, or polymeric N-acetyl-glucosamine residues. In aldehyde-fixed Peyer's patches of adult mice and rats, concanavalin A and the horseradish peroxidase-labelled conjugates of wheat germ agglutinin, Ricinus communis agglutinin, and peanut agglutinin bind to the M cell surfaces with the same binding pattern to the surfaces of absorptive cells.[59] In experiments using routine aldehyde fixation of intestinal tissue, staining with ruthenium red suggested that M cells have a less elaborate glycocalyx than absorptive cells.[55] When the tissue is fixed with aldehyde and ferrocyanide-reduced OsO_4, however, the glycocalyx on the apical membrane of M cells is as abundant as that on the apical membrane of absorptive cells,[42] suggesting that an artifactual decrease in the glycocalyx was found by the other investigators.[55]

Comparisons of freeze fracture replicas of M cell and absorptive cell apical membranes show that membranes of M cells contain relatively few intramembrane particles compared to those of absorptive cells on the patch or villous.[38] These intramembrane particles are thought to represent integral membrane proteins,[61-64] although in the adult mammalian intestine the identity of the proteins represented by the integral membrane particles is not known. In addition, the M cell apical membranes are rich in morphologically detectable cholesterol, represented by a ratio of 1:1 complexes of the polyene antibiotic filipin with cholesterol. The number of intramembrane particles and filipin-sterol complexes in the apical membranes of immature M cells, as compared with mature ones, was the same.[38]

Function

M cells transport many macromolecules and organisms from the lumen to the underlying lymphoid tissue (Table 5-1). Why substances are "attracted" to the apical surface of the M cell and whether M cells act only as passive conduits for these antigens or process antigens as do macrophages, is not known. M cells in the chicken bursa of Fabricius, rabbit appendix, mouse Peyer's patches,[30] and the bronchial-associated lymphoid tissue (BALT) of rats transport native ferritin,[65] and in all but the latter also have been shown to transport carbon particles of India ink to the underlying lymphoid follicles. Horseradish peroxidase has been shown to bind to the apical surface of the epithelium of bronchial-associated lymphoid tissue,[66,67] of intestinal M cells, and of absorptive cells, to enter M cells via apical vesicles, and to be transported to the extracellular space between M cells and the enfolded intrusive cells in the central hollow.[39,43] The peroxidase then binds to the surfaces of lymphocytes and macrophages, and is taken up by macrophages. Bidirectional transport of horseradish peroxidase by M cells occurs. Horseradish peroxidase injected intravenously or into the spleen is found within absorptive cells and M cells, and in the intestinal lumen after 10 to 15 minutes.[45,68] The membrane-bound tracers, cationized ferritin, lectins Ricinus communis agglutinin I and II, and wheat germ agglutinin (which bind to the apical surfaces of both M cells and absorptive cells in rab-

TABLE 5-1 *Substances transported by M cells.*

Macromolecules	Viruses	Bacteria	Parasites
Native ferritin	Reovirus type 1	Mycbacteria	Cryptosporidium
Cationized ferritin	Reovirus type 3	Chlamydia	
Horseradish peroxidase		Vibrio cholera	
Ricinus communis agglutinin I			
Ricinus communis agglutinin II		(Escherichia coli RDEC-1)[a]	
Wheat Germ agglutinin			
Cholera toxin			

[a]Adheres to M cells, but has not been shown to be transported by M cells.
(Adapted from Wolf, J. L., and Bye, W. A.: The membranous epithelial (M) cell and the mucosal immune system. Ann. Rev. Med., *35*:101, 1984).

bit Peyer's patches), are transported across the epithelium *only* by M cells.[44,60] Cholera toxin, which binds to the ganglioside GM_1 on the apical surface of intestinal absorptive cells, is endocytosed by guinea pig M cells.[69]

Not only macromolecules but also living organisms are transported by M cells across the intestinal epithelium. Wolf et al. showed that M cells are the sites where reoviruses, (segmented double-strand RNA viruses that infect the brain[46,47] and other distant tissues in infant mice),[70-72] penetrate the intestinal epithelium. Thirty minutes after inoculation of an ileal loop in 10-day-old BALB/cJ or C3H/HeJ mice with reovirus type 1, viruses selectively adhere to the surfaces of M cells, but not to those of other epithelial cells (Fig. 5-2). In adult C3H/HeJ mice, reovirus type 1 adheres to M cells as well as to a minority of absorptive cells on Peyer's patches, but not to absorptive cells on the villi. Within one hour of the time of inoculation, reoviruses are found in M cell cytoplasmic vesicles, in the intercellular spaces adjacent to the M cell, below the basement membrane, and within mononuclear cells and macrophages (Wolf, J.L., and Bye, W.A.: unpublished data) (Fig. 5-2).[46,47]

In young suckling mice 2 to 7 days of age, reovirus type 1 adheres to the apical surface of M cells and is transported by M cells into the cytoplasm.[73] Although it was not until animals were 5 days of age that reovirus type 1 was seen definitively to be transported through M cells, reovirus was endocytosed by M cells in 2-day-old mice. In 2-day-old mice only rare absorptive cells endocytosed reovirus type 1 into the apical cytoplasm. Adherence to M cell surfaces was greater than 50% at all ages. At 7 days of age, only occasional villous absorptive cells and 11% of Peyer's patch absorptive cells had reovirus adherent to their apical surfaces. In 10-day-old suckling mice, reovirus type 3 also adhered to and was endocytosed by M cells.[47] In contrast to type 1, type 3 reovirus adhered to, and was endocytosed by, absorptive cells, in which it accumulated in lysosome-like bodies. Using reassortants of reovirus types 1 and 3, Wolf et al. showed that σ_1, the viral hemagglutinin, determines whether a reovirus will nonselectively adhere to and be endocytosed by absorptive cells.[47] Dissemination of reovirus to distant sites after penetration of the gastrointestinal tract in 10-day-old or adult mice is also determined by the viral hemagglutinin.[74]

Not only does dissemination of reovirus type 1 to distant sites occur following M cell transport, but reovirus type 1 causes enteritis both in suckling and adult mice.[75,76] In mice inoculated at 10 days of age, viral factories, in which viral particles are made, occur in M cells, Peyer's patch dome, villus absorptive cells and crypt cells by 4 to 6 hours, and persist until at least 72 hours after inoculation. M cells contain virions in endocytic vesicles and/or viral factories, probably representing both endocytosis of reovirus by the M cell and the M cell's coincident infection by the reovirus. The percentage of M cells in the epithelium of proximal Peyer's patches was decreased from 4 to 6 hours until 72 hours postinoculation (1.22 ± 0.65% vs 5.7 ± 1.30%). By 6 days after viral inoculation, there was an increase in the percentage of M cells, most of which appeared immature as compared to the dome epithelium of control animals (15% vs 6 %). By 13 days after inoculation, both control and infected mice had similar percentages of M cells in the dome (13%). This decrease in M cell number following reovirus type 1 infection and probably other infectious enteritides, and the subsequent overpopulation of the dome epithelium by immature M cells that do not transport reovirus,[42] may have profound effects on antigen sampling and on the host response to

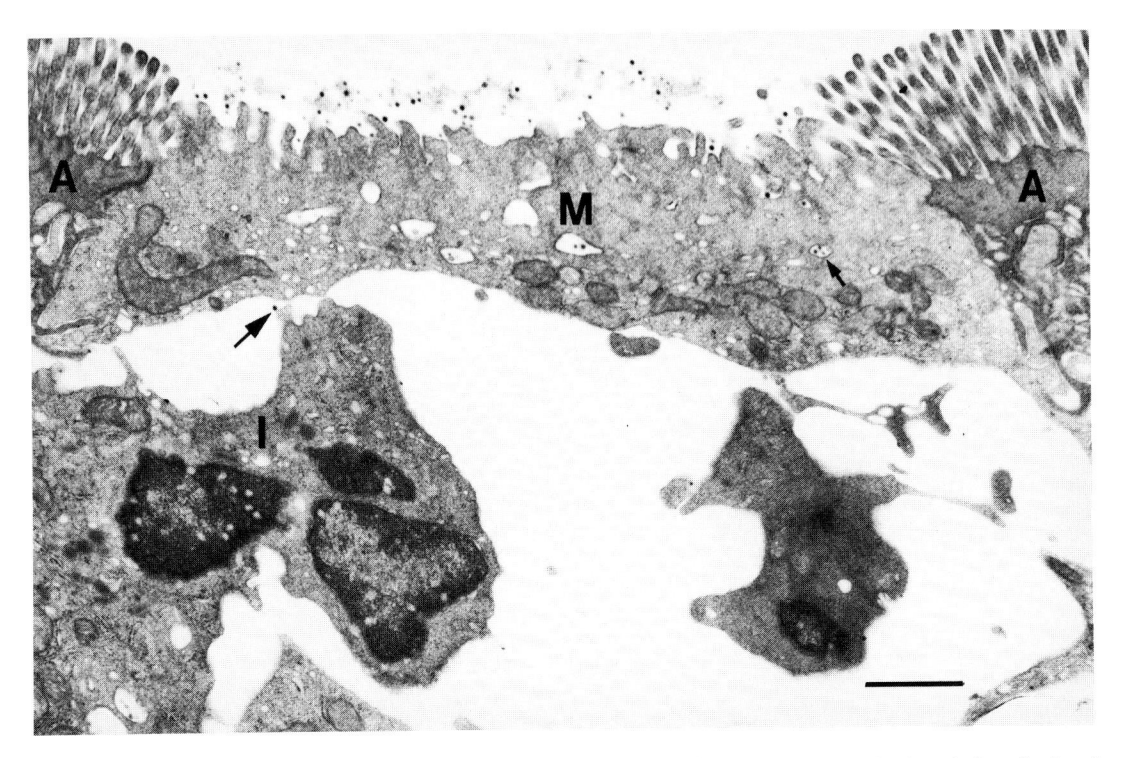

Fig. 5-2. Ileal epithelium overlying a Peyer's patch of a 10-day-old C3H/HeJ mouse obtained 1 hour after inoculation of a closed loop with reovirus type 1. Virions are seen adherent to the luminal surface of an M cell (M), within vesicles of the M cell (small arrow), and within the extracellular space (large arrow) in close proximity to an intrusive cell (I), possibly a macrophage. The adjacent absorptive cells (A) have no adherent virus. Bar equals 1 μm. (Reprinted with permission, from Wolf, J. L. et al.: Determinants of reovirus interaction with the intestinal M cells and absorptive cells of murine intestine. Gastroenterology, 85:294. Copyright © 1983 by The American Gastroenterological Association.)

pathogens during these viral diseases. If the major mode of intestinal epithelial penetration by some or many pathogens prior to local or distant spread is via the M cell, then a change in the M cell population might modify the diseases caused by two distinct viruses inoculated within 1 week of each other. Such disease modification occurring with viral coinfection is seen in the coinfection of newborn mice by lethal intestinal virus of infant mouse (LIVIM) infection (a coronavirus), and by epizootic diarrhea of infant mouse (EDIM) infection (a rotavirus).[77] Newborn mice are usually killed by LIVIM infection, but when coinfected with EDIM, a virus that infects M cells and absorptive cells, most of the animals live and the disease is substantially modified (Wolfe, J.L.: unpublished data). Antibody responses to antigens may also be affected when the M cell population changes.

Several types of bacteria adhere to and/or are transported by M cells (see Table 5-1). Although initially thought to be restricted to the intestinal lumen, intact Vibrio cholerae are endocytosed and transported within vesicles into ileal Peyer's patches by rabbit M cells.[48,49] Within the patch the bacteria are endocytosed by lymphoblasts and macrophages. This epithelial penetration by the Vibrios may be important in initiating an immune response. Chlamydia have been found within intestinal M cells of calves with diarrhea.[37] Escherichia coli RDEC-1, an enteroadherent bacterium that causes a diarrhea in rabbits that is similar to that caused by enteropathogenic Escherichia coli in humans, adheres to the M cells of ileal Peyer's patches within four hours of oral inoculation, but it does not appear to be transported.[55,78] Not until three days after inoculation do E. coli adhere to the absorptive cells of ileal, cecal, and colonic mucosae.[78] Whether the initial specific adherence to M cells is important in the subsequent colonization of the bowel and in the pathogenesis of the diarrhea, or whether it is important for the development of an immune response to the organism, needs to be clarified. Other organisms shown to be endocytosed by M cells are the mycobacterium Bacillus Calmette Guérin (BCG),[67] and cryptosporidium.[50]

Not all organisms penetrate the intestinal barrier via the M cell. Some invasive organisms such as Salmonella typhimurium penetrate the mucosa by disrupting the surface of the villous absorptive cells.[79] Giardia muris neither adheres to M cells nor penetrates the epithelium via the M cell. The trophozoites probably enter the mucosa through breaks in the epithelium or at sites of absorptive cell desquamation.[80]

It is unknown whether M cells have any digestive or nutrient absorptive function. After exposure of an ileal loop of mouse intestine to micellar lipid solution, neither mature nor immature-appearing M cells showed histologic evidence of lipid absorption.[42] This lack of lipid uptake by M cells contrasted with the lipid uptake by surrounding absorptive cells in which the smooth endoplasmic reticulum was distended with lipid droplets, the golgi complexes were prominent with dilated cysternae and vesicles filled with lipoprotein particles. Amino acid uptake by M cells has not been directly examined. However, valine and alanine absorption by follicle-associated epithelium is less than that by villous epithelium.[81,82] In the microvilli and microfolds, the relative paucity of intramembrane particles,[38] and the relative lack of staining for alkaline phosphatase of the M cell apical membrane compared to that of the absorptive cell,[26,58,59] suggest that the M cell apical membrane does not contain the extensive enzymatic machinery for the terminal digestion and absorption of nutrients that characterizes absorptive cells.

Another role for the M cell might be to facilitate the egress of lymphocytes into the gut lumen where such cells may have important immunologic functions. Lymphocytes have been shown to pass between M cells and enterocytes, between adjacent M cells, and through gaps in the apical cytoplasm of M cells into the intestinal lumen.[56,57,83]

The other substances transported by M cells are not known. Transport from the M cell basolateral surface to the apical surface of such lymphocyte products as IgA may occur, but has not been demonstrated. According to my results and those of others,[38,60] the presence of coated pits along M cell basolateral and apical membranes, and of a clathrin-like coat on some M cell endosomes, suggests that some receptor-mediated endocytosis takes place (Wolfe, J. L.: unpublished data).

Origin

Many investigators have attempted to identify the precursor cell from which the M cell develops. The available data support the hypothesis that many, if not all, M cells develop directly from undifferentiated crypt cells. The supporting data are: (1) the nuclei of a few immature-appearing M cells label 24 hours after ^{3}H-thymidine injection of adult mice, in concert with the appearance of labeling of absorptive cell nuclei;[42] (2) mature M cells appear at the crypt mouth and do not appear to be more concentrated higher on the dome;[42] (3) immature and mature M cells have a paucity of intramembrane particles and are rich in cholesterol, compared to absorptive cells;[38] and (4) mature and immature M cells do not endocytose lipid, in contrast to follicle-associated absorptive cells.[42] Specialized intestinal epithelial cells, such as the absorptive cells, goblet cells, Paneth cells, and enteroendocrine cells, also arise from precursor, undifferentiated cells in the crypt.[84-90] An alternative hypothesis is that M cells differentiate from mature absorptive cells on the upper part of the dome.[39,40,52,56,59] This hypothesis is based on the facts that some investigators[40] have found the majority of M cells to be located on the upper part of the lymphoid follicle rather than near the crypt mouth;[40] and that the nuclei of M cells do not label until 72 hours after ^{3}H-thymidine administration, whereas the nuclei of some absorptive cells label by 24 hours.[52]

The Distribution and Renewal of M Cells on Peyer's Patch Domes

The process of cell renewal in the epithelium of Peyer's patches is similar to that of the villi, with migration of maturing cells onto the dome epithelium. Following administration of ^{3}H-thymidine, autoradiographic light microscopic studies show that epithelial cell proliferation is confined to the crypts surrounding the follicle-associated epithelium.[52,91,92] As many as 30 crypts may supply a single dome with cells.[52] Labelling of absorptive cells is seen within 24 hours after ^{3}H-thymidine injection.[52] Labelling of immature cells occurs at 24 hours and of mature M cells at 48 hours.[42] In one strain of mice, M cells were distributed evenly throughout the upper part of the follicle-associated epithelium, but were uncommon over the lower part of the dome,[40] while in another strain, mature and immature M cells were distributed in more or less equal numbers on all parts of the dome, including the extreme base near the mouth of the crypt.[42]

There are species differences in the absolute numbers and percentages of M cells in the follicle-associated epithelium of Peyer's patches. While only about 10% of cells of the ileal follicle-associated epithelium of the mouse are M cells,[91] in the rabbit approximately 50% of cells are M cells (Bye, W. A., and Trier, J. S.: unpublished data).[57] For most species it is not known when, during fetal and neonatal development of the gut, M cells first appear. In chick fetuses, M cells of the bursa of Fabricius have been observed on day 15 of incubation, three days after lymphocytes first appear in the submucosal region.[30] In rabbits, M cells are present at birth.[30] A putative M cell has been noted overlying submucosal lymphoid cells in the small intestine of a 17-week-old human fetus.[93] M cells were reported to be present in the follicle-associated epithelium of newborn rats.[94] In mice, mature M cells are seen by 2 days after birth.[73]

What factors stimulate M cell development are not known but it has been speculated that lymphocytes or macrophages stimulate M cell development.[40,52,56] During the recovery phase of experimentally-induced reovirus type 1 enteritis of 10-day-old mice, a proliferation of immature M cells occurs, such that the M cell population numbers two and one half times that of uninfected animals of the same age.[75]

Importance

The relative importance of the M cell in macromolecular and antigen transport is not known. In suckling animals, absorptive cells transport macromolecules across the gastrointestinal tract mucosa, but at weaning, absorptive cells from rat and mouse pups greatly decrease in their ability to do this.[95,96] Absorptive cells of adult animals have been reported to transport only limited amounts of macromolecules.[96-104] However, whether absorptive-cell transport in adult animals occurs under physiologic circumstances or is a result of the experimental conditions used has been questioned.[105] In contrast, transport of macromolecules by M cells occurs in suckling animals and continues in adult animals.[30,46,47]

Because of the M cell's proximity to the lymphoid follicle, entry of antigens via the M cell may be the route necessary for immunologic processing. It is not known if M cells transport all antigens unchanged via the same pathway or if they have more than one pathway and modify antigens during their passage through the cell. Should different M cell pathways exist, or should antigen processing take place, the subsequent interactions of the antigen with the cells in the lymphoid follicles may be affected. Thus, it is conceivable that the M cell plays a role in determining whether IgA secretion, induction of systemic tolerance, and/or other immunologic reactions occur.

In summary, the M cells transport macromolecules and antigens to the underlying lymphoid tissue. In their location in the epithelium overlying the tonsils, Peyer's patches, aggregated lymphoid tissue of the bronchus, and in the bursa of Fabricius, the M cells are exposed to antigens that are aspirated or swallowed. The M cells provide a conduit to the underlying lymphoid tissue for antigens where an immune response can be stimulated. Whether M cells can also affect the immune response by processing antigens, transporting antigens via different pathways, or acting as antigen-presenting cells is unknown.

Some antigens use M cells as portals of entry into the host, escape from the local immunologic defenses, and cause disease. Such is the case with reovirus type 1, which enters the Peyer's patch,[29,30,74] probably via M cells, disseminates, and causes local and systemic disease.[70-72,74-76] Mycobacteria penetrate the rabbit gastrointestinal tract in the appendix and Peyer's patches, and are also taken up by the M cells of the bronchial-associated lymphoid tissue.[67]

The etiology of idiopathic inflammatory bowel disease is unknown. It may be initiated by antigen uptake via the M cell, leading to sensitization and an immune and/or inflammatory response that is damaging to the host. Whether or not disease ensues following uptake of a specific antigen may be determined by a number of factors, including genetic predisposition, the immunologic status of the host, characteristics of the antigen, or the presence of a promoter substance.

Future studies of the M cell may make it possible to affect transport of noxious substances or infectious organisms and/or affect the subsequent stimulation of an immune response. Such studies might have an impact on the development and treatment of inflammatory bowel disease.

REFERENCES

1. Chiodini, R. J., et al.: The possible role of mycobacteria in inflammatory bowel disease—an unclassified Mycobacterium species isolated from patients with Crohn's disease. Dig. Dis. Sci., *29*:1073, 1984.
2. Chiodini, R. J., et al.: Characteristics of an unclassified Mycobacterium species isolated from patients with Crohn's disease. J. Clin. Microbiol., *20*:966, 1984.
3. Parent, K., and Mitchell, P.: Cell wall-defective variants of pseudomonas-like (group Va) bacteria in Crohn's disease. Gastroenterology, *75*:368, 1978.
4. Graham, D. Y., Yoshimura, H. H., and Estes, M. K.: The role of cell-wall defective bacteria in the pathogenesis of Crohn's disease. Gastroenterology, *78*:1175, 1980.
5. Gitnick, G. L., and Rosen, V. J.: Electron microscopic studies of viral agents in Crohn's disease. Lancet, *2*:217, 1976.
6. Gitnick, G. L., Rosen, V. J., Arthur, M. S., and Hertweck, S. A.: Evidence for the isolation of a new virus from ulcerative colitis patients: comparison with virus derived from Crohn's disease. Dig. Dis. Sci., *24*:609, 1979.
7. Aronson, M. D., Phillips, C. A., Beeken, W. L., and Forsyth, B. R.: Isolation and characterization of a viral agent from intestinal tissue of patients with Crohn's disease and other intestinal disorders. Prog. Med. Virol., *21*:165, 1975.
8. Elson C. O., Graeff, A. S., James, S. P., and Strober, W.: Covert suppressor T cells in Crohn's disease. Gastroenterology, *80*:1513, 1981.
9. Hodgson, H. J. F., Wands, J. R., and Isselbacher, R. J.: Decreased suppressor cell activity in inflammatory bowel disease. Clin. Exp. Immunol., *32*:451, 1978.
10. Ginsburg, C. H., and Falchuk, Z. M.: Defective autologous mixed-lymphocyte reaction and suppressor cell generation in patients with inflammatory bowel disease. Gastroenterology, *83*:1, 1982.
11. Goodacre, R. L., and Bienenstock, J.: Reduced suppressor cell activity in intestinal lymphocytes from patients with Crohn's disease. Gastroenterology, *82*:653, 1982.
12. MacDermott, R. P., et al.: Alterations of IgM, IgG, and IgA synthesis and secretion by peripheral blood and intestinal mononuclear cells from patients with ulcerative colitis and Crohn's disease. Gastroenterology, *81*:844, 1981.
13. Barre-Sinoussi, et al.: Isolation of a T-lymphotropic retrovirus from a patient at risk for acquired immunodeficiency syndrome (AIDS). Science, *220*:868, 1983.
14. Gallo, R. C., et al.: Frequent detection and isolation of cytopathic retroviruses (HTLV-III) from patients with AIDS and at risk for AIDS. Science, *224*:500, 1984.
15. Klatzmann, D., et al.: Selective tropism of lymphadenopathy associated virus (LAV) for helper-inducer T lymphocytes. Science, *225*:59, 1984.
16. Lane, H. C.: Immunologic abnormalities in the acquired immunodeficiency syndrome. *In* The acquired immunodeficiency syndrome: An update. Edited by A. S. Fauci. Ann. Intern. Med., *102*:809, 1985.
17. Cornes, J. S.: Number, size, and distribution of Peyer's patches in the human small intestine. Gut, *6*:225, 1965.
18. Owen, R. L., and Nemanic, P.: Antigen processing structures of the mammalian intestinal tract: An SEM study of lymphoepithelial organs. Scan. Electron Microsc., *2*:367, 1978.
19. Bienenstock, J., Johnston, N., and Perey, D. Y. E.: Bronchial lymphoid tissue. II. Functional characteristics. Lab. Invest., *28*:693, 1973.
20. Kumagai, K.: über den Resorptionsuorgang der corpusculären Bestandteile im Darm. Kekkaku-Zassi, *4*:429, 1922. (Abstracted in Ber. Gesamte Physiol. Exp. Pharmacol., *17*:414, 1922.
21. Bodian, D.: Emerging concept of poliomyelitis infection. Science, *122*:105, 1955.
22. Gaines, S., Sprinz, H., Tully, J. G., and Tigertt, W. D.: Studies on infection and immunity in experimental typhoid fever. VII. The distribution of Salmonella typhi in chimpanzee tissue following oral challenge, and the relationship between the numbers of bacilli and morphologic lesions. J. Infect. Dis., *118*:293, 1968.
23. Hohmann, A. W., Schmidt, G., and Rowley, D.: Intestinal colonization and virulence of Salmonella in mice. Infect. Immun., *22*:763, 1978.
24. Carter, P. B., and Collins, F. M.: The route of enteric infection in normal mice. J. Exp. Med., *139*:1189, 1974.
25. Carter, P. B., Woolcock, J. B., and Collins, F. M.: Involvement of the upper respiratory tract in orally induced Salmonellosis in mice. J. Infect. Dis., *131*:570, 1975.
26. Schmedtje, J. F.: Some histochemical characteristics of lymphoepithelial cells of the rabbit appendix. Anat. Rec. *151*:412, 1965.
27. Schmedtje, J. F.: Fine structure of intercellular lymphocyte clusters in the rabbit appendix epithelium. Anat. Rec. *154*:417, 1966.
28. Shimizu, Y., and Andrew, W.: Studies on the rabbit appendix. I. Lymphocyte-epithelial relations and the transport of bacteria from the lumen to lymphoid nodule. J. Morphol., *123*:231, 1967.
29. Oláh, I., Surjan, L., Jr., and Törö, I.: Electronmicroscopic observations on the antigen reception in the tonsillar tissue. Acta Biol. Acad. Sci. Hung., *23*:61, 1972.
30. Bockman, D. E., and Cooper, M. D.: Pinocytosis by epithelium associated with lymphoid follicles in the bursa of fabricius, appendix, and Peyer's patches. An electron microscopic study. Am. J. Anat., *136*:455, 1973.
31. Owen, R. L., and Jones, A. L.: Epithelial cell specialization within human Peyer's patches: An ultrastructural study of intestinal lymphoid follicles. Gastroenterology, *66*:189, 1974.
32. Bockman, D. E., and Cooper, M. D.: Early lymphoepithelial relationships in human appendix. A combined light- and electron-microscopic study. Gastroenterology, *68*:1160, 1975.
33. Chu, R. M., Glock, R. D., and Ross, R. F.: Gut-associated lymphoid tissues of young swine with emphasis on dome epithelium of aggregated lymph nodules (Peyer's patches) of the small intestine. Am. J. Vet. Res., *40*:1720, 1979.
34. Torres-Medina, A.: Morphologic characteristics of the epithelial surface of aggregated lymphoid follicles (Peyer's patches) in the small intestine of newborn gnotobiotic calves and pigs. Am. J. Vet. Res., *42*:232, 1981.
35. Landsverk, T.: The gastrointestinal mucosa in young milk-fed calves. A scanning electron and light microscopic investigation. Acta Vet. Scand., *20*:572, 1979.
36. Landsverk, T.: The epithelium covering Peyer's patches in young milk-fed calves. An ultrastructural and enzyme histochemical investigation. Acta Vet. Scand., *22*:198, 1981.
37. Landsverk, T.: Peyer's patches and the follicle-associated epithelium in diarrheic calves. Pathomorphology, morphometry and acid phosphatase histochemistry. Acta Vet. Scand., *22*:459, 1981.
38. Madara, J. L., Bye, W. A., and Trier, J. S.: Structural features of and cholesterol distribution in M-cell mem-

branes in guinea pig, rat, and mouse Peyer's patches. Gastroenterology, 87:1091, 1984.
39. Owen, R. L.: Sequential uptake of horseradish peroxidase by lymphoid follicle epithelium of Peyer's patches in the normal unobstructed mouse intestine: An ultrastructural study. Gastroenterology, 72:440, 1977.
40. Smith, M. W., and Peacock, M. A.: M cell distribution in follicle-associated epithelium of mouse Peyer's patch. Am. J. Anat., 159:167, 1980.
41. Bye, W. A., Allan, C. H., Madara, J. L., and Trier, J. S.: Mature and immature M cells-morphology and distribution. Gastroenterology, 84:1118, 1983.
42. Bye, W. A., Allan, C. H., and Trier, J. S.: Structure, distribution, and origin of M cells in Peyer's patches of mouse ileum. Gastroenterology, 86:789, 1984.
43. von Rosen, L., Podjaski, B., Bettman, I., and Otto, H. F.: Observations on the ultrastructure and function of the so-called "microfold" or "membranous" cells (M cells) by means of peroxidase as a tracer. Virchows Arch. A, 390:289, 1981.
44. Neutra, M. R., Guerina, N. G., Hall, T. -L., and Nicolson, G. L.: Transport of membrane-bound macromolecules by M cells in rabbit intestine. Gastroenterology, 82:1137, 1982.
45. Bockman, D. E., and Stevens, W.: Gut-associated lymphoepithelial tissue: Bidirectional transport of tracer by specialized epithelial cells associated with lymphoid follicles. J. Reticuloendothel. Soc., 21:245, 1977.
46. Wolf, J. L., et al.: Intestinal M cells: A pathway for entry of reovirus into the host. Science 212:471, 1981.
47. Wolf, J. L., et al.: Determinants of reovirus interaction with the intestinal M cells and absorptive cells of murine intestine. Gastroenterology, 85:291, 1983.
48. Owen, R. L., Pierce, N. F., Apple, R. T., and Cray, W. D., Jr.: Phagocytosis and transport by M cells of intact Vibrio cholerae into rabbit Peyer's patch follicles. J. Cell Biol. 95:446a, 1982.
49. Owen, R. L., Pierce, N. F., and Cray, W. C., Jr.: Autoradiographic analysis of M cell uptake and transport of cholera vibrios into follicles of rabbit Peyer's patches. Gastroenterology, 84:1267, 1983.
50. Marcial, M. A., and Madara, J. L.: Cryptosporidium: Cellular localization, structural analysis of absorptive cell-parasite membrane-membrane interactions in guinea pigs, and suggestion of protozoan transport by M cells. Gastroenterology, 90:583, 1986.
51. Owen, R. L., Apple, R. T., and Bhalla, D. K.: Cytochemical identification and morphometric analysis of lysosomes in "M" cells and adjacent columnar cells of rat Peyer's patches. Gastroenterology, 80:1246, 1981.
52. Bhalla, D. K., and Owen, R. L.: Cell renewal and migration in lymphoid follicles of Peyer's patches and cecum—an autoradiographic study in mice. Gastroenterology, 82:232, 1982.
53. Atsushi, K.: The epithelial-macrophagic relationship in Peyer's patches: An immunopathological study. Bull. Osaka Med. Sch., 23:67, 1977.
54. Abe, K., and Ito, T.: Fine structure of the dome in Peyer's patches of mice. Arch. Histol. Jpn., 41:195, 1978.
55. Inman, L. R., and Cantey, J. R.: Specific adherence of Escherichia coli (Strain RDEC-1) to membranous (M) cells of the Peyer's patch in Escherichia coli diarrhea in the rabbit. J. Clin. Invest., 71:1, 1983.
56. Smith, M. W., and Peacock, M. A.: Lymphocyte induced formation of antigen transporting "M" cells from fully differentiated mouse enterocytes. In Intestinal Adaptation and its Mechanisms. Edited by J. W. L. Robinson, R. H. Dowling, and E. D. Riecken. Lancaster, MTP Press Ltd, 1982.
57. Owen, R. L., Bhalla, D. K., and Apple, R. T.: Migration of Peyer's patch lymphocytes through intact M cells into the intestinal lumen in mice, rats and rabbits. J. Cell Biol. 95:332a, 1982.
58. Owen, R. L., and Bhalla, D. K.: Cytochemical characterization of enzyme distribution over M cell surfaces in rat Peyer's patches. Gastroenterology, 82:1144, 1982.
59. Owen, R. L., and Bhalla, D. K.: Cytochemical analysis of alkaline phosphatase and esterase activities and of lectin-binding and anionic sites in rat and mouse Peyer's patch M cells. Am. J. Anat., 168:199, 1983.
60. Neutra, M. R., Phillips, T. L., Meyer, E. L., and Fishkind, D. J.: Transport of membrane-bound macromolecules by M cells in follicle-associated epithelium of rabbit Peyer's patch. Cell Tissue Res., 247:537, 1987.
61. Pinto da Silva, P., and Nicholson, G. L.: Freeze-etch localization of concanavalin A receptors to the membrane intercalated particles of human erythrocyte ghost membranes. Biochim. Biophys. Acta, 363:311, 1974.
62. Tillack, T. W., Scott, R. E., and Marchesi, V. T.: The structure of erythrocyte membranes studied by freeze etching. II. Localization of receptors for phytohemagglutinin and influenza virus to the intramembranous particles. J. Exp. Med., 135:1209, 1972.
63. Segrest, J. P., Gulik-Kryzwicki, T., and Sardet, C.: Association of the membrane-penetrating polypeptide segment of the human erythrocyte HN glycoprotein with phospholipid bilayers. I. Formation of freeze-etch intramembranous particles. Proc. Nat. Acad. Sci. USA, 71:3294, 1974.
64. Vail, W. J., Papahadjopoulos, D., and Moscarello, M. A.: Interaction of a hydrophobic protein with liposomes. Evidence for particles seen in freeze-fracture as being proteins. Biochim. Biophys. Acta., 345:463, 1974.
65. Fournier, M., Vai, F., Derenne, J. P. H., and Pariente, R.: Bronchial lymphoepithelial nodules in the rat. Morphologic features and uptake and transport of exogenous proteins. Am. Rev. Respir. Dis., 116:685, 1977.
66. Racz, P., Tenner-Racz, K., Myrvik, Q. N., and Fainter, L. K.: Functional architecture of bronchial associated lymphoid tissue and lymphoepithelium in pulmonary cell-mediated reactions in the rabbit. J. Reticuloendothel. Soc., 22:59, 1977.
67. Myrvik, Q. N., Racz, P., and Racz, K. T.: Ultrastructural studies of bronchial-associated lymphoid tissue (BALT) and lymphoepithelium in pulmonary cell-mediated reactions in the rabbit. In Macrophages and Lymphocytes: Nature, Functions, and Interaction. Edited by M. R. Escobar, and H. Friedman. New York, Plenum, 1980.
68. Hampton, J. C., and Rosario, B.: The passage of exogenous peroxidase from blood capillaries into the intestinal epithelium. Anat. Rec., 159:159, 1967.
69. Shakhlamov, V. A., Gaidar, V. A., and Baranov, U. N.: Electron-cytochemical investigation of cholera toxin absorption by epithelium of Peyer's patches in guinea pigs. Bull. Exp. Biol. Med., 90:1159, 1981.
70. Joklik, W. K.: Reproduction of reoviridiae. In Comprehensive Virology. Edited by H. Fraenkel-Conrat, and R. Wagner. New York, Plenum, 1974.
71. Gonatas, N. K., Margolis, G., and Kilham, L.: Reovirus type III encephalitis: observations of virus-cell interactions in neural tissues. Lab. Invest., 24:101, 1971.
72. Margolis, G., and Kilham, L.: Hydrocephalus in hamsters, ferrets, rats and mice following inoculations with reovirus type 1: pathologic studies. Lab. Invest., 21: 189, 1969.

73. Wolf, J. L., Dambrauskas, R., Sharpe, A. H., and Trier, J. S.: Reovirus penetration of the gastrointestinal tract in neonatal mice. Gastroenterology, 88:1634, 1985.
74. Kauffman, R. S., et al.: The σ_1 protein determines the extent of spread of reovirus from the gastrointestinal tract of mice. Virology, 124:403, 1983.
75. Bass, D., Dambrauskas, R., Trier, J., and Wolf, J.: Reovirus Type 1 enteritis depletes M cells overlying Peyer's patches. Gastroenterology, 90:1338, 1985.
76. Rubin, D. H., Kornstein, M. J., and Anderson, A. O.: Reovirus serotype 1 intestinal infections: A novel replicative cycle with ileal disease. J. Virol., 53:391, 1985.
77. Kraft, L. M.: Epizootic diarrhea of infant mice and lethal intestinal virus infection of infant mice. In Viruses of Laboratory Rodents. Natl. Cancer Inst. Monogr., 20:55, 1966.
78. Cantey, J. R., and Inman, L. R.: Diarrhea due to Escherichia coli strain RDEC-1 in the rabbit: The Peyer's patch as the initial site of attachment and colonization. J. Infect. Dis., 143:440, 1981.
79. Takeuchi, A.: Electron microscope studies of experimental salmonella infection. I. Penetration into the intestinal epithelium by Salmonella typhimurium. Am. J. Pathol., 50:109, 1967.
80. Owen, R. L., Namanic, P. L., and Stevens, D. P.: Ultrastructural observations on giardiasis in a murine model. I. Intestinal distribution, attachment and relationship to the immune system of Giardia muris. Gastroenterology, 76:757, 1979.
81. Smith, M. W., and Syme, G.: Functional differentiation of enterocytes in the follicle-associated epithelium of rat Peyer's Patches. J. Cell Sci., 55:147, 1982.
82. Hajjar, J. J., Hawrani, M., and Khuri, R. N.: Alanine flux across rabbit Peyer's patches. Comp. Biochem. Physiol., 43A:723, 1972.
83. Owen, R. L., and Heyworth, M. F.: Lymphocyte migration from Peyer's patches by diapedesis through M cells into the intestinal lumen. In Microenvironments in the Lymphoid System. Edited by G. G. B. Klause. New York, Plenum Publishing Corp., 1985.
84. Leblond, C. P.: Life history of renewing cells. Am. J. Anat., 160:113, 1981.
85. Cheng, H., and Leblond, C. P.: Origin, differentiation and renewal of the four main epithelial cell types in the mouse small intestine. I. Columnar cell. Am. J. Anat., 141:461, 1974.
86. Cheng, H.: Origin, differentiation and renewal of the four main epithelial cell types in the mouse small intestine. II. Mucous cells. Am. J. Anat., 141:481, 1974.
87. Cheng, H., and Leblond, C. P.: Origin, differentiation and renewal of the four main epithelial cell types in the mouse small intestine. III. Entero-endocrine cells. Am. J. Anat., 141:503, 1974.
88. Cheng, H.: Origin, differentiation and renewal of the four main epithelial cell types in the mouse small intestine. IV. Paneth cells. Am. J. Anat., 141:521, 1974.
89. Cheng, H., and Leblond, C. P.: Origin, differentiation and renewal of the four main epithelial cell types in the mouse small intestine. V. Unitarian theory of the origin of the four epithelial cell types. Am. J. Anat., 141:537, 1974.
90. Troughton, W. D., and Trier, J. S.: Paneth and goblet cell renewal in mouse duodenal crypts. J. Cell Biol., 41:251, 1969.
91. Smith, M. W., Jarvis, L. G., and King, I. S. Cell proliferation in follicle-associated epithelium of mouse Peyer's patch. Am. J. Anat., 159:157, 1980.
92. Faulk, W. P., et al.: Peyer's patches: Morphologic studies. Cell. Immunol., 1:500, 1971.
93. Moxey, P. C., and Trier, J. S.: Specialized cell types in the human fetal small intestine. Anat. Rec., 191:269, 1978.
94. Wilders, M. M., Sminia, T., and Janse, E. M.: Ontogeny of non-lymphoid and lymphoid cells in the rat gut with special reference to large mononuclear Ia-positive dendritic cells. Immunology, 50:303, 1983.
95. Clark, S. L., Jr.: The ingestion of proteins and colloidal materials by columner absorptive cells of the small intestine in suckling rats and mice. J. Biophys. Biochem. Cytol., 5:41, 1959.
96. Halliday, R.: The absorption of antibodies from immune sera by the gut of the young rat. Proc. R. Soc. Lond. Ser. B, 143:408, 1955.
97. Walker, W. A., and Isselbacher, K. J.: Uptake and transport of macromolecules by the intestine. Possible role in clinical disorders. Gastroenterology, 67:531, 1974.
98. Ono, K.: Absorption of horseradish peroxidase by the small intestinal epithelium in postnatal developing rats. Z. Mikrosk. Anat. Forsch., 89:870, 1975.
99. Williams, E. W.: Transmission of dietary proteins through the adult rat gut. In Protein Transmission through Living Membranes. Edited by W. A. Hemmings. New York, Elsevier Horth Holland Biomedical, 1979.
100. Udall, J. N., et al.: Development of gastrointestinal mucosal barrier. I. The effect of age on intestinal permeability to macromolecules. Pediatr. Res., 15:241, 1981.
101. Bockman, D. E., and Winborn, W. B.: Light and electron microscopy of intestinal ferritin absorption. Observations in sensitized and non-sensitized hamsters (Mesorcricetus auratus). Anat. Rec., 155:603, 1966.
102. Cornell, R., Walker, W. A., and Isselbacher, K. J.: Small intestinal absorption of horseradish peroxidase. A cytochemical study. Lab. Invest., 25:42, 1971.
103. Warshaw, A. L., Walker, W. A., Cornell, R., and Isselbacher, K. J.: Small intestinal permeability to macromolecules. Transmissions of horseradish peroxidase in mesenteric lymph and portal blood. Lab. Invest., 25:675, 1971.
104. Williams, E. W., and Hemmings, W. A.: Intestinal uptake and transport of proteins in the adult rat. Proc. R. Soc. London Ser. B, 203:177, 1978.
105. Rhodes, R. S., and Karnovsky, M. J.: Loss of macromolecular barrier function associated with surgical trauma to the intestine. Lab. Invest. 25:220, 1971.

6 · Genetic Aspects of Idiopathic Inflammatory Bowel Disease

RICHARD B. McCONNELL, M.D., F.R.C.P.

The observations on idiopathic regional ileitis made by Dr. Crohn 50 years ago were in a 14-year-old boy whose 32-year-old sister developed the condition soon afterwards.[1] Dr. Crohn commented that "the occurrence may be purely accidental or it may have significance as to a congenital predisposition or a transmissible causative agent in this disease." A familial occurrence of chronic ulcerative colitis (CUC) was recognized early in this century,[2] and since then there have been numerous case reports of idiopathic inflammatory bowel disease (IBD) occurring in families. However, such reports are rarely of value in trying to evaluate the genetic factors involved in IBD, because if a disease is moderately common in the population, as is the case with IBD, large family aggregations can be expected by mere chance alone. Although some clues to genetic and other factors of the condition can be gained from the observations on the types of intra-familial disease relationships and their relative frequencies, the main value of these case reports has been to stress the frequency with which Crohn's disease and ulcerative colitis occur in the same family.

Distribution of Cases Within Families

Kirsner reviewed the literature up to 1973 on CUC or Crohn's disease (CD) occurring in three or more members of the same family,[3] and Table 6-1 is an extension of this that includes the familial cases reported up to 1978. It is immediately apparent that parent-child and sib-sib combinations are much more common than those involving more distant relatives. As well as the familial occurrence of either CUC or CD, Table 6-1 enumerates the reported cases of the two diseases intermingled in the same family. Unfortunately, the latter are of little epidemiologic merit because a clinician probably would report these as examples of intermingling as opposed to those instances in which families show two or more cases of CUC or two or more cases of Crohn's disease.

Of greater interest than these various case reports are the studies from the detailed single-series data collected by Korelitz in New York City.[4] Because the probands were his own patients, the observations show the distribution of

TABLE 6-1. *Numbers of familial occurrences of IBD reported prior to 1978.*

	Ulcerative Colitis	Crohn's Disease	Intermingled Ulcerative Colitis and Crohn's Disease
Parent-Offspring	43	18	7
Sib-Sib	51	27	12
Collateral relatives	13	14	9
Concordant twins	5	7	0
Discordant twins	6	1	0
Husband and Wife	1	1	1

TABLE 6-2. *Inflammatory bowel disease in the first-degree relatives of the 838 Cleveland Clinic patients in whom the onset of the disease occurred before 21 years of age.*

Relationship	Ulcerative Colitis Patients[*]	Crohn's Disease Patients[**]
Father-Son	4 (1.3%)	14 (2.7%)
Father-Son	8 (2.5%)	6 (1.1%)
Mother-Son	10 (3.2%)	14 (2.7%)
Mother-Daughter	9 (2.8%)	14 (2.7%)
Parent-Offspring	31 (9.8%)	48 (9.2%)
Sib-Sib	19 (6.0%)	39 (7.5%)
Total	50 (15.8%)	87 (16.7%)

Total number of examples of familial inflammatory bowel disease = 137 of 838 = 16.3%.
[*]n = 316
[**]n = 522
(Adapted from Farmer, R. G., Michener, W. M., and Mortimer, E. A.: Clin. Gastroenterol., *9*: 271, 1980.)

intra-familial relationships free from the possible bias introduced by the irregular ascertainment of isolated reports. His 353 index patients all had Crohn's disease, and 72 of them (20.4%) had one or more relatives who also suffered from either CD or CUC. The parent-offspring occurrences were slightly more frequent than sib-sib combinations, and the number of affected first cousins, uncles, and aunts was much greater than previous reports in the literature had indicated. Even though Korelitz found as many as eight affected people in a single family, his data do not suggest either a dominant or recessive inheritance, or even a major gene contribution. They indicate that quantitative multifactorial heredity may be operating, rather than family environmental factors.

The Cleveland Clinic data,[5] shown in Table 6-2 are not directly comparable with those of Korelitz as the series of 838 inflammatory bowel disease patients all had the onset of their disease before 21 years of age. Although the number of affected parents was more than the number of affected sibs, it can be anticipated that more sibs subsequently will develop the disease because of the youth of the propositi. On the whole, however, these Cleveland findings lend support to Korelitz's,[4] and support the concept that polygenic inheritance is important in the etiopathogenesis of IBD.

Our study of the families of 336 Liverpool (UK) families produced somewhat different results, as can be seen in Table 6-3. Sib-sib combinations were found more frequently than parent-child combinations, compared to the preponderance of the latter in the New York and Cleveland series,[4,5] and a report from the Netherlands also provided similar results.[6] Though the Liverpool study found a marked "same-generation" distribution, it provided no evidence for a strong single-gene inheritance, and the data suggest that polygenic influences, infective influences, or both, are operating in IBD.

Twins*

Table 6-1 lists the information published up to 1977 on IBD occurring in twins. Among the monozygotic twins there was a high concordance rate for Crohn's disease (7 of 8) but not for CUC (5 of 11). Because it is difficult to imagine why clinicians would more readily report a pair of twins when only one has CUC than when only

TABLE 6-3. *Inflammatory bowel disease among first-degree relatives of 336 Liverpool (U.K.) patients with Crohn's disease or ulcerative colitis.*

	Ulcerative Colitis patients[*]	Crohn's Disease patients[**]
With affected relative	20	31
One generation only affected	13	17
Two generations affected	7	14
Relationships:		
Father-offspring	2	6
Mother-offspring	5	8
Sib-sib	16	27
Number of relatives:		
Parents	342	330
Sibs	533	487
Offspring	251	254

[*]n = 171
[**]n = 165

*See also Chapter 1.

one is affected by Crohn's disease, these data support a theory that while heredity is important in IBD, it is more important in CD than in CUC. Since 1977, there has been a further report of discordance of CUC in identical twins, and another concerning monozygotic twin boys who developed Crohn's disease affecting the terminal ileum, colon, and rectum within eight months of each other.[7,8] Other authors reviewed 11 sets of twins with CD and found that all became symptomatic within 6 years of each other, and in seven, the interval between the disease onset in each of the twin pairs was less than one year.[9] While four pairs were living in the same environment, two pairs were living apart, in one instance for ten years.

There has not yet been a report of twins in which one has Crohn's disease and the other CUC, even though the two diseases are so often found in sib pairs and in parent-child combinations. This provides further evidence that the two conditions may have a quantitative genetic relationship.

The family studies in IBD have yielded no evidence to suggest that a "typical" infectious agent is operating etiopathogenetically either in CUC or CD, because the diseases may occur in family members widely separated geographically and socially, and it does not seem that any nonhuman species is serving as a reservoir for a microbial agent(s).

Spouses

According to Table 6-1, until 1976 there had only been three examples of both spouses in a marriage being affected by IBD, and since then, only five more have been reported.[4,10-13] Although in some instances one spouse had Crohn's disease and the other CUC, which might indicate that the two conditions involve the same exogenous agent, it is more likely that this was a chance occurrence. In one such example, the wife developed ulcerative colitis, then 7 years later her son developed ulcerative proctitis, and 2 years after that her husband developed Crohn's disease of the distal ileum.[10] It is reasonable to conclude that the paucity of spouse-spouse cases does not favor the involvement of a "typical" infectious agent in the etiopathogenesis of IBD.

Positive Family History

The numbers with a positive family history in the reported series of inflammatory bowel disease patients vary, ranging between 10 and 40%.[14] In an early study in the United Kingdom, Paulley reviewed the family histories of 169 cases of ulcerative colitis and found that 19 (11.3%) had an affected first-degree relative, while 98 controls had only 2 sibs with ulcerative colitis.[15] In a slightly later report on patients with CUC from the United States, a smaller percentage had a positive family history, but in this study the patients' relatives were not interviewed,[16] as they had been by Paulley.[15] When such interviewing is done, the percentage with idiopathic inflammatory bowel disease is higher than when only the patients are questioned, because individuals can be quite ignorant of the state of health of other family members, even their brothers and sisters living in the same town.

Data from Kirsner's clinic in Chicago show several features that are of interest (Table 6-4).[17] One is that out of the 1084 cases of ulcerative colitis, there were 66 (6.1%) with a positive family history of IBD, while in those with Crohn's disease, 20 out of 185 (10.8%) had a positive family history. Later, the same author reported that of 103 families with more than one case of inflammatory bowel disease, 31 contained intermingled examples, that is, one member with CUC and another with CD.[3] In addition, although the differential diagnosis of Crohn's disease and ulcerative colitis can be difficult and there may be uncertainty about the diagnosis in relatives, some families may have members with "classic"

TABLE 6-4. *Inflammatory bowel disease—affected relatives (Chicago).*

Disease	Number of Patients	Numbers with Positive Family	Ulcerative Colitis in Relatives	Crohn's Disease in Relatives
Ulcerative colitis	1084	66	75	13
Crohn's disease	185	20	9	12

(Adapted from Kirsner, J. B., and Spencer, J. A.: Ann. Intern. Med., 59:133, 1963.)

TABLE 6-5. *Inflammatory bowel disease in relatives of Cleveland Clinic patients.**

	Number of Patients	Positive Family History	First-degree Relatives
Ulcerative colitis	316	93 (29.4%)	50 (15.8%)
Crohn's disease	522	187 (35.8%)	87 (16.7%)

*All the propositi had the onset of IBD prior to age 21 years. (Adapted from Farmer, R. G., Michener, W. M., and Mortimer, E. A.: Clin. Gastroenterol., 9:271, 1980.)

Crohn's disease affecting the small bowel and a colitis that lacks the features of Crohn's disease, which relates directly to reports documenting that CUC and CD may coexist in an individual.[18]

More recent data from the Cleveland Clinic relate only to patients with an onset of IBD before the age of 21 (Table 6-5).[5] Of their 316 ulcerative colitis patients, no less than 29% had a positive family history of inflammatory bowel disease. In those with Crohn's disease it was even higher, with 35% having a positive family history, and in both forms of IBD there was an unusually high incidence of affected second degree relatives, including grandparents. This high incidence and type of positive family history is similar to that seen in "early onset" cases of other diseases in which a polygenic basis is involved. For instance, patients in whom duodenal ulcer develops under the age of 15 have a high incidence of duodenal ulcer in both their parents.[19]

Table 6-6 shows data from Broadgreen Hospital and the Colon Clinic of the Royal Liverpool Hospital, in which the patients and their relatives were investigated in some detail. The results show the same trends as those in Chicago. Among the 171 ulcerative colitis patients, there were 25 (14.6%) who had relatives with inflammatory bowel disease, while in the 165 Crohn's patients, 35 (21.2%) had affected family members. Again, note the higher incidence of a positive family history among the Crohn's disease patients, and that there was an intermingling of ulcerative colitis and Crohn's disease among the relatives. Of the affected relatives of the patients with CD there were 18 who had ulcerative colitis, but there were only 3 cases of Crohn's disease in the 30 affected relatives of those with CUC.

The data presented in Table 6-7 show that in a Liverpool family study, no significant clinical differences were found between patients with a positive family history and those who had no known affected relative. In particular, those with an affected family member, who perhaps might be expected to have a stronger genetic component in their etiology, did not have either

TABLE 6-6 *Results of study of families of 348 Liverpool patients with inflammatory bowel disease. The numbers are given of the patients with a positive family history of inflammatory bowel disease in first-degree or second-degree relatives. The numbers with at least one first-degree relative affected, and the conditions found in the first-degree relatives are tabulated.*

	Ulcerative Colitis	Crohn's Disease	Unclassified Inflammatory Bowel Disease
Probands (numbers studied)	171	165	12
Positive family history of inflammatory bowel disease			
Number	25	35	1
Percentage	14.6	21.2	8.3
First-degree relative affected:			
Number	20	31	1
Percentage	11.7	18.8	8.3
Disease in first-degree relatives:			
Ulcerative colitis	17	19	1
Crohn's disease	2	21	0
Unclassified inflammatory bowel disease	4	2	0

TABLE 6-7. *Analysis of 336 IBD patients in Liverpool: Family History of Inflammatory Bowel Disease.*

	Crohn's Disease			Ulcerative Colitis		
	Number	Positive Family History	Percentage	Number	Positive Family History	Percentage
Total:	165	35	21.2	171	25	14.6
Males	58	12	20.7	67	8	11.9
Females	107	23	21.5	104	17	16.3
Age at diagnosis:						
0 to 25 years	83	19	22.9	68	9	13.2
26 to 99 years	82	16	19.5	103	16	15.5
Extent at diagnosis:						
Small bowel	27	6	22.2	0	0	—
Small bowel and colon	68	13	19.1	0	0	—
Colon	57	13	22.8	171	25	14.6
Anus affected	47	10	21.3	8	1	12.5
Religion:						
Anglican	93	19	20.4	91	9	9.9
Roman Catholic	51	6	11.8	55	11	20.0
Jewish	5	5	100.0	3	1	33.3
Complications	56	8	14.3	59	11	18.6
No complications	111	26	23.4	121	14	11.6
Remissions	50	10	20.0	99	16	16.2
No remissions	115	25	21.7	72	9	12.5
Severity:						
Mild	40	8	20.0	76	9	11.8
Moderate	42	8	19.0	55	10	18.2
Severe	83	19	22.9	40	6	15.0

an earlier age at onset, or more severe or extensive disease than the nonfamilial cases.

There have been a number of reports of relatives who have developed the same type or distribution of IBD, or the same complication. For instance, toxic dilatation of the colon has been observed in two relatives with Crohn's disease.[20] This might suggest that a familial tendency exists for this infrequent complication, but to establish whether or not this is true would entail a detailed clinical comparison of familial cases within a large series of patients. However, in a study of 10 families in which 32 cases of inflammatory bowel disease developed, it was noted that 3 of 4 affected sib pairs with identical HLA haplotypes had similar disease patterns.[7] The remaining HLA identical pair had one sib with Crohn's of the small bowel and the other with classic ulcerative colitis. In 6 of the 10 families, those affected either all had Crohn's disease or ulcerative colitis. In the other 4 families, the two diseases were intermingled.

Genetic Markers

The discovery of some mark of individual susceptibility would be a considerable asset to advancing the understanding of idiopathic inflammatory bowel disease. Statistical associations such as those between duodenal ulcer, the ABO blood groups, and the salivary secretor status,[21] while not of importance in any individual case, taken overall in a group of affected patients indicate that inherited factors are involved in the disease. Furthermore, when the association is as strong as that between duodenal ulcer and hyperpepsinogenemia,[22] or that between ankylosing spondylitis and HLA-B27, it can contribute in differential diagnosis.

Unfortunately, although there have been many attempts to find blood group associations with inflammatory bowel disease, none has been successful. The distributions of the ABO and Rhesus blood groups and the secretor and nonsecretor frequency either in ulcerative colitis or Crohn's disease do not differ from population controls.[23-27]

Reports of abnormal distributions of HLA-A and HLA-B antigens in some series of inflammatory bowel disease patients have not been confirmed by others.[27-35] There is certainly no strong association between CUC or CD and any particular A or B antigen comparable to that of HLA-B8 with celiac disease.

Kemler et al. studied 15 sib pairs with inflammatory bowel disease and found no support for the hypothesis that a gene locus close to the HLA-A or HLA-B loci predisposes to its development.[7] Four pairs shared both HLA haplotypes compared with 3.75 expected by chance, seven pairs shared one HLA haplotype compared to 7.5 expected by chance, and 4 shared no haplotype compared to 3.75 expected by chance.

In another study of 10 sib pairs, the ratios of HLA-identical-to-haplo-identical-to-HLA-difference were 2:7:1, which is random (2.5:5:2.5 expected). The haplotypes carried by the probands were distributed equally between affected and nonaffected sibs, namely 13:11.[37] Thus, in both of these sib pair studies there was no indication that the inheritance of the disease is linked to HLA-A or HLA-B loci.* There have only been a few studies of HLA-DR antigens in inflammatory bowel disease, and these have been provocative but inconclusive. For example, a Japanese series of only 40 ulcerative colitis patients showed an excess of DR2,[38] while a Belgian study of 206 Crohn's disease patients found a deficiency of DR3 compared with 180 normal controls.[39] Although Burnham et al. reported a significant reduction in the overall incidence of HLA-DR2 in their series of patients with IBD, when CUC and CD were considered separately, the reduction was not significant in either disease.[36]

Associations with Other Disorders†

Several curious associations have been noted between IBD and other conditions in which heredity is involved; such as Hermansky-Pudlak syndrome, which is completely genetic in etiology; ankylosing spondylitis, which has a strong genetic basis with a major gene; and Turner's syndrome, in which there is an abnormal X chromosome.

The Hermansky-Pudlak syndrome is characterized by tyrosine-positive albinism with a defect in the second phase of platelet aggregation, widespread accumulation of a ceroid-like pigment in tissue, and interstitial pulmonary fibrosis with pulmonary insufficiency also has been noted to occur.[40] Schinella et al. diagnosed idiopathic colitis in five of nine albinos in two Puerto Rican families living in New York City.[41] One woman with severe colitis had a brother who died of severe colitis at the age of 17. In the other family, a female albino had required colectomy and two of her albino sisters also had colitis requiring partial colectomy. In each instance, while the clinical diagnosis was ulcerative colitis, the resected colon showed long linear ulcerations, focal mucosal, and noncaseating granulomas, considered typical of Crohn's colitis. Unfortunately, any direct significance of these findings to the etiopathogenesis of IBD remains obscure.

The proportion of CUC and CD patients who have ankylosing spondylitis is much higher than one would expect to find in a random sample of the population.[42-44] The magnitude of the association varies with the diagnostic criteria and the epidemiologic techniques used,[45] but in a Leeds (U.K.) series nearly 20% of male colitics and over 7% of female colitics had ankylosing spondylitis (AS).[46]

It is not certain whether the AS is a complication of inflammatory bowel disease or an associated disease. Because the spondylitis sometimes develops before the bowel disease (see Chapter 16), this may make it more difficult to regard the disease as a complication of IBD, but this point will be referred to later. It is pertinent that when 47 patients whose only diagnosis was ankylosing spondylitis were investigated by sigmoidoscopy, rectal biopsy, and barium enema, 8 had evidence of colitis, and of these, 3 had no gastrointestinal symptoms.[47] Among the first degree relatives of a series of 142 patients in the United Kingdom who had IBD,[48] there were 3 with ankylosing spondylitis, but they had no evidence of inflammatory bowel disease either clinically or on barium enema examination and sigmoidoscopy. Macrae and Wright also found ankylosing spondylitis in some relatives of patients with colitis,[46] and an association between AS and IBD in the families of patients with IBD had been noted previously. Ankylosing spondylitis is strongly familial, and about 90% of the patients

---

*Editors's note: See also Biemond, L., et al.: Gut, 27:934, 1986. HLA-A2 was associated with risk of Crohn's disease while HLA-A11 was associated with a decreased risk. HLA-B27 and HLA-Bw35 showed increased risk of CUC in Caucasians; risk was increased in Japanese patients with HLA-B5.

†See also Chapter 1.

are HLA-B27 positive compared to less than 10% of the general population.[49] Although some have reported that of patients with spondylitis who have IBD only 60 to 80% have HLA-B27,[50-53] the inclusion of patients with sacroiliitis rather than true ankylosing spondylitis is probably the explanation for these lower figures. In support of this suggestion, in a small group of IBD patients who were HLA tested, all 4 of the patients with spondylitis had HLA-B27, and they were among the total of 9 who had HLA-B27. Of 5 patients possessing HLA-B27 but without spondylitis, 3 were female and therefore perhaps less likely to develop the condition. Of the 6 male IBD patients with HLA-B27, 4 had already developed ankylosing spondylitis. The high frequency (66%) of ankylosing spondylitis in this small series of HLA-B27-positive inflammatory bowel disease patients stands in sharp contrast to a prevalence of ankylosing spondylitis of about 5% in HLA-B27-positive people in the general population. This suggests that IBD may be a potent initiating or potentiating factor in the development of ankylosing spondylitis, and that possibly the latter is a complication of IBD. Perhaps there is already subclinical but nevertheless active bowel disease in those patients in whom ankylosing spondylitis appears to develop first, and perhaps the same applies to the relatives with spondylitis who were unable to demonstrate bowel disease.[48] These meager data also suggest that by HLA typing of all ulcerative colitis and Crohn's disease patients, it may be possible to identify the few who have a 66% likelihood of developing ankylosing spondylitis.

Several reports of IBD in patients with Turner's syndrome have been documented, so perhaps its incidence in this syndrome is higher than in the general population.[54-56] If so, this would imply not only a true association between the conditions, but also that the abnormal state of the single X chromosome perhaps increases a genetic predisposition to IBD. It is interesting that in one Turner's syndrome patient with CD reported by Kohler and Grant, there was an unusually high prevalence of karyotypes featuring a structurally abnormal X chromosome;[56] conceivably, this might be part of the cause of the patient's Crohn's disease, or be a result of the Crohn's disease itself. In a study of 50 Crohn's disease patients, Emerit and Michelson found a significant increase in the incidence of chromosomal breaks in all of them compared to 50 controls.[57] Not only was an increased chromosome breakage rate found in lymphocyte cultures from the patients with Crohn's disease, but also contact with the patients' lymphocytes produced chromosome breaks in normal lymphocytes, suggesting that a chromosome damaging agent was released by the patients' cells. While these findings are interesting, further studies are needed to explore their significance.

Although there have been examples of IBD occurring in patients with certain inherited immunologic deficiencies, the significance of these associations is unknown.[58-61]

Genetic Susceptibility

When it became clear some years ago that there are strong familial associations of ulcerative colitis with Crohn's disease, a theoretic explanation was advanced that the two diseases had certain genes in common in their genotypes.[62] It was speculated that if about 10 gene loci were involved in polygenic systems determining a quantitative liability to develop either of these diseases, 3 or 4 of the genes might be common to the two genotypes. As more data have accumulated, however, particularly the repeated demonstration of a stronger family history in CD than in CUC, this theory of overlapping genotypes became inadequate to explain all the family findings.

A more likely explanation for the association between Crohn's disease and ulcerative colitis in their familial occurrences is that there is one genotype, with perhaps 10 or 15 genes, making individuals liable to develop inflammatory bowel disease.[63] If a person possesses only a few of these genes, he or she is more liable to develop ulcerative colitis; however, if he or she has many of the genes (a more complete genotype), then Crohn's disease is more likely. This would explain why relatives of patients with Crohn's disease are more prone to develop inflammatory bowel disease than relatives of individuals with ulcerative colitis. In our present state of knowledge, this seems to be the most likely explanation for the familial patterns of IBD.

Environment and Heredity

It cannot be ruled out that the reason for the occurrence of Crohn's disease and ulcerative colitis in the same family is not primarily genetic, but rather that both conditions have the same environmental cause. If this were the case, however, a more even geographic distribution of the two diseases would be expected, and what evidence there is suggests that the incidence of ulcerative colitis is fairly uniform in the western world, whereas that of Crohn's disease is variable (see Chapter 1).[14] Also, if the two diseases were a result of the same environmental agent, why should the true incidence of Crohn's disease have increased in some areas of the western world in the past 25 years, while that of ulcerative colitis has remained static?[14] One possible response is that the environmental factors are different, and those that cause ulcerative colitis are steadily being "outstripped" in some regions by the factors that cause Crohn's disease. Alternatively, while both diseases may involve the same primary agent, the development of Crohn's disease may also require the action of second (additive) environmental agents, the presence of which have increased in some environments in recent years. This could also explain why many clinicians have patients who had all the criteria of ulcerative colitis ten years ago, and now have Crohn's disease.

Whether the two diseases have different or the same exogenous causes, their relationship in families must have some genetic basis. It is a reasonable hypothesis that all diseases without a simple mendelian pattern of inheritance are caused by a mixture of environmental factors acting on people with various susceptibilities that are genetically determined. Such states are difficult to analyze because both the environmental cause and the degree of genetic susceptibility can vary quantitatively. In some diseases heredity is the more important factor, whereas in others an environmental "attack" may be the major cause. The evidence points to both environment and heredity as being involved in the etiology of CUC and Crohn's disease, and the various interpretations of current epidemiologic and other data are summarized in Table 6-8.

TABLE 6-8. *Possible Bases for the Familial Relationship of Ulcerative Colitis and Crohn's Disease.*

Genetic	Environmental	Fit with Epidemiologic and Other Data
Different	Different	No
Same	Different	Poor
Different	Same	Poor
Same	Same	Poor
Shared*	Different	Possible
	Two factors+	Best

*Crohn's disease developing with fuller genotype; ulcerative colitis with partial genotype.
+One factor for inflammatory bowel disease and an additional one for Crohn's disease

REFERENCES

1. Crohn, B. B.: The broadening concept of regional ileitis. Am. J. Dig. Dis., *1*:97, 1934.
2. Allchin, W. H.: Ulcerative colitis. Proc. R. Soc. Med., *2*:59, 1909.
3. Kirsner, J. B.: Genetic aspects of inflammatory bowel disease. Clin. Gastroenterol., *2*:557, 1973.
4. Korelitz, B. I.: Epidemiological evidence for a hereditary component in Crohn's disease. *In* Recent Advances in Crohn's Disease. Edited by A. S. Peña, I. T. Weterman, C. C. Booth, and W. Strober. Boston, Martinus Nijhoff, 1981.
5. Farmer, R. G., Michener, W. M., and Mortimer, E. A.: Studies of family history among patients with inflammatory bowel disease. Clin. Gastroenterol., *9*:271, 1980.
6. Weterman, I. T., and Peña, A. S.: Familial incidence of Crohn's disease in the Netherlands and a review of the literature. Gastroenterology, *86*:449, 1984.
7. Kemler, B. J., Glass, D., and Alpert, E.: HLA studies of families with multiple cases of inflammatory bowel disease (IBD). Gastroenterology, *78*:1194, 1980.
8. Klein, G. L., Ament, M. E., and Sparkes, R. S.: Monozygotic twins with Crohn's disease: a case report. Gastroenterology, *79*:931, 1980.
9. Morichau-Beauchant, M., et al.: Entérite Régionale chez des jumeaux homozygotes. Revue de la littérature á propos du IIe cas rapporté. Gastroenterol. Clin. Biol., *1*:783, 1977.
10. Rosenberg, J. C., Kraft, S. C., and Kirsner, J. B.: Inflammatory bowel disease in all three members of one family. Gastroenterology, *70*:759, 1976.
11. Zetzel, L.: Crohn's disease in a husband and wife. Lancet, *2*:583, 1978.
12. Whorwell, P. J., Eade, O. E., Hossenbocus, A., and Bamforth, J: Crohn's disease in a husband and wife. Lancet, *2*:186, 1978.
13. Mayberry, J. F., Rhodes, J., and Newcombe, R. G.: Familial prevalence of inflammatory bowel disease in relatives of patients with Crohn's disease. Br. Med. J., *1*:84, 1980.
14. Kirsner, J. B., and Shorter, R. G.: Recent developments in "nonspecific" inflammatory bowel disease. N. Engl. J. Med., *306*:775, 837, 1982.
15. Paulley, J. W.: Ulcerative colitis. Gastroenterology, *16*:566, 1950.
16. Banks, B. M., Korelitz, B. J., and Zetzel, L.: The course of nonspecific ulcerative colitis: review of twenty years experience and late results. Gastroenterology, *32*:983, 1957.
17. Kirsner, J. B., and Spencer, J. A.: Family occurrences of ulcerative colitis, regional enteritis and ileocolitis. Ann. Intern. Med., *59*:133, 1963.
18. Hamilton, S. R.: Diagnosis and comparison of ulcerative colitis and Crohn's disease involving the colon. *In* Pathology of the Colon, Small Intestine and Anus. Edited by H. T. Norris. New York, Churchill Livingstone, 1983.
19. Cowan, W. K.: Genetics of duodenal and gastric ulcer. Clin. Gastroenterol., *2*:539, 1973.
20. Mallinson, C. N., Candy, J. C., Cowan, R., and Prior, A.: Two first degree relatives with dilatation of the colon due to Crohn's disease. Guy's Hosp. Rep., *22*:211, 1973.
21. McConnell, R. B.: The Genetics of Gastrointestinal Disorders. London, Oxford University Press, 1966.
22. Rotter, J. I., et al.: Genetic heterogeneity of hyperpepsinogenemic I and normopepsinogenemic I duodenal ulcer disease. Ann. Intern. Med., *91*:372, 1979.
23. Birnbaum, D., and Menczel, J.: ABO blood group distribution in ulcerative and malignant diseases of the gastrointestinal tract. Gastroenterology, *37*:210, 1959.

24. Smith, R. S., and Truelove, S. C.: Blood groups and secretor status in ulcerative colitis. Br. Med. J., *1*:870, 1961.
25. Winstone, N. E., Henderson, A. J., and Brooke, B. N.: Blood groups and secretor status in ulcerative colitis. Lancet, *2*:64, 1960.
26. Atwell, J. D., Duthie, H. L., and Goligher, J. C.: The outcome of Crohn's disease. Br. J. Surg., *52*:966, 1965.
27. Biemond, I., et al.: Search for genetic markers associated with Crohn's disease in the Netherlands. *In* Recent Advances in Crohn's Disease. Edited by A. S. Peña, I. T. Weterman, C. C. Booth, and W. Strober. Boston, Martinus Nijhoff, 1981.
28. Asquith, P., et al.: Histocompatibility antigens in patients with inflammatory bowel disease. Lancet, *1*:113, 1974.
29. Gleeson, M. H., et al.: Human leucocyte antigens in Crohn's disease and ulcerative colitis. Gut, *13*:438, 1972.
30. Delpre, G., et al.: HLA antigens in ulcerative colitis and Crohn's disease in Israel. Gastroenterology, *78*:1452, 1980.
31. Tsuchiya, M., et al.: HLA antigens and ulcerative colitis in Japan. Digestion, *15*:286, 1977.
32. Lewkonia, R. M., Woodrow, J. C., McConnell, R. B., and Evans, D. A. P.: HL-A antigens in inflammatory bowel disease. Lancet, *1*:574, 1974.
33. Thorsby, E., and Lie, S. O.: Relationship between the HL-A system and susceptibility to diseases. Transplant. Proc., *3*:1305, 1971.
34. Woodrow, J. C., et al.: HLA antigens in inflammatory bowel disease. Tissue Antigens, *11*:147, 1978.
35. Cohen, Z., McCulloch, P., Leung, M. K., and Mervart, H.: Histocompatibility antigens in patients with Crohn's disease. *In* Recent Advances in Crohn's Disease. Edited by A. S. Peña, I. T. Weterman, C. C. Booth, and W. Strober. Boston, Martinus Nijhoff, 1981.
36. Burnham, W. R., Gelsthorpe, K., and Langman, M. J. S.: HLA-D related antigens in inflammatory bowel disease. *In* Recent Advances in Crohn's Disease. Edited by A. S. Peña, I. T. Weterman, C. C. Booth, and W. Strober. Boston, Martinus Nijhoff, 1981.
37. Allan, R. N.: Personal communication.
38. Asakura, H., et al.: Association of the human lymphocyte -DR2 antigen with Japanese ulcerative colitis. Gastroenterology, *82*:413, 1982.
39. Fiasse, R., et al.: Etude des antigénes HLA dans la maladie de Crohn. Acta Gastroenterol. Belg. *47*:137, 1984.
40. Witkop, C. J., White, J. G., and King, R. A.: Oculocutaneous albinism. *In* Heritable Disorders of Amino Acid Metabolism: Patterns of Clinical Expression and Genetic Variation. Edited by W. L. Nyhan. New York, John Wiley and Sons, 1974.
41. Schinella, R. A., et. al.: Hermansky-Pudlak syndrome with granulomatous colitis. Ann. Intern. Med., *92*:20, 1980.
42. Acheson, E. D.: An association between ulceration colitis, regional enteritis and ankylosing spondylitis. Q. J. Med., *29*:489, 1960.
43. Haslock, I., Macrae, I. F., and Wright, V.: Arthritis and intestinal diseases: a comparison of two family studies. Rheumatol. Rehabil., *13*:135, 1974.
44. McBride, J. A., et al.: Ankylosing spondylitis and chronic inflammatory diseases of the intestines. Br. Med. J., *2*:483, 1963.
45. Haslock, I.: Arthritis and Crohn's disease. A family study. Ann. Rheum. Dis., *32*:479, 1973.
46. Macrae, I., and Wright, V.: A family study of ulcerative colitis: with particular reference to ankylosing spondylitis and sacroiliitis. Ann. Rheum. Dis., *32*:16, 1973.
47. Jayson, M. I. V., Salmon, P. R., and Harrison, W. J.: Inflammatory bowel disease in ankylosing spondylitis. Gut, *11*:506, 1970.
48. Lewkonia, R. M., and McConnell, R. B.: Familial inflammatory bowel disease–hereditary or environment? Gut, *17*:235, 1976.
49. Emery, A. E. H., and Lawrence, J. S.: Genetics of ankylosing spondylitis. J. Med. Genet., *4*:239, 1967.
50. Mallas, E. G., Mackintosh, P., Asquith, P., and Cooke, W. T.: Histocompatibility antigens in inflammatory bowel disease. Their clinical significance and their association with arthropathy with special reference to HLA-B27 (W27). Gut, *17*:906, 1976.
51. Russell, A. S., et al.: Transplantation antigens in Crohn's disease: Linkage of associated ankylosing spondylitis with HL-Aw27. Am. J. Dig. Dis., *20*:359, 1975.
52. Dekker-Saeys, B. J., et al.: Clinical characteristics and results of histocompatibility typing (HLA-B27) in 50 patients with both ankylosing spondylitis and inflammatory bowel disease. Ann. Rheum. Dis., *37*:36, 1978.
53. Huaux, J. P., Fiasse, R., de Bruyere, M., and Nagant de Deuxchaisnes, C.: HLA-B27 in regional enteritis with and without ankylosing spondylitis or sacroiliitis. J. Rheumatol. (4th Suppl.), *3*:60, 1977.
54. Price, W. H.: A high incidence of chronic inflammatory bowel disease in patients with Turner's syndrome. J Med. Genet., *16*:263, 1979.
55. Arulantham, K., Kramer, M. S., and Gryboski, J. D.: The association of inflammatory bowel disease and X chromosomal abnormality. Pediatrics, *66*:63, 1980.
56. Kohler, J. A., and Grant, D. B.: Crohn's disease in Turner's syndrome. Br. Med. J., *282*:950, 1981.
57. Emerit, I., and Michelson, A. M.: Chromosomal breakage in Crohn's disease. *In* Recent Advances in Crohn's Disease. Edited by A. S. Peña, I. T. Weterman, C. C. Booth, and W. Strober. Boston, Martinus Nijhoff, 1981.
58. Parker, J. E., and Thomas, J. W.: Regional ileitis, leukaemia and humoral immune deficiencies in a family. Lancet, *2*:1038, 1972.
59. Korsmeyer, S. J., Williams, R. C., Jr., Wilson, I. D., and Strickland, R. G.: Lymphocytotoxic antibody in inflammatory bowel disease. A family study. N. Engl. J. Med., *293*:1117, 1975.
60. Engstrom, J. F., Arvanitakis, C., Sagawa, A., and Abdou, N. I.: Secretory immunoglobulin deficiency in a family with inflammatory bowel disease. Gastroenterology, *74*:747, 1978.
61. Slade, J. D., et al.: Inherited deficiency of second component of complement and HLA haplotype A10, B18 associated with inflammatory bowel disease. Ann. Intern. Med., *88*:796, 1978.
62. McConnell, R. B.: Genetics of Crohn's disease. Clin. Gastroenterol., *1*:321, 1972.
63. McConnell, R. B.: Inflammatory bowel disease: newer views of genetic influence. *In* Developments in Digestive Disease. Edited by J. E. Berk. Philadephia, Lea & Febiger, 1980.

7 · The Immunology of Inflammatory Bowel Disease

CHARLES O. ELSON, M.D.

The immune system has long been suspected of playing a major role in inflammatory bowel disease.[1,2] This belief is based on the pathology of the lesions, the response of the disease to immunosuppressive drugs, the systemic complications of immune etiology, and a variety of laboratory observations of immune abnormalities. Of these, perhaps the strongest evidence in favor of this hypothesis is the pathology of the lesions. In Crohn's disease, the bowel wall is infiltrated with lymphocytes, plasma cells, macrophages, neutrophils, and mast cells. There is lymphangiectasia, lymphedema, and lymph node hyperplasia, with granulomas frequently present in the bowel wall and to a lesser extent in the lymph nodes. In ulcerative colitis a similar infiltration of acute and chronic inflammatory cells occurs in the mucosal layer. The prominence of cells of the immune system in the lesions and a general correlation between the degree of such infiltration with disease activity, would seem to implicate the immune system in at least the pathogenesis of these diseases and perhaps in their etiology.

Before discussing the immunologic aspects of inflammatory bowel disease it is appropriate first to consider the possible role of genes that affect immune responsiveness in these diseases, particularly major histocompatibility complex genes that encode cell surface antigens important in both the induction and effector phases of the immune response.

Immunogenetics

The tendency for ulcerative colitis and Crohn's disease to occur in families is high, as is the high rate of concordance for disease among monozygotic twins,[3] indicating that there is a genetic component operative in these diseases. Considering the apparent involvement of the immune system in these diseases, this genetic factor may be one that alters immune responsiveness in a manner that leads to disease. This has prompted a number of studies on the relationship between IBD and genes known to affect immune responsiveness. Most of these studies have looked for a possible role of the human major histocompatibility complex (MHC) or HLA genes in patients with IBD.

Although MHC antigens were first discovered in relation to transplantation, hence the term major histocompatibility complex for the genes that encode them, it was subsequently learned that MHC genes control the ability of experimental animals to respond to certain antigens.[4,5] The structure of the MHC-gene products or HLA antigens is now known, and many of the genes that encode them have been identified and isolated. The MHC antigens can be divided into several classes based on their structure. Class I MHC molecules, which include the HLA-A, HLA-B, and HLA-C antigens, are composed of a single 45 kD glycoprotein associated with β-2 microglobulin on the surface of cells. Class I molecules are present on all nucleated cells and are important in the presentation of viral and other cell-surface-associated antigens to T cells. Class II MHC molecules, which include the HLA-DR, HLA-DP, and HLA-DQ antigens, encoded at three genetic loci termed DR, DP and DQ,[9] are composed of a 34 kD α chain and 29 kD β chain. Class II MHC molecules are present on B cells, macrophages, Kupffer cells, and activated T cells. Class II MHC molecules can also be expressed on other cell types, such as intestinal epithelial cells.[6-8] An individual inherits a set of alleles of HLA antigens (or haplotypes) from each parent and these alleles are co-dominant. Thus, all nucleated cells have six class I molecules, a set of three from each parent; the cells that express class II molecules have an additional six class II molecules. We now recognize that the purpose of these class I and class II MHC molecules is not to frustrate transplantation, but that they are involved in cell-to-cell recognition and signaling among lymphoid cells. For example, T cells can be divided into two broad groups. One group of T cells recognizes cell-surface-associated antigens in conjunction with class I MHC molecules. These T cells bear the CD8 antigen (formerly termed OKT8 or Leu 2) on their cell surface,[10] and most of these T cells have cytotoxic or suppressor functions. A second group of T cells recognizes soluble antigens in conjunction with class II MHC molecules. These T cells bear the CD4 antigen (formerly called OKT4 or Leu 3) on their cell surface; most of these T cells have helper or inducer functions. The CD4 and CD8 T cell molecules are thought to be important associative recognition structures that stabilize binding of T cell receptors to antigen that is associated with class I or class II MHC molecules, respectively.[11] Thus, MHC molecules play a central role in the triggering of T cells to foreign substances and in self-nonself recognition.

Considering the central role for MHC molecules in the induction and regulation of the immune system, it is not surprising that there has been a great deal of interest in the association of HLA antigens with human diseases.[12] Certain alleles of both class I and class II MHC molecules are associated with human disease, that is, these alleles occur more frequently in patients than would be expected by their distribution in the normal population. The best example regarding class I MHC molecules is the striking association of HLA-B27 with ankylosing spondylitis.[12] Note that this disease association is not with the HLA-B gene locus itself, but with one of approximately 40 allelic HLA-B antigens. An example of an association between class II MHC molecules and human disease is the association of HLA-DR3 with a variety of disorders, including celiac disease, dermatitis herpetiformis, chronic active hepatitis, and Graves disease. The disease association may also occur with more than one class II allele, for example, there is a much stronger association of type I diabetes mellitus with a combination of both DR3 and DR4 than is seen with either of these antigens alone.[5] Lastly, disease associations in which both a class I and class II allele seem to be involved have been noted. For example, B8 and DR3 are frequently associated in individuals with the diseases mentioned above for DR3 alone, although the association is stronger for the DR3 allele than it is for the B8 allele. Associations of two or more alleles with a disease usually occur when the alleles involved are in linkage disequilibrium, that is, they occur together more often than would be expected from their independent frequencies in the general population. Linkage disequilibrium among HLA alleles occurs in all populations studied to date, and although the alleles involved vary from population to population, they are quite consistent within a given population.[13]

The exact reasons for the association between a given disease and one or more HLA antigens is unknown. A number of theories exist, most of them based on what is known about the immunologic function of class I and class II MHC molecules.[12] One major theory is that certain immune response genes important to a disease are linked (not necessarily physically) to HLA. This theory assumes that an MHC-linked immune response gene controls the ability of the host to respond to an agent, such as a virus, etiologic for that disease. A second hypothesis postulates that HLA antigens act as receptors for agents that are etiologic for certain diseases. A third hypothesis is that certain HLA antigens might be structurally and therefore antigenically similar to an etiologic agent, that is, that there is "molecular mimicry" between the etiologic agent and the HLA antigen. According to this explanation, an agent might appear to the host as a self antigen, with the host therefore not responding, leaving the agent free to cause damage. Alternatively, the agent might elicit a response against itself, and thus trigger an autoimmune response to the host's self MHC antigen. A fourth hypothesis relates to the function of class I molecules in presenting viral antigens to cytotoxic T cells. It postulates that certain class I molecules are deficient in such presentation, thus allowing the infection to proceed and tissue damage to occur. More explanations exist, but their abundance indicates that the answer simply is not known.

Dausset has pointed out that diseases associated with HLA share some common features.[13] These include an unknown etiologic agent, an unknown pathophysiology, a hereditary tendency with no simple mendelian segregation, immunologic abnormalities, a subacute or chronic course, and little or no effect on reproduction. Inflammatory bowel disease certainly fits this description. Both population studies and family studies have been done in patients with inflammatory bowel disease to determine whether there is any association between HLA antigens and IBD. In population studies the frequency of HLA antigens in a patient group is compared to that of a reference group without the disease. Because the null hypothesis is that one or more antigens may be associated with the disease, the accepted statistical analysis is to correct the p values for the number of antigens tested. This statistical treatment has not been applied to all the studies done on patients with inflammatory bowel disease. Therefore, a distinction is made below between statistically significant associations that are based on corrected p values and those that are not.

The reported studies on HLA antigens in patients with Crohn's disease are listed in Table 7-1. The HLA-A, HLA-B, and HLA-C antigen frequencies have been measured in some 20 studies from different regions of the world.[14-33] Only three of these studies have shown any statistically significant associations of the HLA-A, HLA-B, or HLA-C antigens with Crohn's disease when the statistical analysis has been corrected for the number of antigens tested.[21,25,33] Even these positive results have been weak ones, with a relative risk of only 2 to 4, that is, the risk that an individual with that HLA antigen will get the disease relative to the risk that individuals lacking that HLA antigen will get the disease. By comparison, the association of HLA-B27 with ankylosing spondylitis has a relative risk of approximately 90. Other studies from the same geographic regions have not confirmed any of these HLA associations with Crohn's disease (Table 7-1). A number of HLA associations have been reported in which less stringent statistical analysis was used (Table 7-1, last column). These associations are inconsistent and frequently conflicting. Six studies have examined HLA-DR antigens. In four of these, no significant associations were found.[23-25,31] One study from Sicily found a weak but significant negative association with DR1 and DQw1 (formerly MT1/MB1) and a positive association with DRw53 (formerly MT3) in a small number of patients.[27] Another study from Japan found a positive association with DR4 and DR5.[33] These associations were not noted in the other four studies,[23-25,31] thus they remain unconfirmed.

The data on HLA antigens in patients with ulcerative colitis are summarized in a similar manner in Table 7-2. Again, most of the reports have found no association with HLA-A, HLA-B, or HLA-C antigens.[15,17-22,24,25,32,34-36,38,39] The four studies finding some statistically significant associations do not agree with one another (Table 7-2, sixth column,)[21,22,26,37] and have not been confirmed by a number of other studies from the same countries or geographic areas. HLA-DR antigens have been tested in five studies, four of which found no association.[24,25,34,36] One report of a positive association of ulcerative colitis with DR2 from Japan awaits confirmation.[38] In ulcerative colitis, as in Crohn's disease, a number of HLA associations have been found using a statistical analysis that did not correct for the number of antigens tested (Table 7-2, last column). No consistent pattern emerges from a consideration of these associations, and they most likely represent the "background noise" of the assay.

Thus, the population studies have not shown any consistent and statistically significant association between HLA-A, HLA-B, or HLA-C antigens in either Crohn's disease or ulcerative colitis*. The studies on the HLA-D region are fewer in number and incomplete, particularly because the HLA-D region is still being defined. New loci have been identified that have not been tested as yet, including alleles encoded in the DP locus, a locus that seems not to be in linkage disequilibrium with the other HLA antigens. In addition, heterogeneity has been identified within currently recognized DR antigens, indicating that the DR specificities may be supertypic ones common to a cluster of alleles, rather than being alleles themselves. It is possible that an association could be significant with one of the subtypic specificities in the DR locus where none was seen with the DR supertypic specificity, but the association is not likely to be strong in the ab-

---

*Editor's note: See also Biemond, I., et al.: Gut, 27:934, 1985, increased risk of Crohn's disease with HLA-A2, decreased risk with HLA-All; increased risk of CUC with HLA-B27 and HLA-BW35 in Caucasian patients; risk of colitis increased with HLA-B5 in Japanese patients.

TABLE 7-1. *HLA Antigens in Crohn's Disease.*

Author	Year	Country	Number of Patients	Locus, Number of Antigens Tested	Statistically Significant HLA Associations Corrected p Values*	Uncorrected p Values
Thorsby[14]	1971	Norway	19	A, 8; B, 12	None	Decrease in A3 (RR = 0.42) increase in B12 (RR = 2.1)
Gleeson[15]	1972	England	18	A, 6; B, 9	None	Increase in A3 (RR = 3.1)
Jacoby[16]	1974	England	74	A, 10; B, 16	None	—
Asquith[17]	1974	England	56	A, 6; B, 6	None	—
Lewkonia[18]	1974	England	30	A, 6; B, 4	None	—
Mallas[19]	1976	England	100	A, 8; B, 16	None	—
Bergman[20]	1976	Sweden	62	A, 8; B, 16	None	Increase in A17 (RR = 3.4)
Berg-Loonen[21]	1977	Holland	51	A, 3; B, 5; C, 3	Increase in B18 (RR = 3.7)	—
Woodrow[22]	1978	England, Holland	100	A, 10; B, 13	None	—
Peña[23]	1980	Holland	149	A, 8; B, 16; DR, 8	None	Decrease in DR2 (RR = 0.6)
			65		None	
Burnham[24]	1981	England	67	A, 11; B, 17; DR, 7	None	—
Smolen[25]	1982	Austria	27	A, 14; B, 17; C, 5; DR, 7	Increase in B12 (RR = 4.1)	—
Delpre[26]	1980	Israel	18	A, 14; B, 16	None	—
Caruso[27]	1983	Sicily	28	A, 2; B, 2; C, 2; DR, 9; MT/MB, 3	Decrease in DR1 (RR = 0.04) and MT1/MB1 (RR = 0.24); increase in MT3 (RR = 4.1)	—
Russell[28]	1975	Canada	77	A, 10; B, 15	None	—
Schwartz[29]	1980	USA	22	A, 9; B, 14	None	—
Eade[30]	1980	USA	64	A, 13; B, 15	None	—
Cohen[31]	1981	Canada	47	DR, 7;	None	—
		Europe	48	A, 15; B, 20	None	—
Hiwatashi[32]	1980	Japan	10	A, 8; B, 15	None	—
Fujita[33]	1984	Japan	62	A, 9; B, 24; C, 7; DR, 8	Increase in Bw46 (RR = 2.6), Bw51 (RR = 2.5), DR4 (RR = 4.8), DR5 (RR = 5.0)	—

*Statistically significant HLA associations using p values corrected for the number of antigens tested. HLA associations: when uncorrected, but not if corrected, p values were significant. RR = relative risk; "—" = not reported.

TABLE 7-2. *HLA Antigens in Ulcerative Colitis.*

Author	Year	Country	Number of Patients	Locus, Number of Antigens Tested	Statistically Significant HLA Associations Corrected p Values*	Uncorrected p Values
Gleeson[15]	1972	England	16	A, 6; B, 9	None	—
Asquith[17]	1974	England	48	A, 6; B, 6	None	Decrease in A3 (RR = 0.31); increase in A11 (RR = 3.2), A7 (RR = 2.1)
Lewkonia[18]	1974	England	37	A, 6; B, 4	None	—
Mallas[19]	1976	England	100	A, 8; B, 16	None	—
Bergman[20]	1976	Sweden	51	A, 8; B, 16	None	Increase in A1 (RR = 1.9), A8 (RR = 2.0)
Berg-Loonen[21]	1977	Holland	58	A, 3; B, 5; C, 3	Increase in A11 (RR = 3.0)	—
Woodrow[22]	1978	England, Holland	145	A, 10; B, 13	Increase in B27 (RR = 2.1)	Increase in B27 (RR = 2.1)
Burnham[24]	1981	England	75	A, 11; B, 17; DR, 7	None	Decrease in DR2 (RR = 0.6)
Smolen[25]	1982	Austria	30	A, 11; B, 17; C, 5; DR, 7	None	—
Schrumpf[34]	1982	Norway	54	A, 13; B, 21; C, 4; DR, 8	None	Increase in B8 and DR3 in hepatobiliary disease
Cottone[39]	1985	England	56	A, 13; B, 20; C, 2; DR, 9	None	—
Nahir[35]	1976	Israel	30	A, 8; B, 9	—	Increase in A2 (RR = 2.6), Bw40 (RR = 4.8); decrease in A10 (RR = 0.1)
Delpre[26]	1980	Israel	60	A, 14; B, 16	Increase in Bw35 (RR = 2.6)	Increase in Aw24 (RR = 2.1)
Caruso[36]	1985	Sicily	28	A, 9; B, 18; C, 4; DR, 9; MT/MB, 3	None	Increase in B5 (RR = 2.4) DR2 (RR = 2.3); decrease in DR3 (RR = 0.14)
Tsuchiya[37]	1977	Japan	44	A, 16; B, 20	Increase in B5 (RR = 3.9)	Decrease in Bw35 (RR = 0.2), Aw30/31 (RR = 0.04)
Hiwatashi[32]	1980	Japan	60	A, 8; B, 15	None	Increase in B5 (RR = 2.4); decrease in B7 (RR = 0.34)
Asakura[38]	1982	Japan	40	A, 11; B, 16; C, 7; DR, 12	Increase in DR2 (RR = 5.1)	—

*Statistically significant HLA associations using p values corrected for the number of antigens tested. HLA associations where uncorrected, but not corrected, p values were significant. RR = relative risk; "—" = not reported.

sence of at least a weak association with the presently known supertypic specificity. Any new HLA-D-locus determinants that are in linkage disequilibrium with the HLA-A, HLA-B, or HLA-C locus antigens already examined probably are not strongly associated with IBD, because one should see at least a weak association of the latter with IBD, for example, such as is seen between HLA-B8 and DR3. Because there are instances in which a strong association exists between a disease and the presence at the same time of two HLA-DR antigens, these sorts of associations will need to be sought in patients with inflammatory bowel disease. For example, juvenile diabetes is weakly associated with DR3 and DR4, but strongly associated with a combination of both DR3 and DR4 in the same individual.[5] Again, one would expect at least a weak association with each of DR alleles separately. A possibly confounding technical factor is that a class II molecule specificity that is important in the disease may not be recognized by currently available antibody reagents.[5] For example, the regions of class II molecules that antibodies recognize are not the same determinants that the T cell receptor recognizes.[9] New approaches to this problem involving the use of DNA gene probes and restriction fragment length polymorphism techniques may allow the identification of HLA or other genes important in these diseases.[5]

HLA antigens have also been studied in families with multiple-affected members. These sorts of studies provide different information from the population studies described above. In this type of study, one looks for a concordant or discordant segregation of HLA within the affected and unaffected members of a family. From this, one is able to tell whether a "disease gene" is physically present close to the HLA genes on the sixth chromosome. If so, the disease and a particular HLA haplotype should segregate together within a family more often than would be expected. Indeed, Schwartz et al. reported a striking association of disease and HLA haplotype in families with multiple-affected members, in which affected siblings shared identical HLA haplotypes in four out of five instances.[29] A number of other studies have now been reported, however, and none have confirmed this observation.[23,30,37,40,41] When one combines the data from all the reports, the frequency of IBD-IBD sibling pairs sharing two, one, or no haplotypes is approximately what would be expected by chance and is no different from the frequencies among IBD-nonIBD sibling pairs. These data argue that there is no IBD disease gene closely linked to the HLA genes on the sixth chromosome.

Not all immune response genes reside within the major histocompatibility complex.[4] Genes either in or close to the immunoglobulin-heavy-

TABLE 7-3 *Serum Antibodies in Inflammatory Bowel Disease.*

Antibodies to	Crohn's Disease	Ulcerative Colitis
Viruses	N	N
Mycoplasma	N	N
Chlamydiae	N	N
Bacteria		
Aerobic flora		
E. Coli	↑	↑
Lipid A	↑	↑
Anaerobic flora	↑	↑
Pathogens		
Mycobacteria	N	N
Others	↑	—
Food		
Milk proteins	N, ↑	N, ↑
BSA	N, ↑	N, ↑
Autoantigens		
Colon	↑	↑
Lymphocyte	↑	↑
Others	N	N

See text for references and specifics.
N = normal; ↑ = increased; — = not reported; BSA = bovine serum albumin.

chain-constant-region gene have been found experimentally to determine immune responsiveness to a number of protein and carbohydrate antigens. Thus, it is interesting that an association has been found between Crohn's disease and a particular IgG-heavy-chain allotype. Kagnoff et al. have reported a significantly increased frequency of the phenotype Gm (a,x,f; b,g) and the haplotype Gm$^{a,x;\,g}$, an association not evident in patients with ulcerative colitis.[42] A study of immunoglobulin allotypes performed on Dutch patients with Crohn's disease has not found a similar association; however, the population groups tested appear to be different.[43] The significance of a possible association between a Gm allotype and Crohn's disease is unknown, but one can speculate that the association involves a putative immune-response-gene locus that may be important in the disease.*

Despite having many features in common with diseases that do have HLA associations, there has been no consistent association demonstrated between inflammatory bowel disease and the HLA-A, HLA-B, HLA-C, or HLA-DR antigens tested, although the number of studies on HLA-DR antigens are relatively few. Studies on multiple-affected families do not support the presence of a disease gene closely linked physically to the MHC gene on chromosome 6. A report of a significant association between Crohn's disease and an immunoglobulin-heavy-chain allotype remains to be confirmed, but illustrates the point that genes outside the MHC locus can influence the immune response. The genes that might be involved in IBD have not yet been identified, but those genes that control or alter the immune response will continue to be a fruitful area on which to focus the search.

Systemic Humoral Immunity

The immune system can be divided conceptually in a variety of ways. One is a division into an afferent (induction) phase and an efferent (effector) phase. The induction of an immune response is a complex process requiring interactions among T cells, B cells, and antigen presenting cells such as macrophages. Clones of cells whose specific receptors are stimulated in these interactions expand logarithmically in number under the influence of growth-promoting lymphokines. In this way, clones that are originally present in only a small number expand sufficiently to effectively deal with the antigenic stimulus. Although the induction phase of the immune response is important to the understanding of IBD, it has not been studied sufficiently in such patients. Most available studies have addressed the effector phases of immunity. The effector phase will be divided into two systems in this chapter, humoral or cellular (Fig. 7-1). The humoral effector system consists of antibodies, complement, and neutrophils. Each of these components of humoral immunity can function alone, but they are most effective when acting in concert. The humoral effector system is involved in host defense against a wide variety of gram-positive and gram-negative bacteria. The cellular effector system consists of antigen-specific lymphocytes, lymphokines, and macrophages/cytotoxic T cells. The cellular effector system is important in host defenses against facultative intracellular bacteria, many fungi, and most viruses. A third effector system may soon need to be added, the natural killer (NK) cell, a lymphocyte that is spontaneously cytotoxic for certain target cells in the absence of prior sensitization. The factors that determine specificity and amplification of NK cells are still being defined. In both the humoral and cellular systems, the first component determines the specificity of the response, the second acts as an amplifier and cell recruiter, and the third consists of a potent nonspecific phagocytic cell. Although this division of the immune system is a useful framework for this discussion, this does not imply that only one or the other effector system operates in a given immune or inflammatory response. Frequently, both systems are activated and operative at the same time, although to varying degrees. An important additional division of the immune system that will be used in this chapter is that of systemic versus mucosal immunity. This division is artificial because these overlap, but mucosal immunity does appear to have some unique features which need to be understood and considered in studies on the immunology of inflammatory bowel disease. For our purposes here, this latter division will be used to distinguish studies done on peripheral blood, which will be assumed to pertain to the systemic immune system, from those done on intestinal tissues or cells, which will be assumed to pertain to the mucosal immune system.

---

*Editor's note: See also Gudjnsson, H., et al.: Gastroenterology, 92:1417, 1987; according to this study, no evidence exists that immunoglobulin allotypes can be used as genetic linkage markers in inflammatory bowel disease.

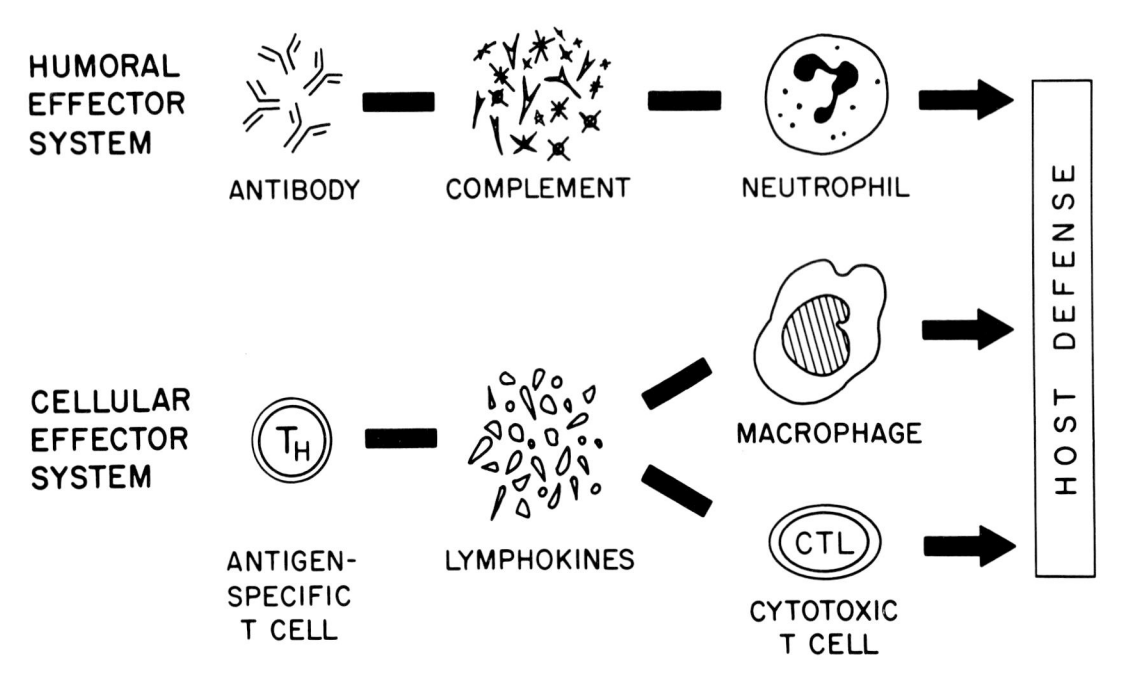

FIG. 7-1. Components of the humoral and cellular effector systems. The first component in each determines the specificity of the response, the second acts to amplify it, and the third is an effector cell.

Circulating Cells

The white blood cell count is frequently elevated in patients with inflammatory bowel disease. This increase is almost entirely a result of an increase in polymorphonuclear leukocytes,[44-46] although an increase in monocytes may also contribute.[44,46,47] The focus of most studies of circulating cells has been the lymphocyte. The total lymphocyte count in patients with Crohn's disease has been found to be either normal,[44,48-50] or decreased.[45,46,51-53] In contrast, the total lymphocyte count in patients with ulcerative colitis has generally been found to be normal,[45,49,50,51,53] with the exception of one study that found decreased lymphocyte counts only in patients with pancolitis.[44] The reason for the decreased lymphocyte counts in some patients with Crohn's disease is often multifactorial, including sequestration of lymphocytes in the lesions, loss of lymphocytes into the bowel lumen, and decreased production of lymphocytes because of malnutrition. This presumably explains why some investigators have found decreased lymphocyte counts only in patients with active Crohn's disease,[50,53,55] whereas others have found decreased counts only in patients with Crohn's disease of long duration and activity was not a factor per se.[46,52] One interesting report found that a low preoperative lymphocyte count (<1000/mm³) was significantly more frequent among patients with Crohn's disease who had early recurrences (<3 years) after surgery.[57]

LYMPHOCYTE SUBSETS. Lymphocytes can be divided into several major, functionally distinct subpopulations, such as T cells, B cells, and null cells. These subpopulations have been measured in the peripheral blood in a variety of diseases of apparent immunologic pathogenesis. Although this may be helpful in some diseases, it should be noted that the number of cells of a given subset present in the blood does not reflect the cells functional ability, nor is their number a measure of either pool size or turnover rate. For instance, the number of T cells and B cells is roughly equivalent in the body, but because B cells tend to be localized to tissues, whereas T cells recirculate constantly, the number of T cells in the peripheral blood is larger than the number of B cells.

Numerous measurements of lymphocyte subsets have been done in patients with inflammatory bowel disease. In patients with Crohn's disease the numbers of T cells, as measured by sheep erythrocyte rosetting (E^+), have been found to be decreased[46,48,49,51-53,56,58,59] more frequently than they have been found to be normal.[44,60-62] In contrast, in patients with ulcerative colitis, T cell numbers have been found more commonly to be normal[44,51,56,58,60] than they have been found to be decreased.[63,64] These results parallel those for total lymphocyte counts, and probably the E^+ T cells are decreased in some patients with Crohn's disease for the same reasons as discussed above. The average decrease in E^+ T cells in patients with Crohn's disease is relatively small and, although significantly different from normal, may not be physiologically significant.

The numbers of B cells present in peripheral blood have also been enumerated in patients with inflammatory bowel disease, usually by incubating peripheral blood lymphocytes with a fluorescein-labelled antiserum to human immunoglobulin. B cells have immunoglobulin molecules inserted in their surface membrane, and thus the antiserum will bind to their surface, allowing them to be counted. However, this type of antiserum can also bind nonspecifically to receptors for the Fc portion of immunoglobulin, a receptor that is present in not only B cells but also monocytes and null cells.[65] Using this method, the number of B cells in patients with inflammatory bowel disease has been found to be normal,[44,46,48,54-56,65] with some exceptions.[49,51] Because B cells also have receptors for the C3 component of complement, another technique used to enumerate them is to rosette peripheral blood cells with antibody-coated and complement-coated red blood cells (EAC). This technique is complicated by the presence of complement receptors on other cells, such as neutrophils and monocytes, that will also score positive. Although there was an early report that the numbers of such EAC-rosetting cells were decreased in both Crohn's disease and ulcerative colitis,[44] this result has not been confirmed by subsequent studies.[55,64,67,68] The number of B cells has also been enumerated using newer methods in which fluorescein-labelled F(ab^1)$_2$ anti-immunoglobulin reagents have been used, a technique in which only B cells are positive. Again, the numbers of B cells are essentially normal in Crohn's disease,[47,52,53,60,67] and also ulcerative colitis,[60] with the exception of one study that found decreased B cell numbers only in patients with Crohn's disease of long duration.[52]

T CELL SUBSETS. T cells with different functional activities can be distinguished by distinct surface glycoprotein markers. This was first demonstrated in experimental animals, and prompted a search for similar markers in man. An early attempt to find such markers was to subdivide T cells according to whether they had Fc receptors for IgM or Fc receptors for IgG. The former were thought to represent helper cells, the latter, suppressor cells. Decreases in the numbers of one,[69] or both,[53] of these subsets were found in patients with inflammatory bowel disease. It was subsequently learned, however, that these Fc receptors do not distinguish helper cells from suppressor cells,[70] and this technique has largely been supplanted by the advent of highly specific monoclonal antibodies that bind to various glycoproteins on the T cell surface membrane. Some of these monoclonal antibodies bind to a glycoprotein present on all T cells (CD3 or pan T cell marker; formerly OKT3, Leu-4), others to a glycoprotein only on helper/inducer cells (CD4; formerly OKT4, Leu-3), and others to a marker present on suppressor/cytotoxic cells (CD8; formerly OKT8, Leu-2).[10] T cells separated using these monoclonal antibodies have been shown to have distinct regulatory functions.[71] In recent years, these monoclonal antibodies have been used to enumerate the absolute number and proportion of T cell subsets present in the peripheral blood of patients with inflammatory bowel disease. Both the total number of T cells and the proportions among T cell subsets have been found to be normal in patients with IBD, whether the disease is active or inactive.[55,64,67,68,72] The one exception was a study in which patients with active Crohn's disease or ulcerative colitis had decreased absolute numbers of total T cells, helper T cells, and suppressor T cells without any change in the relative proportions among them.[50]

Interestingly, the normal number of T cells in patients with Crohn's disease in these recent studies using monoclonal antibodies conflicts with the decreased numbers of T cells found when sheep red blood cell rosetting was used to enumerate the T cells. The reasons for this are not clear and could include technical problems with sheep cell rosetting,[73] a change in the patient population (which seems unlikely), or the possibility that the sheep red blood cell receptor itself is decreased on T cells in patients with Crohn's disease while the total number of T cells remains normal. This latter is an interesting possibility, considering data indicating that the sheep erythrocyte receptor molecule (T11) is important in T cell activation.[74]

Enumeration of T cells and T cell subsets with monoclonal antibodies is a more sophisticated and reliable technique than what has been previously used, but these data must be interpreted with some caution. Although T cell subset markers generally correlate with certain T cell functions, the simple measurement of the number of T cells bearing a given marker cannot predict how such T cells actually function in vitro or in vivo. For example, patients with Crohn's disease with a potent circulating suppressor T cell had normal numbers and ratios of T cell subset markers.[75] Secondly, it is now evident that there is a good deal of functional heterogeneity among cells bearing either the CD4 helper/inducer (OKT4/Leu-3) or the CD8 suppressor/cytotoxic (OKT8/Leu-2) glycoproteins. Within the CD4⁺ T cell population, inducer T cells can be distinguished from helper T cells by the Leu-8 monoclonal antibody,[76] and CD4⁺ T cells that can suppress immunoglobulin synthesis have been identified functionally.[76,77] Within the CD8⁺ T cell population, suppressor T cells can be distinguished from cytotoxic T cells by the 9.3 monoclonal antibody,[76] and cells that contrasuppress (inhibit suppression) have been identified functionally.[78]

This functional heterogeneity makes the information that the numbers and proportion of the CD4⁺ and CD8⁺ T cell subsets are normal in patients with IBD less useful. The identification of diverse, smaller, more functionally homogenous T cell subsets will probably continue, particularly because techniques are now available to simultaneously identify and enumerate cells bearing two different cell surface markers. For example, cells bearing both the HNK-1 and Leu-2 marker have been found to be increased in patients with Crohn's disease,[75] and this small subset contains the "covert" suppressor T cell previously identified in these patients.[79] Continued identification of such subsets, coupled with the study of their functional properties in vitro, is likely to yield important new information about the immune system in general, particularly about how it might be malfunctioning in diseases such as Crohn's disease and ulcerative colitis.

The study of T cell activation antigens in patients with inflammatory bowel disease also appears promising. It was recently reported that T cells of patients with active Crohn's disease express the OKT9 surface antigen to a greater degree than either patients with inactive Crohn's disease or healthy controls.[80] The OKT9 antigen, or transferrin receptor,[81] is expressed on a variety of activated or proliferating cells. Not surprisingly, an increased expression of OKT9 antigen on T cells has been found also in patients with ulcerative colitis, sarcoidosis, systemic lupus erythematosus, rheumatoid arthritis, and after organ transplantation.[82] A possible feature distinguishing patients with Crohn's disease or ulcerative colitis from those with these other diseases may be an increased expression of Fc receptors for IgA on T cells that are also OKT9⁺ in IBD but not in the other diseases.[82] A second activation antigen, 4F2, has also been reported to be increased on peripheral blood T cells from patients with Crohn's disease.[59,83] Previous attempts at demonstrating peripheral T cell activation by testing for the presence of HLA-DR or Ia molecules on circulating T cells was largely negative both in Crohn's disease[47,50,60] and ulcerative colitis.[50] However, we are still beginning to understand the sequence of events that follows triggering of the T cell receptor.[84,85] A stereotypic sequence does appear to occur following such triggering that includes modulation of the T cell receptor itself, expression of receptors for interleukin-2, and expression of a variety of cell activation antigens, such as the transferrin receptor (OKT9), Ia antigens, and others.[84,85] As this process becomes better understood, more sensitive and specific reagents will probably become available that may allow us to better understand and follow T cell activation in IBD.

EFFECT OF TREATMENT ON CIRCULATING CELLS. Auer et al. showed that newly diagnosed but untreated patients with Crohn's disease did not have the decreased number of peripheral blood E⁺ T cells found in those with treated Crohn's disease of longer duration,[46,52] suggesting that treatment itself may affect the circulating cell populations. Few studies have been directed at this point. Sulfasalazine appears to have no major effect on circulating populations.[64,86] Corticosteroids are known to affect circulating cells acutely by altering margination and circulation patterns,[87,88] but there is currently no evidence that chronic therapy with corticosteroids alters the numbers or proportions of circulating cells in patients with IBD.[49,56,66,68] Azathioprine treatment does result in decreased total lymphocyte numbers with a proportionate decline both in T cells and B cells.[89,90] Peripheral blood antibody-dependent-cellular-cytotoxicity (ADCC) and the numbers of plasma cells in rectal biopsies are significantly reduced by azathioprine treatment, but return toward normal after cessation of therapy.[89]

In summary, the frequent elevation of the white blood cell count is a result of increases in neutrophils, and, to a lesser extent, monocytes. The total lymphocyte count may be decreased in patients with Crohn's disease, but is usually normal in patients with ulcerative colitis. The decreased lymphocyte counts seem to be primarily caused by a decrease in E^+ T cells, although recent studies using monoclonal antibodies have found normal numbers of T cells and normal proportions among T cell subsets. B cell numbers, using a variety of techniques to determine them, are normal. Circulating T cells express a number of activation antigens during disease activity, but not during remission. Treatment with azathioprine can decrease the lymphocyte count, but chronic corticosteroid or sulfasalazine treatment seems to have little or no effect on the number of circulating cells.

Serum Immunoglobulins

Serum immunoglobulins represent the total of all the preformed, circulating specific antibodies in the body. Thus, the serum immunoglobulin level is a rough measure of how much antibody the body has produced and has available to serve in host defense. Like other serum proteins, the serum immunoglobulin level represents an equilibrium between synthesis and catabolism; the level can be changed by an alteration in either parameter.[91] Serum immunoglobulin levels are nonspecific, crude evaluators of immunologic competency, but can be helpful and diagnostic in some disorders. For example, they are elevated in monoclonal gammopathies, a number of chronic infections, liver disease, collagen disorders, sarcoidosis, and AIDS; they are reduced in immunodeficiency disorders, protein losing enteropathies, burns, and the nephrotic syndrome.[92]

SERUM IMMUNOGLOBULIN LEVELS. The majority of patients with ulcerative colitis,[64,93-101] or Crohn's disease,[95,99,100,102-105] have normal levels of serum IgG, IgA, IgM, and IgE. In some series, a subset of patients has shown elevations in the serum level of one or more of these isotypes sufficient to increase the mean for the group to a statistically significant level.[101,106-110] These elevations have been found more frequently in ulcerative colitis,[106-110] than in Crohn's disease.[101,106,107] Among the isotypes, serum IgG has been reported as elevated most frequently,[105-110] followed by IgA,[106,107,109,110] and then IgM.[106,107] In the studies reporting elevations in serum immunoglobulins, often the highest levels have been found in patients with associated liver disease.[106,107] Because liver disease can elevate serum immunoglobulin levels by itself, and because patients with inflammatory bowel disease may have cryptic liver disease, this remains a possible confounding factor in such studies. Some investigators have noted a tendency for IgM to rise when patients go into remission,[107] receive corticosteroid therapy,[107] are treated with total parenteral nutrition,[111] or have diseased bowel resected.[112] These are not universal observations;[113] moreover, any such increase in IgM may be nonspecific, because patients with other diseases may also have elevations of IgM after intestinal resection.[114] Increases in the serum IgM level in patients with inflammatory bowel disease after intestinal resection did not correlate with any increase in the anticolon antibody titer, although there were increases in antibodies to the normal bacterial flora of the intestine.[114]

IMMUNOGLOBULIN TURNOVER. As mentioned above, serum immunoglobulin levels represent an equilibrium between synthesis and catabolism.[91] Although serum immunoglobulin levels are normal in most patients with inflammatory bowel disease, studies using radiolabelled immunoglobulin have demonstrated an abnormal increase in IgG and IgM turnover in most patients with Crohn's disease or ulcerative colitis.[93,94,102,103] The catabolic rate for IgG and IgM was increased in virtually every patient with Crohn's disease who was tested.[93,94] A concomitant increase in the catabolic rate for albumin and an increase in the loss of intestinal protein was often present at the same time, but the increased catabolic rate for IgG and IgM could not be explained solely by intestinal protein loss.[94] The synthetic rate for IgG was elevated in 18 of 21 patients with Crohn's disease, while the synthetic rate for IgM was elevated in 2 of 4 of the Crohn's disease patients tested. Similar studies have been done in patients with ulcerative colitis, showing comparable results.[102,103] Moreover, Jensen et al. have shown that the increase in catabolic rate and synthetic rate for IgG in patients with ulcerative colitis correlates directly with disease activity.[103] However, the percentage of patients with ulcerative colitis showing increased catabolism and synthesis of IgG is somewhat less than that found in Crohn's disease patients. Furthermore, the degree of increase in the catabolic rate is not as high in patients with ulcerative colitis as in those with Crohn's disease.[102] Thus, IgG turnover appears to be stimulated more consistently and to a greater degree in Crohn's disease than in ulcerative colitis. It bears mentioning that the serum immunoglobulin levels remained in the normal range in most patients in these studies showing increased IgG and IgM turnover, illustrating how the serum immunoglobulin levels themselves are an insensitive reflection of the dynamic changes in humoral immunity that are occurring in these patients.

IMMUNOGLOBULIN DEFICIENCY. Serum immunoglobulin measurements have identified rare patients with inflammatory bowel disease and concomitant hypogammaglobulinemia. Hypogammaglobulinemia has been identified in patients with Crohn's disease,[94,115-119] or ulcerative colitis.[120-123] Hypogammaglobulinemia itself is frequently associated with intestinal lesions, so one has to be careful about attributing intestinal inflammation to a second, distinct disease process in hypogammaglobulinemic patients.[122] This is particularly true in relation to ulcerative colitis, because rectal biopsies in patients with congenital hypogammaglobulinemia have revealed histologic colitis in the absence of any symptoms.[122] Nevertheless, the clinical course and the distinctive transmural lesions in the cases of concomitant hypogammaglobulinemia and Crohn's disease indicate that these diseases do occur together in rare instances. Selective IgA deficiency has also been reported in patients with Crohn's disease,[97,107,116,123] or ulcerative colitis,[102] as has selective IgG deficiency.[93] Too few cases of concomitant inflammatory bowel disease and immunoglobulin deficiency have been reported to determine whether the humoral deficiency alters the clinical course. Nor can one claim that such cases indicate that humoral immunity is not involved in the pathogenesis of the disease,[118] because in at least two recent cases the hypogammaglobulinemia occurred after the onset of the Crohn's disease and appeared to be a result of the generation of a suppressor T cell secondary to their Crohn's disease.[117] Patients with concomitant inflammatory bowel disease and immunoglobulin deficiency do represent an experiment of nature that might well yield new insights into the pathogenesis of inflammatory bowel disease, and such cases should be studied extensively whenever they occur.

Thus, serum immunoglobulin levels are normal in most patients with Crohn's disease or ulcerative colitis. The normal serum levels do not reflect the increased catabolism and synthesis of IgG and IgM that occur during active inflammatory bowel disease. The turnover of these immunoglobulins is stimulated more consistently and to a greater degree in Crohn's disease than in ulcerative colitis.

Serum Antibodies

Determining whether patients with inflammatory bowel disease have increased antibody levels to a given antigen would seem to be extremely straightforward: either antibody titers are increased or they are not. Many different techniques can be used to measure antibodies, however; techniques based on different properties, for example, agglutination, precipitation, and complement fixation, that are optimal for the detection of certain types of antibodies and may not be optimal for others. This is one explanation why reports of serum antibodies to the same antigen in patients with IBD have been conflicting.

Numerous reports are available on antibody titers to a wide variety of antigens, microbial and otherwise. Many are from studies where an etiologic agent was being sought. These reports are summarized in Table 7–3, clustered according to antigen category. The trend apparent in the table is that patients have increased serum antibody titers to antigens that normally encounter the immune system via the intestine, and have normal titers of serum antibody to antigens encountered outside the intestine.

ANTIBODIES TO VIRUSES, MYCOPLASMA, AND CHLAMYDIA. Patients with inflammatory bowel disease do not have an increase in antibody titers to enteric viruses such as rotavirus,[125-127] or to a variety of other, nonenteric viruses, with the exception of cytomegalovirus.[128,129] The latter has been isolated from the bowel of some patients with inflammatory bowel disease where it seems to be a superinvader. Serum antibodies to mycoplasma are also normal.[128] Although antibodies to Chlamydia trachomatis were reported to be increased in Crohn's disease,[130] this has subsequently been disproven; these patients do not have any increased antibody reactivity against C. trachomatis or other types of Chlamydia.[129,131–133]

ANTIBODIES TO FOOD ANTIGENS. Increased titers of antibodies to casein and β-lactoglobulin, measured with a tanned red cell hemagglutination technique, have been reported in patients with ulcerative colitis,[134] but not in patients with Crohn's disease.[135] No correlation of the antibody titer with the activity of the colitis was found. These results were not confirmed in subsequent studies using the same technique,[136–138] in which antibodies to these milk antigens were detectable in patients with ulcerative colitis or Crohn's disease but were not increased, although they were increased in patients with celiac disease.[136,138] Antibodies to bovine serum albumin have been reported to be normal or increased both in ulcerative colitis and Crohn's disease.[139,140] A possibly confounding factor in such studies relates to the ages of the patient and control groups, because the incidence of demonstrable antibodies to bovine serum albumin in normal individuals declines with age.[141] Thus, a control group significantly older than the patient group could yield a positive result based on the age difference alone. It is not clear that all studies have age-matched the control and patient groups. Recently, patients with ulcerative colitis or Crohn's disease have been found to have increased serum antibodies to β-lactoglobulin,[142] wheat,[143,144] and maize,[144] but no increase in antibodies to soya,[145] or to gliadin.[146,147]

ANTIBODIES TO BACTERIA. These include aerobic bacterial flora, anaerobic bacterial flora, enteric bacterial pathogens, and Mycobacteria.

Aerobic Bacterial Flora. Antibodies to aerobic bacteria in the intestine, such as E. coli, are detectable in the serum of normal individuals, but are increased above the normal background level in many patients with Crohn's disease or ulcerative colitis,[148–151] with a tendency for the antibody levels to be higher in the serum of patients with Crohn's disease than in those with ulcerative colitis.[149,151,152] Not all patients with inflammatory bowel disease have increased antibodies to E. coli, however; a number of negative studies have been reported,[152–155] although most of these concern patients with ulcerative colitis. Serum antibodies to the normal aerobic flora are directed toward different bacterial strains in different patients, and do not correlate with the site or severity of disease.[149] These antibodies may not represent the types of antibodies being produced locally in the intestine: local IgG antibodies to fecal anaerobic bacteria, but not to fecal aerobic bacteria, were detected in rectal biopsy homogenates from ulcerative colitis patients. The reverse was true in the serum, that is, serum antibodies were detected to fecal aerobic but not to fecal anaerobic bacterial species.[156] Considering the extent of ulceration that can occur in ulcerative colitis, it is surprising that high antibody titers are not found more often in these patients. An increased penetration of the mucosal barrier by bacteria, the normal explanation for increases in such serum antibodies, would seem to be a necessary but not sufficient condition, with the ability of the individual to respond to the bacterial antigen and the influences of regulatory cells also being required factors.

Bacterial endotoxin, or lipopolysaccharide, has, as the name implies, both a polysaccharide and a lipid component. The latter, known as lipid A, is responsible for most of the biologic effects of endotoxin. The structure of lipid A is fairly constant among Enterobacteriaceae, whereas the polysaccharide component varies. Antibodies to lipid A occur normally in man, being detectable in 10 to 34% of individuals by using a passive hemolysis method, and in even more when an ELISA is used.[157] Patients with Crohn's disease, but not those with ulcerative colitis, have been found to have increased titers of complement-fixing antibodies to lipid A when tested by passive hemolysis,[152,158] although the total IgG anti-lipid A levels, as measured by ELISA, was lower than normal both in Crohn's disease and ulcerative colitis.[157] Thus, the pattern of response to lipid A is similar to that previously noted for antibodies to E. coli: that is, increased in Crohn's disease and either normal or increased in ulcerative colitis.

Anaerobic Bacterial Flora. Sera from patients with inflammatory bowel disease have been tested for reactivity to various species of anaerobic intestinal bacteria, quantitatively the major component of the normal bacterial flora. Increased titers of serum agglutinins to B. fragilis and B. vulgatis have been found in patients with Crohn's disease.[159,160] Patients with Crohn's disease also have an increased prevalence of detectable agglutinins toward four species of anaerobic coccoid rods that are members of the normal bacterial flora. These four, belonging to the Eubacterium, Peptostreptococcus, and Coprococcus species, are increased in fecal isolates from patients with Crohn's disease.[161] Agglutinins to these four strains are detectable in some 60% of patients with Crohn's disease, although they are not detectable in normal individuals.[162–166] These strain-specific antibodies are of the IgG and IgM class and occur in low titer.[165] Sera positive for one strain tend to be positive for one or more of the others.[167] No correlation exists between these agglutinins and disease activity or other clinical parameters.[167] Agglutinins were detectable in coded sera from patients with Crohn's disease from all parts of the world.[168] The agglutination pattern of sera for these four strains has been proposed as a test to distinguish Crohn's disease from other disorders,[163] and it does seem to distinguish Crohn's disease from normal individuals,[164,166,168] with a sensitivity of only 54% but a high specificity.[165] The agglutinin pattern cannot distinguish Crohn's disease from ulcerative colitis, however,[166] because sera from patients with ulcerative colitis have an increased prevalence of agglutinins (11 to 51%), although not to as high a degree as sera from patients with Crohn's disease (35 to 83%).[168] Thus, the pattern of patients with Crohn's disease having a higher serum antibody response toward normal bacterial flora than do patients with ulcerative colitis holds true for antibodies to anaerobic bacteria as well. The usual explanation that these antibodies are simply caused by increased mucosal permeability is difficult to accept. Serum agglutinins were not found in patients with acute and chronic infectious diarrhea in India,[169] who would be expected to have an increased permeability, and they were more prevalent in patients with Crohn's disease of the small intestine than they were in those with ulcerative colitis.[168] Perhaps the nature of the ulceration is more important; patients with Crohn's disease may have higher antibody titers because their fissuring type of ulceration may allow bacteria to penetrate deeper into the bowel wall. Consistent with this idea, a patient with Crohn's disease was found to have increased agglutinins to bacterial strains cultured from a draining fistula,[170] and IgG-producing plasma cells seem to predominate along fissures and fistulae.[171] Another possibility is that patients with Crohn's disease simply have higher responses toward enteric antigens in general, perhaps because of alterations in local immunoregulatory mechanisms.

Enteric Bacterial Pathogens. Antibody titers to a variety of enteric pathogens have been measured as part of an attempt to define their possible role in inflammatory bowel disease. Most of these studies have been negative. Thus, no evidence is available that enteric pathogens such as Y. enterocolitica or C. jejuni are involved in inflammatory bowel disease.[172,173] Nevertheless, patients with active Crohn's disease have increased antibody titers to a variety of enteric pathogens that are not normally resident in the intestine.[174] This has been interpreted as a nonspecific sensitization to cross reacting antigens, perhaps resulting from an increased permeability of the mucosa to bacteria resident in the gut, with a resulting polyclonal B cell stimulation. An alternative is that these cross reacting antibodies may reflect an alteration of immunoregulatory mechanisms that normally dampen immune responses to enteric antigens.

Mycobacteria. Serum antibodies to a variety of mycobacterial antigens have been sought in patients with inflammatory bowel disease. No increase in IgG antibodies to M. tuberculosis antigens was detected by ELISA,[175,176] although patients with tuberculosis did have increased titers.[175] Patients with Crohn's disease do not have any increased reactivity to arabinomannin, a purified antigen common to most mycobacteria.[174] Thayer et al. have reported a small but statistically significant increase in the serum antibody titer of patients with Crohn's disease, but not of patients with ulcerative colitis, to M. paratuberculosis, a mycobacterium that cross reacts with a putative etiologic agent, M. linda.[176] This has not been confirmed in a study using the same assay, however,[177] nor has it been confirmed in another study using an agglutination assay.[162] In all, patients with inflammatory bowel disease seem to have a normal level of serum antibodies to mycobacteria.

AUTOANTIBODIES. Antibodies to colonic epithelial cells have been consistently identified in patients with ulcerative colitis or Crohn's disease by many investigators in reports that span two decades.[178–186] These antibodies will be discussed at greater length in the section on etiologic theories that follows.

Antibodies to Lymphocytes. Autoantibodies to lymphocyte surface membrane antigens occur in two major forms. One type, of the IgM class, is cytotoxic for lymphocytes when cultured with them in the cold while in the presence of complement. Other antibodies, usually of the IgG class, are identified by their ability to bind to, and interfere with, lymphocyte function in vitro. Cold-reactive lymphocytotoxins bind both to B cells and T cells, but appear to be predominantly directed at the former.[187] The target antigen on

B cells may be surface immunoglobulin.[187] Cold-reactive lymphocytotoxins have been found in 20 to 40% of patients with either Crohn's disease or ulcerative colitis.[188–192] Similar lymphocytotoxic antibodies have been found in 30% of family members of patients with either Crohn's disease or ulcerative colitis, a significant increase compared to family members of control patients. In these families, household contacts of patients, including spouses, were more often positive than non-household contact family members.[190] In addition, 19% of family members of Crohn's disease patients had a higher proportion of antibodies-to-synthetic RNA,[190,193] while none of the family members of ulcerative colitis patients did. These data have been taken to suggest a possible infectious etiology of inflammatory bowel disease. The presence of lymphocytotoxins does not correlate with age, sex, disease activity, drug therapy, prior allogenic sensitization via transfusion or pregnancy, peripheral blood lymphocyte counts, or antibodies to microbes.[188,191,194] The IgG class of anti-lymphocyte antibodies has not been specifically studied in inflammatory bowel disease, except that serum antibodies reactive with T cells have been found to bind to T cells of both helper and suppressor subsets.[192,195]

Anti-lymphocyte antibodies have been found to occur in a wide variety of diseases or conditions, including primary biliary cirrhosis, acute glomerulonephritis, malaria, old age, multiple sclerosis, Graves' disease, after organ transplantation, and after vaccination, to name a few. They occur most often in systemic lupus erythematosus (SLE) and rheumatoid arthritis.[196] In SLE, antibodies have been identified that react with a variety of different lymphocyte subsets, including T cells, B cells, NK cells, monocytes, and lymphoblasts. Some of the lymphocyte binding antibodies cross react with other tissue antigens, including neuronal and hemopoietic cell antigens, and some recognize Class I and Class II HLA molecules. Lymphocytotoxic antibodies reactive with suppressor T cells might contribute to the defect in this cell subset in SLE patients, but no evidence has been found that this occurs in vivo. Anti-lymphocyte antibodies consistently occur in a small, but not insignificant, percentage of normal controls (about 4%). Because of the larger number of normal individuals in the population, the total number of normal individuals with these antibodies is larger than the total number of patients with them in any given disease. The one common theme among all the diverse disorders that have an increased proportion of anti-lymphocyte antibodies is an active immune response. It seems likely that these antibodies represent an exaggeration of an homeostatic immunoregulatory mechanism normally operative during an immune response. They do not seem to be specific for viral infection or autoimmunity. Their role in vivo has yet to be determined in any disease, including inflammatory bowel disease.

Other Autoantibodies. Antibodies to thyroglobulin,[197–200] and to gastric parietal cell antigen,[198,199,201] are not increased in patients with inflammatory bowel disease. Thus, IBD does not fit into the cluster of autoimmune diseases known as the "thyrogastric complex," a group that includes autoimmune thyroiditis, Graves' disease, and atrophic gastritis. Serum from patients has no increased binding capacity for isolated human DNA,[193] and antinuclear antibodies generally have been negative.[198–201] Antibodies binding to human leukocyte nuclei have been reported in a variable number of patients.[197,198,202,203] Whether these are true autoantibodies or are a cross reactivity, for example between a bacterial antigen and some as yet undefined antigen in human granulocyte nuclei, is unknown. The latter possibility is suggested by the recent finding that some anti-DNA antibodies react with bacteria.[204] Anti-smooth muscle cell and anti-mitochondrial antibodies are not detectable in patients with IBD.[201] There are conflicting reports on antibodies to reticulin,[201,205] and isolated reports of antibodies to other putative autoantigens such as intestinal brush border,[201] cytoskeletal antigens,[206] and portal tract antigens.[186] The same question about cross-reactivity applies to these. In all, no convincing, consistent increase in antibodies to autoantigens is apparent other than to colonic epithelial cells and lymphocytes in IBD.

RESPONSE TO IMMUNIZATIONS. Few studies have been made of the response of patients to deliberate immunization. The primary and secondary response to a particulate viral antigen given intravenously was normal in a small number of patients with Crohn's disease or ulcerative colitis,[207,208] except for those who had decreased responses in the setting of known hyposplenism.[208] In contrast, patients with Crohn's disease or ulcerative colitis had significantly depressed IgG responses to a booster immunization with tetanus and diphtheria toxoids given intramuscularly, although the peripheral blood lymphocytes had a normal proliferative response to tetanus toxoid in vitro.[209] The decrease of in vitro IgG anti-tetanus lymphoblastoid B cell responses in this setting may be because of an increased activity by one or more of the suppressor cells that are known to regulate the lymphoblastoid B cells that are stimulated by booster immunization.[210] How these findings relate to the pathogenesis of IBD is unknown, but the use of immunization with defined antigens in these patients is an attractive approach that may reveal important information about the immune system, information that is unlikely to be forthcoming from the study of serum antibodies to a remote or assumed antigen exposure. The response of patients to defined antigens administered via the intestine has never been reported, but is a particularly important question considering the increase in serum antibodies to intestinal antigens (Table 7–3).

In summary, antigens that normally encounter the immune system via the intestine are the predominant ones to which patients with inflammatory bowel disease have increased antibody levels. A general trend is noted for patients with Crohn's disease to have higher antibody levels toward enteric antigens than patients with ulcerative colitis. Whether these antibodies play a role in disease pathogenesis is uncertain because similar antibodies are often present in normal individuals. Autoantibodies to colon epithelium and lymphocytes have been found, but the majority of patients do not have other types of autoantibodies. The anti-colon antibodies may represent a cross reaction with certain E. coli antigens, and the anti-lymphocyte antibodies a homeostatic immunoregulatory mechanism, so the term autoantibody may, in fact, be a misnomer. The spectrum of antibody specificities detected in patients with IBD suggests that the humoral immune response to most exogenous and endogenous antigens is normal, except for antigens encountered via the intestine. The explanation for this latter point is unknown at present. The usual explanation for increased antibodies to intestinal antigens is an increase in mucosal permeability caused by ulceration. However, the trend to higher levels of antibacterial antibodies in patients with Crohn's disease compared to ulcerative colitis, and the presence of antibodies to food antigens that should be digested long before reaching sites of ulceration in the colon, are difficult to fit into this explanation. Moreover, an increased influx of antigen into the body does not automatically equate with a serum response to it. For example, normal adults injected parenterally with the food antigen bovine serum albumin did not develop increased antibody titers,[141] suggesting a state of oral tolerance similar to that found in experimental animals fed soluble proteins. An alternative hypothesis is that these patients have an increased responsiveness to antigens that they encounter via the intestinal tract.

Complement

GENERAL BACKGROUND. The complement system consists of at least 20 glycoproteins that together comprise some 3 to 4% of the total serum proteins. Most circulate in an inactive precursor form. The concentration of the different components varies, with some being present in substantial amounts, for example, C3, C4, factor B, and others only at low concentrations. Most complement components are synthesized by the liver, but some are also synthesized by macrophages. The components can be clustered according to the phase of the complement cascade in which they are involved: the recognition or attachment phase, the activation and amplification phase, or the membrane attack phase.[211,212] Two independent pathways exist for the first two phases, the classic and the alternate, each of which has distinct components and activation requirements. However, both pathways use the same terminal membrane attack mechanism. The general scheme of the two pathways and the substances that activate each of them are shown in Figure 7–2. The complement system is controlled both by spontaneous decay or dissociation of activated components and by inhibitors to crucial components such as C1 and C3.

Although complement is associated with cell lysis, this is only one of many biologic functions mediated by the complement system, and its lytic capability is probably not its most biologically important function. Low molecular weight fragments of C3, C4, and C5, that is, C3a, C4a, C5a, are known as anaphylatoxins. These substances enhance vascular permeability, cause the release of vasoactive amines such as histamine from mast cells and basophils, induce lysosomal enzyme release from granulocytes, and cause smooth muscle contraction (Fig. 7–2). C3b can also enhance phagocytosis via interactions with C3b receptors on phagocytic cells. C5a has additional important properties, including potent neutrophil chemotactic activity, granulocyte aggregation, and granulocyte activation, the latter eventuating in the release of lysosomal enzymes, reactive oxygen metabolites, and leu-

Classic Pathway
IgM, IgG-antigen complexes
Aggregated immunoglobulin
Staphylococcal protein A
C-reative protein
polyanions, polycations
proteolytic enzymes

Alternate Pathway
IgA, IgG-antigen complexes
Bacterial cell walls
Endotoxic lipopolysaccharides
Yeast wall extracts (zymosan)
Cobra venom factor

C1, C4, C2

C3*, Factor B, Factor D, Properdin

C3

C3a [anaphylatoxin]

C5

C5a [anaphylatoxin, chemotaxin]

C5b-C9
membrane attack complex

cell lysis

Stimulation of mast cells to release
   histamine, platelet activating factor, etc
Enhanced vascular permeability, edema
Smooth muscle contraction
Neutrophil aggregation
Enhanced phagocytosis
Activation of neutrophil to release
   lysosomal enzymes, leukotrienes,
   oxygen metabolites

F1G. 7-2. Summary of the classic and alternate complement pathways and the substances that can activate each.

kotrienes. Thus, the low molecular weight fragments of C3, C4, and C5 are important mediators and amplifiers of the inflammatory response. This amplification of the inflammatory response is probably at least as important in the localization and destruction of pathogens as is direct microbial lysis. The importance of complement in inflammation makes it of obvious interest in the study of chronic inflammatory bowel disease.

LEVELS OF COMPLEMENT COMPONENTS IN INFLAMMATORY BOWEL DISEASE. Increased levels of complement components are commonly found in a variety of infectious and inflammatory disorders. Many of the complement components behave as acute phase reactants, increasing as much as two to three fold because of an increase in synthesis.[211] The levels of complement components found in patients with inflammatory bowel disease fit this pattern in that they are either normal or elevated, with elevations occurring predominantly in patients with active disease. The levels of C1q and C5 have been found to be normal in both Crohn's disease and ulcerative colitis.[213–215] The levels of C4, C3, and Factor B have been found to be normal,[214,216–218] or increased,[218,219,222] particularly in patients with active disease.[213,217,220,221,224] The CH_{50} titer, which is a reflection of all the complement components, has most frequently been normal.[214,217,218] The levels of the complement inhibitors C1 INH and Factor I (C3b INA), which are known to be acute phase reactants, are increased in active disease but are normal otherwise, whereas the inhibitor Factor H (β1H-globulin) is normal even in active disease.[223] That these elevations in complement components are part of the acute phase reaction is supported by the finding that elevations of C3 and C4 levels occur in controls with other diseases,[213,219] and the finding of a positive correlation between the levels of C3, C4, and Factor B with serum orosomucoid in patients with ulcerative colitis.[221]

COMPLEMENT METABOLISM AND ACTIVATION. The metabolism of complement components has been measured in normal individuals and in patients with a variety of diseases in which complement or immune complexes are thought to play a role. Complement components are the most rapidly metabolized of the serum proteins, with approximately 50% of the plasma pool being replaced daily.[225] It is not clear where these proteins are catabolized, but their catabolism does not appear to involve complement system activation in normal individuals.[211] An increased catabolism of C3 has been found in selected patients with glomerulonephritis, systemic lupus erythematosus, or seropositive rheumatoid arthritis, diseases in which complement or immune complexes are thought to play a pathogenetic role.[225] Both C1q and C3 metabolism have been studied in patients with inflammatory bowel disease.[223,226] The synthetic rate and the fractional catabolic rate of both were found to be increased compared to normal, despite normal to increased serum levels of C1q and C3 in all patients. Moreover, there was evidence that a fraction of the C1q and C3 was being sequestered in an extravascular compartment. These findings occurred both in patients with ulcerative colitis and in patients with Crohn's disease, most of whom had active disease at the time of study. In order to control for a spuriously increased catabolism resulting from protein losing enteropathy, albumin metabolism was measured simultaneously in each patient. Although the fractional catabolic rate for albumin was also generally increased, consistent with intestinal protein loss, this was not of a sufficient degree to account for the increased complement catabolism.

Although not formally proven, the increased catabolism of complement components presumably is caused by activation of complement in the inflamed intestine. In support of this, an increase in circulating C3 activation products has been found in patients with inflammatory bowel disease.[215,216,218,221,227] Activation products of Factor B of the alternate complement pathway have also been identified.[216,221] Taken together with the metabolism data, these results suggest that activation of both the classic and the alternate pathways occurs in patients with inflammatory bowel disease. The report of a case of C2 deficiency in a patient with Crohn's disease,[228] a component of the classic pathway, implies that the availability of only the alternate pathway is sufficient for inflammation to occur.

Defects in the in vitro activation of the complement cascade via the alternate pathway have been reported, mainly in patients with Crohn's disease. In one study, this occurred with cobra venom as the alternate pathway activator but not with zymosan or rabbit cells.[217] In other studies, defective activation of the alternate pathway has occurred with either nylon fibers or with zymosan as the activator.[214,227] One explanation for these results is that circulating complement activation products are interfering in such in vitro activation assays. In one study, however, a similar defect was identified in the first degree relatives of patients with Crohn's disease, but only in the families of patients who themselves had the defect, suggesting some kind of predisposing genetic factor.[227] The exact significance of such a genetic trait in disease pathogenesis is unknown until further studies are done, including ones with other inflammatory diseases included as disease controls.

IMMUNE COMPLEXES IN INFLAMMATORY BOWEL DISEASE. Although there is evidence that the complement system is activated in patients with inflammatory bowel disease, the mechanism of this activation has yet to be elucidated. A major mechanism of complement activation is through the formation of antigen-antibody immune complexes (Fig. 7–2). Because patients with inflammatory bowel disease have a variety of circulating antibodies to enteric bacteria and to certain foods, and frequently have increased intestinal permeability in the form of ulcerations, it seems logical that immune complexes would be found circulating in their blood. Although this seems a simple question, it has been quite difficult to resolve. Part of the problem lies with the multiple factors that determine the formation and fate of immune complexes in vivo, including the concentration, size, and valence of the antigen, the avidity, isotype, and concentration of the antibody, the resulting size of the complexes, and the clearance of complexes by the reticuloendothelial system. Many of these factors can and do change continuously. Therefore, the formation and disposition of immune complexes is a dynamic process, whereas the methods available to measure this process are by their nature static, looking at a single point in time. The large number of methods available to test for immune complexes reflects that no single method is sufficient to demonstrate all immune complexes.[229] Each assay detects immune complexes of a certain size or property, and each can give false-positive and false-negative results.[230] For example, endotoxin, free DNA, and anti-lymphocyte antibodies can give positive results in some assays, and nonspecifically aggregated immunoglobulin can cause positive results in all assays, although the size and concentration of aggregates that are detected varies among them. Immune complex assays can be grouped according to the property of immune complexes that they detect. These groups include methods based on nonspecific precipitation, on complement-protein interactions, on reactions with antiglobulins, on reactions with cellular complement receptors, and on reactions with cellular Fc receptors.[229] Because of these considerations, at the present time an adequate demonstration of circulating immune complexes in a given disease requires that more than one assay be used, that these assays detect several different properties of immune complexes, that more than one assay be positive, that the result of positive assays correlate with one another to at least some extent, and that similar results be found by different laboratories.

In light of the above criteria, have circulating immune complexes been adequately demonstrated in patients with inflammatory bowel disease? The available studies are summarized in Table 7–4. Many of the early studies, most based on a single assay or two, reported positive results in an appreciable but widely varying percentage of patients.[218,231–235,237,240–243] In some of these studies, there was a good correlation with disease activity;[231–235] in others there was not.[236–238] However, the studies that best fit the criteria described above have not found circulating immune complexes in patients with inflammatory bowel disease,[230,238,239] and other reports have also been entirely negative.[236,242,244] It is difficult to explain or reconcile such divergent results. Soltis et al. have demonstrated that sera from patients with IBD have an increased tendency for nonspecific immunoglobulin aggregation, and this may have played a role in some of the positive studies.[239] Another study found positive results not only in patients with ulcerative colitis or Crohn's disease but also in those with other intestinal diseases to a relatively equivalent extent, indicating a lack of specificity for inflammatory bowel disease.[235] This important group of patient controls was not included in many of the positive reports. Lastly, a difference in patient populations may also be involved. Nevertheless, in view of the complexities involved in tests for immune complexes as described above, and the potential for false-positives to occur, one must conclude that circulating immune complexes occur either infrequently or only in a minority of patients with inflammatory bowel disease.

Immune Complex Disease

LOCALIZED IMMUNE COMPLEX DISEASE. Immune complexes formed locally in the intestinal lesions may contribute to disease pathogenesis. Experimentally, the classic example of this type

TABLE 7-4. *Results of Assays for Circulating Immune Complexes in Patients With Inflammatory Bowel Disease.*

Author	Number of Assays	Type(s) of Assay*	Group/ Number	Percentage Positive	Comment
Doe[240]	1	2	CD/21	57	
			UC/10	20	
			Celiac/91	30	
Jewell[231]	1	5	CD/18	44	Positive correlation with disease activity
			UC/24	16	
Lurhuma[241]	2	2, 3	CD/66	88	SLE 55% and ITP 83% positive
			NL/20	20	
Hodgson[232]	2	2	CD/64	5 to 27	One assay correlated with disease activity and extraintestinal; complications
			UC/92	13 to 32	
Fiasse[233]	2	2, 3	CD/59	61	Positive correlation with disease activity
			NL/100	14	
Nielsen[234]	2	2, 3	UC/22	36	Positive correlation with disease activity
Lambert[230]	17	2, 3, 4, 5	CD/11	0	3 of 17 assays had some positives; no correlation among them
Einstein[242]	1	2	CD/31	0	37% rheumatoid arthritis patients positive
			UC/24	12.5	
Soltis[239]	4	1, 2	CD/34	0	
			UC/17	0	
Kemler[237]	1	4	CD/54	18	18% IBD positive; no correlation with activity or extraintestinal complications
			UC/32	18	
			"itis"/18	0	
Bradby[236]	1	2	CD/18	0	Letter; serial study over 20 months
Pallone[243]	2	2	CD/119	38 to 51	One assay correlated with disease activity
Richens[218]	1	2	CD/55	14	
Learmonth[244]	1	2	UC/40	0	Letter
Danis[235]	1	2	CD/76	26 to 74	Range of % positive represents inactive vs. active disease
			UC/72	15 to 33	
			GI Dis/68	44	
Knoflach[238]	4	1, 2, 4	CD/78	0	No correlation with disease activity. Dis = SLE, PBC, RA
			UC/53	0	
			Dis/74	"+"	

*1 = nonspecific precipitation assays; 2 = complement-protein interactions; 3 = reactions with anti-globulins; 4 = complement receptor reactions; 5 = Fc receptor-dependent reactions (Lawley, 1980)
CD = Crohn's disease; UC = ulcerative colitis; NL = normal controls; celiac = celiac disease; "itis" = patients with enteritis but not Crohn's disease or ulcerative colitis; GI Dis = control patients with gastrointestinal disorders; dis = disease controls; SLE = systemic lupus erythematosus; ITP = idiopathic thrombocytopenic purpura; IBD = inflammatory bowel disease; PBC = primary biliary cirrhosis; RA = rheumatoid arthritis.

of tissue injury is the Arthus reaction. This reaction can be produced by injecting antigen parenterally into the tissues of sensitized animals. If sufficient circulating antibody is available to complex with this antigen, an intense inflammation occurs within a few hours, initially involving infiltration almost exclusively by neutrophils. As blood vessel walls are disrupted, red blood cells also infiltrate the lesions, and later monocytes, lymphocytes, and plasma cells can be found. If either neutrophils or complement are depleted, the Arthus reaction does not occur. Tissue damage is primarily caused by the neutrophil, attracted to the site and activated by complement components such as C5a and C3a (Fig. 7–2). Examples of diseases in man in which localized immune complex mechanisms may contribute to tissue damage include hypersensitivity pneumonitis, Goodpasture's syndrome, rheumatoid arthritis, and Hashimoto's thyroiditis. Inflammatory bowel disease seems to be a good candidate for localized immune complex disease, considering that patients have circulating antibodies to a variety of enteric constituents and appear to synthesize IgG antibodies to bacterial antigens locally in the gut.[156,245] Also favoring this idea are the experiments of Hodgson et al., who induced colitis in animals by using a combination of circulating immune complexes and colonic irritation with dilute formalin.[246] However, immune complex deposits have never been convincingly demonstrated to occur in the tissues of patients with inflammatory bowel disease,[247] although such was claimed in one study.[248] These latter findings were challenged by Baklien and Brandtzaeg[249] who pointed out that both IgG and C3 are present extravascularly in the normal intestine and that inflamed intestine may have increased amounts because of transudation, making identification of deposits of IgG and C3 difficult, particularly in fixed tissue.

The type of vasculature in a tissue is another important determinant of the occurrence of localized immune complex disease. In a study of intestinal lesions caused by circulating immune complexes in rabbits, only half of the animals with immune complex deposits in glomeruli and glomerulonephritis had immune complex deposits in the intestine.[250] Furthermore, only half of those with intestinal deposits had any histologic abnormalities.[250] Presumably differences in vasculature account for such a divergence, with the intestinal vasculature being less susceptible to immune complex deposition than that of the glomerulus. This may contribute to the difficulty in demonstrating immune complex deposits in inflammatory bowel disease. The absence of proof of localized immune complexes in inflammatory bowel disease tissue is not proof that they are absent or that such deposits do not play a significant role in the disease. Indeed, considering the increased complement metabolism and circulating complement split products in patients with inflammatory bowel disease, and the marked infiltration by neutrophils in the lesions, it seems likely that at least the acute inflammatory response in the intestine might involve this mechanism. Considering the continuous antigenic exposure in the gut, immune complexes may be continually formed, generating complement activation products and thus polymorphonuclear infiltration, but also continuously being cleared. Thus, actual deposits of immune complexes, as demonstrable on tissue sections, might not be found even though major tissue damage was occurring in the intestine because of this mechanism. Moreover, direct activation of the alternate pathway by endotoxin bacterial cell walls would cause many of the same effects as immune complexes and might explain apparent localized immune complex disease without immune complexes being demonstrable. A different approach to demonstrating the importance of complement activation locally in the intestinal lesions would be to use antibodies that recognize only activated complement components as immunohistochemical reagents. Such antibodies are presently available, and one would hope that the studies might clarify this question in the future.

SYSTEMIC IMMUNE COMPLEX DISEASE. The classic example of a systemic immune complex disease is serum sickness that occurs when patients are given a substance to which they have (or to which they develop) antibody. The resulting deposition of immune complexes in vessels throughout the body results in fever, lymphadenopathy, arthritis, urticaria, glomerulonephritis, and vasculitis. This type of reaction is felt to occur to varying degrees in persistent bacterial or parasitic infections, Epstein-Barr virus and hepatitis B virus infections, and some autoimmune diseases, especially systemic lupus erythematosus. Systemic immune complex disease has been invoked as an explanation for the extraintestinal complications of inflammatory bowel disease. Some studies have found a correlation between positive tests for circulating immune complexes and extraintestinal complications,[232] but others have not.[237,238] Considering that few patients are positive in tests for circulating immune complexes, even in studies that have found them, most patients with extraintestinal complications must not have them. Moreover, the mere presence of circulating immune complexes does not mean that the immune complexes are pathogenic. For example, patients with primary biliary cirrhosis have a high rate of circulating immune complexes, yet these patients rarely have any evidence of systemic immune complex disease.[229] No direct evidence is presently available that immune complexes are involved in the pathogenesis of any of the extraintestinal complications of IBD. Clearly, these extraintestinal complications are heterogeneous. The pathogenesis is not understood in any of these complications, but complications such as pyoderma gangrenosum, sclerosing cholangitis, or iritis are not seen in diseases such as systemic lupus erythematosus, where good evidence exists that systemic immune complexes are playing a pathogenic role. Among the extraintestinal complications of inflammatory bowel disease, the ones in which immune complexes are most likely to be involved pathogenetically include glomerulonephritis, vasculitis, and arthritis. Cases of glomerulonephritis with IgG deposits in the glomeruli have been reported both in Crohn's disease and ulcerative colitis, although this is a rare complication of either disease.[251,252] One report involved two patients with IgA nephropathy, one with Crohn's disease and the other with ulcerative colitis, whose nephropathy improved with treatment of their intestinal disease, suggesting that IgA immune complexes may have played a role in this complication.[253] Arteritis is also a rare complication of either Crohn's disease or ulcerative colitis, but it does occur and may be a result of systemic deposits of immune complexes.[254–256] Arthritis is a far more common complication of inflammatory bowel disease and is a common feature of systemic immune complex disease, but direct evidence that immune complexes play a role in the arthritis of inflammatory bowel disease is lacking. For example, no reports are available of immune complex deposits in the joints of such patients, and one study found normal synovial fluid CH_{50} titers in a small number of inflammatory bowel disease patients with arthritis, which would not be expected if locally deposited immune complexes were playing a role in the arthritis.[257] On the other hand, a clinically similar type of arthritis occurs in some patients who have had intestinal bypass operations. These individuals often have serum immune complexes in the form of cryoprecipitates containing immunoglobulins, complement components, and bacterial antigens. Deposits of these complexes have been identified in the joints as well as in other tissues,[258] supporting the idea that immune complexes originating in the gut can be deposited in the joints, triggering an arthritis. Whether this is the explanation of the arthritis seen in patients with inflammatory bowel disease is unknown; at present it is only an interesting but unproven hypothesis. Other possibilities exist, for example the deposition of bacterial cell wall peptidoglycans in the joints,[258a] which is known to cause an arthritis in experimental animals. Resolution of these and other hypotheses will require direct examination of the synovial fluid, cells, and tissues of IBD patients with arthritis.

Neutrophils

The third component of humoral immunity is the neutrophil (Fig. 7-1). Although the neutrophil can act independently, it functions best in concert with antibody and complement.[259] The neutrophil is a short-lived cell produced in large numbers.[260] Its half-life is only 6 to 7 hours in blood and 2 to 3 days in the tissues. Large reserves of neutrophils that are in the bone marrow can be mobilized on demand, but even lacking this, some 10^{11} neutrophils are produced per day. The neutrophil has been called a "professional phagocyte." Its phagocytic activity can be separated into multiple distinct phases, including chemotaxis, recognition or binding, ingestion, respiratory burst, degranulation, and killing. The first of these, chemotaxis, simply means a directed movement of neutrophils toward a stimulus. After they have moved to the site of the stimulus, neutrophils bind to particles to be ingested. The presence of immunoglobulin and/or C3b on the particle greatly facilitates this binding by interacting with receptors for the Fc regions of IgG or the C3b component of complement present on the neutrophil surface. Such perturbation of the surface membrane causes an increase in oxidative metabolism that is known as the respiratory burst. The particle is ingested by sequential binding of neutrophil surface Fc and C3b receptors to their ligands around the circumference of the particle, a process similar to zipping a zipper. During and after particle ingestion, neutrophil granules are discharged into the endocytic vesicle or phagozome, forming a phagolysozome, and into the surrounding milieu outside the cell as well. Under some conditions, granule contents can be released externally after surface membrane perturbation but in the absence of phagocytosis.[261] Considering the destructive power of the granule contents, release in either instance is likely to do damage to surrounding tissues. The actual destruction of an ingested particle or organism proceeds by both oxygen-dependent and oxygen-independent mechanisms.[262] Each of these phases of neutrophil function can be measured in assays;[259] many of them have been applied to circulating neutrophils obtained from patients with inflammatory bowel disease. Neutrophils are prevalent in the active lesions of IBD,[263] thus studies on neutrophil function are of obvious relevance to the understanding of these diseases.

Numerous assays of chemotaxis have been performed on neutrophils from patients with inflammatory bowel disease. Chemotaxis means the directed migration of cells toward a stimulus. Chemokinesis, which is an increase in random locomotion,[264] is a different type of cellular response to a stimulus that needs to be differentiated from chemotaxis, but not always is. Two types of assays are in common use. The first of these is the Boyden chamber assay, in which neutrophils are put in a chamber separated by a filter from a second chamber containing a chemotactic substance. The distance the neutrophils move into the filter is measured. This assay cannot distinguish chemotaxis from chemokinesis unless there is an independent assessment of the latter.[264] A second method involves the migration of neutrophils under an Agarose gel toward a chemotactic stimulus placed nearby in the gel. Peripheral blood neutrophils from patients with inflammatory bowel disease have been tested in both of these assays. Neutrophils from patients with Crohn's disease have shown normal chemotaxis in vitro.[265–270] Neutrophils from patients with ulcerative colitis have shown in vitro chemotaxis that was either normal,[266,269,270] or decreased.[271-274] In some of the latter studies showing decreased chemotaxis, this was associated with active colitis.[271,274] Neutrophils from patients with active colitis frequently demonstrated increased unstimulated chemokinesis,[271,272] and increased adhesiveness,[273] suggesting that the cells were being activated in vivo and were thus less responsive to in vitro stimuli.

Neutrophil migration in vivo is studied by creating an abrasion of the skin and measuring the numbers of neutrophils that migrate into the resulting "skin window" over a defined length of time. The neutrophils migrating into the skin abrasion can be quantitated by counting the numbers that stick to an overlying glass slide or that are present in a fluid filled chamber applied to the abrasion. Most of the studies in patients with IBD have used the latter technique. Interestingly, and opposed to the belief that chemotaxis in vitro is the same process as in vivo migration,[264] the results in vivo have been nearly the reverse of the results in vitro. Patients with Crohn's disease have had significantly decreased migration of neutrophils into skin windows despite concomitant normal chemotactic responses in vitro.[265,266,268] In contrast, patients with ulcerative colitis have been found to have normal numbers of neutrophils entering skin windows,[266,274,275] despite their sometimes having decreased chemotaxis in vitro.[271,272,274] An early report of increased numbers of basophils in glass slide (Rebuck) skin windows in patients with ulcerative colitis,[275] has not been described in more recent studies using the chamber technique.[266,274] The apparent defect of in vivo motility of neutrophils in Crohn's disease has brought forth the hypothesis that a defect in the ability of neutrophils to accumulate at sites of inflammation in the intestine may be involved in the pathogenesis of the disease. The migration of neutrophils to the intestinal lesions in patients with Crohn's disease, however, appears to be unimpaired when directly measured in vivo by gamma camera after the injection of ^{111}Indium-labelled leukocytes.[276] Possibly, the abnormal chemotaxis into skin windows reflects a competitive inhibition, with the stimulus provided at the skin surface being unable to compete with the much stronger stimulus provided by the inflammation in the intestine.

Neutrophils are clearly under complex influences in vivo, particularly in patients with inflammatory diseases, and the findings of apparent defects in neutrophil motility need to be interpreted with caution. An acquired defect in neutrophil chemotaxis has been reported in many disorders, including diabetes, overwhelming bacterial infections, trauma, burns, and malignancies. The diversity of these disorders suggests that defective chemotaxis is frequently nonspecific and can be multifactorial. One example of an acquired defect in chemotaxis that has been well studied is the defect that can occur during hemodialysis. Cellophane membranes used in hemodialysis can activate the C5 component of complement generating C5a,[277] a potent chemotaxin that acts on circulating neutrophils, causing increased adherence to endothelium and leukostasis, particularly in the lungs, and neutropenia.[278] This margination and aggregation reverses over a period of hours. Interestingly, at this point, neutrophils tested in vitro for chemotaxis are refractory to C5a.[279] By analogy, one explanation of an apparent defect in in vitro chemotaxis in ulcerative colitis patients might be that the neutrophils exposed in vivo to complement components become refractory to in vitro stimulation involving similar stimuli. In fact, a refractoriness to C5a has been found in patients with Crohn's disease or ulcerative colitis.[270] Secondly, drugs used to treat the disease might have effects on chemotaxis. Third, immature neutrophils have a lower chemotactic ability; thus, an increased turnover of neutrophils in patients might result in an apparently defective chemotaxis. Lastly, circulating inhibitors of chemotaxis might explain some of the instances of apparent defective chemotaxis in patients with diseases such as inflammatory bowel disease.[273,280]

Neutrophil functions other than motility have been examined also. Although a number of studies have been reported, few of them have used exactly the same assays, so a comparison of the results is difficult. A variety of different types of assays have assessed the intracellular killing ability of neutrophils. The most commonly performed test of this type is the nitroblue tetrazolium (NBT) dye reduction test. NBT is a water soluble compound that becomes dark blue on reduction. Neutrophils can reduce this dye following ingestion and the oxidative burst. The proper reduction of the dye appears to require a variety of metabolic events, including increased HMP shunt activity, increased oxygen consumption, and increased hydrogen peroxide and superoxide radical formation.[259] A deficiency in NBT dye reduction is found in patients with chronic granulomatous disease. This test has been performed frequently in patients with IBD, and has been found to be either normal,[265,281–283] or increased,[268,281,284] with the exception of one study that found decreased stimulated NBT reduction in patients with Crohn's disease.[268] Chemiluminescence is an assay similar to the NBT test, and measures similar events in the cells, but the final determination is the amount of light generated during phagocytosis. Apparently, a good correlation exists between the light emission and antimicrobial activity. Two studies have measured chemiluminescence in neutrophils from patients with Crohn's disease, with conflicting results. One found chemiluminescence stimulated by S. aureus to be decreased in Crohn's disease,[282] whereas the other found both resting and zymosan-stimulated chemiluminescence to be increased significantly.[285] Oxygen consumption during phagocytosis has been measured in a substantial number of patients with Crohn's disease and found to be normal.[266] The actual production of superoxide radicals and H_2O_2 by neutrophils was normal when concanavalin A or cytochalasin E was used as a stimulant, but decreased when phorbol myristic acetate was used as a stimulant.[286] The significance of this latter finding is unknown. A direct assessment of bacteriocidal activity has only been reported once in patients with Crohn's disease, and it was found to be decreased in three of nine patients.[282] The small number of patients involved in this study warrants caution in its interpretation. In summary, most of the assays examining these aspects of neutrophil function have been largely normal, with some of the reports of abnormalities involving small numbers of patients or involving results conflicting with those of other laboratories. The evidence favors the opinion that these functions are either normal in patients with inflammatory bowel disease or may be increased during active disease.

A somewhat different approach to the study of neutrophil function has been the measurement of neutrophil enzyme markers either in the blood or in the intestinal tissues. Peripheral blood neutrophil alkaline phosphatase content was found to be increased in both diseases.[288] Serum total B_{12} binding capacity (transcobalamins) and lysozyme levels have been found to be elevated in both ulcerative colitis and Crohn's disease.[287,288] The former is thought to reflect the total neutrophil blood pool, the latter the neutrophil (and monocyte) turnover. However, the total pool size and turnover of neutrophils has not been directly measured as yet in patients with IBD. Various neutrophil enzyme markers have been measured in biopsies of the intestinal lesions. Both the total vitamin B_{12} binding capacity and lysozyme activity were significantly increased in biopsies from areas of active colitis.[287,290] The transcobalamins and lysozymes are stored in the secondary (specific) granules, along with other substances. The contents of these granules, including substances that can cleave C5 to C5a and substances chemotactic for monocytes, seem to be preferentially released during the evolution of the inflammatory response,[261] probably serving to amplify the inflammatory response further. Enzymes present in the primary (azurophil) granules have been measured in the same mucosal biopsies, but the results have been more variable. For example, myeloperoxidase has been found to be increased in areas of active inflammation in two studies,[289,290] although the increase reached statistical significance in only one.[290] Other constituents of primary granules such as α-chymotrypsin, elastase, and cathepsin D were found to be normal or decreased rather than increased,[289] but technical factors, such as autoinactivation by the primary granule products themselves, may partly explain this discrepancy.[261] Biopsies of noninflamed or inactive areas of colitis did not have any increases in either secondary or primary granule contents. These studies are consistent with the large numbers of neutrophils present in the lesions of IBD and do not support the concept of a defect in neutrophil function in IBD.

Drugs known to be clinically useful in the treatment of IBD are inhibitors of neutrophil function, further disputing the pathogenetic importance of a defect in neutrophil function in IBD. Corticosteroids decrease the margination of neutrophils, inhibit neutrophil aggregation, inhibit the chemotactic response to complement components, and decrease cell migration into skin windows in vivo.[291,292] Corticosteroids also interfere with neutrophil eicosonoid metabolism, decreasing prostaglandin and leukotriene synthesis via stimulation of lipomodulin, an inhibitor of phospholipase A.[293] Sulfasalazine and its components, sulfapyridine and 5-ASA, have been found to inhibit a variety of neutrophil functions in vitro, such as superoxide generation, lysosomal enzyme release, and myeloperoxidase-mediated cytotoxicity.[294] Sulfasalazine and 5-ASA inhibited neutrophil chemotaxis in vitro, although indomethacin, used at doses that completely inhibited prostaglandin production, did not.[295] These results are perhaps explained by the observation that sulfasalazine and 5-ASA inhibit neutrophil production of the chemotactic leukotriene metabolites, 5-HETE and 5,12-diHETE,[296] at concentrations achieved in the intestinal lumen of patients being given therapeutic doses,[297] although these levels are much higher than the concentrations present in the blood.[298] The dose achieved in the mucosa itself is unknown, but it is presumably closer to the level in the intestinal lumen than that in the blood. If one postulates that a defect in neutrophil function underlies inflammatory bowel disease, then drugs that inhibit neutrophil function should make the disease worse, not better. This point plus the results of other studies reviewed above make this hypothesis seem unlikely. Perhaps future work should focus on the potential destructive capability of the neutrophil in the pathogenesis of the disease, at least in the active stages, rather than on putative defects in neutrophil function.

Intestinal Humoral Immunity

The Mucosal Immune System

Lymphoid cells constitute about 25% of the cells present in the intestine, therefore gut-associated lymphoid tissue (GALT) represents a major component of the immune system.[299–302] GALT is organized in at least three interconnecting cell populations or compartments: Peyer's patches, lamina proprial lymphoid cells, and intraepithelial lymphoid cells (Fig. 7-3). The mesenteric lymph nodes, although outside the intestine proper, are frequently considered a fourth compartment. The different cell compartments are distinguished not only by differences in physical location and structure, but also in the types of cells present within them and in their functions. The antigenic challenge to GALT is enormous. It has been estimated that the number of microbial cells in the body, most of them in the intestine, exceeds the total number of cells in the body.[303] One can add to these bacterial antigens those antigens present in food, drink, and ingested chemicals. Exactly how the mucosal system deals with this challenge is not yet known; however, it is apparent that GALT is in a constant state of response, as witnessed by the large number of plasma cells present throughout the intestine and by studies on germ-free animals in whom the various cell populations of GALT are poorly developed.[304–306] These observations have led to the concept of "physiologic inflammation," in which the "normal" intestine is viewed as being in a state of mild inflammation.[306]

PEYER'S PATCHES. Peyer's patches are organized lymphoid aggregates with one or more lymphoid follicles that extend from the epithelial layer into the lamina propria, and sometimes the submucosa. Although Peyer's patches usually are thought of as visible, macroscopic structures, clustered in certain regions such as the ileum in man, they are frequently microscopic in size with a single follicle and are dispersed throughout the intestine.[307,308] A typical colonic Peyer's patch-like lymphoid follicle is shown in Figure 7-4.[308a] Peyer's patches differ from other peripheral lymphoid tissues by the lack of afferent lymphatics, although they do have efferent lymphatics. Instead of afferent lymphatics, they have a specialized epithelium that is able to "pinocytose" materials in the intestinal lumen and deliver these into the Peyer's patch.[309] Distinguishing features of this specialized follicle-associated epithelium (FAE) include a relative lack of goblet cells, a lack of secretory component, and the presence of M or membrane cells (see Chap. 5).[302,310,311] The M cell serves as an important first step in the induction of intestinal immune responses, but relatively little is known about the factors determining its function. At present, we know of no selectivity exerted by

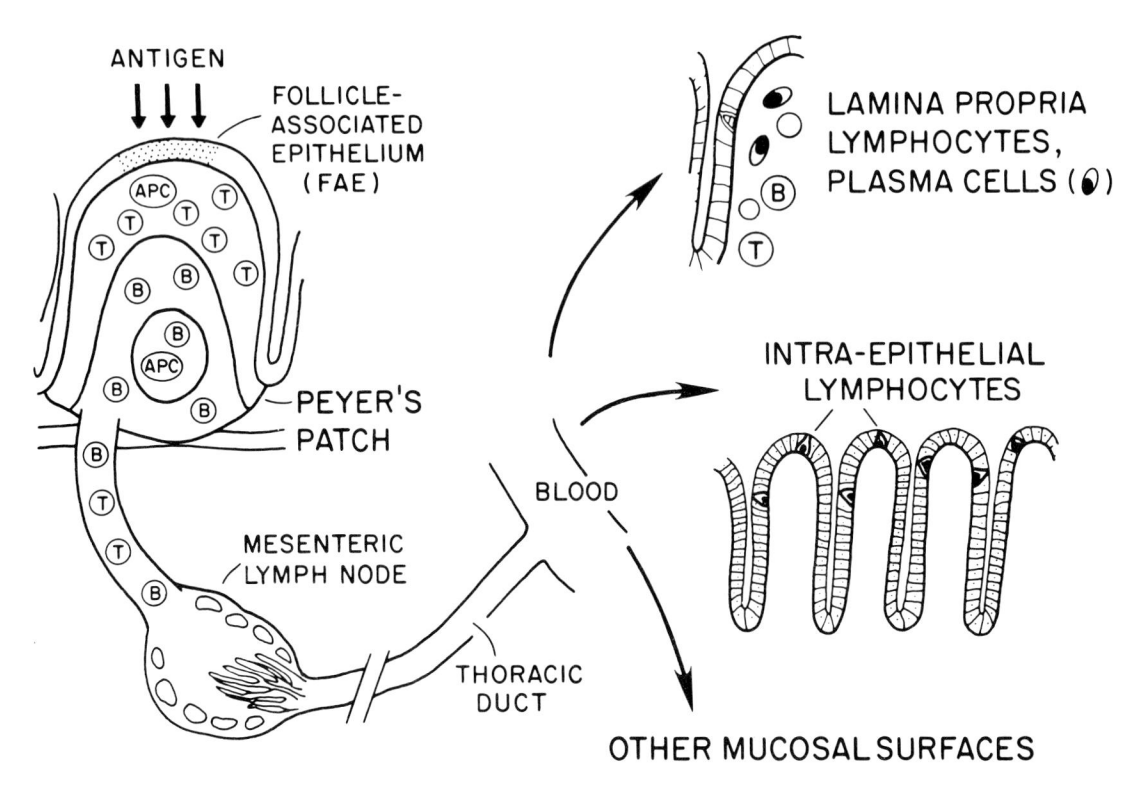

FIG. 7-3. The organization of gut-associated-lymphoid tissue (GALT) into three major compartments.

the M cell in the material that it will "pinocytose." Presumably, the only limiting factor is the size of the material; particles as large as whole bacteria can be taken up.[312] Human M cells may express HLA-DR molecules,[302] thus potentially presenting antigen directly to the lymphocytes infiltrating the dome epithelium.

Consistent with the antigen sampling by their dome epithelium, Peyer's patches serve as sites for the induction of immune responses. It is now recognized that the Peyer's patch contains all the cells needed for immune induction, that is, B cells, T cells, and antigen presenting cells (macrophages and dendritic cells). These cell types are structured in B cell dependent and T cell dependent areas similar to other peripheral lymphoid tissues (Fig. 7-3).[302,313] B cells predominate in the follicles, while T cells predominate in the interfollicular areas and beneath the dome epithelium; macrophages appear to be scattered both beneath the dome epithelium and in the follicles.[302,309,315] Quantitatively, B cells predominate overall in the adult Peyer's patch, consisting of about 60 to 70% of total cells, while T cells, including both helper and suppressor cells, comprise about 20% of the total. Although T cells are present in relatively smaller numbers, the rudimentary Peyer's patches and the deficient IgA responses found in T cell deficient mice indicate that Peyer's patch function is highly dependent upon T cells.[315] A curious feature of Peyer's patch cells is that they appear to represent precursor rather than effector cells. For example, although the Peyer's patch contains many B cells, few or no plasma cells are present, even after extensive immunization.[316] The same ap-

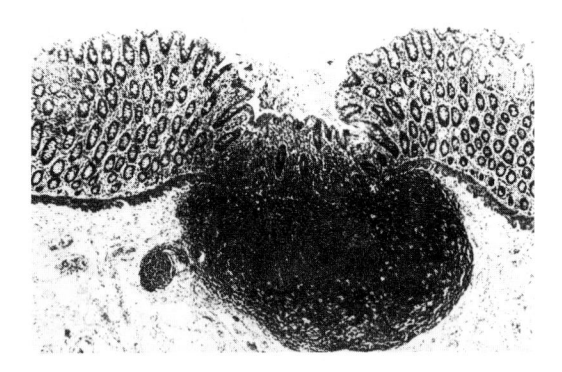

FIG. 7-4. A typical small Peyer's patch-like lymphoid follicle in the human colon, also referred to as 'lymphoepithelial' or 'lymphoglandular complexes'. (Courtesy of Dr. Desmond O'Leary, Oslo, Norway.)

pears to be true for cytotoxic T cells, the Peyer's patch contains precursors rather than effectors.[317] One explanation is that differentiating B cells and T cells leave Peyer's patches and migrate to the gut and other lymphoid tissues.[318,319] A second important feature of Peyer's patches is that the induction of immune responses there is highly dependent on the route of antigen exposure. Peyer's patches respond predominantly, if not exclusively, to antigen presented via the intestinal lumen, that is, via M cells.[304–306] The Peyer's patch is not only a site of immune induction but also a major site for the induction of IgA responses, an important function considering that IgA is the major immunoglobulin in mucosal secretions. Peyer's patch cells are enriched for IgA B cell precursors relative to other lymphoid tissues,[320,321] particularly IgA B cell precursors specific for antigens present in the intestine.[322] The reasons for this preferential expression of IgA responses by Peyer's patch B cells is not clear, but microenvironment-B cell interactions,[323] and the effects of an unusual Peyer's patch switch T cell,[324] are two possible explanations. Switch T cells, cloned from the murine Peyer's patch, have been shown to cause B cells to change or switch from the production of IgM to the production of IgA. T cells that specifically regulate mature B cells already expressing IgA have been found in the Peyer's patch as well.[325–327] These and other aspects of the T cell regulation of IgA have been reviewed recently.[328,329]

Lymphocytes induced in the Peyer's patches leave these structures via efferent lymphatics that drain into mesenteric lymph nodes where these cells may undergo further division and perhaps maturation.[330] From there they travel via the thoracic duct into the circulation and are dispersed widely in the body to a variety of lymphoid tissues.[331] However, they tend to selectively accumulate back (or "home") to the intestine and other mucosal sites such as the lactating breast.[332,333] The ability of mesenteric lymphoblasts to populate mucosal sites other than the intestine has given rise to the concept of a mucosa-associated-lymphoid-tissue or MALT, a more generalized system that would encompass GALT, bronchus-associated-lymphoid tissue (BALT), and other mucosa (Fig. 7-3).[334] The mechanism of selective localization in mucosa is unknown; however, a similar type of cell trafficking also occurs with peripheral lymph node cells, that is, lymphoblasts from peripheral lymph nodes tend to selectively traffic back to peripheral lymph nodes,[333,335] thus this type of preferential cell trafficking is not peculiar to GALT. Organ specific localization of lymphocytes may be directed by receptors on the lymphocytes that recognize distinct molecules in the endothelium that are distinctive to the organ. For instance, the high endothelial venules in Peyer's patch and peripheral lymph nodes appear to have distinct structures that are recognized by lymphoid cells from these sites.[335,336] High endothelial venules are not present in the intestinal lamina propria, but perhaps similar structures exist in the endothelium of the intestine that serve this function.

LAMINA PROPRIAL LYMPHOCYTES. The intestinal lamina propria contains an abundance of B cells, plasma cells, T cells, and macrophages as well as a lesser number of other cells such as eosinophils and mast cells.[302] The intestinal lamina propria is the only place in the body where large numbers of plasma cells are present continuously as a normal event. Approximately 70 to 90% of the plasma cells in the intestine produce IgA.[337] The next most common isotype produced is IgM, representing 5 to 15% of the plasma cells, followed by IgG, representing only 3 to 5%. IgE and IgD plasma cells are infrequent. Plasma cells are terminally differentiated, end-stage cells whose half-life is approximately five days,[338] indicating that there must be a dynamic, continuous repopulation of lamina proprial B cells. It has recently become possible to isolate lamina proprial lymphocytes and study their functions in vitro.[339] In such isolates B cells comprise some 15 to 40% of the total cells with IgA producing cells predominating.[339] Considerable numbers of T cells are present also, ranging from 40 to 90% in different reports.[340–342] Approximately two-thirds of lamina proprial T cells have the helper/inducer phenotype and one-third the suppressor/cytotoxic phenotype, similar to what is found in peripheral blood.[343] Macrophages make up about 10% of lamina proprial isolates,[339] and mast cells from 1 to 3%.[344] Interestingly, cells with neither B cell or T cell markers, that is, null cells, and cells with natural killer cell markers seem to be deficient in the intestinal lamina propria,[339,345,346] although lymphokine-activated killer (LAK) cells seem to be well represented.[348]

Lamina proprial lymphocytes are functional cells, that is, they are not all terminally differentiated, end-stage cells. They respond to a variety of stimuli in vitro and probably also do so in vivo. It is not clear whether induction of immune responses occurs in the lamina propria; although all the cells required for immune induction are present there, they are physically dispersed and the types of cell-to-cell interactions necessary for immune induction would seem less likely to occur there than in organized lymphoid tissues such as Peyer's patches, lymph nodes, or the spleen. The functional activities of T cells in the lamina propria have not yet been studied extensively. These T cells do appear to have a variety of regulatory functions that are still being defined.[349–351] They may also be more activated than their counterparts circulating in the peripheral blood.[352] Consistent with deficiency of certain markers among lamina proprial cells, certain cytotoxic activities, such as antibody dependent cellular cytotoxicity (ADCC) and natural killer (NK) cell activity, seem to be diminished.[345,346] Defective generation of T cell killing of allogeneic targets has also been reported.[353]

INTRAEPITHELIAL LYMPHOCYTES (IEL). The third compartment of GALT is represented by lymphocytes that are physically located within the epithelial layer, numbering one out of every six cells in the epithelium. Although these cells have been a source of fascination to immunologists and gastroenterologists for some time, surprisingly little is known about what they do.[354–356] The cellular composition of this compartment is different from that in either the Peyer's patch or the lamina propria. Plasma cells are not present, and B cells are absent or infrequent. The predominant cell type is the T cell, and most of these have the suppressor/cytotoxic phenotype. These T cells appear to originate in the Peyer's patch and traffic to the epithelium via the lamina propria.[357] In many species, a large proportion of the IEL contain granules that stain metachromatically and resemble mast cell granules, but contain little or no histamine.[358] It has been proposed that these cells become intestinal mast cells,[357] but little evidence is available to support this hypothesis.[356] In most species, IEL also differ greatly from LPL in their functional properties. IEL have full cytotoxic capabilities including NK, ADCC, and T cell cytotoxicity.[359] Because IEL increase in number after roundworm infestations, they might serve a cytotoxic function directed primarily at parasites. Secondly, IEL are increased in experimental graft versus host disease, prompting the suggestion that an increase in IEL may be a marker for cell-mediated immune responses in the intestine.[360] Thirdly, IEL might defend the epithelium against viral infections by secreting interferon,[361] and perhaps by direct cytotoxicity. Although we know little about their precise function in GALT, IEL are situated in a site that would render them exposed to a variety of antigenic stimuli. They appear to turn over rapidly, suggesting they are responding to such stimuli.[355] The numbers of IEL have been reported to be increased in some human diseases including celiac disease, dermatitis herpetiformis, and tropical sprue, but whether these increases are real and whether IEL play a role in these diseases has been questioned.[355] IEL are not increased in number in IBD, and whether they play any role in IBD is also unknown; however, the cytotoxic capabilities of IEL would seem to give them at least pathogenic potential if their cytotoxic activity were directed against adjacent epithelial cells.

SECRETORY IgA AND ITS TRANSPORT SYSTEM. Most plasma cells at mucosal sites are producing IgA. The transport of this IgA into the intestinal lumen has recently been unravelled.[362–364] IgA is produced both as a monomer of 150 KD plus a dimer of 320 KD. IgA dimer is covalently coupled to a 15 KD protein, known as J-chain, prior to secretion from plasma cells. Dimeric IgA, but not monomeric IgA, is able to bind to secretory component (SC), a 70 KD receptor molecule produced by, and present on, the surface membrane of epithelial cells. J-chain appears to be required for this binding of dimeric IgA to secretory component.[365] After binding to SC, the complex is endocytosed in a coated pit-type of vesicle. These vesicles do not fuse with lysosomes but are transported to the apical membrane via a microtubular dependent process, where the IgA-SC complex is released into the lumen. Polymeric IgM is transported in a similar manner. In addition to transporting IgA into the lumen, secretory component confers on IgA a certain resistance to proteolysis.[366] In man, IgA consist of two subclasses, IgA_1 and IgA_2. IgA_1 comprises about 90% of the IgA in serum, but only 40 to 50% of IgA in secretions. The expression of IgA_1 appears to predominate in the proximal intestine, whereas IgA_2 is expressed mainly in the distal intestine.[367] Once released into the lumen, secretory IgA has antiviral, antitoxin, and antibacterial functions, primarily by decreasing the ability of such cells or substances to bind to mucosa. In recent years it has been learned that the liver can also transport IgA,[368,369] as well as IgA immune complexes.[370,371] This pathway is particularly important in certain rodents, such as the rat, which transports 90% of its intestinal secretory IgA through the liver.[369] In man, this pathway appears to be of minor importance;[372] moreover, IgA transport occurs in man through bile ductular cells rather than through the hepatocyte.[373,374] Transport of IgA immune complexes through bile ductular cells has not been demonstrated in man, but this may be the link between IBD and bile duct complications such as pericholangitis and sclerosing cholangitis.

REGULATION OF THE RESPONSE TO ANTIGENS IN THE INTESTINE. Immunity to an antigen after an intestinal exposure is well documented following natural infections in man and oral immunization regimens in experimental animals.[328] Natural antibodies, such as hemagglutinins, are an example of immunization at an intestinal surface.[375] Such exposure can also result in a state of unresponsiveness or "oral tolerance."[328] The factors determining which result predominates are not understood, but presumably the answer lies in complex regulatory cell interactions within the GALT. Oral tolerance has been demonstrated in animals after the feeding of a variety of antigens, including proteins,[376,377] contact allergens,[378,379] heterologous erythrocytes,[380,381] and viral hemagglutinin.[382] Some evidence exists demonstrating that bacterial lipopolysaccharide may sensitize GALT in a manner that predisposes to the development of oral tolerance,[383] and to nonspecific suppression.[384] Multiple mechanisms of tolerance have been demonstrated,[385] but the most common one is the generation of suppressor T cells in GALT.[328] These suppressor T cells are currently thought to affect only systemic immune responses, allowing secretory IgA responses to the fed antigen to continue,[386] but this may not be true.[387] The demonstration of oral tolerance in a wide variety of species makes it likely that oral tolerance occurs in man, although little evidence supports this.[388] Could the increased titers of serum antibodies to a variety of enteric antigens in IBD (see "Serum Antibodies" section) or increased intestinal cellular reactivity be explained by defects in oral tolerance in these patients? We can only speculate on this at present, but it seems to be an important question that needs to be addressed.

Mucosal Immune System in Inflammatory Bowel Disease

With this overview of the structure and function of gut associated lymphoid tissue in mind, some important questions arise: How does GALT contribute to inflammatory bowel disease; and, conversely, how is the normal functional activity of GALT altered by these diseases? We cannot answer these questions yet. Most of the information available relates to cells in the lamina propria. The numbers and morphology of cells present in this compartment have been described, and analysis of the functional capacity of isolated lamina propria cells has begun. However, information about the morphology or functional abilities of intraepithelial or Peyer's patch lymphocytes in inflammatory bowel disease is almost nonexistent.

IMMUNOPATHOLOGY OF THE INTESTINAL LESIONS: LIGHT AND ELECTRON MICROSCOPIC STUDIES. The pathology of ulcerative colitis and Crohn's disease is covered in detail elsewhere (see Chap. 18). Only the features important for an understanding of the immunopathogenesis will be considered here. These two diseases share certain pathologic features. In both diseases the inflammatory lesions are restricted essentially to the intestine, the active lesions are infiltrated by both acute and chronic inflammatory cells, with neutrophils being the hallmark of acute activity,[389] and the lesions can relapse and remit spontaneously. They also have some distinct pathologic features. Ulcerative colitis is limited to the rectum and colon and the inflammation involves only the mucosa, whereas Crohn's disease can occur anywhere in the intestine and the inflammatory process involves the entire wall of the bowel. In ulcerative colitis, the epithelial layer itself seems to be the target (or at least the scene of the battle) because electron microscopic studies reveal signs of injury diffusely in the epithelium coincident with both an intercellular and intracellular infiltration with neutrophils.[389–391] In Crohn's disease, the epithelium itself is largely normal except for limited areas of full thickness ulceration,[390,392] or focal cellular infiltration;[393] consistent with this, neutrophils are present subepithelially in nonulcerated areas,[390] but not generally in the epithelium itself,[391] and not in the deeper layers of the bowel wall.[394] These various common and distinct features need to be considered and explained in theories of immune pathogenesis.

One of the puzzling aspects of these diseases, from an immunologic standpoint, is that the lesions of IBD are often localized, whereas immune cells are distributed diffusely throughout the intestine (Fig. 7-3). Ulcerative colitis is usually localized to the rectum and to variable amounts of the colon. Crohn's disease is usually grossly localized to limited segments of the intestine, with the segments not uncommonly being discontinuous. Both diseases can have an abrupt transition from diseased to apparently normal tissue. If immune cells are involved in the pathogenesis why are the lesions so sharply localized? The answer may be that the intestine is involved diffusely in both Crohn's disease and ulcerative colitis. This is most obvious in Crohn's disease, in which focal areas of chronic inflammation and increased numbers of plasma cells have been identified in apparently uninvolved areas in the mouth,[395] upper gut,[396–398] and rectum.[393] Rare cases of "metastatic" Crohn's disease in skin, bone, and other extraintestinal tissues have even been reported. In ulcerative colitis, remote involvement of the intestine is not as prominent as in Crohn's disease, but abnormalities of villous architecture and infiltration with plasma cells have been found in the small intestine of these patients.[396,399–401] If sensitized lymphoid cells are present diffusely in the gut, then local factors must determine the restriction of inflammation to limited segments. These local factors are not yet understood, but some of the possibilities include colon specific antigens in ulcerative colitis,[402] lymphatic drainage in Crohn's disease,[403] tropism of an infectious agent, or failure of as yet ill-defined local immunoregulatory mechanisms.

One of the lesions occurring in remote, uninvolved intestine that should be mentioned is the aphthous ulcer in Crohn's disease. Although not specific to Crohn's disease,[404] this lesion seems to be one of the earliest lesions identifiable in this disease.[405,406] These small lesions may be evident for some years before the development of the characteristic transmural involvement of Crohn's disease.[407] Aphthoid ulcers are interesting immunologically because they are ulcers of the epithelium covering Peyer's patch-like lymphoid follicles such as the one shown in Figure 7-4. As mentioned above, such follicle-associated-epithelium contains specialized M cells that pinocytose materials present in the intestinal lumen, delivering them into the lymphoid tissue below.[307,309–312] If this is one of the earliest lesions of Crohn's disease, ulceration of this epithelium implies that an agent or antigen is being taken up from the lumen by M cells into these Peyer's patch-like follicles and that the immune response to it begins in this compartment of GALT. This idea would fit with the well known salutary effects of diversion of the fecal stream in Crohn's disease, a maneuver that should reduce the uptake and transport of luminal antigens. Although this is only supposition, it underscores the importance of having more information about the morphology and function of lymphoid follicles in Crohn's disease, currently a major void in our knowledge.

Detailed electron microscopic studies of the lesions of Crohn's disease have identified and emphasized the involvement of a variety of nonlymphoid cells. Increased secretion of mucus by goblet cells, an increased number of Paneth's cells in the epithelium, focal venular necrosis, an abundance of platelets packed in the lumen of many venules, prominent numbers of mast cells in diseased areas, the presence of numerous eosinophils with depleted central cores (implying granule secretion), and abnormalities of neurons and smooth muscle cells, have all been noted.[392,394,408–410] The involvement of neurons and smooth muscle cells is notable because these cells may have a significant role in the course of Crohn's disease.[408] The damage and regeneration that have been identified in neuronal axons in diseased intestine may affect interactions that are now recognized to occur between the nervous and immune systems.[411] For example, T lymphocytes have receptors for the neurotransmitter vasoactive intestinal peptide (VIP).[412–414] One effect of the binding of VIP to this receptor on T cells is the inhibition of mitogen-stimulated T cell proliferation.[412] Thus, an increased number of VIP-containing neurons in the lesions of Crohn's disease has the potential to interact with and alter the function of T cells in the lesions.[415] Whether this actually occurs in vivo is unknown, but the modulation of immune function by neuropeptides is an interesting and exciting area of current research that may eventually explain the relationship between stress and flares of disease activity, a relationship well known to the clinician. A second nonlymphoid cell involved in the lesions of Crohn's disease that may have pathogenic importance is the smooth muscle cell. Smooth muscle cells show morphologic changes consistent with proliferation, hypercontraction, focal necrosis, and myofibroblastic transformation. The last change refers to the cells in the lesions being closely related to and producing new collagen fibers.[408] This last morphologic observation has now been confirmed biochemically. The types of collagen present in the strictures of Crohn's disease have been analyzed and an increase in type V collagen has been found, a type produced by smooth muscle cells but not generally by fibroblasts.[416,417] In addition, in vitro cultures of human smooth muscle cells produce large amounts of collagen, including type V and the other types found in the intestinal strictures of Crohn's disease.[416,418] The factors that stimulate and control collagen production by smooth muscle cells are unknown. One hypothesis is that mediators released by inflammatory cells in the intestinal lesions stimulate smooth muscle cells to proliferate and produce collagen, eventually resulting in stricture formation.[416] If this is true, the identification of the inflammatory factors involved may lead to therapies aimed at preventing stricture formation.

Regional Lymph Nodes. Lymph nodes isolated from colectomy specimens from patients with ulcerative colitis or Crohn's disease have been examined to see whether they had any characteristic involvement of either the B cell or T cell dependent areas.[419] B cell areas, such as the cortical follicles, were found to be activated in both diseases. In addition, the number of plasma cells in the lymph node was increased more than ten-fold for IgA, and between one- and ten-fold for IgG and IgM. In both diseases, T cell areas, such as the paracortex, showed activation also. Crohn's disease did have a higher frequency of granulomas, but overall the lymph nodes did not differ significantly in the two diseases. This study suggests that both the cellular and humoral immune systems are activated in the regional lymph nodes, implying that the same is true in the bowel lesions that these lymph nodes drain.

IMMUNOHISTOCHEMISTRY OF THE INTESTINAL LESIONS. *Plasma Cells in the Lamina Propria.* Immunohistochemistry has been aptly described as a technique that is easy to do but difficult to do well. A variety of technical factors need to be carefully considered.[420] The antisera used in the immunohistochemical analysis of the plasma cells in a tissue like the intestine need to be independently verified using sensitive immunohistochemical techniques, such as the staining of cell lines known to produce a single immunoglobulin isotype. A variety of controls are required to ensure that unexpected and unwanted antibodies are not present in the antisera. These controls should include blocking of specific staining by an excess of the purified relevant immunoglobulin isotype. The method used to quantify the data can be an important variable;[421] most studies have expressed the results as cells per unit area of lamina propria, a method that does not account for the two-to-four-fold increase in lamina propria area that occurs in IBD. An expression of results as cells per unit length of intestine seems preferable. Plasma cells of different isotypes can be distributed inhomogenously in the lamina propria, and can vary a great deal according to the degree of histologic inflammation,[247,421–423] so the selection of areas to count and the types of tissue samples analyzed can influence the results considerably. These technical factors may account for some of the discrepant results among immunohistochemical studies of the intestinal lamina propria in inflammatory bowel disease. The results with IgE plasma cells are particularly conflicting and will be covered in a separate section. However, despite these potential pitfalls and some continuing discrepancies,[424–426] a fairly consistent pattern of changes in the number and composition of plasma cells has emerged.

In Crohn's disease the total number of plasma cells is increased in the active lesions, including cells producing IgA, IgM, and IgG.[247,421–423,427–429] Cells producing IgD are scarce in the lamina propria of patients with Crohn's disease just as they are in controls. IgA remains the predominant isotype, but the relative increase in IgG and IgM is greater than the relative increase in IgA. The increase in cells producing IgG correlates positively with the degree of histologic inflammation.[247,421–423,429] In the most severely inflamed areas, adjacent to fissuring ulceration, cells producing IgG can become the predominant cell type.[422] In areas with only slight inflammation, IgA and IgM are increased but IgG is not.[422] These changes in the number and isotypes of plasma cells tend to recede with receding inflammatory activity. Differences in the rate of resolution, and in how one defines activity, probably account for the variable results obtained on tissue from uninvolved areas or 'inactive' patients with Crohn's disease. The plasma cells in such mucosa have been reported to be normal,[423,425] to have an increase in all isotypes,[429] or to have an increase only in cells producing IgM.[247,398,421]

In ulcerative colitis, the total number of plasma cells is increased also, including cells producing IgA, IgM, and IgG, but not IgD.[247,248,421,423,428,430,431] Similar to what has been found in Crohn's disease, IgA plasma cells are predominant but the relative increase is greatest for IgG, and then IgM. The infiltration with IgG plasma cells also correlates positively with the degree of histologic inflammation.[247,421,423,431] Although it has been claimed that ulcerative colitis and Crohn's disease can be distinguished immunohistochemically, based on an increase in IgM producing cells in Crohn's disease but not in ulcerative colitis,[421] this has not been supported by the results of other studies,[171,247,423,428] in which the immunohistochemical findings have been compared and do not differ significantly between the two diseases. The similarities between the two include the results on tissue from uninvolved mucosa or from inactive patients, results that are as variable in ulcerative colitis as they are in Crohn's disease. Plasma cells in the lamina propria have been reported to be increased in all isotypes,[432] increased only in IgM cells,[247] and increased only in IgG cells[248,430] One interesting preliminary report indicated that an increase in rectal mucosal plasma cell numbers, especially IgG cells, occurred 3 to 5 weeks before clinical relapses of ulcerative colitis.[432] Although this observation is awaiting confirmation, it indicates that changes in mucosal plasma cells are important prognostically and may also be important pathogenetically in this disease.

Changes in the numbers and composition of mucosal plasma cells are not unique to inflammatory bowel disease, because they occur in other intestinal diseases. A relative increase in IgG cells occurs in the lamina propria in celiac disease,[433] gastritis, and uninvolved mucosa adjacent to colon cancer,[434] although these increases are not as marked as those seen in IBD. These alterations have been thought to represent a generalized mechanism of response of the intestine to a variety of inflammatory stimuli. Brandtzaeg et al. have proposed that the initial intestinal reaction to an inflammatory stimulus is an increase in IgA and IgM plasma cells, and thus local IgA and IgM synthesis.[434] Because both isotypes can be transported into the intestinal lumen via secretory component, thereby increasing secretory antibodies there and decreasing further uptake of the stimulus, this phase is seen as "immune exclusion." If this mechanism is ineffective or overwhelmed, a second phase, called "immune elimination," is triggered, resulting in an increase in IgG plasma cells and local IgG synthesis in the intestine. The latter event may result in a self-perpetuating process because the IgG antibody,[435] and the inflammatory response that it stimulates, can cause more damage to the intestinal barrier, more leakage of antigens into lamina propria, and more IgG production, setting up a repeating cycle. At least some of the IgG produced in the intestinal lesions in IBD may be directed at fecal bacteria.[156,245] With this hypothesis in mind, it is interesting that acute bacterial colitis has been reported to have an increase in IgA plasma cells and a variable increase in IgM plasma cells in the lamina propria, but no increase in IgG plasma cells.[423,436,437a] It is unclear from these reports whether the degree of histologic inflammation of the mucosa was comparable to that seen in IBD, but if so this would seem to be an important distinguishing feature between acute self-limited infectious colitis and chronic idiopathic colitis. Moreover, it tends to support the idea that local IgG production is important in the pathogenesis of IBD.[434] Alternatively, the increase in IgG plasma cells in the lesions of IBD might be reflecting a heightened overall humoral and cellular response in the intestine, the other aspects of which are not as apparent but of more pathogenic importance. The former alternative raises some questions concerning the harmful qualities of local IgG production. The properties of IgG and IgM are not that different. Both can act as opsonins and agglutinins, and although both fix complement, IgM is far more effective in this regard. IgG does mediate ADCC more effectively than IgM. Whatever the reasons, the relative lack of IgG plasma cells in the normal lamina propria suggests that this deficiency is advantageous to the host, and that an increase in the number of IgG plasma cells is not.

Plasma Cells in Deeper Layers of the Bowel Wall. Lymphoid follicles are abundant in the submucosa in inflammatory bowel disease. The central areas of these follicles consist almost exclusively of B cells and antigen presenting cells, most of the B cells having IgM on their surface.[422,429] In Crohn's disease, B cells are found to represent a substantial, that is 60% or more, component of the lymphoid infiltration in the deeper layers of the intestinal wall, when one includes cells in the follicles in the calculation.[429] The mantle zone surrounding the follicles contains many T cells,[426] as well as B cells producing IgG.[171,422] In ulcerative colitis, increased numbers of IgG plasma cells are concentrated in the upper submucosa just below the muscularis mucosa, but not in the lower submucosa, the muscularis, or the subserosa.[431] In contrast, in Crohn's disease significant numbers of IgG plasma cells occur scattered throughout the submucosa, in the muscularis propria, and in the subserosa.[422,429] This infiltration of the deep bowel layers with plasma cells (and other types of cells) distinguishes Crohn's disease from ulcerative colitis.

T Cells in the Intestinal Lesions. T cells constitute a large proportion of the lymphoid cells present in the epithelium and lamina propria of the normal intestine. Immunohistochemical studies on T cells in intestinal lesions are much more limited than those on plasma cells, because reagents capable of identifying subtypes of T cells have only recently become available. As described earlier, most of the cells in the normal epithelium are T cells and most of these have the CD8 (OKT8; Leu 2) antigen. The number of intraepithelial cells is not increased in inflammatory bowel disease, except perhaps in Crohn's ileitis,[437] nor is the proportion of cells that are CD8$^+$ increased.[436a,437,438] In the lamina propria in both Crohn's disease and ulcerative colitis the total number of T cells is increased, but the ratio of the CD4$^+$ helper to the CD8$^+$ suppressor T cell subset is unchanged,[437,438] that is, two-thirds of the lamina propria T cells remain CD4$^+$ (OKT4; Leu 3). The number of T cells expressing HLA-DR class II molecules is not increased.[437,438] The mantle zone surrounding lymphoid follicles consists mainly of T cells, which are 75 to 80% CD4$^+$, as well as scattered HLA-DR$^+$ interdigitating antigen-presenting cells.[439] Lymphoid follicles in the lamina propria in Crohn's disease and ulcerative colitis do not differ from noninflamed control specimens in the types of cells present nor in the ratios among them.[438] In Crohn's disease, but not in ulcerative colitis, T cells have been shown to infiltrate the deeper layers of the bowel wall, including the submucosa, muscularis propria, and subserosa; in certain areas of these layers, T cells are the predominant cell type.[426,440] The T cell subsets present in these deeper bowel layers have not been characterized. Again, the presence of T cells in the deeper layers in Crohn's disease (along with the IgG$^+$ plasma cells, as already noted) distinguishes Crohn's disease from ulcerative colitis.

Antigen-presenting Cells. Little information is available concerning antigen-presenting cells in the intestine.[439,441,442] The intestine has been postulated to contain at least two types of antigen-presenting cells (APC), both having HLA-DR class II MHC molecules on their surfaces.[439] One type is small and stellate, strongly ATPase positive, and weakly positive or negative for acid phosphatase and nonspecific esterase. These are the features of an interdigitating cell. APC in the small intestine appear to be predominantly this cell type.[439] The second type of APC is large and round, strongly acid phosphatase positive, nonspecific esterase positive, but weakly positive or negative for ATPase. These are the characteristics of a tissue macrophage. This type of APC appears to predominate in the colon. In inflammatory bowel disease, increased numbers of APC are present, and a hybrid-type of APC appears in the colon that has stellate processes but is strongly acid phosphatase positive.[439] This heterogeneity among APC in the lamina propria was not noted in a recent immunohistochemical study,[442] and not enough information is available to determine whether these distinctions are more apparent than real.

Another cell type that could potentially act as an antigen-presenting cell in the intestine is the epithelial cell. Epithelial cells on the small intestinal villi normally express HLA-DR$^+$ class II MHC molecules.[6,7] Although epithelial cells in the colon normally do not express HLA-DR antigens,[343,442,443] those overlying inflamed areas do.[442,444,445] In theory, HLA-DR$^+$ epithelial cells could present antigen to intestinal lymphoid cells, although this has not been proven. Expression of DR antigens by inflamed colonic mucosa is not a specific feature of Crohn's disease or ulcerative colitis because it occurred in four out of five biopsies from patients with infectious colitis.[445] The consequences of antigen presentation by colon epithelial cells in areas of inflammation are unknown, but one could speculate that this might greatly amplify immune reactions in these sites, making reestablishment of local immunologic homeostasis more difficult.

THE SECRETORY IgA SYSTEM IN INFLAMMATORY BOWEL DISEASE. Despite abundant immunohistochemical data on the increased numbers of IgA plasma cells in inflammatory bowel disease, little is known about the general competency of the secretory IgA system in these disorders. A local deficiency in the transport of IgA across the epithelium has been postulated, based on immunohistochemical studies in which the epithelial content of secretory component and IgA appeared to be decreased in inflamed areas,[425,446] and even in more proximally uninvolved mucosa.[446] Others have found the numbers of fecal bacteria coated with secretory IgA to be consistently and significantly reduced in patients with Crohn's disease or ulcerative colitis, again suggesting a defective secretory IgA system.[447] These observations are in conflict with the more common immunohistochemical finding that the expression of secretory component and IgA content of epithelial cells are unaltered in inflammatory bowel disease.[171,424,428,431] Moreover, the lack of any known increase in IBD among patients with IgA deficiency may prove that IgA has little or nothing to do with disease pathogenesis. These discrepancies highlight how little we know about the secretory IgA system in IBD. Secretory IgA in the intestine has rarely been measured directly. In serum, where low but detectable levels of sIgA occur, no characteristic alteration has been found in patients with either Crohn's disease or ulcerative colitis.[448–450] Salivary IgA was increased in patients with Crohn's disease,[451] suggesting a general activation of the IgA system in this disease, but was normal in patients with ulcerative colitis.[452,453] Jejunal fluid IgA was normal in Crohn's disease,[454] but decreased in patients with ulcerative colitis;[452] however, IgA levels in feces were normal in four children with ulcerative colitis in remission.[455] These studies on small numbers of patients are insufficient to permit conclusions other than that we know too little about the secretory IgA system in these diseases. Some of the gaps in our knowledge include: the quantity of sIgA in the intestinal lumen, particularly in areas of inflammation; the qualitative composition of that sIgA (it might be abnormal because cells isolated from the lesions of IBD secrete an increased amount of monomeric IgA and IgA of the IgA1 subclass);[456] the antigen specificities of intestinal sIgA in IBD as compared to normal; and the response of the sIgA system to test antigens given via the intestine. Technical factors have limited the study of these questions,[457] but methods are becoming available that will allow some of them to be answered.[458]

IgE, Allergy, and Mast Cells. IgE-producing plasma cells are present in the normal intestinal lamina propria.[459] Some workers have found them to represent a significant fraction of the plasma cells present in the normal intestinal lamina propria,[460] and to be increased in inflammatory bowel disease.[423,461,462] This has prompted the suggestion that IgE-mediated reactions may be important in disease pathogenesis. However, many researchers have found IgE plasma cells to be infrequent in normal lamina propria and to be unchanged in number in inflammatory bowel disease.[420–422,425,428,430,431] It is hard to reconcile such directly divergent results. A number of sources of error are possible in the proper identification of IgE plasma cells, including nonspecific staining of eosinophils by IgE antisera,[420] and the misidentification of mucosal mast cells as IgE plasma cells.[463,464] The number of negative findings by experienced investigators and the many possible confounding technical factors,[420] make it unlikely that significant numbers of IgE plasma cells are present in either the normal or inflamed intestinal lamina propria. This does not preclude a role for IgE-mediated allergic mechanisms in inflammatory bowel disease, but simply indicates that any IgE involved is probably not produced locally within the intestine.

Some forms of colitis or proctitis may be allergic,[465] particularly colitis occurring in infants,[466] although this has never been proven in older children or adults. Eosinophils have been noted to be increased in the lamina propria in ulcerative colitis, and this increase has been postulated to be an attempt at suppression of the inflammation, because the increased numbers of rectal eosinophils were good prognostic indicators in some studies,[467,468] although not in others.[469] Observations like these suggesting that allergy may be contributing to the tissue reaction in inflammatory bowel disease have prompted a number of therapeutic trials with disodium cromoglycate, an inhibitor of mast cell mediator release that is efficacious topically in allergic asthma. Although two early reports were positive,[470,471] disodium cromoglycate has been shown to be of no benefit in inflammatory bowel disease.[469,472-474] The results with disodium cromoglycate in food allergy itself are somewhat equivocal and mucosal mast cells are probably resistant to this drug.[329] More direct assessments of IgE and allergy have been made in patients with inflammatory bowel disease. The serum IgE level is consistently normal,[475-479] as are IgE levels in jejunal secretions.[454,460] Serum IgE antibodies specific for food antigens are not increased.[476,477,479,480] Serum IgE antibodies specific for bacterial antigens or other enteric nonfood antigens have not been reported, although there is one report that peripheral blood basophils of patients with ulcerative colitis did have an increased histamine release (a measure of cell-bound specific IgE) when exposed to colon mucosal homogenates.[478] Lastly, neither IBD patients nor their families have any increased history of atopy as compared to control.[476] Thus, at present no evidence is available that IgE-mediated allergic mechanisms are playing a major role in idiopathic inflammatory bowel disease, and in fact the weight of the evidence is rather against this idea.

The lack of evidence that IgE and allergy are playing a role in inflammatory bowel disease does not imply that mast cells are not involved. Mast cell numbers have been noted to be increased in the intestine in both Crohn's disease[394,410] and ulcerative colitis.[389] In Crohn's disease significant numbers of mast cells are present in the deeper layers of the bowel wall, and mast cells appear to be degranulating.[394] The role that mast cells play in the pathogenesis of inflammatory bowel disease is undefined. Mast cells do respond to a variety of stimuli other than IgE, however, such as C3a and C5a anaphylotoxins and neutrophil cationic protein, among others, and are involved in reactions other than immediate hypersensitivity.[481] Mast cells produce a variety of potent mediators including histamine, prostaglandins, and leukotrienes that can greatly affect cells in the surrounding tissues. The existence of a mucosal mast cell subset in man, similar to what has been described in the rat, has been suspected as a result of differences in formalin fixation of mucosal vs. nonmucosal mast cells.[464] This has now been firmly established: human mucosal mast cells contain only tryptase in their granules, whereas nonmucosal mast cells contain both tryptase and chymotryptase.[482] Of note, formalin poorly fixes both types of mast cell, but particularly mucosal mast cells, thus the number of these cells has probably been underestimated in histologic sections. Mast cell concentration in the small bowel, using immunoperoxidase staining with a tryptase-specific monoclonal antibody after proper fixation, was approximately 20,000 per cubic mm in mucosa and 85,000 per cubic mm of submucosa,[483] a significant number. It is unknown at present whether both or only one of these mast cell subsets is increased in inflammatory bowel disease tissue. This will be important because there are major differences in responsiveness to secretagogues and inhibitors between mucosal and peritoneal mast cells in the rat, and the same may be true in man. These points and others regarding recent progress in our understanding of mast cell structure and function have been recently reviewed.[329] These advances, including the ability to isolate intestinal mucosal mast cells in vitro,[484] hold great promise for rapid expansion of our knowledge in this important area.

ISOLATED LAMINA PROPRIAL CELLS. A recent advance in the study of the immunology of inflammatory bowel disease has been the development of techniques allowing isolation of lymphoid cells from the intestinal lamina propria.[339] Cells isolated from lamina propria include T cells, B cells, and macrophages; the average recoveries of these different cell types are shown in Table 7-5. Although this technique is a major advance, it does have some limitations that need to be understood. First, the technique selects for certain types of cells and against others,[485] for example, almost no plasma cells are recovered using this technique, although they are abundant in the intestine.[339,342,486] Moreover, cell selection appears to vary in different laboratories, perhaps because most workers use their own modifications of the method; the wide range in the percentage of different cells recovered attests to this point (Table 7-5). It is unclear what the ideal ratio among T cells, B cells, and macrophages should be. Second, lamina proprial isolates contain cells from both the Peyer's patch and lamina proprial compartments of GALT (Fig. 7-3). In man, the Peyer's patches are small, dispersed, and not evident to the naked eye, thus they are included in the mucosal layer that is subjected to the separation procedure. Third, "collagenase" is a lyophilized bacterial supernatant that contains multiple enzymes, many of them unidentified. Crude collagenase preparations in particular have significant toxicity. Those preparations that are not directly toxic to cells may yet impair cell function in unexpected ways. At a minimum, one must show that the immune function being studied is unaffected by putting peripheral blood lymphocytes through the entire procedure. Mechanical techniques have been tried but appear to have no advantages;[340,487,488] in fact, they seem more adversely to affect cell function.[487,488]

In the studies reported to date few differences have been revealed between isolated lamina proprial cells from inflamed vs. noninflamed mucosa. What differences have been demonstrated have been quantitative rather than qualitative, for example, the lamina proprial isolates

TABLE 7-5. *Cell types found in intestinal lamina proprial isolates.*

	Percentage	
	Mean	Range
T cells	59	38 to 90
CD4+	58	53 to 64
CD8+	42	36 to 47
B cells	24	7 to 40
Macrophages	10	7 to 14
Fc+ cells	3	0 to 7
"Null" cells	?	0 to 26
Plasma cells	<1	0 to 7

from the intestinal lesions of IBD contain 2 to 5 times more lymphoid cells than those from normal mucosa. Isolated lamina proprial cells from IBD mucosa have been reported to contain more B cells, particularly B cells producing IgG,[489] compared to noninvolved IBD mucosa or control mucosa. Although lamina proprial isolates contain some cells that seem to have been activated in vivo, these isolates also contain resting cells that can be activated to proliferate when stimulated with mitogens,[340,341,352,490] alloantigens,[340,341,353] and at least some bacterial antigens.[352] In general, no difference has been found between the proliferative responses of lamina proprial cells isolated from inflamed vs. noninflamed mucosa, although there have been differences between lamina proprial cells vs. peripheral blood cells, with a tendency for lamina proprial cells to respond less well. This may be caused by an alteration in the kinetics of the response, however,[340] rather than a real difference. Lamina propria appears to be deficient in or lack some cell types that are present in the peripheral blood, for example, cells with Fc receptors, a subset that encompasses certain types of cytotoxic cells.[339,489] Some controversy exists about the presence and function of Fc bearing cells in the intestinal lamina propria, a subject that will be covered in detail in the following section. Suppressor-inducer and suppressor-effector T cell subsets may also be deficient in intestinal lamina propria relative to peripheral blood.[491] The findings of more differences between lamina proprial and peripheral blood cells than between lamina proprial cells from inflamed vs. noninflamed mucosa has been surprising. It might be a result of cell selection or assays simply not looking in the right direction. Another explanation is that cells in the "normal" intestinal mucosa are continuously in a state of activation or inflammation that is held in check by as yet undefined regulatory mechanisms, with IBD representing a state in which these regulatory mechanisms are less able to limit this activation. This would account for the lack of qualitative differences in inflamed vs. non-inflamed lamina proprial cells.

Cultures of isolated lamina proprial cells synthesize and secrete immunoglobulin to a much greater degree than do peripheral blood lymphocytes, and at least some of the IgA and IgG antibodies produced by isolated lamina proprial cells are directed at intestinal bacteria.[492] Immunoglobulins synthesized include IgA, IgM, and IgG.[339,349,489,493] In short-term cultures, cells from inflamed mucosa produced much more IgG than did cells from noninflamed mucosa,[489] although this was not evident when cells were cultured for longer periods.[493,494] In longer-term cultures, less spontaneous immunoglobulin was produced in isolates from inflamed mucosa than was evident in isolates from noninflamed lamina propria.[493] Moreover, an increased percentage of monomeric IgA and of IgA1 was produced by lymphocytes from inflamed mucosa,[456] suggesting a subtle alteration in the IgA system in IBD. Lamina proprial T cells that regulate immunoglobulin synthesis have begun to be studied: consistent with the preceding observations, helper activity predominates in lamina proprial isolates, and little suppressor activity is evident in either control or inflamed lamina proprial cells.[349,350]

Systemic Cellular Immunity

The cellular immune system is particularly important in host defense against intracellular pathogens such as viruses and mycobacteria, in the immune response to contact allergens, and in the immune reactions to tumors and transplanted organs. The specificity of the cellular immune system resides in antigen-specific T lymphocytes (Fig. 7-5), a role played by antibody in the humoral immune system. T cells that initiate and regulate cellular immunity bear the helper CD4 antigen. Similar to other CD4$^+$ cells, antigen is recognized in association with Class II MHC molecules. Once stimulated by antigen, these T cells release lymphokines such as interleukin 2, gamma interferon, macrophage chemotactic factor, macrophage inhibitory factor, and macrophage activating factor, and they begin to proliferate. The released lymphokines recruit macrophages to sites of antigen deposition and also activate them. Cytotoxic T cells (CTL), which bear the CD8 antigen, are also affected by the released lymphokines, particularly interleukin 2. Cytotoxic T cells proliferate and clonally expand when they are both stimulated by antigen in association with Class I MHC molecules and are exposed to interleukin 2, and they are particularly important in the host defense against virally infected cells. In the sections that follow, cells that mediate other types of cytotoxicity, such as natural killing (NK) and antibody dependent cellular cytotoxicity (ADCC), will be discussed under cellular immunity, although these cells appear to represent a distinct lineage.

It has long been suspected that cellular immunity plays a role, perhaps a major one, in the pathogenesis of inflammatory bowel disease.

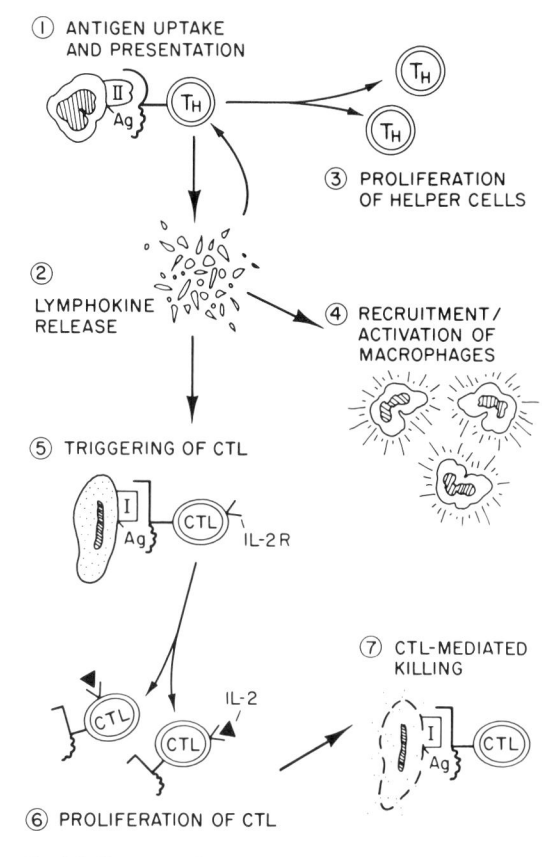

FIG. 7-5. Sequence of events required for the activation of the cellular effector system. Ag, antigen; II, class II MHC molecules; I, class I MHC molecules; IL-2R, interleukin-2 receptors, IL-2, interleukin-2; T_H, helper T lymphocytes; CTL, cytotoxic T lymphocytes.

This belief stems partly from the resemblance of Crohn's disease to intestinal tuberculosis, an infection in which cellular immunity has a major role in host defense. In addition, the suspicion that a virus may cause inflammatory bowel disease also tends to implicate cellular immunity in IBD, because this effector system plays a major role in clearance of virally infected cells from the body. Lastly, the hallmark of cellular immune reactions is the presence in tissues of an abundance of activated macrophages, sometimes forming granulomas. Crohn's disease would certainly seem to fit into this type of tissue reaction, and, to a lesser extent, so would ulcerative colitis. The following discussion of assays of cellular immunity in inflammatory bowel disease will follow the sequence of events shown in Figure 7-5, that is, lymphocyte proliferation, lymphokine release, macrophage function and activation, delayed skin test responses, and cytotoxic cells.

LYMPHOCYTE PROLIFERATION. The ideal situation would be the testing of the proliferative capacity of patients' lymphocytes to the agent or antigen that is causing inflammatory bowel disease. With this in mind, some workers have incubated patient peripheral blood lymphocytes with extracts of intestinal contents or with extracts of gut homogenates, achieving essentially negative results.[494,495] Lymphocytes from patients with Crohn's disease do not have any increased reactivity to the Kveim antigen isolated from sarcoidosis tissue.[496] The proliferative response to extracts of E.coli bacteria is normal in most patients with ulcerative colitis,[497] but may be decreased in active cases.[498] The proliferative response to antigens other than these has not been tested extensively. A decreased proliferative response to a "cocktail" of common environmental antigens (streptococcal varidase, trichophyton, candida, mumps, and PPD) was found in patients with Crohn's disease as compared to normal controls;[499] however, little subsequent work is available to compare with this study. The proliferative response to streptococcal varidase alone was decreased in Crohn's patients;[500] however, the response to PPD was normal.[501,502] Overall, little evidence is available to suggest that the proliferative response of peripheral blood lymphocytes to either intestinal or nonintestinal common environmental antigens is altered.

An alternative method for examining the proliferative capacity of lymphocytes is to use mitogenic lectins. Mitogenic lectins will stimulate lymphocyte proliferation in most individuals, although the response of any given individual can be variable. Some of the mitogens appear specific for T cells, such as phytohemagglutinin (PHA) and concanavalin A (ConA), others for both T cells and B cells, such as pokeweed mitogen (PWM), and yet others for B cells alone, such as staphylococcus protein A (SAC). Among the available mitogens, the one most widely applied to the study of inflammatory bowel disease has been PHA. This is perhaps a fortunate choice because PHA has recently been found to bind to a subunit of the T3 molecule that forms a complex with the T cell receptor.[503] The proliferative response to PHA has been consistently normal in patients with ulcerative colitis,[494,497,498,500,504,505] except for a single report of decreased responsiveness.[506] Results in patients with Crohn's disease are more variable. Some have reported a 25 to 60% decrease in the proliferative response to PHA,[494,500,506,507] whereas others have found normal responses.[499,501,504,505,508-510] The responses to mitogens such as ConA and pokeweed mitogen have not been as extensively studied, but have been generally normal in both Crohn's disease and ulcerative colitis.[499,500,504,505,507,509] The response to B cell mitogens such as staphylococcal protein A has not yet been reported. In sum, the majority of patients have normal proliferative responses to mitogens. However, a subset of patients with Crohn's disease, perhaps as many of one-third,[506] may have decreased proliferative responses to PHA. The significance of the decreased PHA responsiveness in this subset of patients and whether the decrease is biologically important are unclear.

A third approach to studying lymphocyte proliferation in inflammatory bowel disease has been the response of T cells to nonself alloantigens on other lymphoid cells. The mixed lymphocyte reaction (MLR) assay consists of culturing peripheral blood lymphocytes of two different individuals together in vitro. The lymphocytes used to stimulate are usually irradiated or treated with mitomycin C to prevent them from responding (one-way MLR). The results of such MLR assays in patients with inflammatory bowel disease have been conflicting. A decreased MLR response has been described in patients with Crohn's disease and in ulcerative colitis.[511,512] In one of these studies much of the reduced responsiveness could be reversed by removal of adherent cells, presumably macrophages, so it is unclear whether the T cells themselves were impaired. Other workers have found normal MLR responses both in Crohn's disease,[507,508,513,514] and also ulcerative colitis.[507,514] In recent years, it has become apparent that T cells will proliferate when cultured with autologous B cells, null cells, or macrophages. This response is called the autologous mixed lymphocyte reaction or AMLR. The AMLR has memory and specificity,[515] two hallmarks of an immune response. Xenogeneic antigens found on sheep red blood cells and in fetal calf serum seem to boost the AMLR,[516,517] but even in their absence a relatively smaller but significant response occurs. The AMLR may be involved in generating immunoregulatory cells, particularly suppressor cells.[518-520] Only a few studies are available on the AMLR done in patients with inflammatory bowel disease and they are conflicting, with two showing a decreased response,[521,522] and the other showing normal results.[507] This divergence may be caused by differences in the patients studied or their treatments. The AMLR in normal individuals is sensitive to corticosteroids,[523] and this represents a pitfall in studies on patients with IBD who are often treated with this medication.

In summary, little evidence exists for an altered proliferative response to enteric or nonenteric antigens, mitogens, or alloantigens in the majority of patients with inflammatory bowel disease. A subset of patients with a diminished lymphocyte proliferative response to antigens or mitogens may occur. This latter subset of patients may be seen more frequently at certain major referral centers, and thus be represented disproportionately in studies done at these centers. This might explain some of the divergent reports in the literature.

LYMPHOKINES. Cells of the immune system interact extensively. Most of this interaction occurs via the release of and response to soluble mediators or lymphokines. Some coherence has recently been brought to the lymphokine field by the purification and biochemical characterization of a number of important lymphokines. This, in turn, has led to the recognition that the same lymphokine can have multiple activities in different assay systems. Thus, what were thought to be multiple different lymphokines are now recognized to be multiple different activities of a few molecules. Four lymphokines in particular have been extensively characterized and the genes encoding them isolated. Interleukin-1 is a soluble mediator released by activated macrophages that acts on T lymphocytes, inducing the production of both interleukin-2 and interleukin-2 receptors. Interleukin-2, produced by activated T cells, is essential for T cell proliferation and clonal expansion. Interleukin-3 is a lymphokine produced by T cells that acts as a colony stimulating factor for mast cells and a variety of hematopoietic cells. Lastly, the interferons are a group of inducible molecules that can be clustered into three classes: alpha, beta, and gamma. The last of these, gamma or immune interferon, is produced by T cells and has a variety of effects on other cells in the immune system, particularly on cells involved in cellular immunity, as well as on cells outside the immune system.[329]

As noted in Figure 7–5, lymphokines are released by T cells when the latter are stimulated by specific antigens or by nonspecific mitogens. Lymphokines thus released can be measured indirectly by their effects on other cells. When antigen is used as the stimulant, lymphokine release can be used to determine whether cells sensitized to that antigen are present. This has been the rationale for testing peripheral blood lymphocytes of IBD patients for sensitivity to mucosal or fecal antigens in macrophage- or leukocyte-migration inhibition tests. In ulcerative colitis patients, leukocyte migration was inhibited upon exposure to extracts of allogeneic fetal colon or fetal small intestine,[524] suggesting the presence of lymphocytes sensitized to mucosal antigens. In another study, however, leukocyte migration inhibition was not evident when autologous mucosal antigens were used.[525] Peripheral blood cells of patients with both ulcerative colitis and Crohn's disease do appear to release migration inhibition factor upon exposure to enterobacterial common antigen, with cells from ulcerative colitis patients responding more frequently than those from Crohn's disease patients.[526,527] This is not specific for IBD, however, because patients with cirrhosis have a similar responsiveness.[527a] Mitogens can also be used to stimulate lymphokine release, but few studies of this type have been done. One report is available of deficient IL-2 production by PHA-stimulated peripheral blood cells in patients with Crohn's disease.[522] This observation needs to be confirmed, but may partly explain the decreased lymphocyte proliferation seen in a subset of patients with Crohn's disease. Lastly, one can try to directly measure lymphokines in body fluids, such as plasma. Using this last approach, elevated levels of circulating interferon have been demonstrated in the blood of patients with ulcerative colitis and Crohn's disease.[528-530] The type of interferon that is elevated and the biologic effects of this elevation have yet to be defined. Few conclusions can be drawn from the limited number of studies in this area, other than the fact that much of the recent progress in lymphokine research has yet to be applied to the study of inflammatory bowel disease.

MONOCYTES/MACROPHAGES. Lymphokines released by antigen specific T cells act upon local tissue macrophages and also recruit and retain new macrophages into the area from the circulating precursor pool, the blood monocytes (Fig. 7–5). In this way the effects of a relatively small number of antigen specific T cells are greatly amplified. Lymphokines also activate the macrophages, that is, convert them from relatively quiescent cells into actively phagocytic, bacteriocidal cells that synthesize literally dozens of biologically active substances. The monocyte/macrophage has a variety of other functions other than as a nonspecific effector cell, for example, in antigen presentation, but these are beyond the scope of this chapter.[531-533]

Macrophages are prominent in the intestinal lesions of Crohn's disease and ulcerative colitis. Because tissue macrophages are largely derived from circulating blood monocytes, circulating monocytes have been examined with the rationale that the function of the precursor cell should approximate that of the tissue macrophage. Monocyte numbers, response to activators, motility, phagocytosis, bacteriocidal ability, and the synthesis of various monokines and other bioactive compounds have all been assessed. The absolute number of circulating monocytes is increased in both ulcerative colitis and Crohn's disease.[44,46,534,535] In the only study of its kind, the production of monocytes in the bone marrow was moderately increased in both Crohn's disease and ulcerative colitis, being 1.4 times and 1.7 times the level of normal controls, respectively.[536] This level of monocyte production in IBD is similar to that found in sarcoidosis, a granulomatous disease distinguished by relatively low macrophage turnover. Despite the prominence of granulomata in Crohn's disease, monocyte production in patients with this disease was not significantly different from that in patients with ulcerative colitis.

Monocyte motility has been tested in vitro using the same methods applied to neutrophils. Random macrophage motility (chemokinesis) was significantly increased both in patients with ulcerative colitis[269,537] and in patients with Crohn's disease.[537] Monocyte chemotaxis in vitro was normal or increased.[269,537] Monocyte motility in vivo has not received much attention,[255,275] but is thought to be normal despite the demonstration of circulating inhibitors to chemotaxis.[280] Monocyte phagocytosis of C. albicans,[537] and of opsonized S. aureus, was significantly and comparably increased both in ulcerative colitis and Crohn's disease, with no evident relationship to disease activity or duration.[538] Intracellular killing of phagocytosed S. aureus was normal.[538] The cellular content and secretion of a number of monocyte lysosomal enzymes was increased in patients with ulcerative colitis or Crohn's disease,[534,539] as were other synthetic products such as transcobalamin II,[540] plasminogen activator,[541] but spontaneous monocyte prostanoid synthesis was not increased.[535] Although not directly tested in vitro, increased production of lysozyme by monocytes may partly explain the elevated serum levels of this enzyme found in IBD.[542,543] Despite this evidence of in vivo activation, patient blood monocytes remain able to respond normally to activation by endotoxin and immune complexes.[544]

In summary, the number and production of blood monocytes is increased. Monocytes show increases in random motility, in phagocytosis, and in the synthesis of a number of bioactive substances, all indicating that some activation of these cells occurs in vivo. Not every aspect of their function has been assessed, but the results are remarkably consistent. No differences in monocyte function between ulcerative colitis and Crohn's disease are apparent, despite the frequent presence of granulomata in the latter. From these studies, little is found to support the speculation of deficient macrophage function as a primary factor in the pathogenesis of IBD.[545] Another point that tends to contradict this idea is that drugs effective in the treatment of IBD inhibit monocyte/macrophage function.[295,533,535,546]

CYTOTOXIC CELLS. The second major effector cell of the cell-mediated immune system is the cytotoxic T lymphocyte (CTL). In contrast to activated macrophages, CTL are highly specific. Cytotoxic T lymphocyte receptors recognize, and CTL are thus activated by, allogeneic class I MHC molecules or by other cell surface antigens, such as viral antigens, in conjunction with autologous class I MHC molecules (Fig. 7–5). Clonal expansion of antigen-activated CTL precursors is highly dependent upon the secretion of interleukin-2 by inducer T cells. In addition to CTL there are two other major classes of cytotoxic cells. Although these are not generally considered part of the cell-mediated immune system, they will be discussed here for convenience. Antibody dependent cellular cytotoxicity (ADCC) can be mediated by lymphocytes, granulocytes, or macrophages that have Fc receptors for IgG.[547] Among lymphocytes, a non-T cell, non-B subset with high affinity Fc receptors is the major cell type mediating ADCC. This cell frequently has been called a killer (K) cell. The specificity of this type of cytotoxicity is determined by the antibody rather than by any specific receptor on the effector cell. Cytotoxicity occurs when antibody bridges the target to the effector cell. A third type of cytotoxic cell is the natural killer (NK) cell. Natural killer cells are large granular lymphocytes that have high affinity Fc receptors. Although functional heterogeneity occurs within the NK cell subset, these cells do appear to be a distinct lineage that expresses distinct membrane glycoproteins, such as those recognized by monoclonal antibodies Leu 7 or Leu 11. The distinguishing feature of NK cells is that they require no induction but are spontaneously cytotoxic to certain types of target cells. Recognition of the target does not involve either antibody or MHC molecules. Natural killer cells are postulated to be involved in host resistance to viral infections and in tumor surveillance, and may also have noncytotoxic functions such as regulation of hematopoiesis and of B cell proliferation and function.[329]

Each of these various types of cytotoxicity has been examined in peripheral blood mononuclear cells of IBD patients. In this section the general functional ability of these types of cytotoxic cells in patients will be covered. The role of cytotoxic cells specific for intestinal epithelial cells in IBD will be addressed in the "Etiologic Theories" section. Cytotoxic T cell-mediated cytotoxicity to allogeneic target cells is normal in patients with ulcerative colitis or Crohn's disease who have inactive or only mild disease activity.[507,522] It may be decreased in those with active disease, however;[514,522] this reduction may be partly caused by a decrease in the production of or response to interleukin-2.[522] ADCC have been tested in a variety of systems, and no two are alike. Peripheral blood ADCC has been largely normal in Crohn's disease,[548–550] and in ulcerative colitis,[550] with the exception of one study that found increased ADCC in Crohn's disease patients using an unusual plaque assay,[551] an assay that has been criticized.[548] Patients with active Crohn's disease tend to have lower levels of ADCC as compared to patients with inactive disease.[548,550] Natural killer cell cytotoxicity has been measured by a variety of workers with more divergent results. Auer first described a significantly decreased peripheral blood NK cell activity against the LIK lymphoblastoid cell line in patients with Crohn's disease.[552] This was subsequently confirmed by others using the K562 human erythroleukemia cell line as a target,[553,554] as well as the human colon cancer cell line, RPMI 4788.[555] Normal NK cell activity toward K562 cells has also been found in patients with Crohn's disease, however.[550,556,557] Peripheral blood lymphocytes from patients with ulcerative colitis have also been noted to have NK cell activity that is either decreased,[553] or normal.[550,556] These discrepancies may be related to differences in disease activity among the types of patients studied. For example, MacDermott et al., using a variety of cell targets, found that patients with active Crohn's disease had decreased natural killing to all the targets, although the overall group of patients with Crohn's disease was not significantly different from controls.[550] Interestingly, NK cells from IBD patients were relatively hyporesponsive to stimulation with gamma interferon. The numbers of circulating NK cells are not reduced in IBD patients,[533,557] thus a relative hyporesponsiveness of NK cells to activators, perhaps because of prior in vivo exposure to activating signals, is attractive as a possible explanation of reduced NK cell activity in this disease. Another factor might be the treatments being used to control the disease. Brogan et al. found a statistically significant but slight decrease in NK cell activity in patients with Crohn's disease, while they found a greatly decreased NK cell activity in patients with Crohn's disease who were being treated with 6-Mercaptopurine.[558] Peripheral blood cytotoxic cell function appears to be intrinsically normal in these patients; however, each type of cytotoxicity may be reduced, particularly when the disease is active. Natural killer cell activity seems to be the most prone to reduction by disease activity and by drug treatment.

SKIN TEST RESPONSES AND ANERGY. Intradermal injection of an antigen to determine whether an individual is sensitive to it is a well-known and apparently simple clinical test. A complex series of interactions and events must occur, however, before the familiar erythema and induration occur. Circulating, antigen-specific lymphocytes must be triggered by the antigen to release lymphokines that, in turn, must act upon circulating monocytes, causing them to accumulate locally in the skin and become activated, releasing a variety of monokines and other biologically active molecules (Fig. 7–5, steps 1 to 4). An interruption in any step of this process can result in a deficient skin test response to the antigen. Early studies of skin test responses in patients with inflammatory bowel disease found that many patients with Crohn's disease or ulcerative colitis had reduced responses to tuberculin as compared to historic controls.[502,559-561] When appropriate concurrent controls were done, however, tuberculin responses were found to be normal;[501,562,563] only patients with Crohn's disease who were ill and receiving steroids had reduced responses.[563] Skin test responses to recall antigens other than tuberculin have also been examined. Meuwissen et al. found a significant increase in the number of Crohn's disease patients who failed to respond to any of five common skin test antigens, although no difference was found in the mean number of positive skin reactions in the Crohn's disease group as compared to controls.[499] These results conflict with the more common observation of normal skin test responses to common environmental antigens in Crohn's disease and ulcerative colitis,[509,564,565] with the exception of Crohn's disease patients receiving immunosuppressive therapy who had decreased responses.[509] Patients with IBD were skin tested both before and 6 to 18 months after an intestinal resection. Some 40% of patients with Crohn's disease or ulcerative colitis were anergic prior to surgery. Almost all of the anergic patients responded when tested postoperatively, however.[566] This reversion to responsiveness was attributed to the removal of diseased intestine, cessation of steroids, and improved nutrition.

Because of reports of decreased responsiveness to recall antigens, patients with inflammatory bowel disease have been tested for their ability to respond in a primary, delayed-type hypersensitivity response to the contact allergen, dinitrochlorobenzene (DNCB). The response of patients to DNCB has been found to be significantly decreased,[63,561,567] to be normal except in patients with active Crohn's disease on steroids,[563] and to be normal in nonimmunosuppressed patients but deficient in those receiving immunosuppressive medications.[509] The response to DNCB sensitization was normal among relatives and spouses of IBD patients.[567] Although no correlation appeared to exist between a diminished DNCB responsiveness and either the extent, activity, or duration of the disease,[63,561] this conclusion is based on a comparison of different patient subgroups and not a comparison of the same patients followed at different stages of their disease. Of note, the report that skin test anergy to recall antigens resolves after intestinal resection comes from one of the centers reporting that diminished responses to DNCB sensitization were apparently unrelated to disease activity.[63,566,567] This conclusion deserves to be reexamined because it seems likely that the same factors that restore skin test responses to recall antigens would also restore responsiveness to DNCB sensitization.

The occurrence of sarcoid-like noncaseating granulomata in the lesions of Crohn's disease and the reports of anergy in Crohn's disease have prompted the testing of Crohn's disease patients with the Kveim antigen.[568] Although initial reports were positive,[569,570] this could not be confirmed,[496,571-573] even when the same Kveim antigens were used.[571] Thus, patients with

Crohn's disease do not react to the Kveim antigen, nor do they have a positive skin response to Crohn's disease tissue homogenates.[560]

Anergy occurs in a subgroup of patients with Crohn's disease and ulcerative colitis. Considering that malnutrition,[574] immunosuppressive therapy, and lymphocyte sequestration can all decrease skin test responses,[575] it is not surprising that these may be diminished in patients with inflammatory bowel disease. The anergy that occurs in patients with inflammatory bowel disease is probably caused by a combination of these factors; it appears to resolve in most patients after intestinal resection,[566] when these factors are reversed or inoperative. Thus, anergy does not equate with a primary underlying immunodeficiency in these patients. Lastly, reactions occurring in the skin are not an accurate reflection of immune responses occurring in other organs. This is true in sarcoidosis where anergic skin test responses do not accurately reflect the presence of sensitized lymphocytes in the blood or an abundance of activated T cells in the lung.[576,577] It is also likely to be true in inflammatory bowel disease.

Intestinal Cellular Immunity

Little is known about cellular immunity either in the normal or inflamed intestine. All the necessary cell types are present in the intestine, however, and cell-mediated immune reactions occur in the intestine in experimental animals.[578] Cell-mediated immune reactions undoubtedly occur in the human intestine, and have long been postulated to be involved in inflammatory bowel disease,[579] but the extent to which they occur and their importance compared to other types of immune reactivity has yet to be defined either in health or disease.

MUCOSAL LYMPHOCYTE PROLIFERATION. Lamina proprial cells both from control and inflammatory bowel disease patients show evidence of in vivo activation. For example, they have been noted to have a higher rate of spontaneous proliferation than is seen with peripheral blood lymphocytes.[352,580] Lamina proprial lymphocytes have also been found to proliferate when cultured in vitro with interleukin-2 under conditions in which peripheral blood lymphocytes do not respond.[581] Interestingly, lamina proprial cells from the uninvolved resection margin in Crohn's disease responded similarly to those from non-IBD controls, whereas those from the active lesions of Crohn's disease had a reduced, rather than increased, response.[581] Cells that have already been activated respond poorly, if at all, to cellular activators such as mitogenic lectins; for example, IL-2 dependent T cells do not proliferate when reexposed to mitogens in the absence of IL-2. In addition to containing cells that have been activated in vivo, however, lamina proprial isolates also contain resting cells that can proliferate when stimulated in vitro with mitogens,[341,352,353,490] allo-antigens,[341,353] or selected bacterial antigens.[352] Lamina proprial cells tend to respond less well to mitogens than peripheral blood lymphocytes,[352,490] although the peak response may not be different.[352] In the few studies that have been done, little difference has been found in the proliferative response to mitogens or alloantigens by lamina proprial cells isolated from either inflammatory bowel disease or control specimens.[341,352,353,490] The response of lamina proprial cells to specific antigens, such as those likely to be present in the gut lumen, has rarely been examined. In the one study available, lamina proprial cells from Crohn's disease specimens had a statistically significant increase in proliferative response to E. coli lipopolysaccharide and to Staphylococcus aureus, but no increased response to Bacteroides antigens, lipid A, or enterobacterial common antigen.[352] Overall, this aspect of cellular immunity appears intact in both IBD and control mucosa, with the exception of some impairment related to deficient IL-2 production or responsiveness in actively inflamed mucosa.

LYMPHOKINES AND INFLAMMATORY MEDIATORS IN THE INTESTINE. Considering the central role that lymphokines play in the immune system, they probably also play an important role in normal mucosal immunologic homeostasis and in diseases such as inflammatory bowel disease. Disorders of lymphokine function have been observed in a number of diseases such as immunodeficiency, systemic lupus erythematosus, rheumatoid arthritis, and others,[329] suggesting that abnormal lymphokine function could be important in inflammatory bowel disease. This question has only recently been addressed and the data available are sketchy. No reports are available yet on the production of or response to interleukin-1 in the intestinal mucosa. From the large numbers of macrophages present in the normal gut and increased numbers present in inflammatory bowel disease, however, one can surmise that interleukin-1 will be an important mediator in the mucosa. Interleukin-2 is produced by intestinal lamina proprial cells when they are stimulated by phorbol myristic acetate (PMA), a protein kinase-C activator, or by phytohemagglutinin.[582] Interestingly, lamina proprial cells from inflamed mucosa from patients with Crohn's disease or ulcerative colitis had a reduced production of interleukin-2 when stimulated with PMA but not with PHA,[582] suggesting some reduction of IL-2 production in the active lesions in vivo. Thus, both the production of and response to IL-2 by lamina proprial cells from inflamed intestine appear to be impaired.[581] The role of interferon in intestinal immunity remains to be defined. Interferon causes an increase in class II MHC expression by a variety of cells, including human epithelial cells.[583] An increase in interferon production may help explain the increased class II MHC expression by epithelial cells in areas of active colitis.[444,445] Only a single, preliminary report on interferon production by mucosal cells is available, and decreased rather than increased production was found in human intestinal lamina proprial cells isolated from patients with inflammatory bowel disease when they were stimulated with IL-2.

In addition to lymphokines, such as interleukin-1 and interferon, a variety of molecules promote or "mediate" the inflammatory response. These include substances such as histamine, serotonin, bradykinin, C3a and C5a anaphylotoxins, neutrophil chemotactic factor, platelet activating factor, and a variety of arachidonic acid metabolites (the prostaglandins and leukotrienes).[585] Little is known about whether or how these inflammatory mediators might mediate inflammation in the intestine, but interest has been expressed in the possible role of arachidonic acid metabolites in IBD.[586,587] Arachidonic acid in membrane phospholipids is released into its free form by the action of phospholipases; free arachidonic acid is then metabolized by oxygenation through two distinct pathways, the cyclooxygenase pathway resulting in various prostaglandins and thromboxanes, or the lipoxygenase pathway resulting in the leukotrienes. Prostaglandins, in particular PGE_2,[586-589] and leukotrienes, in particular LTB_4,[584,590] are increased in the mucosa and blood during active colitis. The observation that sulfasalazine and prednisone decrease rectal mucosal and serum levels of prostaglandins[588,591] has prompted the suggestion that prostaglandins are the major inflammatory mediators of inflammatory bowel disease.[588] Drugs such as indomethacin that are much more potent inhibitors of the cyclooxygenase pathway are not efficacious in inflammatory bowel disease,[592] however, raising doubts about this hypothesis. Recent interest has shifted to the leukotrienes, particularly LTB_4, as important mediators of inflammation in inflammatory bowel disease. Sulfasalazine and prednisone also decrease leukotriene levels in inflamed mucosa.[590,593,594] Inhibitors specifically for the leukotriene pathway are not yet available but are being developed; the response of patients to such inhibitors should tell us a great deal about the role of leukotrienes in inflammatory bowel disease. The entire area of inflammatory mediators remains a fertile, but as yet undeveloped, area of research in inflammatory bowel disease. Although these mediators are clearly secondary rather than primary in these diseases, the term secondary does not mean unimportant. Clearly, a better understanding of the final common pathway of inflammation in these diseases should permit the fashioning of new therapies that might be just as efficacious as H-2 blockers have been in peptic ulcer disease.

INTESTINAL MACROPHAGES. Macrophages form a significant proportion of the cells present in both the noninflamed and inflamed intestinal lamina propria, but little information about them is available. Histochemical stains suggest that intestinal macrophages are heterogeneous,[439] with cells resembling interdigitating cells predominating in the small intestine and cells resembling tissue macrophages predominating in the colon. A third type of cell, one with features of both of the other types, has been identified in inflamed colonic mucosa.[439] It is uncertain whether this third type represents the veiled cells reported by Wilders and colleagues.[441]

Further understanding of the intestinal macrophage will require its isolation and study in vitro.[595] Approximately 10 to 50% of isolated lamina proprial cells are macrophages. These appear to be larger and more phagocytic than blood monocytes,[339,596] and are esterase positive and peroxidase negative, similar to alveolar macrophages.[597] Most have surface HLA-DR class II molecules, and about half have surface Fc receptors for IgG.[598] Intestinal macrophages actively synthesize and secrete lysozyme during culture,[589] which may be related to the increased levels of serum and fecal lysozyme that have been noted in patients.[542,543] Intestinal mononuclear cells from IBD mucosa, presumably macrophages, secrete increased amounts of prostanoids into the culture media.[599] No other data are available about other secretory products of macrophages isolated from IBD mucosa.

One of the problems in this area is the lack of a reliable technique to purify intestinal macrophages without altering their function.[595] For example, adherence to plastic or glass, commonly used to purify blood monocytes, is variable with intestinal macrophages;[595] moreover, adherence itself can activate macrophages. A second problem relates to the interpretation of various assays that compare macrophages from noninflamed and inflamed mucosa. Prior activation in vivo may render the cells relatively refractory or unresponsive in some in vitro assays; cells from inflamed mucosa may thus appear less functional in vitro, whereas the reverse may be true in vivo. Careful attention to the effects of activation itself on the functional ability of blood monocytes in in vitro assays will be needed in order to allow proper interpretation.

MUCOSAL CYTOTOXIC CELLS. Cytotoxic cells in the intestine have drawn a lot of attention because they seem to be likely candidates as mediators of tissue damage in inflammatory bowel disease,[329] especially because lymphocytes that are cytotoxic for intestinal epithelial cells are present in the peripheral blood of patients,[600] a subject that will be covered in the Etiologic Theories section. Cytotoxic T cells generated in mixed lymphocyte reactions in vitro are deficient in lamina proprial cell isolates from both control and inflamed intestine.[353] T cells with the surface markers of cytolytic effector cells (Leu 2+, 9.3+) are present in lamina proprial cells and are isolated from both control and Crohn's disease intestine, however.[601] Thus, the deficient cytotoxic T cell response to mixed lymphocyte stimulation may be caused by deficient interleukin-2 production or responsiveness rather than by the absence of cytotoxic T cell precursors in the lamina propria. Consistent with this notion, significant mitogen-induced cellular cytotoxicity (MICC) is present in lamina proprial cells from controls and patients with IBD.[345,488,602] MICC is a type of cytotoxicity in which the effector cells and target cells are bridged by a T cell mitogen such as PHA, and presumably reflects cytotoxic T cell capability. MICC in lamina proprial cells from inflamed intestine has not been different from that in lamina proprial cells from noninflamed control intestine, although both have tended to be lower than MICC activity present in the peripheral blood.[345,488,602]

Antibody-dependent cellular cytotoxicity (ADCC) to nucleated target cells is not demonstrable using lamina proprial cells isolated from either control or IBD intestine.[341,345,488,489,550,604] Positive ADCC activity to a nucleated target cell was reported,[605] but could not be confirmed by subsequent work done in the same laboratory.[488] Lamina proprial cell ADCC can be demonstrated when more sensitive target cells, antibody-coated chicken erythrocytes, are used.[345,488] The level of this type of ADCC is similar in lamina proprial cells from IBD and control intestine; however, both are significantly less than that present in peripheral blood lymphocytes. The biologic significance of this low-level ADCC activity is uncertain. It does seem that if ADCC is an important mechanism in intestinal host defense or disease, attention should shift to other cell types such a neutrophils, eosinophils, and macrophages, that bear Fc receptors for IgG and can mediate ADCC.[547] All three of these cells are present in the normal and/or inflamed mucosa, but the ability of these cells to mediate ADCC there has never been examined. Nor has the possible synergy of IgA with IgG antibody in ADCC reactions been explored.[605]

NK cell cytotoxicity in human intestinal lamina proprial cells has either been absent,[345,602,604,606,607] or detectable at low levels,[488,550,608-610] levels considerably below those found in peripheral blood. Demonstration of even those low amounts of NK cell activity has frequently required technical manipulations such as effector cell enrichment,[608] or high effector to target cell ratios.[610] These low levels of NK cell activity in lamina proprial cells appear to reflect low numbers of NK effector cells in the human intestinal mucosa: cells with the NK antigens recognized by the monoclonal antibodies Leu-7 and Leu-11 are infrequent in both the lamina propria and the epithelium.[606,611] Natural killer cells are correspondingly infrequent in lamina proprial isolates whether measured as Leu-7+ cells[609,610] or as large granular lymphocytes.[607] The NK cell activity that is detectable in lamina proprial cells appears to respond to stimulators such as interferon,[608,610] although lamina proprial cells from some patients with IBD or other diseases may be hyporesponsive.[550,610] When NK cell activity has been detectable, no difference has been found between it in lamina proprial cells from control or IBD intestine.[488,550,608,610] Not only does NK cell activity not increase in inflamed mucosa but, in an animal model of colitis in monkeys, it decreased during active inflammation.[612] These points have raised major doubts about any role for NK cells in human disease.[613] Most of the studies on NK cell activity in the intestine have used nonepithelial human tumor cells as targets, however, which may be inappropriate for the detection of intestinal NK cell activity. For example, NK cell activity for the human colon cancer cell line, RPMI 4788, has been identified in human lamina proprial cells that have no demonstrable NK cell activity toward the more commonly used target, K562 erythroleukemia cells.[614] It is also possible that the primary role of NK cells in the intestine is the immunoregulation of differentiated B cells rather than cytotoxicity.[329]

Recently, the intestinal lamina propria has been found to contain precursors for a newly described type of cytotoxicity, the lymphokine-activated killer (LAK) cell.[606,607] These cells are generated by incubating cells in interleukin-2 for two or more days. Lymphokine-activated killer cells are able to lyse both NK sensitive and NK resistant cultured tumor cell lines, as well as a variety of fresh primary or metastatic tumor cells, but they do not kill normal cells. The cytotoxic capabilities of LAK cells is thus much broader than those of NK cells, and they have been receiving much attention as a potential therapy in cancer.[615] The lineage of LAK cells is still being defined, but they are probably primitive T lymphocytes.[615] Freshly isolated human lamina proprial cells, even from inflamed intestine, do not show LAK cell activity. Thus, inflammation by itself does not seem to activate these LAK cell precursors in the mucosa. Lamina proprial cells do develop substantial LAK cell cytotoxicity after culture in interleukin-2, however.[606,607] Both the effector cell and precursor cell of LAK cell activity in the intestine appear to be OKT11$^+$, OKT3$^-$, Leu-7$^-$, and Leu-11$^-$.[607] As with other forms of cytotoxicity, no difference in mucosal LAK cell precursors was evident between lamina proprial cells from IBD or from control intestine.[606] The exact role of LAK cells in IBD, if any, remains to be defined.

In summary, all types of cytotoxicity are reduced in the intestinal lamina propria relative to activities found in the peripheral blood.* T cell cytotoxicity, as measured by MICC, is only moderately reduced but ADCC and NK cell cytotoxicity are greatly diminished. The results appear to reflect the numbers of cytotoxic effector cells in the mucosa; that is the type of cell mediating ADCC or NK cell cytotoxicity is infrequent. No differences in any type of cytotoxicity have been evident in lamina proprial cells from IBD vs. noninflamed control intestine.

Etiologic Theories

THE IMMUNOLOGIC HYPOTHESIS. Many theories have been put forward on the causes of inflammatory bowel disease. The two current ones are the infectious and immunologic hypotheses. The immunologic hypothesis in its simplest form proposes that the immune system in patients is reacting abnormally or inappropriately against an agent(s) or antigen(s) to which everyone is commonly exposed.[579] Bacterial antigens present in the intestine are frequently thought to be the "common" antigens involved.[579] The infectious hypothesis proposes that some as yet undiscovered pathogen is causing the disease and that the immune system is simply responding appropriately to it. The immunologic and infectious hypotheses are compared in Table 7-6. This table is liberally adapted from a summary of a workshop on infectious agents in IBD.[616] It was meant only to compare the features expected if the putative infectious agent was rare as opposed to common; however, it is also a comparison of the infectious (rare agent) and immunologic (common agent) theories on the causes of IBD. It is not known which of these hypotheses is correct, and it is possible to fashion hypotheses intermediate between these two. Note that the immune system plays a role in both hypotheses, not only as a primary factor in the immunologic hypothesis, but also as an element in the pathogenesis of disease caused by a putative rare infectious agent. Unless this postulated rare pathogen has direct cytopathic effects, the immune system is probably the mediator of most

*Editors' note: See also Shanahan, F., et al.: Gastroenterology, 92:1635, 1987.

TABLE 7-6. *A comparison of the infectious and immunologic hypotheses concerning the etiology of IBD.*

	Infectious Hypothesis	Immunologic Hypothesis
1. Agent	Rare	Common
2. Exposure leads to disease	Most individuals	Few individuals
3. Isolation of agent	Only those affected	Many unaffected
4. Susceptibility	Less important	Very important
5. Host immune response	Appropriate	Inappropriate
6. Genetic factors	Unlikely	Likely

of the tissue damage under either hypothesis. A number of specific theories exist on exactly how the immune system is responding inappropriately in inflammatory bowel disease. These will be covered in the sections that follow.

IMMUNODEFICIENCY. One immunologic theory of disease holds that a deficiency of some aspect of the immune system is the primary cause of IBD. This deficiency is seen as either allowing microbes to damage the intestine, or as skewing the immune response in such a way as to cause tissue damage during attempts to compensate for the defect and protect the host. Various deficiencies have been postulated. A defect in cell-mediated immunity has been proposed based on the decreased T lymphocyte counts,[49] decreased proliferative response to mitogens,[499,500,507] and anergy found in some patients with IBD.[499,567] Others have postulated defects in neutrophils,[255] macrophages,[545] and in the secretory IgA system.[425,446] In support of this theory, a histologic colitis resembling ulcerative colitis does occur in some patients with immunodeficiency,[122] and granulomatous inflammation occurs in the intestine of those with the neutrophil disorder, chronic granulomatous disease. Several problems do exist with this theory: (a) many of these "defects" in the immune system do not stand up to critical scrutiny, as previously noted, and those that do occur at most in a minority of patients with IBD; (b) patients with IBD do not have increased susceptibility to infections with any known pathogens, whether viral, bacterial, fungal, or parasitic, so the postulated defect would have to be a small chink in the armor of immunity, which would be difficult to reconcile with the fairly extensive immune reactions occurring in the active lesions in IBD; and, (c) treatments that are effective in IBD are immunosuppressive. Agents such as sulfasalazine and corticosteroids have profound effects on neutrophils and monocytes, and agents such as azathioprine or 6-mercaptopurine have major effects on various lymphocyte populations. It is hard to envision how immunosuppression would be beneficial in an immunodeficiency disorder.

AUTOIMMUNITY—ANTI-COLON ANTIBODIES. The idea that inflammatory bowel disease might be some form of an autoimmune reaction has been under consideration for several decades. This idea is particularly attractive in relation to ulcerative colitis confined to the colonic epithelium. Antibodies able to bind to colon epithelial cells were first described in 1959.[617] This initial finding has been confirmed and expanded upon by many investigators in the decades since. The characteristics of anti-colon antibodies are given in Table 7-7. The antigen recognized by serum from patients with IBD is a lipopolysaccharide extractable from human fetal colon using the Westphal technique.[178,617] Similar cross-reacting antigens can be extracted from germ-free rat colon or feces,[178,179,618] and these

TABLE 7-7. *Characteristics of anti-colon antibodies.*

Serum Anti-colon lipopolysaccharide:

1. Present in many but not all patients with IBD.
2. Equally common in ulcerative colitis and Crohn's disease.
3. Organ specific, but cross react with enterobacterial common antigen and with human blood group ABH antigens.
4. Do not correlate with disease activity, duration, or extent.
5. No evidence of antibody binding in vivo.
6. Do not mediate complement lysis of cells or ADCC.
7. Present in many illnesses other than IBD, that do not have intestinal involvement.

Colitis colon-bound antibody (CCA-IgG):

1. Elutable from ulcerative colitis but not Crohn's colitis or control tissue.
2. Recognizes a 40 kD protein that is present on the plasma membrane only of colon epithelial cells, i.e., a colon specific antigen.
3. Antibody to this 40 kD protein found only in patients with ulcerative colitis.
4. A related serum IgG antibody that mediates ADCC to colon epithelial targets.
5. This serum ADCC-mediating antibody activity correlates with disease activity.

Anti-epithelial cell-associated components:

1. Antibody mediating ADCC present in serum in both ulcerative colitis and Crohn's disease.
2. Similar antibody found in 50% of IBD family members' sera.

have frequently been substituted for human material in assays. The colon lipopolysaccharide antigen is related to, but distinct from, the common enterobacterial antigen of Kunin,[618] and human ABH blood group antigens.[619] Serum antibodies have most often been detected by hemagglutination of antigen-coated red blood cells, a method that detects mainly antibodies of the IgM class, but antibodies of the IgG and IgA class are also present.[185,620] These antibodies can also be demonstrated by indirect immunofluorescence,[179,180,181] where the staining is most prominent on goblet cells and the mucous coat.[180,619] Antibodies are equally common in patients with ulcerative colitis and Crohn's disease. No correlation with disease localization or extent has been found. Patients with small bowel vs. colonic Crohn's disease and patients with proctitis vs. pancolitis all have an equal frequency of antibodies.[148,179] Nor does any correlation exist between age, disease activity, or duration and the presence of antibodies.[176,620] No direct evidence that these antibodies bind to colon cells in vivo is available. In fact, these antibodies seem to have a singular lack of effector activity, that is, they do not appear to fix complement,[622] nor, in one assay, could they mediate ADCC.[623] Moreover, they do not appear to be disease specific, because they are found in reasonably high titer in a variety of autoimmune diseases,[199,264] as well as other illnesses,[182] that do not have intestinal involvement. The mere presence of these antibodies is not sufficient to cause inflammatory bowel disease. The role of these antibodies in IBD remains uncertain even after several decades of interest in them. Furthermore, considering their lack of effector functions, it is possible that these antibodies function to down-regulate the immune response to the colon, and thus are beneficial rather than harmful.

One inherent problem with serum anti-colon antibodies has been the question of whether they have anything to do with the initiation or pathogenesis of the disease in the intestinal mucosa. Das and co-workers, reasoning that if an antibody were important in the disease it should be present in the mucosa, acid-eluted an IgG antibody from ulcerative colitis tissue (Table 7-7); similar treatment did not recover the antibody from Crohn's disease or control tissues.[183] Although the IgG antibody eluted from ulcerative colitis tissue (CCS-IgA) was initially thought to detect an antigen present only in ulcerative colitis mucosa,[183,184] subsequently it has been found to bind to an antigen present in all colonic mucosa, inflamed or not.[625] The CCA-IgG antibody has been found only in ulcerative colitis tissue and not in Crohn's colitis or other controls, however; thus the antibody appears to be disease specific. The antigen recognized by CCA-IgG has been identified as a 40 kD protein present on all colon epithelial cells.[625] Immunohistochemical staining using monoclonal antibodies to this 40 kD protein show that it is localized to the plasma membrane of colon epithelial cells and is not present in stomach, small intestine, liver, or pancreas.[626] An antibody similar to CCA-IgG may be circulating. Serum IgG from ulcerative colitis patients, but not from Crohn's disease or control patients, mediates ADCC against the RPMI 4788 human colon cancer cell line.[627] The serum antibody mediating this ADCC reactivity is significantly decreased during clinical remission or after colectomy,[628] thus there appears to be a close correspondence between the presence of this antibody in the circulation and clinical disease.

A different approach has been taken by Roche and co-workers, who have been purifying and immunologically characterizing various epithelial cell-associated antigens (ECAC) and then determining whether patients with inflammatory bowel disease react to them (Table 7-7). Indeed, a circulating antibody to certain ECAC is demonstrable in patients with ulcerative colitis and Crohn's disease, using an ADCC assay in which the target is an ECAC-coated red blood cell.[629] It has recently been shown that approximately half of family members of patients with IBD have a similar circulating antibody to ECAC.[630,631] Antibody to ECAC may therefore represent a marker for genetic susceptibility to the development of IBD.

These new developments in which the colon antigens are being carefully identified are welcome, but it is still unknown whether CCA-IgG or anti-ECAC will have any more disease specificity than anti-colon lipopolysaccharide. The role of antibodies to any of these antigens is uncertain. Both CCA-IgG and anti-ECAC seem to be able to mediate ADCC by lymphocytes; however this subset of lymphocytes is poorly represented in both the inflamed and non-inflamed intestine. This does not preclude a role for these antibodies in IBD, however. They may mediate cytotoxicity via complement activation, or they may mediate ADCC by cells other than lymphocytes. Macrophages and neutrophils can act as effector cells in ADCC, and both are increased in the mucosa in IBD. A massive infiltration of the epithelium with neutrophils is a hallmark of active IBD. Curiously, neither neutrophils nor macrophages have ever been tested for ADCC using those types of anti-colon antibodies.

AUTOIMMUNITY—CELLS CYTOTOXIC FOR COLONIC EPITHELIAL CELLS. Cells cytotoxic for colonic epithelial cells were first found in the peripheral blood of patients with ulcerative colitis,[632,633] and were subsequently found in the peripheral blood of patients with Crohn's colitis.[634-641] The existence of such cells raises the possibility that a cellular autoimmune reaction to the colonic epithelium may be involved in the pathogenesis of inflammatory bowel disease. Again, this is an attractive notion from the standpoint of explaining why ulcerative colitis remains confined to the colonic mucosa. Because long-term cultures of human epithelial cells are not available, the targets of these assays have been either fetal or adult colonic epithelial cells freshly isolated by trypsinizing minced colonic mucosa. Such cells have a limited life span in culture, a factor that has greatly limited the numbers of studies done, and the numbers of investigators involved in this area. The characteristics of this cytotoxicity are given in Table 7-8. The major points are that these cytotoxic cells are found in most patients with chronic inflammatory bowel disease but not in most normal individuals or individuals with other diseases. The cell mediating this cytotoxicity is neither a T cell nor a B cell, but it is in the K cell or the NK cell subset.[642,643] Thus, the cytotoxicity represents either ADCC or NK cell cytotoxicity. This is consistent with the observation that a high molecular weight factor is in the serum of patients with IBD that can induce cytotoxicity in lymphocytes of normal individuals.[638,639,641] Although this material has never been conclusively identified, it is thought to be some type of cytophilic antibody or small immune complexes that "arms" the K cells. A similar type of cytotoxicity has been identified in the lamina proprial cells of patients with inflammatory bowel disease.[643] It is also present in patients with colon cancer, although less activity is present in these patients than in IBD patients.[643] The finding of these cells in the mucosa strengthens the possibility that they play a role in disease pathogenesis, converting them from a status of guilt by association to one of being at the scene of the crime.

A number of features about this cytotoxicity remain unexplained or puzzling, however. The disease and tissue specificities of the cytotoxicity remain uncertain. If a circulating anti-colon antibody mediates this ADCC, patients with illnesses other than IBD that are known to have a high incidence of anti-colon antibody should be tested. These would include patients with cirrhosis of the liver and pyelonephritis.[182] These groups have not been included to date; therefore the disease specificity of this cytotoxicity remains unproven. Similarly, the data on tissue specificity are based on the results of small numbers of experiments and are unclear. The demonstration of a lymphotoxin only in lysates of lymphocytes from patients with inflammatory bowel disease is puzzling because the K cell or NK cell subset is present in normal peripheral blood,[640] and the cytotoxins of these cells are stored in preformed granules.[644] The mechanism by which E. coli lipopolysaccharide stimu-

TABLE 7-8. *Characteristics of lymphocyte cytotoxicity for colonic epithelial cells in inflammatory bowel disease.*

1. Cytotoxic cells occur in peripheral blood of most patients with either ulcerative colitis or Crohn's disease.
2. Cytotoxic cells not found in normals or a variety of other diseases.
3. Cytotoxicity present in remission but gone 10 days after a resection.
4. Cytotoxicity not related to disease severity but may be decreased by steroid therapy.
5. Cytotoxic cell is not a T cell or a B cell but is in the K or NK cell subset (E^-, sIg^-, FcR^+, non-phagocytic, or trypsin sensitive).
6. Cell free lysates of lymphocytes from IBD patients, but not from normals, are cytotoxic. The lysate is toxin inactivated by extremes of pH heating to 90°C for 30 minutes, and by trypsin.
7. Normal lymphocytes can become cytotoxic through preincubation in IBD serum, or with E. coli LPS.
8. Inflammatory bowel disease lymphocytes lose cytotoxicity through preincubation in other IBD serum, or with E. coli LPS.
9. The cytotoxicity-inducing factor in IBD sera is in the high fractions, that is, >500 kD.
10. Cells cytotoxic for autologous colon cells are found in the colonic lamina propria in ulcerative colitis, Crohn's colitis, and in normal mucosa adjacent to colon cancer. The activity is higher in IBD than in colon cancer. These cells are FcR^+ and trypsin sensitive, similar to those found in the blood.

lates this type of cytotoxicity in normal peripheral blood lymphocytes is unclear because no specific receptor for antigen on the lymphocyte subset mediates ADCC or NK cell activity.[636] One possible explanation is that this lipopolysaccharide induced interferon secretion that, in turn, increased NK cell activity in normal peripheral blood lymphocytes. If so, other types of lipopolysaccharide should work just as well. The finding of substantial lamina proprial cell ADCC (or NK cell) cytotoxicity toward autologous epithelial cells is at odds with the relative lack of K or NK effector cells in the mucosa or immunohistochemical staining and the deficient ADCC and NK cell activity by lamina proprial cells (see Mucosal Cytotoxic Cells section). It is possible that a small subset of lamina proprial lymphocytes, that is Leu-7$^-$ and Leu-11$^-$ but has high efficiency cytotoxicity toward epithelial cells, exists, however, and is mediating these effects.

A related, but somewhat different, approach has been taken by Roche and co-workers.[629,630] As mentioned previously these workers have isolated and partially characterized biochemically a number of murine epithelial cell-associated components (ECAC) that have antigenic determinants specific for the intestine. Patients with inflammatory bowel disease show evidence of sensitization to these antigens because peripheral blood mononuclear cells plus serum from IBD patients specifically lyse red blood cells coated with ECAC.[629] Autosensitization to these epithelial antigens has also been shown using lamina proprial mononuclear cells. Lamina proprial mononuclear cells from abnormal segments from 71% of patients with inflammatory bowel disease were directly cytotoxic for ECAC-coated red blood cells.[645] In contrast, lamina proprial mononuclear cells from control intestinal segments did not lyse these targets. Serum did not enhance the lamina proprial cell cytotoxicity, but the latter was significantly reduced by preincubation of the cells with ECAC antigen.[645] The effector cell involved seemed to be a nonadherent, T11$^+$, T3$^+$ lymphocyte. The mechanism of cytotoxicity is unclear, because the target in this instance (red blood cells) lacks class I MHC determinants, and this would preclude the involvement of classic cytotoxic T cells.

The role that cells cytotoxic for colon cells play in inflammatory bowel disease remains unknown. Although such cytotoxicity could explain the localization of disease to the colonic mucosa in ulcerative colitis, the role of cytotoxic cells in the transmural damage seen in Crohn's colitis, or in Crohn's disease of the small bowel, is problematic. Further progress in this area will depend on the development of techniques allowing for long-term culture of human intestinal epithelial cells. The availability of such cells as targets in these types of assays will permit a better definition of disease specificity and tissue specificity, precise identification of the antigens and cytotoxic effector cells involved, and ultimately the definition of the role that these cells play in inflammatory bowel disease.

ABNORMAL IMMUNOREGULATION. The possibility that an abnormality in immunoregulation might be involved in inflammatory bowel disease stems from a consideration of the large antigenic load encountered in the intestine and the complexity of immunoregulatory mechanisms. The immune system is tightly regulated. In fact, the majority of lymphocytes seem to be in the business of regulating other lymphocytes. For example, in an antibody response, regulatory cells, particularly regulatory T cells, not only determine how much antibody will be produced, but what isotypes and even what antibody combining sites (idiotypes) will be synthesized. Regulatory T cells interact in complex circuits, which in man are only beginning to be defined.[646] In fact, an analogy has been drawn between lymphocyte circuits and those of the nervous system.[647] Both display considerable complexity, integrative functions such as memory and self-recognition, and flexibility and precision of response. Much of the interaction between the various lymphocyte sets seems to be mediated by soluble factors that are released by one set and act upon another. The regulatory mechanisms that operate in the human intestinal lamina propria are virtually unknown. It is clear from studies in experimental animals that the immune response to many intestinal antigens is predominantly inhibitory, however. For example, the feeding of protein antigens to animals frequently results in a state of oral tolerance or unresponsiveness to that specific antigen.[328] Multiple mechanisms may come into play in oral tolerance, but one of the major ones is inhibition by suppressor T cells that arise initially in GALT and then disseminate to other tissues. It is not difficult to envision that a defect in immunoregulatory mechanisms, together with the large and continuous antigenic exposure normally present in the intestine, could result in chronic inflammation and disease. In fact, studies with germ-free animals would suggest that the normal intestinal mucosa is in a state of "physiologic" inflammation (this might explain why only quantitative differences exist between lamina proprial cells obtained from control and inflamed mucosa). Inflammatory bowel disease might be a state in which these as yet undefined local regulatory mechanisms are less able to limit this inflammation. In this regard, the situation in inflammatory bowel disease might be analogous to the situation in allergy in which the disease represents a type of immunologic hypereactivity to multiple environmental antigens.

Abnormalities in regulatory T cell function have been identified in a number of human diseases. For example, in some diseases suppressor T cell function appears to be deficient, whereas in others excessive suppressor T cell activity has been identified.[79] In addition, it has been reported that abnormal immunoregulation within in an organ may contribute to disease localized within that tissue. Support for this comes from work done in sarcoidosis, a condition that shares some pathologic features with Crohn's disease; lung lymphocytes obtained from patients with pulmonary sarcoidosis contain a higher fraction of T cells, and these T cells appear to be more activated than peripheral blood T cells.[648] Furthermore, lung T cells, but not peripheral blood T cells, have increased helper activity for IgG and IgM synthesis by B cells.[649]

Does abnormal immunoregulation exist in inflammatory bowel disease patients? One approach to answering this question has been to measure the proportion of cells that bear the CD4 helper/inducer or the CD8 suppressor/cytotoxic antigens. Such analyses have been consistently normal in patients with the exception of one study in which patients with active, untreated inflammatory bowel disease had decreased absolute numbers of $CD8^+$ cells in the peripheral blood.[652] The proportion of cells with these two markers is not altered either in the lamina propria, even when intense inflammation is present.[437,438] This last finding has been interpreted as indicating that no immunoregulatory abnormality exists in inflammatory bowel disease.[438] That conclusion is premature for a number of reasons. We know, for instance, that there are morphologic and functional subsets within both the CD4 and $CD8^+$ T cell subsets. Thus, helper T cells are $CD4^+$, $Leu\text{-}8^-$, inducer T cells are $CD4^+$, $Leu\text{-}8^+$, suppressor T cells are $CD8^+$, 9.3^-, and cytolytic T cells are $CD8^+$, 9.3^+.[76,653] It is also clear that regulatory T cells are heterogeneous.[77,78] Cells that regulate delayed hypersensitivity responses are distinct from those that regulate immunoglobulin synthesis. Moreover, those that would regulate any particular antigen-specific response would constitute a small fraction of the total number of T cells bearing a particular marker. Thus, data on the proportions of cells bearing particular markers have limited usefulness.

More direct functional assays of immunoregulatory cell activity have been done. Assays looking at the regulation of lymphocyte proliferation have been used most often. In these assays, cells activated in vitro with a polyclonal mitogen are tested for suppressor activity against fresh responder cells stimulated by mitogens or alloantigens. Peripheral blood lymphocytes from patients with IBD have been found to have decreased,[521,654-656] or normal,[650,656,657] suppressor activity for lymphocyte proliferation. In a number of instances, the decreased suppression was restricted to patients with clinically active disease,[650,654,656] although this was not a universal finding.[521] In the most extensive study of this kind to date, Auer and co-workers, using multiple different assays of lymphocyte proliferation, found patients in remission to be largely normal.[650] Only patients with active disease had selective, moderate defects in suppression of lymphocyte proliferation. Similarly, lamina proprial cells have been reported to have increased and reduced suppression for autologous peripheral blood lymphocyte proliferative responses.[658,659] These results are, at the least, "inconclusive." This particular assay of immune regulation probably will not shed much light on the situation. Although this assay is the easiest to do, it is the least informative. The identity of the cells suppressing and of the cells being suppressed is usually left to the imagination. Furthermore, it is unclear whether this assay is measuring any physiologically relevant immunoregulatory event, or whether it is simply an assay in which activated cells absorb out important lymphokines such as IL-2.

A second major avenue of approach has been to measure the effects of immunoregulatory cells that control immunoglobulin synthesis. In the initial studies of this kind, patients with mild or inactive Crohn's disease, not on corticosteroids, were found to have a circulating, potent suppressor T cell for immunoglobulin synthesis.[79] This cell was termed a "covert" suppressor because it was not evident until peripheral blood lymphocytes were purified into T cell and B cell fractions. A cell similar to this one was identified in two patients with Crohn's disease who developed hypogammaglobulinemia,[117] suggesting that this cell could have major effects in vivo. The suppressor cell was subsequently identified in the small subset of peripheral blood lymphocytes bearing both the CD8$^+$ and Leu-7$^+$ (HNK-1) antigens.[75] Although the presence of this suppressor cell in patients with active disease has not been studied, the evidence of B cell activation in such patients suggests that it is not present during active disease.[492,651] Suppressor T cell activity has not been evident in lamina proprial cells,[349,350] which may be because active disease is present in most patients going to surgery, or may be because distinct immunoregulatory mechanisms exist in the lamina propria that are not present in blood. Regulatory T cells are present in the lamina propria and they exhibit functional heterogeneity, although this is still being defined.[351,660] For example, a contrasuppressor activity appears to be present in lamina propria but not blood CD8$^+$ cells.[351] Whether this is a separate cell type or an activity expressed by activated CD8$^+$ T cells in the lamina propria is unclear. It is clear that the predominant net regulatory activity for immunoglobulin synthesis among lamina proprial T cells is "help." This in itself may be an inhibitory immunoregulatory activity, because the majority of plasma cells in the lamina propria secrete IgA, an isotype lacking most effector functions; therefore, local secretion of IgA could inhibit a variety of immune reactions that would be more harmful to the host. No explanation has been found yet from in vitro studies on lamina proprial regulatory T cells for the lack of IgG and the abundance of IgA plasma cells in the lamina propria, and its reversal in inflammatory bowel disease. Lamina proprial helper activity, at least in pokeweed mitogen assays, has not been isotype specific.

The available data are inconclusive. No "global" defect appears in T cell regulation of lymphocyte proliferation. Because the immune system in inflammatory bowel disease appears to be largely intact, global defects in immunoregulation would seem unlikely. This presents a difficulty, because the assays presently available probably only detect global defects. Further resolution of this hypothesis will require the fashioning of new assays and new approaches. The regulation of responses to specific antigens needs to be studied in patients with inflammatory bowel disease. Antigens encountered in the intestine would be of particular interest because the defect in inflammatory bowel disease may be evident only when this route of antigen exposure is used. The mechanisms that maintain normal homeostasis in the intestine in the face of huge antigenic challenge, and the mechanisms that reestablish this homeostasis after epithelial cell injury, need to be defined. In regard to the latter point, experience with animal models of IBD shows that although acute inflammation can be easily induced, normal homeostasis is quickly reestablished when the irritant or stimulus is withdrawn.[661] Chronic intestinal inflammation has been remarkably difficult to induce. The mechanisms that reestablish homeostasis in this setting are unknown and probably multiple, but one of these will probably be local immunoregulation.

Comparison of the Immunologic Features of Ulcerative Colitis and Crohn's Disease

For the most part, extensive homology exists between the immunologic features of these two diseases, despite their different natural histories. Most of the differences are quantitative rather than qualitative. Thus a decreased total lymphocyte count, a higher rate of IgG turnover, higher levels of serum antibodies to anaerobic intestinal bacteria, and decreased immigration of neutrophils into skin windows has been found more often in Crohn's disease than in ulcerative colitis. The major distinguishing immunologic difference between them is the presence of chronic inflammatory cells in the deeper layers of the bowel wall in Crohn's disease but not in ulcerative colitis. Perhaps a closer examination of cells in these deeper layers might be advantageous. The reasons for this lack of differences where some would be expected is unknown. One explanation is that the two diseases share a final common pathway, although they are initiated by different stimuli, analogous to the complement system (Fig. 7-2). Another explanation is that many assays are detecting aspects of an activated immune system rather than distinct abnormalities of immunity. Because the immune system is activated in both diseases, patients with either disease would appear similar. Lastly, all the immunologic abnormalities may represent epiphenomena that would occur in any chronic inflammatory process involving the intestine, but because chronic inflammatory bowel disease resulting from specific causes is fairly rare, we have no way to judge whether this is the case.

REFERENCES

1. Kraft, S. C., and Kirsner, J. B.: The immunology of ulcerative colitis and Crohn's disease: clinical and humoral aspects. *In* Inflammatory Bowel Disease. Edited by J. B. Kirsner, and R. G. Shorter. Philadelphia, Lea & Febiger, 1980.
2. Watson, D. W., Bartnik, W., and Shorter, R. G.: Lymphocyte function and chronic inflammatory bowel disease. *In* Inflammatory Bowel Disease. Edited by J. B. Kirsner, and R. G. Shorter. Philadelphia, Lea & Febiger, 1980.
3. Weterman, I. T., and Peña, A. S.: Familial incidence of Crohn's disease in the Netherlands and a review of the literature. Gastroenterology, 86:449, 1984.
4. Zaleski, M. B., Dubiski, S., Niles, E. G., and Cunningham, R. K.: Biologic function and significance of the MHC. *In* Immunogenetics. Boston, Pitman, 1983.
5. Stobo, J. D.: The human major histocompatibility complex (MHC) and disease. *In* Gastrointestinal Immunity for the Clinician. Edited by R. G. Shorter, and J. B. Kirsner. Orlando, Grune & Stratton, 1985.
6. Scott, H., Solheim, B. G., Brandtzaeg, P., and Thorsby, E.: HLA-DR-like antigens in the epithelium of the human small intestine. Scand. J. Immunol., 12:77, 1980.
7. Selby, W. S., Janossy, G., Goldstein, G., and Jewell, D. P.: T lymphocyte subsets in human intestinal mucosa: The distribution and relationship to MHC-derived antigens. Clin. Exp. Immunol., 44:453, 1981.
8. Selby, W. S., Janossy, G., Mason, D. Y., and Jewell, D. P.: Expression of HLA-DR antigens by colonic epithelium in inflammatory bowel disease. Clin. Exp. Immunol., 53:614, 1983.
9. Bach, F. H.: The HLA class II genes and products: the HLA-D region. Immunol. Today, 5:89, 1985.
10. IUIS-WHO Nomenclature Subcommittee. Announcement. J. Immunol., 134:659, 1985.
11. Reinherz, E. L., Meuer, S. C., and Schlossman, S. F.: The delineation of antigen receptors in human T lymphocytes. Immunol. Today, 4:5, 1983.
12. Schwartz, B. D., and Shreffler, D. C.: Genetic influences on the immune response. *In* Clinical Immunology. Edited by C. W. Parker. Philadelphia, W. B. Saunders Co., 1980.
13. Dausset, J.: Clinical implications (nosology, diagnosis, prognosis, and preventive therapy). *In* HLA and Disease. Edited by J. Dausset, and A. Svejgaard. Copenhagen, Munksgaard, 1977.
14. Thorsby, E., and Lie, S. O.: Relationship between HL-A system and susceptibility to diseases. Transplant. Proc., 3:1305, 1971.
15. Gleeson, F. C., et al.: Human leucocyte antigens in Crohn's disease and ulcerative colitis. Gut, 13:438, 1972.
16. Jacoby, R. K., and Jayson, M. I.: HLA-27 in Crohn's disease. Ann. Rheum. Dis., 33:422, 1974.
17. Asquith, P., et al.: Histocompatibility antigens in patients with inflammatory bowel disease. Lancet, 1:113, 1974.
18. Lewkonia, R. M., Woodrow, J. C., McConnell, R. B., and Price-Evans, D. A.: HL-A antigens in inflammatory bowel disease (letter). Lancet, 1:574, 1974.
19. Mallas, E. G., et al.: Histocompatibility antigens in inflammatory bowel disease. Their clinical significance and their association with arthropathy with special reference to HL-A B27. Gut, 17:906, 1976.
20. Bergam, L., et al.: HLA frequencies in Crohn's disease and ulcerative colitis. Tissue Antigens, 7:145, 1976.
21. Berg-Loonon, E. M. V. D., et al.: Histocompatibility antigens and other genetic markers in ankylosing spondylitis and inflammatory bowel disease. J. Immunogenet. 4:167, 1977.
22. Woodrow, J. C., et al.: HLA antigens in inflammatory bowel disease. Tissue Antigens, 11:147, 1978.
23. Peña, A. S., et al.: HLA antigen distribution and HLA haplotype segregation in Crohn's disease. Tissue Antigens, 16:56, 1980.
24. Burnham, W. R., Gelsthrope, K., and Langman, M. J. S.: HLA-D related antigens in inflammatory bowel disease. *In* Recent Advances in Crohn's Disease. Edited by A. S. Peña, I. T. Weterman, C. C. Booth, and W. Strober. The Hague, Martinus Nijhoff, 1981.
25. Smolen, J. S., et al.: HLA antigens in inflammatory bowel disease. Gastroenterology, 82:34, 1982.
26. Delpre, G., et al.: HLA antigens in ulcerative colitis and Crohn's disease in Israel. Gastroenterology, 78:1452, 1980.
27. Caruso, C., Oliva, L., Palmeri, P., and Cottone, M.: B cell alloantigens in Sicilian patients with Crohn's disease. Tissue Antigens, 21:170, 1983.
28. Russell, A. S., Percy, J. S., and Schlaut, J.: Transplantation antigens in Crohn's disease. Am. J. Dig. Dis., 20: 359, 1975.
29. Schwartz, S. E., et al.: Regional enteritis: evidence for genetic transmission by HLA typing. Ann. Intern. Med., 93:424, 1980.
30. Eade, O. E., et al.: Discordant HLA haplotype segregation in familial Crohn's disease. Gastroenterology, 79:271, 1980.
31. Cohen, Z., McCulloch, P., Leung, M. K., and Mervart, H.: Histocompatibility antigens in patients with Crohn's disease. *In* Recent Advances in Crohn's Disease. Edited by A. S. Peña, I. T. Weterman, C. C. Booth, and W. Strober, The Hague, Martinus Nijhoff, 1981.
32. Hiwatashi, N., et al.: HLA antigens in inflammatory bowel disease. Tohoku J. Exp. Med., 131:381, 1980.
33. Fujita, K., Naito, S., Okabe, N., and Yao, T.: Immunological studies in Crohn's disease. I. Association with HLA systems in the Japanese. J. Clin. Lab. Immunol., 14:99, 1984.
34. Schrumpf, E., et al.: HLA antigens and immunoregulatory T cells in ulcerative colitis associated with hepatobiliary disease. Scand. J. Gastroenterol., 17:187, 1982.
35. Nahir, M., Gideoni, D., Edielman, S., and Barzilai, A.: HLA antigens in ulcerative colitis. Lancet, 2:573, 1976.
36. Caruso, C., et al.: HLA antigens in ulcerative colitis: a study in the Sicilian population. Tissue Antigens, 25:47, 1985.
37. Tsuchiya, M., et al.: HLA antigens and ulcerative colitis in Japan. Digestion, 15: 286, 1977.
38. Asakura, H., et al.: Association of human lymphocyte-DR2 antigen with Japanese ulcerative colitis. Gastroenterology, 82:413, 1982.
39. Cottone, M., et al.: Ulcerative colitis and HLA phenotype. Gut, 26:952, 1985.
40. Kemler, G. L., Glass, D., and Alpert, E.: HLA studies of families with multiple cases of inflammatory bowel disease (IBD). Gastroenterology, 78:1194, 1980.
41. Achord, J. L., Gunn, C. H., Jr., and Jackson, J. F.: Regional enteritis and HLA concordance in multiple siblings. Dig. Dis. Sci., 27:330, 1982.
42. Kagnoff, M. F., Brown, R. J., and Schanfield, M. S.: Association between Crohn's disease and immunoglobulin heavy chain (Gm) allotypes. Gastroenterology, 85:1004, 1983.
43. Ockhuizen, T. H., et al.: Immunoglobulin allotypes are not involved in systemic amyloidosis. J. Rheumatol., 12:742, 1985.
44. Thayer, W. R., Jr., Charland, C., and Field, C. E.: The subpopulations of circulating white blood cells in inflammatory bowel disease. Gastroenterology, 71:379, 1976.

45. Mutchnick, M. G., White, D. S., and Dopp, A. C.: Influence of SRBC/lymphocyte ratio on T-cell rosettes in alcoholic liver disease and inflammatory bowel disease.Clin. Exp. Immunol., 30:277, 1977.
46. Auer, I. O., et al.: Immune status in Crohn's disease. I. Leukocyte and lymphocyte subpopulations in peripheral blood. Scand. J. Gastroenterol., 13:561, 1978.
47. Pfreundschuh, M., Bader, B., and Feurle, G. E.: T-lymphocyte subpopulations in Crohn's disease: definition by monoclonal antibodies. Klin. Wochenschr., 60:1369, 1982.
48. Strickland, R. G., and Williams, R. C., Jr.: Letter: T-cells in Crohn's disease. Gastroenterology, 69:275, 1975.
49. Sachar, D. B., et al.: T and B lymphocytes and cutaneous anergy in inflammatory bowel disease. Ann. NY Acad. Sci., 278:99, 1976.
50. Selby, W. S., and Jewell, D. P.: T lymphocyte subsets in inflammatory bowel disease: peripheral blood. Gut, 24:99, 1983.
51. Sorensen, S. F., and Hoj, L.: Lymphocyte subpopulations in Crohn's disease and chronic ulcerative colitis. Acta Pathol. Microbiol. Scand. [C], 85:41, 1977.
52. Auer, I. O., et al.: Immune status in Crohn's disease. 3. Peripheral blood B lymphocytes, enumerated by means of F(ab)$_2$-antibody fragments, Null and T lymphocytes. Gut, 20:261, 1979.
53. Pfreundschuh, M., et al.: T-lymphocyte subpopulations in the peripheral blood of patients with Crohn's disease. Scand. J. Gastroenterol., 16:845, 1981.
54. Learmonth, R. P., et al.: Altered blood lymphocyte subclasses in patients with ulcerative colitis. Aust. N Z J. Surg., 54:265, 1984.
55. Yuan, S. Z., Hanauer, S. B., Kluskens, L. F., and Kraft, S. C.: Circulating lymphocyte subpopulations in Crohn's disease. Gastroenterology, 85:1313, 1983.
56. Strickland, R. G., et al.: Peripheral blood T and B cells in chronic inflammatory bowel disease. Gastroenterology, 67:569, 1974.
57. Heimann, T. M., and Aufses, A. H., Jr.: The role of peripheral lymphocytes in the prediction of recurrence in Crohn's disease. Surg. Gynecol. Obstet., 160:295, 1985.
58. Dopp, A. C., Mutchnick, M. G., and Goldstein, A. L.: Thymosin-dependent T-lymphocyte response in inflammatory bowel disease. Gastronenterology, 79:276, 1980.
59. Pallone, F., et al.: Studies of peripheral blood lymphocytes in Crohn's disease. Circulating activated T cells. Scand. J. Gastroenterol., 18:1003, 1983.
60. Roche, J. K, Watkins, M. H., and Cook, S. L.: Inflammatory bowel disease: prevalence and level of activation of circulating T-lymphocyte subpopulations mediating suppressor/cytotoxic and helper function as defined by monoclonal antibodies. Clin. Immunol. Immunopathol., 25:362, 1982.
61. Bird, A. G., and Britten, S.: No evidence for decreased lymphocyte reactivity in Crohn's disease. Gastroenterology, 67:926, 1974.
62. Makiyama, K., Selby W. S., and Jewell, D. P.: E rosetting lymphocytes in inflammatory bowel disease. An analysis using monoclonal antibodies. Clin. Exp. Immunol., 52:350, 1983.
63. Meyers, S., Sachar, D. B., Taub, R. N., and Janowitz, H.D.: Anergy to dinitrochlorobenzene and depression of T-lymphocytes in Crohn's disease and ulcerative colitis. Gut, 17:911, 1976.
64. Rubenstein, A., Das, K. M., Melamed, J., and Murphy, R. A.: Comparative analysis of systemic immunological parameters in ulcerative colitis and idiopathic proctitis: effects of sulfasalazine in vivo and in vitro. Clin. Exp. Immunol., 33:217, 1978.
65. Winchester, R. J., Fu, S. M., Hoffman, T., and Kunkel, H. G.: IgG on lymphocyte surfaces; technical problems and the significance of a third cell population. J. Immunol., 114:1210, 1975.
66. Richens, E. R., Thorp, C. M., Bland, P. W., and Gough, K. R.: Peripheral blood and mesenteric lymph node lymphocytes in Crohn's disease. Gut, 21:507, 1980.
67. Pepys, E. D., et al: Enumeration of lymphocyte populations defined by surface markers in the whole blood of patients with Crohn's disease. Gut, 23:766, 1982.
68. Lyanga, J. J., Davis, P., and Thomson, A. B. R.: In vitro testing of immunoresponsiveness in patients with inflammatory bowel disease: prevalence and relationship to disease activity immunoresponsiveness in IBD. Clin. Exp. Immunol., 37:120, 1979.
69. Victorino, R. M., and Hodgson, H. J. F.: Alteration in T lymphocyte subpopulations in inflammatory bowel disease. Clin. Exp. Immunol., 41:156, 1980.
70. Reinherz, E. L., et al.: Human T lymphocyte subpopulations defined by Fc receptors and monoclonal antibodies. A comparison. J. Exp. Med., 151:969, 1980.
71. Reinherz, E. L., et al.: Regulation of B cell immunoglobulin secretion by functional subsets of T lymphocytes in man. Eur. J. Immunol., 10:570, 1980b.
72. Brown, T. E., Bankhurst, A. D., and Strickland, R. G.: Natural killer cell function and lymphocyte subpopulation profiles in inflammatory bowel disease. J. Clin. Lab. Immunol., 11:113, 1983.
73. Dwyer, J. M.: Identifying and enumerating human T and B lymphocytes. A review of techniques, problems, and progress in clinical studies. Prog. Allergy, 21:178, 1976.
74. Meuer, S. C., et al.: An alternative pathway of T cell activation: a functional role for the 50 KD T 11 sheep erythrocyte receptor protein. Cell, 36:897, 1984.
75. James, S. P., et al.: Suppression of immunoglobulin synthesis by lymphocyte subpopulations in patients with Crohn's disease. Gastroenterology, 86:1510, 1984.
76. Damle, N. K., Mohagheghpour, N., and Engleman, E. G.: Soluble antigenprimed inducer T cells antigen-specific suppressor T cells in the absence of antigen-pulsed accessory cells: phenotypic definition of suppressor-inducer and suppressor-effector cells. J. Immunol., 132:644, 1984.
77. Thomas, Y., et al.: Functional analysis of human T cell subsets defined by monoclonal antibodies. IV. Induction of suppressor cells within the OKT4$^+$ population. J. Exp. Med., 154:459, 1981.
78. Thomas, Y., et al.: Functional analysis of human T cell subsets defined by monoclonal antibodies. VI. Distinct and opposing immunoregulatory functions within the OKT8$^+$ population. J. Mol. Cell. Immunol., 1:103, 1984.
79. Elson, C. O., Graeff, A.S., James, S. P., and Strober, W.: Covert suppressor T cells in Crohn's disease. Gastroenterology, 80:1513, 1980.
80. Raedler, A., et al.: Involvement of the immune system in the pathogenesis of Crohn's disease. Expression of the T9 antigen on peripheral immunocytes correlates with the severity of the disease. Gastroenterology, 88:978, 1985.
81. Goding, J. W., and Burns, G. F.: Monoclonal antibody OKT9 recognizes the receptor for transferrin on human acute lymphocytic leukemia cells. J. Immunol., 127:1256, 1981.
82. Raedler, A., Fraenkel, S., Klose, G., and Thiele, H. G.: Elevated numbers of peripheral T cells in inflammatory bowel disease displaying T9 antigen and Fc alpha receptors. Clin. Exp. Immunol., 60:518, 1985.
83. Fais, S., Pallone, F., Squarcia, O., Boirvant, M., and Pozzilli, P.: T cell early activation antigens expressed by pe-

ripheral lymphocytes in Crohn's disease. J. Clin. Lab. Immunol., *16*:75, 1975.
84. Hercend, T., Ritz, J., Schlossman, S. F., and Reinherz, E.L.: Comparative expression of T9, T10, and Ia antigens on activated human T cell subsets. Hum. Immunol., *3*:247, 1981.
85. Romaine, P. L., and Schlossman, S. F.: Human T lymphocyte subsets. Functional heterogeneity and surface recognition structures. J. Clin. Invest., *74*:1559, 1984.
86. Thayer, W. R., Jr., Charland, C., and Field, C. E.: Effects of sulfasalazine in selected lymphocyte subpopulations in vivo and in vitro. Am. J. Dig. Dis., *24*:672, 1979.
87. Dale, D. C., Fauci, A. S., and Wolff, S. M.: Alternate day prednisone leukocyte kinetics and susceptibility to infections. N. Engl. J. Med. *291*:1154, 1974.
88. Claman, H. N.: Anti-inflammatory effects of corticosteroids. Clin. Immunol. Allergy, *4*:317, 1984.
89. Campbell, A. C., et al.: Immunosuppression in the treatment of inflammatory bowel disease. I. Changes in lymphoid sub-populations in the blood and rectal mucosa following cessation of treatment with azathioprine. Clin. Exp. Immunol., *12*:521, 1974.
90. Campbell, A. C., et al.: Immunosuppression in the treatment of inflammatory bowel disease. II. The effects of azathioprine on lymphoid cell populations in a double blind trial in ulcerative colitis. Clin. Exp. Immunol., *24*:249, 1976.
91. Waldmann, T. A., and Strober, W.: Metabolism of immunoglobulins. Prog. Allergy, *13*:1, 1969.
92. Stites, D. P.: Clinical laboratory methods for detection of antigens and antibodies. *In* Basic and Clinical Immunology. 5th Ed. Edited by D. P. Stites, J. D. Stobo, H. H. Fudenberg, and J. V. Wells. Los Altos, CA, Lange Medical Publications, 1984.
93. Bendixen, G., et al.: IgG and albumin turnover in Crohn's disease. Scand. J. Gastroenterol., *3*:481, 1968.
94. Jensen, B. G., et al.: IgM turnover in Crohn's disease. Gut, *11*:223, 1970.
95. Weeke, B., and Jarnum, S.: Serum concentrations of 19 serum proteins in Crohn's disease and ulcerative colitis. Gut, *12*:297, 1971.
96. Persson, S.: Studies on Crohn's disease. III. Concentrations of immunoglobulins G, A, M in the mucosa of the terminal ileum. Acta Chir. Scand., *140*:64, 1974.
97. Bergman, L., Johansson, S. G., and Krause, U.: The immunoglobulin concentrations in serum and bowel secretions in patients with Crohn's disease. Scand. J. Gastroenterol., *8*:401, 1973.
98. MacPherson, B. R., Alberini, R. J., and Beeken, W. L.: Immunological studies in patients with Crohn's disease. Gut, *17*:100, 1976.
99. El Khatib, O. S., et al.: Serum lysozyme, serum proteins, and immunoglobulin determinations in nonspecific inflammatory bowel disease. Am. J. Dig. Dis., *23*:297, 1978.
100. Kraft, S. C., et al.: Serum immunoglobulin levels in ulcerative colitis and Crohn's disease. Gastroenterology, *54*:1251, 1968.
101. Jones, E. G., Beeken, W. L., Roessner, K. D., and Brown, W. A.: Serum and intestinal fluid immunoglobulins and jejunal IgA secretion in Crohn's disease. Digestion, *14*:12, 1976.
102. Bendixen, G., et al.: Immunoglobulin and albumin turnover in ulcerative colitis. Scand. J. Gastroenterol., *5*:433, 1970.
103. Jensen, K. B., Jarnum, S., Kondahl, G., and Kristensen, M.: Serum orosomucoid in ulcerative colitis. Its relation to clinical activity, protein loss, and turnover of albumin and IgG. Scand. J. Gastroenterol., *11*:177, 1976.
104. Nielson, H., et al.: Variations in plasma protein concentrations in individuals with ulcerative colitis: analytical and biological factors. Scand. J. Clin. Lab. Invest., *39*:495, 1979.
105. Brown, W. R., Lansford, C. L., and Hornbrook, M.: Serum immunoglobulin E (IgE) concentrations in patients with gastrointestinal disorders. Am. J. Dig. Dis., *18*:641, 1973.
106. Deodhar, S. D., Michener, W. M., and Farmer, R. G.: A study of the immunologic aspects of chronic ulcerative colitis and transmural colitis. Am. J. Clin. Pathol., *51*:591, 1969.
107. Hodgson, H. J. F., and Jewell, D. P.: The humoral immune system in inflammatory bowel disease. II. Immunoglobulin levels. Am. J. Dig. Dis., *23*:123, 1978.
108. Weeke, B., and Bendixen, G.: Serum immunoglobulins and organ-specific, cellular hypersensitivity in ulcerative colitis and Crohn's disease. Acta Med. Scand., *186*:87, 1969.
109. LoGrippo, G. A., et al.: Immunologic competence in idiopathic ulcerative colitis: humoral aspects of immunity. Henry Ford Hosp. Med. J., *18*:249, 1970.
110. Hardy-Smith, A., and Macphee, I. W.: A clinico-pathological study of ulcerative colitis and ulcerative proctitis. Gut, *12*:20, 1971.
111. Jacobson, S., and Kallner, A.: Effect of total parenteral nutrition on serum concentrations of eight proteins in Crohn's disease. Am. J. Gastroenterol., *79*:501, 1984.
112. Gelernt, I. M., Present, D. H., and Janowitz, H.D.: Alterations in serum immunoglobulins after resection of ulcerative and granulomatous disease of the intestine. Gut, *13*:21, 1972.
113. Marner, I. L., Friborg, S., and Simonsen, E.: Disease activity and serum proteins in ulcerative colitis. Scand. J. Gastroenterol., *10*:537, 1975.
114. Soltis, R. D., and Wilson, I. D.: Serum immunoglobulin M concentrations following bowel resection in chronic inflammatory bowel disease. Gastroenterology, *69*:885, 1975.
115. Fillit, H., et al.: Primary acquired hypogammaglobulinemia and regional enteritis. Arch. Intern Med., *137*:1251, 1977.
116. Soltoft. J., Peterson, L., and Kruse, P.: Immunoglobulin deficiency and regional enteritis. Scand. J. Gastroenterol., *7*:233, 1972.
117. Elson, C. O., et al.: Hypogammaglobulinemia due to abnormal suppressor T-cell activity in Crohn's disease. Gastroenterology, *86*:569, 1984.
118. Eggert, R. C., Wilson, I. D., and Good, R. A. Agammaglobulinemia and regional enteritis. Ann. Intern Med., *71*:581, 1969.
119. Waldmann, T. A., and Schwab, P. J.: IgG (7S gammaglobulin) metabolism in hypogammaglobulinemia: studies in patients with defective gammaglobulin synthesis, gastrointestinal protein loss, or both. J. Clin. Invest., *44*:1523, 1965.
120. Kirk, B. W., and Freedman. S. O.: Hypogammaglobulinemia, thymoma, and ulcerative colitis. Can. Med. Assoc. J., *96*:1272, 1967.
121. Kopp, W. L., Trier, J. S., Steihm, E. R., and Forozoan, P.: Acquired agammaglobulinemia with defective delayed hypersensitivity. Ann. Intern. Med., *69*:309, 1968.
122. Ament, M. E., Ochs, H. D., and Davis, S. D.: Structure and function of the gastrointestinal tract in primary immunodeficiency syndromes. Medicine, *52*:227, 1973.
123. Matuchansky, C., et al.: Ulcerative colitis in a patient with anti-B lymphocytotoxin and hypogammaglobulinemia. Gastroenterology, *73*:578, 1977.
124. Falchuk, K. R., and Falchuk, Z. M.: Selective immuno-

globulin A deficiency, ulcerative colitis, and gluten-sensitive enteropathy—a unique association. Gastroenterology, 69:503, 1975.
125. DeGroote, G., Desmyter, J., Vantrappen, G., and Phillips, C. A.: Rotavirus antibodies in Crohn's disease and ulcerative colitis. Lancet, 1:1263, 1977.
126. Greenberg, H. B., et al.: Antibodies to viral gastroenteritis viruses in Crohn's disease. Gastroenterology, 76:349, 1979.
127. Gebhard, R. L., et al.: Acute viral enteritis and exacerbations of inflammatory bowel disease. Gastroenterology, 83:1207, 1982.
128. Beeken, W. L.: Evidence of virus infection as a cause of Crohn's disease. Z. Gastroenterol (Suppl.)., 17:101, 1979.
129. Swarbrick, E. T., et al.: Chlamydia, cytomegalovirus, and Yersinia in inflammatory bowel disease. Lancet, 2:11, 1979.
130. Schuller, J. L., et al.: Antibodies against Chlamydia of lymphogranuloma venereum type in Crohn's disease. Lancet, 1:19, 1979.
131. Taylor-Robinson, D., O'Morain, C. A., Thomas, B. J., and Levi, A. J.: Low frequency of chlamydial antibodies in patients with Crohn's disease and ulcerative colitis. Lancet, 1:1162, 1979.
132. Mardh, P. A., Ursing, B., and Sandgren, E.: Lack of evidence for an association between infection with Chlamydia trachomatis and Crohn's disease, as indicated by micro-immunofluorescence antibody tests. Acta Pathol. Microbiol. Scand. [B], 88:57, 1980.
133. Elliott, P. R., et al.: Chlamydiae and inflammatory bowel disease. Gut, 22:25, 1981.
134. Taylor, K. B., and Truelove, S. C.: Circulating antibodies to milk proteins in ulcerative colitis. Br. Med. J., 2:924, 1961.
135. Taylor, K. B., Truelove, S. C., and Wright, R.: Serologic reactions to gluten and cow's milk proteins in gastrointestinal disease. Gastroenterology, 46:99, 1964.
136. Sewell, P., Cooke, W. T., Cox, E. V., and Meynell, M. J.: Milk intolerance in gastrointestinal disorders. Lancet, 2:1132, 1963.
137. Dudek, B., Spiro, H. M., and Thayer, W. R., Jr.: A study of ulcerative colitis and circulating antibodies to milk proteins. Gastroenterology, 49:544, 1965.
138. Jewell, D. P., and Truelove, S. C.: Circulating antibodies to cow's milk proteins in ulcerative colitis. Gut, 13:796, 1972.
139. McCaffery, T. D., Jr., Kraft, S. C., and Rothberg, R.M.: The influence of different techniques in characterizing human antibodies to cow's milk proteins. Clin. Exp. Immunol., 11:225, 1972.
140. Falchuk, K. R., and Isselbacher, K. J.: Circulating antibodies to bovine albumin in ulcerative colitis and Crohn's disease. Characterization of the antibody response. Gastroenterology, 70:5, 1976.
141. Korenblatt, P. E., Rothberg, R. M., Minden, P., and Farr, R. S.: Immune responses of human adults after oral and parenteral exposure to bovine serum albumin. J. Allergy, 41:226, 1968.
142. Paganelli, R., et al.: Isotypic analysis of antibody response to a food antigen inflammatory bowel disease. Int. Arch. Allergy Appl. Immunol., 78:81, 1985.
143. Eterman, K. P., and Feltkamp, T. E. W.: Antibodies to gluten and reticulin in gastrointestinal diseases. Clin. Exp. Immunol., 31:92, 1978.
144. Davidson, I.W., Lloyd, R. S., Whorwell, P. J., and Wright, R.: Antibodies to maize in patients with Crohn's disease, ulcerative colitis and coeliac disease. Clin. Exp. Immunol., 35:147, 1979.

145. Heaney, M. R., et al.: Soya protein antibodies in man: their occurrence and possible relevance in coeliac disease. J. Clin. Pathol., 35:319, 1982.
146. Koninckx, C. R., Giliams, J. P., Polanco, I., and Peña, A. S.: IgA antigliadin antibodies in celiac and inflammatory bowel disease. J. Pediatr. Gastroenterol. Nutr., 3:676, 1984.
147. Rawcliffe, P. M., Jewell, D. P., and Faux, J. A.: Specific IgG subclass antibodies, IgE and IgG S-TS antibodies to wheat gluten fraction B in patients with coeliac disease. Clin. Allergy, 15:155, 1985.
148. Thayer, W. R., et al.: Escherichia coli 0:14 and colon hemagglutinating antibodies in inflammatory bowel disease. Gastroenterology, 57:311, 1969.
149. Tabaqchali, S., O'Donoghue, D. P., and Bettelheim, K. A.: Escherichia coli antibodies in patients with inflammatory bowel disease. Gut, 19:108, 1978.
150. Bartnik, W., and Kauzewski, S.: Cellular and humoral response to Kunin antigen (CA) in ulcerative colitis and Crohn's disease. Arch. Immunol. Ther. Exp. (Warsz.), 27:531, 1979.
151. Mattsby-Baltzer, I., et al.: Studies of antibodies to lipid A and Tamm-Horsfall in patients with inflammatory bowel disease. Scand. J. Gastroenterol, 18:305, 1983.
152. Marget, W., et al.: Is the pathogenesis of Crohn's disease similar to that in juvenile recurrent pyelonephritis? A study of lipid A antibody titers in Crohn's disease. ulcerative colitis and acute enteritis. Infection, 4:110, 1976.
153. Brown, W. R., and Lee, E. M.: Radioimmunologic measurements of naturally occurring bacterial antibodies. I. Human serum antibodies reactive with Escherichia coli in gastrointestinal and immunologic disorders. J. Lab. Clin. Med., 82:125, 1973.
154. Kovacs, A.: Titre of anti-E. coli antibodies in ulcerative colitis. Digestion, 10:205, 1974.
155. Heddle, R. J., and Shearman, D. J.: Serum antibodies to Escherichia coli in subjects with ulcerative colitis. Clin. Exp. Immunol., 38:22, 1979.
156. Monteiro, E., et al.: Antibacterial antibodies in rectal and colonic mucosa in ulcerative colitis. Lancet, 1:249, 1971.
157. Mattsby-Baltzer, I., and Alving, C. R.: Antibodies to lipid A: occurrence in humans. Rev. Infect. Dis., 6:553, 1984.
158. Kruis, W., et al.: Circulating lipid A antibodies despite absence of systemic endotoxemia in patients with Crohn's disease. Dig. Dis. Sci., 29:502, 1984.
159. Persson, S., and Danielsson, D.: On the occurrence of serum antibodies to Bacteroides fragilis and serogroups of E.coli in patients with Crohn's disease. Scand. J. Infect. Dis. [Suppl.], 19:61,1979.
160. Helpingstine, C. J., et al.: Antibodies detectable by counterimmuno-electrophoresis against Bacteroides antigens in serum of patients with inflammatory bowel disease. J. Clin. Microbiol., 9:373, 1979.
161. Wensinck, F. et al.: The faecal flora of patients with Crohn's disease. J. Hyg. (Lond.) 87:1, 1981.
162. Matthews, N.: Agglutinins to bacteria in Crohn's disease. Gut, 21:376, 1980.
163. Van de Merwe, J. P., Schmitz, P. I., and Wensinck, F.: Antibodies to Eubacterium and Peptostreptococcus species and the estimated probability of Crohn's disease. J. Hyg. (Lond.), 87:25, 1981.
164. Mayberry, J., Rhodes, J., Matthews, N., and Wensinck, F.: Serum antibodies to anaerobic coccoid rods in patients with Crohn's disease or ulcerative colitis, and in medical and nursing staff. Br. Med. J. [Clin. Res.], 282:108, 1981.
165. Wensinck, F., and Van de Merwe, J. P.: Serum agglutinins to Eubacterium and Peptostreptococcus species in Crohn's and other disease. J. Hyg. (Lond.), 87:13, 1981.

166. Auer, I. O., et al.: Selected bacterial antibodies in Crohn's disease and ulcerative colitis. Scand. J. Gastroenterol., 18:217, 1983.
167. Van de Merwe, J. P., et al.: Factors determining the occurrence of serum agglutinins to Eubacterium and Peptostreptococcus species in patients with Crohn's disease and ulcerative colitis. Digestion, 23:104, 1982.
168. Wensinck, F., Van de Merwe, J. P., and Mayberry, J. F.: An international study of agglutinins to Eubacterium, Peptostreptococcus and Coprococcus species in Crohn's disease, ulcerative colitis, and control subjects. Digestion, 27:63, 1983.
169. Howells, B., Matthews, N., Mayberry, J. F., and Rhodes, J.: Agglutinins to anaerobic bacteria in Crohn's disease and in Indian patients with diarrhea. J. Med. Microbiol., 17:207, 1984.
170. Danielsson, D., Kjellander, J., Persson, S., and Wallensten, S.: Investigation of the immune response to aerobic and anaerobic intestinal bacteria in a patient with Crohn's disease. Scand. J. Infect. Dis. [Suppl.], 19:52, 1979.
171. Baklien, K., and Brandtzaeg, P.: Comparative mapping of the local distribution of immunoglobulin-containing cells in ulcerative colitis and Crohn's disease of the colon. Clin. Exp. Immunol., 22:197, 1975.
172. Persson, S., Danielsson, D., Kjellander, J., and Wallensten, S.: Studies on Crohn's disease. I. The relationship between Yersinia enterocolitica infection and terminal ileitis. Acta Chir. Scand., 142:84, 1976.
173. Blaser, M. J., et al.: Studies of Campylobacter jejuni in patients with inflammatory bowel disease. Gastroenterology, 86:33, 1984.
174. Blaser, M. J., Miller, R. A., Lacher, J., and Singleton, J. W.: Patients with active Crohn's disease have elevated serum antibodies to antigens of seven enteric bacterial pathogens. Gastroenterology, 87:888, 1984.
175. Grange, J. M., Gibson, J., Nassau, E., and Kardjito, T.: Enzyme-linked immunosorbent assay (ELISA): a study of antibodies to Mycobacterium tuberculosis in the IgG, IgA, and IgM classes in tuberculosis, sarcoidosis and Crohn's disease. Tubercle, 61:145, 1980.
176. Thayer, W. R., Jr., et al.: Possible role of mycobacteria in inflammatory bowel disease. II. Mycobacterial antibodies in Crohn's disease. Dig. Dis. Sci., 29:1080, 1984.
177. Cho, S., Brennan, P. J., Yoshimura, H. H., and Graham, D. Y.: Mycobacterial etiology of Crohn's disease: serologic study using common mycobacterial antigens and the species-specific glycolipid antigen from M. Paratuberculosis. Gastroenterology, 88:1348, 1985.
178. Perlmann, P., Hammarstrom, S., Lagercrantz, R., and Gustafsson, B. E.: Antigen from colon of germfree rats and antibodies in human ulcerative colitis. Ann. NY Acad. Sci., 124:377, 1965.
179. Lagercrantz, R., Hammarstrom, S., Perlmann, P., and Gustafsson, B. E.: Immunological studies in ulcerative colitis. 3. Incidence of antibodies to colon-antigen in ulcerative colitis and other gastrointestinal diseases. Clin. Exp. Immunol., 1:263, 1966.
180. Marcussen, H., and Nerup, J.: Fluorescent anti-colon and organ-specific antibodies in ulcerative colitis. Scand. J. Gastroenterol., 8:9, 1973.
181. Marcussen, H.: Fluorescent anti-colonic and E.coli antibodies in ulcerative colitis. Scand. J. Gastroenterol., 13:277, 1978.
182. Carlsson, H. E., Lagercrantz, R., and Perlmann, P.: Immunological studies in ulcerative colitis. VIII. Antibodies to colon antigen in patients with ulcerative colitis, Crohn's disease, and other diseases. Scand. J. Gastroenterol., 12:707, 1977.
183. Das, K. M., Dubin, R., and Nagai, T.: Isolation and characterization of colonic tissue-bound antibodies from patients with idiopathic ulcerative colitis. Proc. Natl. Acad. Sci. USA, 75:4528, 1978.
184. Nagai, T., and Das, K. M.: Detection of colonic antigen(s) in tissues from ulcerative colitis using purified colitis colon tissue-bound IgG (CCA-IgG). Gastroenterology, 81:463, 1981.
185. Hibi, T., et al.: Circulating antibodies to the surface antigens on colon epithelial cells in ulcerative colitis. Clin. Exp. Immunol., 54:163, 1983.
186. Chapman, R. W., et al.: Serum antibodies, ulcerative colitis, and primary sclerosing cholangitis. Gut, 27:86, 1986.
187. Ozturk, F., and Terasaki, P. I.: Non-HLA lymphocyte cytotoxins in various diseases. Tissue Antigens, 14:52, 1979.
188. Strickland, R. G., et al.: Serum lymphocytotoxins in inflammatory bowel disease. Studies of frequency and specificity for lymphocyte subpopulations. Clin. Exp. Immunol., 21:384, 1975.
189. Korsmeyer, S. J., et al.: Differential specificity of lymphocytotoxins from patients with systemic lupus erythematosus and inflammatory bowel disease. Clin. Immunol. Immunopath., 5:67, 1976.
190. Korsmeyer, S. J., Williams, R. C., Jr., Wilson, I. D., and Strickland, R. G.: Lymphocytotoxic and RNA antibodies in inflammatory bowel disease: a comparative study in patients and their families. Ann. NY Acad. Sci., 278:574, 1976.
191. Brown, D. J. C., and Jewell, D. P.: Cold-reactive lymphocytotoxins in Crohn's disease and ulcerative colitis. I. Incidence and characterization. Clin. Exp. Immunol., 49:67, 1982.
192. Abe, T., et al.: Functional differences of anti-T-cell antibody in patients with systemic lupus erythematosus and ulcerative colitis. Scand. J. Immunol., 18:521, 1983.
193. DeHoratius, R. J., et al.: Antibodies to synthetic polyribonucleotides in spouses of patients with inflammatory bowel disease. Lancet, 1:1116, 1978.
194. Gump, D., et al.: Lymphocytotoxic and microbial antibodies in Crohn's disease and matched controls. Antonie Van Leeuwenhoek, 47:455, 1981.
195. Aiso, S., et al.: Characterization of thymus cells in hyperplastic thymuses in patients with myasthenia gravis and ulcerative colitis with monoclonal antibodies. J. Clin. Lab. Immunol., 13:137, 1984.
196. Searles, R. P., and Williams, R. C., Jr.: Lymphocyte-reactive antibodies in SLE. Clin. Rheum. Dis., 8:1, 1982.
197. Calabresi, P., Thayer, W. R., Jr., and Spiro, H. M.: Demonstration of circulating anti-nuclear globulins in ulcerative colitis. J. Clin. Invest., 40:2126, 1961.
198. Harrison, W. J.: Thyroid, gastric (parietal cell) and nuclear antibodies in ulcerative colitis. Lancet, 1:1350, 1965.
199. Deodhar, S. D., Michener, W. M., and Farmer, R. G.: A study of the immunologic aspects of chronic ulcerative colitis and transmural colitis. Am. J. Clin. Pathol., 51:591, 1969.
200. Fujita, K., Okabe, N., and Yao, T.: Immunological studies on Crohn's disease. II. Lack of evidence for humoral and cellular dysfunctions. J. Clin. Lab. Immunol., 16:155, 1985.
201. Skogh, T., Heuman, R., and Tagesson, C.: Anti-brush border antibodies (ABBA) in Crohn's disease. J. Clin. Lab. Immunol., 9:147, 1982.
202. Nielsen, H., Wiik, A., and Elmgreen, J.: Granulocyte specific antinuclear antibodies in ulcerative colitis. Aid in differential diagnosis of inflammatory bowel disease. Acta Pathol. Microbiol. Immunol. Scand. [C], 91:23, 1983.

203. Elmgreen, J., et al.: Type I allergy to normal cellular constituents in chronic inflammatory bowel disease? Results from basophil histamine release test compared with total IgE and antinuclear antibodies. Allergy, *39*:23, 1984.
204. Schwartz, R. S., and Stollar, B. D.: Origins of anti-DNA antibodies. J. Clin. Invest., *75*:321, 1985.
205. Alp, M. H., and Wright, R.: Autoantibodies to reticulin in patients with idiopathic steatorrhoea, coeliac disease, and Crohn's disease, and their relation to immunoglobulins and dietary antibodies. Lancet, *2*:682, 1971.
206. Zauli, D., et al.: Antibodies to the cytoskeleton components and other autoantibodies in inflammatory bowel disease. Digestion, *32*:140, 1985.
207. Bucknall, R. C., Jones, J. V., and Peacock, D. B.: The immune response to phi chi 174 in man. II. Primary and secondary antibody production in patients with Crohn's disease. Am. J. Dig. Dis., *20*:430, 1975.
208. Ryan, F. P., Jones, J. V., Wright, J. K., and Holdsworth, C. D.: Impaired immunity in patients with inflammatory bowel disease and hyposplenism: the response to intravenous phi chi 174. Gut, *22*:187, 1981.
209. Stevens, R., et al.: Defective generation of tetanus-specific antibody-producing B cells after in vivo immunization of Crohn's disease and ulcerative colitis patients. Gastroenterology, *88*:1860, 1985.
210. Brieva, J. A., Targan, S., and Stevens, R. H.: NK and T cell subsets regulate antibody production by human in vivo antigen-induced lymphoblastoid B cells. J. Immunol., *132*:611, 1984.
211. Atkinson, J. P., and Frank, M. M.: Complement. *In* Clinical Immunology. Edited by C. W. Parker. Philadelphia, W. B. Saunders Co., 1980.
212. Cooper, N.: The complement system. *In* Basic and Clinical Immunology. Edited by D. P. Stites, J. D. Stobo, H. H. Fudenberg, and J. V. Wells. Los Altos, CA, Lange, 1984.
213. Hodgson, H. J. F., Potter, B. J., and Jewell, D. P.: Humoral immune system in inflammatory bowel disease: I. Complement levels. Gut, *18*:749, 1977a.
214. Elmgreen, J., Berkowicz, A., and Srensen, H.: Defective release of C5a related chemo-attractant activity from complement in Crohn's disease. Gut, *24*:525, 1983.
215. Elmgreen, J., Berkowicz, A., and Srensen, H.: Hypercatabolism of complement in Crohn's disease-assessment of circulating C3c. Acta Med. Scand., *214*:403, 1983. 1983.
216. Teisberg, P., and Gjone, E.: Humoral immune system activity in inflammatory bowel disease. Scand. J. Gastroenterol., *10*:545, 1975.
217. Lake, A. M., et al.: Complement alterations in inflammatory bowel disease. Gastroenterology, *76*:1374, 1979.
218. Richens, E. R., Thorp, C. M., Bland, P. W., and Hall, N. D.: Circulating immune complexes in Crohn's disease. Their characterization and interrelationship with components of the complement system. Dig. Dis. Sci, *27*:129, 1982.
219. Ross, I. N., Thompson, R. A., Montgomery, R. D., and Asquith, P.: Significance of serum complement levels in patients with gastrointestinal disease. J. Clin. Pathol., *32*:798, 1979.
220. Ward, M., and Eastwood, M. A.: Serum C3 and C4 complement components in ulcerative colitis and Crohn's disease. Digestion, *13*:100, 1975.
221. Nielsen, H., Petersen, P. H., and Svehag, S. E.: Circulating immune complexes in ulcerative colitis—II. Correlation with serum protein concentrations and complement conversion products. Clin. Exp. Immunol., *31*:81, 1978.
222. Feinstein, P. A., Kaplan, S. R., and Thayer, W. R., Jr.: The alternate complement pathway in inflammatory bowel disease. Quantitation of the C3 proactivator (factor B) protein. Gastroenterology, *70*:181, 1976.
223. Potter, B. J., Hodgson, H. J. F., Mee, A. S., and Jewell, D. P.: C1q metabolism in ulcerative colitis and Crohn's disease. Gut, *20*:1012, 1979.
224. Potter, B. J., Brown, D. J., Watson, A., and Jewell, D. P.: Complement inhibitors and immunoconglutinins in ulcerative colitis and Crohn's disease. Gut, *21*:1030, 1980.
225. Ruddy, S., et al.: Human complement metabolism: an analysis of 144 studies. Medicine, *54*:165, 1975.
226. Hodgson, H. J. F., Potter, B. J., and Jewell, D. P.: C3 metabolism in ulcerative colitis and Crohn's disease. Clin. Exp. Immunol., *28*:490, 1977.
227. Elmgreen, J., Both, H., and Binder, V.: Familial occurrence of complement dysfunction in Crohn's disease: correlation with intestinal symptoms and hypercatabolism of complement. Gut, *26*:151, 1985.
228. Slade, J. D., et al.: Inherited deficiency of second component of complement and HLA haplotype A10, B18 associated with inflammatory bowel disease. Ann. Intern. Med., *88*:796, 1978.
229. Lawley, T. J., James, S. P., and Jones, E. A.: Circulating immune complexes: their detection and potential significance in some hepatobiliary and intestinal diseases. Gastroenterology, *70*:626, 1976.
230. Lambert, P. H., et al.: A WHO collaborative study for the evaluation of eighteen methods for detecting immune complexes in serum. J. Clin. Lab. Immunol., *1*:1, 1978.
231. Jewell, D. P., and MacLennon, I. C. M.: Circulating immune complexes in inflammatory bowel disease. Clin. Exp. Immunol., *14*:219, 1973.
232. Hodgson, H. J. F., Potter, B. J., and Jewell, D. P.: Immune complexes in ulcerative colitis and Crohn's disease. Clin. Exp. Immunol., *29*:187, 1977.
233. Fiasse, R., et al.: Circulating immune complexes and disease activity in Crohn's disease. Gut, *19*:611, 1978.
234. Nielsen, H., Peterson, P. H., and Svehag, S. E.: Circulating immune complexes in ulcerative colitis—I. Correlation to disease activity. Clin. Exp. Immunol., *31*:72, 1978.
235. Danis, V. A., Harries, A. D., and Heatley, R. V.: Antigen-antibody complexes in inflammatory bowel disease. Scand. J. Gastroenterol., *19*:603, 1984.
236. Bradby, G. V. H., and Hawkins, C. F.: Detection and significance of immune complexes. Gastroenterology, *79*:601, 1980.
237. Kemler, B. J., and Alpert, E.: Inflammatory bowel disease associated circulating immune complexes. Gut, *21*:195, 1980.
238. Knoflach, P., Vladutiu, A. O., Weiser, M. M., and Albini, B.: Circulating immune complexes in ulcerative colitis and Crohn's disease. Clin. Res., *33*: 3322, 1985.
239. Soltis, R. D., Hasz, D., Morris, M. J., and Wilson, I. D.: Evidence against the presence of circulating immune complexes in chronic inflammatory bowel disease. Gastroenterology, *76*:1380, 1979.
240. Doe, W. F., Booth, C. C., and Brown, D. L.: Evidence for complement-binding immune complexes in adult coeliac disease, Crohn's disease, and ulcerative colitis. Lancet, *1*:402, 1973.
241. Lurhuma, A. Z., Cambiaso, C. L., Masson, P. L., and Heremans, J. F.: Detection of circulating antigen-antibody complexes by their inhibitory effect on the agglutination of IgG-coated particles by rheumatoid factor of C1q. Clin. Exp. Immunol., *25*:212, 1976.
242. Einstein, E., Charland, C., and Thayer, W. R., Jr.: Circulating C1q binding complexes in inflammatory bowel diseases. Digestion, *19*:65, 1979.
243. Pallone, F., et al.: New evidence of circulating immune complexes in Crohn's disease using two sensitive methods. J. Clin. Lab. Immunol., *5*:23, 1981.

244. Learmonth, R. P., Pihl, E., and Johnson, W. R.: Immune complexes in ulcerative colitis. Dig. Dis. Sci., 29:381, 1984.
245. Folkerson, J., Sfeldt, S., and Svehag, S. E.: Application of electroblotting technique to studies of the intestinal antibody response to extractable fecal antigens. Scand. J. Gastroenterol., 20:247, 1985.
246. Hodgson, H. J. F., Potter, B. J., Skinner, J., and Jewell, D. P.: Immune complex mediated colitis in rabbits. An experimental model. Gut, 19:225, 1978.
247. Keren, D. F., et al.: Correlation of histopathologic evidence of disease activity with the presence of immunoglobulin-containing cells in the colons of patients with inflammatory bowel disease. Hum. Pathol., 15:757, 1984.
248. Ballard, J., and Shiner, M.: Evidence of cytotoxicity in ulcerative colitis from immunofluorescent staining of the rectal mucosa. Lancet, 1:1014, 1974.
249. Baklien, K., and Brandtzaeg, P.: Letter: Local immunity and ulcerative colitis. Lancet, 2:411, 1974.
250. Accinni, L., et al.: Deposition of circulating antigen-antibody complexes in the gastrointestinal tract of rabbits with chronic serum sickness. Am. J. Dig. Dis. 23:1098, 1978.
251. Schofield, P. M., and Williams, P. S.: Proliferative glomerulonephritis associated with Crohn's disease. Br. Med. J. [Clin. Res.], 289:1039, 1984.
252. O'Loughlin, E. V., et al.: Membranous glomerulonephritis in a patient with Crohn's disease of the small bowel. J. Pediat. Gastroenterol. Nutr., 4:135, 1985.
253. Hubert, D., Beautils, M., and Meyrier, A.: Immunoglobulin A glomerular nephropathy associated with inflammatory colitis. A propos of 2 cases. Presse Med., 13:1083, 1984.
254. Solley, G. O., Winkelmann, R. K., and Rovelstad, R. A.: Correlation between regional enterocolitis and cutaneous polyarteritis nodosa. Gastroenterology, 69:235, 1975.
255. Kahn, E. L., Daum, F., Riges, H. W., and Silverberg, M.: Cutaneous polyarteritis nodosa associated with Crohn's disease. Dis. Colon. Rectum, 23:258, 1980.
256. Slater, D. N., Waller, P. C., and Reilly, G.: Cutaneous granulomatous vasculitis: presenting feature of Crohn's disease. J. R. Soc. Med., 78:589, 1985.
257. Bunch, T. W., et al.: Synovial fluid complement determination as a diagnostic aid in inflammatory joint disease. Mayo Clin. Proc., 49:715, 1974.
258. Good, A. E. and Utsinger, P. D.: Enteric arthropathies. In Textbook of Rheumatology. Edited by W. N. Kelley, E. D. Harris, S. Ruddy, and C. B. Sledge. Philadelphia, W. B. Saunders, Co., 1984.
258a. Sartor, R. B.: Animal model of granulomatous enterocolitis induced by bacterial cell wall polymers. In Inflammatory Bowel Disease. Edited by D. Rachmilewtiz. Dordrecht, Martinus Nijhoff, In Press, 1987.
259. Stites, D. P.: Clinical laboratory methods for detection of cellular immune function. In Basic and Clinical Immunology. Edited by D. P. Stites, J. D. Stobo, H. H. Fudenberg, and J. V. Wells. Lange, Los Altos, CA, 1984.
260. Cline, M. J., and Territo, M. C.: Phagocytosis. In Clinical Immunology. Edited by W. A. Parker. Philadelphia, W. B. Saunders, Co., 1980.
261. Gallin, J. L.: Neutrophil specific granules: a fuse that ignites the inflammatory response. Clin. Res., 32:320, 1984.
262. Drutz, D. J., and Mills, J.: Immunity and infection. In Basic and Clinical Immunology. Edited by D. P. Stites, J. D. Stobo, H. H. Fudenberg, and J. V. Wells. Lange, Los Altos, CA, 1984.

263. Dobbins, W. O., 3rd: Colonic epithelial cells and polymorphonuclear leukocytes in ulcerative colitis. An electron-microscopic study. Am. J. Dig. Dis., 20:236, 1975.
264. Ward, P. A.: Chemotaxis. In Clinical Immunology. Edited by W. A. Parker. Philadelphia, W. B. Saunders, Co., 1980.
265. Segal, A. W., and Loewi, G.: Neutrophil dysfunction in Crohn's disease. Lancet, 2: 219, 1976.
266. O'Morain, C. O., Segal, A. A., Walker, D., and Levi, A. J.: Abnormalities of neutrophil function do not cause the migration defect in Crohn's disease. Gut, 22:817, 1981.
267. D'Amelio, R., et al.: In vitro studies on cellular and humoral chemotaxis in Crohn's disease using the agarose gel technique. Gut, 22:466, 1981.
268. Wandall, J. H., and Binder, V.: Leukocyte function in Crohn's disease. Studies on mobilization using a quantitative skin window technique and on the function of circulating polymorphonuclear leukocytes in vitro. Gut, 23:173, 1982.
269. Rhodes, J. M., and Jewell, D. P.: Motility of neutrophils and monocytes in Crohn's disease and ulcerative colitis. Gut, 24:73, 1983.
270. Elmgreen, J.: Subnormal activation of phagocytes by complement in chronic inflammatory bowel disease? Neutrophil chemotaxis to complement split product C5a. Gut, 25:737, 1984.
271. Binder, V., and Riis, P.: The leukocyte chemotactic function in patients with ulcerative colitis. Scand. J. Gastroenterol., 12:141, 1977.
272. Hermanowicz, A., and Nawarska, Z.: Chemotaxis and random migration of polymorphonuclear leukocytes in ulcerative colitis examined by the agarose method. Scand. J. Gastroenterol., 16:961, 1981.
273. Kirk, A. P., et al.: Polymorphonuclear leukocyte function in ulcerative colitis and Crohn's disease. Dig. Dis. Sci., 28:236, 1983.
274. Elmgreen, J., and Binder, V.: The chemotactic function of neutrophils in ulcerative colitis. Scand. J. Gastroenterol., 17:561, 1982.
275. Priest, R. J., Rebuck, J. W., and Havey, G. T.: A new qualitative defect of leukocyte function in ulcerative colitis. Gastroenterology, 38:715, 1960.
276. Saverymuttu, S. H., et al.: In vivo assessment of granulocyte migration to diseased bowel in Crohn's disease. Gut, 26:378, 1985.
277. Craddock, P., et al.: Hemodialysis leukopenia: pulmonary vascular leukostasis resulting from complement activation by dialyzer cellophane membranes. J. Clin. Invest., 59:879, 1977.
278. O'Flaherty, et al.: Effect of intravascular complement activation on granulocyte adhesiveness and distribution. Blood, 51:731, 1978.
279. Skubitz, K. M., and Craddock, P. R.: Reversal of hemodialysis granulocytopenia and pulmonary leukostasis. J. Clin. Invest., 67:1383, 1981.
280. Rhodes, J. M., Potter, B. J., Brown, D. J. C., and Jewell, D. P.: Serum inhibitors of leukocyte chemotaxis in Crohn's disease and ulcerative colitis. Gastroenterology, 82:1327, 1982.
281. Koldkjaer, O., Klitgaard, N. A., and Schmidt, K. G.: Cellular and humoral indices of disease activity in inflammatory bowel disease. Digestion, 17:387, 1978.
282. Worsaae, N., Staehr Johansen, K., and Christensen, K. C.: Impaired in vitro function of neutrophils in Crohn's disease. Scand. J. Gastroenterol., 17:91, 1982.
283. Krause, U., Michaelsson, G., and Juhlin, L.: Skin reactivity and phagocytic function of neutrophil leukocytes in Crohn's disease and ulcerative colitis. Scand. J. Gastroenterol., 13:71, 1978.

284. Ward, M., and Eastwood, M. A.: The nitroblue tetrazolium test in Crohn's disease and ulcerative colitis. Digestion, *14*:179, 1979.
285. Faden, H., and Rossi, T. M.: Chemiluminescent response of neutrophils from patients with inflammatory bowel disease. Dig. Dis. Sci., *30*:139, 1985.
286. Verspaget, H. W., Mieremet Ooms, M. A., Weterman, I. T., and Peña, A. S.: Partial defect of neutrophil oxidative metabolism in Crohn's disease. Gut, *25*:849, 1984.
287. Kane, S. P., Hoffbrand, A. V., and Neale, G.: Indices of granulocyte activity in inflammatory bowel disease. Gut, *15*:953, 1974.
288. Koldkjaer, O., Klitgaard, N. A., and Schmidt, K. G.: Lysozyme in plasma and neutrophilic granulocytes in ulcerative colitis and Crohn's disease. Scand. J. Gastroenterol., *12*:135, 1977.
289. Kane, S. P., and Vincenti, A. C.: Mucosal enzymes in human inflammatory bowel disease with reference to neutrophil granulocytes as mediators of tissue injury. Clin. Sci., *57*:295, 1979.
290. O'Morain, Smethurst, P., Levi, A. J., and Peters, T. J.: Biochemical analysis of enzymic markers of inflammation in rectal biopsies from patients with ulcerative colitis and Crohn's disease. J. Clin. Pathol., *36*:1312, 1983.
291. Claman, H. N.: Anti-inflammatory effects of corticosteroids. Clin. Immunol. Allergy, *4*:317, 1984.
292. Dale, D. C., Fauci, A. S., and Wolff, S. M.: Alternate day prednisone leukocyte kinetics and susceptibility to infections. N. Engl. J. Med., *291*:1154, 1974.
293. Hirata, F.: The regulation of lipomodulin, a phospholipase inhibitory protein, in rabbit neutrophils by phosphorylation. J. Biol. Chem., *256*:7730, 1981.
294. Molin, L., and Stendahl, O.: The effect of sulfasalazine and its active components on human polymorphonuclear leukocyte function in relation to ulcerative colitis. Acta Med. Scand., *206*:451, 1979.
295. Rhodes, J. M., Bartholomew, T. C., and Jewell, D. P.: Inhibition of leukocyte motility by drugs used in ulcerative colitis. Gut, *22*:642, 1981.
296. Stenson, W. F., and Lobos, E.: Sulfasalazine inhibits the synthesis of chemotactic lipids by neutrophils. J. Clin. Invest., *69*:494, 1982.
297. Peppercorn, M. A., and Goldman, P.: Distribution studies of salicylazosulfapyridine and its metabolites. Gastroenterology, *64*:240, 1973.
298. Das, K. M., Eastwood, M. A., McManus, J. P. A., and Sircus, W.: The metabolism of salicylazosulphapyridine in ulcerative colitis. I. The relationship between metabolites and the response to treatment in inpatients. Gut, *14*:631, 1973.
299. Strober, W., Hanson L. A., and Sell K. W., (Eds.): Recent Advances in Mucosal Immunity. New York, Raven Press, 1982.
300. McGhee, J. R., and Mestecky, J.: The secretory immune system. Ann. NY Acad. Sci., *409*:1, 1983.
301. Kagnoff, M. F.: Immunology of the digestive system. *In* Physiology of the Gastrointestinal Tract. Edited by L. R. Johnson. New York, Raven Press, 1981.
302. Brandtzaeg, P.: Research in Gastrointestinal immunology. State of the Art. Scand. J. Gastroenterol. [Suppl.], *20*:137, 1984.
303. Savage, D. C.: Microbial ecology of the gastrointestinal tract. Annu. Rev. Microbiol., *31*:107, 1977.
304. Crabbe, P. A., Bazin, H., Eyssen, H., and Heremans, J. F.: The normal microbial flora as a major stimulus for proliferation of plasma cells synthesizing IgA in the gut. The germ-free intestinal tract. Int. Arch. Allergy, Appl. Immunol., *34*:362, 1968.
305. Glaister, J. R., et al.: Factors affecting the lymphoid cells in the small intestinal epithelium of the mouse. Int. Arch. Allergy. Appl. Immunol., *45*:719, 1973.
306. Abrams, G. D., Bauer, H., and Sprinz, H.: Influence of the normal flora on mucosal morphology and cellular renewal in the ileum. Lab. Invest., *12*:355, 1963.
307. Keren, D. F., et al.: The role of Peyer's patches in the local immune response of rabbit ileum to live bacteria. J. Immunol., *120*:1892, 1978.
308. Cornes, J. S.: Number, size, and distribution of Peyer's patches in the human small intestine. I. The development of Peyer's patches. Gut, *6*:225, 1965.
308a. O'Leary, A. D., and Sweeney, E. C.: Lymphoglandular complexes of the colon: structure and distribution. Histopathology, *10*:267, 1986.
309. Bockman, D. E., Boydston, W. R., and Beezhold, D. H.: The role of epithelial cells in gut-associated immune reactivity. Ann. NY Acad. Sci., *409*:129, 1983.
310. Owen, R. L., and Jones, A. L.: Epithelial cell specialization within human Peyer's patches: an ultrastructural study of intestinal lymphoid follicles. Gastroenterology, *66*:189, 1974.
311. Owen, R. L.: Sequential uptake of horseradish peroxidase by lymphoid follicle epithelium of Peyer's patches in the normal unobstructed mouse intestine: an ultrastructural study. Gastroenterology, *72*:440, 1977.
312. Owen, R. L., Pierce, N. F., Juhasz, E. P., and Cray, W. C., Jr.: Attachment and transport of Vibrio cholerae in Peyer's patches of adult rabbits despite oral immunization. Gastroenterology *86*:1204, 1984.
313. Faulk, W. P., et al.: Peyer's patches: morphologic studies. Cell Immunol., *1*:500, 1971.
314. Sobhon, P.: The light and electron microscopic studies of Peyer's patches in non-germ-free adult mice. J. Morphol., *135*:457, 1971.
315. Guy-Grand, D., Griscelli, C., and Vassalli, P.: Peyer's patches, gut IgA plasma cells and thymic function: Study in nude mice bearing thymic grafts. J. Immunol., *115*:361, 1975.
316. Bienenstock, J., and Dolezel J.: Peyer's patches: lack of specific antibody-containing cells after oral and parenteral immunization. J. Immunol., *106*:938, 1971.
317. Kagnoff, M. F.: Effects of antigen feeding on intestinal and systemic immune responses. I. Priming of precursor cytotoxic T cells by antigen feeding. J. Immunol., *120*:395, 1978.
318. Kagnoff, M. F.: Functional characteristics of Peyer's patch cells. IV. Effect of antigen feeding on the frequency of antigen-specific B cells. J. Immunol., *118*:992, 1977.
319. Guy-Grand, D., Griscelli, C., and Vassalli, P.: The gut-associated lymphoid system: nature and properties of the large dividing cells. Eur. J. Immunol., *4*:435, 1974.
320. Craig, S. W., and Cebra, J. J.: Peyer's patches: an enriched source of precursors for IgA-producing immunocytes in the rabbit. J. Exp. Med., *134*:188, 1971.
321. Tseng, J.: Transfer of lymphocytes of Peyer's patches between immunoglobulin allotype congenic mice: repopulation of the IgA plasma cells in the gut lamina propria. J. Immunol., *127*:2039, 1981.
322. Gearhart, P. J., and Cebra, J. J.: Differentiated B lymphocytes. Potential to express particular antibody variable and constant regions depends on site of lymphoid tissue and antigen load. J. Exp. Med., *149*:216, 1979.
323. Cebra, J. J., Komisar, J. L., and Schweitzer, P. A.: CH isotype switching during normal B-lymphocyte development. Annu. Rev. Immunol., *2*:493, 1984.
324. Kawanishi, H., Saltzman, L. E., and Strober, W.: Mecha-

nisms regulating IgA class-specific immunoglobulin production in murine gut-associated lymphoid tissues. I. T cells derived from Peyer's patches that switch sIgM B cells in vitro. J. Exp. Med., *157*:433, 1983.
325. Elson, C. O., Heck, J. A., and Strober, W: T-cell regulation of murine IgA synthesis. J. Exp. Med., *149*:632, 1979.
326. Kiyono, H., et al.: Murine Peyer's patch T cell clones. Characterization of antigen-specific helper T cells for immunoglobulin A responses. J. Exp. Med., *156*:1115, 1982.
327. Kiyono, H., et al.: Isotype-specific immunoregulation: IgA binding factors produced by Fcα receptor-positive T cell hybridomas regulate IgA responses. J. Exp. Med., *161*:731, 1985.
328. Elson, C. O.: Induction and control of the gastrointestinal immune system. Scand. J. Gastroenterol., *20*:1, 1985.
329. Elson, C. O., et al.: Intestinal immunity and inflammation: recent progress. Gastroenterology, *91*:746, 1986.
330. Lamm, M. E., et al.: Differentiation and migration of mucosal plasma cell precursors. *In* Recent Advances in Mucosal Immunity. Edited by W. Strober, L. A. Hanson, and K. W. Sell. New York, Raven Press, 1982.
331. Lamm, M. E.: Cellular aspects of immunoglobulin A. Adv. Immunol., *22*:223, 1976.
332. Lamm, M. E., et al.: Mode of induction of an IgA response in the breast and other secretory sites by oral antigen. *In* Immunology of Breast Milk. Edited by P. Ogra, and D. Dayton. New York, Raven Press, 1979.
333. McWilliams M., Phillips-Quagliata, J. M., and Lamm, M. E.: Characteristics of mesenteric lymph node cells homing to gut-associated lymphoid tissue in syngeneic mice. J. Immunol., *115*:54, 1975.
334. Bienenstock, J., McDermott, M., Befus, D., and O'Neill, M.: A common mucosal immunologic system involving the bronchus, breast and bowel. Adv. Exp. Med. Biol., *107*:53, 1978.
335. Butcher, E. C., Scollay, R. G., and Weissman, I. L.: Organ specific lymphocyte migration: mediation by highly selective lymphocyte interaction with organ-specific determinants on high endothelial venules. Eur. J. Immunol., *10*:556, 1980.
336. Chin, Y. H., Rasmussen, R. A., Woodruff, J. J., and Easton, T. G.: A monoclonal anti-HEBF antibody with specificity for lymphocyte surface molecules mediating adhesion to Peyer's patch high endothelium of the rat. J. Immunol., *136*:2556, 1986.
337. Brandtzaeg, P., et al.: The human gastrointestinal secretory immune system in health and disease. Scand J. Gastroenterol., *20*:17, 1985.
338. Mattioli, C. A., and Tomasi, T. B., Jr.: The life span of IgA plasma cells from the mouse intestine. J. Exp. Med., *138*:452, 1973.
339. Bull, D. M., and Bookman, M. A.: Isolation and functional characterization of human intestinal mucosal lymphoid cells. J. Clin. Invest., *59*:966, 1979.
340. Goodacre, R., Davidson, R., Singal, D., and Bienenstock, J.: Morphologic and functional characteristics of human intestinal lymphoid cells isolated by a mechanical technique. Gastroenterology, *76*:300, 1979.
341. Fiocchi, C., Battisto, J. R., and Farmer, R. G.: Gut mucosal lymphocytes in inflammatory bowel disease: isolation and preliminary functional characterization. Dig. Dis. Sci., *24*:705, 1979.
342. Eade, O. E., et al.: Lymphocyte subpopulations of intestinal mucosa in inflammatory bowel disease. Gut, *21*:675, 1980.
343. Selby, W. S., Janossy, G., Goldstein, G., and Jewell, D. P.: T lymphocyte subsets in human intestinal mucosa: the distribution and relationship to MHC-derived antigens. Clin. Exp. Immunol., *44*:453, 1981.
344. Fox, C. C., et al.: Isolation and characterization of human intestinal mucosal mast cells. J. Immunol., *135*:483, 1985.
345. MacDermott, R. P., et al.: Human intestinal mononuclear cells. I. Investigation of antibody-dependent, lectin-induced, and spontaneous cell-mediated cytotoxic capabilities. Gastroenterology, *78*:47, 1980.
346. Targan, S., et al.: Isolation of spontaneous and interferon inducible natural killer-like cells from human colonic mucosa: lysis of lymphoid and autologous epithelial target cells. Clin. Exp. Immunol., *54*:14, 1983.
347. Fiocchi, C., Tubbs, R. R., and Youngman, K. R.: Human intestinal mucosal mononuclear cells exhibit lymphokine-activated killer cell activity. Gastroenterology, *88*:625, 1985.
348. Hogan, P. G., Hapel, A. J., and Doe, W. F.: Lymphokine-activated and natural killer cell activity in human intestinal mucosa. J. Immunol., *135*:1731, 1985.
349. Elson, C. O., Machelski, E., Weiserbs, D. B.: T cell-B cell regulation in the intestinal lamina propria in Crohn's disease. Gastroenterology, *89*:321, 1985.
350. James, S. P., Fiocchi, C., Graeff, A. S., and Strober, W.: Immunoregulatory function of lamina propria T cells in Crohn's disease. Gastroenterology, *88*:1143, 1985.
351. Lee, A., Sugerman, H., and Elson, C. O.: A comparison of the functional properties of the T8$^+$ T cell subset in human intestinal lamina propria (LP) and peripheral blood (PB). Gastroenterology, *88*:1469, 1985.
352. Fiocchi, C., Battisto, J. R., and Farmer, R. G.: Studies on isolated gut mucosal lymphocytes in inflammatory bowel disease. Detection of activated T cells and enhanced proliferation to Staphylococcus aureus and lipopolysaccharides. Dig. Dis. Sci., *26*:728, 1981.
353. MacDermott, R. P., et al.: Human intestinal mononuclear cells. II. Demonstration of a naturally occurring subclass of T cells which respond in the allogeneic mixed lymphocyte reaction but do not effect cell mediated lympholysis. Gastroenterology, *80*:748, 1981.
354. Ferguson, A.: Intraepithelial lymphocytes of the small intestine. Gut, *18*:921, 1977.
355. Marsh, M. N.: Functional and structural aspects of the epithelial lymphocyte, with implications for coeliac disease and tropical sprue. Scand. J. Gastroenterol., *20*:55, 1985.
356. Ernst, P. B., Befus, A. D., and Bienenstock, J.: Leukocytes in the intestinal epithelium: an unusual immunological compartment. Immunol. Today, *6*:50, 1985.
357. Guy-Grand, D., Griscelli, C., and Vassalli, P.: The mouse gut T lymphocyte, a novel type of T cell. Nature, origin, and traffic in mice in normal and graft-versus-host conditions. J. Exp. Med., *148*:1661, 1978.
358. Cerf-Bensussan, N., Guy-Grand, D., and Griscelli, C.: Intraepithelial lymphocytes of human gut: isolation, characterisation and study of natural killer activity. Gut, *26*:81, 1985.
359. Arnaud-Battandier, F., et al.: Cytotoxic activities of gut mucosal lymphoid cells in guinea pigs. J. Immunol., *121*:1059, 1978.
360. Ferguson, A. Mowat, A. M., Strobel, S., and Barnetson, R. St. C.: Induction and expression of cell-mediated immunity in the small intestine. *In* Regulation of the Immune Response, 8th International Convocation of Immunology. Edited by P. L. Ogra, and D. M. Jacobs. Basel, Karger, 1983.
361. Cerf-Bensussan, N., Quaroni, A., Kurnick, J. T., and Bhan, A. K.: Intraepithelial lymphocytes modulate Ia expres-

sion by intestinal epithelial cells. J. Immunol., *132*:2244, 1984.
362. Brandtzaeg, P., and Baklien, K.: Intestinal secretion of IgA and IgM: a hypothetical model. Ciba Found. Symp., *46*:77, 1977.
363. Ahnen, D. J., Brown, W. R., and Kloppel, T. M.: Secretory component: The polymeric immunoglobulin receptor. What's in it for the gastroenterologist and hepatologist? Gastroenterology, *89*:667, 1985.
364. Solari, R., and Kraehenbuhl, J. P.: The biosynthesis of secretory component and its role in the transepithelial transport of IgA dimer. Immunol. Today, *6*:17, 1985.
365. Brandtzaeg, P., and Prydz, H.: Direct evidence for an integrated function of J chain and secretory component in epithelial transport of immunoglobulins. Nature, *311*:71, 1984.
366. Brown, W. R., Newcomb, R. W., and Ishizaka, K.: Proteolytic degradation of exocrine and serum immunoglobulins. J. Clin. Invest., *49*:1374, 1970.
367. Crago, S.S., et al.: Distribution of IgA1-, IgA2-, and J chain-containing cells in human tissues. J. Immunol., *132*:16, 1984.
368. Lemaitre-Coelho, I., Jackson, G. D. F., and Vaerman, J. P.: Relevance of biliary IgA antibodies in rat intestinal immunity. Scand. J. Immunol., *8*:459, 1978.
369. Jackson, G. D. F., et al.: Rapid disappearance from serum of intravenously injected rat myeloma IgA and its secretion into bile. Eur. J. Immunol., *8*:123, 1978.
370. Peppard, J., Orlans, E., Payne, A. W. R., and Andrew, E.: The elimination of circulating complexes containing polymeric IgA by excretion into the bile. Immunology, *42*:83, 1981.
371. Russell, M. W., Brown, T. A., and Mestecky, J.: Role of serum IgA. Hepatobiliary transport of circulating antigens. J. Exp. Med., *153*:968, 1981.
372. Delacroix, D. L., et al.: Selective transport of polymeric immunoglobulin A in bile. Quantitative relationships of monomeric and polymeric IgA, IgM, and other proteins in serum, bile, and saliva. J. Clin. Invest., *70*:230, 1982.
373. Smith, P. D., Nagura, H., Nakane, P. K., and Brown, W. R.: IgA in human hepatic bile and liver. J. Immunol., *80*:1476, 1981.
374. Brown, W. R.: Ultrastructural studies on the translocation of polymeric immunoglobulins by intestinal epithelium and liver. In Recent Advances in Mucosal Immunity. Edited by W. Strober, L. A. Hanson, and K. W. Sell. New York, Raven Press, 1982.
375. Springer, G. F.: Importance of blood-group substances in interactions between man and microbes. Ann. NY Acad. Sci., *169*:134, 1970.
376. Hanson, D. G., et al.: Inhibition of specific immune responses by feeding protein antigens. Int. Arch. Allergy Appl. Immunol., *55*:526, 1977.
377. Richman, L. K., et al.: Enterically induced immunologic tolerance. I. Induction of suppressor T lymphocytes by intragastric administration of soluble proteins. J. Immunol., *121*:2429, 1978.
378. Chase, M. W.: Inhibition of experimental drug allergy by prior feeding of the sensitizing agent. Proc. Soc. Exp. Biol. Med., *61*:257, 1946.
379. Asherson, G. L., et al.: Production of immunity and unresponsiveness in the mouse by feeding protein sensitizing agents and the role of suppressor cells in the Peyer's patches, mesenteric lymph nodes and other lymphoid tissues. Cell. Immunol., *33*:145, 1977.
380. Kagnoff, M. F.: Effects of antigen feeding on intestinal and systemic immune responses. III. Antigen-specific serum-mediated suppression of humoral antibody responses after antigen feeding. Cell. Immunol., *40*:186, 1978.
381. Mattingly, J. A., and Waksman, B. H.: Immunologic suppression after oral administration of antigen. I. Specific suppressor cells formed in rat Peyer's patches after oral administration of sheep erythrocytes and their systemic migration. J. Immunol., *121*:1878, 1978.
382. Rubin, D., Weiner, H. L., Fields, B. N., and Greene, M. I.: Immunologic tolerance after oral administration of reovirus: requirement for two viral gene products for tolerance induction. J. Immunol., *127*:1697, 1981.
383. Michalek, S. M., et al.: The IgA response: inductive aspects, regulatory cells, and effector functions. Ann. NY Acad. Sci., *409*:48, 1983.
384. Mattingly, J. A., Eardley, D. D., Kemp, J. D., and Gershon, R. K.: Induction of suppressor cells in rat spleen: influence of microbial stimulation. J. Immunol., *122*:787, 1979.
385. Vives, J., Parks, D. E., and Weigle, W. O.: Immunologic unresponsiveness after gastric administration of human gammaglobulin: antigen requirements and cellular parameters. J. Immunol., *125*:1811, 1980.
386. Challacombe, S. J., and Tomasi, T. B., Jr.: Systemic tolerance and secretory immunity after oral immunization. J. Exp. Med., *152*:1459, 1980.
387. Woogen, S., Ealding, W., and Elson, C. O.: Lack of secretory IgA response after feeding protein antigens able to bind to intestinal mucosa. Gastroenterology, *88*:1636, 1985.
388. Korenblatt, P. E., Rothberg, R. M., Minden, P., and Farr, R. S.: Immune responses of human adults after oral and parenteral exposure to bovine serum albumin J. Allergy, *41*:226, 1968.
389. Gonzalez-Licea, A., and Yardley, J. H.: Nature of the tissue reaction in ulcerative colitis: light and electron microscopic findings. Gastroenterology, *51*:825, 1966.
390. O'Connor, J. J.: An electron microscope study of inflammatory colonic disease. Dis. Colon Rectum, *15*:265, 1972.
391. Dobbins, W. O., III: Colonic epithelial cells and polymorphonuclear leukocytes in ulcerative colitis. An electron-microscopic study. Am. J. Dig. Dis., *20*:236, 1975.
392. Dvorak, A. M., Osage, J. E., Monahan, R. A., and Dickerson, G. R.: Crohn's disease: transmission electron microscopic studies. I. Barrier function, possible changes related to alterations of cell coat, mucous coat, epithelial cells, and Paneth cells. Hum. Pathol., (Suppl.) *11*:561, 1980.
393. Hamilton, S. R., Bussey, H. J. R., Boitnott, J. K., and Morson, B. C.: Active inflammation and granulomas in grossly uninvolved colonic mucosa of Crohn's disease resection specimen studied with an en face histologic technique. Gastroenterology, *80*:1167, 1981.
394. Dvorak, A. M., Monahan, R. A., Osage, J. E., and Dickerson, G. R.: Crohn's disease: transmission electron microscopic studies. II. Immunologic inflammatory response. Alterations of mast cells, basophils, eosinophils, and the microvasculature. Hum. Pathol., *11*:606, 1980.
395. Crama-Bohbouth, G., et al.: Immunohistochemical findings in lip biopsy specimens from patients with Crohn's disease and healthy subjects. Gut, *24*:202, 1983.
396. Ferguson, R., Allan, R. N., and Cooke, W. T.: A study of the cellular infiltrate of the proximal jejunal mucosa in ulcerative colitis and Crohn's disease. Gut, *16*:205, 1975.
397. Goodman, M. J., Kent, P. W., and Truelove, S. C.: Abnormalities in the apparently normal bowel mucosa in Crohn's disease. Lancet, *1*:275, 1976.
398. VanSpreeuwel, J. P., et al.: Morphological and immuno-

histochemical findings in upper gastrointestinal biopsies of patients with Crohn's disease of the ileum and colon. J. Clin. Pathol., 35:934, 1982.
399. Salem, S. M., and Truelove, S. C.: Small intestinal and gastric abnormalities in ulcerative colitis. Br. Med. J., 1:827, 1965.
400. Jankey, N., and Price, L. A.: Small intestinal histochemical and histological changes in ulcerative colitis. Gut, 10:267, 1969.
401. Binder, V., Soltoft, J., and Gudmand-Hoyer, E.: Histological and histochemical changes in the jejunal mucosa in ulcerative colitis. Scand. J. Gastroenterol., 9:293, 1974.
402. Nagai, T., and Das, K. M.: Detection of colonic antigen(s) in tissue from ulcerative colitis using purified colitis colon tissue-bound IgG (CCA-IgG). Gastroenterology, 81:463, 1981.
403. Bargen, J. A., Wesson, H. R., and Jackman, R. J.: Studies on the ileocecal junction (ileocecus). Surg. Gynecol. Obstet., 71:33, 1940.
404. Lusk, L. B., Reichen, J., and Levin, J. S.: Aphthous ulceration in diversion colitis. Clinical Implications. Gastroenterology, 87:1171, 1984.
405. Morson, B. C.: The early histological lesion of Crohn's disease. Proc. R. Soc. Med., 65:71, 1972.
406. Rickert, R. R., and Carter, H. W.: The early ulcerative lesion of Crohn's disease: correlative light- and scanning electron-microsopic studies. J. Clin. Gastroenterol., 2:11, 1980.
407. Morson, B. C.: Pathology of Crohn's disease. Clin. Gastroenterol., 1:265, 1972.
408. Dvorak, A. M., Osage, J. E., Monahan, R. A., and Dickerson, G. R.: Crohn's disease: transmission electron microscopic studies. III. Target tissues, proliferation of the injury to smooth muscle and the autonomic nervous system. Hum. Pathol., 11:620, 1980.
409. Dvorak, A. M.: Ultrastructural evidence for release of major basic protein-containing crystalline cores of eosinophil granules in vivo: cytotoxic potential in Crohn's disease. J. Immunol., 125:460, 1980.
410. Ranlov, P., Nielsen, M. H., and Wanstrup, J.: Ultrastructure of the ileum in Crohn's disease. Immune lesions and mastocytosis. Scand. J. Gastroenterol., 7:471, 1972.
411. Payan, D. G., and Goetzl, E. J.: Modulation of lymphocyte function by sensory neuropeptides. J. Immunol. (2 Suppl.), 135:783S, 1985.
412. Ottaway, C. A., and Greenberg, G. R.: Interaction of vasoactive intestinal peptide with mouse lymphocytes: specific binding and the modulation of mitogen responses. J. Immunol., 132:417, 1984.
413. Ottaway, C. A., Bernaerts, C., Chan, B., and Greenberg, G. R.: Specific binding of vasoactive intestinal peptide to human circulating mononuclear cells. Can. J. Physiol. Pharmacol., 61:664, 1983.
414. O'Dorisio, M. S., Wood, C. L., and O'Dorisio, T. M.: Vasoactive intestinal peptide and neuropeptide modulation of the immune response. J. Immunol. (2 Suppl.), 135:792S, 1985.
415. Bishop, A. E., et al.: Abnormalities of vasoactive intestinal polypeptide-containing nerves in Crohn's disease. Gastroenterology, 79:853, 1980.
416. Graham, M. F., et al.: Abnormal accumulation of basement membrane (type IV) and cytoskeletal (type V) collagens in the strictures of Crohn's disease: the probable role of smooth muscle cells. Ann. NY Acad. Sci., 460:439, 1985.
417. Graham, M. F., Elson, C. O., and Diegelmann, R. F.: Increased proportions of type V and type I trimer collagens in the intestinal strictures of Crohn's disease. Gastroenterology, 90:1436, 1986.
418. Graham, M. F., et al.: Isolation and culture of human intestinal smooth muscle cells. Proc. Soc. Exp. Biol. Med., 176:503, 1984.
419. Skinner, J. M., and Whitehead, R.: A morphological assessment of immunoreactivity in colonic Crohn's disease and ulcerative colitis by a study of the lymph nodes. J. Clin. Pathol., 27:202, 1974.
420. Brandtzaeg, P., and Baklien, K.: Inconclusive immunohistochemistry of IgE in mucosal pathology. Lancet, 1:1297, 1976.
421. Rosekrans, P. C., et al.: Immunoglobulin containing cells in inflammatory bowel disease of the colon: a morphometric and immunohistochemcial study. Gut, 21:941, 1980.
422. Brandtzaeg, P., and Baklien, K.: Immunohistochemical characterization of local immunoglobulin formation in Crohn's disease of the ileum. Scand. J. Gastroenterol, 11:447, 1976.
423. Scott, B. B., Goodall, A., Stephenson, P., and Jenkins, D.: Rectal mucosal plasma cell in inflammatory bowel disease. Gut, 24:519, 1983.
424. Gelzayd, E. A., Kraft, S. C., Fitch, F. W., and Kirsner, J. B.: Distribution of immunoglobulins in human rectal mucosa. II. Ulcerative colitis and abnormal mucosal control subjects. Gastroenterology, 54:341, 1968.
425. Green, F. H. Y., and Fox, H.: The distribution of mucosal antibodies in the bowel of patients with Crohn's disease. Gut, 16:125, 1974.
426. Meuwissen, S. G., et al.: Analysis of the lympho-plasmacytic infiltrate in Crohn's disease with special reference to identification of lymphocyte-subpopulations. Gut, 17:770, 1976.
427. Persson, S., and Danielson, D.: Studies on Crohn's disease. II. Immunoglobulin-containing cells in the terminal ileum. Acta Chir. Scand., 139:735, 1973.
428. Skinner, J. M., and Whitehead, R.: The plasma cells in inflammatory disease of the colon: a quantitative study. J. Clin. Pathol., 27:643, 1974.
429. Meijer, C. J., Bosman, F. T., and Lindeman, J.: Evidence for predominant involvement of the B-cell system in the inflammatory process in Crohn's disease. Scand. J. Gastroenterol., 14:21, 1979.
430. Soltoft, J., Binder, V., and Gudmand-Hoyer, E.: Intestinal immunoglobulins in ulcerative colitis. Scand. J. Gastroenterol., 8:293, 1974.
431. Brandtzaeg, P., Baklien, K., Fausa, O., and Hoel, P. S.: Immunohistochemical characterization of local immunoglobulin formation in ulcerative colitis. Gastroenterology, 66:1123, 1974.
432. Lopes Pontes, E., et al.: Changes in the population of mucosal immunoglobulin-containing cells preceding a relapse of ulcerative colitis. Gut, 22:A421, 1981.
433. Baklien, K., Brandtzaeg, P., and Fausa, O.: Immunoglobulin in jejunal mucosa and serum from patients with adult coeliac disease. Scand. J. Gastroenterol., 12:149, 1977.
434. Brandtzaeg, P., et al.: The human gastrointestinal secretory system in health and disease. Scand. J. Gastroenterol. (Suppl.), 20:17, 1985.
435. Brandtzaeg, P., and Tolo, K.: Mucosal penetrability enhanced by serum-derived antibodies. Nature, 266:262, 1977.
436. van Spreeuwel, J. P., Lindeman, J., and Meijer, C. J.: A quantitative study of immunoglobulin containing cells in the differential diagnosis of acute colitis. J. Clin. Pathol., 38:774, 1985.
436a. Selby, W. S., Janossy, G., and Jewell, D. P.: Immunohistological characterization of intraepithelial lymphocytes of the human gastrointestinal tract. Gut, 22:169, 1981.

437. Hirata, I., et al.: Immunohistochemical characterization of intraepithelial and lamina propria lymphocytes in control ileum and colon and in inflammatory bowel disease. Dig. Dis. Sci., *31*:593, 1986.

437a. van Spreeuwel, J. P., et al.: Campylobacter colitis: histological, immunohistochemical and ultrastructural findings. Gut, *26*:945, 1985.

438. Selby, W. S., Janossy, G., Bofill, M., and Jewell, D. P.: Intestinal lymphocyte subpopulations in inflammatory bowel disease: an analysis by immunohistological and cell isolation techniques. Gut, *25*:32, 1984.

439. Selby, W. S., et al.: Heterogeneity of HLA-DR-positive histiocytes in human intestinal lamina propria: a combined histochemical and immunohistological analysis. J. Clin. Pathol. (Suppl. R. Coll. Pathol.) *36*:379, 1983.

440. Strickland, R. G., Husby, G., Black, W. C., and Williams, R. C., Jr.: Peripheral blood and intestinal lymphocyte sub-populations in Crohn's disease. Gut, *16*:847, 1975.

441. Wilders, M. M., et al.: Veiled cells in chronic idiopathic inflammatory bowel disease. Clin. Exp. Immunol., *55*:377, 1984.

442. Hirata, I., et al.: Immunoelectron microscopic localization of HLA-DR antigen in control small intestine and colon and in inflammatory bowel disease. Dig. Dis. Sci., *31*:1317, 1986.

443. Scott, H., Solheim, B. G., Brandtzaeg, P., and Thorsby, E.: HLA-DR-like antigens in the epithelium of the human small intestine. Scand. J. Immunol., *12*:77, 1980.

444. Selby, W. S., Janossy, G., Mason, D. Y., and Jewell, D. P.: Expression of HLA-DR antigens by colonic epithelium in inflammatory bowel disease. Clin. Exp. Immunol., *53*:614, 1983.

445. McDonald, G. B., Gatter, K. C., and Jewell, D. P.: Immune-associated antigen (HLA-DR) expression by epithelial cells in inflammatory colitis. Clin. Res., *33*:96A, 1985.

446. Das, K. M., Erber, W. F., and Rubenstein, A.: Immunohistochemical changes in morphologically involved and uninvolved colonic mucosa of patients with idiopathic proctitis. J. Clin. Invest., *59*:379, 1977.

447. Van Saene, H. F. K., and van der Waaij, D.: Fluorescence immuno-assay for monitoring of activity of gut associated lymphoid tissue. *In* Recent Advances in Crohn's Disease. Edited by A. S. Peña, I. T. Weterman, C. C. Booth, and W. Strober. The Hague, Martinus Nijhoff, 1981.

448. Delacroix, D., and Vaerman, J. P.: Reassessment of levels of secretory IgA in pathologic sera using a quantitative radioimmunoassay. Clin. Exp. Immunol., *43*:633, 1981.

449. Thompson, R. A., Asquith, P., and Cooke, W. T.: Secretory IgA in the serum. Lancet, *2*:517, 1969.

450. Asquith, P., Thompson, R. A., and Cooke, W. T.: Quantitation of secretory IgA in the serum of patients with gastrointestinal diseases. Gut, *11*:368, 1970.

451. Crama-Bohbouth, G., et al.: Immunological findings in whole and parotid saliva of patients with Crohn's disease and healthy controls. Dig. Dis. Sci., *29*:1089, 1984.

452. Soltoft, J., Binder, V., and Gudmand-Hoyer, E.: Intestinal immunoglobulins in ulcerative colitis. Scand. J. Gastroenterol., *8*:293, 1973.

453. Morris, T. J., Matthews, N., and Rhodes, J.: Serum and salivary immunoglobulin A and free secretory component in ulcerative colitis. Clin. Allergy, *11*:561, 1981.

454. Jones, E. G., Beeken, W. L., Roessner, K. D., and Brown, W. A.: Serum and intestinal fluid immunoglobulins and jejunal IgA secretion in Crohn's disease. Digestion, *14*:12, 1976.

455. Haneberg, B., and Aarskog, D.: Human faecal immunoglobulins in healthy infants and children, and in some with disease affecting the intestinal tract or immune system. Clin. Exp. Immunol., *22*:210, 1975.

456. MacDermott, R. P., et al.: An increased percentage of monomeric IgA and IgA subclass (IgA1) is present in the IgA spontaneously secreted by isolated intestinal mononuclear cells from inflammatory bowel disease patients. Gastroenterology, *86*:1169, 1984.

457. Samson, R. R., McClelland, D. B. L., and Shearman, D. J. C.: Studies on the quantitation of immunoglobulin in human intestinal secretions. Gut, *14*:616, 1973.

458. Gaspari, M. M., and Elson, C. O.: A method of obtaining, processing and analyzing human intestinal secretions for antibody content. Gastroenterology, *90*:1454, 1986.

459. Patterson, S., et al.: IgE plasma cells in human jejunum demonstrated by immune electron microscopy. Clin. Exp. Immunol., *46*:301, 1981.

460. Brown, W. R., Borthistle, B. K., and Chen, S. T.: Immunoglobulin E (IgE) and IgE-containing cells in human gastrointestinal fluids and tissues. Clin. Exp. Immunol., *20*:227, 1975.

461. Heatley, R. V., et al.: Immunoglobulin E in rectal mucosa of patients with proctitis. Lancet, *2*:1010, 1975.

462. O'Donahue, D. P., and Kumar, P.: Rectal IgE cells in inflammatory bowel disease. Gut, *20*:149, 1979.

463. Mayrhofer, G., Bazin, H., and Gowens, J. L.: Nature of cells binding anti-IgE in rats immunized with Nippostrongylus brasiliensis: IgE synthesis in regional nodes and concentration in mucosal mast cells. Eur. J. Immunol., *6*:537, 1976.

464. Befus, A. D., et al.: Mast cell heterogeneity in man. I. Histological studies of the intestine. Int. Arch. Allergy Appl. Immunol., *76*:232, 1985.

465. Rosekrans, P. C., Meijer, C. J., van der Wal, A. M., and Lindeman, J.: Allergic proctitis, a clinical and immunopathological entity. Gut, *21*:1017, 1980.

466. Jenkins, H. R., et al. Food allergy: the major cause of infantile colitis. Arch. Dis. Child., *59*:326, 1984.

467. Heatley, R. V., and James, P. D.: Eosinophils in rectal mucosa. Gut, *20*:787, 1978.

468. Willoughby, C. P., Piris, J., and Truelove, S. C.: Tissue eosinophils in ulcerative colitis. Scand. J. Gastroenterol., *14*:395, 1979.

469. Binder, V., et al.: Disodium cromoglycate in the treatment of ulcerative colitis and Crohn's disease. Gut, *22*:55, 1981.

470. Heatley, R. V., et al.: Disodium cromoglycate in the treatment of chronic proctitis. Gut, *16*:559, 1975.

471. Mani, V., Green, F. H. Y., Floyd, G., and Fox, H.: Treatment of ulcerative colitis with oral disodium cromoglycate. Lancet, *1*:439, 1976.

472. Dronfield, M. W., and Langman, M. J. S.: Controlled comparison of sodium cromoglycate and sulphasalazine in the maintenance of remission in ulcerative colitis. Gut, *19*:973, 1977.

473. Buckell, N. A., et al.: Controlled trial of disodium cromoglycate in chronic persistent ulcerative colitis. Gut, *19*:1140, 1978.

474. Willoughby, C. P., Heyworth, M. F., Piris, J., and Truelove, S. C.: Comparison of disodium cromoglycate and sulphasalazine as maintenance therapy for ulcerative colitis. Lancet, *1*:119, 1979.

475. Brown, W. R., Lansford, C. L., and Hornbrook, M.: Serum immunoglobulin E (IgE) concentrations in patients with gastrointestinal disorders. Am. J. Dig. Dis., *18*:641, 1973.

476. Mee, A. S., Brown, D., and Jewell, D. P.: Atopy in inflammatory bowel disease. Scand. J. Gastroenterol., *14*:743, 1979.

477. Becker, S. A., Bass, D. D., Weissglas, L., and Cohen, D.:

IgE in inflammatory bowel disease. Isr. J. Med. Sci., 19:1105, 1983.
478. Elmgreen, J., et al.: Type I allergy to normal cellular constituents in chronic inflammatory bowel disease? Results from basophil histamine release test compared with total IgE and antinuclear antibodies. Allergy, 39:23, 1984.
479. Jones, D. B., Kerr, G. D., Parker, J. H., and Wilson, R. S. E.: Dietary allergy and specific IgE in ulcerative colitis. J. R. Soc. Med., 74:292, 1981.
480. Jewell, D. P., and Truelove, S. C.: Reaginic hypersensitivity in ulcerative colitis. Gut, 13:903, 1972.
481. Schleimer, R. P., et al.: Human mast cells and basophils - structure, function, pharmacology, and biochemistry. Clin. Rev. Allergy, 1:327, 1983.
482. Irani, A. A., et al.: Two human mast cell subsets with distinct protease composition. Proc. Natl. Acad. Sci. USA, 83:4464, 1986.
483. Craig, S. S., DeBlois, G., and Schwartz, L. B.: Mast cells in human keloid, small intestine and lung by an immunoperoxidase technique using a murine monoclonal antibody against tryptase. Am. J. Pathol., 124:427, 1986.
484. Fox, C. C., et al.: Isolation and characterization of human intestinal mucosal mast cells. J. Immunol., 135:483, 1985.
485. Selby, W. S., Janossy, G., Bofill, M., and Jewell, D. P.: Intestinal lymphocyte subpopulations in inflammatory bowel disease: an analysis by immunohistochemical and cell isolation techniques. Gut, 25:32, 1984.
486. Bartnik, W., et al.: Isolation and characterization of colonic intra-epithelial and lamina proprial lymphocytes. Gastroenterology, 78:976, 1980.
487. Bland, P. W., Richens, E. R., Britton, D. C., and Lloyd, J. V.: Isolation and purification of human large bowel mucosal lymphoid cells: effect of separation technique on functional characteristics. Gut, 20:1037, 1979.
488. Chiba, M., et al.: Human colonic intraepithelial and lamina propria lymphocytes: cytotoxicity in vitro and the potential effects of the isolation method on their functional properties. Gut, 22:177, 1981.
489. Bookman, M. A., and Bull, D. M.: Characteristics of isolated intestinal mucosal lymphoid cells in inflammatory bowel disease. Gastroenterology, 77:503, 1979.
490. Brown, H. A., Douglas, J., Williams, C. B., and Walker Smith, J. A.: A method for isolation and culture of lymphocytes from endoscopic biopsies: J. Immunol. Methods, 54:55, 1982.
491. James, S. P., Fiocchi, C., Graeff, A. S., and Strober, W.: Lamina propria lymphocytes contain cells having phenotypic markers of cytolytic effector T cells but a diminished proportion of cells having phenotypes of suppressor-inducer and suppressor-effector cells. Gastroenterology, 88:1430, 1985.
492. Heddle, R. J., LaBrooy, J. T., and Shearman, D. J.: Escherichia coli antibody-secreting cells in the human intestine. Clin. Exp. Immunol., 48:469, 1982.
493. MacDermott, R. P., et al.: Alterations of IgM, IgG, and IgA synthesis and secretion by peripheral blood and intestinal mononuclear cells from patients with ulcerative colitis and Crohn's disease. Gastroenterology, 81:844, 1981.
494. Parent, K., Barrett, J., and Wilson, I. D.: Investigation of the pathogenetic mechanisms in regional enteritis with in vitro lymphocyte cultures. Gastroenterology, 61:431, 1971.
495. Weinstock, J. V., and Simon, M. R.: Lymphocyte reactivity to Crohn's ileal homogenates. J. Clin. Lab. Immunol., 9:77, 1982.
496. Simon, M. R., Weinstock, J. V., and Kataria, Y. P.: Kveim lymphocyte-reactivity in patients and household contacts of patients with Crohn's disease. J. Clin. Lab. Immunol., 3:175, 1980.
497. Hinz, C. F., Jr., Perlmann, P., and Hammerstrom, S.: Reactivity in vitro of lymphocytes from patients with ulcerative colitis. J. Lab. Clin. Med., 70:752, 1967.
498. Stefani, S., and Fink, S.: Effect of E. coli antigens, tuberculin, and phytohemagglutinin upon ulcerative colitis lymphocytes. Gut, 8:249, 1967.
499. Meuwissen, S. G. M., Schellekens, P. T. A., Huismans, L., and Tytgat, G. N.: Impaired anamnestic cellular immune response in patients with Crohn's disease. Gut, 16:854, 1975.
500. Lyanga, J. J., Davis, P., and Thomson, A. B.: In vitro testing of immunoresponsiveness in patients with inflammatory bowel disease: prevalence and relationship to disease activity immunoresponsiveness in IBD. Clin. Exp. Immunol., 37:120, 1979.
501. Ropke, C.: Lymphocyte transformation and delayed hypersensitivity in Crohn's disease. Scand. J. Gastroenterol., 7:671, 1972.
502. Bird, A. G., and Britten, S.: No evidence for decreased lymphocyte reactivity in Crohn's disease. Gastroenterology, 67:926, 1974.
503. Valentine, M. A., et al.: Phytohemagglutinin binds to the 20-kDa molecule of the T3 complex. Eur. J. Immunol., 15:851, 1985.
504. Aas, J., et al.: Inflammatory bowel disease: lymphocyte responses to non-specific stimulation in vitro. Scand. J. Gastroenterol., 7:299, 1972.
505. Asquith, P., Kraft, S. C., and Rothberg, R. M.: In vitro lymphocyte response to non-specific mitogens in inflammatory bowel disease. Gastroenterology, 65:1, 1973.
506. Sachar, D. B., et al.: Impaired lymphocyte responsiveness in inflammatory bowel disease. Gastroenterology, 64:203, 1973.
507. MacDermott, R. P., Bragdon, M. J., and Thurmond, R. D.: Peripheral blood mononuclear cells from patients with inflammatory bowel disease exhibit normal function in the allogeneic and autologous mixed leukocyte reaction and cell-mediated lympholysis. Gastroenterology, 86:476, 1984.
508. MacLaurin, B. P., Cooke, W. T., and Ling, N. R.: Impaired lymphocyte reactivity against tumour cells in patients with Crohn's disease. Gut, 13:614, 1972.
509. MacPherson, B. R., Albertini, R. J., and Beeken, W. L.: Immunological studies in patients with Crohn's disease. Gut, 17:100, 1976.
510. Simon, M. R., et al.: Increased spontaneous morphological blast transformation in patients with Crohn's disease. Clin. Immunol. Immunopath., 13:426, 1979.
511. Richens, E. R., Williams, M. J., Gough, K. R., and Ancill, R. J.: Mixed-lymphocyte reaction as a measure of immunological competence of lymphocytes from patients with Crohn's disease. Gut, 15:24, 1974.
512. Fiske, S. C., and Falchuk, Z. M.: Impaired mixed-lymphocyte culture reactions in patients with inflammatory bowel disease. Gastroenterology, 79:682, 1980.
513. Auer, I. O., Buschmann, C., and Ziemer, E.: Immune status in Crohn's disease. 2. Originally unimpaired cell mediated immunity in vitro. Gut, 19:618, 1978.
514. Auer, I. O., Schmidt, A., Ziemer, E., and Frolich, J.: Impaired cell mediated lympholysis in Crohn's disease. Immunobiology, 160:3, 1981.
515. Weksler, M. E., and Kozak, R.: Lymphocyte transformation induced by autologous cells. V. Generation of immunologic memory and specificity during autologous

mixed lymphocyte reaction. J. Exp. Med., *146*:1833, 1977.
516. Huber, C., et al.: Human autologous mixed lymphocyte reactivity is primarily specific for xenoprotein determinants adsorbed to antigen-presenting cells during rosette formation with sheep erythrocytes. J. Exp. Med., *155*:1222, 1982.
517. MacDermott, R. P., and Bragdon, M. J.: Fetal calf serum augmentation during cell separation procedures accounts for the majority of human autologous mixed lymphocyte reactivity. Behring Inst. Mitt., *72*:122, 1983.
518. Smith, J. B., and Knowlton, R. P.: Activation of suppressor T cells in human autologous mixed lymphocyte culture. J. Immunol., *123*:419, 1979.
519. Innes, J. B., Kuntz, M. M., Kim, Y., and Weksler, M. E.: Induction of suppressor activity in the autologous mixed lymphocyte reaction and in cultures with concanavalin A. J. Clin. Invest., *64*:1608, 1979.
520. James, S. P., et al.: Immunoregulatory function of T cells activated in the autologous mixed lymphocyte reaction. J. Immunol., *127*:2605, 1981.
521. Ginsburg, C. H., and Falchuk, Z. M.: Defective autologous mixed-lymphocyte reaction and suppressor cell generation in patients with inflammatory bowel disease. Gastroenterology, *83*:1, 1982.
522. Ebert, E. C., Wright, S. H., Lipshutz, W. H., and Hauptman, J. P.: T cell abnormalities in inflammatory bowel disease are mediated by interleukin 2. Clin. Immunol. Immunopath., *33*:232, 1984.
523. Hahn, B. H., et al.: Immunosuppressive effects of low doses of glucocorticoids: effect on autologous and allogeneic mixed lymphocyte reactions. J. Immunol., *24*:2812, 1980.
524. Bendixen, G.: Cellular hypersensitivity to components of intestinal mucosa in ulcerative colitis and Crohn's disease. Gut, *10*:631, 1969.
525. Astrup, L., Rasmussen, S. N., and Binder, V.: Leukocyte migration test with autologous colonic mucosa as antigen in patients with ulcerative colitis. Scand. J. Gastroenterol., *12*:765, 1977.
526. Bull, D. M., and Ignaczak, T. F.: Enterobacterial common antigen-induced lymphocyte reactivity in inflammatory bowel disease. Gastroenterology, *64*:43, 1973.
527. Bartnik, W., Swarbrick, E. T., and Williams, C.: A study of peripheral leukocyte migration in agarose medium in inflammatory bowel disease. Gut, *15*:294, 1974.
527a. Eckhardt, R., Heinisch, M., and Meyer zum Buschenfelde, K. H.: Cellular immune reactions against common antigen, small intestine and colon antigen in patients with Crohn's disease, ulcerative colitis and cirrhosis of the liver. Scand. J. Gastroenterol., *11*:49, 1976.
528. Strickland, R. G., Robinson, J. M., Greenlee, L. S., and McLaren, L. C.: Circulating interferon in active inflammatory bowel disease. Gastroenterology, *78*:1271, 1980.
529. Simon, M. R., et al.: Antiviral activity in sera of patients with Crohn's disease. Am. J. Med. Sci., *286*:21, 1983.
530. Stalnikowicz, R., et al.: (2′-5′) Oligo adenylate synthetase activity in leukocytes of patients with inflammatory bowel disease. Gut, *26*:556, 1985.
531. Nelson, D. S.: Immunobiology of the Macrophage. New York, Academic Press, 1976.
532. Adams, D. O., and Hamilton, T. A.: The cell biology of macrophage activation. Ann. Rev. Immunol., *2*:283, 1984.
533. Tanner, A. R., Arthur M. J., and Wright, R.: Macrophage activation, chronic inflammation and gastrointestinal disease. Gut, *25*:760, 1984.
534. Ganguly, N. K., et al.: Acid hydrolases in monocytes from patients with inflammatory bowel disease, chronic liver disease, and rheumatoid arthritis. Lancet, *1*:1073, 1978.
535. Rachmilewitz, D., Ligumsky, M., Haimovitz, A., and Treves, A. J.: Prostaglandin synthesis by cultured peripheral blood mononuclear cells in inflammatory diseases of the bowel. Gastroenterology, *82*:673, 1982.
536. Meuret, G., Bitzi, A., and Hammer, B.: Macrophage turnover in Crohn's disease and ulcerative colitis. Gastroenterology, *74*:501, 1978.
537. Whorwell, P. J., Bennett, P., Tanner, A. R., and Wright, R.: Monocyte function in Crohn's disease and ulcerative colitis. Digestion, *22*:271, 1981.
538. Mee, A. S., Szawatakowski, M., and Jewell, D. P.: Monocytes in inflammatory bowel disease: phagocytosis and intracellular killing. J. Clin. Pathol., *33*:94, 1980.
539. Mee, A. S., and Jewell, D. P.: Monocytes in inflammatory bowel disease: monocyte and serum lysosomal enzyme activity. Clin. Sci., *58*:295, 1980.
540. Rachmilewitz, D., et al.: Transcobalamin II level in peripheral blood monocytes—a biochemical marker in inflammatory disease of the bowel. Gastroenterology, *78*:43, 1980.
541. Doe, W. F., and Dorsman, B.: Chronic inflammatory bowel disease—increased plasminogen activator secretion by mononuclear phagocytes. Clin. Exp. Immunol., *48*:256, 1982.
542. Falchuk, K. R., Perrotto, J. L., and Isselbacher, K. J.: Serum lysozyme in Crohn's disease and ulcerative colitis. N. Engl. J. Med., *292*:395, 1975.
543. Klass, H. J., and Neale, G.: Serum and faecal lysozyme in inflammatory bowel disease. Gut, *19*:233, 1978.
544. Mee, A. S., Nuttall, L., Potter, B. J., and Jewell, D. P.: Studies on monocytes in inflammatory bowel disease: factors influencing monocyte lysosomal enzyme activity. Clin. Exp. Immunol., *39*:785, 1980.
545. Ward M.: The pathogenesis of Crohn's disease. Lancet, *2*:903, 1977.
546. Hermanowicz, A., Gibson, P. R., and Jewell, D. P.: The role of phagocytes in inflammatory bowel disease. Clin. Sci., *69*:241, 1985.
547. Shaw, G. M., Levy, P. C., and LoBuglio, A. F.: Human lymphocyte, monocyte, and neutrophil antibody-dependent cell-mediated cytotoxicity toward human erythrocytes. Cell. Immunol., *41*:122, 1978.
548. Auer, I. O., and Ziemer, E.: Immune status in Crohn's disease. 4. In vitro antibody dependent cell mediated cytotoxicity in peripheral blood. Klin. Wochenschr., *58*:779, 1980.
549. Britton, S., Eklund, A. E., and Bird, A. G.: Appearance of killer (K) cells in the mesenteric lymph nodes in Crohn's disease. Gastroenterology, *75*:218, 1978.
550. MacDermott, R. P., Bragdon, M. J., Kodner, I. J., and Bertovich, M. J.: Deficient cell-mediated cytotoxicity and hyporesponsiveness to interferon and mitogenic lectin activation by inflammatory bowel disease peripheral blood and intestinal mononuclear cells. Gastroenterology, *90*:6, 1986.
551. Eckhardt, R., Kloos, P., Dierich, M. P., and Meyer zum Buschenfelde, K. H.: K-lymphocytes (killer-cells) in Crohn's disease and acute virus B-hepatitis. Gut, *18*:1010, 1977.
552. Auer, I. O., Ziemer, E., and Sommer, H.: Immune status in Crohn's disease. V. Decreased in vitro natural killer cell activity in peripheral blood. Clin. Exp. Immunol., *42*:41, 1980.
553. Ginsburg, C. H., Dambrauskas, J. T., Ault, K. A., and Falchuk, Z. M.: Impaired natural killer cell activity in pa-

tients with inflammatory bowel disease: evidence for a qualitative defect. Gastroenterology, 85:846, 1983.
554. Okabe, N., Fujita, K., and Yao, T.: Immunological studies on Crohn's disease. III. Defective natural killer activity. J. Clin. Lab. Immunol., 17:143, 1985.
555. Beeken, W. L., et al.: Depressed spontaneous cell-mediated cytotoxicity in Crohn's disease. Clin. Exp. Immunol., 51:351, 1983.
556. Brown, T. E., Bankhurst, A. D., and Strickland, R. G.: Natural killer cell function and lymphocyte subpopulation profiles in inflammatory bowel disease. J. Clin. Lab. Immunol., 11:113, 1983.
557. James, S. P., et al.: Suppression of immunoglobulin synthesis by lymphocyte subpopulations in patients with Crohn's disease. Gastroenterology, 86:1510, 1984.
558. Brogan, M., et al.: The effect of 6-mercaptopurine on natural killer-cell activities in Crohn's disease. J. Clin. Immunol., 5:204, 1985.
559. Phear, D. N.: The relation between regional ileitis and sarcoidosis. Lancet, 2:1250, 1958.
560. Williams, W. J.: A study of Crohn's syndrome using tissue extracts and the Kveim and Mantoux tests. Gut, 6:503, 1965.
561. Jones, J. V., Housley, J., Ashurst, P. M., and Hawkins, C. F.: Development of delayed hypersensitivity to dinitrochlorobenzene in patients with Crohn's disease. Gut, 10:52, 1969.
562. Fletcher, J., and Hinton, J. M.: Tuberculin sensitivity in Crohn's disease. Lancet, 2:753, 1967.
563. Bolton, P. M., et al.: The immune competence of patients with inflammatory bowel disease. Gut, 15:213, 1974.
564. Binder, H. J., Spiro, H. M., and Thayer, W. R., Jr.: Delayed hypersensitivity in regional enteritis and ulcerative colitis. Am. J. Dig. Dis., 11:572, 1966.
565. Krause, U., Michaelsson, G., and Juhlin, L.: Skin reactivity and phagocytic function of neutrophil leukocytes in Crohn's disease and ulcerative colitis. Scand. J. Gastroenterol., 13:71, 1978.
566. Heimann, T., et al.: Surgical treatment, skin test reactivity, and lymphocytes in inflammatory bowel disease. Am. J. Surg., 145:199, 1983.
567. Meyers, S., Sachar, D. B., Taub, R. N., and Janowitz, H. D.: Significance of anergy to DNCB in inflammatory bowel disease: family and post-operative studies. Gut, 19:249, 1978.
568. Anderson, R., et al.: The Kveim test in sarcoidosis. Lancet, 2:650, 1963.
569. Mitchell, D. N.: The Kveim test in Crohn's disease. Proc. R. Soc. Med., 64:164, 1971.
570. Karlish, A. J., et al.: Kveim test in Crohn's disease. Lancet, 2:977, 1970.
571. Siltzbach, L. E., et al.: Is there Kveim responsiveness in Crohn's disease? Lancet, 2:634, 1971.
572. Hannuksela, M., Alkio, H., and Selroos, O.: Kveim reaction in Crohn's disease. Lancet, 2:974, 1971.
573. Williams, W. J.: The Kveim controversy. Lancet, 2:926, 1971.
574. Forse, R. A., et al.: Reliability of skin testing as a measure of nutritional state. Arch. Surg. 116:1284, 1981.
575. Schlossman, S. F., et al.: The compartmentalization of antigen-reactive lymphocytes in desensitized guinea pigs. J. Exp. Med., 134:741, 1971.
576. Caspary, E. A., and Field, E. J.: Lymphocyte sensitization in sarcoidosis. Br. Med. J., 2:143, 1971.
577. Crystal, R. G., et al.: Pulmonary sarcoidosis: a disease characterized and perpetuated by activated lung T-lymphocytes. Ann. Intern. Med., 94:73, 1981.
578. Ferguson, A., Mowat, A. M., Strobel, S., and Barnetson, R. St. C.: Induction and expression of cell-mediated immunity in the small intestine In Regulation of the Immune Response, 8th International Convocation of Immunology. Edited by P. L. Ogra, and D. M. Jacobs. Basel, Karger, 1983.
579. Shorter, R. G., Huizenga, K. A., and Spencer, R. J.: A working hypothesis for the etiology and pathogenesis of non-specific inflammatory bowel disease. Am. J. Dig. Dis., 17:1024, 1972.
580. Clancy, R.: Isolation and kinetic characteristics of mucosal lymphocytes in Crohn's disease. Gastroenterology, 70:177, 1976.
581. Weiserbs, D. B., and Elson, C. O.: Abnormal T cell-T cell communication in the lesions of active Crohn's disease. Gastroenterology, 84:1145, 1983.
582. Fiocchi, C., et al.: Interleukin 2 activity of human intestinal mucosa mononuclear cells. Decreased levels in inflammatory bowel disease. Gastroenterology, 86:734, 1984.
583. Mayer, L., and Schlien, R.: Function of Ia molecules on epithelial cells of the GI tract. Gastroenterology, 90:1540, 1986.
584. Fiocchi, C., Lieberman, B. Y., Youngman, K., and Proffitt, M. R.: Decreased production of interleukin 2-induced interferon by human intestinal mucosal mononuclear cells in inflammatory bowel disease. Gastroenterology, 88:1383, 1985.
585. Larsen, G. L., and Henson, P. M.: Mediators of inflammation. Ann. Rev. Immunol., 1:335, 1983.
586. Donowitz, M.: Arachidonic acid metabolites and their role in inflammatory bowel disease. An update requiring addition of a pathway. Gastroenterology, 88:580, 1985.
587. Rampton, D. S., and Hawkey, C. J.: Prostaglandins and ulcerative colitis. Gut, 25:1399, 1985.
588. Sharon, P., Ligumsky, M., Rachmilewitz, D., and Zor, U.: Role of prostaglandins in ulcerative colitis. Enhanced production during active disease and inhibition by sulfasalazine. Gastroenterology, 75:638, 1978.
589. Lauritsen, K., Laursen, L. S., Bukhave, K., and Rask-Madsen, J.: Effect of topical 5-aminosalicylic acid (5-ASA) and prednisolone on prostaglandin (PG)E2 and leukotriene (LT)B4 levels determined by equilibrium in vivo dialysis of rectum in relapsing ulcerative colitis. Gastroenterology, 88:1466, 1985.
590. Sharon, P., and Stenson, W. F.: Enhanced synthesis of leukotriene B4 by colonic mucosa in inflammatory bowel disease. Gastroenterology, 86:453, 1984.
591. Hawkey, C. J., and Truelove, S. C.: Effect of prednisolone on prostaglandin synthesis by rectal mucosa in ulcerative colitis: investigation by laminar flow bioassay and radioimmunoassay. Gut, 22:190, 1981.
592. Gould, S. R., Brash, A. R., Conolly, M. E., and Lennard-Jones, J. E.: Studies of prostaglandins and sulphasalazine in ulcerative colitis. Prostaglandins Med., 6:165, 1981.
593. Stenson, W. F.: Pharmacology of sulfasalazine. Viewpoints Dig. Dis., 16:13, 1984.
594. Lauritsen, K., Laursen, L. S., Bukhave, K., and Rask-Madsen, J.: Effects of systemic prednisolone on arachidonic acid metabolites determined by equilibrium in vivo dialysis of rectum in severe relapsing ulcerative colitis. Gastroenterology, 88:1466, 1985.
595. Verspaget, H., and Beeken, W.: Mononuclear phagocytes in the gastrointestinal tract. Acta Chir. Scand. [Suppl.], 525:113, 1985.
596. Beeken, W. L., St. Andre Ukena, S., and Gundel, R. M.: Comparative studies of mononuclear phagocyte function in patients with Crohn's disease and colon neoplasms. Gut, 24:1034, 1983.

597. Winter, H. S., et al.: Isolation and characterization of resident macrophages from guinea pig and human intestine. Gastroenterology, 85:358, 1983.
598. Golder, J. P., and Doe, W. F.: Isolation and preliminary characterization of human intestinal macrophages. Gastroenterology, 84:795, 1983.
599. Zifroni, A., Treves, A. J., Sachar, D. B., and Rachmilewitz, D.: Prostanoid synthesis by cultured intestinal epithelial and mononuclear cells in inflammatory bowel disease. Gut, 24:659, 1983.
600. Shorter, R. G., Cardoza, M., and Huizenga, K. A.: Further studies of in vitro cytotoxicity of lymphocytes from patients with ulcerative and granulomatous colitis for allogeneic colonic epithelial cells including the effects of colectomy. Gastroenterology, 56:304, 1969.
601. James, S. P., Fiocchi, C., Graeff, A. S., and Strober, W.: Lamina propria lymphocytes contain cells having phenotypic markers of cytolytic effector T cells but a diminished proportion of cells having phenotypes of suppressor-inducer and suppressor-effector cells. Gastroenterology, 88:1430, 1985.
602. Falchuk, Z. M., Barnhard, E., and Machado, I.: Human colonic mononuclear cells: studies of cytotoxic function. Gut, 22:290, 1981.
603. Clancy, R., and Pucci, A.: Absence of K cells in human gut mucosa. Gut, 19:273, 1978.
604. Bland, P. W., Britton, D. C., Richens, E. R., and Pledger, J. V.: Peripheral, mucosal, and tumor-infiltrating components of cellular immunity in cancer of the large bowel. Gut, 22:744, 1981.
605. Shen, L., and Fanger, M. W.: Secretory IgA antibodies synergize with IgG in promoting ADCC by human polymorphonuclear cells, monocytes, and lymphocytes. Cell. Immunol., 59:75, 1981.
606. Fiocchi, C., Tubbs, R. R., and Youngman, K. R.: Human intestinal mucosal mononuclear cells exhibit lymphokine-activated killer cell activity. Gastroenterology, 88:625, 1985.
607. Hogan, P. G., Hapel, A. J., and Doe, W. F.: Lymphokine-activated and natural killer cell activity in human intestinal mucosa. J. Immunol., 135:1731, 1985.
608. Targan, S., et al.: Isolation of spontaneous and interferon inducible natural killer like cells from human colonic mucosa: lysis of lymphoid and autologous epithelial target cells. Clin. Exp. Immunol., 54:14, 1983.
609. Gibson, P. R., et al.: Natural killer cells and spontaneous cell-mediated cytotoxicity in the human intestine. Clin. Exp. Immunol., 56:438, 1984.
610. Gibson, P. R., and Jewell, D. P.: Local immune mechanisms in inflammatory bowel disease and colorectal carcinoma. Natural killer cells and their activity. Gastroenterology, 90:12, 1985.
611. Gibson, P. R., Verhaar, H. J. J., Selby, W. S., and Jewell, D. P.: The mononuclear cells of human mesenteric blood, intestinal mucosa and mesenteric lymph nodes: compartmentalization of NK cells. Clin. Exp. Immunol., 56:445, 1984.
612. James, S. P., Graeff, A. S., Quinn, T. C., and Strober, W.: Natural killer [NK] cell activity is decreased in lamina propria lymphocytes [LPL] isolated from non-human primates with colitis due to lymphogranuloma venereum [LGV]. Gastroenterology, 88:1430, 1985.
613. James, S. P., and Strober, W.: Cytotoxic lymphocytes and intestinal disease. Gastroenterology, 90:235, 1986.
614. Beeken, W. L., et al.: In vitro cellular cytotoxicity for a human colon cancer cell line by mucosal mononuclear cells of patients with colon cancer and other disorders. Cancer, 55:1024, 1985.
615. Rosenberg, S. A., and Lotze, M. T.: Cancer immunotherapy using interleukin-2 and interleukin-2 activated lymphocytes. Ann. Rev. Immunol., 4:681, 1986.
616. Thayer, W. R., Jr.: Executive summary of the AGA-NFIC sponsored workshop on infectious agents in inflammatory bowel disease. Dig. Dis. Sci., 24:781, 1979.
617. Broberger, O., and Perlmann, P.: Autoantibodies in human ulcerative colitis. J. Exp. Med., 110:657, 1959.
618. Lagercrantz, R. S., Hammerstrom, S., Perlmann, P., and Gustafsson, B. E.: Immunological studies in ulcerative colitis. IV. Origin of autoantibodies. J. Exp. Med., 128:1339, 1968.
619. Hammarstrom, S., Lagercrantz, R., Perlmann, P., and Gustafsson, B. E.: Immunological studies in ulcerative colitis. II. Colon antigen and human blood group A- and H-like antigens in germfree rats. J. Exp. Med., 122:1075, 1965.
620. Marcussen, H.: Anti-colon antibodies in ulcerative colitis. A clinical study. Scand. J. Gastroenterol., 11:763, 1976.
621. Zeromski, J., et al.: Immunological studies in ulcerative colitis. VII. Anticolon antibodies of different immunoglobulin classes. Clin. Exp. Immunol., 7:468, 1970.
622. Broberger, O., and Perlmann, P.: In vitro studies of ulcerative colitis. I. Reactions of patient's serum with human fetal colon cells in tissue cultures. J. Exp. Med., 117:705, 1963.
623. Thayer, W. R., and Perlmann, P.: Inability to demonstrate antibody-dependent cell cytotoxicity against colon lipopolysaccharide antigen by inflammatory bowel disease sera. In Recent Advances in Crohn's Disease. Edited by A. S. Peña, I. T. Weterman, C. C. Booth, and W. Strober. The Hague, Martinus Nijhoff, 1981.
624. Asherson, G. L., and Broberger, O.: Incidence of hemagglutinating and complement-fixing antibodies. Br. Med. J., 1:1429, 1961.
625. Takahashi, F., and Das, K. M.: Isolation and characterization of a colonic autoantigen specifically recognized by colon tissue bound immunoglobulin G from idiopathic ulcerative colitis. J. Clin. Invest., 76:311, 1985.
626. Vecchi, M., Sakamaki, S. B., Diamond, K. M., and Das, A.: Human colon specific antigen reactive with ulcerative colitis colon tissue-bound IgG: immunohistochemical localization by the use of a monoclonal antibody. Gastroenterology, 90:1679, 1986.
627. Nagai, T., and Das, K. M.: Detection of colonic antigen(s) in tissues from ulcerative colitis using purified colitis colon tissue-bound IgG (CCA-IgG). Gastroenterology, 81:463, 1981.
628. Das, K. M., Kadano, Y., and Fleischner, G. M.: Antibody-dependent cell-mediated cytotoxicity in serum samples from patients with ulcerative colitis. Relationship to disease activity and response to total colectomy. Am. J. Med., 77:791, 1984.
629. Aronson, R. A., Cook, S. L., and Roche, J. K.: Sensitization to epithelial antigens in chronic mucosal inflammatory disease. I. Purification, characterization, and immune reactivity of murine epithelial cell-associated components (ECAC). J. Immunol., 131:2796, 1983.
630. Fiocchi, C., Roche, J. K., Paul, W., and Sapatnekar, W.: Familial immune reactivity to intestinal epithelial cell-associated components (ECAC) in inflammatory bowel disease (IBD). Gastroenterology, 90:1415, 1986.
631. Edison, J.: Immunoregulation of anti-epithelial cell responses: study of epithelial cell-associated antigens and antibodies in the peripheral blood of families with a genetic predisposition to chronic inflammatory bowel disease. Gastroenterology, 90:1788, 1986.
632. Perlmann, P., and Broberger, O.: In vitro studies of ulcerative colitis. II. Cytotoxic action of white blood cells

from patients on human fetal colon cells. J. Exp. Med., 117:717, 1963.
633. Watson, D. W., Quigley, A., and Bolt, R. J.: Effect of lymphocytes from patients with ulcerative colitis on human adult colon epithelial cells. Gastroenterology, 51:985, 1966.
634. Shorter, R. G., et al.: Inhibition of in vitro cytotoxicity of lymphocytes from patients with ulcerative colitis and granulomatous colitis for allogenic colonic epithelial cells using horse anti-human thymus serum. Gastroenterology, 54:227, 1968.
635. Shorter, R. G., et al.: Further studies of in vitro cytotoxicity of lymphocytes from patients with ulcerative and granulomatous colitis for allogeneic colonic epithelial cells including the effects of colectomy. Gastroenterology, 56:304, 1969.
636. Shorter, R. G., et al.: Further studies of in vitro cytotoxicity of lymphocytes for colonic epithelial cells. Gastroenterology, 57:30, 1969.
637. Shorter, R. G., et al.: Modification of in vitro cytotoxicity of lymphocytes from patients with chronic ulcerative colitis or granulomatous colitis for allogenic colonic epithelial cells. Gastroenterology, 58:692, 1970.
638. Shorter, R. G., et al.: Effects of preliminary incubation of lymphocytes with serum on their cytotoxicity for colonic epithelial cells. Gastroenterology, 58:843, 1970.
639. Shorter, R. G., et al.: Cytophilic antibody and the cytotoxicity of lymphocytes for colonic cells in vitro. Am. J. Dig. Dis., 16:673, 1971.
640. Shorter, R. G., et al.: Inflammatory bowel disease: the role of lymphotoxin in the cytotoxicity of lymphocytes for colonic epithelial cells. Am. J. Dig. Dis., 18:79, 1972.
641. Kemler, B. J., and Alpert, E.: Inflammatory bowel disease: study of cell mediated cytotoxicity for isolated human colonic epithelial cells. Gut, 21:353, 1980.
642. Stobo, J. D., et al.: In vitro studies of inflammatory bowel disease. Surface receptors of the mononuclear cell required to lyse allogeneic colonic epithelial cells. Gastroenterology, 70:171, 1976.
643. Shorter, R. G., McGill, D. B., and Bahn, R. C.: Cytotoxicity of mononuclear cells for autologous colonic epithelial cells in colonic diseases. Gastroenterology, 86:13, 1984.
644. Herberman, R. B., Reynolds, C. W., and Ortaldo, J. R.: Mechanism of cytotoxicity by natural killer (NK) cells. Ann. Rev. Immunol., 4:651, 1986.
645. Roche, J. K., Fiocchi, C., and Youngman, K.: Sensitization to epithelial antigens in chronic mucosal inflammatory disease. Characterization of human intestinal mucosa-derived mononuclear cells reactive with purified epithelial cell-associated components in vitro. J. Clin. Invest., 75:522, 1985.
646. Broder, S., et al.: Characterization of a suppressor cell leukemia. Evidence for the requirement of an interaction of two T cells in the development of human suppressor effector cells. N. Engl. J. Med., 298:66, 1978.
647. Mitchison, N. A.: Differentiation within the immune system: the importance of cloning. In Isolation, Characterization, and Utilization of T Lymphocyte Clones. Edited by C. G. Fathman, and F. W. Fitch. New York, Academic Press, 1982.
648. Crystal, R. G., et al.: Pulmonary sarcoidosis: a disease characterized and perpetuated by activated lung T-lymphocytes. Ann. Int. Med., 94:73, 1981.
649. Hunninghake, G. W., and Crystal, R. G.: Pulmonary sarcoidosis. A disorder mediated by excess helper T-lymphocyte activity at sites of disease activity. N. Engl. J. Med., 305:429, 1981.
650. Auer, I. O., Roder, A., and Frohlich, J.: Immune status in Crohn's disease. VI. Immunoregulation evaluated by multiple distinct T suppressor cell assays of lymphocyte proliferation, and by enumeration of immunoregulatory T lymphocyte subsets. Gastroenterology, 86:1531, 1984.
651. Sieber, G., et al.: Abnormalities of B-cell activation and immunoregulation in patients with Crohn's disease. Gut, 25:1255, 1984.
652. Godin, N. J., et al.: Loss of suppressor T-cells in active inflammatory bowel disease. Gut, 25:743, 1984.
653. Damle, N. K., Mohagheghpour, N., Hansen, J. A., and Engleman, E. G.: Alloantigen-specific cytotoxic and suppressor T lymphocytes are derived from phenotypically distinct precursors. J. Immunol., 131:2296, 1983.
654. Hodgson, H. J. F., Wands, J. R., and Isselbacher, K. J.: Decreased suppressor cell activity in inflammatory bowel disease. Clin. Exp. Immunol., 32:451, 1978.
655. Victorino, R. M., and Hodgson, H. J. F.: Spontaneous suppressor cell function in inflammatory bowel disease. Dig. Dis. Sci., 26:801, 1981.
656. Knapp, W., et al.: Con A induced suppressor activity in IBD and other inflammatory conditions. In Recent Advances in Crohn's Disease. Edited by A. S. Peña, I. T. Weterman, C. C. Booth, and W. Strober. Martinus Nijhoff Publishers, Hague, 1981.
657. Holdstock G., Chastenay, B. F., and Krawitt, E. L.: Functional suppressor T cell activity in Crohn's disease and the effects of sulfasalazine. Clin. Exp. Immunol., 48:619, 1982.
658. Fiocchi, C., Youngman, K. R., and Farmer, R. G.: Immunoregulatory function of human intestinal mucosa lymphoid cells: evidence for enhanced suppressor cell activity in inflammatory bowel disease. Gut, 24:692, 1983.
659. Goodacre, R. L., and Bienenstock, J.: Reduced suppressor cell activity in intestinal lymphocytes from patients with Crohn's disease. Gastroenterology, 82:653, 1982.
660. Lee, A., Sugerman, H., Hempfling, S. H., and Elson, C. O.: A functional comparison of human intestinal lamina and peripheral blood CD4 (OKT4) helper T cells. Gastroenterology, 90:1514, 1986.
661. Strober, W.: Animal models of inflammatory bowel disease—an overview. Dig. Dis. Sci., 30:38, 1985.

Section 3 · *Clinical Aspects*

8 · Clinical Features, Course, and Laboratory Findings in Ulcerative Colitis

JOHN W. SINGLETON, M.D.

Idiopathic ulcerative colitis is an inflammatory disease of the colonic mucosa of unknown etiology. The disease is variable both in the extent and the severity of involvement of the colon. In its most limited extent it may affect only the distal rectum, often only the most distal centimeter or two. In its most extensive form, the entire colon is involved, with secondary changes of so-called "backwash ileitis" extending into the distal ileum. The spectrum of severity extends from inflammation so mild that it is undetectable except by biopsy, to florid ulceration and hemorrhage extending into, and sometimes through, the full thickness of the colonic wall and leading to perforation. As might be expected, the clinical and laboratory manifestations of the disease closely parallel the variation in extent and severity of colonic involvement. The course of the disease is also somewhat predictable from its initial presentation (see the following section and Chap. 21).

Ulcerative Proctitis

When the mucosal inflammation of idiopathic ulcerative colitis is confined to the rectum, with the upper limit of disease visible using the conventional sigmoidoscope, the disease is called ulcerative proctitis. This mild variant of ulcerative colitis represents approximately 30% of the ulcerative colitis population at diagnosis in population-based surveys,[1] and approximately 25% in hospital-based series.[2,3] The age distribution of patients with ulcerative proctitis is similar to that of ulcerative colitis,[4] with peak age of onset in the second and third decades (see also Chap. 1).

The presenting symptoms of ulcerative proctitis all refer to the affected rectum. Rectal bleeding is present in over 90% of patients, and change in bowel habit in over 50%.[5] Either diarrhea or constipation may occur, and the latter is frequently present. Urgency and tenesmus occur in approximately 30% of patients. About 10% of patients have lower abdominal or sacral pain.[4] Systemic symptoms of fever, malaise, and weight loss are absent.

General physical examination is normal in ulcerative proctitis. On digital rectal examination, rectal tenderness may be present. Anal or perianal lesions are rare and should suggest Crohn's disease as the diagnosis. Proctosigmoidoscopy reveals an inflamed mucosa (see also Chap. 19).[4] Edema is evident in the early stages, recognized by loss of the vascular pattern. With more severe involvement, mucopus appears on the surface and bleeding may be spontaneous or induced by the minor trauma of wiping. Frank ulceration is rare and suggests another diagnosis, for example Crohn's disease or infectious proctitis (see Chap. 10). As the disease becomes chronic, the mucosa remains thickened and opaque while also becoming granular.

The laboratory abnormalities seen with more extensive ulcerative colitis are rare in ulcerative proctitis. Thus, the patient is rarely anemic or hypoalbuminemic. The erythrocyte sedimentation rate is only minimally elevated, if at all.

The course of ulcerative proctitis usually is benign. Few data are available on the untreated course. Placebo-controlled studies indicate that spontaneous remissions do occur in approximately 20% of episodes.[6] Medical treatment with sulfasalazine and local steroids leads to remission in 75 to 80% of first attacks. Approximately 40% of patients have permanent remission of disease after the first attack subsides.[7] The majority of patients run a relapsing course following the first episode of ulcerative proctitis. Munro found that approximately one-fourth of patients had at least one relapse each year over a seven year period (see also Chaps. 21, 32).[8]

Extension to involve more proximal colon occurs in approximately 15% of patients followed for 10 years,[7] with extension as far as the hepatic flexure in 7% of these patients. In a follow-up of 20 years or more, extension to the sigmoid probably occurs in at least 20% of the patients. Only a tiny proportion of those with ulcerative proctitis require surgical treatment, almost always as a result of proximal extension of the disease process. In the St. Mark's Hospital series, surgical treatment had been performed in less than 5% of cases in the five years following diagnosis,[2] and in hardly more after 10 years.[7] These results reflect medical therapy as carried out in specialty clinics in the past ten years. An earlier series reported a less favorable course for ulcerative proctitis (see also Chap. 32).[9]

Ulcerative Colitis

Symptoms

The cardinal sign of ulcerative colitis involving any portion or extent of the colon is hematochezia or visible blood in the stool. This is present in 80 to 90% of patients at the onset of their disease.[1,10] When the bowel involvement is confined to the rectum or rectum and distal sigmoid, the blood is seen in association with bowel movements, streaking the outside of the stool. If more of the colon is involved, the blood will be mixed with a soft, pultaceous or liquid stool. If the colonic inflammation is severe, blood may be mixed with mucopurulent exudate, and, rarely, almost pure blood may be passed.

The most characteristic symptom is diarrhea, present at onset in more than 80% of patients.[1,10,11] Diarrhea may vary from a change in character of the stool toward softer, less well formed movements, to the passage of small amounts of mucopus and blood as frequently as every few minutes. Because ulcerative colitis always involves the distal colon no matter how far upward it extends, the diarrhea occurs frequently and usually in small amounts, reflecting the irritability of the affected rectum. When only the distal rectum is involved, constipation may be present as the solid stool formed in the descending and sigmoid colon is blocked by painful rectal spasm.

Abdominal pain or rectal cramps occur in approximately one-half of the patients at the time of diagnosis,[9] as does fever. About 40% of the patients also suffer noticeable weight loss at this time.

Initial Attack

The onset of ulcerative colitis may be sudden, with bloody diarrhea appearing within a few days. The usual mode of onset is more gradual, however, with diarrhea progressing from increased frequency of stool to frequent bloody liquid movements over a period of several weeks. Watts et al. found that in about 40% of their patients the symptoms of the first attack reached the maximum severity in less than a month, and developed more slowly for the remainder of the study.[12]

The extent of colonic involvement in the first attack has been reasonably uniform in several large series of referred patients.[3,12] Approximately 30% of ulcerative colitis patients have disease limited to the rectum, about 40% have disease extending above the rectum but not beyond the hepatic flexure (so-called substantial disease), and the remaining 30% have total colitis at their first attack. In a population-based survey,[13] which included a large number of patients with mild disease, 74% of the patients had disease limited to the rectum or rectosigmoid.

The more colon that is involved, the more likely are systemic symptoms to be present. The scheme introduced by Truelove and Witts for classifying severity of attacks of ulcerative colitis (Table 8-1) has been widely adopted and confers some uniformity on the clinical description of attacks.[14] Only 10 to 15% of those with ulcerative proctitis have disease categorized as severe at the time of diagnosis,[11,12] whereas over 50% of the patients with disease extending at least to the splenic flexure have severe disease by the

Table 8-1. *Truelove and Witts Classification of Ulcerative Colitis.*

Severe:	Diarrhea: 6 or more motions per day, with blood
	Fever: mean evening temperature over 37.5° C, or any time of day over 37.7° C on at least 2 out of 4 days
	Tachycardia: Mean pulse rate over 90 per minute
	Anemia: Hemoglobin of 75% or less, allowing for recent transfusions
	Sedimentation rate: more than 30 mm in one hour
Mild:	Mild diarrhea: less than 4 motions per day, with only small amounts of blood
	No fever
	No tachycardia
	Mild anemia
	Sedimentation rate: below 30 mm in one hour
Moderately Severe:	Intermediate between mild and severe

(Adapted from Truelove, S.C., and Witts, L.J.: Br. Med. J., *2*:1041, 1955.)

Truelove criteria.[11] Edwards and Truelove, in their classic description of ulcerative colitis,[15] found that the first attack was severe in 19%, moderate in 27%, and mild in 54% of the patients studied. Twenty years later, the Danish investigators Both et al. reported that 70% of their patients had active or very active disease at the time of diagnosis, 28% had mild disease, and 2% inactive disease.[1] A typical pattern of distribution of disease severity at diagnosis is shown in Figure 8-1.

PHYSICAL FINDINGS. During an acute attack of ulcerative colitis, physical findings also depend upon both extent and severity of colonic involvement. Fever, prostration, dehydration, and postural hypotension accompany the most severe involvement. The abdomen may be protruberant as a result of colonic atony and distention. Abdominal tenderness over the course of the colon is an ominous sign, particularly when rebound tenderness is present, and should suggest the possibility of toxic dilatation or early perforation. Bowel sounds are usually hypoactive in severe attacks of ulcerative colitis; disappearance of bowel sounds is another ominous sign. Milder involvement will be manifest on examination as pallor, low-grade fever, evident weight loss, and mild abdominal tenderness.

EXTRAINTESTINAL MANIFESTATIONS. These are present in less than 10% of patients at the time of initial diagnosis.[1,11] The most common are arthralgia or mild arthritis. Aphthous stomatitis, eye inflammation (iritis, uveitis, and conjunctivitis), and skin rash are each present in 1 to 2% of first attacks (see also Chap. 16 and the sections that follow).

ENDOSCOPIC EXAMINATION. Endoscopy is the most accurate method for determining the extent of disease in the colon. Early in the course of ulcerative colitis, the mucosa shows edema (evident as loss of vascular pattern) and friability, with bleeding on minor trauma. With progression, or in more severe cases, granular, spontaneously hemorrhagic mucosa appears, with overlying mucopurulent exudate. The lumen seems narrowed and straightened, and the normal thin mucosal folds are lost. In the most severe episodes, the mucosa may be diffusely hemorrhagic and frank ulceration with loss of mucosal integrity may be seen. Powell-Tuck et al. have presented a useful scheme for classifying the endoscopic appearance of affected mucosa (Table 8-2).[16] A more detailed description of the endoscopic appearance of ulcerative colitis is given in Chapter 19.

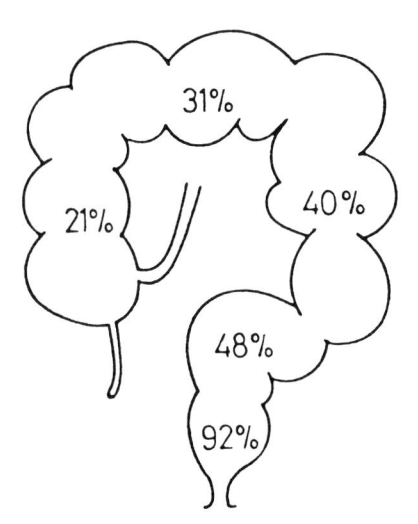

FIG. 8-1. Localization of disease at diagnosis in 783 patients with ulcerative colitis. (Reproduced with permission from Both, H., et al.: Scand. J. Gastroenterol., *18*:987, 1985.)

TABLE 8-2. *Classification of Sigmoidoscopic Appearance of Ulcerative Colitis.*[*]

Grade 0—Nonhemorrhagic: No bleeding, either spontaneously or on light touch
Grade 1—Hemorrhagic: Bleeding on light touch, but no spontaneous bleeding seen ahead of instrument
Grade 2—Hemorrhagic: Spontaneous bleeding seen ahead of instrument at initial inspection, with bleeding on light touch

(Adapted from Descos, L., et al.: Digestion, 28:148, 1983.)
[*]See also Chapter 19.

RADIOLOGIC FINDINGS. Although these are covered in Chapter 20 of this volume, some mention must be made here of the findings on supine and upright plain films of the abdomen. This examination should be part of the evaluation of every patient with moderate or severe symptoms of ulcerative colitis (see Table 8-1) in order to recognize dilatation of the colon and incipient or established perforation (see also Chaps. 14 and 20). Approximately 10 to 20% of patients with severe attacks of colitis demonstrate colonic dilatation (transverse diameter of the transverse colon 5.5 cm or greater).[17] An equally important and more ominous sign recognizable on plain abdominal film is the irregular mucosal edge as outlined by intraluminal gas in the dilated segment. This finding has been named "mucosal islands," and it indicates ulceration that extends through the mucosa and submucosa into the muscularis propria, threatening perforation.[18]

LABORATORY FINDINGS. Studies in ulcerative colitis in the laboratory also parallel the extent and severity of the bowel disease. Table 8-1 demonstrates that decreased hemoglobin level and elevated sedimentation rate have been used for over 30 years as indicators of the severity of ulcerative colitis. Anemia, hypoalbuminemia, and electrolyte imbalance also accompany severe colitis. Hypokalemia and metabolic acidosis can be particularly severe as the result of diarrheal loss of potassium and bicarbonate. Serum orosomucoid is the acute phase reactant that most closely parallels clinical activity in ulcerative colitis.[13]

Course[*]

Since Edwards and Truelove's classic study of the course of ulcerative colitis,[15] advances in diagnosis and management of the disease have substantially altered its natural history. As one example of this, whereas Edwards and Truelove found that their patients had an excess mortality of 20% in the 10 years following diagnosis in

[*]See also Chapters 21 and 32.

comparison with an age- and sex-matched general population group, Ritchie et al., reporting 15 years later from a comparably expert clinic, found no excess mortality in their patients.[2] This striking improvement in the course of disease is evident both in the outcome of acute attacks and in the long-term morbidity and mortality. In the discussion that follows, the course of the disease in response to modern medical and surgical therapy will be described, with occasional reference to the "natural history" of untreated disease, as demonstrated by the placebo group in controlled therapeutic trials and clinical data collected prior to the introduction of modern medical and surgical treatment.

OUTCOME OF FIRST ATTACK. For all degrees of severity of disease and patterns of colonic involvement, the overall outcome of the first attack of ulcerative colitis is presented in Table 8-3. Note that the sex of the patient has no influence on outcome.

The outcome of the first attack is greatly influenced by the extent of colonic involvement, the severity of the attack, and the age of the patient. The extent of disease is highly correlated with severity; typical figures are shown in Table 8-4, taken from data of Watts et al. gathered in a referral hospital.[12] Data from the best recent population-based survey are given in Tables 8-5 and 8-6. These demonstrate that the first attack of mild disease carries negligible mortality, no recourse to surgery, and a 91% rate of remission with medical therapy. None of the deaths in patients with mild disease was caused by colitis. For severe first attacks, colectomy was necessary in 29% of the patients and death occurred in 23% of them. These results can be compared to those cited by Edwards and Truelove for the presteroid era (1938 to 1952), when 43% of all patients referred in severe first attacks died and the overall mortality with first attacks was 14%.[15]

Although colonic dilatation is not included in the Truelove scheme for classifying severity of disease activity (Table 8-1), its occurrence has

TABLE 8-3. *Outcome of First Attack of Ulcerative Colitis.*[13]

	Death	Remission	Surgical Treatment	Continuous Symptoms	Unknown
Female	9 (3%)	225 (86%)	6 (2%)20 (8%)	1	0
Male	8 (3%)	240 (87%)	9 (3%)	21 (8%)	0
Total	17 (3%)	465 (87%)	15 (8%)	41 (8%)	1

(Adapted from Sinclair, T. S., Brunt, P. N., and Mowat, N. A. G.: Gastroenterology, 85:1, 1983.)

TABLE 8-4. *Incidence of Severe First Attacks Related to Clinical Extent of Disease.*

Extent of Disease	Total Number of patients	Number of Patients with Severe Attacks	Incidence of Severe Attacks
Rectum	72	9	12.5%
Sigmoid-splenic flexure	75	28	37.3%
Total colon	41	24	58.5%

(Adapted from Watts, J. McK., et al.: Gut, 7:16, 1966.)

TABLE 8-5. *Outcome of First Attack vs. Severity.*

	Mild	Moderate	Severe
Total patients	364	138	33
Remission	333 (91.5%)	118 (84.9%)	13 (38.2%)
Surgical treatment	0 (0.0%)	5 (3.6%)	10 (29.0%)
Continuing symptoms	29 (8.0%)	11 (7.9%)	1 (2.9%)
Death (total)	5 (1.4%)	4 (2.9%)	8 (23.0%)
Death caused by colitis	0 (0.0%)	1 (0.7%)	8 (23.0%)

(Adapted from Sinclair, T. S., Brunt, P. W., and Mowat, N. A. G.: Gastroenterology, 85:1, 1983.)

TABLE 8-6. *Outcome of First Attack vs. Age.*

	AGE			
	0-29	30-49	50-69	70+
Total patients	172	161	145	59
Remission	151 (87.8%)	143 (88.8%)	126 (86.9%)	44 (74.6%)
Surgical Treatment	7 (4.0%)	3 (2.0%)	4 (3.0%)	1 (2.0%)
Continuing symptoms	15 (8.7%)	12 (7.5%)	10 (6.9%)	4 (6.8%)
Death (total)	0 (0.0%)	2 (1.2%)	4 (2.7%)	11 (19.2%)
Death caused by colitis	0 (0.0%)	2 (1.2%)	2 (1.4%)	5 (8.0%)

(Adapted from Sinclair, T. S., Brunt, P. N., and Mowat, N. A. G.: Gastroenterology, 85:1, 1983.)

an ominous prognostic effect. In Binder's series,[19] colonic perforation followed recognition of dilatation in 20% of cases (see also Chap. 14).

As might be expected, age has an effect on the outcome of the first attack. Five of the nine deaths resulting from colitis shown in Table 8-6 occurred in patients 70 years of age or older. In part, this is caused by the increased severity of first attacks in older patients. Patients younger than 20 and older than 70 are twice as likely to have a severe first attack, in comparison with patients 20 to 59 years of age.[12]

Data from earlier series indicate that the mode of onset (rapid vs. gradual) also affects the outcome of the first attack. In the series reported by Watts et al.,[12] patients whose disease reached maximum severity in less than a month had a two fold greater rate of failure of medical therapy than did patients whose disease was of more gradual onset.

The course of the acute attack is highly dependent upon the therapy chosen. The recommendation of Truelove and Jewell,[20,21] that surgical therapy be undertaken if a severe attack does not respond to maximum medical therapy after five days, undoubtedly has saved lives but may have resulted in more colectomies than when more "conservative" regimens were followed. More recent data from Sweden and the United States suggest that a somewhat longer trial of medical therapy with close observation may be equally safe and less likely to lead to surgical therapy (see also Chap. 21)[22,23] Continuing maximum medical therapy beyond 10 days may not yield success.[23]

Course following the first attack*

Accurate representation of the long-term course of any disease is obtained only by using actuarial (life-table) methods. Only studies using such methods will be cited in this section.

Edwards and Truelove characterized the course of ulcerative colitis, as shown in Table 8-7.[15] Despite the current use of steroids for treatment of the acute attack and sulfasalazine in prophylaxis of recurrent attacks, the distribution of clinical patterns shown remains approximately accurate. Most patients who survive an acute attack subsequently experience recurrent attacks. A small minority never achieve a satis-

*See also Chapters 21 and 32.

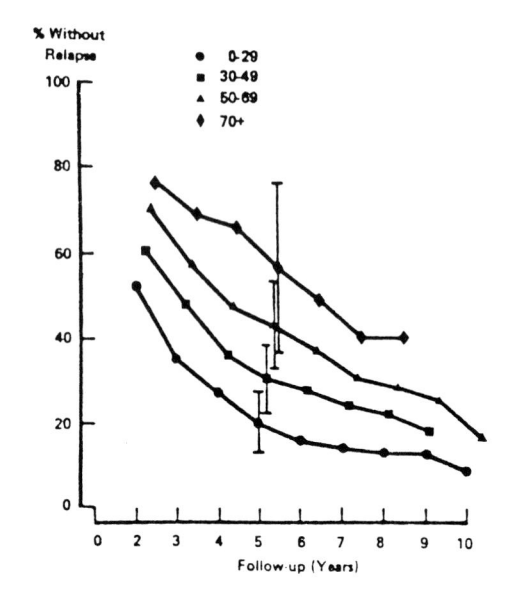

FIG. 8-2. Risk of relapse following first attack versus age. (Reproduced with permission from Sinclair, T. S., Brunt, P. W., and Mowat, N. A. G.: Gastroenterology, 85:1, 1983.)

factory remission and continue with symptoms of greater or lesser degree. Approximately one-fifth of patients never experience another attack during 10 years, or more, of follow-up.

REMISSION AND RELAPSE. Edwards and Truelove found that the severity of the first attack had no influence on the subsequent pattern of the disease. Sinclair et al. have confirmed this finding in their population-based survey.[13] The extent of colonic involvement at diagnosis has no effect on frequency of recurrence.[13] The patient's age at diagnosis does affect the likelihood of relapse, however, as shown in Figure 8-2. These data show an inverse linear correlation of age

TABLE 8-7. *The Clinical Course of Ulcerative Colitis.*

Clinical Course	Number of Patients	Percentage
Acute fulminating	20	8.0
Chronic intermittent	161	64.4
Chronic continuous	18	7.2
One attack only	45	18.0
Total colectomy in first attack	2	0.8
Died in first attack of other causes	1	0.4
Unknown	2	0.8
Total	249	100.0

(Adapted from Edwards, E. C., and Truelove, S. C.: Gut, 4:299, 1963.)

*See also Chapters 21 and 32.

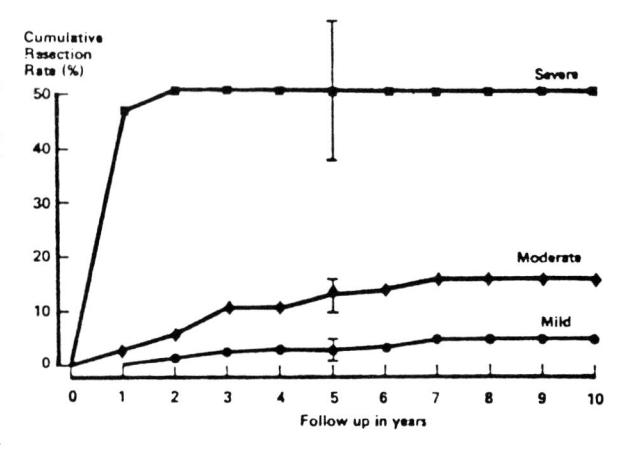

FIG. 8-3. Cumulative resection rate versus severity of first attack. (Reproduced with permission from Sinclair, T. S., Brunt, P. W., and Mowat, N. A. G.: Gastroenterology, 85:1, 1983.)

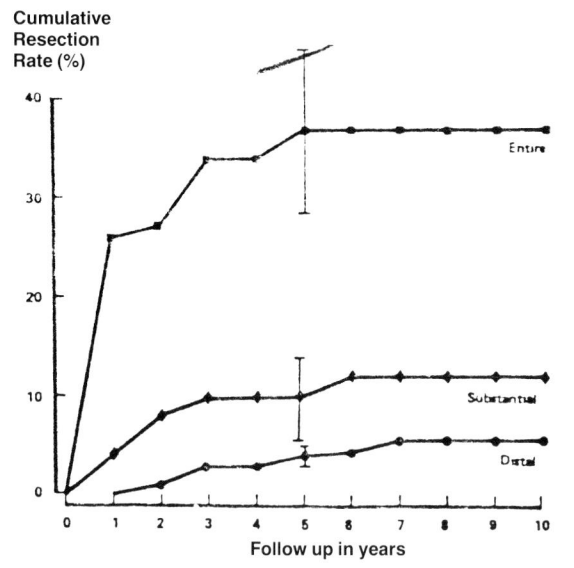

FIG. 8-4. Cumulative resection rate versus extent at onset. (Reproduced with permission from Sinclair, T. S., Brunt, P. W., and Mowat, N. A. G.: Gastroenterology, 85:1, 1983.)

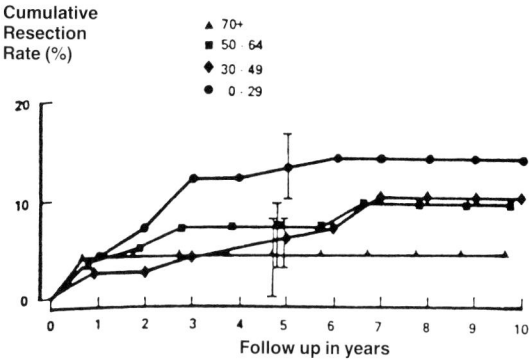

FIG. 8-5. Cumulative resection rate versus age at onset. (Reproduced with permission from Sinclair, T. S., Brunt, P. W., and Mowat, N. A. G.: Gastroenterology, 85:1, 1983.)

with occurrence of relapse. At five years following the first attack, 60% of patients who were septuagenarians had not had a relapse, while only 20% of those patients who were under 30 at the time of their first attack were still without relapse. The effect of prophylactic use of sulfasalazine is not reported in these series. Prospective controlled trials have shown that sulfasalazine reduces the likelihood of relapse by 75% in the first year of use, however, and this effect appears to persist indefinitely.[24,25]

EXTENSION OF DISEASE. Good data are available on the likelihood of extension of disease with time. The chance of spread of proctitis to involve the sigmoid colon is about 12% after five years,[13] and after 10 years it is 30%.[2] The risk of spread from proctitis to the whole colon is between 5% and 10% in 10 years.[2]

NEED FOR SURGICAL TREATMENT* Of patients who survive their first attack of ulcerative colitis without requiring surgical treatment, about 8% will have had a colectomy after 5 years and about 11% after 10 years.[13] The need for surgical treatment subsequent to the first attack depends on both the severity of the first attack and the extent at diagnosis. Age at onset also affects need for surgical treatment. These relationships are graphically explained by Figures 8-3, 8-4, and 8-5. Clearly, the patients most likely to require surgical treatment are young people whose first attack is severe and involves the entire colon. The need for surgical treatment diminishes rapidly after the first few years of disease.

EXTRAINTESTINAL MANIFESTATIONS.* A minority of patients with ulcerative colitis develop one or more extraintestinal manifestations of the disease during the life-long course. Unfortunately, no population-based data exist on prevalence of these symptoms. The largest collection of patients in whom extraintestinal manifestations have been carefully recorded is shown in Table 8-8.[26] Bear in mind that this select group of patients was referred to hospitals and doctors famous for management of inflammatory bowel disease. A population-based series, if such were

*See also Chapters 25 and 26.

*See also Chapter 18.

TABLE 8-8. *Extraintestinal Manifestations in 202 Patients with Ulcerative Colitis.*

Organ Involved	Number of Patients	Percentage of Total
Joint:	53	26%
Polyarthralgia	27	13%
Spine	8	4%
Extremities	18	9%
Skin:	39	19%
Erythema nodosum	9	4%
Pyoderma gangrenosum	10	5%
Other	20	10%
Mouth	8	4%
Eye	9	13%
Total patients	202	

(Adapted from Greenstein, A. J., Janowitz, H. D., and Sachar, D. B.: Medicine, 55:401, 1976)

*See also Chapter 16.

available, might show a different pattern of distribution of extraintestinal manifestations. A detailed description of these phenomena is given in Chapter 16.

References

1. Both, H., et al.: Clinical appearance at diagnosis of ulcerative colitis and Crohn's disease in a regional patient group. Scand. J. Gastroenterol., *18*:987, 1983.
2. Ritchie, J. K., Powell-Tuck, J., and Lennard-Jones, J. E.: Clinical outcome of the first ten tears of ulcerative colitis and proctitis. Lancet, *1*:1140, 1978.
3. Lanfranchi, G. A., et al.: Clinical course of ulcerative colitis in Italy. Digestion, *20*:106, 1980.
4. Lennard-Jones, J. E., et al.: Observations on idiopathic proctitis. Gut, *3*:201, 1962.
5. Myers, A., Humphreys, D. M., and Cox, E. V.: A ten-year follow-up of hemorrhagic proctitis. Postgrad. Med. J., *52*:224, 1976.
6. Lennard-Jones, J. E., et al.: A double-blind controlled trial of prednisolone-21-phosphate suppositories in treatment of idiopathic proctitis. Gut, *3*:207, 1962.
7. Powell-Tuck, J., Ritchie, J. K., and Lennard-Jones, J. E.: The prognosis of idiopathic proctitis. Scand. J. Gastroenterol., *12*:727, 1977.
8. Ritchie, J. K., and Hawley, P. R.: Idiopathic proctitis. *In* Inflammatory Bowel Diseases. Edited by R. N. Allan, et al. New York, Churchill Livingstone, 1983.
9. Sparberg, M., Fennessy, J., and Kirsner, J. B.: Ulcerative proctitis and mild ulcerative colitis: a study of 220 patients. Medicine, *45*:391, 1966.
10. Gilat, T., et al.: Ulcerative colitis in the Jewish population of Tel-Aviv Yafo. III. Clinical course. Gastroenterology, *70*:14, 1976.
11. Wright, J. P., et al.: Inflammatory bowel disease in Cape Town, 1975-1980. Part I. Ulcerative Colitis. S. Afr. Med. J., *63*:223, 1983.
12. Watts, J. McK., et al.: Early course of ulcerative colitis. Gut, *7*:16, 1966.
13. Sinclair, T. S., Brunt, P. W., and Mowat, N. A. G.: Nonspecific proctocolitis in northeastern Scotland: a community study. Gastroenterology, *85*:1, 1983.
14. Truelove, S. C., and Witts, L. J.: Cortisone in ulcerative colitis. Final report on a therapeutic trial. Br. Med. J., *2*:1041, 1955.
15. Edwards, E. C., and Truelove, S. C.: The course and prognosis of ulcerative colitis. Gut, *4*:299, 1963.
16. Powell-Tuck, J., et al.: Correlations between defined sigmoidoscopic appearances and other measures of disease activity in ulcerative colitis. Dig. Dis. Sci., *27*:533, 1982.
17. Binder, S. C., Patterson, J. F., and Glotzer, D. J.: Toxic megacolon in ulcerative colitis. Gastroenterology, *66*:909, 1974.
18. Buckell, N. A., et al.: Depth of ulceration in acute colitis. Correlation of outcome and clinical and radiologic feature. Gastroenterology, *79*:19, 1980.
19. Descos, L., et al.: Assessment of appropriate laboratory measurements to reflect the degree of activity of ulcerative colitis. Digestion, *28*:148, 1983.
20. Truelove, S. C., and Jewell, D. P.: Intensive intravenous regimen for severe attacks of ulcerative colitis. Lancet, *1*:1067, 1974.
21. Truelove, S. C., et al.: Further experience in the treatment of severe attacks of ulcerative colitis. Lancet, *2*:1086, 1978.
22. Järnerot, G., Rolny, P., and Sandberg-Gertzén, H.: Intensive intravenous treatment of ulcerative colitis. Gastroenterology, *89*:1005, 1985.
23. Lever, P., et al.: Predicting therapeutic outcomes of severe ulcerative colitis. Gastroenterology, *88*:1471, 1985.
24. Misiewicz, J. J., et al.: Controlled trial of sulphasalazine in maintenance therapy for ulcerative colitis. Lancet, *1*:185, 1965.
25. Dissanayake, A. S., and Truelove, S. C.: A controlled therapeutic trial of long-term maintenance treatment of ulcerative colitis with sulphasalazine. Gut, *14*:923, 1973.
26. Greenstein, A. J., Janowitz, H. D., and Sachar, D. B.: The extra-intestinal complications of Crohn's disease and ulcerative colitis: a study of 700 patients. Medicine, *55*:401, 1976.

9 · Clinical Features, Laboratory Findings, and Course of Crohn's Disease

RICHARD G. FARMER, M.D.

Historic Overview

As is well known, the clinical features of what is now called Crohn's disease were described by Crohn, Ginsberg, and Oppenheimer in a landmark article in 1932. They called the disease "regional ileitis" and described most of the clinical features found in the disease, even today.[1] The first clinical description of Crohn's disease however, was probably by Dalzeil who, in Glasgow, Scotland in 1913, described nine patients with the illness now known as Crohn's disease.[2] Because the disease was recognized as involving more than just the terminal ileum, the term "regional enteritis" was popularized by Bargen and his colleagues, who reported some 600 cases in 1954.[3] Further progress in defining the disease was made in 1960 with the finding by Lockhart-Mummery and Morson that gross lesions of Crohn's disease could present in the large intestine only.[4] Over the next decade, much confusion existed, particularly in differentiating Crohn's disease of the large intestine from chronic ulcerative colitis (CUC). Several additional studies provided some clinical and pathologic differentiation between the two diseases, however, so that clarity, at least regarding the clinical features, began to emerge.[5,8] This experience continued into the following decade, and in some geographic locations remarkable increases occurred in the number of patients with Crohn's disease.[9-11] Thus, what was once considered a rare intestinal disease has emerged as one of the major digestive disorders encountered in clinical practice, particularly in North America and Western Europe (see also Chap. 1). The nature of the disease makes it socioeconomically important because it affects a predominantly young population, it is chronic and recurrent, the therapy is often unpredictable, responses may be suboptimal, operations are frequently needed, and recurrences may follow. This chapter will deal with many of the clinical and laboratory features of Crohn's disease; however, some aspects of differential diagnosis, many of its local and systemic complications, the specific problems in children, and the radiologic and endoscopic features and therapy are considered in detail elsewhere (see Chaps. 10, 14–16, 19–23, and 27).

Symptoms and Signs

Approximately 90% of patients with Crohn's disease have a triad of features that are persistent and progressive, namely diarrhea, abdominal pain, and weight loss.[12-14] In our study of 615 consecutive new patients seen from 1966 to 1969,[13] the mean age was 32 years (range 5 to 83 years) and 26% of the patients were under the age of 20 at the time of diagnosis. Although the mean duration of symptoms from onset to diagnosis was five years, 30% of the patients had had symptoms for less than one year. The National Cooperative Crohn's Disease Study (NCCDS),[14] a multicenter therapeutic trial involving 14 institutions and 569 patients, found mean ages at the time of diagnosis ranging from 31.5 to 33.7 years in the various clinical categories, and the average duration from onset of symptoms to diagnosis was 35 months. Because the onset of the disease usually is ill-defined, persistent and progressive symptoms exist over a variable period of time prior to diagnosis.

Most patients with Crohn's disease have a gradual onset of loose bowel movements that increase both in frequency and in the lack of stool consistency. Some patients may have ten or more watery bowel actions in a 24 hour period, and diarrhea typically occurs after eating, although it also may occur at night. The volume of stool in patients with Crohn's disease relates to the anatomic location of disease, being greater with proximal intestinal involvement and loss of absorptive surface, although gross steatorrhea is unusual. Fat soluble vitamin deficiencies may occur, and serious losses of protein may be present in the stool, which then leads to edema. Although virtually all patients with Crohn's disease have diarrhea, bleeding occurs only in about half of the patients with colonic Crohn's disease, and in less than 25% of those with ileocolic or "pure" small intestinal involvement.[13]

Abdominal pain is present in essentially all patients with Crohn's disease, but because it is a subjective phenomenon it is impossible to quantify. Typically, the pain is described as cramping, extending across the lower abdomen, with maximum referral to the right lower quadrant. It may occur after eating, and usually is not described as severe.

Weight loss is also a common feature and generally is in the range of 10 to 20% of body weight, depending on a variety of factors. Importantly, an estimation of the degree of weight loss must be based on the patient's ideal weight, the patient's weight prior to the onset of symptoms, or on the anticipated weight (for example, in a child or teenager in a growth phase). Although weight loss may correlate with the degree of abdominal pain and diarrhea, it usually relates to the severity of anorexia and malaise. A general feeling of "loss of well-being" is a common complaint, and, less frequently, low grade fever may be present. Vomiting may be a feature, but more commonly the intestinal symptoms are referable to the lower rather than the upper intestinal tract. In general, the clinical picture is dominated by the triad of diarrhea, abdominal pain, and weight loss, as emphasized previously.

The next most common manifestation of Crohn's disease is perianal involvement, and a wide spectrum of this may be found, from tenderness of the anal sphincter to fistula formation and perirectal abscess (see also Chap. 14).[15] About one-third of all patients with Crohn's disease have such lesions, which may consist of: (1) edematous skin tags around the anal sphincter, (2) fissuring and ulceration in the anal sphincter itself, (3) the presence of a fistulous tract extending from the anus into the perineum or vagina, and (4) development of a perirectal abscess.[15,16]

A Scandinavian study of 185 patients with newly diagnosed Crohn's disease showed the following frequencies of features: diarrhea 96%, abdominal pain 76%, weight loss 54%, rectal bleeding 51%, fever 34%, and perianal manifestations 23%.[17] Extraintestinal complications represent a systemic aspect of the disease and are described in detail elsewhere (see also Chap. 14). Our experience in a long-term follow-up has been that between 10 and 20% of patients with Crohn's disease have such manifestations.[16] Even though it may be virtually impossible to differentiate CUC from Crohn's disease when the latter presents clinically in the large intestine alone (see also Chap. 10), if the patient is observed over a period of several months the diagnosis usually becomes apparent,[18,19] because during this time the clinical features of Crohn's disease usually are divergent from those of ulcerative colitis.[16,19,20]

Because of the increased incidence of Crohn's disease in various parts of the world (see also Chap. 1) and its socioeconomic significance, a great deal of interest in the disease internationally has emerged in recent years, with the formation of an International Organization for the Study of Inflammatory Bowel Disease (IOIBD), and considerable activity by the World Organization of Gastroenterology (OMGE). The OMGE Research Committee has reported clinical data obtained from 2,657 patients in 35 centers from 16 different countries.[21] In Crohn's disease, they found that right lower quadrant abdominal pain was by far the most important symptom for helping to discriminate between it and ulcerative colitis, and a history of anal fissure was the next most important distinction. Lesser degrees of difference (favoring Crohn's disease) were the absence of gross blood and mucus from the stools, and a history of appendectomy. No significant differential diagnostic features were apparent in terms of age, the duration of symptoms, or the degree of diarrhea. Unfortunately, the relative lack of specificity of symptoms for patients with early Crohn's disease continues to be a diagnostic problem.

By far the most important physical features in patients with Crohn's disease (in addition to pallor and weight loss) are the presence of a right lower quadrant abdominal mass with tenderness and a perianal fistula.[14,21,22] Typically, the rectal mucosal changes in ulcerative colitis are distinct enough from those in Crohn's disease to make a visual distinction,[23] because the earliest lesion in Crohn's disease is seen endoscopically as a mucosal aphthous ulcer (see also Chap. 18).[21]

Clinical Patterns and Disease Locations

The clinical features of Crohn's disease relate to the anatomic location of disease at presentation, which has been designated the clinical pattern.[13] As our studies have emphasized, the location of disease at the time of diagnosis plays a significant role not only in the clinical features,[13] but also in the complications, indications for surgery,[23] and long-term prognosis.[16] The findings in Hellers' study from Stockholm and the report from the National Cooperative Crohn's Disease Study (NCCDS) are in broad agreement with our experience at the Cleveland Clinic (Table 9-1).[12,14] The three major clinical patterns in Crohn's disease are: ileocolic location of the gross disease, small intestinal location, and large intestinal location. Approximately 40% of patients have the ileocolic pattern, that is, disease involving the distal ileum and proximal colon. Approximately 30% of patients have "pure" small intestinal disease and the vast majority of these have distal ileal involvement, similar to that originally reported by Crohn et al.;[1] fewer than 10% of those with the small intestinal pattern have disease confined proximally to the ileum.[13] Only about 5% of all patients have primary jejunal, gastroduodenal, or perianal involvement, while about 25% have "pure" large bowel Crohn's disease, which can be confused with ulcerative colitis. About two-thirds of those with the colonic pattern of disease have diffuse involvement of the entire large intestine, while segmental involvement is present in the other one-third.[13,16]

As previously stated, defining the clinical pattern is important because the clinical features, complications, and indications for surgery relate directly to the initial location of disease (Table 9-2).[13,16,23] Perianal lesions are more frequent in patients with colitis or ileocolitis than in those with only small intestinal involvement.[13,14,15] Patients with ileocolitis more commonly have internal fistulae than those in the other categories, and intestinal obstruction is more frequent in those with "pure" small intestinal disease.[13,16]

In recent years, because of an increasing number of patients with Crohn's disease, various other initial anatomic locations of the disease have been reported. It is emphasized, however, that collectively, clinical patterns other than the three major ones already described encompass less than 5% of those with Crohn's disease.

From studies of patients with perianal Crohn's disease,[24,25] ileal involvement,[26] or large bowel involvement,[19,27] a general statement can be made that ileal disease is most associated with abdominal pain, while in the large bowel, disease has a greater association with systemic symptoms, extracolonic manifestations,[13] and chronic diarrhea.

Although it is rare, Crohn's disease may occur in more proximal portions of the gastrointestinal tract, with a predilection for the buccal cavity, but when the latter site is involved by "true" Crohn's lesions and not simply by aphthous stomatitis, usually overt disease is elsewhere in the tract. Esophageal involvement is uncommon, but Crohn's disease of the stomach and duodenum has been reported relatively frequently, and its endoscopic characteristics have been described.[28,29] Duodenal disease occurs in about 2% of cases and may involve the proximal (first and second) portions, frequently with stenosis,[30] and may extend into the gastric antrum. Our experience has indicted that the majority of such patients require surgical treatment because of progressive obstruction, weight loss, and postprandial vomiting, and that gastrojejunostomy without resection is often beneficial (see also Chaps. 25 and 27).[32] Duodenal Crohn's disease is almost invariably associated with gross lesions in other sites in the gastrointesti-

TABLE 9-1. *Crohn's Disease, Initial Location of Disease.*

Series	Ileocolic	Small Intestine	Colon	Other
Cleveland Clinic[13]	41%	29%	27%	3%
NCCDS[26]	55%	30%	14%	1%
Stockholm[12]	41%	41%	17%	1%
Oxford[57]	42%	30%	26%	2%

TABLE 9-2. *Initial Symptoms of Crohn's Disease Related to Location of Disease.*

	NCCDS (569 Cases)		Cleveland Clinic (615 Cases)		
	Total	Colon	Ileocolic Location	Colonic Location	Small Intestine Location
Diarrhea	92%	92%	Virtually all patients		
Abdominal pain	95%	93%	65%	62%	55%
Bleeding	41%	62%	22%	10%	46%
Weight loss	85%	88%	12%*	19%	22%
Perianal disease	36%	47%	21%	5%	19%
Arthritis	19%	22%	4%	4%	16%

*Loss of 20% of body weight or more
(Adapted from Farmer, R. G., Hawk, W. A., and Turnbull, R. B.: Gastroenterology, 68:627, 1975; and Mekhijian, H. S., et al.: Gastroenterology, 77:898, 1979.)

nal tract, as is Crohn's disease of the esophagus.

"Appendicitis-like" symptoms are known to occur in patients with Crohn's disease; although the disease may involve the vermiform appendix itself,[33] this is more a curiosity than a frequent finding.

Some differential considerations in the diagnosis of Crohn's enteritis are listed in Table 9-3 (those in Crohn's colitis are discussed in Chapter 10). Fortunately, in many instances this diagnosis can be made readily, based on the history and the characteristic radiographic appearances. Certain diseases, however, such as tuberculous enteritis, which is seen particularly in immigrants from underdeveloped countries in the United States and Western Europe, and Yersinial infections with a chronic course, may cause diagnostic problems and laparoscopy or laparotomy, and appropriate microbiologic studies may be necessary.

Laboratory Features

No laboratory markers exist that are either specifically indicative of Crohn's disease, define its activity, or predict its course, and this is a considerable clinical handicap. The OMGE Research Committee surveyed five tests to evaluate their differential diagnostic significance between Crohn's disease and ulcerative colitis, and did not find any that gave clear distinctions between the two diseases.[21] The features considered were a circulating hemoglobin of less than 10 g%, leukocytosis of greater than 20,000/mm^3, a serum albumin level of less than 3.5 g%, platelet counts of less than 150,000/mm^3, or

TABLE 9-3. *Differential Considerations in the Diagnosis of Crohn's Enteritis.*

Inflammatory	Vascular	Neoplastic	Other
Yersinia enterocolitica infections	Ischemic enteritis (especially those caused by vasculitis)	Metastatic deposits in small bowel	Nodular lymphoid hyperplasia
Ileocecal tuberculosis		Primary lymphoma of small bowel	Amyloid
Acute appendicitis; appendiceal abscess		Carcinoma of small bowel	Fabry's disease
Tubovarian abscess Cecal diverticulitis		Carcinoid of small bowel	
Radiation enteritis Anisakiasis of bowel		Mucocele of the vermiform appendix	
Ameboma Eosinophilic gastroenteritis		Carcinoma of the cecum Ovarian tumors	
Chronic ulcerative, non-granulomatous jejunoileitis			

greater than 400,000, and serum iron levels of 20 to 40 μg/dl. Unfortunately, these were of little help either to diagnose Crohn's disease, differentiate it from ulcerative colitis, or assess its prognosis.

André and colleagues, from France, have had a particular interest in various laboratory measurements in inflammatory bowel disease, particularly as these relate to evaluating disease activity.[34] They studied the following serologic or hematologic determinations: hematocrit, sedimentation rate, C-reactive protein, serum albumin, serum iron, serum IgM, IgG and IgA values, circulating immune complexes, alpha-1 antitrypsin, serum orosomucoids, as well as the hemoglobin concentration and the leukocyte count. They concluded that the serum orosomucoid level and the hematocrit correlated well with a simple clinical index of disease activity. The serum orosomucoid is extensively used in Europe but not in the United States and appears to be similar to C-reactive protein in its nonspecificity as a marker for inflammation generally. Despite André's conclusions, the use of laboratory data to assist in the evaluation of disease activity continues to be disappointing.

Other features of Crohn's disease that are difficult to evaluate quantitatively are abdominal tenderness and/or an abdominal mass. Although the radiographic features of Crohn's disease are described elsewhere (Chap. 20), it is worth noting here that both ultrasonography and computerized tomography have been used to estimate bowel wall thickness (and, therefore, presumably the degree of disease activity) in patients with Crohn's disease. These studies have shown promise in solving the difficult problem of finding an objective measure for assessing the clinical status of a patient with Crohn's disease.[35-38]

Disease Activity Indices

The NCCDS developed and popularized the concept of a Crohn's Disease Activity Index (CDAI) for evaluating the clinical responses of patients in a large therapeutic trial.[39] This index was heavily influenced by subjective factors, however, and subsequently it was re-evaluated, based on data from 1,058 patients.[40] The factors reviewed included: (1) the number of liquid or soft stools, (2) the degree of abdominal pain, (3) the patient's feeling of general well-being, (4) systemic manifestations, (5) the need for diphenoxylate or opiates to control diarrhea, (6) the presence of an abdominal mass, (7) the hematocrit, and (8) the body weight (Table 9-4). Unfortunately, although the CDAI in either its original or rederived form appeared to be satisfactory for the NCCDS therapeutic trial, it is cumbersome and ineffective in clinical practice.[40] Therefore, attempts have been made to develop other indices that might be useful, resulting in the Dutch Activity Index,[41] which is objective, uses 18 variables, and is cumbersome, and the so-called "simple" Index of Crohn's Disease Activity.[42] In the latter, only five factors are used, and each is "quantified," although some only in a subjective fashion. The five are: (1) the patient's well-being, (2) abdominal pain, (3) the number of liquid stools per day, (4) the presence of an abdominal mass and (5) the existence of complications, including various systemic and extraintestinal features (Table 9-5).

Cooke and Prior compared hemoglobin concentrations, sedimentation rates, and the serum concentrations of albumin and orosomucoids when patients were both seriously ill and later,

TABLE 9-4. *Crohn's Disease Activity Index (CDAI) from the National Cooperative Crohn's Disease Study (NCCDS).*

1. Liquid or soft stools—sum in one week
2. Abdominal pain—sum of seven daily ratings
3. General well-being—sum of seven daily ratings
4. Symptoms or findings presumed to be related to Crohn's disease
   a. Arthritis or arthralgia
   b. Skin or mouth lesions, pyoderma gangrenosum, or erythema nodosum
   c. Iritis or uveitis
   d. Anal fissure, fistula, or perirectal abscess
   e. Other bowel-related fistulae, such as enterovesical
   f. Febrile episode exceeding 100°F (37.8°C) during past week.
5. Taking diphenoxylate or opiates for diarrhea
6. Abdominal mass
7. Hematocrit
8. Body weight

(Adapted from Best, W.R., Becktel, J.M., Singleton, J.W.: Gastroenterology, 70:439, 1976.)

TABLE 9-5. *The Simple Index of Crohn's Disease Activity.*

1. General well-being
2. Abdominal pain
3. Number of liquid stools per day
4. Abdominal mass
5. Complications—arthralgia, uveitis, erythema nodosum, aphthous ulcers, pyoderma gangrenosum, anal fissure, new fistula, and abscess

(Adapted from Harvey, R.G., and Bradshaw, J.M.: Lancet, 1:514, 1980.)

when they were well.[43] Only the serum albumin and orosomucoid levels showed clear separation between the two situations, while the hemoglobin values and sedimentation rates showed significant overlap. The OMGE Research Council and the IOIBD reevaluated disease activity indices in an attempt to correlate the severity with the short-term outcome.[21] The ten factors considered were (1) pain; (2) six or more bowel movements a day, or blood and mucus in the stools; (3) perianal complications; (4) fistulae; (5) other complications; (6) abdominal mass; (7) wasting or emaciation; (8) temperature above 38°C; (9) abdominal tenderness; and (10) a hemoglobin concentration below 10 g/100 ml (Table 9-6). Other experienced clinicians also have tackled the problem of quantifying activity,[43] but, unfortunately, all the numerical indices are of limited value in clinical practice. Nevertheless, attempts to correlate various indices with each other, with clinical characteristics, with severity of disease, with complications, with short-term prognosis as it relates to indication for surgical treatment, and with long-term outcome are continuing because a reliable numerical index would be of obvious clinical help in assessing the disease activity and response to therapy in patients with Crohn's disease, and predicting the prognosis for these patients.†

Indications for Surgical Treatment and Post-surgical Recurrences

Although specific surgical indications are considered in detail elsewhere both from the medical and surgical viewpoints (see Chaps. 25 and

†See also Chapter 33.

TABLE 9-6. *IOIBD Rating System.*

Clinical assessment of disease activity in Crohn's disease

1. Pain present
2. Bowel movements six or more times a day, or blood and mucus in stools
3. Perianal complications
4. Fistula
5. Other complications
6. Mass present
7. Wasting, emaciation
8. Temperature above 38°C
9. Abdominal tenderness
10. Hemoglobin below 10 g/100 ml

(Adapted from Myren, J., et al.: Scand. J. Gastroenterol. [Suppl.], 95:1, 1984.)

TABLE 9-7. *Comparison of Disease Location with Indication for Surgical Treatment in Crohn's Disease.*

Indication for Surgical Treatment	Colon	Small intestine	Ileocolic
Perianal disease	++	-	+
Intestinal obstruction	±	+++	++
Internal fistula and abscess	±	+	++
Toxic megacolon	+	-	-
Poor response to medical therapy	+	-	-

(Adapted from Farmer, R. G., Hawk, W. A., and Turnbull, R. G.: Gastroenterology, 71:245, 1976.)

26), post-surgical recurrences and some aspects of prognosis will be briefly mentioned here (see also Chaps. 22, 27, and 32), because these are parts of the clinical continuum of the disease. Following studies that indicated the importance of the initial clinical pattern in Crohn's disease,[20] the indications for surgical treatment were assessed as they related to such patterns (see also Chaps. 25 and 26). (Table 9-7).[23] It was found that the most common indication for surgical treatment in patients with the small intestine pattern was intestinal obstruction, with this being the indication in over 50% of such cases.[23] For patients with the ileocolic location of disease, a combination of perforation with abscess and/or intestinal obstruction was the most common surgical indication, accounting for almost 90% of the surgical interventions in this group. In those patients with colonic Crohn's disease the indications were diverse, however, with perianal manifestations being the most frequent, while chronic illness and failure to respond to medical therapy were other factors. The incidences of surgical intervention in the various clinical patterns are shown in Table 9-8.

Recurrence following surgical intervention (see also Chap. 32) is one of the major problems in the long-term care of patients with Crohn's disease, and has been the subject of intense clinical interest for many years.[44-46] Studies have tried to identify risk factors in patients that might either predict recurrence or determine that clinical setting in which recurrence occurs. These have included that location of disease,[47] and the type of operation as compared to the location of disease.[48-51] The reason for this interest is the magnitude of the problem: over two-

TABLE 9-8. *Crohn's Disease Study from the Cleveland Clinic.*

Clinical Pattern	Original Diagnosis— 1966-1969	Follow-up[*]	Patients with Operations
Ileocolic	252	246 (41.5%)	225 (91.5%)
Small intestine	176	165 (28%)	108 (65.5%)
Colon/ anorectal	187	181 (30.5%)	105 (58%)
Total	615	592 (96.3%)	438 (74%)

[*]Mean duration exceeded 13 years; minimum 7 years
(Adapted from Farmer, R. G., Whelan, G., and Fazio, V. W.: Gastroenterology, 88:1818, 1985.)

thirds of all patients with Crohn's disease require an operation,[16,52] and recurrences occur in as many as 50% of those who have undergone surgical treatment.[44-47] In general, recurrences are more common in patients with the ileocolic location of disease initially than in patients with either "pure" small or large bowel disease,[47] and they are more common following resection with anastomosis than after resection with the creation of a stoma.[51] Such recurrences are more common proximal to the anastomosis than distally,[49] and the degree of sepsis and inflammation present prior to the original surgical intervention seems to be an important factor.[52] In our latest review of recurrences, those patients with the surgical indications of internal fistula/perforation and abscess formation had a higher recurrence rate than did those in whom the surgical indication was intestinal obstruction.[53] Although after a certain time recurrences seem to become less frequent as the disease becomes "burned out," it is not unusual for patients to require several operations because of a series of proximal recurrences at the anastomosis.[47,51-53] Sachar and colleagues found that recurrences were less common if the patient had a long preoperative duration of disease and interpreted this to "reflect persisting differences between inherently more aggressive versus more indolent forms" of the disease.[51] This suggestion is in keeping with the finding that when fistula/perforation with abscess formation is the surgical indication, a higher recurrence rate exists.[53]

To obviate the development of short bowel syndrome, surgical procedures now are more conservative, with less bowel being removed (see also Chap. 27).[50,53] Two studies have evaluated the prognostic significance of the histologic features at the surgical margins at the time of resection. In a Swedish study, the histopathologic appearance of the resection margin seemed to influence the prognosis, and the presence of ulcers and/or granulomas correlated with a significantly increased recurrence rate.[54] The opposite was found by Hamilton and colleagues, however, who concluded that the postsurgical recurrence rates did not differ whether the resected margins were histologically involved or uninvolved.[55] They felt that their findings supported conservative resection leaving grossly uninvolved margins rather than using multiple frozen tissue sections and more extensive resection to achieve margins free from histologic changes.[*]

The definition of recurrence continues to be imprecise, varying from that proved by subsequent resection and histology,[47] to that diagnosed endoscopically.[56] To illustrate this, in a Dutch study of 114 patients one year after "curative" resection of the terminal ileum and a portion of the ascending colon for Crohn's disease, "early" endoscopic signs of recurrence were found in 70% of these patients, regardless of their symptoms. The primary visual appearance was that of aphthous ulcers occurring in clusters or in a linear fashion in hyperemic, friable mucosa.[56] For comparison, in a recent study of recurrences with histologic confirmation,[53] 438 patients who had undergone an operation were followed and it was found that patients with ileocolic location of disease (clinical pattern) had the highest recurrence rate, 53%, compared with 45% for patients with the colonic pattern, and 44% in those with the small intestinal pattern. The median times of recurrence in the three major clinical groups ranged from 66 to 116 months, values that were not significantly different. Second recurrences were likewise relatively high (the mean follow-up period being over 13 years), with similar incidences in all three clinical patterns and one-third of patients in each pattern requiring yet another operation.

In a study of long-term prognosis for patients with Crohn's disease we found a 6% mortality rate during a mean follow-up of over 13 years.[16] Of course, this is significant, particularly when one remembers that the disease predominantly affects a young population. This finding occasioned Sachar to title his editorial "Crohn's disease in Cleveland: A matter of life and death,"[52] and to conclude that "the fact remains that a specifically disease associated mortality rate of 6% is a sobering statistic, flying in the face of the old adage that nobody ever dies from Crohn's disease." The two major factors contributing to

[*]Editors' note: see also Geboes, K, et al.: Gut, 27:A610, 1986.

mortality in our series were sepsis and malnutrition.[16]

Others have also looked at the long-term prognosis with special regard to mortality, and in the report by Trnka and colleagues a calculated cumulative 30 year mortality was 16% disease-related.[50] Studies from Oxford and Birmingham in the United Kingdom found mortality rates of 12% and 13% respectively, the latter being some three to four times higher than expected.[57,58] Two Scandinavian studies emphasized that the mortality rate is highest early in the course of the disease,[59,60] particularly in the first year or two, a finding also noted in our study.[16] In the most recent Scandinavian report, however, the mortality rate was not excessive compared to an age- and sex-matched control population.[61] The latter study was of a regional group of 185 patients seen in Copenhagen between 1960 and 1978, and all were followed in the same gastroenterology unit for periods ranging from 1 to 18 years. This experience reflects our own in that the mortality rate appears to be less in the past decade, perhaps because of improved therapeutic (including nutritional) measures.[16]

Quality of Life

As noted repeatedly, Crohn's disease is a chronic disease so it is important for the managing physician to appreciate the impact of its long-term nature on the patient and his or her family, and its particular significance in young patients. This impact reflects the severity of illness, the need for long-term use of medication, frequent operations and recurrences, and its interference with personal growth and development, economic productivity, and general wellbeing. Studies that have assessed the quality of life of patients over the long-term have found that this is frequently suboptimal,[16,18,52,62,63] particularly in those who have required resection of gut for ileocolic disease.[16] The suboptimal quality of life was specifically commented upon by Sachar who emphasized that "we certainly must start by paying more attention to their psychosocial needs and concerns."[52] This is particularly true of patients in whom the onset of the disease is in childhood.[18,63,64]

While many of the features considered under "quality of life" have been felt in the past to be "psychological," the managing physician must appreciate the seriousness of their ramifications in order to maintain an appropriate empathy with the patient. Frustration caused by the lack of a simple cure can be felt by the patient, the family, and the attending physician, and this may have a negative effect not only on the patient and his or her ability to function, but also on the physician in his or her clinical analysis and decision making. The ability to maintain the patient's social and economic function, optimal nutritional and other therapy in a disease which is unpredictable is a great challenge, and re-emphasizes the importance of Crohn's disease as a major chronic digestive disease in the Western World today.[65]

REFERENCES

1. Crohn, B. B., Ginsberg, L., and Oppenheimer, G. D.: Regional ileitis. A pathological and clinical entity. J. Am. Med. Assoc., 99:1323, 1932.
2. Dalzeil, T. K.: Chronic interstitial enteritis. Br. Med. J., 2:1068, 1913.
3. Van Patter, W. N., et al.: Regional enteritis. Gastroenterology, 26:347, 1954.
4. Lockhart-Mummery, H. E., and Morson, B. C.: Crohn's disease (regional enteritis) of the large intestine and its distinction from ulcerative colitis. Gut, 1:87, 1960.
5. Janowitz, H. D., and Present, D. H.: Granulomatous colitis—pathogenetic concepts. Gastroenterology, 51:788, 1966.
6. Lennard-Jones, J. E., Lockhart-Mummery, H. E., and Morson, B. C.: Clinical and pathological differentiation of Crohn's disease and proctocolitis. Gastroenterology, 54:1162, 1968.
7. Farmer, R. G., Hawk, W. A., and Turnbull, R. B.: Regional enteritis of the colon. A clinical and pathologic comparison with ulcerative colitis. Am. J. Dig. Dis., 13:501, 1968.
8. Glotzer, D. J., et al.: Comparative features and course of ulcerative and granulomatous colitis. N. Engl. J. Med., 282:582, 1970.
9. Calkins, B. M., Lilienfeld, A. M., Garland, O. F., and Mendeloff, A. I.: Trends in incidence rates of ulcerative colitis and Crohn's disease. Dig. Dis. Sci., 29:913, 1984.
10. Mayberry, J. F., and Rhodes, J.: Epidemiological aspects of Crohn's disease: a review of literature. Gut, 25:886, 1984.
11. Langman, M. J. S.: Recent changes in the patterns of chronic digestive disease in the United Kingdom. Postgrad. Med. J., 60:733, 1984.
12. Hellers, G.: Crohn's disease in Stockholm County, 1955-1974. A study of epidemiology, results of surgical treatment and longterm prognosis. Acta Chir. Scand. [Suppl.], 490:1, 1979.
13. Farmer, R. G., Hawk, W. A., and Turnbull, R. B.: Clinical patterns in Crohn's disease: A statistical study of 615 cases. Gastroenterology, 68:627, 1975.
14. Mekhjian, H. S., et al.: Clinical features and natural history of Crohn's disease. Gastroenterology, 77:898, 1979.
15. Rankin, G. B., Watts, H. D., Melnyk, C. S., and Kelley, M. L. Jr.: National Cooperative Crohn's Disease Study: Extraintestinal manifestations and perianal complications. Gastroenterology, 77:914, 1979.
16. Farmer, R. G., Whelan, G., and Fazio, V. W.: Long-term follow-up of patients with Crohn's disease. Relationship between the clinical pattern and prognosis. Gastroenterology, 88:1818, 1985.
17. Both, H., et al.: Clinical appearance at diagnosis of ulcerative colitis and Crohn's disease in a regional patient group. Scand. J. Gastroenterol., 18:987, 1983.

18. Michener, W. M., Greenstreet, R. L., and Farmer, R. G.: Comparison of the clinical features of Crohn's disease and ulcerative colitis with onset in childhood and adolescence. Cleve. Clin. Q., *49*:13, 1983.
19. Lennard-Jones, J. E., Ritchie, J. K., and Zohrab, W. J.: Proctocolitis and Crohn's disease of the colon. A comparison of the clinical course. Gut, *17*:477, 1976.
20. Farmer, R. G., and Michener, W. M.: The prognosis of Crohn's disease with onset in childhood and adolescence. Dig. Dis. Sci., *24*:752, 1979.
21. Myren, J., et al.: The O.M.G.E. Multinational Inflammatory Bowel Disease Survey, 1976-1982. A further report of 2657 cases. Scand. J. Gastroenterol. [Suppl.], *95*:1, 1984.
22. Farmer, R. G.: Clinical features and natural history of inflammatory bowel disease. Med. Clin. North Am., *64*:1103, 1980.
23. Farmer, R. G., Hawk, W. A., and Turnbull, R. G.: Indications for surgery in Crohn's disease. An analysis of 500 cases. Gastroenterology, *71*:245, 1976.
24. Buchmann, P., et al.: Natural history of perianal Crohn's disease. Ten year follow-up: a plea for conservativism. Am. J. Surg., *140*:642, 1980.
25. Hellers, G., Bergstrand, O., Ewerth, S., and Holmstrom, B.: Occurrence and outcome after primary treatment of anal fistulae in Crohn's disease. Gut, *21*:525, 1980.
26. Higgens, C. S., and Allan, R. N.: Crohn's disease of the distal ileum. Gut, *21*:933, 1980.
27. Ritchie, J. K., and Lennard-Jones, J. E.: Crohn's disease of the distal large bowel. Scand. J. Gastroenterol., *11*:433, 1976.
28. Beardin, D., et al.: Crohn's disease of the stomach. A case report and review of the literature. Am. J. Dig. Dis., *18*:623, 1973.
29. Danzi, J. T., Farmer, R. G., Sullivan, B. H., and Rankin, G. B.: Endoscopic features of gastroduodenal Crohn's disease. Gastroenterology, *70*:9, 1976.
30. Farmer, R. G., Hawk, W. A., and Turnbull, R. B.: Crohn's disease of the duodenum (Transmural duodenitis). Clinical manifestations. Report of 11 cases. Am. J. Dig. Dis., *17*:191, 1972.
31. Nugent, F. W., Richmond, M., and Park, S. K.: Crohn's disease of the duodenum. Gut, *18*:115, 1977.
32. Ross, T. M., Fazio, V. W., and Farmer, R. G.: Long term results of surgical treatment for Crohn's disease of the duodenum. Ann. Surg., *197*:399, 1983.
33. Yang, S. S., et al.: Primary Crohn's disease of the appendix. Report of 14 cases and review of the literature. Ann. Surg., *189*:334, 1979.
34. André, C., Descos, L., Landais, P., and Fermanian, J.: Assessment of appropriate laboratory measurements to supplement the Crohn's disease activity index. Gut, *22*:571, 1981.
35. Dubbins, P. A.: Ultrasound demonstration of bowel wall thickness in inflammatory bowel disease. Clin. Radiol., *35*:227, 1984.
36. Kaftori, J. K., Menucha, P., and Kleinhaus, U.: Ultrasonography in Crohn's disease. Gastrointest. Radiol., *9*:137, 1984.
37. Kerber, G. W., Greenberg, M., and Rubin, J. M.: Computed tomography evaluation of local and extraintestinal complications of Crohn's disease. Gastrointest. Radiol., *9*:143, 1984.
38. Gore, M. R., et al.: CT findings in ulcerative, granulomatous and indeterminate colitis. Am. J. Radiol., *143*:279, 1984.
39. Best, W. R., Becktel, J. M., and Singleton, J. W.: Development of a Crohn's Disease Activity Index: National Cooperative Crohn's Disease Study. Gastroenterology, *70*:439, 1976.
40. Best, W. R., Becktel, J. M., and Singleton, J. W.: Rederived values of the eight coefficients of Crohn's Disease Activity Index (CDAI). Gastroenterology, *77*:843, 1979.
41. Van Hees, P. A. M., Van Elteren, P. H., Van Lier, H. J. J., and Van Tongeren, J. H. M.: An index of inflammatory activity in patients with Crohn's disease. Gut, *21*:279, 1980.
42. Harvey, R. G., and Bradshaw, J. M.: A simple index of Crohn's disease activity. Lancet, *1*:514, 1980.
43. Cooke, W. T., and Prior, P.: Determining disease activity in inflammatory bowel disease. J. Clin. Gastroenterol., *6*:17, 1984.
44. Lennard-Jones, J. E., and Stalder, G. A.: Prognosis after resection of chronic ileitis. Gut, *8*:332, 1967.
45. de Dombal, F. T., Burton, I., and Golligher, J. C.: Recurrence of Crohn's disease after primary excisional surgery. Gut, *12*:519, 1971.
46. Greenstein, A. J., Sachar, D. B., Pasternack, B. S., and Janowitz, H. D.: Reoperation and recurrence in Crohn's colitis and ileocolitis. N. Engl. J. Med., *292*:685, 1975.
47. Lock, M. R., et al.: Recurrences and reoperation for Crohn's disease: The role of disease location in prognosis. N. Engl. J. Med., *304*:1585, 1981.
48. Mekhijian, H. S., et al.: National Cooperative Crohn's Disease Study: Factors determining recurrence of Crohn's disease after surgery. Gastroenterology, *77*:907, 1979.
49. Lock, M. R., et al.: Proximal recurrence and the fate of the rectum following excisional surgery for Crohn's disease of the large bowel. Ann. Surg., *194*:754, 1981.
50. Trnka, Y. M., et al.: The long-term outcome of restorative operation in Crohn's disease: Influence of location, prognostic factors, and surgical guidelines. Ann. Surg., *196*:345, 1982.
51. Sachar, D. B., et al.: Risk factors for postoperative recurrence of Crohn's disease. Gastroenterology, *85*:917, 1983.
52. Sachar, D. B.: Crohn's disease in Cleveland: A matter of life and death (editorial). Gastroenterology, *88*:1996, 1985.
53. Whelan, G., Farmer, R. G., Fazio, V. W., and Goormastic, M.: Recurrence after surgery in Crohn's disease. Relationship to location of disease (clinical pattern) and surgical indication. Gastroenterology, *88*:1826, 1985.
54. Lindhagen, T.: Recurrence rate after surgical treatment of Crohn's disease. Scand. J. Gastroenterol., *18*:1037, 1983.
55. Hamilton, S. R., et al.: The role of resection margin frozen section in the general surgical management of Crohn's disease. Surg. Gynecol. Obstet., *160*:57, 1985.
56. Rutgeerts, P., et al.: Natural history of recurrent Crohn's disease at the ileocolic anastomosis after curative surgery. Gut, *25*:665, 1984.
57. Truelove, S. C., and Peña, A. S.: Course and prognosis of Crohn's disease. Gut, *17*:192, 1976.
58. Prior, P., et al.: Mortality in Crohn's disease. Gastroenterology, *80*:307, 1981.
59. Storgaard, L., et al.: Survival rate in Crohn's disease and ulcerative colitis. Scand. J. Gastroenterol., *14*:255, 1979.
60. Bergman, L., and Krause, U.: Crohn's disease and the long-term study of the clinical course of 186 patients. Scand. J. Gastroenterol., *12*:937, 1977.
61. Binder, V., Hendriksen, C., and Kreiner, S.: Prognosis in Crohn's disease—based on results from a regional patient group from the county of Copenhagen. Gut, *26*:146, 1985.
62. Meyers, S., et al.: Quality of life after surgery for Crohn's disease. Gastroenterology, *78*:1, 1980.
63. Gazzard, B. G., Price, H. L., Libby, G. W., and Dawson, A. M.: Social toll of Crohn's disease. Br. Med. J., *2*:1117, 1978.
64. Sales, D. J., and Kirsner, J. B.: The prognosis of inflammatory bowel disease. Arch. Intern. Med., *143*:294, 1983.
65. Sorensen, V. Z., Olsen, B. G., and Binder, V.: Life prospects and quality of life in patients with Crohn's disease. Gut, *28*:382, 1987.

10 · Differential Diagnosis of Chronic Ulcerative Colitis and Crohn's Disease of the Colon

F. WARREN NUGENT, M.D., AND PETER F. KOLACK, M.D.

Nonspecific chronic inflammatory disease of the colon is, largely, a diagnosis of exclusion. This diagnosis can only be made when all other etiologic factors have been ruled out. Careful history taking and physical examination, and laboratory, radiographic, endoscopic, and histologic studies must be performed before the diagnosis of nonspecific inflammatory bowel disease can be made. Even then, in the majority of instances the diagnosis is an assumption. The finding of noncaseating granulomas in a setting of inflammation of the colon does, of course, suggest Crohn's disease. On the other hand, in the case of chronic ulcerative colitis, not even the histologic findings allow the diagnosis to be made with certainty. The diagnosis of these diseases can be made with a high degree of probability, but this diagnosis is often a "soft" one, and a careful watch must be kept for new information as the course of the disease is followed.

Ulcerative Colitis[*]

Ulcerative colitis may be divided into three degrees of severity based on the extent of involvement of the colon. The disease always involves the rectum and may extend for a variable distance proximally in the colon. Although the extent of disease may be greater when measured either endoscopically or histologically than when measured either radiographically or endoscopically, a general clinical assessment of the extent of disease can almost always be made by using a radiographic examination with or without endoscopy. In this way, patients may be divided into three groups: those with proctosigmoiditis, those with left-sided colitis involving the descending colon and perhaps the distal transverse colon, and those with universal disease extending proximally throughout most of the colon. On the whole, the course of the disease is much milder in patients with proctosigmoiditis than in patients with left-sided disease, and it is milder in patients with left-sided disease than in those with universal disease.

In distal disease, that is, disease endoscopically involving part or all of the rectum with or without involvement of the sigmoid, the patient is rarely ill. The disease may extend only a few centimeters from the anal verge and never involve more of the colon at any time during a prolonged course. In this case, the primary, and often the only, symptom is rectal bleeding. Stools may be formed, and the patient is often constipated with a paucity of systemic symptoms and signs, such as fever, weight loss, and anemia, all of which are commonly seen in more extensive disease. If the entire rectum is involved with or without all or a portion of the sigmoid colon, the patient may have loose stools or diarrhea, and systemic symptoms and signs may be present. Pain is not a prominent symptom of

[*]See also Chapter 8.

disease confined to the distal rectum, although some rectal discomfort, and tenesmus, and left lower quadrant or suprapubic discomfort may be present. When the disease extends into the sigmoid, pain is more noticeable. Small amounts of mucus or frequent passage of mucus, almost always accompanied by blood, may be a prominent symptom. When taking a history it is important to understand precisely what patients mean when they report multiple stools daily. With distal disease they may be referring to one or two formed or hard stools and the passage of numerous globs of mucus, blood, or both. When the rectum is severely inflamed, even though the disease may be limited in extent, tenesmus, urgency, and incontinence may be prominent and, at times, disabling symptoms.

Distal disease tends to be mild, and in some series makes up the large proportion of patients with ulcerative colitis. Sinclair et al. reported that in a 5-year follow-up study of 537 patients with ulcerative colitis in a Scottish community, 74% of them had only distal colitis.[1]

Others have reported on large series of patients with distal colitis followed up over long periods of time.[2-4] This form of ulcerative colitis has been shown to be mild. In one large series,[4] only 12% of patients had extension of disease into more proximal parts of the colon over an 8-year follow-up period, and only 4% of patients required proctocolectomy over this period.

As the disease extends more proximally to involve the left colon or all of the colon, the severity of the illness is usually much greater. In addition to diarrhea and bleeding, abdominal pain and systemic symptoms are common and may even be life threatening. Weight loss, fever, and generalized nutritional depletion are often present with acute exacerbations, and in severe disease abdominal distention and clinical signs of peritoneal irritation may herald the onset of a toxic megacolon. In this instance, the disease is life threatening, with extension of the inflammatory process and necrosis of the deeper layers of the bowel wall.[5]

Crohn's Colitis[*]

The symptoms and signs of Crohn's colitis are less predictable than those of ulcerative colitis. The right colon is a common site, of this disease

[*]See also Chapter 9.

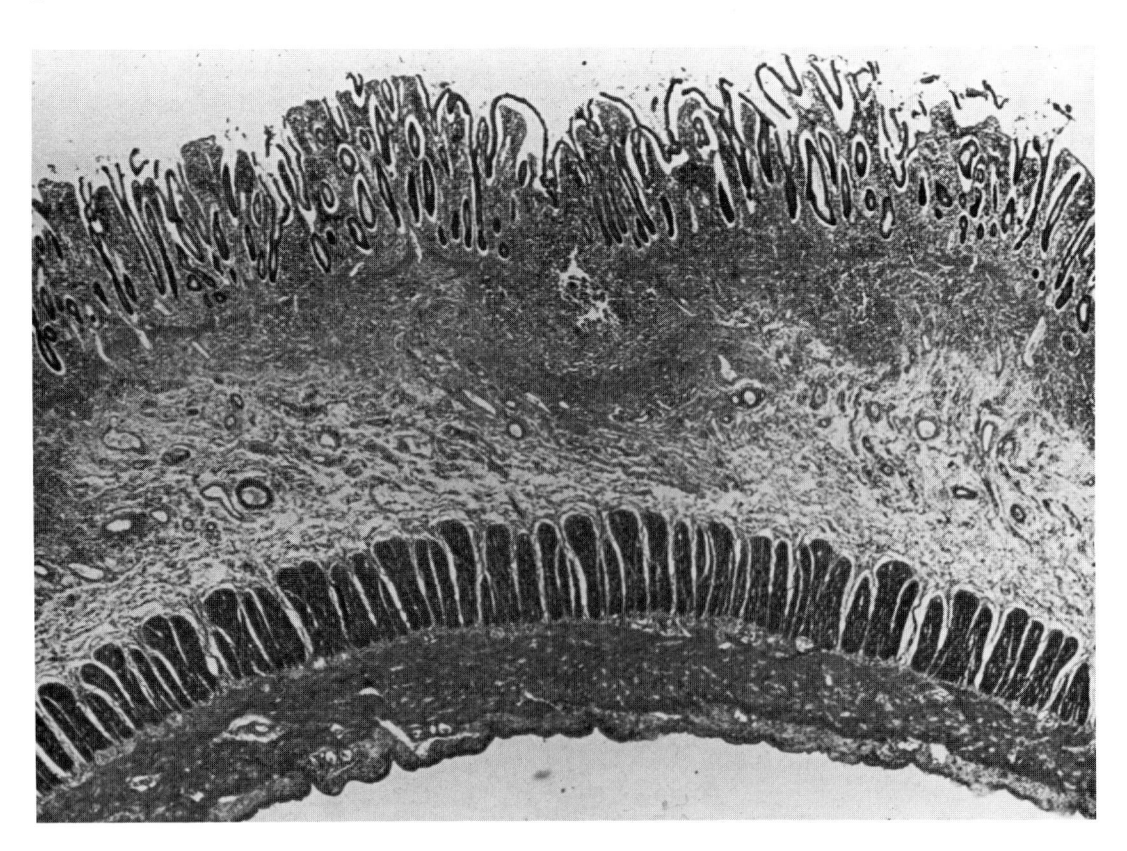

FIG. 10-1. Ulcerative colitis; the inflammatory process is confined to the mucosa and submucosa.

often in association with disease of the distal ileum.[6] Any part of the colon may be involved, however, and the area involved may be extensive or short. Segmental disease is common. Because of this wide variation in distribution, the symptoms also differ. Abdominal pain is a frequent complaint. Diarrhea may be present to any degree, or it may be absent. Rectal bleeding may be a finding, but on the other hand, it is often intermittent or absent, despite activity of the disease. An abdominal mass may be palpable, particularly when the right colon and terminal ileum are involved. Abscesses and fistulas involving the perineum, rectovaginal septum, or urinary tract are present in approximately 30% of patients with colonic Crohn's disease. Systemic signs and symptoms, such as weight loss and fever, are commonly seen. Fistulas from the colon to the skin or to other loops of bowel, including the duodenum, may occur.[7]

When approaching the differential diagnosis between ulcerative colitis and Crohn's colitis, one must keep in mind the basic anatomic and histologic differences between the two diseases. Ulcerative colitis is a disease of the colonic mucosa (Fig. 10-1). The pathologic process is almost entirely confined to the mucosa, except in severe disease where it may penetrate into the deeper layers, as seen in the "toxic colon" (see also Chap. 18). Ulcerative colitis begins at the anorectal margin and involves a variable extent of the colon in continuity. It is diffuse, symmetric, and circumferential, and may extend proximally from the anorectal margin for a few centimeters or may involve the entire colon. The disease is not spotty or segmental unless it is under treatment or in a healing stage. Because it is a mucosal disease, bleeding is almost universally present with all or most stools during activity of the process.

Crohn's disease, on the other hand (see also Chap. 18), involves all layers of the bowel wall (Fig. 10-2). Although it may have an appearance similar to ulcerative colitis at times, it is often spotty, segmental, and asymmetric. In approximately 50% of patients, the rectum is spared or relatively spared in distinction to ulcerative colitis. It may involve a short segment of any part of the colon or the entire colon (Fig. 10-3). When the right colon is involved, the distal ileum is frequently affected as well.[8] Farmer et al. described the following patterns of Crohn's disease: distal

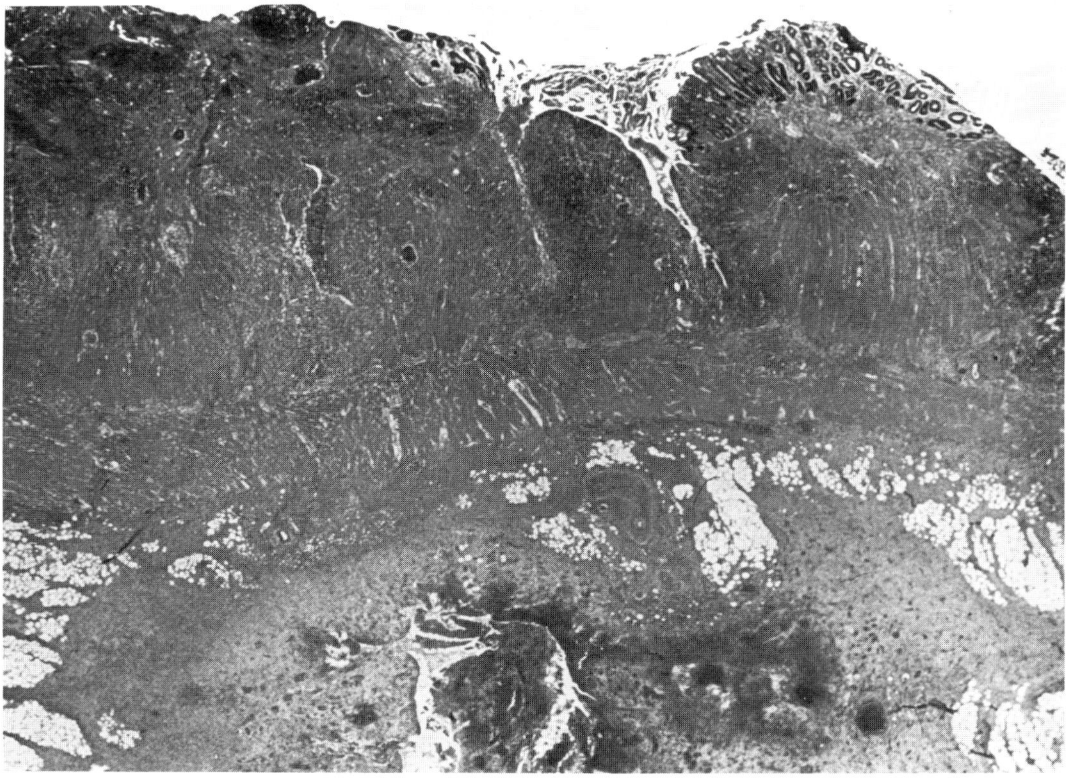

Fig. 10-2. Crohn's colitis; transmural inflammation and deep fissures are prominent.

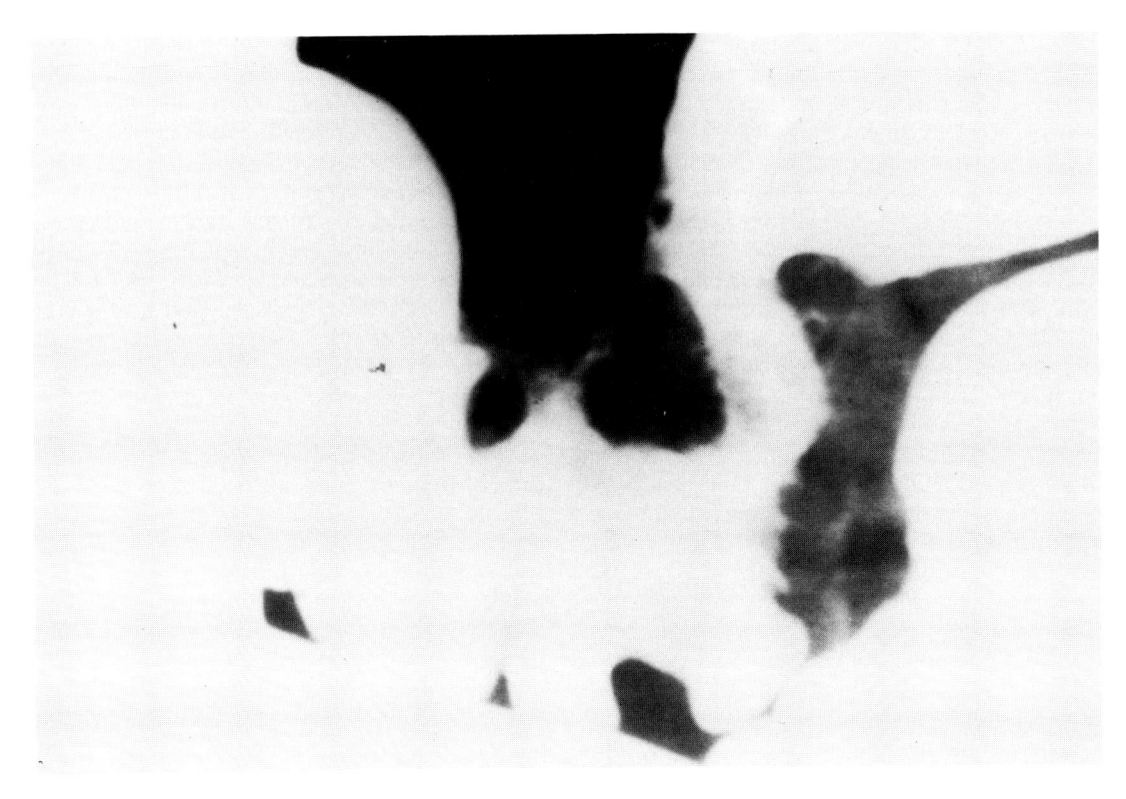

FIG. 10-3. Short area of Crohn's colitis with small colocolonic fistulas.

ileum and right colon, 41%; small intestine, 28.6%; colon only, 27%; and anorectum, 3.4%.[6] The differential diagnostic criteria of ulcerative colitis and Crohn's colitis from the World Organization of Gastroenterology Survey are listed in Table 10-1.[9]

Although anal complications, such as hemorrhoids, fissures, acute inflammation, and excoriation, may be present in patients with either ulcerative colitis or Crohn's disease, chronic inflammatory disease of the anus or perineum is rarely seen in ulcerative colitis (see also Chap. 14). The stigmata of Crohn's disease include perianal abscesses, fistulas, and chronic inflammation and induration of the anal canal and perianal tissues. The perineal fistulas may involve the rectovaginal septum.

Keeping in mind the basic histologic differences between these two diseases is helpful in understanding the different symptoms and signs that may be seen. When clinical, endoscopic, and radiographic findings are assessed, it is possible to differentiate ulcerative colitis from Crohn's colitis in at least 80% of patients.[10] A scoring system has been reported by Clamp et al. with an accuracy in excess of 90% in the differential diagnosis of these two diseases.[11] The two diseases are unlikely to coexist in the same patient, but the possibility has been suggested in case reports.[12]

TABLE 10-1. *Diagnostic Features: Views of More Than 100 Clinicans.*

Diagnostic Mode	Favors Crohn's Disease	Favors Ulcerative Colitis
Clinical	Severe pain; complications; Tenderness/ wasting; Mass/ distention	6 + Bowel actions per day Blood + +per rectum Mucus + +per rectum
Radiography	Segmental change; stenosis; dilatation; fistulas; skip lesions	
Endoscopy	Normal findings; patchy changes;	Continuous changes Ulcers/contact bleeding
Biopsy	Transmural changes; giant-cell- noncaseating granulomas	Mucosal changes Ulcers

Laboratory Findings

No specific laboratory determinations confirm the diagnosis of ulcerative colitis or Crohn's colitis. Standard laboratory tests should be carried out, of course, to aid in establishing the severity of the disease, the presence of complications, and the nutritional status of the patient.

Stool examinations for culture and for ova and parasites should be performed on all patients with new disease. No general agreement exists on whether these examinations should be repeated, or how often they should be requested as the course of the disease continues. They should be repeated under suspect circumstances, such as after foreign travel. The toxin level of Clostridium difficile should be determined, particularly when antibiotics have been prescribed. Although C. difficile infection may cause reactivation of nonspecific inflammatory disease of the colon,[13,14] it has rarely been found unless the patient had recently been taking antibiotics or sulfasalazine.[15] In one study,[15] the incidence of the C. difficile toxin in ulcerative colitis or Crohn's colitis was no higher than in a variety of other nonspecific diarrheal illnesses. The finding of the C. difficile infection in inflammatory bowel disease seems fortuitous.

Endoscopy[*]

Endoscopic examination is often helpful in the diagnosis and differential diagnosis of nonspecific inflammatory disease of the colon. In ulcerative colitis, during activity, a diffuse confluent inflammatory process begins at the anorectal margin and extends proximally for a variable length. Sizable individual ulcerations are not seen. A degree of unevenness of inflammation may be apparent if the colitis is under active treatment or is healing. Otherwise, segmental disease is not found. The normal vascular pattern is lost; degrees of friability of the mucosa are noted. At times a purulent exudate, as well as blood and mucus, is present. Pseudopolyps may be seen.

In Crohn's colitis, endoscopic findings may reveal segmental disease. The rectum may be completely or relatively spared. Longitudinal stellate or "rake" ulcerations may be seen and are pathognomonic of Crohn's disease. On the other hand, diffuse confluent disease indistinguishable from ulcerative colitis may be present in Crohn's disease, and in this instance the endoscopic picture may not help in the differential diagnosis. Endoscopic findings in colonic in-

TABLE 10-2. *Colonoscopic Mucosal Features and Their Diagnostic Specificity in Inflammatory Bowel Disease.*[*]

Lesion	Ulcerative Colitis	Crohn's Disease
Inflammation		
Distribution		
Colon		
Contiguous	+ + +	+
Symmetric	+ + +	+
Rectum	+ + +	+
Friability	+ + +	+
Topography		
Granularity	+ + +	+
Cobblestoned	+	+ + +
Ulceration		
Location		
Overt colitis	+ + +	+
Ileum	0	+ + + +
Discrete lesion	+	+ + +
Features		
Size > 1 cm	+	+ + +
Deep	+	+ +
Linear	+	+ + +
Aphthoid	0	+ + + +
Bridging	+	+ +

*Specificity index range: 0 (not seen) to 4 + (diagnostic). (Reprinted from Hogan, W. J., Hensley, G. T., and Geenen, J. E.: Med. Clin. North Am., 64:1084, 1980.)

flammatory bowel disease are summarized in Table 10-2.[16]

Radiography[*]

Barium studies of the colon are best performed when the colonic disease is quiescent. If proctosigmoidoscopy shows inflammatory disease and laboratory studies do not reveal a specific cause, a diagnosis of nonspecific inflammation of the colon can be assumed. Barium studies may be carried out at this time if the symptoms are mild and the patient is not systemically ill. Otherwise, the performance of a barium enema may aggravate the disease and even precipitate a toxic megacolon. In ulcerative colitis the barium study will show a diffuse, confluent, symmetric disease involving the colon. When the disease is confined to the rectum, sigmoid colon, or both, the rectum may be narrowed and the sigmoid colon shortened (Fig. 10-4). The colon may be shortened and narrowed in long-standing disease, and pseudopolyps may be seen (Fig. 10-5). In extreme cases, pseudopolyps may obstruct the colon (Fig. 10-6). In universal colitis some degree of "backwash" ileitis may be seen involving a few centimeters of the terminal ileum, and in this case the ileum may be mildly dilated with a smooth loss of the normal mark-

---

[*]See also Chapter 19.

[*]See also Chapter 20.

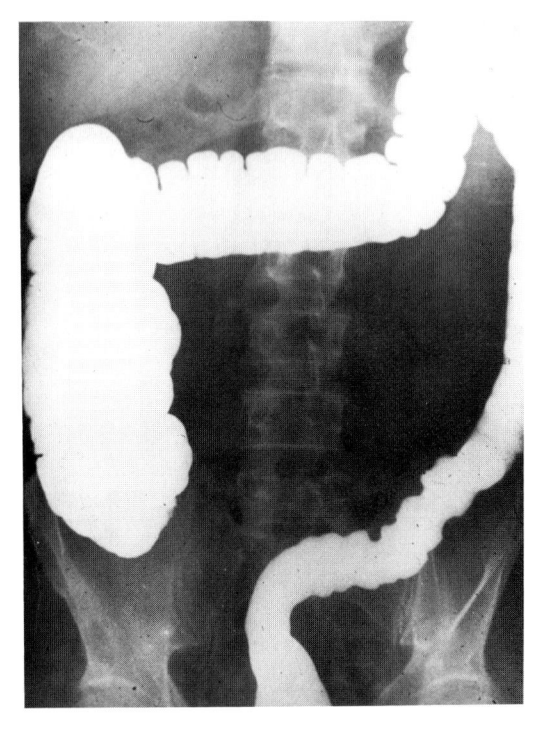

FIG. 10-4. Distal ulcerative colitis (proctosigmoiditis) with narrow rectum and loss of sigmoid curve.

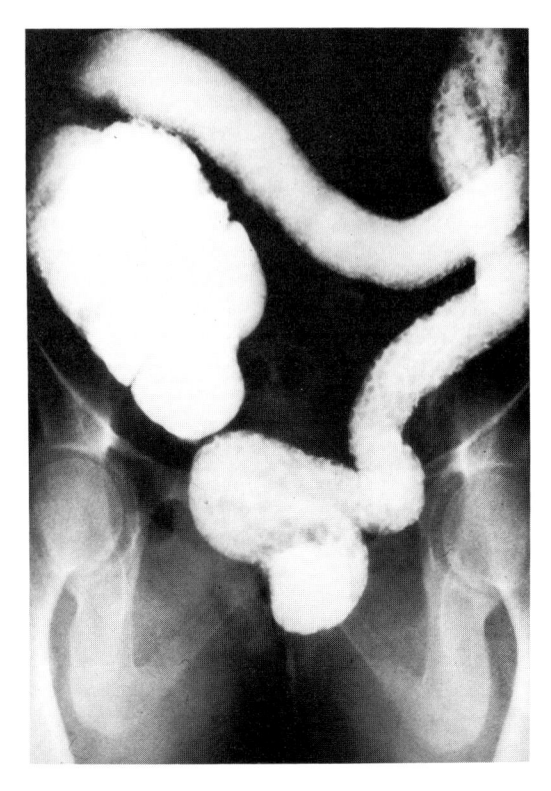

FIG. 10-5. Ulcerative colitis involving most of the colon with significant pseudopolyposis.

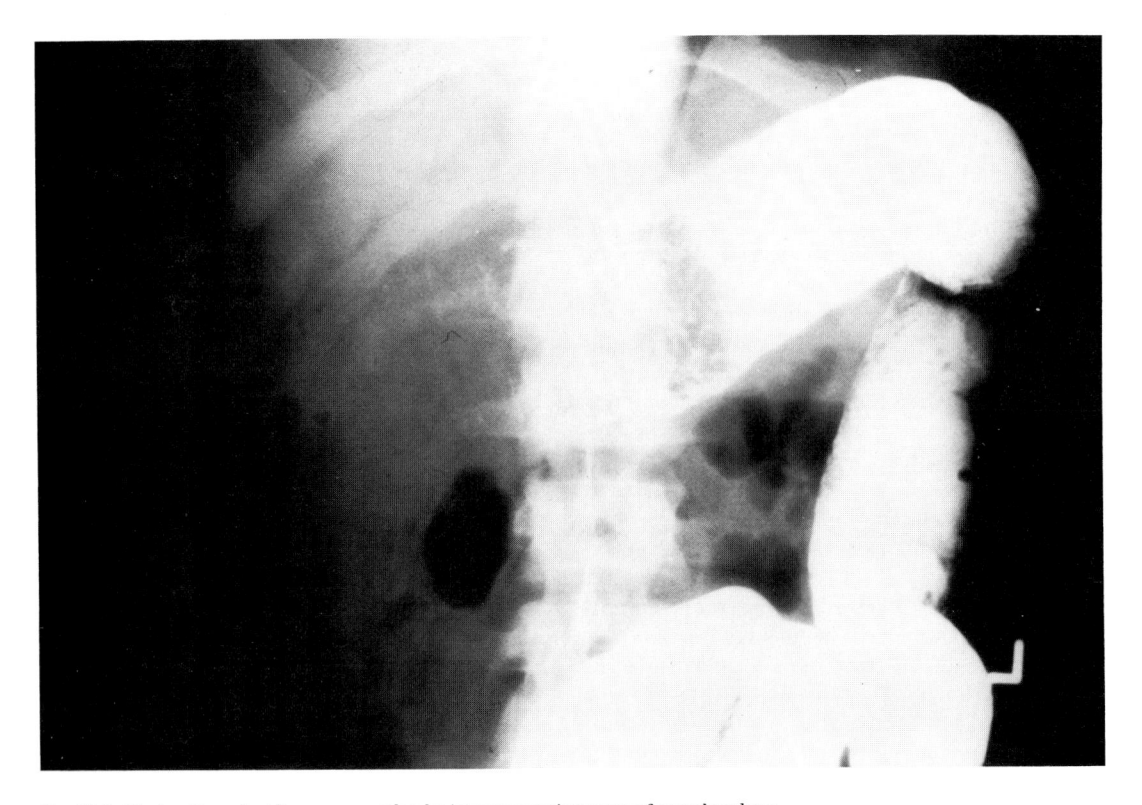

FIG. 10-6. Obstruction of midtransverse colon by intussuscepting mass of pseudopolyps.

ings. Deep "collar button" ulcerations may be seen with severe disease. However, a barium enema study is ill-advised at this time. While the radiographic findings usually reflect the severity of the disease, this is not always the case.[17] Toxic megacolon, although more commonly described with ulcerative colitis, may also be seen in Crohn's colitis (see also Chap. 14).[18]

In Crohn's colitis the rectum is spared radiographically in approximately 50% of patients. Segmental changes are not uncommon with an abnormal area "bracketed" by more normal areas (Fig. 10-7A). Strictures are common, and mucosal relief films may show cobblestoning of the mucosal pattern. Pseudopolyps may be present as in ulcerative colitis. The terminal ileum is commonly involved, usually by narrowing with irregularity and cobblestoning of the mucosa. Fistulas may be seen between the colon and the skin, vagina, or the urinary tract, or between the colon and loops of small intestine, particularly from the sigmoid colon or from he cecal area to the distal ileum. Adjacent deep ulcerations in the bowel wall may coalesce to form intramural fistulas, a radiographic finding highly suggestive of Crohn's colitis (Figs. 10-7B and 10-8).

Pathology

The pathology of ulcerative colitis and Crohn's colitis is dealt with in depth in Chapter 18. Suffice it to say here that biopsies taken at the time of endoscopy are superficial and usually show nonspecific changes of acute and chronic inflammation. On occasion, the inflammatory change is focal in character, suggesting Crohns disease. Noncaseating granulomas may be seen, although not frequently, and these may be pathognomonic of Crohn's disease.

Diverticulitis

When inflammatory bowel disease occurs in patients older than 50 years of age, diverticular disease may also be a finding. It should not be difficult to distinguish ulcerative proctitis or proctosigmoiditis from diverticulitis. Endoscopically, involvement of the distal rectum is not seen in diverticulitis as it is in ulcerative colitis. Differentiating diverticulitis from Crohn's disease may be more difficult, however, when Crohn's disease develops in this older age group. It is less likely to involve the small intestine than in the younger patient, frequently involving the

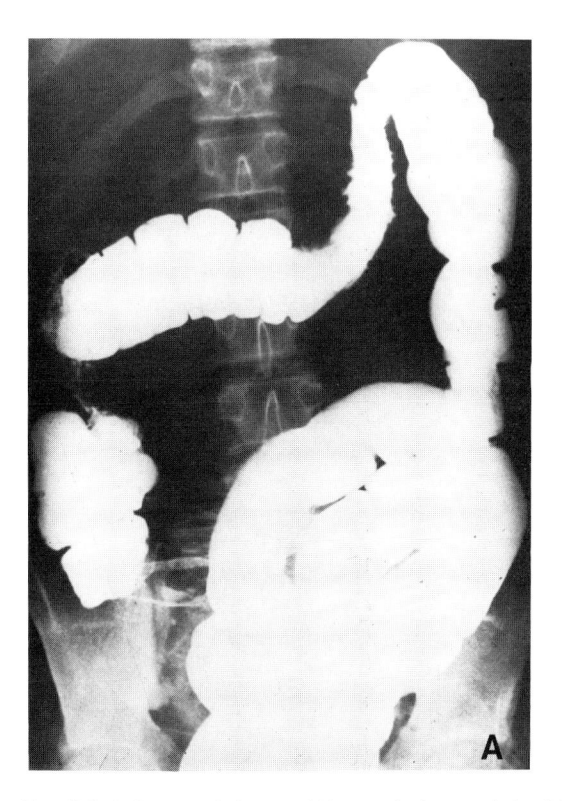

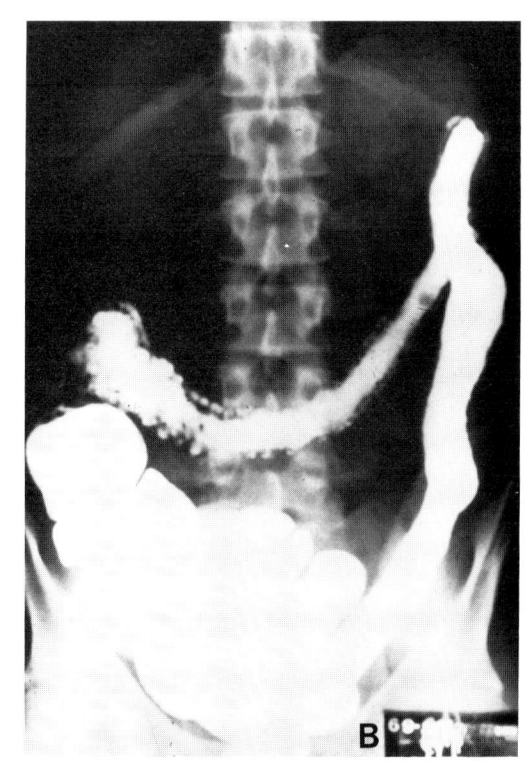

FIG. 10-7. A. Segmental changes (skip areas) characteristic of Crohn's colitis. B. Crohn's colitis; deep ulcers in the transverse colon that coalesce in areas.

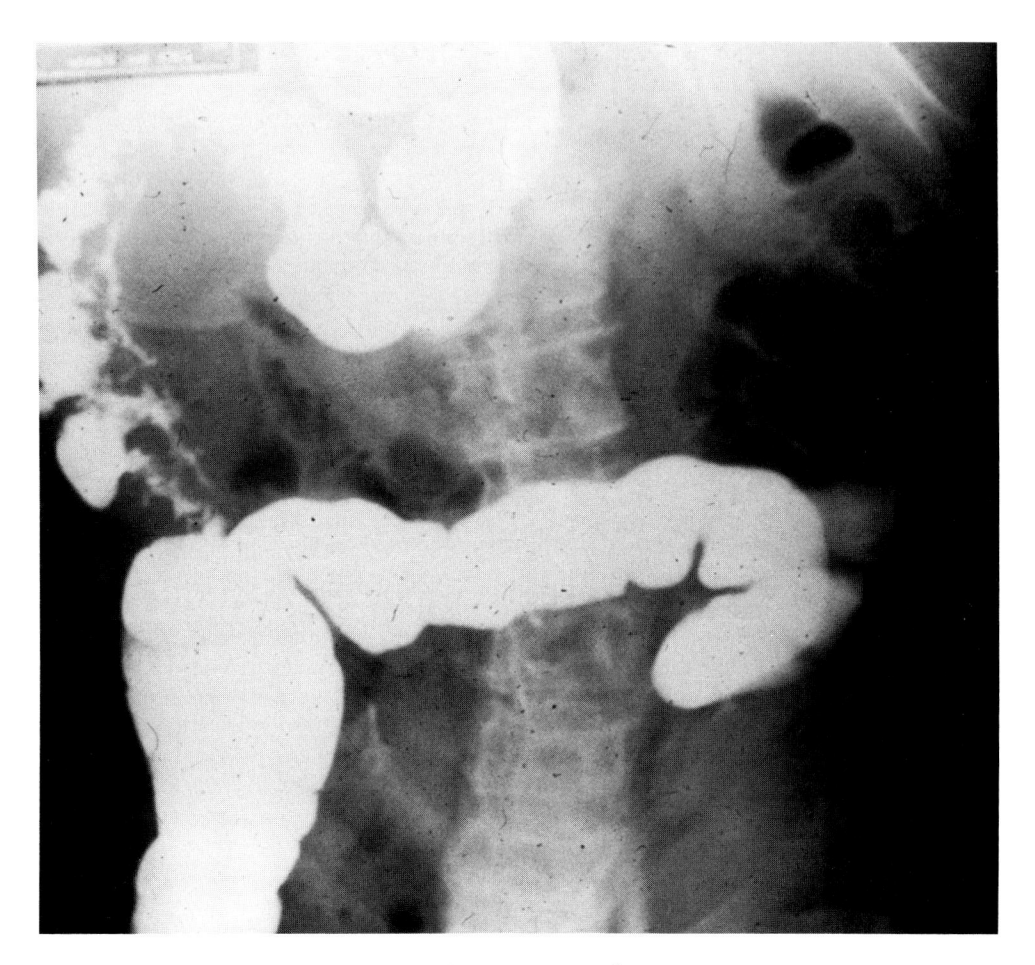

FIG. 10-8. Crohn's colitis; long intramural fistula "second lumen sign."

left colon, particularly the sigmoid.[19,20] Many patients 60 years of age or older presenting with Crohn's disease have involvement of the colon. In many of these patients, the differential diagnoses between Crohn's disease, diverticulitis, and ischemic disease are not easy to establish. The differential diagnosis of Crohn's disease versus diverticulitis is particularly difficult at times, but clinical clues frequently aid in this regard. Crohn's disease of the sigmoid tends to be a more chronic, low-grade process clinically, while diverticulitis probably presents as recurrent acute attacks.

Most series report a preponderance of women with both Crohn's disease and diverticular disease, while the sexual incidence associated with Crohn's disease in general is equal.[20,21] Perhaps the most characteristic differential findings are the presence of rectal bleeding, disease of the rectal mucosa, and anal or perianal disease, all frequently present in colonic Crohn's disease. Although patients with diverticular disease may experience significant bleeding at times, it is rare to have small amounts of rectal bleeding on an almost daily basis over long periods, such as is seen often in patients with Crohn's disease of the distal colon. The frequency of bleeding in Crohn's disease associated with diverticulitis has been reported to be as high as 77%.[22,23] Chronic anal and perianal disease of the type associated with Crohn's disease are not found in diverticular disease, another important differential diagnostic clue.[21,22] The perineal disease may antedate colonic Crohn's disease by months or years (see also Chap. 14).

Berman et al. reported an incidence of bleeding in 52% of 25 patients with Crohn's disease and diverticulitis, and 88% of this same group had either rectal bleeding, perianal disease, or both.[22] Fistulas other than in the perineum may occur with either Crohn's disease or diverticulitis and are not helpful in the differential diagnosis.

Extracolonic manifestations, such as enteropathic arthropathy, stomatitis, erythema nodosum, or pyoderma gangrenosum, are not found with diverticulitis, and if they are present this suggests coincidental Crohn's disease (see also Chap. 16).

Patients requiring more than one resection for diverticulitis may have Crohn's disease, because recurrence of diverticulitis after resection is rare.[19]

Endoscopically, inflammatory change with ulceration in the rectum where no diverticula are present militates against the diagnosis of diverticulitis. The typical longitudinal rake ulcerations of Crohn's disease are a pathognomonic finding. Biopsies may show granulomas, which are rarely found in diverticulitis. Although a longitudinal intramural fistulous tract, seen histologically and radiographically, can occur in diverticulitis, it is more common in Crohn's disease and is usually longer than that seen in diverticulitis.[24,25]

Collagenous Colitis

In 1976, Lindström first described a colitis characterized by a thick collagen deposition in the subepithelial layer of the colonic mucosa.[26] It was thought that this layer of collagen impaired absorption of water and electrolytes, thus producing watery diarrhea. Approximately 48 cases have been reported since that time. Almost all patients have had watery diarrhea, but in some the diarrhea has been intermittent or it eventually disappeared, and in one patient the diarrhea and the collagenous band resolved spontaneously without therapy.[27] The presence of such a thick collagen layer has not been described in other inflammatory processes in the colon. For the most part, the cases reported have had a benign clinical course. The cause is unknown, but both inflammatory and toxic factors have been suggested. Treatment with steroid enemas, sulfasalazine, or both, has been reported to resolve the collagen deposition.[28,29]

Teglbjaerg and Thaysen described the microscopic progression of this unusual form of colitis,[30] beginning with acute nonspecific inflammation, followed by an intermediate stage of edema and slight fibrosis in the subepithelial layer, and ending with the development of the thick collagenous layer. They suggested that this change may develop because of a functional disturbance in the maturation of the pericryptal fibroblasts, resulting in an overproduction of collagen. In turn, this maturation disturbance might be triggered by an inflammatory or toxic stimulus.*

*Editors' note: See also Rams, H., et al.: Ann. Intern. Med., *106*:108, 1987.

Diversion Proctitis

A nonspecific inflammatory process can occur in the rectum and distal colon after surgical diversion has been performed for a variety of entities, usually after diversion for diverticulitis or Crohn's disease.[31,32] Ulceration of the mucosa in the diverted section, similar to that seen in inflammatory bowel disease, may develop in previously normal-appearing mucosa. Macroscopically and microscopically, it is most frequently a nonspecific inflammation,[31,32] although the histologic finding of Crohn's disease may be seen in patients whose operation was performed for more proximal Crohn's disease. In diversion proctitis, resolution of the inflammation with restoration of a normal-appearing rectum endoscopically after reanastomosis has been reported.[31,32] Diversion proctitis takes approximately three months to develop after an operation, and resolution of the inflammation following reanastomosis takes approximately the same length of time.

Allergic Proctitis

In 1980, Rosekrans et al. described 12 patients with the typical clinical histologic picture of distal colitis with intermittent fluctuating symptoms over an average of seven years.[33] Immunoperoxidase staining revealed a substantial increase in the number of cells in the lamina propria containing IgE. Of the 12 patients, eight were treated with orally administered disodium cromoglycate, and all improved. It has been thought that this might be a different form of proctitis and suggested the term allergic proctitis. Others have reported large numbers of eosinophils in biopsies of rectal mucosa,[34] suggesting to them that an allergic phenomenon was present. Our experience suggests that plentiful eosinophils are a common finding in mucosal biopsies of inflammatory bowel disease.

Infectious Colitis

The typical patient with moderately severe ulcerative colitis or Crohn's colitis presents with chronic, watery diarrhea, that is large in volume, lasting weeks rather than days at a time, often associated with some lower abdominal cramping and intermittent low-grade fever. Occasionally, red blood may be present in the stool. Other conditions, which may mimic inflammatory bowel disease, exist, however. In infectious colitis (especially that caused by Shigella, Amoeba, or Campylobacter), symptoms may occur that, although similar to those that occur with inflammatory bowel disease (Fig. 10-9), are not usually chronic. Ischemic colitis may present with hematochezia and diarrhea, its course usually being self-limited, although repeated bouts of ischemia may appear over several months. The well-known irritable colon is characterized by a similar course of chronic, intermittent diarrhea with cramps, but in this disorder stools are usually small in volume, and low-grade fever and hematochezia are not features.

In acute severe ulcerative colitis or Crohn's colitis, bloody diarrhea, fever, dehydration, and even prostration are common, making differentiation from acute infectious colitis a major problem at times. Sigmoidoscopy often confirms the presence of colitis but may not distinguish between idiopathic and infectious colitis. As will be reviewed in the following, acute salmonellosis, shigellosis, or amebiasis may be ruled out within 24 to 48 hours by microscopy of aspirates and stool cultures; Campylobacter infection also can be excluded by culture. Pseudomembranous colitis is another entity that must be differentiated from severe idiopathic colitis.

Greater variation in sexual practices has been recognized as a factor in urban transmission of bacterial, protozoal, and viral enteric diseases.[35] Atypical infections must also be considered, such as herpes simplex, lymphogranuloma venereum, and even rectal syphilis. These agents, along with Shigella, Entamoeba histolytica, and Campylobacter, are being found with increased frequency in the homosexual population. The gay bowel syndrome will be discussed in detail as a separate entity.

Specific Infections of the Colon
Salmonellosis

Involvement of the colon in the course of Salmonella gastroenteritis is common, at least with experimental animal studies and proctoscopic examinations in selected patients.[36] Although most patients with Salmonella present with mild diarrhea and watery bowel movements, colonic involvement dominates the clinical picture in a small but important group. Patients with Salmonella colitis typically have diarrhea for 10 to 15 days before the diagnosis is established. In the colonic form, the diarrhea is more persistent than it is in Salmonella gastroenteritis even though the organism may have disappeared from the feces.[37] Bowel movements are bloody in approximately half the patients.

Diagnosis is best made by culture of the stool on specific media, such as bismuth sulfite and MacConkey agar.[38] Available antigenic tests are of little or no value in the diagnosis of the gastroenteric form of salmonellosis.[39]

Proctoscopic findings include hyperemia, granularity, friability, and ulcerations. A biopsy of the rectum reveals mucosal ulceration, hemorrhage, and crypt abscesses.

In the acute form, idiopathic ulcerative colitis cannot reliably be distinguished from Salmonella colitis other than by stool culture.[40] Patients with an acute onset of colitis, who have no past history of colitis, and have symptoms of less than three weeks' duration, should be considered to have an infectious form of colitis, and Salmonella, Shigella, and Campylobacter should be important considerations.

The course of Salmonella colitis varies, ranging from one week to two or three months. The average duration of illness is three weeks, and it may be complicated by bleeding, sepsis, or development of a megacolon.

Some studies have shown a 3 to 5% incidence of Salmonella cultured from stools of patients with ulcerative colitis either at the onset or during exacerbation;[36] however, manifestations of inflammatory bowel disease persisted despite eradication of the Salmonella. The usual carrier rate for Salmonella is only 0.2%, and the signifi-

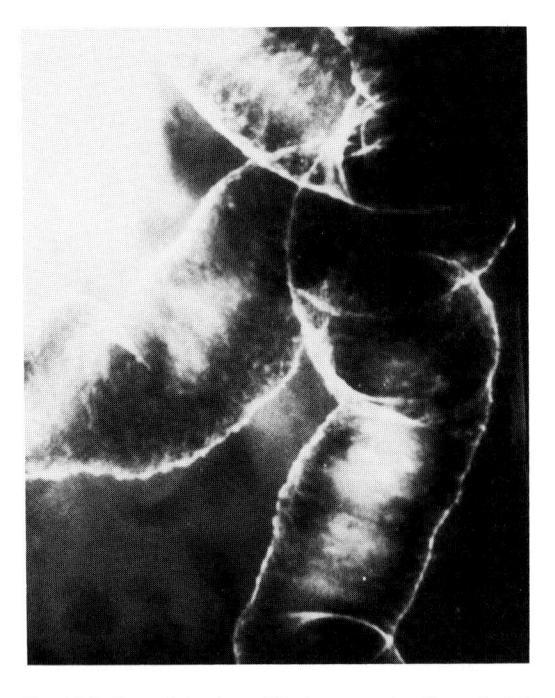

FIG. 10-9. Campylobacter colitis; hazy margins, fine spiculations, and secretions indicate edema and inflammatory reaction. Initially this was thought to be ulcerative colitis.

cance of the higher rate in inflammatory bowel disease is not understood. Two theories have been proposed. Hook has postulated that inflammatory bowel disease is one of the underlying diseases that predisposes patients to Salmonella infections.[41] On the other hand, Shorter and associates have postulated that inflammatory bowel disease may be caused by a hypersensitivity reaction to bacterial antigens (see also Chap. 4).[42]

Shigellosis

Shigellosis, commonly known as bacillary dysentery, is caused by a gram-negative organism that primarily involves the large intestine. Common symptoms are fever, crampy abdominal pain, tenesmus, and mucoid bloody diarrhea. In the United States, the highest incidence occurs in warm humid climates with overcrowding and poor sanitary conditions. The handling of food and water by infected persons is a common source of infection. Sigmoidoscopically, the findings may vary from erythematous and somewhat granular mucosa to extreme hyperemia, friability, and superficial ulceration. Wright's stain of the stool reveals polymorphonuclear leukocytes. The diagnosis is usually made by culture of the mucus and fecal material obtained by swabbing the ulcerated area during proctosigmoidoscopy. A culture plate should be incubated as soon as possible, and MacConkey's agar is the recommended medium.[38]

Campylobacter Fetus Subspecies Jejuni

Although C. fetus subspecies jejuni has been recognized as a common cause of bacterial diarrhea, only recently have investigators described a clinical syndrome including abdominal pain, diarrhea (which may be bloody or mucopurulent), and, occasionally, peritoneal irritation.[43] Sigmoidoscopic findings vary from mucosal edema, erythema, and contact friability to exudation, granularity, and spontaneous bleeding. These findings are indistinguishable from ulcerative colitis (Fig. 10-9). Barium enema studies may reveal pancolitis.

Histologically, biopsies vary from nonspecific inflammatory changes to acute inflammation with crypt abscesses suggestive of ulcerative colitis. The diagnosis usually can be made by isolating the organism from fecal specimens, which are cultured on the selective medium of vancomycin, polymyxin B sulfate, and trimethoprim lactate, and incubated at 43° C in an atmosphere of 5% oxygen, 10% carbon dioxide, and 85% hydrogen. Agglutinating antibodies may appear during the clinical syndrome, but this test is not widely available.

Tuberculosis

Any region of the gastrointestinal tract may be involved by tuberculosis. This disease is rarely diagnosed in developed nations, but tuberculosis is still seen in third world countries where it continues to be a health problem. Before the early 1930s, ileocecal granulomatous disease was assumed to arise from tuberculosis despite lack of bacteriologic confirmation. Crohn et al. separated the entity of regional enteritis, and since then cases of tuberculous enterocolitis have been diagnosed much less frequently.[44]

Before the development of effective treatment, autopsies on patients with pulmonary tuberculosis demonstrated intestinal involvement in 55 to 90% of such patients.[45] The frequency of intestinal disease was related to the severity of the pulmonary involvement. Gastrointestinal infection occurred in 1% of patients with minimal pulmonary tuberculosis, compared with 4.5% of patients with moderately advanced pulmonary disease and 25% with far-advanced disease.[46] A higher risk of intestinal involvement was also present with pulmonary cavitation and positive sputum smears, reflecting the risk of a high inoculum of swallowed organisms. Over the past 20 years, however, pulmonary involvement has been seen in less than 20% of patients with intestinal tuberculosis.[47] In fact, radiographs of the chest may reveal normal findings in patients with intestinal tuberculosis. Suspicion should be aroused, however, when pulmonary or other extraintestinal forms of tuberculosis are found.[48,49] Today, tuberculosis is usually secondary to pulmonary disease with the frequency paralleling the stage of disease, being most frequent in positive sputum smears and advanced cavitary disease.[47]

The cecum is the most common site of intestinal involvement in 85 to 90% of patients. The ileum is the next most common site, followed by, in order, ascending colon, jejunum, appendix, duodenum, stomach, sigmoid colon, and rectum.[47]

The macroscopic appearance of intestinal tuberculosis reveals three patterns: ulcerative, occurring in about 60% of patients, with multiple superficial lesions confined largely to the epithelial surface; hypertrophic, seen in approximately 10% of patients, with scarring, fibrosis, and heaped up mass lesions mimicking cancer; and ulcerohypertrophic, present in about 30% of patients, with mucosal ulcerations combined with healing and scar formation.[50] These patterns are recognized simply as different stages of the same disease.

The diagnosis of ileocecal tuberculosis is difficult to establish. Chronic abdominal pain is reported in about 90% of patients. A right lower quadrant abdominal mass, deep and posterior, is palpated in approximately two-thirds of patients. Diarrhea, weight loss, malaise, and low-grade fever may be seen. The tubercle bacillus may be isolated from stool in about one-third of the patients, but this finding is not helpful in patients with coexisting pulmonary tuberculosis because it may represent only swallowed organisms.

The definitive diagnosis of intestinal tuberculosis is made by identifying the organism in tissue either by light microscopy (acid-fast stain) or by culture. The finding of caseation necrosis in granulomas of the bowel or lymph nodes establishes the tuberculous basis of the intestinal disease. A presumptive diagnosis can be established in a patient with active pulmonary tuberculosis who has radiographic and clinical findings suggestive of intestinal involvement. The PPD test is not helpful because a positive result does not mean active disease. Many patients, especially when malnourished, have a negative result on skin test with active intestinal tuberculosis.

When the ileum is involved, the segment of tuberculosis is usually shorter than in regional enteritis. Ileal involvement alone suggests regional enteritis, while cecal involvement alone may suggest tuberculosis.[47] Radiographic examination may help in the distinction between these two diseases and reveals a thickened mucosa with distortion of the mucosal folds, ulcerations, varying degrees of thickening and stenosis of the bowel, and pseudopolyp formation.[51,52] The cecum is contracted with disease on both sides of the valve, and the valve itself is often distorted and incompetent. Tuberculosis tends to involve small segments of the intestine with stenosis and fistula formation. In the hypertrophic form, a mass that resembles a cecal cancer can be seen. The presence of calcified mesenteric lymph nodes is yet another sign aiding in the diagnosis.

Gonorrheal Proctitis

Rectal gonorrhea has been recognized since the late 19th century. With the discovery of Gram's stain in 1884, the organism was demonstrated in rectal smears. Over the past 20 years, rectal gonorrhea has been acknowledged as a public health problem with asymptomatic rectal carriers, both women and homosexual men, providing a reservoir for its perpetuation. Today, most rectal infections in men and many in women result from rectal sexual practices.[53] In general, rectal gonorrhea in men is contracted solely by anal intercourse.[54] In women, 90% of cases are believed to be secondary to genital-anal spread, and the other 10% are acquired by anal intercourse. As many as two-thirds of persons are asymptomatic, and disease is discovered by tracing a contact.

The clinical picture is not characteristic. Some patients have rectal burning, itching, a bloody or mucoid discharge, or diarrhea, but most have no symptoms.[53,55,56] When present, symptoms can be similar to ulcerative proctitis, with a purulent anal discharge, tenesmus, blood and mucus in the stools, dyschezia, and anal pruritus. Any homosexual patient with rectal complaints should be considered as possibly having gonorrhea. The sigmoidoscopic appearance is indistinguishable from that of ulcerative proctitis.[57] Generalized erythema with a mucopurulent exudate is most commonly seen. Edema, friability, superficial erosion, and fissures may be present but do not correlate well with a positive result on culture.[56] Abnormal findings in the mucosa are most prominent near the anorectal junction at the site of the anal crypts and columns of Morgagni,[58] sparing the distal stratified squamous portion that is resistant to gonococcal infection. Changes rarely extend beyond the rectum into the sigmoid colon. Differentiation from ulcerative proctitis can best be achieved by performing tests with Gram's stain and selective culturing of the purulent exudate.[57] The concomitant presence of genital gonorrhea may be found in 90% of women but in a much smaller percentage of men.[58] Patients with symptomatic rectal gonorrhea often will have other rectal conditions, such as condyloma acuminatum, anal fissures, fistulas, or inflamed hemorrhoids.[54]

Barium enema examination in rectal gonorrhea shows edematous mucosa, small ulcerations, and mild loss of distensibility, all nonspecific findings of inflammatory proctitis.[59]

Differentiation from inflammatory bowel disease is by selective culturing, response to specific therapy, and epidemiologic history of rectal intercourse in men.

Histoplasmosis

Histoplasmosis is a common disease, with 500,000 new cases occurring annually in the United States. The incidence is highest in the south central and southeastern sections of the United States. Its manifestations resemble tuberculosis in both the lung and the gastrointestinal tract.

Direct invasion of the alimentary tract has been postulated but never documented, and is uncommon, if it occurs at all. Direct hematogenous involvement of the gastrointestinal tract may occur in disseminated histoplasmosis. While oropharyngeal ulcerations are perhaps the most common, ulcerative lesions in the ileocecal and rectal area have also been described.[60] These ulcerations resemble tuberculosis or large amebic ulcers, with normal mucosa present between lesions.

Often the first clue to the diagnosis of histoplasmosis is the finding of splenic calcification on radiographs of the abdomen or the suggestion of pulmonary tuberculosis on the chest film. The oldest diagnostic test, the histoplasmin skin test, is sensitive, but the incidence of positivity in endemic areas is extremely high. The gastrointestinal manifestations may be caused by residual mediastinal disease and not become apparent until years later. Thus, it is not surprising that results of the skin test may be negative when the patient presents with gastrointestinal symptoms.

Serologic tests for the diagnosis of acute histoplasmosis are well-developed. The mainstay of diagnosis is the complement fixation test. The test reveals positive findings approximately 3 weeks after the primary infection, and the titers begin to diminish after 6 to 12 months. In disseminated histoplasmosis, serologic testing is helpful if the complement fixation titers are high or rising. A positive result is not diagnostic of dissemination, however, and a negative result does not rule it out.[61] The agar gel immunodiffusion test using histoplasmin as the antigen is frequently used as a screening test. It is an easy test to perform, but it is not sensitive.

Ultimately, the proved standard for the diagnosis is culture of the fungus on specially enriched peptone or meat infusion broth, or visualization of small, single budding yeasts in histopathologic sections, particularly stained by the periodic acid-Schiff method.

Lymphogranuloma Venereum

Lymphogranuloma venereum is an infectious disease caused by a microbe of the Chlamydia group. It is usually transmitted venereally. Infection with lymphogranuloma venereum may be divided into the anorectal (usually women) and genitoinguinal adenitis (mostly men) groups. The former can be subdivided into those causing proctocolitis (37%) and anorectal strictures (73%).[62] The proctocolitis stage occurs approximately six weeks after exposure.[63] Clinical symptoms of this acute illness include passage of blood and pus, diarrhea, constipation, tenesmus, and rectal pain. Inguinal adenitis is rarely encountered.[62-64] The rectal mucosa is granular, ulcerated, and edematous. Barium studies disclose a nonspecific appearance resembling colitis with mucosal edema and spastic narrowing. Fistulas (frequently to the vagina), perirectal abscesses, and edematous perianal tags are seen. Involvement of the colon diffusely or in a multifocal pattern is also frequently noted, but the rectum is always the most severely affected. Rectal strictures are late sequelae of untreated disease, and these may be tubular or diaphragmatic (Fig. 10-10). Early disease is usually confined to the rectum, but left-sided colitis and universal colitis may occur. Similar to inflammatory bowel disease, systemic signs and symptoms, such as fever, malaise, arthralgias, and erythema nodosum, may occur.

Lymphogranuloma venereum may be diagnosed three ways. First, through the isolation of the organism, which is difficult but can be accomplished by major laboratories.[65] Second, by using the Frei test, which uses commercially available antigen and gives positive results 12 to 40 days after signs of infection appear (this test has a relatively high false-negative rate in early disease).[63,65] If results are negative, the test should be repeated in three weeks. When results are positive, they usually remain positive for the life of the patient, although the titer may fall with treatment.[64] The third way to diagnose lymphogranuloma venereum is with a complement fixation test, which is the most sensitive diagnostic test, and is usually available from state laboratories. Spontaneous conversion of a positive result to a negative one has been observed.

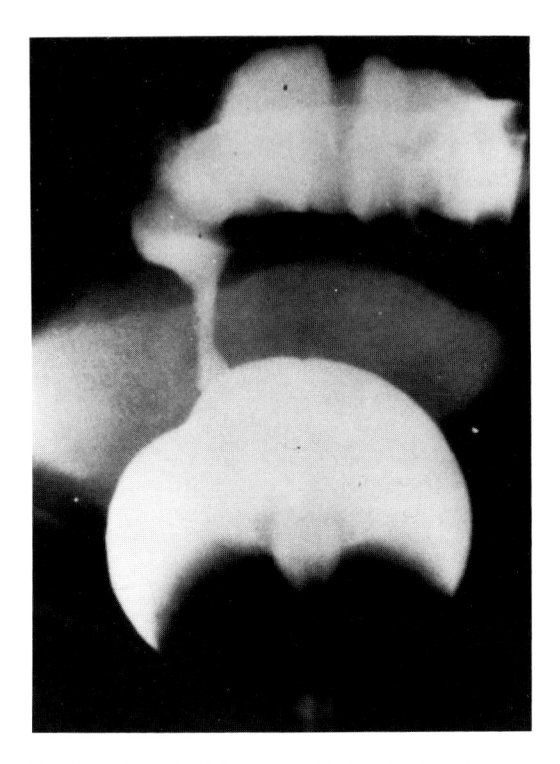

Fig. 10-10. Rectal stricture caused by lymphogranuloma venereum.

Cytomegalovirus Occlusion Disease

Cytomegalovirus infection occurs in adults more often as a late complication of other serious illnesses, such as malignant disease or chronic infection, or in patients who are transplant recipients or who are receiving cytotoxic drugs or steroids. Recently, concern over cytomegalovirus infection of the bowel has heightened with the development of the acquired immunodeficiency syndrome epidemic. Patients from this select population may present with abdominal pain and severe diarrhea, which may be bloody. Endoscopically, the mucosa appears granular, erythematous, and friable. Discrete ulcerations, both punched out and linear, may be noted. Barium enema studies may show extensive ulceration throughout the colon. The sigmoidoscopic findings and radiographic picture can closely mimic those of ulcerative colitis. Cytomegalic inclusion cells may be observed on routine hematoxylin-eosin staining of tissue obtained at rectal biopsy.[66]

Amebiasis

Amebiasis, an acute and chronic disease caused by the organism Entamoeba histolytica, may present with a variety of clinical patterns, including asymptomatic carriers, noninvasive diarrhea, amebic dysentery, and extraintestinal manifestations. Although multiple organs may be involved, the colon is the usual site of initial disease. The clinical manifestations vary from the asymptomatic carrier state to severe fulminating illness with mucosal inflammation and ulceration, occasionally with a fatal outcome.

Amebic dysentery may simulate nonspecific inflammatory bowel disease clinically, and differentiation by sigmoidoscopy may be difficult. Examination by sigmoidoscopy may reveal the characteristic isolated ulcers, 5 to 15 mm in diameter, covered with small yellow hemispheric elevations of exudate, with intervening normal mucosa (Fig. 10–11 A). These ulcers, which are scattered throughout the large intestine, most frequently involve the cecum and ascending colon, with the descending colon, sigmoid, rectum, and hepatic flexure following in frequency. Rarely, the disease may involve the terminal ileum. As the disease progresses, the ulcers may grow to 2 cm or more in diameter, the edges become more undermined, and the base may extend from the submucosa into the muscular coat. Undermining of the irregular margins of these discrete ulcers produces a rolled edge, and the base may be covered with a necrotic eschar. On rare occasions, involvement of the blood vessels at the base of the ulcer may produce brisk bleeding. More rarely, the colon may perforate. In contrast to bacillary dysentery and ulcerative colitis, the intervening mucosa may appear relatively normal. This is not seen in ulcerative colitis, but differentiation between amebic and Crohn's colitis may be impossible sigmoidoscopically. Amebic dysentery may have remissions and exacerbations as seen in inflammatory bowel disease, confusing the differentiation. Histologically, a diffuse inflammatory lesion is indistinguishable from the nonspecific inflammation seen in other types of colitis. Amebae may be found at the surface or in the adjacent exudate. Changes seen on electron microscopic examination include extensive damage to the microvillous border, which may account in part for the diarrhea of amebic colitis. With advanced disease, the classic flask-shaped ulcer with undermined edges may be seen (Fig. 10–11 B).

The diagnosis of amebiasis is important not only because it is readily made in most acute cases, but also because therapy is highly effective. It is necessary to distinguish amebiasis from inflammatory bowel disease because steroids are often prescribed in the latter but may be lethal in patients with acute invasive amebia-

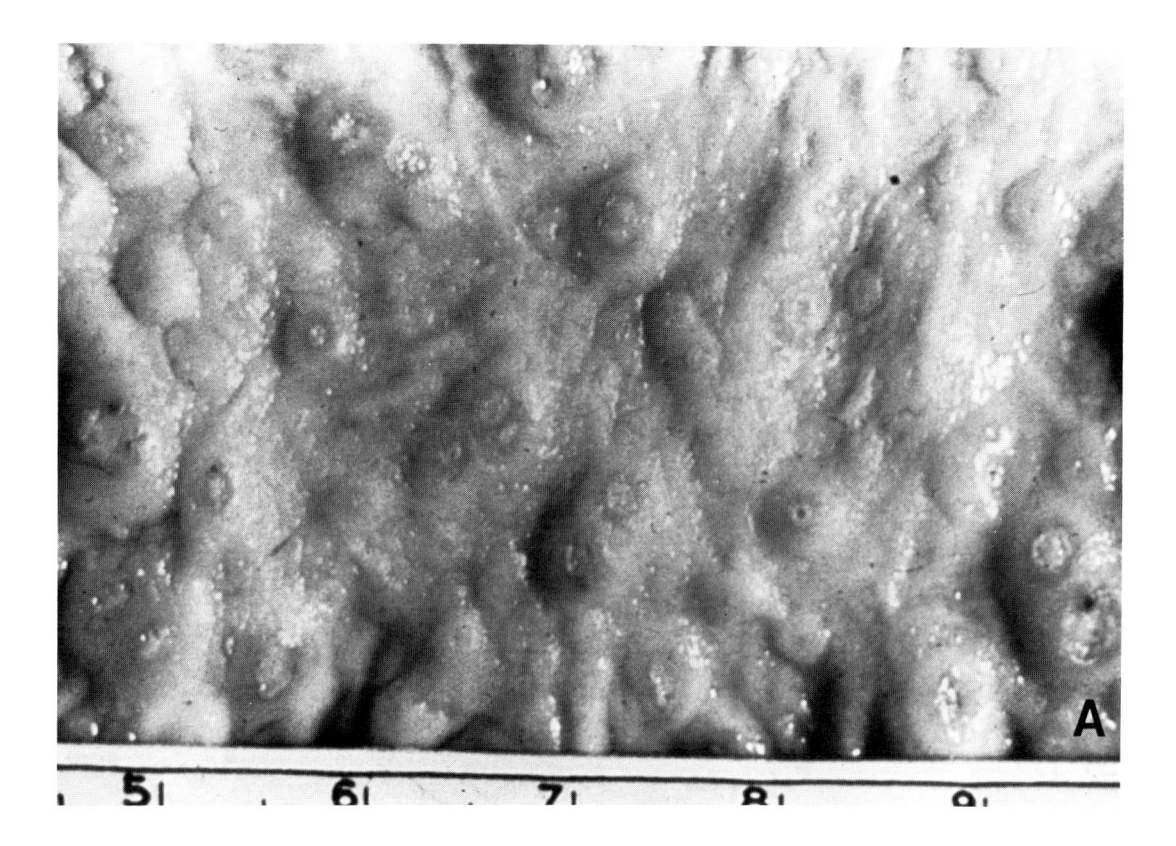

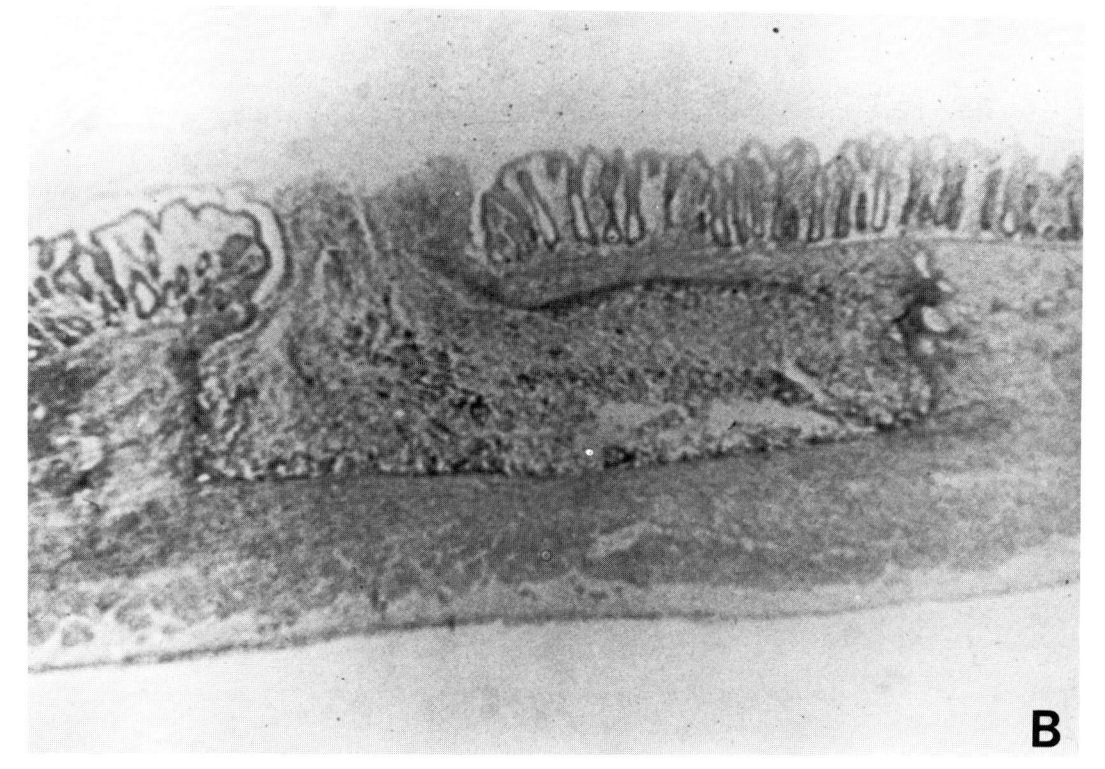

FIG. 10-11. A. Amebiasis of the colon, dysentery type; multiple amebic ulcers are seen. B. Amebic ulceration of the colon with the classic flask-shaped ulceration.

sis. Microscopic examination of repeated (three to six) fresh stool specimens, if performed correctly, will reveal trophozoites and establish a diagnosis in 90% of patients with asymptomatic amebiasis.[67] In acute infection with E. histolytica, trophozoites will be seen to contain ingested red blood cells when invasion of the bowel wall has occurred. Stool examination should be completed before barium studies, because the yield is greatly decreased after introduction of barium into the colon.[68]

Sigmoidoscopy is helpful in some, but not all, patients with acute amebiasis because the rectum is involved less frequently than the cecum. The examination should be performed initially without preparing the bowel before therapy. Choosing material directly from the ulcers through a sigmoidoscope may increase the diagnostic yield. Certain serologic tests, particularly the indirect hemagglutination test, counterimmunoelectrophoresis, and the latex agglutination test, are useful in the diagnosis of invasive disease. Healy and Kraft showed that no etiologic relationship existed between inflammatory bowel disease and amebic dysentery by using the findings of indirect hemagglutination test titers in a group of 511 patients with inflammatory bowel disease.[69] These results were not different in the false-positive rate from a normal control group.[69] In contrast, 30% of patients with amebic dysentery had positive titers.[70]

The radiographic features of enteric amebiasis are many, varied, and nonspecific. With severe involvement, abdominal films may show toxic dilatation of the colon. Mucosal changes on barium enema study vary from fine granularity and irregularity of the bowel margins to collar button ulcers, that is, deep, spike-like penetrating ulcers. Pseudopolyps, cobblestoning, and thumbprinting may be seen. Haustral changes include spasm, irritability, and stricture formation (Fig. 10–11 C). The cecum, involved in 90% of patients with chronic amebiasis, can become concentrically narrowed, that is, the "cone cecum." Any portion of the colon, including the appendix, may be involved, and multiple skip lesions are found in 50% of patients. Other findings may be perforation, fistulas, and pericolic abscesses. Rarely, an ameboma appears as a mass lesion, often impossible to distinguish from a neoplasm.

The entity of ulcerative postdysenteric amebic colitis is even more difficult to distinguish from nonspecific colonic inflammatory bowel disease. The usual setting is one of severe amebic colitis, with slow resolution lasting up to nine months or longer, whereas in most cases of amebic dysentery, healing is seen usually in ten days or less.[71] Amebae will not be seen in the stool in the chronic form, and a condition simulating inflammatory bowel disease, with fever, leukocytosis, anemia, and an elevated erythrocyte sedimentation rate, may occur. The changes seen radiographically will probably suggest chronic ulcerative colitis when the lesions of amebiasis are diffuse, whereas when skip lesions are produced, the radiographic findings may mimic Crohn's disease. Distinguishing features include the recent past history of amebic dysentery, with steady recovery and lack of intestinal manifestations. In general, steroid therapy is considered less effective in postdysenteric colitis than in nonspecific colonic inflammatory bowel disease.[71]

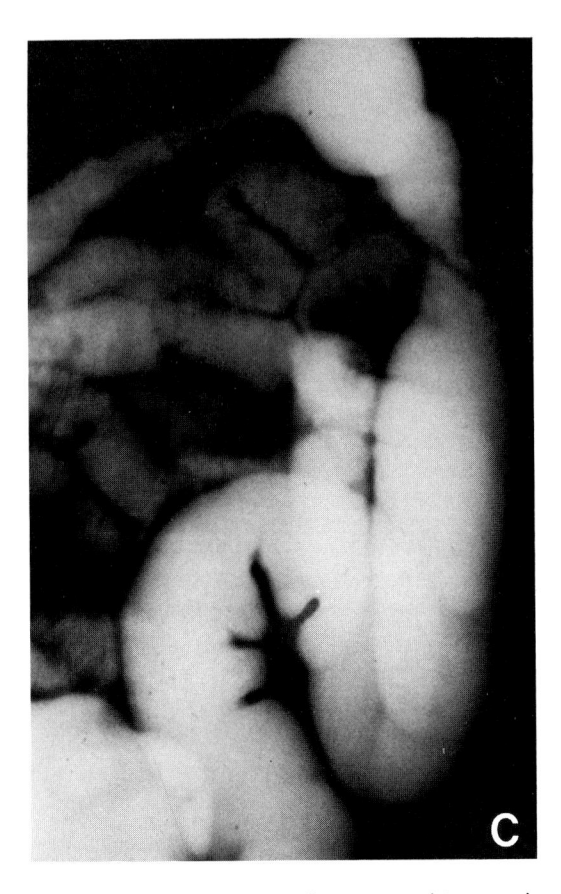

FIG. 10-11. (*continued*) C. The inflammatory stricture seen in the distal transverse colon is secondary to infection with E. histolytica.

The Gay Bowel Syndrome

Sexual transmission of enteric pathogens in homosexual men was first recognized in 1967. Over the past ten years, the incidence of reported symptomatic intestinal amebiasis among homosexual men living in San Francisco who are 20- to 39-years-old has increased by 1000%. Other studies following these reports have confirmed these high prevalence rates among homosexual men residing in major urban areas of the United States, England, Europe, and Canada.[72]

Now, however, with the recognition of the acquired immunodeficiency syndrome, other enteric pathogens are also being identified in homosexual men with gastrointestinal symptoms. These pathogens include cryptosporidia, Isospora, Mycobacterium avium, Mycobacterium intracellulare, and cytomegalovirus. In addition, such classic sexually transmitted pathogens as Neisseria gonorrhoeae, Chlamydia trachomatis, herpes simplex virus, Treponema pallidum, and papilloma virus are known to cause rectal disease. Thus, the microbial cause of intestinal disease in most homosexual men is complex.[73]

Proctocolitis is usually caused by enteric organisms, such as Campylobacter, Shigella, Salmonella, or E. histolytica. These organisms may be invasive and may produce ulcerations of the rectum and colon.

Infected patients complain of lower abdominal discomfort, pain, and bloody diarrhea. Colonoscopy may reveal discrete ulcerations, and rectal biopsy may show nonspecific inflammation.

In patients with proctocolitis, stools should be cultured for enteric organisms and examined for ova and parasites. Treatment of patients with these infections depends on the susceptibility of the pathogen to antibiotic agents. This susceptibility may vary from one location of the country to another.

Disease confined to the rectum is most frequently caused by N. gonorrhoeae, herpes simplex, Chlamydia, Trichomonas, and T. pallidum. Rectal infection results from direct inoculation of these organisms from the urethra of the infected person into the rectum of the partner during anal intercourse.

Gonorrheal and chlamydial proctitis may produce a slight mucopurulent discharge and mild anal discomfort. Herpes infection of the rectum or perianal area is associated with severe anorectal pain and the appearance of herpetic vesicles or ulcerations. The presence of a rectal mass or pain with ulcerations suggests anorectal syphilis.

Diffuse rectal inflammation and ulceration are occasionally associated with chlamydial infection of the lymphogranuloma venereum immunotype. Lymphogranuloma venereum infection can easily be confused with granulomatous colitis on rectal biopsy. The diagnosis of lymphogranuloma venereum or chlamydial infection in general can only be made by culture.

Thus, multiple enteric infections are frequently found in homosexual men with and without the acquired immunodeficiency syndrome. The diagnosis of these intestinal diseases requires a systematic approach with the sexual history, predominant symptoms, and findings on physical examination, endoscopy, cultures, and mucosal biopsy guiding the clinician in selecting the specific diagnostic tests and appropriate antimicrobial therapy.

Radiation Colitis

A history of presently undergoing or having undergone radiation therapy is the key to the diagnosis of radiation colitis. The most common clinical setting for radiation colitis is a patient with a history of intra-abdominal or pelvic cancer who is having or has completed radiotherapy. The total dose of radiation usually has exceeded 4000 rad. Symptoms may appear early during therapy, shortly after therapy has been completed, or from months to many years afterward.

EARLY ONSET. During the acute state, usually in the 5th to the 14th day of radiation therapy, mucoid rectal discharge, tenesmus, and rectal bleeding may develop. In many respects, the onset and clinical picture resemble acute idiopathic ulcerative colitis.

Sigmoidoscopy during this period demonstrates dusky, edematous, and inflamed mucosa. Friability is usually not severe, and ulceration is uncommon at this stage. With increasing doses of radiation, however, mucosal ulceration and friability may occur. This may be accompanied by tenesmus and rectal bleeding. The symptoms usually resolve shortly after completion of radiation treatment or when the daily dose is decreased. The severity of early symptoms correlates with the risk of late radiation damage, but the absence of acute symptoms does not indicate protection against late radiation changes.[74]

Radiographically, both the intestinal wall and the mesentery become edematous during the early stage of radiation injury; if extensive, edema may cause separation of intestinal loops and thickening and straightening of the mucosal folds. A spiked appearance of the mucosa may be present. Barium contrast studies of the rectum during the acute phase often demonstrate spasm, and rarely, an isolated ulcer may be present on the anterior rectal wall. If surrounding mucosal edema is present, radiographic changes may suggest cancer. Thumbprint-like indentations of the barium column by edematous mucosa may mistakenly lead to the erroneous diagnosis of a primary ischemic process. When haustral markings are also lost, the radiographic picture may resemble other superficial acute ulcerating mucosal diseases, such as ulcerative colitis.

LATE CHANGES. The pattern of delayed radiation damage to the bowel varies widely. Predisposing factors appear to be the amount of bowel radiated and the total tissue dose. Additionally, fixation of any bowel loop makes an area vulnerable to further radiation damage. Although the onset is usually insidious, clinical manifestations tend to progress relentlessly. Symptoms may begin as early as a few months or as late as many years after treatment has been completed.[75] The variability in the duration of the latent period emphasizes the importance of the medical history in evaluating these patients. Overall frequency of late bowel injury after radiation has been estimated to be at least 10%, especially when the rectum has been irradiated.[76]

Symptoms include tenesmus, rectal bleeding, or a change in bowel habit. Sigmoidoscopy may reveal a granular, friable mucosa. Telangiectasia and ulcerations may be present, and rectal strictures may develop.[77] The characteristic telangiectasias enable the late stage of radiation colitis to be distinguished from ulcerative colitis.

When the rectum is primarily involved, symptoms of proctitis, including tenesmus, bleeding, and a mucoid rectal discharge, develop. Discrete ulcerations of the rectal mucosa occur in about 10% of patients and are often located on the anterior rectal wall, about 4 to 8 cm from the anus.[78] These ulcers vary in size and are frequently transversely oriented. Occasionally, the ulcers may have a neoplastic appearance. Rectal strictures tend to be located higher than the ulceration, usually 8 to 12 cm above the anal verge.[75] A biopsy of the ulcer or the strictured area may be helpful but should be performed with care because bleeding or even perforation of necrotic bowel may occur.

Radiographic changes may show narrowed, straightened, anhaustral segments that may be indistinguishable from those of chronic ulcerative colitis or of Crohn's colitis. A focal collection of barium in the anterior rectal wall may suggest ulceration. Fibrosis of the colon or the rectum may result in long or short narrowed areas that are smooth and symmetric with tapered edges.[79]

Ischemic Disease

The response of the colon to vascular insufficiency depends on several factors, including the location and extent of the occlusive disease and whether or not associated systemic disorders are present.[80] Thus, ischemia of the colon may accompany nonthrombotic infarction of the small bowel in patients with cardiac failure, or it may result from interruption of colonic blood supply during an abdominal aortic aneurysmectomy or abdominoperineal resection.

Colonic ischemia may result from localized occlusive disease in the inferior mesenteric artery or its critical collateral channels.[80,81] Less commonly, it may be associated with hypercoagulable states, amyloidosis, vasculitis, ruptured aortic aneurysm, obstructing colorectal cancer, or with the use of oral contraceptives. Ischemic colitis associated with oral contraceptives is typically segmental in distribution.

The syndrome of ischemic colitis may be variable in its extent, severity, and prognosis. Extensive infarction, gangrene, or perforation may result. Commonly seen are the catastrophic cases, which are usually associated with localized or segmental ischemia. Particularly vulnerable are those parts of the colon that lie in the "watershed" between adjacent arterial supplies, that is, in the splenic flexure (involving the superior and inferior mesenteric arteries) and in the rectosigmoid area (involving the inferior mesenteric and internal iliac arteries).[82] In small vessel disease, any portion of the colon may be affected.

Ischemic disease must be considered in the elderly patient presenting with abdominal pain and hematochezia.[83] Usually the history or physical findings suggest peripheral vascular disease. Pain in the left lower quadrant of the abdomen predominates, and rectal bleeding may be extensive or it may be detected only by occult blood testing. At proctoscopy, blood will be seen coming down from above. Ischemic colitis rarely involves the rectum and distal sigmoid because of its rich vascular supply from collaterals. A plain film of the abdomen may show

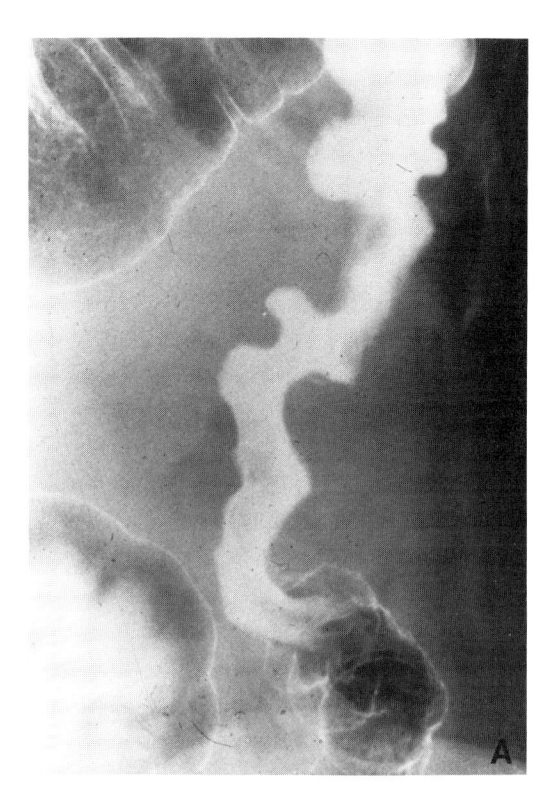

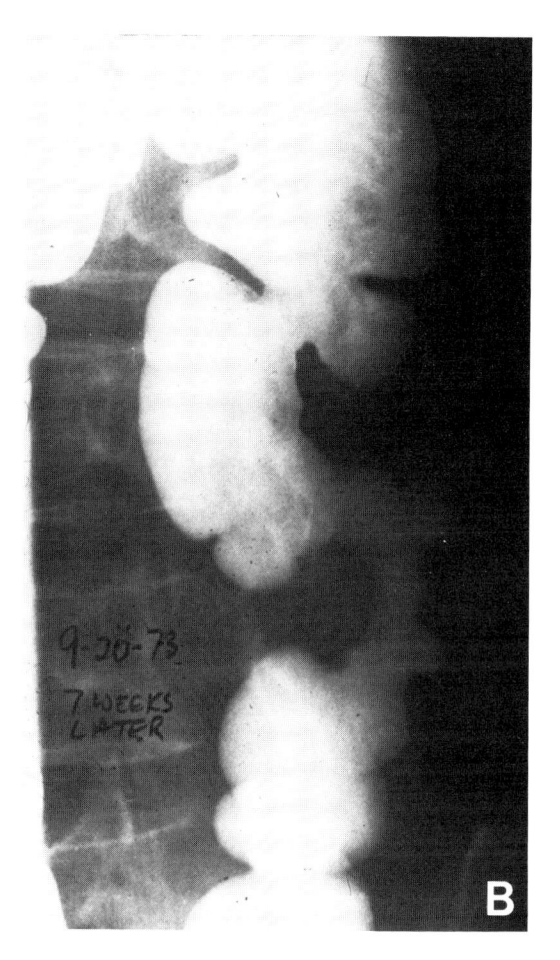

Fig. 10-12. Acute ischemic colitis in early stage (A), and when healed seven weeks later (B).

thumbprinting of the colonic outline, highly suggestive of ischemic disease (see also Chap. 20). A barium enema study will usually distinguish ischemic disease from ulcerative colitis, although radiographs may show findings consistent with either diagnosis (Fig. 10-12A, B). Rarely, the severity of the clinical picture suggests local or generalized peritonitis.

Ischemic disease may also affect the rectosigmoid area.[84] These patients, who are usually older, present with abdominal pain, rectal bleeding, and a change in bowel habit. Unlike those with more proximal involvement, however, signs of peritonitis are unusual. Sigmoidoscopic findings are variable and may include a picture suggestive of nonspecific proctitis, multiple discrete ulcers, or nodular lesions that occasionally are blue-black (reflecting underlying hemorrhage).[84]

The differentiation of ischemic colitis from nonspecific ulcerative colitis, proctitis, or Crohn's disease of the colon may be difficult or impossible to establish on the basis of the clinical evidence alone. Ischemic colitis can occur in younger patients, not all of whom have an apparent predisposing cause. Furthermore, ischemic colitis has even been reported to resemble "toxic dilatation."[83] Histologic examination may also fail to differentiate these various diseases. Obviously, it is important to consider the diagnosis of ischemic colitis in older patients who present with what appears to be an initial episode of acute ulcerative colitis. Angiography may be helpful in establishing the presence of vascular disease, but occlusions that are localized to smaller vessels may not be detectable. Thus, angiography is of limited value in the evaluation of patients with ischemic colitis.

Pseudomembranous Enterocolitis

Pseudomembranous enterocolitis of the colonic and rectal mucosa is characterized by the formation of elevated yellow-white plaques, varying in diameter from a few millimeters to a few centimeters. The plaques usually are separated from one another by mucosa that is usually inflamed

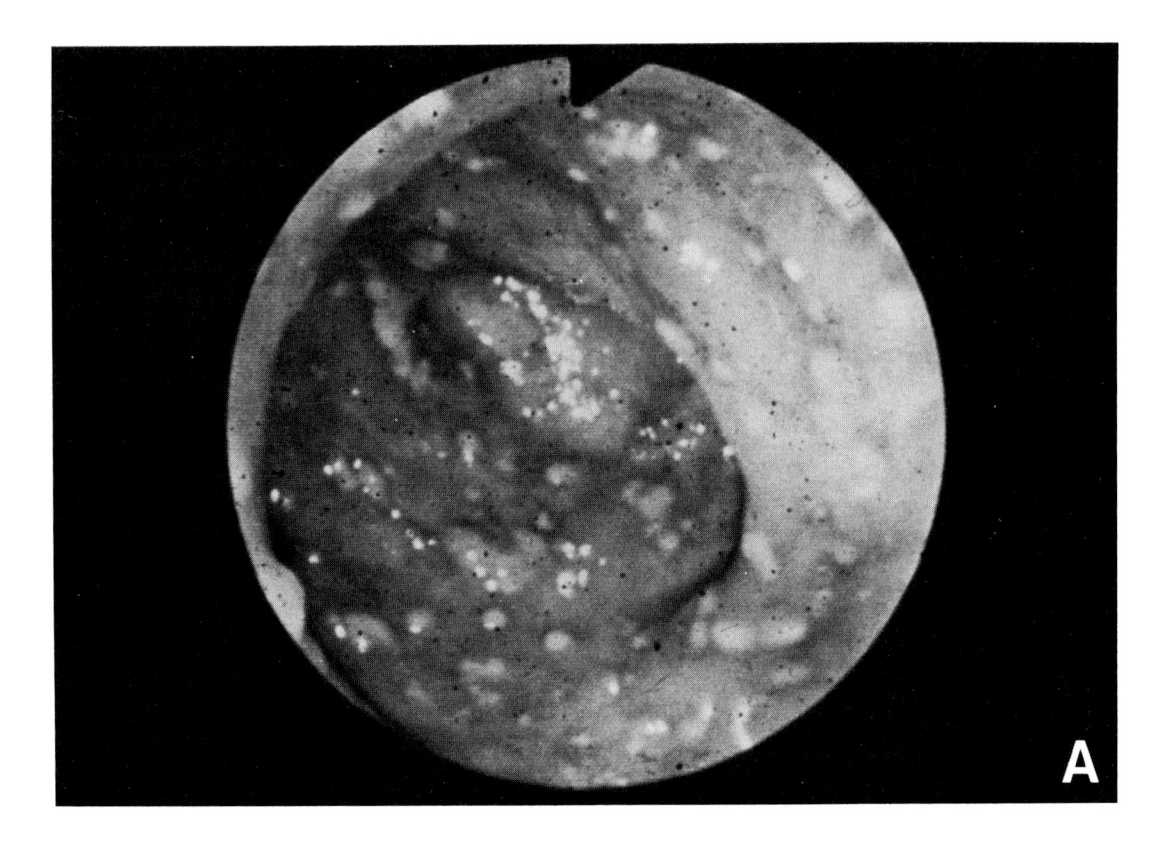

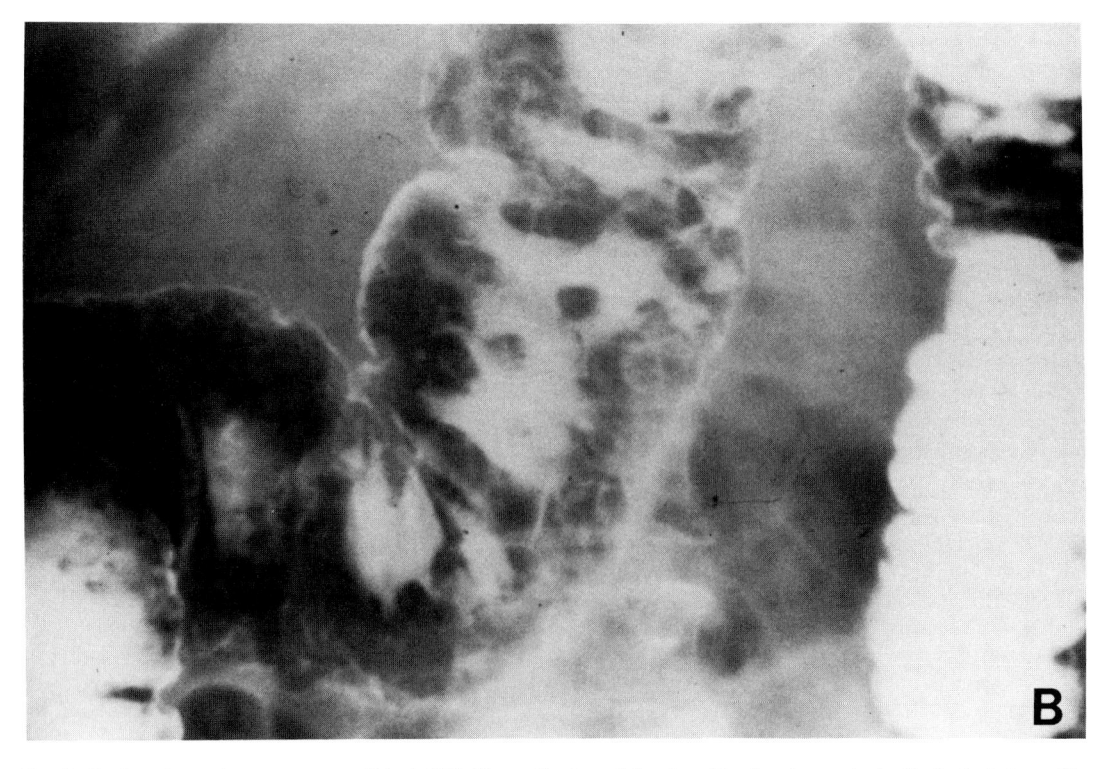

Fig. 10-13. Pseudomembranous enterocolitis. A. This fiberoptic view of the sigmoid colon demonstrates the typical plaque-like membranes. B. Persistent filling defects in the transverse colon caused by the pseudomembrane.

and covered with mucus, but may be normal. Clinically, the dominant symptom is diarrhea, ranging in severity from soft stools to frequent and incapacitating watery motions. The duration of illness is also variable and may be as short as two days or as long as two months. This disease usually occurs during or after antibiotic therapy, especially with lincomycin, clindamycin, ampicillin, or the cephalosporins. Substantial evidence now shows this disorder is caused by toxins elaborated within the colon by C. difficile. Both acquisition of the organism and toxin production are promoted by alteration of the normal colonic flora. The original detection of C. difficile as an important intestinal pathogen was observed in a hamster model of antibiotic-induced colitis.

Improved diagnostic methods have followed the implication of C. difficile toxins as the cause of the disease and have revealed a wider spectrum of disease than was hitherto recognized, creating problems defining it. Illness caused by C. difficile now appears to include diarrhea in patients who do not have pseudomembranes and in whom nonspecific inflammatory changes may or may not be found histologically in the colonic or rectal mucosa. Suitable nomenclature in such patients might be antibiotic-associated, C. difficile colitis or diarrhea. It is almost impossible to distinguish these two patterns with confidence in the absence of a complete colonoscopic examination, however. Consequently, the appropriate diagnostic label for many patients with diarrhea and C. difficile toxins in their feces is uncertain. For convenience, this whole spectrum of disease will be referred to under the sometimes misleading heading of pseudomembranous colitis.

The clinical features of pseudomembranous colitis have been well-defined.[85–88] The principal symptom, watery diarrhea, is associated with intermittent fever in many patients. Some patients experience colicky abdominal pain and, in severe disease, intense pain that may simulate an acute abdominal emergency. Toxic megacolon is a rare complication. Diarrheal stool often contains excess mucus, and pus or blood may or may not be found.[88] Nausea and vomiting accompany the diarrhea in some patients. Other findings include leukocytosis in excess of 15,000 mm^3 in 40% of patients, and a low serum albumin level in 76% of patients.[88]

Duration of symptoms in patients who are not given specific treatment may be as short as 48 hours or as long as 50 days, but, in the majority of patients, resolution of symptoms is complete within 10 to 14 days of stopping antibiotics.[85] Symptoms may commence as early as the second day of antibiotic treatment but usually begin a few days after completion of a course of therapy. Symptoms sometimes may be delayed by as much as three weeks after institution of antibiotic therapy, however.

DIAGNOSIS. The sigmoidoscopic appearance is of small plaques of membrane adherent to the mucosa, with intervening areas that appear normal. Performing sigmoidoscopy combined with a biopsy is the most widely used clinical procedure in the diagnosis of pseudomembranous colitis (Fig. 10-13A). When diarrhea is profuse or abundant mucus obscures the rectal mucosa, visualization of the pseudomembranes may be difficult, and the findings may be inconclusive. If the results are negative, sigmoidoscopy should be repeated daily until the results of the stool cytotoxin tests are available because the typical morphologic appearance of pseudomembrane may not be present initially.[88] The main limitation to the use of sigmoidoscopy is that in some patients with pseudomembranous colitis the rectum is spared, while patchy or sometimes extensive involvement is present in the more proximal colon. These patients can be identified by using colonoscopy.[85]

The histologic criteria for pseudomembranous colitis and a scheme for grading them have been well-defined.[89] Characteristic changes are seen in Figure 10-13B. Frozen sections have been shown to be a reliable alternative to conventional paraffin sections and have the advantage of providing a more rapid diagnosis in patients with nonvisible mucosal plaque.[90]

A barium enema study is recommended for the diagnosis of pseudomembranous colitis.[91] Reports of exacerbation of symptoms after a barium enema study suggest caution, however.[87]

The discovery of a fecal cytotoxin initially provided an obvious diagnostic test for pseudomembranous colitis. The test is easy to perform in a laboratory with facilities for tissue cultures. The most recent data on C. difficile toxins indicate, however, that both diarrhea and the mucosal lesions are probably caused by the enterotoxin, and that the cytotoxin has only a minor role in the pathogenesis of the colitis.

References

1. Sinclair, T. S., Brunt, P. W., and Mowat, N. A. G.: Nonspecific proctocolitis in northeastern Scotland: A community study. Gastroenterolgy, 85:1, 1983.

2. Farmer, R. G., and Brown, C. H.: Ulcerative proctitis: Course and prognosis. Gastroenterolgy, *51*:219, 1966.
3. Sparberg, M., Fennessy, J., and Kirsner, J. B.: Ulcerative proctitis and mild ulcerative colitis: A study of 220 patients. Medicine, *45*:391, 1966.
4. Nugent, F. W., et al.: The clinical course of ulcerative proctosigmoiditis. Am. J. Dig. Dis., *15*:321, 1970.
5. Truelove, S. C., and Marks, C. G.: Toxic megacolon: Part I. Pathogenesis, diagnosis and treatment. Clin. Gastroenterol., *10*:107, 1981.
6. Farmer, R. G., Hawk, W. A., and Turnbull, R. B., Jr.: Clinical patterns in Crohn's disease: A statistical study of 615 cases. Gastroenterology, *68*:627, 1975.
7. Jacobson, I. M., Schapiro, R. H., and Warshaw, A. L.: Gastric and duodenal fistulas in Crohn's disease. Gastroenterology, *89*:1347, 1985.
8. Truelove, S. C., and Peña, A. S.: Course and prognosis of Crohn's disease. Gut, *17*:192, 1976.
9. Myren, J., Bouchier, I. A. D., Watkinson, G., and de Dombal, F. T.: Inflammatory bowel disease—An O. M. G. E. survey. Scand. J. Gastroenterol. (Suppl.), *14*:1, 1979.
10. Kirsner, J. B.: Problems in the differentiation of ulcerative colitis and Crohn's disease of the colon: The need for repeated diagnostic evaluation (editorial). Gastroenterology, *68*:187, 1975.
11. Clamp, S. E., et al.: Diagnosis of inflammatory bowel disease: An international multicentre scoring system. Br. Med. J., *284*:91, 1982.
12. Eyer, S., et al.: Simultaneous ulcerative colitis and Crohn's disease: Report of a case. Am. J. Gastroenterol., *73*:345, 1980.
13. Bolton, R. P., Sherriff, R. J., and Read, A. E.: Clostridium difficile associated diarrhea: A role in inflammatory bowel disease? Lancet, *1*:303, 1980.
14. LaMont, J. T., and Trnka, Y. M.: Therapeutic implications of Clostridium difficile toxin during relapse of chronic inflammatory bowel disease. Lancet, *1*:381, 1980.
15. Meyers, S., et al.: Occurrence of Clostridium difficile toxin during the course of inflammatory bowel disease. Gastroenterology, *80*:697, 1981.
16. Hogan, W. J., Hensley, G. T., and Geenen, J. E.: Endoscopic evaluation of inflammatory bowel disease. Med. Clin. North Am., *64*:1083, 1980.
17. De Dombal, F. T., et al.: Radiological appearances of ulcerative colitis: An evaluation of their clinical significances. Gut, *9*:157, 1968.
18. Buzzard, A. J., Baker, W. N. W., Needham, P. R. G., and Warren, R. E.: Acute toxic dilatation of the colon in Crohn's colitis. Gut, *15*:416, 1974.
19. Leigh, J. E., Judd, E. S., and Waugh, J. M.: Diverticulitis of the colon: Recurrence after apparently adequate segmental resection. Am. J. Surg., *103*:51, 1962.
20. Meyers, M. A., Alonso, D. R., Morson, B. C., and Bartram, C.: Pathogenesis of diverticulitis complicating granulomatous colitis. Gastroenterology, *74*:24, 1978.
21. Carr, N., and Schofield, P. F.: Inflammatory bowel disease in the older patient. Br. J. Surg., *69*:223, 1982.
22. Berman, I. R., Corman, M. L., Coller, J. A., and Veidenheimer, M. C.: Late onset Crohn's disease in patients with colonic diverticulitis. Dis. Colon Rectum, *22*:524, 1979.
23. Schmidt, G. T., Lennard-Jones, J. E., Morson, B. C., and Young, A. C.: Crohn's disease of the colon and its distinction from diverticulitis. Gut, *9*:7, 1968.
24. Marshak, R. H., Lindner, A. E., Pochaczevsky, R., and Maklansky, D: Longitudinal sinus tracts in granulomatous colitis and diverticulitis. Semin. Roentgenol., *11*:101, 1976.
25. Marshak, R. H., Janowitz, H. D., and Present, D. H.: Granulomatous colitis in association with diverticula. N. Engl. J. Med., *283*:1080, 1970.
26. Lindström, C. G.: 'Collagenous colitis' with watery diarrhoea—A new entity? Pathol. Eur., *11*:87, 1976.
27. Pieterse, A. S., Hecker, R., and Rowland, R.: Collagenous colitis: A distinctive and potentially reversible disorder. J. Clin. Pathol., *35*:338, 1982.
28. Farah, D. A., et al.: Collagenous colitis: Possible response to sulfasalazine and local steroid therapy. Gastroenterology, *88*:792, 1985.
29. Weidner, N., Smith, J., and Pattee, B.: Sulfasalazine in treatment of collagenous colitis: Case report and review of the literature. Am. J. Med., *77*:162, 1984.
30. Teglbjaerg, P. S., and Thaysen, E. H.: Collagenous colitis: An ultrastructural study of a case. Gastroenterology, *82*:561, 1982.
31. Glotzer, D. J., Glick, M. E., and Goldman, H.: Proctitis and colitis following diversion of the fecal stream. Gastroenterology, *80*:438, 1981.
32. Korelitz, B. I., Cheskin, L. J., Sohn, N., and Sommers, S. C.: Proctitis after fecal diversion in Crohn's disease and its elimination with reanastomosis: Implications for surgical management. Gastroenterology, *87*:710, 1984.
33. Rosekrans, P. C. M., Meijer, C. J. L. M., van der Wal, A. M., and Lindeman, J.: Allergic proctitis, a clinical and immunopathological entity. Gut, *21*:1017, 1980.
34. Heatley, R. V., and James, P. D.: Eosinophils in rectal mucosa: A simple method of predicting the outcome of ulcerative proctocolitis? Gut, *20*:787, 1978.
35. Owen, R. L.: Sexually transmitted enteric disease. *In* Current Clinical Topics in Infectious Diseases. 3rd Vol. Edited by J. S. Remington, and M. N. Swartz. New York, McGraw-Hill, 1982.
36. Lindeman, R. J., Weinstein, L., Levitan, R., and Patterson, J. F.: Ulcerative colitis and intestinal salmonellosis. Am. J. Med. Sci., *254*:855, 1967.
37. Mandal, B. K., and Mani, V.: Colonic involvement in salmonellosis. Lancet, *1*:887, 1976.
38. Zinsser Microbiology. 12th Ed. New York, Appleton-Century-Crofts, 1960.
39. Viranuvatti, V.: Infectious diarrheas. Part II. Cholera, salmonellosis, and shigellosis. *In* Gastroenterology. 12th Vol. Edited by H. L. Bockus. Philadelphia, W. B. Saunders, 1976.
40. Dronfield, M. W., Fletcher, J., and Langman, M. J. S.: Coincident salmonella infections and ulcerative colitis: Problems of recognition and management. Br. Med. J., *1*:99, 1974.
41. Hook, E. W.: Salmonellosis: Certain factors influencing the interactions of Salmonella and the human host. Bull. NY Acad. Med., *37*:499, 1961.
42. Shorter, R. G., Huizenga, K. A., and Spencer, R. J.: A working hypothesis for the etiology and pathogenesis of nonspecific inflammatory bowel disease (editorial). Am. J. Dig. Dis., *17*:1024, 1972.
43. Lambert, M. E., Schofield, P. F., Ironside, A. G., and Mandal, B. K.: Campylobacter colitis. Br. Med. J., *1*:857, 1979.
44. Crohn, B. B., Ginzburg, L., and Oppenheimer, G. D.: Regional ileitis: A pathologic and clinical entity. J. Am. Med. Assoc., *99*:1323, 1932.
45. Hordan, G. L., Jr., and Debakey, M. E.: Complications of tuberculous enteritis occurring during antimicrobial therapy. Arch. Surg., *69*:688, 1954.
46. Mitchell, R. S., and Bristol, L. J.: Intestinal tuberculosis: An analysis of 346 cases diagnosed by routine intestinal radiography on 5,529 admissions for pulmonary tuberculosis, 1924–49. Am. J. Med. Sci., *227*:241, 1954.
47. Abrams, J. S., and Holden, W. D.: Tuberculosis of the gastrointestinal tract. Arch. Surg., *89*:282, 1964.
48. Bentley, G., and Webster, J. H. H.: Gastrointestinal tuberculosis: A 10-year review. Br. J. Surg., *54*:90, 1967.

49. Schulze, K., Warner, H. A., and Murray, D.: Intestinal tuberculosis: Experience at a Canadian teaching institution. Am. J. Med., 63:735, 1977.
50. Hoon, J. R., Dockerty, M. B., and Pemberton, J. de J.: Collective review: Ileocecal tuberculosis including comparison of this disease with nonspecific regional enterocolitis and noncaseous tuberculated enterocolitis. Int. Abstr. Surg., 91:417, 1950.
51. Werbeloff, L., Novis, B. H., Banks, S., and Marks, I. N.: The radiology of tuberculosis of the gastro-intestinal tract. Br. J. Radiol., 46:329, 1973.
52. Kolawole, T. M., and Lewis, E. A.: A radiologic study of tuberculosis of the abdomen (gastointestinal tract). Am. J. Roentgenol. Radium Ther. Nucl. Med., 123:348, 1975.
53. Klein, E. J., Fisher, L. S., Chow, A. W., and Guze, L. B.: Anorectal gonococcal infection. Ann. Intern. Med., 86:340, 1977.
54. Catterall, R. D.: Anorectal gonorrhoea. Proc. R. Soc. Med., 55:871, 1962.
55. Owen, R. L., and Hill, J. L.: Rectal and pharyngeal gonorrhea in homosexual men. J. Am. Med. Assoc., 220:1315, 1972.
56. Lebedeff, D. A., and Hochman, E. B.: Rectal gonorrhea in men: diagnosis and treatment. Ann. Intern. Med., 92:463, 1980.
57. Kilpatrick, Z. M.: Gonorrheal proctitis. N. Engl. J. Med., 287:967, 1972.
58. Scott, J., and Stone, A. H.: Some observations on the diagnosis of rectal gonorrhoea in both sexes using a selective culture medium. Br. J. Vener. Dis., 42:103, 1966.
59. Goodman, K. J.: Radiologic findings in anorectal gonorrhea. Gastrointest. Radiol., 3:223, 1978.
60. Henderson, R. G., Pankerton, H., and Moore, L. T.: Histoplasma capsulatum as a cause of chronic ulcerative enteritis. J. Am. Med. Assoc., 118:885, 1942.
61. Goodwin, R. A., Jr., and Des Prez, R. M.: State of the art: Histoplasmosis. Am. Rev. Respir. Dis., 117:929, 1978.
62. Annamunthodo, H.: Rectal lymphogranuloma venereum in Jamaica. Dis. Colon Rectum, 4:17, 1961.
63. Grace, A. W.: Anorectal lymphogranuloma venereum. J. Am. Med. Assoc., 122:74, 1943.
64. Abrams, A. J.: Lymphogranuloma venereum. J. Am. Med. Assoc., 205:199, 1968.
65. Schachter, J., et al.: Lymphogranuloma venereum: I. Comparison of the Frei test, complement fixation test, and isolation of the agent. J. Infect. Dis., 120:372, 1969.
66. Tamura, M.: Acute ulcerative colitis associated with cytomegalic inclusion virus. Arch. Pathol., 96:164, 1973.
67. Healy, G. R.: Laboratory diagnosis of amebiasis. Bull. NY Acad. Med., 47:478, 1971.
68. Juniper, K.: Amoebiasis. Clin. Gastroenterol., 7:3, 1978.
69. Healy, G. R., and Kraft, S. C.: The indirect hemagglutination test for amebiasis in patients with inflammatory bowel disease. Am. J. Dig. Dis., 17:97, 1972.
70. Kotcher, E., Miranda, M., and de Salgado, V. G.: Correlation of clinical, parasitological, and serological data of individuals infected with Entamoeba histolytica. Gastroenterology, 58:388, 1970.
71. Powell, S. J., and Wilmot, A. J.: Ulcerative post-dysenteric colitis. Gut, 7:438, 1966.
72. Quinn, T. C., et al.: The etiology of anorectal infections in homosexual men. Am. J. Med., 71:395, 1981.
73. Quinn, T. C., et al.: The polymicrobial origin of intestinal infections in homosexual men. N. Engl. J. Med., 309:576, 1983.
74. Kline, J. C., et al.: The relationship of reactions to complications in the radiation therapy of cancer of the cervix. Radiology, 105:413, 1972.
75. DeCosse, J. J., et al.: The natural history and management of radiation induced injury of the gastrointestinal tract. Ann. Surg., 170:369, 1969.
76. Novak, J. M., et al.: Effects of radiation on the human gastrointestinal tract. J. Clin. Gastroenterol., 1:9, 1979.
77. Wellwood, J. M., and Jackson, B. T.: The intestinal complications of radiotherapy. Br. J. Surg., 60:814, 1973.
78. Strockbine, N. F., Hancock, J. E., and Fletcher, G. H.: Complications in 831 patients with squamous cell carcinoma of the intact uterine cervix treated with 3,000 rads or more whole pelvis irradiation. A. J. R., 108:293, 1970.
79. Mason, G. R., Dietrich, P. C. H., Friedland, G. W., and Hanks, G. E.: The radiological findings in radiation-induced enteritis and colitis: A review of 30 cases. Clin. Radiol., 21:232, 1970.
80. Fagin, R. R., and Kirsner, J. B.: Ischemic diseases of the colon. Adv. Intern. Med., 17:343, 1971.
81. Williams, L. F., Jr.: Vascular insufficiency of the bowels. D. M., August:1, 1970.
82. Marston, A., Pheils, M. T., Thomas, M. L., and Morrison, B. C.: Ischaemic colitis. Gut, 7:1, 1966.
83. Miller, W. T., et al.: Ischemic colitis with gangrene. Radiology, 94:291, 1970.
84. Kilpatrick, Z. M., Farman, J., Yesner, R., and Spiro, H. M.: Ischemic proctitis. J. Am. Med. Assoc., 205:74, 1968.
85. Tedesco, F. J.: Clindamycin-associated colitis: Review of the clinical spectrum of 47 cases. Am. J. Dig. Dis., 21:26, 1976.
86. Bartlett, J. G., and Gorbach, S. L.: Pseudomembranous enterocolitis (antibiotic-related colitis). Adv. Intern. Med., 22:455, 1977.
87. Kappas, A., et al.: Diagnosis of pseudomembranous colitis. Br. Med. J., 1:675, 1978.
88. Mogg, G. A. G., et al.: Antibiotic-associated colitis—A review of 66 cases. Br. J. Surg., 66:738, 1979.
89. Price, A. B., and Davies, D. R.: Pseudomembranous colitis. J. Clin. Pathol., 30:1, 1977.
90. Slater, D., Corbett, C., Underwood, J., and Richards, D.: Rapid frozen section diagnosis of pseudomembranous colitis (letter). Lancet, 1:10, 1981.
91. Shimkin, P. M., and Link, R. J.: Pseudomembranous colitis: A consideration in the barium enema differential diagnosis of acute generalized ulcerative colitis. Br. J. Radiol., 46:437, 1973.

11 · Psychosocial Aspects of Ulcerative Colitis and Crohn's Disease

DOUGLAS A. DROSSMAN, M.D.

The Challenge

Psychosocial factors are acknowledged to be important influences in patients with chronic ulcerative colitis (CUC) or Crohn's disease, but for decades the challenge has been twofold: to determine *how* these factors contribute to our understanding of these disorders, and, particularly for physicians, how this information can be applied to clinical care. Consider the following case report:

> Ms. G., a 29-year-old single woman, has had Crohn's disease for 15 years, with frequent hospitalizations because of rectovaginal fistulas and perianal abscesses. She claims these complications limit her social activities and she is reluctant to reveal her condition to others. Despite clinical remissions for years at a time, she does not seek employment and remains on full medical disability. Because her prognosis is uncertain, she fears that she will never be able to hold a job. Her latest admission was for new symptoms of epigastric pain, nausea, and vomiting.
>
> The current medical evaluation was unchanged from recent previous outpatient visits, except she had lost 5 kg over 6 weeks. Radiologic studies showed continued involvement of the jejunum, ileum, and colon, but no evidence of disease progression or complications such as obstruction or abscess. Her condition improved slightly with increased doses of prednisone and sulfasalazine. After several days of treatment she was told she could leave the hospital, but then the symptoms worsened.
>
> The resident physician told Ms. G. that no more hospital treatment was needed. Her mother, who maintained bedside vigil, angrily questioned the resident's decision and requested another physician be consulted. Her son (who also has Crohn's disease) was once sent home only to be readmitted for emergency bowel resection and drainage of an abscess. The physician carefully explained to the mother the reasons for discharging her daughter, and said that she could get another opinion if she chose. Trying to help the patient, the physician rebuked the mother for "smothering" the daughter, that is, not permitting her to make her own decisions.
>
> Over the next few days the pain worsened and prednisone was increased. Ms. G. became tearful, slept and ate poorly, and continued to lose weight, though physical examination and laboratory studies were unchanged. Central hyperalimentation was begun but was complicated by hemomediastinum during the catheter line placement. Over the next few weeks, Ms. G. increasingly requested narcotics and extra bedside care

that led to repeated confrontations with the nurses who viewed her as demanding, dependent, and immature. A psychiatric consult was requested.

The psychiatric interview yielded additional important information. Ms. G.'s parents had been divorced for 15 years. Early in the illness, her hospitalizations brought the parents together to care for her. Her father died of cirrhosis one year ago with symptoms of pain, nausea, and vomiting, and she harbored ambivalent feelings about his death. The previous good relationship with him deteriorated when his progressive alcohol consumption led to frequent verbal and physical abuse. Eight weeks prior to admission, on the one year anniversary of his death, she began having recurrent dreams of him, and soon thereafter her present symptoms began.

The psychiatrist made a diagnosis of unresolved grief that was manifest as a somatizing clinical depression, and recommended a tricyclic antidepressant. He believed the patient was intelligent though emotionally immature and, like many patients with inflammatory bowel disease (he had been taught), had little insight or capacity to work through the psychodynamic aspects of her condition. The mother's overinvolvement compensated for her guilt for bearing two children with this disease. The mother-daughter interdependence ("enmeshment") maintained the patient in an emotionally regressed state. Supportive psychotherapy was also recommended.

Several questions typically arise: Are the present symptoms "functional" or "organic?" What drugs (steroids, narcotics, or antidepressants) should she take? When would you stop hyperalimentation and discharge her? Should she be on disability? Is the patient's psychological state a cause or effect of the disease? Could the "stresses" of the previous divorce and the deteriorating relationship with the father contribute to the onset of illness? If so, how? Does a unique personality exist among patients with inflammatory bowel disease (IBD)? Finally, how should the physician achieve a better working relationship with the patient and the mother?

To effectively answer the questions in this complex case history, the physician must be familiar with the psychosocial literature and then be able to apply this information in treatment. Through the literature review in the first part of this chapter, evidence will be presented to show that illness is best understood as the *interaction* of biologic, psychologic, and sociocultural processes. The application of this framework to patients with IBD makes good clinical sense because it is unlikely that specific etiologies, if or when they are identified, will be sufficient to explain the timing of disease onset, the experience of the illness, or the patient's clinical response. The second part of this chapter will show how to elicit, establish a priority, and incorporate this information in the treatment to obtain an optimal response. Finally, through use of this more comprehensive understanding of illness, the case of Ms. G. will be discussed.

Literature Review

Our present understanding of the relationships between psychosocial phenomena and disease is incomplete. Psychosocial data are more difficult to obtain and validate than biologic data. Table 11-1 lists some of the methodologic problems. Because psychosocial and environmental influences on the individual's behavior and gut function are complex, completely controlled studies are beyond present capability. Clinicians are responsible for evaluating the total context of the patient's illness, however, even if the validity of the clinical data is not well established. Subtle and complex psychologic information may be obtained through clinical training and experience, but this information is not easily verified by experimental technique. With this understanding I will attempt to answer the previous questions through review of the research studies and by reporting my own observations and those of experts.

What do Doctors Think?

Through the mail, a random sample of 1,000 members of the American Gastroenterological Association was taken to determine their knowledge of, attitudes toward, and practice patterns regarding IBD.[1] Over 70% responded; 53.4% were in clinical practice, 33.3% in academic practice, and 11.1% were in training. Of those who responded, 14% of their patients had IBD (6.8% UC, 7.1% Crohn's disease).

In general, these physicians agreed that psychosocial factors did not contribute to the etiology or pathogenesis of IBD but did contribute to the clinical exacerbation of symptoms (more so in UC than in Crohn's disease). Their belief (from clinical experience) in the role of psycho-

TABLE 11-1. *Methodologic Problems in Behavioral Research.*

A. Behavioral Research in General
  1. Lack of agreement as to terminology, conceptualization, and research design among the behavioral disciplines.
  2. Difficulties in obtaining relevant psychosocial data:
     a. Behavioral factors are subjective—cannot easily be defined or measured (e.g., pain, stress, social support, and illness behavior).
     b. Information from questionnaires or interviews may not be reliable or valid (e.g., do not account for denial and social compliance).
     c. Information from physician case reports is not easily verified by experimental technique (retrospective, uncontrolled, may be biased).
  3. Inability to control for numerous psychosocial variables.
  4. Retrospective data (therefore, association does not mean causation).
B. Related to Inflammatory Bowel Disease
  1. Early studies were unable to distinguish between CUC and Crohn's disease.
  2. Assessments made without healthy or medical comparison groups.
  3. Symptom severity or illness chronicity not considered as confounding variables.
  4. Conclusions erroneously obtained through improper use of investigative instruments (e.g., use of unskilled interviewers or questionnaires to obtain sensitive or deep-seated psychologic data).

social factors in IBD exceeded what they learned from the scientific literature. Of interest, older physicians placed more importance on psychosocial factors in the etiology-pathogenesis and exacerbation of these disorders than did younger physicians. All responders did not believe their IBD patients had a characteristic personality style, and the psychosocial impact of IBD was considered no more or less than with other chronic disease (such as diabetes mellitus or arthritis).

Regarding treatment, personal psychosocial support was provided over 75% of the time, and involvement of the family was considered an important part of patient care. Educational resources (brochures, films) and support groups (the National Foundation for Ileitis and Colitis [NFIC] and ostomy clubs) were frequently recommended. These physicians were moderately interested in furthering their education and developing clinical skills in this area.

The data suggest the following:

1. Physicians consider psychosocial factors to be an important influence on IBD symptoms and apply this understanding in their practice.
2. Further scientific inquiry is needed to explain the discrepancy between what physicians experience (that is, a greater role for psychosocial factors) and what they have read in the literature.
3. Physicians do not consider their patients with IBD to be psychologically unique or different from patients with other chronic diseases.
4. Older physicians ascribe greater importance to psychosocial factors in these illnesses. Whether this reflects the benefit of experience, or results from educational beliefs prevalent in the past cannot be determined.

Relationship of Psychosocial Factors to Symptom Onset and Exacerbation

Is there evidence that antecedent psychosocial events lead to disease onset or exacerbation? Support for this relationship comes from several types of investigation.

ANIMAL STUDIES With animal research, confounding social and biologic factors are minimized; animals are more biologically similar and more likely to exhibit inbred behavioral patterns. Altering the social environment of animals effects mortality rates and the incidence of disease. For example, physical restraint or premature weaning may result in "stress ulcers" in rats.[2,3] Chronic gastrointestinal lesions, primarily gastroduodenitis, were reported in 11/19 Rhesus monkeys either restrained in chairs or placed in a conditioned anxiety situation, and two of these monkeys developed a wasting syndrome and chronic colitis.[4]

Of special interest to this discussion is the social setting of the spontaneous development of fatal colitis in 4 Siamang gibbons.[5] Six weeks after the death of her mate, a previously healthy female died with extensive ulceration of the colon and rectum. Within 5 days of being introduced into a cage containing a resident gibbon of the opposite sex who was acclimated to the environment, the three other gibbons developed bloody diarrhea and died. In each case, the resident animal indicated behaviorally that the cage was his territory. Bacterial cultures were negative and the resident and adjacent animals did not develop the disease. In an accompanying editorial by Engel,[6] the stress was interpreted to be the disruption of the supporting aspects of the environment with an inability of the organism to cope. A similarity to the psychosocial setting of the onset of human ulcerative colitis was noted by Engel, who previously had studied these issues in his medical patients.[7]

An animal model to study the effects of social or environmental change on the development of IBD is desirable and now may be possible. The cotton-topped tamarin, a New World monkey, was noted to develop colitis and also to have a high incidence of colon carcinoma.[8] Some evidence exists that these diseases may increase when the animal is captured, and behavioral as well as biologic influences may contribute. A field study of a related tamarin species suggests that in the feral state these animals exist in a communal social unit consisting of one breeding female, several nonbreeding females, and 1 to 3 reproductively active males who care for the offspring.[9] Therefore, the routine of placing the tamarin species in cages containing one adult male and female would require social readjustment. If it is possible to control for dietary and other physical effects associated with captivity, then this possible disruption of the social environment might be a natural stress, thereby establishing a behavioral model for the study of colitis.[10]

Animal research demonstrates that social alteration can lead to gastrointestinal end-organ damage. The significance of this research to the development of chronic colitis is still under question. While controlled behavioral studies of animals have not been done, informal observation suggests an association between environmental changes requiring social adjustment and the development of colitis in the biologically predisposed host.

EPIDEMIOLOGIC STUDIES IN HUMANS The goal of epidemiologic research is to identify factors that discriminate populations by minimizing the effects of confounding variables statistically or in the study design. The importance of social structure as a factor in human disease susceptibility has been demonstrated in the epidemiologic literature.[11] Persons with marginal status in society who experience social disorganization are more susceptible to a variety of medical disorders. Major changes in a person's lifestyle have been shown to correlate with the subsequent incidence of illness or injury.[12] Similarly, a high pressure job (air traffic controller) was associated with a higher prevalence of hypertension and twice the prevalence of peptic ulcer disease compared to other military workers (second-class airmen).[13]

Few group differences have been found between patients with CUC and those with Crohn's disease. Both diseases are more prevalent among Western or Caucasian than Eastern or noncaucasian populations, urban than rural dwellers, Western (Ashkenazi) urbanized Jews than Eastern (Oriental or Sephardim) Jews or non-Jews; IBD also runs in families (see also Chap. 1).[14]

It is possible that cultural factors may contribute to these differences. It has been proposed that the higher frequency of IBD among Jews may be related to the influence of the strong family structures rather than genetic factors, giving as evidence even higher prevalences of IBD among other religious groups such as Plymouth Brethren who have strong family organizations.[15] The relative influences of environmental factors, genetic factors, and methodologic artifact have not yet been determined.

Few studies have been made regarding the association of psychosocial factors with the onset or exacerbation of inflammatory bowel disease. Of interest is the first report of ulcerative colitis developing in Bedouin Arabs who moved from their nomadic life into government housing,[16] suggesting that the stresses of modern living or the change of lifestyle influenced the development of the disorder.

Though epidemiologic studies are methodologically sound and reliable, the psychosocial content is limited. For example, one study concluded that IBD patients were less likely to report stressful situations preceding hospitalization than patients with irritable bowel syndrome; in fact, the responses of the IBD patients were more similar to the nondisease control population.[17] The limitations of obtaining psychosocial data by lay investigators through a single structured interview have been acknowledged. Furthermore, a selection bias may undermine the validity of these results. While most IBD patients eventually see physicians, most with irritable bowel do not, and those that do appear to have a greater tendency to report complaints.[18] Survey questionnaires and brief interviews are used to compare groups, and it is up to the clinician to determine whether the group under study is appropriate. The study instruments used cannot capture how the information is communicated (nonverbally, by intonation, or with consideration of patient denial or minimization), or whether it is meaningful to the patient. Contextual cues can only be picked up by experienced clinicians.

PSYCHIATRIC/PSYCHOLOGIC DATA. Psychiatrists first observed the psychosocial aspects of IBD among patients referred to them for psychoanalysis or therapy. Karush reviewed the data relating to ulcerative colitis[7,19-24] and the patients were believed to have conflicts relating to an intensely dependent relationship with a controlling and dominating parent (usually the mother) or other key figure. A real or threatened disruption of the dependent relationship (marriage, death of the dominant person, parental disapproval of the patient, or the assumption of greater responsibility or independence), or a fear of failure provoked symptoms. Bleeding and diarrhea were sometimes reported to occur within 24 hours of the stressful event.[7,21]

The conclusions drawn from these data are limited by the selection criteria (patients referred for psychotherapy/analysis), their retrospective nature, and the lack of control/comparison groups. Also, most of the studies were done primarily by psychiatrists at a time when the psychosomatic school of thought was dominant in medical education. Later criticism of the study design was justified, but the authors of the studies were also misunderstood: they did not think psychologic factors caused IBD but contributed to its onset in the biologically predisposed individual.[26] The misconceptions about psychogenic causes of disease probably had more of an effect on physician training and attitudes about psychosomatic research than was warranted. The observations of these skilled clinicians are not to be ignored, but considered for their value among selected patients.

In later years, attempts were made to improve research design via rated interviews, standardized questionnaires, and, sometimes, controlled studies. Table 11-2 shows retrospective studies of at least moderately adequate research design that examine the association of psychosocial events with the onset or exacerbation of IBD symptoms.[27-35] Though varied in method and content, the studies support the contention that stressful life events precede illness onset or exacerbation. Similar research on other diseases suggests that this phenomenon is not unique to IBD.

Mediating Mechanisms

Just how antecedent environmental events influence disease susceptibility or illness onset is not yet established. Immunohistochemical mapping of brain-gut peptides may further our understanding of the associations between the environment, altered psychologic states, and physiologic responses of the intestine. Certain peptides such as the enkephalins, vasoactive intestinal peptide, neurotensin, bombesin, secretin, cholecystokinin, and substance P are also localized in many areas of the brain. Growing evidence exists that these and other peptides may produce different effects on perception, memory, and emotion, based on their location (such as mood-limbic system pain control-periaqueductal gray).[36] Furthermore, the location of these peptide receptors in the gut, on lymphocytes, and other organ systems will probably provide the basis for the observed relationships between behavioral influences, intestinal function, and susceptibility to disease (see also Chap. 7).

Animal research in psychoneuroendocrinology and psychoimmunology supports the prospect that environmental factors influence disease susceptibility via the central nervous system.[37] For example, "stress" is associated with alterations of humoral and cellular immune mechanisms both in laboratory animals and humans. Decreased responsiveness to mitogens and antigens, reduced lymphocyte-mediated cytotoxicity, reduced delayed hypersensitivity, diminished skin graft rejection and graft-vs-host reactivity, and suppressed antibody response have all been observed after stress-inducing experiments. The hypothalamus may interface between environmental input to the brain and peripheral regulatory systems that include immunity, endocrine, and neurotransmitter release.[38]

Central nervous system-mediated alterations in immune function may, in turn, affect host susceptibility to disease. Benzodiazepine receptors have been found on monocytes, suggesting a close association between the regulation of mood and immunity.[39] Behavioral conditioning may affect immune function. In one study, a neutral stimulus (saccharin-flavored drink)

TABLE 11-2. *Association of Significant Life Events with Onset or Exacerbation of Inflammatory Bowel Disease.*

Study	Patients	Method	Percent with Life Events	$P < 0.05^*$	Types of Events
Controlled					
Feldman[27] 1967	34 UC 74 GI	Psychiatric interview	12 (onset) 44 (exacerbation)	− +	Not mentioned
Feldman[28] 1967	19 CD 74 GI	Psychiatric interview	0 (onset) 11 (exacerbation)	− −	Not mentioned
Hislop[29] 1971	50 IBD 50 normal	Interview?	94	+	Birth, death (actual, symbolic, or threatened)
Fava[30] 1976	20 UC 20 IBD 20 Appendicitis	Life Events Scale (Paykel)	1.35[†]	+	Death, divorce, illness, leaving home
Uncontrolled					
Prugh[31] 1951	16 UC (Pediatrics)	Retro/Prospective interview; play therapy	94		Leaving home, punishment, death
Whybrow[32] 1968	39 CD	Chart review	64		Death, marital discord, exams, pregnancy
Ford[33] 1969	17 CD	Psychiatric interviews	82		Illness-relative, loss of self-esteem, conflict
McKegney[34] 1970	21 UC 19 CD	Semistructured interview	86 (UC) 68 (CD)		Death, ill health, life change
Cohn[35] 1970	12 CD	Interview, testing	92		Independence, death, interpersonal conflict

*Significant difference when compared to control group.
†Reported mean number of life events per patient preceding hospitalization.
Key: UC = ulcerative colitis; GI = gastrointestinal; CD = Crohn's disease; IBD = inflammatory bowel disease.

paired with the immunosuppressive effects of cyclophosphamide later produced an attenuated immune response to the drinking solution alone.[40] Later, this conditioned response model was reported to delay the development of murine lupus erythematosus.[41]

In humans, change in in vitro immune function after the effects ("stress") of space flight was reported in the Apollo astronauts.[41] A prospectively studied group of 26 recently bereaved spouses showed impaired in vitro T cell function when compared to a control group, as measured by response to phytohemagglutinin and concanavalin A.[43] Altered immunity might explain the poor health of widows and widowers the year following the death of their spouses.[44]

Recent studies suggest that the effect of stress on immune function and disease susceptibility may be mediated by natural opioid peptides. Opiate drugs or endogenous opioids retard or enhance tumor growth, depending on the agent and route of administration.[45] In vitro studies demonstrate that in the opioid response to footshock stress in rats, natural killer (NK) cell function is suppressed. The same stress-reduced median survival time and percent survival are seen in tumor injection experiments (rat mammary adenocarcinoma), and the effect can be blocked by pre-stress injection of naltrexone, an opiate antagonist.[46] To say, however, that the NK suppressive effects are responsible for decreased survival in stress-induced tumor growth is premature, because interrelated hormonal and neurotransmitter mechanisms may influence this activity (Fig. 11-1).

These in vitro, animal and human observational data do suggest that environmental changes or the organisms' responses to change influence physiologic function and disease susceptibility through effects on neurotransmitter, endocrine, and immune systems. Because the physiologic changes are small, the magnitude of the clinical effects awaits further investigation.

Psychosocial Observations Regarding Patients with Inflammatory Bowel Disease

CHARACTERISTIC PERSONALITY FEATURES. Asked to describe patients with chronic disorders such as IBD, physicians remarkably agree about their behavior, whether these features have diagnostic value or influence disease pathogenesis or not. A major concern of research during the psychoanalytically dominated era of psychosomatic medicine (1920 to 1955) was psychosomatic specificity, that is, whether specific psychologic features were associated with, and necessary for, the development of a particular disease. Beginning with the belief that distinct personality profiles existed,[47] later work was directed at the role for unconscious conflicts in the onset of disease. Based on psychoanalytic study of medical patients, Alexander and his associates identified seven diseases, including ulcerative colitis and peptic ulcer, that were associated with particular psychologic profiles.[48]

The antecedent conflict for patients who develop ulcerative colitis was said to be between the wish to carry out certain obligations and the unwillingness or inability to do so. Disease onset or exacerbation was believed to occur under circumstances when the conflict would be activated; in this case, when the patient was required to accomplish something and felt unprepared. In psychodynamic terms, the patient regresses to the time of the first environmental demand for accomplishment, the period of bowel control development. At this stage of life, the child perceives bowel function and stools as achievements; excretion is both giving up a cherished possession, and an accomplishment. In the biologically susceptible person, the conflict and this regression were believed to activate parasympathetic pathways in the colon, the physiologic effect then being to alter bowel motility (producing diarrhea), while also breaking the protective mucosal barrier and making it vulnerable to digestion and bacterial invasion (with ulceration). A biologic predisposition (X factor) was thought necessary: "some specific local somatic factor may be responsible for the fact that in some patients anal regression produces ulceration in the bowels."[48]

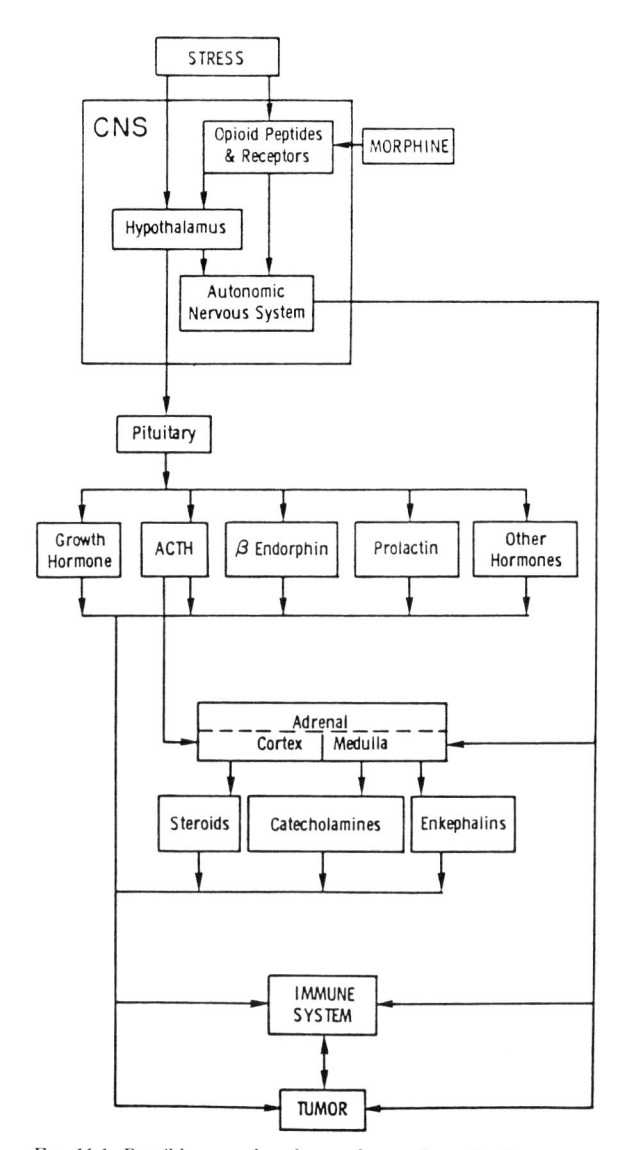

FIG. 11-1. Possible neural and neurohumoral mechanisms mediating the effect of stress on immune function and tumor susceptibility.

Further elaboration of the psychodynamic hypothesis occurred when the research shifted from intrapsychic conflicts to problems with interpersonal relationships. Ulcerative colitis patients were described as dependent, immature, overly attached to parents or parent substitutes, and overly sensitive to interpersonal rejection. Relationship difficulties were manifest either as extreme dependence and unrealistic demands on others, or as reluctance to develop any trusting relationships.[24] Illness exacerbation would occur when a key relationship was lost because of separation or bereavement. Thus, it was concluded that the personality structure and intrapsychic conflicts could cause these people to evolve to certain relationships or gravitate toward certain kinds of life situations, disruption of which may be followed by onset or relapse of the disease. Given this construct, it was recommended that the physician establish a predictable and consistent relationship with such patients.[25]

According to more recent psychosomatic literature, patients with certain medical disorders have difficulty expressing thoughts, moods, or fantasies. Alexithymia, a condition literally meaning "no words for mood," is reported to distinguish patients with inflammatory bowel disease and certain other "psychosomatic" disorders from other medical patients.[49] The term is applied to patients observed to have a concrete cognitive style ("La pensée operatoire"), minimal ability to fantasize, and resistance to traditional psychotherapeutic intervention.[50] Physicians may relate this concept to their experience with patients who appear passive, emotionally unexpressive, and fail to see the connection between their symptoms and any feeling of distress.[51] Whether this concept enhances our understanding of these patients or merely describes patients with chronic disease, is open to further study.[52]

These retrospective reports cannot determine how specific personality profiles are related to IBD. A prospectively designed controlled study, beginning early in the subject's personality development and continuing until disease onset, is necessary. Although there have been attempts to validate the specificity of the personality features,[49,53] the methodology and results are not sufficient to be convincing. This question is less important now, because our concept of illness has moved away from cause-and-effect relationships toward a multidetermined illness system. Earlier reports, by focusing primarily on intrapsychic issues and interpersonal transactions, presented a perspective that was too simplistic. Little attention was paid to influences such as social support, coping, and other sociocultural phenomena. Nevertheless, the work provided a foundation for future study by acknowledging the role for early psychosocial influences on the patient's experience of the illness and susceptibility to disease. Furthermore, it underscores the need to carry out multidisciplinary collaborative work in the behavioral and biologic sciences.

PSYCHIATRIC DIAGNOSES. In the last 25 years, standardized psychologic tests and interviews have been employed to make psychiatric diagnoses. Also, improved medical diagnostic techniques now permit patients with ulcerative colitis and Crohn's disease to be studied separately and compared to other medical populations. A review of 20 Crohn's disease studies concluded that these patients exhibited personality characteristics similar to those with "neurotic, psychosomatic, and other chronic medical conditions," and about a third had psychiatric morbidity (primarily anxiety/depression).[54] Psychiatric morbidity increased with the chronicity and severity of the disease. Consecutive outpatients having CUC or Crohn's disease, and a group of other chronic medical patients were compared on a structured interview and psychometric tests.[55,56] No difference was found in the number of psychiatric disorders among patients with ulcerative colitis, but significantly more (almost half) of the Crohn's group had psychiatric illness, predominantly depression. No relationship between psychiatric morbidity and activity of the disease was found. Psychiatric diagnoses were generally overlooked by the physicians, yet the patients with the psychiatric diagnosis were no more impaired. It cannot be determined from the design of these studies whether the psychiatric disorders precede or are secondary to the disease.

Standardized psychologic scales and structured interviews have not confirmed the psychiatric case data. Self-report research scales show IBD patients to be normal or "hypernormal" compared to other medical patients, and brief, structured interviews fail to identify the range of psychopathology previously reported. On this basis, some have rejected the psychodynamic hypotheses. While offering reliable data, however, the standardized psychologic instruments are not sufficient to evaluate the psychologic information elicited by experienced clinicians. Most of the self-report methods used do not take into consideration issues of denial, minimization, or social compliance. If the psychodynamic formulation is correct, then it is to be expected that these patients would be unwilling to disclose personal information before a trusting relationship is established.[57]

The possibility for such a construct is supported by one study that compared family perceptions and reported differences between IBD patients and their nonaffected siblings.[58] While the patients and their parents perceived an idealized family without conflict, the siblings reported disharmony. The parents perceived the patients as compliant, neither unusual or problematic, and the siblings as rebellious and less accepting of parental values. The siblings were actively resolving identity issues while the patients continued to please and meet the expectations of others. If it is true that the patient's identity depends on approval by and agreement with key figures, the ability to report "unacceptable" thoughts and feelings is limited by parental expectations. In the McMahon study, short self-report tests did not distinguish between patients and siblings, though some of the Minnesota Multiphasic Personality Inventory (MMPI) subscales that take into account patient denial were significantly abnormal. These MMPI results have been replicated elsewhere,[33] and suggest that IBD patients do not differ from patients with other chronic medical disorders;[59] IBD has no distinguishing psychologic features.

In an effort to evaluate research for clinical purposes, the physician must assess whether the information is relevant to the question being asked and whether the method used is appropriate. The inconsistencies obtained from the varying methodologies must, therefore, be understood as different elaborations on the total psychosocial understanding, rather than as evidence that confirms or refutes data obtained by different methods.

Impact of the Disorder

All illness requires psychologic and social adjustment. For the IBD patient these include: (1) coping with chronic or recurrent symptoms such as pain, nausea, diarrhea, incontinence, or the effects of malnutrition; (2) working through fears of possible surgical therapy, early death, cancer, or the unknown; (3) adjusting to the physical changes and psychologic effects of perineal disease, ileostomy/colostomy, or short bowel syndrome; and (4) adjusting to possible financial hardship or limited ability to work or engage in usual social activities. The longer an illness is present, the more adjustments are required, giving the physician a greater role in providing emotional support, education, and counseling. To illustrate what the physician should do, this section discusses how psychosocial factors influence the individual's experience and "illness behaviors," and then discusses the effects of chronic IBD on the patient, family, and society.

PSYCHOSOCIAL INFLUENCES ON THE EXPERIENCE OF ILLNESS Throughout life, personality, family, and society shape an individual's attitudes, expectations, and behaviors. These features influence how the patient experiences and copes with the symptoms, uses medical facilities, and complies with treatment. Over time, the disease itself will contribute to how future illness events are experienced and reported to family, friends, and physicians.

How symptoms are perceived, evaluated, and responded to are designated "illness behaviors."[60] For example, the patient with Crohn's disease who awakens with abdominal pain may not go to the physician if he or she has previously experienced the symptom without consequence, is worried about losing time from work, grew up in a family where attention to illness was minimized, or believes that complaining is a "weakness." Another patient with the same symptom may readily seek medical assistance if he has not experienced the symptom before, perceives it as potentially dangerous, is seeking disability, has established a dependent relationship with the physician, or comes from a family in which greater attention was paid to illness. These factors influence why some patients are considered stoics and others "hypochondriacs."

Social and cultural factors will influence how symptoms are experienced, perceived, and communicated. In China, mental illness is stigmatized and patients with minor psychiatric problems present with physical complaints.[61] Variations in pain behavior among first and second generation ethnic groups have been observed;[62] Jews and Italians more dramatically responded to pain, the Irish denied their symptoms, and the Anglo-Saxon Protestants were stoic. In Western cultures, women with minor complaints are more likely to see physicians,[63] perhaps because males have traditionally been encouraged to be more stoic. When a symptom aberration, such as diarrhea among Mexican Americans in the southwestern United States, is widespread, the recognition of a "disease" with this symptom may not be considered.[64] Awareness of this and similar factors can help to reconcile the great variability that can exist between the patient's symptom reports and the morphologic findings.

While some people with active disease ignore their symptoms, psychologic and social factors influence others with minimal or no disease activity to amplify their symptoms. Motivating "benefits" from the "sick role" include exemption from work or family obligations, avoidance of stressful situations, and gratification of dependency needs by a physician.[65]

Certain personality patterns, psychiatric disorders, and social influences underlie abnormal illness behavior.[66] For example, *hypochondriacal patients* are preoccupied with bodily functions and magnify numerous seemingly innocuous complaints into worries about serious illness. Persistent complaining maintains their self-esteem and provides a means of social communication. *People with histrionic personalities* also develop or amplify their bodily complaints in situations that in others produce mental distress. These patients strongly depend on others for gratification and support, and will readily visit physicians during these periods. *Depressed patients* will exacerbate their physical complaints, and any weight loss may be caused by lack of interest in eating rather than disease activity. To make rational diagnostic and treatment decisions in such cases, the physician must evaluate these psychologic factors along with the biomedical factors.

Once the disorder is manifest, the patient will respond psychologically to the experience and adapt. How the physician assists in this process is crucial to the patient's psychologic well-being and clinical course. The chronically ill individual will often regress and behave in a dependent manner. Continued complaints and the increased caretaking needs may tax family, friends, and physician, all of whom may feel unable to give enough emotional or medical assistance. Other patients will resist the help of others to avoid acknowledging their imposed dependence. The physician must not only respond to these behaviors, realizing the patient's best interests, but also work to reconcile the difficulties among the various individuals. Most often the problems are worked out and the patient learns to cope. If the patient has limited psychologic capacities, if the disorder is particularly incapacitating, or if family relationships are unstable, more physician and ancillary effort (social service, psychologic counseling, and peer support groups such as NFIC) will be required, however, to achieve a satisfactory adjustment.

EFFECT OF INFLAMMATORY BOWEL DISEASE ON THE PATIENT. An area of recent investigation involves assessing the effects of disease on the quality of life and the patient's psychosocial adjustment. Few studies of this type of outcome for IBD patients have been done, but the results are favorable. A large series of ulcerative colitis patients (n = 122) from Copenhagen with a disease duration median of 10 years reported good to excellent outcomes.[67] Fewer than 20% reported sexual problems, family difficulties, or treatment for mental disorders, and over 90% had no work restriction and engaged in moderate to high levels of social and physical activities; the colitis patients did not differ from a group of patients with acute medical problems. Over 90% of Crohn's disease patients reported a fair to good quality of life 13 years later.[68] Patients who did not have surgical therapy, or who had nonrecurrent or localized disease, fared better.

Crohn's disease patients who underwent surgical treatment reported postoperative improvement in interpersonal relationships, recreational capability, sexual function, and body image, with an overall quality of life similar to the previous studies.[69] The outcome was better among patients who had bowel resection rather than bypass, who did *not* have an ileostomy, and who did not have recurrence of disease. In particular, ostomy patients reported a significantly lower adjustment in overall quality of life and body image, but these ratings were improved over the preoperative period. These results are not surprising; those with more severe disease and, therefore, a poorer quality of life, often require surgical intervention and tend to benefit from it.

Besides disease activity, it is important to determine the behavioral factors that are associated with the quality of life. A patient's successful adaptation to Crohn's disease has been shown in one study to be more closely related to certain personality factors than to the severity of the disease itself.[70] Successful adjustment to chronic illness requires the patient to shift from seeing himself as "sick" to seeing himself as "different."[71] The patient must "continue to affirm himself, collaborate in his care through learning, endure certain pathologic and technical givens, and actively negotiate the bargain for his needs."[72] From my personal experience, the best adjustment to the disorder occurs in the patient who accomplishes a degree of control over his illness through education, who participates in the treatment, and who commits himself to a reliable working relationship with the doctor. To accomplish this, the physician must educate the patient and permit him to make decisions, thereby minimizing patient anxiety about lack of control.

Supporting this is a recent survey of a local National Foundation for Ileitis and Colitis (NFIC) group that assessed patients' psychologic adjustment to inflammatory bowel disease.[73] The more information a patient had about IBD, the better he or she reported adapting to living with the disease. Better adjustment occurred among patients who: (1) thought the information they received was useful, (2) believed that being informed about IBD provided a sense of control by preparing them for what was to come, (3) had high self-esteem and social competence, (4) were comfortable talking with their doctors, and (5) felt they had enough time with their doctors. The results must be interpreted in terms of the population studied, however: those who join self-help organizations such as NFIC more often want an active role in managing their disease. Another survey of Crohn's disease patients indicated that successful adaptation to the disease was associated with a perceived sense of control over the disorder and strong social support.[74] It is the patients' beliefs rather than "reality" that determine successful adjustment, and this underscores the importance of trust and communication in the physician-patient interaction.

HEALTH CARE COSTS. IBD also affects the health care system in the community. Hospital costs for inpatients with IBD in the six hospital catchment area of Rochester, N.Y. with a referral base of 1.2 million were compared with other GI disorders, as shown in Table 11-3.[75] More is spent on IBD than on gallbladder operations, appendectomies, or medical treatment of peptic ulcer disease. The total hospital cost for IBD in 1981 was $1,763,484 or approximately $2.50 for each man, woman, and child in the Rochester community. If Rochester, N.Y. is representative, then IBD has a major impact on hospital use and national health costs.

Applying Psychosocial Principles in Diagnosis and Treatment

Most physicians recognize a close association between biologic and psychosocial factors among patients with IBD and, despite certain methodologic limitations of the studies, the scientific literature supports this correlation. Because physicians must address both types of factors in daily medical practice, an integrated treatment approach is needed. This section offers a framework that incorporates rather than separates the biologic and behavioral dimensions of illness, and then makes practical suggestions for patient evaluation and care.

Need for an Integrated Model

The limitations of conceptualizing disease as separate from psychosocial factors is clinically evident. Important life events may precipitate or exacerbate disease, and mood, personality and behavior are altered by the continued presence of disease. The experience of illness and the behaviors of ill people are shaped by intrapsychic determinants, family, culture, and society.

It is helpful to understand these interrelationships through use of a framework, consisting of hierarchical subsystems, that extends from the molecule to the organ, the person, the family, and society.[76] All the subsystems are interrelated so that a change, for example, at the cellular level, such as impaired lymphocyte function from steroid treatment, has the potential of affecting the organ (intestinal abscess), the individual (sepsis/shock), the family (threatened loss of the "breadwinner"), or the community (major health care costs through an extended

TABLE 11-3. *Inpatient Hospital Costs for IBD and Other GI Disorders. ROCHESTER, NEW YORK—1981*

	Inflammatory Bowel Disease	Acute Cholecystitis Surgical Treatment	Acute Cholecystitis No Surgical Treatment	Peptic Ulcer Disease Surgical Treatment	Peptic Ulcer Disease No Surgical Treatment	Appendicitis Surgical Treatment
Number of Cases	320	221	118	285	322	631
Charge/year (million $)	1.763	1.075	0.490	1.949	1.304	1.498
Charge/case ($)	5,510	4,864	4,153	6,839	4,050	2,352

(Modified with permission from Stowe, S. P., et al.: Fiscal and hospital utilization impact of IBD in Rochester New York Community hospitals. Presented at the Second International Symposium for Inflammatory Bowel Disease, Jerusalem, 1985.)

hospitalization). In a clinical setting, information about other systems is obtained from the person via the interview and physical examination. Further evaluation may include gathering data at any other level (culture, tissue biopsy, family interview, or epidemiologic survey).

This model does not increase demands on a physician; rather, it allows him or her to best use what is already known to constitute optimal evaluation and care. Furthermore, by its use, one avoids the pitfalls of trying to decide whether a problem is functional or organic, or of assuming that if the behavioral influences are considered, less attention will be paid to the proper treatment of the disease.

Approach to the Patient

The following guidelines will assist in the assessment of psychosocial factors and behavioral management of patients with IBD. While psychosocial factors contribute to illness in all patients, the degree of physician intervention required will vary. Therefore, these suggestions are to be considered as part of an individualized clinical approach.

DATA GATHERING.
Doctor: How can I help you?
Patient: I developed a flare-up of my Crohn's ... the pain, nausea, and vomiting, when I came back from vacation ... (pause) ... I ...
Doctor: Was the pain like what you had before?
Patient: Yes ... well almost ...
Doctor: Was it made worse by food?
Patient: Yes.
Doctor: Did you have fever? or diarrhea?
Patient: Well yes, I think, but I didn't take my temperature.
Doctor: So you had fever and diarrhea?
Patient: Uh no, well, they were a little loose ... I guess.

In this case, the physician eventually diagnosed partial small bowel obstruction secondary to Crohn's disease. Some relevant information was not elicited by this interview technique, however, and because of the physician's interruptions and use of leading questions the accuracy of the information obtained after the first question is suspect.

The medical history should be obtained by encouraging the patient to tell the story in his or her own way so that the events contributing to the illness unfold naturally;[77] this is called the patient-centered, nondirective interview. Open-ended questions produce the most accurate data. Additional information is obtained with facilitating expressions: "Yes?", "Can you tell me more?", repeating the patient's previous statements, head nodding, or even silence with an expectant look. Avoid rigid (yes-no) questions at first, though they may be used later in the interview to further characterize the symptoms. Never use multiple-choice or leading questions because the patient's desire to comply may bias the responses.

The traditional "medical" and "social" histories should not be separated but elicited together, so the medical problem is described in the context of the psychosocial events surrounding the illness. The setting of symptom onset or exacerbation should always be obtained. At all times, the questions should communicate the physician's willingness to address both biologic and psychologic aspects of the illness:

Patient: I developed a flare-up of my Crohn's ... the pain, nausea, and vomiting, when I came back from vacation ... (pause) ...
Doctor: Yes ... ?
Patient: I was about to start my new position as floor supervisor, and thought I'd take vacation to get prepared ... and then all this happened.
Doctor: Oh, I see ... (pause) ... so then you got sick.
Patient: Yes. I started getting that crampy feeling right here ... and then it got worse after eating. So I knew I'd be obstructed again if I didn't get in to see you.
Doctor: Any other symptoms?
Patient: Well, I felt warm, but didn't take my temperature.
Doctor: What about your bowel pattern?
Patient: They started getting loose when I was on vacation. Now they're slowing down. I haven't gone today.

Here, the association of symptom onset with the beginning of a new job situation was identified. This new information may permit the patient's adjustment to other challenging tasks through self-awareness. If this does not occur, the possibility for treatment strategies (stress reduction techniques, counseling, or job change) may then be considered.

EVALUATING THE DATA. After the history is taken and the physical examination performed, the physician should assess the relative influences of the medical and psychosocial dimensions of the disorder to establish priorities for further evaluation or treatment. It is as inappropriate to obtain psychiatric consultation for a patient with fulminant colitis and toxic megacolon as it is to run tests on a patient with inexplicable symptoms to "rule out disease" without exploring the psychologic context.

The physician should explore the patient's perceptions, fears, and expectations both to understand the illness and to plan an educational and treatment approach:

> Ms. L., a 27-year-old homemaker has had chronic, moderately active ulcerative colitis for 13 years. Colonoscopy on two recent occasions showed high-grade epithelial dysplasia; she refused colectomy. After several unsuccessful attempts to "educate" her as to the reasons for the procedure, the physician asked what she believed would happen if she underwent surgical treatment. For the first time she expressed fear she would be unable to have children, and she and her husband were childless. When these unrealistic fears were addressed, she consented.

A common concern reported by IBD patients is that of fecal incontinence and the associated sense of humiliation. Fears less often reported include loss of physical attractiveness or sexual function, transmitting the disease to others, cancer or premature death, and financial hardship because of inability to work. Such concerns are not always volunteered, and the physician must gain the patient's trust so they can be discussed. Good, nonthreatening questions include: "What led you to come at this time?"; "What do you think is causing this?"; "What concerns do you have?"; and "What do you hope I can do for you?"

It is also important to compare the patient's perception of his or her functional capability with the physician's and family's assessments. Some patients may lose family attention, work relief, or disability/compensation by getting well, so they maintain the "sick role." With these individuals, the physician must realistically appraise the patient of the status of his or her clinical condition and encourage "well" behavior. To some, the benefits derived from being ill exceed the benefits that motivate the patient to return to a state of health.

> Mr. C., a 28-year-old single machinist with a 12 year history of Crohn's colitis, was receiving disability compensation for weight loss from malabsorption caused by a jejunocolic fistula. He moved in with his parents so they could care for him. After several years of poor medical control, he agreed reluctantly to a proctocolectomy and ileostomy that produced weight gain and healing of the perianal disease. Nevertheless, for the next 18 months he complained of lethargy and weakness, increased his alcohol intake, felt unable to work and requested that his disability benefits be continued. Attempts to involve him with vocational rehabilitation were unsuccessful and he remains unemployed.

As part of the evaluation, additional studies are often ordered. Safety, cost-effectiveness, and clinical usefulness (that is, will the results make a difference in treatment?) should be considered. Because the patient's symptom reporting influences clinical decision making, information from the interview must be assessed relative to the objective data. Frightened of the implications of a disease flare-up, some patients minimize or ignore their symptoms; others persistently complain and challenge the physician to "do something!", and may lead him or her to order unnecessary studies or recommend surgical intervention.[78]

TREATMENT APPROACH. The following recommendations can be made using the review of the research and clinical experience:

Establish a Therapeutic Relationship. Treatment must be individualized because patients vary in the degree of negotiation and participation they require. The physician should respond to the patient's needs empathically and nonjudgmentally, though this does not mean "going along" with the patient when it would not be in his or her best interest. For example, disability can be a disincentive for the patient to reestablish "wellness" and return to gainful employment. If the physician thinks the patient does not qualify, he or she should state this clearly and firmly.

As a key figure in the patient's life, it is important for one primary physician to be identified who can behave consistently, respond objectively, and communicate realistic treatment goals. This is a difficult role because at times the patient may bring up inappropriate or idiosyncratic issues that interfere with treatment.

Early in treatment, Ms. G. would not keep regular appointments, but would then visit the emergency room or call on evenings or weekends for "emergencies": she felt there was no reason to attend the appointments when she was feeling well. This behavior resulted from counterproductive dependency needs ("Does he really care, that is, will he *always* be there when I need help?"). She was told that the physician was interested in treating *her*, not the disease, and expected to see her at scheduled times no matter how she felt. Her "emergency" behavior remitted. Years later, she recalled the effect of this discussion. When symptoms developed or worsened, she would decide whether it was a true "emergency," and she could often wait until the next visit knowing that help was available.

Help the Patient Learn. Reassurance, careful explanation, and the provision of relevant educational materials are important components of the treatment plan. Some patients successfully adapt to the disorder once they understand it ("surprises frighten me more than facts").[73] The information provided must be individualized. "Sensitizing" patients want a great deal of information, while "repressors" become anxious if given too much. If, for example, a "repressor" has ulcerative proctitis, a detailed explanation of the cancer risks and of the surgical indications would not be appropriate. The physician can determine what to provide by the nature of the patient's questions and responses.

Prior to full acceptance of the disease, patients with IBD may feel "different" and benefit from talking with others who share the same experiences. I have my "choice" patients with ileostomies or previous surgical intervention who privately meet with any new patient about to undergo similar treatment, and I strongly encourage all new patients and their families to join self-help groups such as the NFIC. A source book for patients that focuses on personal experience of these illnesses is highly recommended.[79]*

Involve the Family. With an adolescent or child, the parents must be involved in all aspects of diagnosis and care; for many adult patients, communication with their spouse is recommended. Family members may feel helpless, guilty, or angry, though expressing such feelings is not usually socially permitted. The physician can play a major role in ameliorating these feelings by acknowledging them, by enlisting the family's participation in the treatment, or by recommending family counseling if necessary. In all cases, the patient's autonomy should be maintained. It is countertherapeutic to work through the family when the patient is an adolescent or adult.

Consider Behavioral Interventions. For most patients, the aforementioned recommendations are sufficient for establishing a successful physician-patient relationship. The following behavior management techniques are particularly helpful for those IBD patients who exhibit chronic illness behaviors, however:

HELP THE PATIENT UNDERSTAND AND ADAPT TO THE IDENTIFIED STRESSES. Many patients recognize that their bowel symptoms follow some psychosocial upset, and this recognition helps them deal with the illness. Others are unwilling or unable to see this association and will not benefit from attempts by the physician to provide "insight," for they may attribute the association to mental illness or some personal "weakness." With such patients, the physician should emphasize that human circumstance and psychologic, social, situational, and interpersonal factors are implicated in every illness; therefore, the issue is *not* whether a mental illness exists. The physician's interest is to understand *all* factors in the illness, including the patient's feelings, to help him or her cope.

HELP THE PATIENT GROW OUT OF THE "SICK ROLE." Many of the "physician behaviors" appropriate for patients with acute illness (including attending to patient complaints to the exclusion of other issues, acting on each complaint without objective clinical changes, and maintaining patient dependency by assuming full responsibility for his well-being), actually reinforce "sick role" behavior among patients with chronic disease. Thus, patients may conclude that physicians attend more to "sick" than "well" behaviors, and that they should be passive and dependent.

When appropriate, the physician should encourage the patient to take responsibility in treatment. For example, an individual with Crohn's disease and an increase in episodes of partial bowel obstruction should be apprised of

---

*Other patient-oriented books, brochures, and videotapes can be obtained from the National Foundation for Ileitis and Colitis, 444 Park Avenue South, New York, N.Y. 10016; (212) 685-3440.

the risks and benefits of small bowel resection. Given the present quality of his or her life, he or she can then help decide whether surgical intervention can be delayed. By giving up some control, the physician encourages patient responsibility and "perceived control."

OBTAIN PSYCHIATRIC REFERRAL WHEN APPROPRIATE. Psychiatric consultation should be considered when a treatment decision depends partially on emotional variables. For example, a concurrent psychiatric illness may require pharmacotherapy (such as a tricyclic agent for depression), or the patient's psychosocial function (such as his or her inability to work) or family interaction may be seriously impaired. Whenever invasive or expensive diagnostic and therapeutic strategies are being considered, based on patient complaints without supportive medical data, psychiatric consultation is also recommended.

Referral for psychiatric treatment will also depend on the consultant's and physician's assessment of whether the symptoms and affective state constitute a personal, social, and economic hardship. The decision should be based on the expectation of a clinical response to some therapeutic intervention rather than the presence of a psychiatric diagnosis. Treatment may include insight-oriented psychotherapy, supportive counseling, family therapy, behavioral modification, relaxation, drugs, or some combination of these. The patient must consider the treatment relevant to personal needs.

CONSIDER YOURSELF. Patients with chronic gastrointestinal disease can tax the physician who expects his or her patient to become symptom free. Therefore, it is important to set realistic treatment goals, such as functional adaptation and symptom improvement (rather than cure). Most treatment decisions are based on "quality of life" rather than complications or emergencies where the choices are clear. Clinical data may not be available or sufficient, and decisions often must be made in the face of uncertainty. Particularly at these times, understanding the psychosocial dimensions of the illness will often help focus the problem.

Case Analysis of Ms. G.

Given a biopsychosocial framework, the question "are the symptoms functional *or* organic?" cannot be answered because Ms. G.'s illness has both medical (Crohn's disease) and behavioral (unresolved grief-depression and chronic illness behavior) components. The medical diagnosis is unquestionable (particularly during the recent hospitalization), though the symptoms sometimes are not fully explained by the disease. Symptom recurrence and complications over the years, along with her brother's medical experience, made her feel uncertain of the future and reluctant to work and thereby lose disability benefits. Symptom flareups were adaptive by bringing both parents together to care for her. Over time, she saw herself as unwell and assumed the "sick role" even when in clinical remission. Furthermore, the social inhibition and reluctance to disclose her condition to others reflected an inner sense of shame and isolation from others. Although her mother's helplessness and guilt can be understood, the consequent overprotectiveness fostered Ms. G.'s regressive and dependent behaviors during hospitalizations when symptoms exacerbated. Chronic illness delays emotional maturation and autonomy by impeding the testing and learning of independent behaviors in the adolescent. At age 29, Ms. G. remains passive and compliant, and lets others make her decisions. When in pain or under stress she is perceived as childish, demanding, and manipulative.

Ms. G.'s disease appeared when her parents divorced, and most recently the symptoms flared on the first anniversary of her father's death. The more than chance association for these occurrences and the possible mediating factors affecting disease susceptibility and symptom exacerbation have been addressed in this chapter. We note more than a significant timing of the most recent event. Her symptoms are similar to her father's and she was ambivalent about their relationship, having been abused by her father as a child. All these factors support the proposition that a psychologic component, unresolved grief, contributed to the symptom complex.[80]

The possible effect of Ms. G.'s behavior on her health care providers must also be understood. The physician's comment about the mother "smothering" the patient, while possibly accurate, is also defensive and challenging, perhaps in response to the mother's request for another opinion. These occasional inappropriate responses to the demands of patients or their families result from feelings of helplessness or inadequacy when the physician's competence is challenged, when he or she feels uncertain, or when patients do not meet expectations to become symptom free and compliant. Awareness of these feelings when they occur is usually sufficient to permit a more objective response. Similarly, the inability to meet the (at times) unrealistic demands of patients may lead to "confrontations," particularly when the legitimacy of the complaints is in question, such as when the patient's behavior is not explained by the apparent disease activity. Rather than challenge the patient's credibility, elicitation of the contributing psychosocial factors can be used to optimize the treatment approach.

Without clear evidence of active disease, the steroid medication was gradually decreased to Ms. G.'s maintenance level. The next day she ate without difficulty and hyperalimentation was stopped. A tricyclic antidepressant to improve her mood, diminish the physical manifestations (anorexia and pain) of the depression, and possibly lessen her need for narcotic analgesia was begun.[81] Ms. G.'s pain and need for assistance was acknowledged, and her unrealistic expectations for care relative to available resources was explained. A treatment plan between Ms. G. and her physician, taking into consideration these factors, was mutually agreed upon and reevaluated daily. In particular, the nursing plan was designed to encourage independent function. At times, when she "tested" the agreement, the responses of the nurses and doctor remained understanding but firmly consistent. The mother participated, but an effort was made not to shift the treatment focus from Ms. G. Over the next several days her condition improved and she was discharged to return to see her physician in two weeks.

On this occasion, the psychosocial influences on Ms. G.'s illness outweighed the biologic ones. This case represents the degree to which such influences can contribute to a patient's illness. The contribution of biologic and behavioral factors in IBD will vary over time and among patients in a medical practice. It makes sense to consider all the variables in diagnosis and treatment, and to attend to both the emotional and medical needs of patients. The research review herein provides some scientific basis for the use of this more comprehensive framework to benefit the individual with IBD.*

References

1. Drossman, D. A., and Broom, C. M.: Report to the Nerve-Gut Council: Results of AGA survey of physician knowledge, attitudes and practice patterns. Digestive Diseases Week, New York, 1985.

*Editors' note: See also Drossman, D. A., et al.: Gastroenterology, *92*:1375, 1987.

2. Ader, R.: Gastric erosions in the rat: Effects of immobilization at different points in the activity cycle. Science, *145*:406, 1964.
3. Ackerman, S. H., Hofer, M. A., and Weiner, H.: Age at maternal separation and gastric erosion susceptibility in the rat. Psychosom. Med., *37*:180, 1975.
4. Porter, R. W., et al.: Some experimental observations on gastrointestinal lesions in behaviorally conditioned monkeys. Psychosom. Med., *20*:379, 1958.
5. Stout, C., and Snyder, R. L.: Ulcerative colitis-like lesions in Siamang gibbons. Gastroenterology, *57*:256, 1969.
6. Engel, G. L.: Psychological factors in ulcerative colitis in man and gibbon. Gastroenterology, *57*:362, 1969.
7. Engel, G. L.: Studies of ulcerative colitis. III. The nature of the psychologic process. Am. J. Med., *19*:231, 1955.
8. Chalifoux, L. V., and Bronson, R. T.: Colonic adenocarcinoma associated with chronic colitis in cotton top marmosets, Saguinus oedipus. Gastroenterology, *80*:942, 1981.
9. Garber, P. A., Moya, L., and Malaga, C.: A preliminary field study of the moustached tamarin monkey (Saguinus mystax) in northeastern Peru: Questions concerned with the evolution of a communal breeding system. Folia Primatol., *42*:17, 1984.
10. Drossman, D. A.: Is the cotton-topped tamarin a model for behavioral research? Dig. Dis. Sci., *30*:24S, 1985.
11. Cassell, J.: The contribution of the social environment to host resistance. Am. J. 'Epidemiol., *104*:107, 1976.
12. Holmes, T. H., and Rahe, R. H.: The social readjustment rating scale. J. Psychosom. Res., *11*:213, 1967.
13. Cobb, S., and Rose, R. M.: Hypertension, peptic ulcer and diabetes in air traffic controllers. J. Am. Med. Assoc., *224*:489, 1973.
14. Mendeloff, A. I.: The epidemiology of inflammatory bowel disease. Clin. Gastroenterol., *9*:259, 1980.
15. Paulley, J. W.: Psychological factors. Br. Med. J., *2*:308, 1963.
16. Salem. S. N., and Shubair, K. S.: Non-specific ulcerative colitis in Bedouin Arabs. Lancet, *1*:473, 1967.
17. Mendeloff, A. I., Monk, M., Siegel, C. I., and Lilienfeld, A.: Illness experience and life stresses in patients with irritable colon and with ulcerative colitis. An epidemiologic study of ulcerative colitis and regional enteritis in Baltimore, 1960–1964. N. Engl. J. Med., *282*:14, 1970.
18. Sandler, R. S., Drossman, D. A., Nathan, H. P., and McKee, D. C.: Symptom complaints and health care seeking behavior in subjects with bowel dysfunction. Gastroenterology, *87*:314, 1984.
19. Karush, A.: A review of the psychosomatic literature on chronic ulcerative colitis. *In* Psychotherapy in Chronic Ulcerative Colitis. Edited by A. Karush. Philadelphia, W. B. Saunders, 1977.
20. Murray, C. D.: Psychogenic factors in the etiology of ulcerative colitis and bloody diarrhea. Am. J. Med. Sci., *180*:239, 1930.
21. Sullivan, A. J.: Psychogenic factors in ulcerative colitis. Am. J. Dig. Dis. Nutr., *2*:651, 1935.
22. Daniels, G. E.: Psychiatric aspects of ulcerative colitis. N. Engl. J. Med., *226*:178, 1942.
23. Lindemann, E.: Modifications in the course of ulcerative colitis in the relationship to changes in life situations and reaction patterns. Proc. Assoc. Res. Nerv. Ment. Dis., *29*:796, 1949.
24. Weiner, H.: Psychobiology and Human Disease. New York, Elsevier Science Publishing, 1977.
25. Engel, G. L.: Studies of ulcerative colitis. V. Psychological aspects and their implications for treatment. Am. J. Dig. Dis., *3*:315, 1958.
26. Drossman, D. A.: The physician and the patient. Review of the psychosocial gastrointestinal literature with an inte-

26. grated approach to the patient. *In* Gastrointestinal Disease: Pathophysiology, Diagnosis, Management. Edited by M. H. Sleisenger and J. S. Fordtran. Philadelphia, W. B. Saunders, 1983.
27. Feldman, F., Cantor, D., Soll, S., and Bachrach, W.: Psychiatric study of a consecutive series of 34 patients with ulcerative colitis. Br. Med. J., *3*:14, 1967.
28. Feldman, F., Cantor, D., Soll, S., and Bachrach, W.: Psychiatric study of a consecutive series of 19 patients with regional ileitis. Br. Med. J., *4*:711, 1967.
29. Hislop, I. G.: Onset setting in inflammatory bowel disease. Med. J. Aust., *1*:981, 1974.
30. Fava, G. A., and Pavan, L.: Large bowel disorders. I. Illness configuration and life events. Psychother. Psychosom., *27*:93, 1976/77.
31. Prugh, D. G.: The influence of emotional factors on the clinical course of ulcerative colitis in children. Gastroenterology, *18*:339, 1951.
32. Whybrow, P. C., Kane, F. J., and Lipton, M. A.: Regional ileitis and psychiatric disorder. Psychosom. Med., *30*:209, 1968.
33. Ford, C. V., Glober, G. A., and Castelnuovo-Tedesco, P.: A psychiatric study of patients with regional enteritis. J. Am. Med. Assoc., *208*:311, 1969.
34. McKegney, F. P., Gordon, R. O., and Levine, S. M.: A psychosomatic comparison of patients with ulcerative colitis and Crohn's disease. Psychosom. Med., *32*:153, 1970.
35. Cohn, E. M., Lederman, I. I., and Shore, E.: Regional enteritis and its relation to emotional disorders. Am. J. Gastroenterol., *54*:378, 1970.
36. Pert, C. B., Ruff, M. R., Weber, R. J., and Herkenham, M.: Neuropeptides and their receptors: A psychosomatic network. J. Immunol., *135*:820, 1985.
37. Ader, R.: Psychoneuroimmunology. New York, Academic Press, 1981.
38. Stein, M., Keller, S., and Schleifer, S.: The hypothalamus and the immune response. *In* Brain, Behavior and Bodily Disease, Vol. 59. Edited by H. Weiner, M. A. Hofer, and A. J. Stunkard. New York, Raven Press, 1981.
39. Ruff, M. R., et al.: Benzodiazepine receptor-mediated chemotaxis of human monocytes. Science, *229*:1281, 1985.
40. Ader, R., and Cohen, N.: Behaviorally conditioned immunosuppression. Psychosom. Med. *37*:333, 1975.
41. Ader, R., and Cohen, N.: Behaviorally conditioned immunosuppression and murine systemic lupus erythematosus. Science, *215*:1534, 1982.
42. Fischer, C. L., Daniels, J. C., and Levin, W. C.: Effects of the space flight environment on man's immune system. II. Lymphocyte counts and reactivity. Aerospace Med., *43*:1122, 1972.
43. Bartrop, R. W., et al.: Depressed lymphocyte function after bereavement. Lancet, *1*:834, 1977.
44. Parkes, C. M.: Health after bereavement. A controlled study of young Boston widows and widowers. Psychom. Med., *34*:449, 1972.
45. Weber, R. J., and Pert, C. B.: Opiatergic modulation of the immune system. *In* Central and Peripheral Endorphins. Basic and Clinical Aspects. Edited by E. E. Muller and A. R. Genazzani. New York, Raven Press, 1984.
46. Shavit, Y., et al.: Stress, opioid peptides, the immune system, and cancer. J. Immunol., *135*:834, 1985.
47. Dunbar, H. F.: Psychosomatic Diagnosis. New York, Hoeber, 1943.
48. Alexander, F.: Psychosomatic Medicine. New York, Norton, 1950.
49. Sifneos, P. E.: The prevalence of 'Alexithymic' characteristics in psychosomatic patients. Psychother. Psychosom., 22:255, 1973.
50. Marty, P., and de M'Uzan, M.: La pensée operatoire. Rev. Fr. Psychoanal. (suppl.), *27*:1345, 1963.
51. Groen, J., and Bastiaans, J.: Studies on ulcerative colitis: Personality structure, emotional conflict, situations and effects of psychotherapy. *In* Modern Trends in Psychosomatic Medicine. Edited by D. F. O'Neil. London, Butterworth Publishing, 1955.
52. Lesser, I. M., and Lesser, B. Z.: Alexithymia: Examining the development of a psychological concept. Am. J. Psychiatry, *140*:1305, 1983.
53. Alexander, F., French, T. M., and Pollack, G.: Psychosomatic specificity: Experimental study and results, Vol. 1. Chicago, University of Chicago Press, 1968.
54. Latimer, P. R.: Crohn's disease: a review of the psychological and social outcome. Psychol. Med., *8*:649, 1978.
55. Helzer, J. E., et al.: A controlled study of the association between ulcerative colitis and psychiatric diagnoses. Dig. Dis. Sci., *27*:513, 1982.
56. Helzer, J. E., et al.: A study of the association between Crohn's disease and psychiatric illness. Gastroenterology, *86*:324, 1984.
57. Engel, G. L., and Salzman, L. F.: A double standard for psychosomatic papers? N. Engl. J. Med., *288*:44, 1973.
58. McMahon, A. W., Schmitt, P., Patterson, J. F., and Rothman, E.: Personality differences between inflammatory bowel disease patients and their healthy siblings. Psychosom. Med., *35*:91, 1973.
59. West, K. L.: MMPI correlates of ulcerative colitis. J. Clin. Psychol., *26*:214, 1970.
60. Mechanic, D.: The concept of illness behavior. J. Chronic. Dis., *15*:189, 1962.
61. Tseng, W. S.: The nature of somatic complaints among psychiatric patients: The Chinese case. Compr. Psychiatry, *16*:237, 1975.
62. Zborosky, M.: Cultural response to pain. J. Soc. Issues, *8*:16, 1952.
63. Verbrugge, L. M.: Sex differentials in morbidity and mortality in the United States. Soc. Biol., *23*:275, 1976.
64. Zola, I. K.: Culture and symptoms—An analysis of patients' presenting complaints. Amer. Sociol. Rev., *31*:615, 1966.
65. Parsons, T.: The Social System. New York, Free Press of Glencoe, 1951.
66. Pilowski, I.: Abnormal illness behavior. Br. J. Med. Psychol., *42*:347, 1969.
67. Hendriksen, C., and Binder, V.: social prognosis in patients with ulcerative colitis. Br. Med. J., *2*:581, 1980.
68. Farmer, R. G., Whelan, G., and Fazio, V. W.: Long-term follow-up of patients with Crohn's disease. Relationship between the clinical pattern and prognosis. Gastroenterology, *88*:1818, 1985.
69. Meyers, S., et. al.: Quality of life after surgery for Crohn's disease: A psychosocial survey. Gastroenterology, *78*:1, 1980.
70. Gazzard, B. G., Price, H. L., Libby, G. W., and Dawson, A. M.: The social toll of Crohn's disease. Br. Med. J., *2*:1117, 1978.
71. Feldman, D. F.: Chronic disabling illness: A holistic view. J. Chronic Dis., *27*:287, 1974.
72. Sadler, H. H., and Gransz, H.: A clinical challenge. West. J. Med., *125*:393, 1976.
73. Olbrisch, M. E., and Ziegler, S. W.: Psychological adjustment to inflammatory bowel disease: informational control and private self-consciousness. J. Chronic Dis., *35*:573, 1982.
74. Schnieder, A. P.: Coping with Crohn's disease: Some of factors contributing to the appraisal of a chronic stressor. Dissertation, Department of Psychology, New York University, 1985.

75. Stowe, S. P., et al.: Fiscal and hospital utilization impact of IBD in Rochester New York community hospitals. Presented at the Second International Symposium for Inflammatory Bowel Disease, Jerusalem, 1985.
76. Engel, G. L.: The clinical application of the biopsychosocial model. Am. J. Psychiatry, 137:535, 1980.
77. Morgan, J., and Engel, G. L.: The Clinical Approach to the Patient. Philadelphia, W. B. Saunders, 1969.
78. DeVaul, R. A., and Faillace, L. A.: Persistent pain and illness insistence. A medical profile of proneness to surgery. Am. J. Surg., 135:828, 1978.
79. Steiner, P., Banks, P. A., and Present, D. H. (eds.): People not patients. A source book for living with inflammatory bowel disease. New York, National Foundation for Ileitis and Colitis, 1985.
80. Drossman, D. A.: Patients with psychogenic abdominal pain: Six years' observation in the medical setting. Am. J. Psychiatry, 139:1549, 1982.
81. Walsh, T. C.: Antidepressants in chronic pain. Clin. Neuropharmacol., 6:271, 1983.

12 · Ulcerative Colitis and Crohn's Disease in Children

KATHLEEN J. MOTIL, M.D., PH.D. AND RICHARD J. GRAND, M.D.

Once considered rare in pediatric practice, chronic inflammatory bowel disease is being recognized with increasing frequency in children. As in adults, ulcerative colitis and Crohn's disease constitute the two major entities. Many characteristics of these diseases in children are similar to those seen in adults (Table 12-1). Similarities include presumed etiology and pathogenesis, an almost equal incidence of disease among males and females, and a distribution ratio of three new cases of Crohn's disease to every one to two new cases of ulcerative colitis. The distribution of involvement throughout the intestine in Crohn's disease and other major clinical features also are similar in adults and children. The response to therapy is comparable, although no controlled trials of pharmacologic agents have been conducted in patients younger than 15 years. The incidence of recurrence of Crohn's disease following surgical treatment appears to be similar among adults and children. Children often have a different presentation and course, however, and may require different methods of management. With respect to differences, the tempo of disease activity, the frequency of complications, and the long-term impact of disease seem to be greater in children than in adults, although this observation has not been documented in a carefully controlled population. Extraintestinal findings tend to be less prevalent in children. On the other hand, growth failure is common in children with inflammatory bowel disease, and little is known of the long-term outcome. The lack of development of secondary sex characteristics, the diminished subcutaneous tissue and muscle bulk, and the clubbing that accompanies malnutrition in inflammatory bowel disease can be reversed by nutritional therapy and appropriate pharmacologic control of the disease. The mechanism by which chronic inflammatory bowel disease induces growth failure is unknown, however. These disorders also can masquerade as juvenile rheumatoid arthritis, idiopathic growth failure,

TABLE 12-1. *Similarities and Differences Between Children and Adults with Inflammatory Bowel Disease.*

Similarities:
   Presumed etiology and pathogenesis
   Sex ratio
   Distribution of cases
   Distribution of intestinal involvement
   Major clinical features
   Recurrence after surgical treatment
Differences:
   Age at onset
   Tempo of disease
   Extraintestinal findings
   Growth failure
   Outcome

or even anorexia nervosa before intestinal manifestations are recognized and a correct diagnosis is made.[1] Moreover, the emotional impact of chronic disease and its complications on the immature patient may add another factor that requires specialized therapy. As in any other chronic illness of childhood, the long-term management of inflammatory bowel disease continues to provide a challenge for the physician and other health care workers who are responsible for these patients.

Epidemiology of Inflammatory Bowel Disease in Children*

Since 1950, a well-recognized increase in the incidence of Crohn's disease has ranged from 100% to 400% in all age groups.[2,3] In Northern Europe and North America, where the incidence of disease is about 4 per 100,000, this trend probably has leveled off, but the incidence still may be rising in less industrialized areas.[4] Two peaks of onset of disease exist, one in early and one in late adult life; however, one-fourth to one-third of patients with Crohn's disease present before the age of 20 years (Table 12-2). In contrast to Crohn's disease, the incidence of ulcerative colitis has not changed significantly (see also Chap. 1). Only 15% of patients with ulcerative colitis present before the age of 20 years, however, usually in adolescence. Although ulcerative colitis may present in infancy, it is likely that inflammatory disease of the colon presenting in the first year of life represents food allergy or other infectious diseases.[8]

Certain groups of children are at greater risk of developing inflammatory bowel disease.[3] Ulcerative colitis and Crohn's disease are more common among Northern European and Anglo-Saxon races, urban rather than rural dwellers, and in Jewish individuals living in Europe and North America (but less common in Israelis).

*See also Chapter 1.

Males and females are equally affected. Multiple familial occurrences occur in 15 to 40% of patients with ulcerative colitis or Crohn's disease,[9] and in one-quarter of these families both forms of inflammatory bowel disease may occur. Inflammatory bowel disease also occurs with greater frequency in children with the histocompatibility marker HLA-B27 and ankylosing spondylitis.[10]

Clinical Presentation of Inflammatory Bowel Disease in Children.

Although 60% of children with ulcerative colitis present with mild diarrhea of insidious onset, with or without blood in the stools, 10% present as a fulminant colitis (Table 12-3). In childhood, ulcerative colitis appears in one of three forms. The most common presentation is the insidious onset of diarrhea and rectal bleeding, without fever or abdominal pain, with disease that remains confined to the distal colon.[12] In the second type of presentation, bloody diarrhea, tenesmus, urgency, low-grade fever, weight loss, and mild anemia are present. Physical findings generally are limited to abdominal tenderness. In severe disease, more than six bloody stools per day, tachycardia, weight loss, anemia, and hypoalbuminemia occur; the abdominal examination reveals diffuse tenderness, but without peritoneal signs. Toxic megacolon is the extreme presentation of this group and represents a true emergency situation.[13,14]

In Crohn's disease, periumbilical abdominal pain, which is colicky in nature and worse after meals, diarrhea, and weight loss are the most common presenting symptoms (Table 12-4). The cause of diarrhea in patients with Crohn's disease is multifactorial; extensive mucosal dysfunction, bile acid malabsorption in terminal ileal disease, bacterial overgrowth secondary to strictures and disordered motility, and protein

TABLE 12-2. *Ages at Onset of Symptoms in Inflammatory Bowel Disease.*

Age at Onset (year)	Ulcerative Colitis (n = 465)	Crohn's Disease (n = 166)	(n = 168)
0-9	2%[5]	—[6]	2%[7]
10-19	14%	19%	30%
20-29	24%	25%	38%
30-39	25%	16%	13%

TABLE 12-3. *Presenting Features in Ulcerative Colitis; Children vs. Adults*

Clinical Finding	Adults[5] (n = 465)	Children[11] (n = 125)
Diarrhea	44%	53%
Rectal bleeding	39%	20%
Weight loss	—	10%
Abdominal Pain	1%	5%
Arthritis	—	4%
Growth failure	—	2%

TABLE 12-4. *Presenting Features in Crohn's Disease; Children vs. Adults.*

Clinical Finding	Combined (n = 175)	Adults (n = 140)	Children (n = 36)
Abdominal pain	52%	85%	82%
Diarrhea	25%	62%	88%
Weight loss	2%	50%	60%
Fever	—	41%	77%
Rectal bleeding	6%	13%	22%
Arthritis	2%	—	23%
Mass	2%	—	10%
Growth failure	—	—	30%

(See also Burbidge, E. J., Huang, S., and Bayless, T. M.: Pediatrics, 55:866, 1975; Kyle, J.: Crohn's Disease. New York, Appleton Century Crofts, 1972; Ehrenpreis, T. H., Gierup, J., and Lageracrantz, R.: Acta Paediatr. Scand., 60:209, 1971; and Korelitz, B. I., Gribetz, D., and Kopel, F. B.: Pediatrics, 42:446, 1968.)

exudation from inflamed surfaces lead to diarrhea. Rectal blood loss may be apparent with colitis. Crohn's disease often is insidious in onset, and extraintestinal symptoms such as intermittent fever, arthritis,[17,18] iridocyclitis, erythema nodosum, or growth retardation may predominate, with few or no symptoms that suggest gastrointestinal involvement.[1,19] In children, malnutrition and abnormalities in growth often are present. With mild, short-term disease, the weight-for-height may be depressed; in severe disease, wasting may be extreme and hypoalbuminemia may be present. In chronic, long-term disease, children may be short in stature, but with a weight appropriate for their height. Anemia is present in as many as 50% of all patients. Not surprisingly, the initial diagnosis in affected children often is incorrect, and conversely, the correct diagnosis may be delayed considerably. In general, the average delay between the onset of symptoms and the diagnosis is 13 months.[1] Moreover, delayed referral may raise this figure to nearly three years.[20] The site and extent of disease have a considerable effect upon the delay in diagnosis; left-sided colonic disease (2 months) is diagnosed more rapidly than either diffuse small bowel disease (5 months) or disease confined to the terminal ileum and right colon (16 months).[1] In children, ileocolitis is the most common (52%), and colitis (9%) is the least common form of disease, with diffuse small bowel disease and ileal involvement each accounting for about 20% of all cases. The importance of seeking diagnostic clues outside the abdomen cannot be overemphasized. Thus, the presence of clubbing, perianal disease including skin tags, fissures, and fistulas,[21] oral ulceration, uveitis, or arthritis provide valuable information on which a clinical diagnosis may be based.

Complications of Inflammatory Bowel Disease in Pediatric Patients*

Intestinal

Anal fissures, intestinal strictures, and fistulas occur less frequently in ulcerative colitis than in Crohn's disease. Hemorrhoids are rarely encountered in children, but when present may be confused with skin tags found in Crohn's disease. Massive hemorrhage may occur during fulminating episodes of ulcerative colitis or, uncommonly, Crohn's disease.[14] Pseudopolyps are a common complication of long-standing disease, but are not frequent sources of bleeding.

The two most important local complications of ulcerative colitis are toxic megacolon and carcinoma. Toxic megacolon occurs in 5% of children, and it represents a medical and surgical emergency.[14] Antidiarrheal agents (opiates and anticholinergics) and an antecedent barium enema have been implicated in this complication. The course is one of progressive deterioration; the child appears severely ill, the temperature rises, bowel sounds diminish, and the abdomen becomes more distended, tender, and tympanitic. Hypoalbuminemia and electrolyte disturbances are invariably present. Gram-negative sepsis, hemorrhage, and perforation are life-threatening complications (see Chap. 14).

Although the incidence of carcinoma complicating pancolitis beginning in childhood was reported to be 20% per decade after the first 10 years of disease,[22] the current risks are probably less.[23] Patients with left-sided colitis or proctitis have a lower risk for the development of carcinoma than those with right-sided disease.[24] In general, epithelial dysplasia precedes the development of invasive carcinoma, and although dysplastic lesions often are patchy, carcinoma without associated dysplasia is rare.[24,25] When carcinoma does complicate colitis, the outlook is the same as that for colorectal carcinoma in general,[24] although the younger patient has a substantially poorer prognosis than the older one (see Chap. 15).[26]

*See also Chapters 14, 15, and 16.

In Crohn's disease, adhesions, strictures with stagnant loop syndrome, fistulas, and abscesses result from the transmural nature of the inflammation. Toxic megacolon may complicate Crohn's colitis, but is less common than that seen in ulcerative colitis (see Chap. 14).

Perianal disease may precede the appearance of the intestinal manifestations of Crohn's disease by several years and is seen most commonly in patients with colitis.[21,27] In one series of children and adolescents with Crohn's disease, 49% had perianal disease, including fissures and skin tags (70%), fistulas (14%), and abscesses (16%).[21] The risk of intestinal and extraintestinal carcinoma is increased in Crohn's disease. In children whose disease is diagnosed before the age of 21 years, the risk of developing carcinoma is twenty times greater than normal.[28] The risk of developing carcinoma still is exceedingly low, however, and does not warrant prophylactic resection of the small or large bowel (see also Chap. 15).

Extraintestinal*

Arthritis and arthralgia are the most common extraintestinal manifestations of inflammatory bowel disease in children. In ulcerative colitis, arthritis occurs in approximately 25% of patients, particularly during exacerbations of disease.[17] Arthritis in Crohn's disease occurs in approximately 11% of children, particularly those with ileocolitis.[29] Typically, arthritis and arthralgia affect the large joints in the lower limbs and may even occur when intestinal disease is in remission. Arthritis may be mono- or polyarticular, and synovitis with an effusion is commonly present. Sacroiliitis and ankylosing spondylitis may occur rarely in children and adolescents who are HLA-B27 positive.

Erythema multiforme, erythema nodosum, pyoderma gangrenosum, or aphthous stomatitis occur in about 10% of pediatric IBD patients, often at times of exacerbation of intestinal disease or when doses of corticosteroids are reduced.[17,19,30]

Acute symptomatic uveitis occurs in only 0.5 to 3% of pediatric patients; however, the incidence of asymptomatic transient uveitis in childhood may be as high as 30%. Uveitis occurs particularly in male patients with colitis and bears no relationship to the duration of disease or the extent of disease activity.[31]

Renal calculi are seen in approximately 5% of children with Crohn's disease;[29] the incidence is increased following colectomy and ileostomy.[32,33] In Crohn's disease, noncalculous hydronephrosis and hydroureter may result from compression of the ureter by an inflammatory mass, fibrosis, or an abscess. Enterovesicular fistulas may present with pneumaturia and recurrent urinary tract infections.

Hepatic dysfunction is found in 8% of patients with inflammatory bowel disease as determined by liver function studies,[34] particularly serum alkaline phosphatase.[35,36] Occasionally, children with inflammatory bowel disease may present primarily with chronic liver disease and minimal gastrointestinal symptoms.[37] Therefore, the diagnosis of inflammatory bowel disease is important to consider in children with chronic liver disease of unknown etiology. The incidence of histologic abnormalities varies from 15 to 19% of adults with biochemical abnormalities.[38] The most common lesion is fatty liver. Cirrhosis, chronic active hepatitis, sclerosing cholangitis, and biliary tract carcinoma are rare. Intensive medical treatment of the intestinal disease or colectomy in patients with Crohn's colitis may halt the pericholangitic process;[35,38] however, surgery in children is not indicated on this basis alone.

Cholelithiasis occurs in one-third of adults with Crohn's disease involving the terminal ileum, secondary to the interruption of the enterohepatic circulation of bile salts.[39,40] Symptomatic cholelithiasis in children with Crohn's disease is rare, however, but may be more common than presumed in long-standing disease.

Growth Failure

Malnutrition and growth arrest are ominous complications of inflammatory bowel disease in children. Protein-energy malnutrition and multiple vitamin (folate and B_{12}; D) and mineral (Ca, Mg, Fe, and Zn) deficiencies may be seen in 30 to 40% of affected children and adolescents.[12] Impairment of linear growth, lack of weight gain, retarded bone development, and delayed onset of sexual maturation occur in 10 to 40% of patients under 21 years of age with inflammatory bowel disease,[1,29,41-44] and nearly 80% of these children and adolescents have Crohn's disease.[1,43,45] One-third of these patients have depressed linear growth rates that range from 1 to 11 years prior to the onset of gastrointestinal symptoms.[43] Moreover, at least 50% of such individuals demonstrate linear growth arrest prior to corticosteroid therapy.[43] Similarly, weight

---

*See also Chapter 16.

losses of 2 to 11 kg or failure to gain weight also are reported at the time of diagnosis.[1,29,41] Thus, linear and ponderal growth abnormalities are significant presenting features of inflammatory bowel disease in childhood.

The impact of growth failure in inflammatory bowel disease is twofold: alterations in body composition and potentially permanent short stature. Abnormalities in body composition have been demonstrated by combined height and weight deficits in almost one-half of the children and adolescents with inflammatory bowel disease.[44] In one study, mid-arm circumference and arm muscle area measurements were less than the fifth percentile in 10% of the group, and the triceps skinfold thickness was reduced in 5% of the patients.[46] Serum total proteins and albumin levels were depressed in nearly 20% of these individuals. Lean body mass and skeletal muscle compartments, measured by whole body potassium (^{40}K) and urinary creatinine excretion, were reduced by 30%.[47] Notably, acute disease activity was present in less than 10% of the patients at the time of the assessment. In another study, long-term follow-up of patients from adolescence to adulthood demonstrated that the average height of these individuals was significantly less than that of the normal population.[41] These observations suggest that alterations in body composition are a prominent feature of chronic inflammatory bowel disease in childhood.

Growth failure associated with inflammatory bowel disease has been attributed to nutritional, hormonal, and disease-related factors.[48] The endocrine status of children with growth failure has been studied extensively. Cortisol levels,[49,50] thyroid function,[49,50] and growth hormone production are normal.[49,51,52] Serum somatomedin-C values may be depressed in some patients with growth failure;[53] however, the levels of these peptide hormones are increased readily with refeeding of adequate dietary protein and energy.[54] Thus, further information is needed regarding the hormonal impact on growth in children with inflammatory bowel disease.

Both the inflammatory process and treatment with corticosteroids have been implicated as contributory factors in growth failure. Nevertheless, some patients with inflammatory bowel disease continue to grow while receiving corticosteroid therapy, presumably because of the suppression of the inflammatory activity[19,29,55,56] and an increase in appetite and nutrient intake. Surgical resection of the affected gut has not been uniformly successful in the restoration of normal growth rates.[19,29,43,56-58] Indeed, in prepubertal patients with Crohn's disease studied 2 to 5 years after removal of all active ileal and colonic disease, only 14 to 18% demonstrated catch-up growth. The other patients either grew slowly in their premorbid growth channels or failed to grow.[29,56]

Presently, the strongest evidence supports the hypothesis that malnutrition is the primary cause of growth delay and altered body composition in inflammatory bowel disease.[46,48,59] The etiology of malnutrition in patients with inflammatory bowel disease is multifactorial and includes inadequate dietary intake, excessive gastrointestinal losses, malabsorption, increased nutritional requirements, and hormonal imbalances (Table 12-5). Inadequate dietary intakes may occur as a result of the anorexia associated with chronic illness, or because of increased diarrhea or abdominal pain associated with the ingestion of food. Dietary records of adolescents with inflammatory bowel disease demonstrated that these children have lower energy intakes (2760 kcal/day) than the average requirements for chronologic age (3180 kcal/day). Similarly, relative deficiencies in dietary vitamin and mineral intakes, particularly folate, pyridoxine, and iron, have been identified.[60]

Excessive losses of nutrients may originate from the gut. Hematochezia, protein-losing enteropathy, and increased fecal losses of cellular constituents are associated with chronic inflammation and damage to the intestinal mucosa.[61,62] Bile salt-losing enteropathy and subsequent fat malabsorption result from ileal resection or from fistulous tracts that bypass the terminal ileum. Furthermore, large doses of corticosteroids,[63,64] or the stress-induced response to

TABLE 12-5. *Causes of Malnutrition in Inflammatory Bowel Disease.*

Inadequate intake:	Excessive Intestinal Losses:
Anorexia	Protein-losing enteropathy
Altered taste	Hematochezia
Abdominal pain	Bile salt-losing enteropathy
Malabsorption:	Increased Requirements:
Protein	Fever
Carbohydrate (xylose, lactose)	Fistulas
	Repletion
	Growth
Fat:	
Minerals (Ca, Mg, Fe, Zn)	Hormonal Imbalances:
Vitamins (folate, B, A, D, K)	Somatomedins
	Insulin
Bacterial overgrowth	
Drug inhibition (folate)	

(Adapted from Motil, K. J., and Grand, R. J.: *In* Nutrition in Pediatrics—Basic Science and Clinical Application. Boston, Little Brown, 1985.)

acute inflammation,[65] lead to increased nutrient losses.

Malabsorption is more common in patients with Crohn's disease than in those with ulcerative colitis.[66] Approximately 16% will have abnormal xylose absorption tests, while one-third will have a moderate degree of steatorrhea and increased bile salt malabsorption.[66–68] Lactose intolerance is present in 30% of patients and is more common than in age-matched controls, except for those with diffuse, small bowel disease.[69] Hypoalbuminemia may be found in at least 50% of patients.[62,67,70] Hypocalcemia and hypomagnesemia have been associated with enteric protein loss or steatorrhea.[67,71–73] Vitamin A and D deficiencies are present in 33% and 25%, respectively, of adults with Crohn's disease,[74,75] and presumably occur in children with long-standing disease. Vitamin K deficiency, when present, is a consequence of steatorrhea.[68] Reductions in serum iron and folate levels are common,[60,67] and in severe ileal disease or resection, vitamin B_{12} deficiency is inevitable.[67,68,76] Some children with Crohn's disease have reduced serum zinc levels, but the role of this trace element in malnutrition and growth failure is unclear.[77–80]

Increased nutrient requirements may be present in response to increased inflammatory activity, fever, intestinal fistulas, or periods of rapid growth, particularly during adolescence. Inflammation leads to negative energy and nitrogen balance as a result of decreased dietary intake and increased metabolic activity.[65,81] Increased urinary losses of vitamins (A and C) and minerals (K, Ca, Mg, P, Zn, and S) also are associated with inflammation.[77,82,83] Additional nutrient requirements occur in response to the demands of growth in children and may average 170 kcal/day. Over the short-term, dietary deficits of small amounts are inconsequential, but over the long-term they are additive and of significant magnitude to account for reduced growth.[84] Thus, on the basis of these observations, nutritional assessment and therapy should be considered for all young patients with inflammatory bowel disease.

Evaluation of the Pediatric Patient

Complete evaluation of the child suspected of having the diagnosis of inflammatory bowel disease depends upon detailed history, physical findings, laboratory and radiographic studies, endoscopic examination, and histologic data (Table 12-6).

History

In ulcerative colitis, the important clinical symptoms to be investigated include diarrhea (particularly nocturnal), abdominal pain, rectal bleeding, tenesmus, anorexia, vomiting, fever, weight loss, linear growth arrest, or delayed puberty. A family history of inflammatory bowel disease should be sought. Travel or exposure to contaminated food or water must be determined because other infectious conditions may mimic ulcerative colitis.

In Crohn's disease, pain may be recurrent, and crampy, may be located predominantly in the periumbilical area or localized to the right lower quadrant or epigastric area, and often is triggered by eating.[29] Diarrhea, with or without rectal blood loss, commonly is prominent. The patient should be questioned regarding low-grade fever late in the afternoon, anorexia, nausea, vomiting, and weight loss. Other symptoms, including urgency, arthralgia, arthritis, recurrent mouth ulcers, skin rashes, anal fissures or abscesses, altered linear growth, malnutrition, or delayed sexual maturation, should alert the physician to the possibility of Crohn's disease.

Physical Examination

The general appearance should be noted for the degree of illness, state of hydration, and nutritional status. Height and weight measurements should be plotted on appropriate growth charts (National Center for Health Statistics). Aphthous stomatitis with superficial and painful ulcerations on the gums and buccal mucosa, or digital clubbing may be present. The abdominal examination should include measurements of the liver span and spleen size, and the assessment of tenderness, masses, and signs of peritoneal irritation. During the rectal examination, the physician should search for skin tags, fissures, fistulas, abscesses, hemorrhoids, or masses. Pallor, skin lesions, joint swelling, or eye changes also should be recorded.

Laboratory Assessment

Laboratory abnormalities commonly found in children with Crohn's disease are shown in Table 12-7. Hematologic examination reveals the presence of an anemia in 38 to 50% of patients, presumably as a result of malabsorption and/or rectal blood loss. An elevated erythrocyte sedimentation rate and a polymorphonuclear leukocytosis may be present, and lymphopenia may result from malnutrition. The degree of hypoal-

TABLE 12-6. *Evaluation of the Child with Inflammatory Bowel disease.*

History:
  Appetite, extracurricular activity
  Type and duration of inflammatory bowel disease, frequency of relapse
  Severity and extent of current symptoms
  Medications
Three-Day Diet Record
Physical Examination:
  Height, weight, arm circumference, triceps skinfold measurements
  Loss of subcutaneous fat, muscle wasting, edema, pallor, skin rash, hepatomegaly
Laboratory Tests:
  CBC and differential, reticulocyte and platelet count, prothrombin time, sedimentation rate, urinalysis
  Stool guaiac, cultures for bacteria, smears for ova, parasites, and fat
  Serum total proteins, albumin, transferrin, immunoglobulins
  Serum electrolytes, calcium, magnesium, phosphate, iron, zinc
  Serum folate, vitamins A, E, D, B_{12}
Special tests:
  Xylose absorption
  72-hour fecal fat, fecal $alpha_1$-antitrypsin
  Lactose breath test
  Schilling's test
Radiographic Studies:
  Upper GI and small bowel series
  Air contrast barium enema
  Intravenous pyelogram or ultrasonography
  Computerized tomography
Colonoscopy with Biopsies

(Adapted from Motil, K. J., and Grand, R. J.: *In* Nutrition in Pediatrics—Basic Science and Clinical Application. Boston, Little Brown, 1985.) Crohn's Disease Activity Index (Gastroenterology, 70:439, 1976) or Lloyd-Still Clinical Scoring System (Dig. Dis. Sci., 24:1979) may be useful.

buminemia,[85] thrombocytosis,[86] or the plasma levels of acute phase reactive proteins,[87] may correlate with disease activity. Fecal examination may reveal the presence of occult or obvious blood. Stools should be obtained for assay of Clostridium difficile toxin or culture of other pathogens such as shigella, salmonella, campylobacter, and yersinia; stool also should be examined for amoebae. Absorptive and secretory functions of the gut may be altered as reflected by decreased values for serum total proteins, albumin, immunoglobulins, folate, vitamin B_{12}, vitamin A, vitamin D, calcium, magnesium, iron, and zinc, and by increased fecal fat and $alpha_1$-antitrypsin content.[62] The significance of the hematologic and biochemical investigation is in the assessment of the severity of the disease; abnormalities of these tests become more pronounced as the inflammatory process worsens.

TABLE 12-7. *Laboratory Abnormalities Found in Inflammatory Bowel Disease.*

Value	Limits	Ulcerative Colitis (n = 22)	Crohn's Disease (n = 52)
Erythrocyte sedimentation rate	> 20mm/hr	90%	67%
Hematocrit	< 33%	38%	50%
Leukocytosis	> 10,000/mm^3	33%	58%
Iron	< 50 μg/dl	68%	55%
Albumin	< 3.3 g/dl	46%	45%
Folate	< 3.6 ng/dl	34%	44%

(Adapted from Gryboski, J., and Hillemeier, C.: Med. Clin. North Am., 64:1185, 1980.)

Radiologic Examination

In mild or moderate ulcerative colitis, a plain film of the abdomen usually is normal, but in severe attacks, extensive ulceration with thumbprinting created by edematous mucosa may be seen. In toxic megacolon, the colon may be dilated grossly, or may at its widest part (transverse colon or splenic flexure) be only 4 cm in diameter (see also Chap. 20).

In Crohn's disease patients with colicky abdominal pain and distention, upright and supine films of the abdomen may reveal the presence of incomplete small intestinal obstruction, distended loops of bowel, and air-fluid levels. Occasionally, an intra-abdominal abscess may be found by displacing the loops of small intestine (see also Chap. 20).

Examination of the small intestine should be performed in all children suspected of having the diagnosis of Crohn's disease. A small bowel study in which barium is introduced directly into the duodenum by a transpyloric tube probably gives more accurate information,[88,89] but is less comfortable for the child. The column of barium should be followed to the cecum, and its passage through the terminal ileum screened, preferably during palpation of the right lower quadrant in an attempt to separate overlying loops of ileum, and also to localize areas of tenderness. Radiologic features of inflammatory bowel disease in children are similar to those in older patients, and are discussed extensively in Chapter 20.

The air contrast barium enema is preferable to the single contrast study because it allows demonstration of mucosal detail of the colon in both ulcerative colitis and Crohn's disease. However, this study is not accomplished easily in children less than 5 years of age. The radiologic features useful in differentiating Crohn's colitis from ulcerative colitis are shown in Table 12-8.

Abdominal Ultrasonography and Computerized Tomography

These procedures are especially valuable for delineation of intra-abdominal masses or abscesses. Both techniques have received wide application in pediatric patients, usually with clear interpretation when studies are performed by qualified pediatric radiologists. These modalities are discussed further in Chapter 20.

^{111}Indium-labeled Leukocyte Scan

Gamma camera scanning following the intravenous injection of ^{111}indium-labeled autologous leukocytes is useful for the assessment of inflammatory bowel disease in adults.[90] This technique also has been used in children.[91] Although apparently accurate in the localization of active disease, the radiographic study involves a relatively high radiation exposure. Therefore, in children with inflammatory bowel disease, an ^{111}indium scan is indicated *only* when other methods have proven unsatisfactory.

Sigmoidoscopy and Colonoscopy*

Sigmoidoscopic examination and rectal biopsies are essential for the diagnosis and management of ulcerative colitis. In active disease, hyperemic, edematous mucosa with spontaneous and induced friability is seen; ulcerations may be present and the vascular pattern is diminished. With inactive disease, the mucosa appears granular and the vascular pattern becomes more prominent, reflecting mucosal atrophy. Sigmoidoscopy in patients with Crohn's disease may be similar to that in ulcerative colitis or may dem-

*See also Chapter 19.

TABLE 12-8. *Radiographic Features Useful in the Differentiation Between Ulcerative Colitis and Crohn's Colitis.*

Feature	Ulcerative Colitis	Crohn's Colitis
Pattern of involvement	Symmetric, contiguous	Asymmetric, eccentric
Sites of involvement	Rectum almost always involved; terminal ileum normal	Rectum involved in 50%, terminal ileum abnormal in majority, right-side colitis in 35%
Mucosal pattern	Diffuse granular mucosa caused by edema and superficial ulceration	Focal aphthous ulcers in more normal adjacent mucosa
Mucosal pattern (chronic)	Coarse granularity caused by deep ulcers in mucosa, loss of haustra, foreshortening	Deep ulcerations with cobblestone pattern, pseudosacculations, skip areas
Abdominal sequelae	Fistulas, abscesses, strictures with or without obstruction	Toxic megacolon, carcinoma, strictures

*See also Chapter 20.

onstrate normal findings when rectal involvement is absent. When present, mucosal abnormalities consist of erythema, edema, increased friability, and linear or aphthous ulcerations. Except for rectal sparing, fissures, and fistulas, sigmoidoscopic findings may not be diagnostic.

The availability of flexible, small-diameter pediatric colonoscopes has provided a safe method of directly examining the entire colon in children and of obtaining adequate biopsies.[92,93] The examination is performed under sedation, or occasionally, general anesthesia. Intravenous meperidine hydrochloride (Demerol) (1 to 2 mg/kg/dose) and diazepam (0.1 to 0.2 mg/kg/dose) are the drugs most commonly administered for sedation during colonoscopy. In ulcerative colitis, loss of the normal vascular pattern is the initial abnormality, followed by hyperemia, granularity of the mucosa, and contact bleeding. These lesions are continuous and predominantly left-sided. Subsequently, the hemorrhagic mucosa becomes superficially ulcerated, but without fissuring. Inflammatory pseudopolyps commonly are seen in the colon.[94] In contrast, Crohn's colitis is characterized initially by well-defined patches of hyperemia and edema with skip areas. The mucosa usually is not friable and may show aphthoid ulcerations with sharply defined craters and thin, erythematous edges. With more advanced disease, deep, linear, serpiginous or flat ulcerations, and cobblestone patterns are present. Colonoscopy is indicated (Table 12-9) in the initial evaluation of the child when the sigmoidoscopic examination and biopsies are normal, when the small bowel and colonic roentgenograph studies fail to identify the etiology of the symptoms and physical findings, or when it is impossible to distinguish between Crohn's disease or ulcerative colitis.[95] Colonoscopy also is useful preoperatively for the determination of the extent of colonic disease. In patients with diffuse small bowel Crohn's disease, in whom the differential diagnosis of lymphoma is difficult to rule out, colonoscopy and biopsies may reveal inflammatory activity in the colon, establishing the diagnosis of inflammatory bowel disease.[96] Finally, in adolescents who present with inflammatory bowel disease at an early age, colonoscopy permits visualization and biopsy of the entire colon in the surveillance for dysplasia.[97]

Pathology

Suction rectal biopsies always should be obtained during sigmoidoscopy. Despite the appearance of normal rectal mucosa, abnormal histologic findings may be present. Details are presented in Chapter 18. In general, rectal biopsies are useful for making the diagnosis of inflammatory bowel disease or for differentiating between ulcerative colitis and Crohn's disease,[98,99] when other diagnostic studies have been normal or inconclusive. Based on gross histologic and radiologic findings, the diagnosis of inflammatory bowel disease can be confirmed in over 90% of children presenting with symptoms.

Differential Diagnosis in Children[*]

Ten percent of children experience recurrent abdominal pain at some time during childhood. A common diagnostic problem is to decide when to investigate such children for possible inflammatory bowel disease (Table 12-10). Children with Crohn's disease or ulcerative colitis rarely present with periumbilical abdominal pain in the absence of other symptoms; thus, pain, diarrhea, weight loss, perianal disease, or mouth ulcers all suggest the need for further investigation.

The presence of small bowel disease often distinguishes patients with Crohn's disease from those with ulcerative colitis. When the disease is confined to the colon, the segmental, predominantly right-sided nature of Crohn's colitis differentiates it from ulcerative colitis in which left-sided disease is usually present and skip lesions are absent. Colonoscopy with biopsies, combined with clinical and radiographic findings, will help distinguish the two diseases.[101,102] Not more than 15% of cases remain indeterminate; the correct diagnosis may become apparent after patients have been followed carefully.

Allergic colitis generally presents in infancy. Although the appearance of the colon in allergic colitis may be indistinguishable from ulcerative colitis, the histology reveals a marked increase in eosinophils in the lamina propria.[8] Symptoms remit promptly with the removal of the allergen (usually casein or soy) from the diet.

TABLE 12-9. *Indications for Colonoscopy in Children.*

Definitive diagnosis when roentgenograms negative or equivocal
Staging colonic disease before surgical treatment
Surveillance for dysplasia
---

[*]See also Chapters 8, 9, and 10.

TABLE 12-10. *Differential diagnosis of Enterocolitis in Children.*

Bacteria:
  Salmonella
  Shigella
  Campylobacter
  Clostridium difficile
  Yersinia
  Tuberculosis
  Gonococcus
Parasites:
  Giardiasis
  Amebiasis
Inflammatory Bowel Disease:
  Ulcerative colitis
  Crohn's disease
Protein Sensitivity:
  Casein
  Soy
Miscellaneous:
  Meckel's diverticulitis
  Hemolytic uremic syndrome
  Severe combined immune deficiency
  Ischemia
  Henoch-Schönlein Purpura

Infectious causes of diarrhea or rectal bleeding such as salmonella, shigella, campylobacter, yersinia, or amoeba should be excluded by appropriately collected stool specimens for routine culture or examination by smear. Pseudomembranous colitis is uncommon in children;[102] usually they have a history of previous exposure to antibiotic therapy, and *Clostridium difficile* toxin is isolated from the stools. Endoscopy reveals raised, adherent, yellow-white mucosal plaques consisting of crypt necrosis and replacement of the epithelium by a pseudomembrane of fibrin, mucus, and inflammatory cells. Oral vancomycin hydrochloride (40 mg/kg/day in four divided doses, maximum 2 g/day),[103] or metronidazole (20 mg/kg/day in three divided doses, maximum 1 g/day) for 7 to 10 days, is effective, although relapse may occur when treatment is discontinued. *Clostridium difficile* colitis may masquerade as a flare-up of disease in patients with known inflammatory bowel disease. Prompt treatment of the condition allows distinction between specific infectious and idiopathic inflammatory bowel diseases.

Abdominal pain and bloody diarrhea accompany the renal failure, hemolytic anemia, and thrombocytopenia of hemolytic-uremic syndrome. Indeed, colitis may dominate the clinical presentation and mimic ulcerative colitis.[104] As mentioned previously, frequently, both ulcerative colitis and Crohn's disease in children may be associated with minimal gastrointestinal symptoms and present with idiopathic, chronic liver disease.[36]

Intestinal tuberculosis may mimic Crohn's disease; however, the two are differentiated most reliably by histologic examination and culture of colonoscopic biopsies. Other granulomatous diseases, such as sarcoidosis and histoplasmosis, are rare in childhood, as are small bowel malignancies. Immunoproliferative disease of the small intestine,[105] although uncommon in children, may present with diarrhea, abdominal pain, and weight loss. Colonoscopy may help in the differentiation of lymphoma from Crohn's disease.[96] The systemic manifestations of inflammatory bowel disease may mimic juvenile rheumatoid arthritis, anorexia nervosa, collagen vascular disease, acute rheumatic fever, or growth hormone deficiency.[1] Thus, the physician must have a high index of suspicion to make the appropriate diagnosis of inflammatory bowel disease in children.

References

1. Burbidge, E. J., Huang, S., and Bayless, T. M.: Clinical manifestations of Crohn's disease in children and adolescents. Pediatrics, 55:866, 1975.
2. Calkins, B. M., Lilienfeld, A. M., Garland, C. F., and Mendeloff, A. I.: Trends in incidence rates of ulcerative colitis and Crohn's disease. Dig. Dis. Sci., 29:913, 1984.
3. Mendeloff, A. I.: The epidemiology of inflammatory bowel disease. Clin. Gastroenterol., 9:259, 1980.
4. Gilat, T.: Incidence of inflammatory bowel disease: Going up or down? Gastroenterology, 85:196, 1983.
5. Goligher, J. C., et al.: Ulcerative Colitis. Baltimore, Williams & Wilkins, 1968.
6. Kyle, J.: Crohn's Disease. New York, Appleton Century Crofts, 1972.
7. Banks, B. M., Zetzel, L., and Richter, H. S.: Morbidity and mortality in regional enteritis: Report of 168 cases. Am. J. Dig. Dis., 14:369, 1969.
8. Jenkins, H. R., et al.: Food allergy: The major cause of infantile colitis. Arch. Dis. Child., 59:326, 1984.
9. Farmer, R. G., Michener, W. M., and Mortimer, E. A.: Studies of family history among patients with inflammatory bowel disease. Clin. Gastroenterol., 9:271, 1980.
10. Kirsner, J. B., and Shorter, R. G.: Recent developments in nonspecific inflammatory bowel disease. N. Engl. J. Med., 306:837, 1982.
11. Michener, W. M.: Ulcerative colitis in children: Problems in management. Pediatr. Clin. North Am., 14:159, 1967.
12. Silverman, A., and Roy, C. C.: Pediatric Clinical Gastroenterology. St. Louis, C. V. Mosby, 1983.
13. Grand, R. J., and Homer, D. R.: Approaches to inflammatory bowel disease in childhood and adolescence. Pediatr. Clin. North Am., 22:835, 1975.
14. Werlin, S. L., and Grand, R. J.: Severe colitis in children and adolescents: Diagnosis, course and treatment. Gastroenterology, 73:828, 1977.

15. Ehrenpresis, T. H. Gierup, J., and Lageracrantz, R.: Chronic regional enterocolitis in children and adolescents. Acta Paediatr. Scand., *60*:209, 1971.
16. Korelitz, B. I., Gribetz, D., and Kopel, F. B.: Granulomatous colitis in children: A study of 25 cases and comparison with ulcerative colitis. Pediatrics, *42*:446, 1968.
17. Lindsley, C. B., and Schaller, J. G.: Arthritis associated with inflammatory bowel disease. J. Pediatr., *84*:6, 1974.
18. Scully, R. E., Mark, E. J., and McNeely, B. U.: Case records of the Massachusetts General Hospital: Case 47-1983. N. Engl. J. Med., *309*:1306, 1983.
19. Gryboski, J., and Hillemeier, C.: Inflammatory bowel disease in children. Med. Clin. North Am., *64*: 1185, 1980.
20. O'Donoghue, D. P., and Dawson, A. M.: Crohn's disease in childhood. Arch. Dis. Child., *52*:627, 1977.
21. Markowitz, J., et al.: Perianal disease in children and adolescents with Crohn's disease. Gastroenterology, *86*:829, 1984.
22. Devroede, G. J., et al.: Cancer risk and life expectancy in children with ulcerative colitis. N. Engl. J. Med., *285*:17, 1971.
23. Lennard-Jones, J. E., et al.: Cancer in colitis: An assessment of the individual risk by clinical and histological criteria. Gastroenterology, *73*:1280, 1977.
24. Butt, J. H., Lennard-Jones, J. E., and Ritchie, J. K.: A practical approach to the risk of cancer in inflammatory bowel disease. Med. Clin. North Am., *64*:1203, 1980.
25. Morson, B. C., and Dawson, I. M. P.: Gastrointestinal Pathology. Oxford, Blackwell, 1979.
26. Hultén, L., Kenenter, J., Aaren, C., and Ojerskög, B.: Clinical and morphological characteristics of colitis, carcinoma and colorectal carcinoma in young people. Scand. J. Gastroenterol., *14*:673, 1979.
27. Buchmann, P., and Alexander-Williams, J.: Classification of perianal Crohn's disease. Clin. Gastroenterol., *9*:323, 1980.
28. Weedon, D. D., et al.: Crohn's disease and cancer. N. Engl. J. Med., *289*:1099, 1973.
29. Gryboski, J. D., and Spiro, H. D.: Prognosis in children with Crohn's disease. Gastroenterology, *74*:807, 1978.
30. Greenstein, A. J., Janowitz, H. D., and Sachar, D. B.: The extraintestinal complications of Crohn's disease and ulcerative colitis: A study of 700 patients. Medicine, *55*:401, 1976.
31. Daum, F., et al.: Asymptomatic transient uveitis in children with inflammatory bowel disease. Am. J. Dis. Child., *133*:170, 1979.
32. Singer, A. M., Bennett, R. C., Carter, N. G., and Hughes, E. S. R.: Blood and urinary changes in patients with ileostomies and ileorectal anastomosis. Br. Med. J., *3*:141, 1973.
33. Brewer, R. I., Gelzayd, E. A., and Kirsner, J. K.: Urinary crystalloid excretion in patients with inflammatory bowel disease. Gut, *11*:314, 1970.
34. Dew, M. J., Thompson, H., and Allan, R. N.: The spectrum of hepatic dysfunction in inflammatory bowel disease. J. Med., *48*:113, 1979.
35. Eade, M. N., Cooke, W. T., Brooke, B. N., and Thompson, H.: Liver disease in Crohn's colitis: A study of 21 consecutive patients having colectomy. Ann. Intern. Med., *74*:518, 1971.
36. Perrett, A. D., et al.: The liver in Crohn's disease. Q. J. Med., *40*:187, 1971.
37. Kane, W., Miller, K., and Sharp, H. L.: Inflammatory bowel disease presenting as liver disease during childhood. J. Pediatr., *97*:775, 1980.
38. Freese, D., et al.: Therapeutic response of the pericholangitis in the liver lesion associated with inflammatory bowel disease (IBD). Gastroenterology, *78*:1168, 1980.
39. Heaton, K. W., and Read, A. E.: Gallstones in patients with disorders of the terminal ileum and disturbed bile salt metabolism. Br. Med. J., *3*:494, 1969.
40. Cohen, S., Kaplan, M., Gottlieb, L., and Patterson, J.: Liver disease and gallstones in regional enteritis. Gastroenterology, *60*:237, 1971.
41. Castille, R. G., et al.: Crohn's disease in children: Assessment of the progression of disease, growth, and prognosis. J. Pediatr. Surg., *15*:462, 1980.
42. Farmer, R. G., and Michener, W. M.: Prognosis of Crohn's disease with onset in childhood or adolescence. Dig. Dis. Sci., *24*:752, 1979.
43. McCaffery, T. D., et al.: Severe growth retardation in children with inflammatory bowel disease. Pediatrics, *45*:386, 1970.
44. Motil, K. J., Grand, R. J., and Davis-Kraft, E.: The epidemiology of growth failure in children and adolescents with inflammatory bowel disease. Gastroenterology, *84*:1254, 1983.
45. Sobel, E. H., Silverman, F. N., and Lee, C. M.: Chronic regional enteritis and growth retardation. Am. J. Dis. Child. *103*:569, 1962.
46. Motil, K. J.: Macronutrient status in inflammatory bowel disease. J. Clin. Nutr., *2*:12, 1983.
47. Motil, K. J., et al.: Whole body leucine metabolism in adolescents with Crohn's disease and growth failure during nutritional supplementation. Gastroenterology, *82*:1359, 1982.
48. Motil, K. J., and Grand, R. J.: Inflammatory bowel disease. *In* Nutrition in Pediatrics-Basic Science and Clinical Application. Edited by W. A. Walker and J. B. Watkins. Boston, Little Brown, 1985.
49. Kelts, D. G., et al.: Nutritional basis of growth failure in children and adolescents with Crohn's disease. Gastroenterology, *76*:720, 1979.
50. Kirschner, B. S., Voinchet, O., and Rosenberg, I. H.: Growth retardation in inflammatory bowel disease. Gastroenterology, *75*:504, 1978.
51. Gotlin, R. W., and DuBois, R. S.: Nyctohemeral growth hormone levels in children with growth retardation and inflammatory bowel disease. Gut, *14*:191, 1973.
52. Tenore, A., Berman, W. F., Parks, J. S., and Bongiovanni, A. M.: Basal and stimulated serum growth hormone concentrations in inflammatory bowel disease. J. Clin. Endocrinol. Metabol., *44*:622, 1977.
53. Kirschner, B. S.: Somatomedin deficiency: A possible cause of growth failure in children with chronic inflammatory bowel disease. Gastroenterology, *80*:1192, 1981.
54. Isley, W. L., Underwood, L. E., and Clemmons, D. R.: Dietary components that regulate serum somatomedin-C concentrations in humans. J. Clin. Invest., *71*:175, 1983.
55. Berger, M., Gribetz, D., and Korelitz, B. I.: Growth retardation in children with ulcerative colitis: The effect of medical and surgical therapy. Pediatrics, *55*:459, 1975.
56. Homer, D. R., Grand, R. J., and Colodny, A. H.: Growth, course and prognosis after surgery for Crohn's disease in children and adolescents. Pediatrics, *59*:717, 1977.
57. Frey, C. F., and Weaver, D. K.: Colectomy in children with ulcerative and granulomatous colitis: Operative indications and results. Arch. Surg., *104*:416, 1972.
58. Harris, B. H., Hollabaugh, R. S., and Clatworthy, H. W.: Surgery for developmental and growth failure in childhood granulomatous colitis. J. Pediatr. Surg., *9*:301, 1974.
59. Motil, K. J., and Grand, R. J.: Nutritional management of inflammatory bowel disease. Pediatr. Clin. North Am., *32*:447, 1985.

60. Hodges, P., et al.: Vitamin and iron intake in patients with Crohn's disease. J. Am. Diet. Assoc., *84*:52, 1984.
61. Andersson, H., Filipsson, S., and Hultén, L.: Determination of the fecal excretion of labeled bile salts after I. V. administration of 14C-cholic acid. Scand. J. Gastroenterol., *13*:249, 1978.
62. Grill, B. B., Hillemeier, A. C., and Gryboski, J. D.: Fecal alpha$_1$-antitrypsin clearance in patients with inflammatory bowel disease. J. Pediatr. Gastroenterol. Nutr., *3*:56, 1984.
63. Wannemacher, R. W.: Protein metabolism. *In* Total Parenteral Nutrition. Edited by H. Ghadimi. New York, John Wiley and Sons, 1975.
64. Young, V. R.: The role of skeletal and cardiac muscle in the regulation of protein metabolism. *In* Mammalian Protein Metabolism. Vol. IV. Edited by H. N. Munro. New York, Academic Press, 1970.
65. Beisel, W. R., Wannemacher, R. W., Jr., and Neufeld, H. A.: Relation of fever to energy expenditure. *In* Assessment of Energy Metabolism in Health and Disease. Edited by J. M. Kinney and E. Lense. Columbus, Ross Laboratories, 1980.
66. Smith, A. N., and Balfour, T. W.: Malabsorption in Crohn's disease. Clin. Gastroenterol., *1*:433, 1972.
67. Beeken, W. L.: Absorptive defects in young people with regional enteritis. Pediatrics, *52*:69, 1974.
68. Gerson, C. D., Cohen, N., and Janowitz, H. J.: Small intestinal absorptive function in regional enteritis. Gastroenterology, *64*:907, 1973.
69. Kirschner, B. S., DeFavaro, M. V., and Jenson, W.: Lactose malabsorption in children and adolescents with inflammatory bowel disease. Gastroenterology, *81*:829, 1981.
70. Beeken, W. L., Bush, H. J., and Sylvester, D. L.: Intestinal protein loss in Crohn's disease. Gastroenterology, *62*:207, 1972.
71. Gerlach, K., Morowitz, D. A., and Kirsner, J. B.: Symptomatic hypomagnesemia complicating regional enteritis. Gastroenterology, *59*:567, 1970.
72. Grand, R. J., and Colodny, A. H.: Increased requirement for magnesium therapy during parenteral therapy for granulomatous colitis. J. Pediatr., *81*:788, 1972.
73. Krawitt, E. L., Beeken, W. L., and Janney, C. D.: Calcium absorption in Crohn's disease. Gastroenterology, *71*:251, 1976.
74. Driscoll, R. H., Jr., et al.: Vitamin D deficiency and bone disease in patients with Crohn's disease. Gastroenterology, *83*:1252, 1982.
75. Schoelmerich, J., et al.: Zinc and vitamin A deficiency in patients is correlated with activity but not with localization or extent of the disease. Hepatogastroenterology, *32*:34, 1985.
76. Filipson, S., Hultén, L., and Lindstedt, G.: Malabsorption of fat and vitamin B$_{12}$ before and after intestinal resection for Crohn's disease. Scand. J. Gastroenterol., *13*:529, 1978.
77. Main, A. N. H., et al.: Clinical experience of zinc supplementation during intravenous nutrition in Crohn's disease: Value of serum and urine zinc measurements. Gut, *23*:984, 1982.
78. McClain, C., Soutor, C., and Zieve, L.: Zinc deficiency: A complication of Crohn's disease. Gastroenterology, *78*:272, 1980.
79. Solomons, N. W., et al.: Growth retardation and zinc nutrition. Pediatr. Res., *10*:923, 1976.
80. Sturniolo, G. C., et al.: Zinc absorption in Crohn's disease. Gut, *21*:387, 1980.
81. Beisel, W. R.: Effect of infection on human protein metabolism. Fed. Proc., *25*:1682, 1966.
82. Motil, K. J., Altchuler, S. I., and Grand, R. J.: Mineral balance during nutritional supplementation in adolescents with Crohn's disease and growth failure. J. Pediatr., *107*:473, 1985.
83. Scrimshaw, N. S.: Effect of infection on nutrient requirements. Am. J. Clin. Nutr., *30*:1536, 1977.
84. Forbes, G. B.: A note on the mathematics of catch-up growth. Pediatr. Res., *8*:929, 1974.
85. Lloyd-Still, J. D., and Green, O. C.: A clinical scoring system for chronic inflammatory bowel disease in children. Dig. Dis. Sci., *24*:620, 1979.
86. Harries, A. D., et al.: Platelet count: A simple measure of activity in Crohn's disease. Br. Med. J., *286*:1476, 1983.
87. Campbell, C. A., Walker-Smith, J. A., Hindocha, P., and Adinolfi, M.: Acute phase proteins in chronic inflammatory bowel disease in childhood. J. Pediatr. Gastroenterol. Nutr., *1*:193, 1982.
88. Nolan, D. J.: Radiology of Crohn's disease of the small intestine: A review. J. R. Soc. Med., *74*:294, 1981.
89. Nolan, D. J.: Barium examination of the small intestine. Gut, *22*:682, 1981.
90. Savery-Muttu, S., et al.: [111]Indium autologous leukocytes in inflammatory bowel disease. Gut, *24*:293, 1983.
91. Gordon, I., and Vivian, G.: Radiolabeled leukocytes: A new diagnostic tool in occult infection/inflammation. Arch. Dis. Child., *59*:62, 1984.
92. Williams, C. B., et al.: Total colonoscopy in childhood. Arch. Dis. Child., *57*:49, 1982.
93. Hassall, E., Barclay, G. N., and Ament., M. E.: Colonoscopy in childhood. Pediatrics, *73*:594, 1984.
94. Rossini, F. P.: Atlas of Colonoscopy. Berlin, Springer-Verlag, 1977.
95. Farmer, R. G., Whelan, G., and Sivak, M. V.: Colonoscopy in distal colon ulcerative colitis. Clin. Gastroenterol., *9*:297, 1980.
96. Hyams, J. S., Goldman, H., and Katz, A. J.: Differentiating small bowel Crohn's disease from lymphoma. Role of rectal biopsy. Gastroenterology, *79*:340, 1980.
97. Blackstone, M. O., Riddell, R. H., Rogers, B. H. G., and Levin, B.: Dysplasia-associated lesion or mass (DALM) detected by colonoscopy in long-standing ulcerative colitis: An indication for colectomy. Gastroenterology, *80*:366, 1981.
98. Goodman, M. J., Kirsner, J. B., and Riddell, R. H.: Usefulness of rectal biopsy in inflammatory bowel disease. Gastroenterology, *72*:952, 1977.
99. Surawicz, C. M., and Belic, L.: Rectal biopsy helps to distinguish acute self-limited colitis from idiopathic inflammatory bowel disease. Gastroenterology, *86*:104, 1984.
100. Kirsner, J. B.: Problems in the differentiation of ulcerative colitis and Crohn's disease of the colon: The need for repeated diagnostic evaluation. Gastroenterology, *68*:187, 1975.
101. Tedesco, F. J.: Differential diagnosis of ulcerative colitis and Crohn's ileocolitis and other specific inflammatory disease of the bowel. Med. Clin. North Am., *64*:1173, 1980.
102. Buts, J. P., Weber, A. A., Roy, C. C., and Morin, C. L.: Pseudomembranous enterocolitis in children. Gastroenterology, *78*:823, 1977.
103. Tedesco, F., et al.: Oral vanomycin for antibiotic-associated pseudomembranous colitis. Lancet, *2*:226, 1978.
104. Berman W.: The hemolytic-uremic syndrome: Initial clinical presentation mimicking ulcerative colitis. J. Pediatr., *81*:275, 1972.
105. Khojastesh, A., Haghshenass, M., and Haghighi, P.: Immunoproliferative small intestinal disease. N. Engl. J. Med., *308*:1401, 1983.

13 · Pathophysiology of Symptoms and Clinical Features of Inflammatory Bowel Disease

SIDNEY F. PHILLIPS, M.D., F.R.A.C.P., F.A.C.P.

For most physicians, the idiopathic inflammatory bowel diseases (IBD) are frustrating enigmas.[1] They present the major clinical challenges common to all chronic, debilitating illnesses; their unknown etiologies raise perplexing differential diagnoses, and the need to rely upon empirical therapies is disquieting. These therapeutic decisions separate naturally into those that attempt to modify the etiopathogenesis of IBD, albeit in an arbitrary fashion, and those that attempt only to reduce the symptoms. The mechanisms underlying the symptoms and clinical features of IBD are hardly understood better than are their etiologies. New insights into human pathophysiology offer a few rudimentary clues into the genesis of these clinical features, however; perhaps, therefore, they also offer better rationales for symptomatic treatment. This chapter addresses those pathophysiologic mechanisms that underlie the clinical features of IBD.

The subject matter includes ulcerative colitis and Crohn's disease of the fore-, mid-, and hindgut. Emphasis will be placed on the presurgical pathophysiology, but reference will also be made to the ileostomist and to ileal resection; however, specific problems of the patient with "short bowel syndrome" are considered elsewhere (see Chaps. 30 and 31). The major symptoms to be covered are anorexia, nausea, and vomiting; under nutrition; diarrhea; abdominal pain; bleeding; and features specific to the postoperative state.

Specific Clinical Features
Anorexia, Nausea, and Vomiting

The sequence, though producing in the patient progressive degrees of discomfort, is of prime interest to the physician as a cause of undernutrition; this clinical feature is exemplified most dramatically by the stunted adolescent with Crohn's disease and growth failure.[2] These tragic circumstances can often be reversed if the disease activity is controlled; control can be by medical or surgical means,[2-4] or by repletion of calories.[3] The problem is that many of these patients cannot eat normal meals, and this failure of adequate intake is caused by severe anorexia, with nausea and/or vomiting. Of greater frequency are less extreme examples of this "upper gut syndrome," in which undernutrition appears to be compromising remission from a debilitating recurrence.

What is the mechanism of the poor intake of food in some patients with IBD? One of the possible answers is that a deficiency of trace minerals reduces the attraction of food. Deficiency of zinc may cause hypogeusia and hyposmia,[5,6] both of which have been incriminated in the anorexia and nausea of inflammatory bowel disease.[7] Because many patients with diarrhea lose important trace elements, including zinc, this hypothesis has intrinsic appeal. Indeed, a reasonably good correlation usually exists between stool volume and fecal losses of zinc.[8] Moreover, when caloric intake is reduced, deficiency states are more likely to develop; thus, zinc deficiency occurs in IBD.[7] Unfortunately, serum levels of zinc have been reported to be normal even in undernourished children,[6] and no correlation was found between serum zinc levels and several indices of nutritional status in patients with IBD.[9] Confounding the interpretation of much data, circulating zinc is bound to albumin, and blood levels do not necessarily reflect body stores.

A more probable cause of these symptoms is direct involvement of the gastroduodenum by inflammatory bowel disease. The National Cooperative Crohn's Disease Study found that 8% of patients had disease of the duodenum, and three times that number had radiologic abnormalities that suggested duodenal Crohn's disease.[10] Systematic diagnostic studies directed towards the incidence of gastroduodenal disease, using endoscopy and histology, were not performed, however, and the true prevalence of gastroduodenal Crohn's disease or its role in the clinical syndrome of anorexia and undernutrition is uncertain. That patients with major symptoms referable to the upper gut may have local disease despite negative barium studies, must be kept in mind. Even if the upper gut is affected by Crohn's disease, the mechanisms producing anorexia remain unclear, unless there is clear evidence of partial intestinal obstruction. It must also be remembered that gastric and duodenal ulceration are common diseases; indeed, the differential diagnosis between duodenal ulcer and Crohn's disease can be difficult. Clearly, either could lead to nausea, vomiting, and anorexia, and either could contribute to undernutrition.

The local or central effects of drugs must also be considered seriously as pathogenic factors in symptoms referable to the upper gut. The list of drugs causing nausea is a long one, but salicylazosulfapyridine needs special consideration in the present context. From 10 to 20% of patients given salicylazosulfapyridine develop nausea and/or vomiting and, at times, this can be severe enough to require that the drug be stopped. Though initially attributed to gastric irritation, possibly because of the salicylic acid moiety, symptoms are more correctly correlated with the circulating levels of sulfapyridine and the patient's status as an acetylator of sulfapyridine.[11-13] Thus, the effect is probably mediated centrally, possibly through the chemosensitive trigger zone of the hindbrain. A schedule of "desensitization" has been proposed for this side effect.[11] The program requires discontinuance of the drug for 2 weeks; medication is recommended at doses up to 0.25 g daily, and increased gradually thereafter at weekly intervals.

Local, obstructive lesions of the ileum can produce nausea and vomiting, and less obvious ileal lesions might lead to milder symptoms, such as anorexia. The recently described "ileal brake" is triggered by excess fat in the ileum.[14,15]* This mechanism, presumably of hormonal mediation, slows the transit of meals through the jejunum and can also delay gastric emptying. Thus, steatorrhea, from any cause, should be considered a potential cause of nausea and vomiting arising from gastric stasis.

In an attempt to evaluate the possible role of delayed gastric emptying in the genesis of a reduced intake of food and, therefore, to underly poor nutrition and growth retardation, a group of young patients with Crohn's disease were studied.[16] The subjects included those with growth retardation, undernutrition, normal development and nutrition, and healthy controls. In this selected population, symptoms of anorexia, nausea, and vomiting were common (Fig. 13-1). Gastric emptying of liquids and solids was quantified scintigraphically. Liquids emptied at the same rate in all groups, and children with growth retardation emptied solids normally. Solids emptied slowly in 5 of 7 patients with malnutrition, however, and the delay could not be correlated with the Crohn's Disease Activity Index. Slow gastric emptying was related to reduced caloric intake, and half of those with delayed emptying had radiologic or endoscopic evidence of nonobstructive lesions of the duodenum. The major findings of this study are given in Figure 13-2. While not indicative of any causal relationship, and raising many questions as to how delayed gastric emptying and symptoms could be related mechanistically, these observations point to a potentially important pathophysiologic process.

CLINICAL APPROACHES. Patients with IBD who complain of nausea, anorexia, and vomiting

*Editors' note: see also Jain, N. K., et al.: Gastroenterology, 92:1450, 1987.

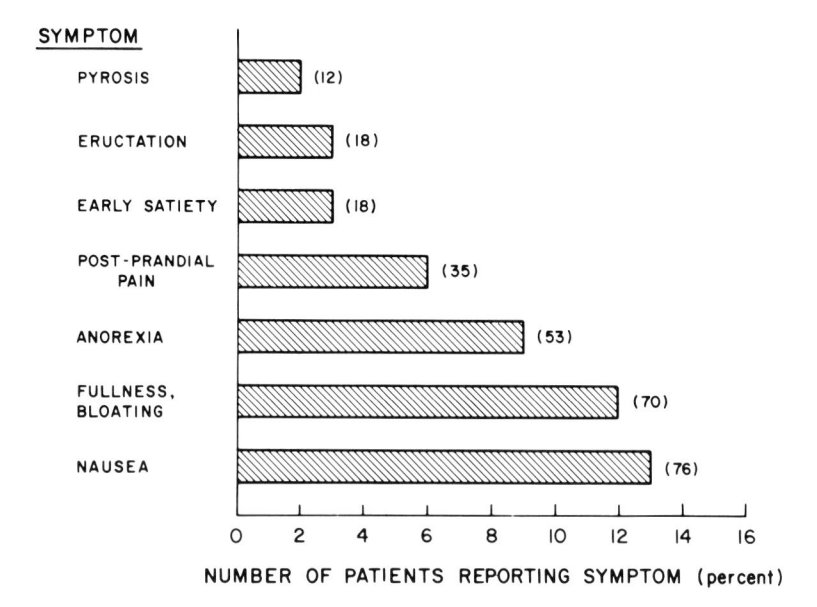

SYMPTOM	
PYROSIS	(12)
ERUCTATION	(18)
EARLY SATIETY	(18)
POST-PRANDIAL PAIN	(35)
ANOREXIA	(53)
FULLNESS, BLOATING	(70)
NAUSEA	(76)

NUMBER OF PATIENTS REPORTING SYMPTOM (percent)

FIG. 13-1. Symptoms in 17 young patients (aged 18 years or less, mean 14 years) with Crohn's disease. (Reproduced with permission from Grill, B. B., et al.: J. Clin. Gastroenterol., 7:216, 1985.

need the encouragement of a diet that is as full and varied as is compatible with their overall clinical status. All unnecessary drugs should be discontinued, and those that need to be continued should be reduced to minimal effective doses. The search for causative factors of these symptoms should include upper gastrointestinal endoscopy with biopsy of any suspicious areas in the stomach and duodenum; an assessment of gastric emptying might also be considered.

The message is clear: correctable causes of anorexia, nausea, and diminished intakes of food exist. Though uncommon, these need to be sought and treated appropriately. When no treatable causes are found, appetite needs to be stimulated by a complete and attractive diet. When the problem is recalcitrant, the stomach may need to be circumvented as an entry point for nutrients by the use of enteral or parenteral nutrition (see Chap. 24).

Undernutrition

Broad license will be taken with this topic. The symptoms to be considered include weight loss, weakness, fatigue, and malabsorption, which extends the subject matter to diarrhea, a feature that will also be considered independently. These complaints are manifested by the laboratory findings of anemia, hypoalbuminemia, and evidence of maldigestion-malabsorption. Of the possible mechanisms underlying these clinical features, the first that should be considered is a decreased intake of nutrients. This will usually be attributable to anorexia, nausea or vomiting (as discussed previously). Though some patients with IBD certainly consume less calories (and presumably less micronutrients also) than they require, the majority do not.[17] Thus, the next question to be posed is, do patients with IBD require larger than anticipated intakes of nutrients?

A wide-spread, but largely unsupported, belief is that patients with IBD have greater than normal expenditures of energy. This appears unlikely, because the observations by Barot and by Fleming's group do not support this assumption.[18,19] Fleming and his colleagues performed indirect calorimetry on 54 patients with Crohn's disease. Actual expenditures of energy, in the basal state as measured by indirect calorimetry, were not greater than those calculated from the nomograms developed by Harris and Benedict (Fig. 13-3), which are based on values for healthy persons. Fleming's patients did not have acute complications, such as fever or active infection, both of which might be expected to increase metabolic requirements. Nevertheless, the results suggest that most patients with IBD are not in a catabolic state.

A second general consideration relates to a putative cycle that links malnutrition with an impairment of digestive-absorptive potential; thus, it could be hypothesized that once established in IBD, from whatever cause, undernutrition leads to less efficient assimilation of nutri-

▲ Crohn's disease with malnutrition
○ Normals
● Crohn's disease without growth retardation or malnutrition
—— Solids
---- Liquids
● = $\bar{x} \pm$ S.E.

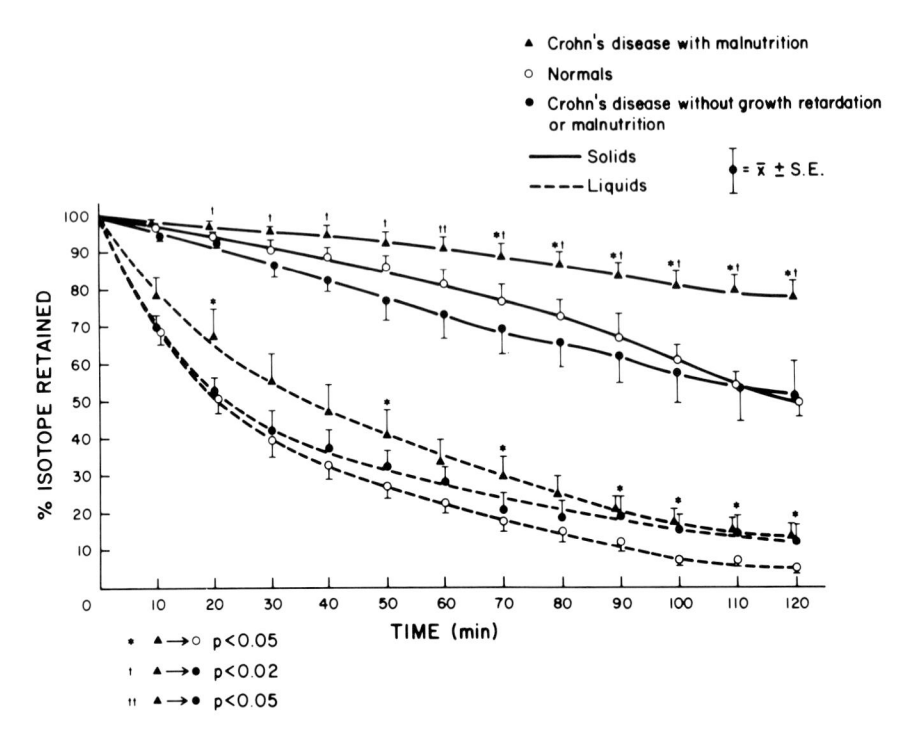

* ▲→○ $p<0.05$
† ▲→● $p<0.02$
†† ▲→● $p<0.05$

FIG. 13-2. Percent of isotope retained in the stomach after a mixed, solid-liquid meal in patients with Crohn's disease; n = 7 for group with malnutrition, n = 6 for those without growth disturbances, n = 13 for controls. (Reproduced with permission from Grill, B. B., et al.: J. Clin. Gastroenterol., 7:216, 1985.)

ents. The relationship between undernutrition and malabsorption has been reviewed,[20] and the following conclusions were reached: (1) the intestine has major needs for metabolic energy, if its rapid turnover of cells is to be maintained; 300 g of cells and 20 g of protein and fat are estimated to be shed from the small intestine alone each day; (2) the small intestine appears to be impaired functionally in severe starvation; for example, the syndrome of protein-calorie malnutrition; and (3) further complicating the bowel's ability to adapt to malnutrition are certain specific defects that result from deficiencies of trace elements or vitamins. Unfortunately, no useful data are available on these points in IBD, but the possibilities should be kept in mind when extreme malnutrition develops.

Of more immediate concern are the direct maldigestive-malabsorptive consequences of IBD. Malabsorption should be anticipated when the small bowel is involved extensively by Crohn's disease or after resection of the ileum. The more subtle question remains unanswered, however: might unsuspected malabsorption contribute to generalized undernutrition and, at the same time, exacerbate diarrhea? Early measurements of intestinal lactase activity in IBD and assessments of lactose malabsorption incriminated maldigestion-malabsorption of milk sugar in the symptoms of IBD.[21] However, this and other reports antedated a full appreciation of the prevalence of lactase deficiency in certain races. Since that time, it has been recognized that, after allowance is made for the racial background of the patient, lactose intolerance is no more frequent in young patients with IBD than in those with nonspecific abdominal symptoms.[22] The clinical message now is different, but is still an important one. Strong, positive evidence should be required before young patients with IBD are denied an attractive and effective nutrient by advising a milk-free diet.[22]

The other major carbohydrate nutrient, starch, has also attracted attention because it is now apparent that even the healthy small intestine does not digest and absorb all starch. Using hydrogen breath tests as an index of carbohydrate malabsorption, up to 20% of a test meal of starch was available for metabolism by the colonic flora.[23,24] These results were supported by recovery of chyme by direct aspiration of the ileum after homogenized test meals containing 20 or 60 g of starch;[25] in these experiments, a mean of 10% of starch was not absorbed.[25] Though comparable studies on ileostomates have yielded conflicting results,[26] significant

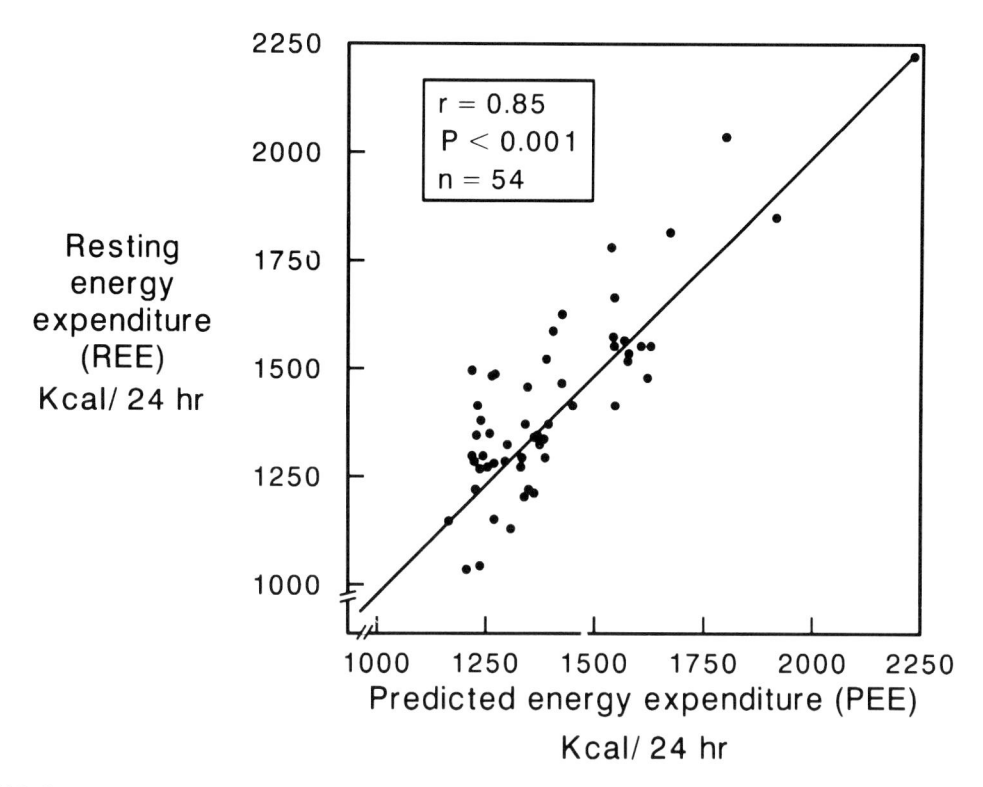

FIG. 13-3. Resting energy expenditure measured by indirect calorimetry plotted against predicted energy expenditure (using the Harris-Benedict formula) in 54 patients with Crohn's disease. Actual expenditure of energy was no greater than values predicted for healthy persons. (Reproduced with permission from Chan, A. T. H., Fleming, C. R., O'Fallon, W. M., and Huizenga, K. A.: Gastroenterology, 91:75, 1986.)

amounts of starch were not recovered in stomal effluents. If the healthy small intestine cannot digest and absorb a starch load, the question as to whether the bowel in Crohn's disease is compromised even further is highly relevant, but still unexplored.

Can unrecognized maldigestion or malabsorption of fat underlie malnutrition, even in circumstances that are not usually associated with such sequelae, such as limited ileocolonic involvement by Crohn's disease or in ulcerative colitis? It could be argued that abnormalities of villous architecture have been reported, even in ulcerative colitis;[27,28] further, because the ileum may be an important site for fat absorption,[29] even in health, mild ileal disease may produce steatorrhea. With more experience in the interpretation of jejunal biopsies, however, the early reports of villous changes in IBD have not been corroborated. Moreover, Felipsson found that most patients, even those with extensive Crohn's disease of the small intestine, did not have significant steatorrhea;[30] only 25% of those with short segments (<30 cm) of disease did, with a few more in those with greater (30 to 60 cm) involvement. Following ileal resection, the correlation between the length of ileum resected and the presence and degree of steatorrhea was better.[30] He concluded, however, that malabsorption of fat per se was not of great importance to the nutritional consequences of Crohn's disease.

Hypoalbuminemia occurs in one-third or more of all patients with Crohn's disease of the small bowel, and is even more common when the colon is extensively involved by Crohn's colitis or ulcerative colitis.[30] While exudative enteropathy can result from any ulcerative lesion, excessive loss of protein through IBD mucosa will be exaggerated by the increased capillary permeability and high blood flow to the mucosa.[31] Though hypoalbuminemia could contribute to undernutrition and weight loss, as unrecognized malabsorption of carbohydrate and fat might, we have not progressed much further than in 1960 when Kalser concluded that the deficient nutritional status of patients with IBD was caused by a combination of anorexia, chronic infection, anemia, and losses of proteins.[32]

The final area to be addressed is the possible effect of drugs on digestion-absorption. The list of drugs that impair the absorption of nutrients is a diverse one and the mechanisms by which drugs cause malabsorption is equally variable. Longstreth and Newcomer listed mucosal damage caused by direct cellular toxicity, inhibition of mucosal enzymes, and alteration of the intraluminal milieu by physicochemical interactions with bile or fatty acids as causes of drug-induced malabsorption.[33] Those particularly pertinent to IBD are listed in Table 13-1, although because many other drugs affect intestinal function, it is reasonable to expect side effects to be even more frequent in an intestine that is already compromised by disease.

Clinical judgment must be the guide to a search for associated infection or the presence of an intra-abdominal abscess in patients with IBD who are not doing as well as would be predicted from the extent and activity of their disease. These complications will be common causes of undernutrition. If no such feature is found, an assessment of activity of the disease will be needed. A careful dietary history and a count of caloric intake under dietary supervision may reveal important but inapparent anorexia. Testing for fecal excretion of fat, other tests of intestinal absorption, and a careful drug history will be necessary. In most instances, it is the severity of the bowel's involvement by IBD that has been underestimated. More aggressive medical, or surgical, therapy is usually needed.

The special problem of growth retardation and delayed sexual development in the adolescent will not be covered here because it is discussed in Chapters 12, 23, and 24. However, this dramatic manifestation of IBD exemplifies well those approaches likely to be successful also in less severe examples of undernutrition. Growth retardation and sexual underdevelopment can be reversed by increased intake of nutrients by any route (meals, enteral feeding, or parenteral nutrition) or by successful control of the disease activity by medical or surgical means.[2-4]

Pathophysiology of Diarrhea in Inflammatory Bowel Disease

A precise description of all the pathogenic mechanisms of diarrhea in inflammatory bowel disease is impossible; the gaps in our understanding of normal physiology are too great. All that is certain is that mucosal inflammation deranges normal mechanisms of absorption and transit quite variably. Moreover, the clinical spectrum of inflammatory bowel disease is broad, anatomically and qualitatively; thus, it is especially important to distinguish clearly between the mechanisms of diarrhea in disease confined to the colon and in disease of the small intestine.

The major clinical features of diarrhea from any cause should also be kept in mind. Increased frequency of excreting stool is the most common complaint, but this index has wide interindividual variations. The consistency of stools is also important clinically, but because it cannot be quantified precisely it is only of subjective value. Rectal discomfort is also a nonspecific feature, albeit this is a frequent complaint of patients with IBD. Fecal weight is perhaps the most objective index; in Western societies, normal stool weight has an upper limit of 200 to 300 g/day.

DIARRHEA IN COLITIS. Diseases confined to the colon include chronic ulcerative colitis and Crohn's disease of the colon, but the category should be subdivided further into proctosigmoiditis, or other localized forms of inflammation, and colitis with total or near total involvement of the large intestine.

Table 13-2 gives results from seven series in which total fecal weight per day was recorded from patients with colitis. When the colon was involved extensively, and especially when the disease was of moderate to high severity, fecal output varied widely but was generally 2 to 3 times the normal value in health. On the other hand, when disease was confined to the rectum, total daily weights were at about the upper limit of normal. These findings in proctitis support our clinical impressions. Thus, it should be noted that in descriptions of idiopathic proctitis, such as that by the group from St. Mark's Hospital,[38] constipation or normal bowel habits were found in approximately two-thirds of patients. Indeed, a syndrome of "fecal stasis in inflammatory bowel disease" has been described.[39] It also has been shown that the potassium-to-sodium ratio in stools from patients with proctosigmoiditis is normal or only slightly elevated.[37] These data can be interpreted as supporting the essentially normal composition of stools in proctosigmoiditis.

Although studies are not available to support the hypothesis that absorption in the small intestine and proximal colon is normal in proctosigmoiditis, this seems to be a reasonable proposal. Thus, the volume of stool presented to the distal colon may not be greatly above normal. On the

TABLE 13-1. *Malabsorption caused by drugs used for IBD.**

Drug	Absorptive Defect	Possible Mechanism
Salicylazosulfapyridine	Folate	Decreased folate uptake by enterocytes
Glucocorticoids	Calcium, iron	Decreased active transport
Cholestyramine	Fat, fat soluble vitamins, fat soluble drugs	Decreased micellar bile acids
Antacids	Phosphorus, drugs	Physicochemical interactions

*Adapted from Longstreth, G. F., and Newcomer, A. D.: Mayo Clin. Proc., 50:284, 1975.

other hand, exudation of blood and mucus from the rectum is to be expected. Thus, the evacuations in proctitis are often bloody mucus and contain little fecal matter. Another interesting speculation is that the sensitivity of the rectum to its contents is increased in proctitis, perhaps because of decreased compliance of the rectal segment.[40] A less compliant rectum might well contribute to the frequency of defecation and the rectal discomfort noted by these patients.

When the colonic involvement is more extensive, the colon absorbs less sodium, chloride, and water. These functions of the diseased colon have been studied in vivo and in vitro; perfusions of the colon in vivo yield results most consistent with a primary defect in the absorption of sodium, chloride, and water (Table 13-3). Observations on colitis tissue in vitro are more limited (Table 13-4). Hawker and Turnberg showed reduced mucosal-to-serosal fluxes of sodium and chloride, but little or no change was present in the serosal-to-mucosal movements of these ions;[45] potassium flux was normal. Archampong showed an increased serosal-to-mucosal flux of sodium; however, the mucosal-to-serosal flux was also increased.[46] Overall, these results are inconclusive, but no overwhelming evidence supports an active process of secretion.

Prostaglandin production by colonic mucosa is increased in colitis, and prostanoids have been implicated in the diarrhea of inflammatory bowel disease as well as in the inflammatory process. Prostaglandins are able to influence electrolyte transport by colonic epithelium in vitro[47] and the possibility that prostaglandins play a role in the diarrhea of IBD remains attractive, but unproven. Moreover, as described earlier, no strong evidence exists of a secretory state in the colon affected by inflammatory bowel disease.

Indeed, perhaps more important are the opposing contributions of the cytoprotective role of certain prostaglandins versus the mediation of inflammation by others (e.g., lipoxygenase products). Other prostanoids certainly have secretory and motility effects on the bowel (for example, E_2 and $F_{2\alpha}$), but their relationship to the pathophysiology of inflammatory bowel disease is uncertain.[48,49] As to how drugs that influence the arachidonic acid cascade (e.g., 5-ASA) act in inflammatory bowel disease is also unclear.[49] ASA is a weak inhibitor of the cyclooxygenase pathway but does block the degradation of some prostaglandins (by inhibiting prostaglandin dehydrogenase); some action against lipoxygenases is also found in certain systems.

DIARRHEA IN DISEASE OF THE SMALL INTESTINE. Two major mechanisms for diarrhea as an accompaniment of severe ileal disease or after ileal resection can be identified.[50] One is induced primarily by malabsorbed bile acids and the other by malabsorbed fat. When the impairment of ileal function is minimal, wastage of bile acids is also small and their increased hepatic synthesis is sufficient to compensate for the fecal losses. Luminal concentrations of bile acids are maintained within the micellar range. When steatorrhea is present, it is of mild degree, but the excess of bile acids that enters the colon impairs electrolyte and water absorption.[51] The term

TABLE 13-2. *Fecal Weight in Inflammatory Bowel Disease.*

	Number	Range	Mean + SEM
Chronic ulcerative colitis (severe)[34]	9	100–1500 g/d	620
Chronic ulcerative colitis (severe)[35]	14	140–870 g/d	384 ± 49
Chronic ulcerative colitis[36]	25	100–1500 g/d	347 ± 77
Chronic ulcerative colitis[37]	10	—	560 ± 63
Chronic ulcerative colitis[37]	13	—	474 ± 60
Proctosigmoiditis[37]	8	—	234 ± 50
Actinic proctitis[36]	5	100–725 g/d	303 ± 125

TABLE 13-3. *Water and Electrolyte Absorption in Colitis: Studies In Vivo.*

	H_2O	Na^+	K^+	Cl^-
Chronic ulcerative colitis (n = 6)[41]	Decreased	Decreased	Normal	—
Chronic ulcerative colitis (n = 4)[42]	Decreased	Decreased	Secretion	—
Crohn's disease (n = 8)[43]	Decreased	Decreased	—	Decreased
Pre vs Post*[43]	No change	No change	—	No change
Proctitis (n = 10)[44]	—	Decreased	—	—

*Pre- versus post-operatively (diverting ileostomy). (—) = not reported.

"bile acid diarrhea" has been applied to this circumstance.[50] On the other hand, when the ileal resection is extensive, hepatic compensation for wastage of bile acids is incomplete and the concentration of bile acids in the lumen is too low for adequate micellar solubilization of fat. This aggravates steatorrhea and, in these circumstances, it is thought that the malabsorbed fat is responsible primarily for diarrhea. Excessive amounts of fatty acids in the colon are known to impair electrolyte and water absorption.[51] Consistent with these proposed pathogenic mechanisms are the therapeutic observations that a reduction in the dietary intake of long chain fats will reduce the severity of diarrhea in the second instance, whereas a sequestrant of bile acids (cholestyramine or aluminum hydroxide) is effective therapy in bile acid diarrhea.

These basic concepts require some modification in the light of other information. One such report emphasized the role of the colon in the diarrhea that follows ileal resection.[52] These investigators reasoned that variable portions of the large bowel are removed in association with resection of the ileum, and they examined independently the role of missing segments of the small and large intestines. The amount of colon removed was an important determinant of the severity of diarrhea, whereas the length of ileal resection was not. On the other hand, fecal excretion of fat correlated well with the length of ileum removed but not with the proportion of the colon resected. These findings were confirmed and extended in a subsequent report.[53]

A second important determinant of bile acid diarrhea, additive to the length of ileal resection, has now been identified. Thus, intracolonic pH is known to influence greatly the solubility of secretory bile acids.[54] Because the potential of dihydroxy bile acids to impair sodium, chloride, and water absorption in the colon must depend on their ability to enter the aqueous phase, factors that modify the solubility of bile acids might influence the propensity of bile acids to provoke diarrhea. Fromm's group showed that the aqueous concentrations of deoxycholic and chenodeoxycholic acids are related to fecal pH;[54] the higher the intraluminal pH, the more dihydroxy bile acids pass into solution and the more their secretory potential should be.

A final point relates to the absorptive capacity of the small intestine. Residual or recurrent Crohn's disease after ileal resection, or extensive proximal disease of the unoperated bowel, must be anticipated to reduce absorption of all components of chyme; water, electrolytes, and nutrients.

Can these observations be linked together? It can be proposed that short chain fatty acids, volatile fatty acids (VFA), might be such a link, because they are important determinants of colonic function.[59] These anions are well-absorbed from the human small and large intestine and, moreover, their presence in the colon facilitates the reabsorption of sodium ions and water. Being acidic radicals, their generation in the lumen will tend to lower the intraluminal pH. Thus, colonic resection and the resultant rapid transit through the remaining large intestine might be anticipated to reduce the opportunities

TABLE 13-4. *Electrolyte Transport in Colitis: Studies In Vitro.*

	Sodium		Chloride		Potassium	
	$M \rightarrow S$	$S \rightarrow M$	$M \rightarrow S$	$S \rightarrow M$	$M \rightarrow S$	$S \rightarrow M$
Crohn's disease (n = 3)*[45]	Decreased	Normal	Decreased	Normal	Normal	Normal
Chronic ulcerative colitis (n = 7)*[45]	Decreased	Normal	Decreased	Normal	Normal	Normal
Crohn's disease (n = 4)[46]	Increased	Increased	—	—	—	—
Chronic ulcerative colitis (n = 4)[46]	Increased	Increased	—	—	—	—

*Healthy controls vs untreated, p < 0.001; healthy controls vs steroid treated, N. S.; M → S = flux from mucosa to serosa, S → M = flux from serosa to mucosa.

for bacterial degradation of unabsorbed carbohydrate. The net result of this paucity of organic anions should be a reduced absorption of electrolytes and water; moreover, the tendency for a less acidic intraluminal environment might facilitate the solubilization of secretory bile acids and hence their diarrheogenic effects. Thus, Cummings showed that the greater the length of colon resected, the lesser the luminal concentration of organic anions.[52] Under these circumstances, a parallel increase in sodium and chloride concentrations in stools occurred, supporting the probability that sodium and chloride were poorly absorbed concurrent with incomplete generation of organic anions. Not surprisingly, transit time was also reduced when the amount of colon resected was larger.

CLINICAL APPROACHES. Important information as to the precise pathophysiology of diarrhea can be obtained from the simplest possible approaches, albeit these are frequently overlooked. A careful history will reveal whether or not the major complaint is actually one of incontinence, pain, or tenesmus rather than large fecal volumes. Similarly, inspection of several stools can be most revealing as to whether frequent, small volume stools are a manifestation of the proctitis syndrome or whether a major defect of small intestinal function, such as malabsorption, should be considered. Daily weighings of stools should also be considered, and, when total collections are made, fecal excretion of fat should be measured. During an exacerbation of IBD, and especially when the direction of medical or surgical therapy might be changed, further exclusion of intercurrent infectious diarrheas (such as Campylobacter or C. difficile) should be considered. The systematic evaluation of diarrhea otherwise is beyond the present scope. Figure 13-4 summarizes the pathophysiology of diarrhea in IBD.

Abdominal Pain

The abdominal viscera are insensitive to many stimuli that are painful if applied to the skin, but the gut is sensitive to stretching of its wall. Increased tension in the wall of the bowel occurs most often in IBD as a consequence of intestinal obstruction. Certain other contractile events, along the whole length of the gut, may be sensed as discomfort or pain, however. Esophageal spasm and the colorectal cramps of dysenteric or ulcerative colitis are good examples. Less well recognized are similar associations in the small intestine. Visceral pain can also be caused by inflammation or irritation of the serosa, and this mechanism can certainly pertain to IBD, if the inflammatory process is transmural. Rectal inflammation can also sensitize the wall of the

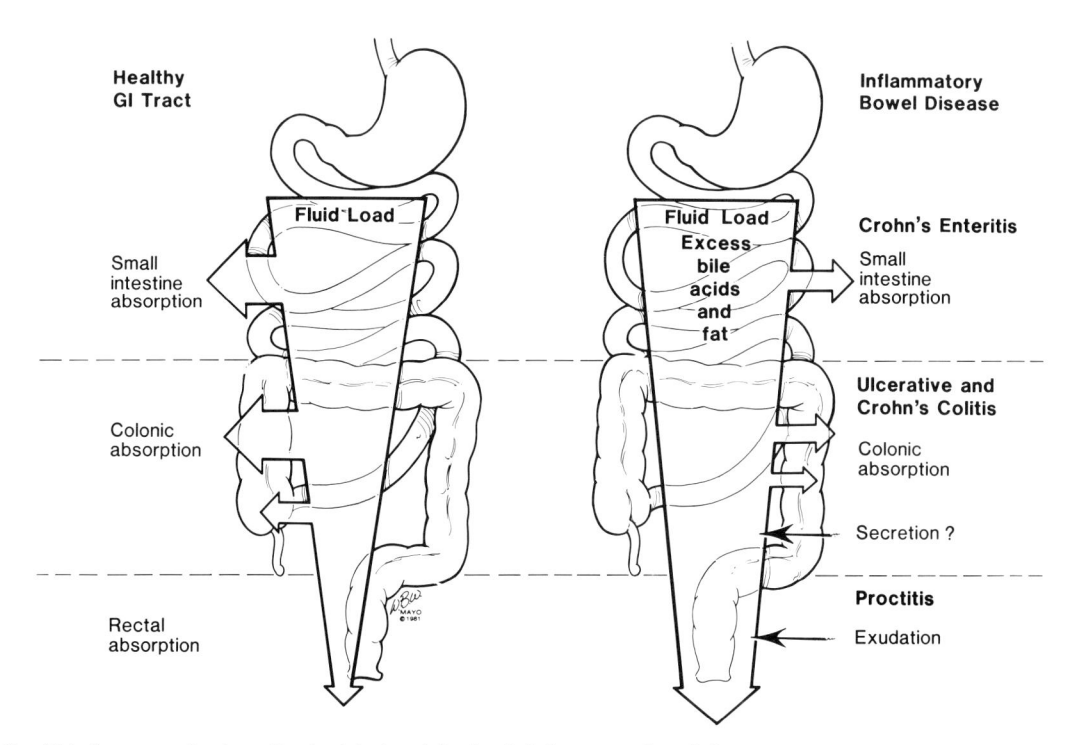

FIG. 13-4. Summary of major pathophysiologies of diarrhea in inflammatory bowel disease.

Fed - Mechanical Obstruction

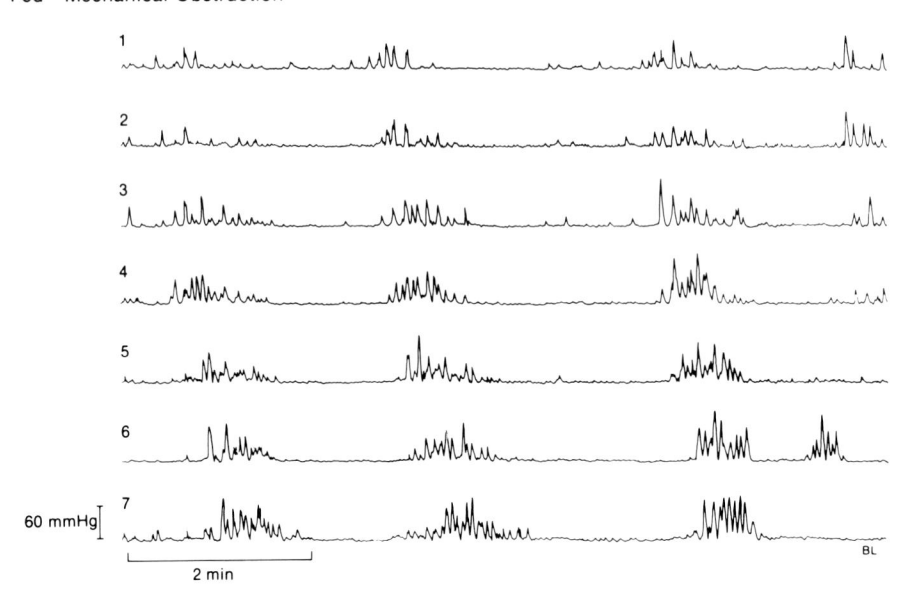

FIG. 13-5. Pattern of jejunal motility in patient with partial ileal obstruction from Crohn's disease. The clusters of phasic waves which appear to migrate distally are abnormal for the postprandial state, though similar patterns can occur in the healthy, fasting bowel. These abnormalities are reversed by relief of obstruction. (Reproduced with permission from Summers, R. W., Anuras, S., and Green, J.: Gastroenterology, 85:1290, 1983.)

bowel to stretch, a mechanism that has been suggested to contribute to the symptom of tenesmus. The remainder of this section will deal with painful sensations related to increased wall tension and powerful contractions of the tunica muscularis.

Pain resulting from distension of the bowel has been examined most closely in relation to the "irritable bowel syndrome," however the observations in symptomless controls provide useful background data.[57] Inflation of a balloon in the sigmoid colon produces pain in some healthy persons at a volume of 80 ml, although some can tolerate 300 ml or more; the D50 is approximately 140 ml. Pain occurs when the retroperitoneal colon is distended, implying that tension in the wall of the bowel, and not of the peritoneum, is involved. Also in the context of irritable bowel syndrome, the localization of pain from distension at different levels of the gut has been examined.[57] In symptomatic patients, the localization of pain was extremely variable, but the results suggest that distension of any segment of large or small bowel has the potential to cause pain.

The small bowel affected by Crohn's disease was studied by Summers who recorded jejunal motility in 9 persons with a clinical syndrome of partial, intermittent obstruction of the ileum.[58] Patterns of motility were considered to be within the wide range of normality during fasting but, after a meal, bursts of "clustered contractions" appeared, and these often migrated, usually in an aborad direction (Fig. 13-5). The overall frequency of these patterns was 9 per hour postprandially, and some, but not all, were associated with cramping pain or peristaltic rushes. It should be noted that most of these patients had definite radiologic evidence of obstruction.

In some healthy subjects painful contractions of the ileum have been observed, and their frequency increases during infusions of CCK-octapeptide (Kellow and Phillips, unpublished data). Thus, it appears that the distal small bowel is also sensitive to powerful contractions, perhaps more so than the proximal gut. The ileum of dog and man exhibits powerful, though infrequent, peristaltic waves. These migrate rapidly through the terminal 15 to 45 cm of small bowel and they empty the ileum more effectively than do other patterns of motility.[59,60] Because these peristaltic sequences often cause pain in healthy subjects, it would not be surprising if patients with ileitis exhibited a similar mechanism.

Strong contractions of the ascending colon may also be sensed as cramps. We infused the proximal colon of healthy subjects with an emulsion of oleic acid, simulating steatorrheal

PROPAGATED PRESSURE WAVES INDUCED BY INTRACOLONIC INFUSION OF OLEIC ACID

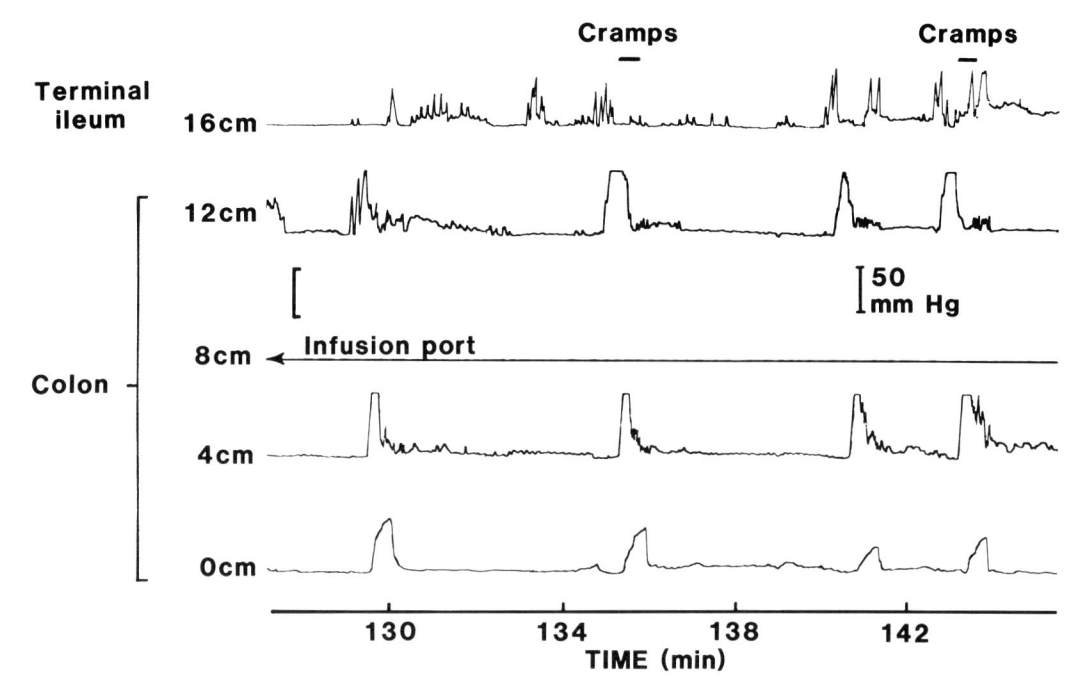

Fig. 13-6. Frequent, high pressure waves in human ascending colon which migrate distally and are associated with cramping pains. The colon was infused with an emulsion of oleic acid, to simulate bowel contents in steatorrhea. Similar patterns were not seen when the colon was perfused with saline. (Reproduced with permission from Spiller, R. C., and Phillips, S. F.: Gastroenterology, *91*:100, 1986.)

chyme; we recorded motility at the same time as the movement of contents was quantified scintigraphically.[61] Infusions of fat were associated with powerful contractions in the ascending colon (Fig. 13-6), decreased capacitance of the proximal large bowel and rapid transit of contents to the rectosigmoid accompanied by abdominal discomfort and/or cramping pain. The urge to defecate followed and, after evacuation, symptoms subsided.

The pathology of partial obstruction of the intestine in Crohn's disease has two major etiopathogeneses; one is an edematous swelling, in relation to the acute or subacute inflammatory process. The importance of this mechanism, because it involves a potentially reversible swelling of the mucosa and submucosa, is that surgical therapy is not essential for alleviation of the symptoms. On the other hand, and usually at a later stage, fibrous strictured areas develop as a chronic response to the disease; little benefit can then be expected from nonsurgical therapy.

Obstructing strictures of the colon are less common in ulcerative colitis than in Crohn's disease, and, when present, always raise the possibility of malignant degeneration. Although benign strictures are uncommon, they do occur in ulcerative colitis, however. Goulston and McGovern performed careful anatomicopathologic dissections and pointed out that the striking feature of CUC strictures is hypertrophy of the muscularis mucosae, which appears to be in a state of spastic contraction.[62] In strictured areas, the inner circular coat appears to be "pulled away from the outer longitudinal coat," resulting in a narrowed segment. It was postulated that narrowing of the lumen from such a mechanism was potentially reversible, unlike a fibrous stricture.

Two other causes of abdominal pain should be mentioned here, though they both relate more to the postoperative state and will be considered in more detail later. These are renal colic from nephrolithiasis, a recognized complication of colectomy, and biliary colic caused by cholelithiasis occurring as a complication of ileal resection.

CLINICAL APPROACHES. Details of the clinical evaluation of abdominal pain will not be given here; however, it should be reemphasized that pain in IBD has more than one potential mechanism.

Rectal Bleeding

That mucosal ulceration, which is invariably the major pathologic expression of ulcerative colitis and is usually a major feature of Crohn's disease, should cause slow bleeding and loss of fresh blood from the rectum, is not surprising. Indeed, the bowel movements of patients with colitis, especially when the disease is distal in its location, may consist almost entirely of blood and mucus with little fecal matter. Thus, these patients may exhibit concurrently fecal stasis in the right colon despite frequent evacuations of blood from the rectum.[39] In general, Crohn's colitis causes less bleeding than does ulcerative colitis and the passage of fresh blood is unusual when Crohn's disease is confined to the small bowel. Occult blood loss is common with all forms of IBD and, though other potential causes for anemia (folate and/or vitamin B_{12} deficiency, hemolysis, and impaired absorption of iron) must be considered, anemia in IBD is essentially always a result of blood loss. As pointed out by Morson, active colitis is always associated with prominent vascularity of all layers of the bowel wall, but this is particularly evident on the mucosal aspect.[63]

The physiology of the colonic microcirculation has been studied in the dog.[64,65] Blood flow to the colon is less than that to the proximal small bowel, and a lesser proportion of total flow is directed to the mucosa. Colonic blood flow is increased little postprandially, in contrast to that of the small bowel. The pathophysiology of the microvasculature in IBD was examined by Hulten.[31] Blood flow was measured at laparotomy and results were compared with a careful histopathologic classification of the stage of the disease. Severe, active colitis (either ulcerative or Crohn's type) was associated with increased total flow to the colon and to the mucosal-submucosal layers; flow to the muscular layers was within normal limits. Inactive, chronic ulcerative colitis and segmental, chronic Crohn's colitis showed normal or even reduced blood flow. Ileitis tissues received normal blood flows, and sometimes these were even reduced in chronic, fibrotic specimens.

Bleeding diatheses are not generally associated with IBD though, in theory, steatorrhea or severe liver disease could lead to malabsorption or impaired synthesis of hemostatic factors. More commonly, however, abnormalities of the hemostatic system in IBD lead to thromboembolic phenomena; these clinical associations with active IBD are well recognized (see Chaps. 8 and 16).

CLINICAL APPROACHES. The plan by which a specific diagnosis can be established involves the systematic investigation of anemia. In addition to a clinical history of overt bleeding and of any medications being used, primary emphasis should be placed on the usual hematologic indices, supplemented by determination of the levels of serum iron, folate, and vitamin B_{12}. A peripheral blood smear should give additional information, as might the Schilling test for vitamin B_{12} absorption. Indeed, it is advisable to assess the ileum's capacity for vitamin B_{12} absorption in all patients after ileal resection.

Post-operative States

ILEOSTOMY. Proctocolectomy and ileostomy returns the majority of patients with ulcerative colitis to excellent health, indeed, when the first postoperative year has passed ileostomists have a life expectancy at least as good as the general population.[66] The loss of the colon, however, leads to inevitable pathophysiologic consequences that obtain whether intestinal continuity is restored with a conventional, incontinent ileostomy or one of the newer procedures, such as the Kock pouch or ileoanal anastomosis (see also Chaps. 30 and 31).

Outputs from an Ileostomy. After an ileostomy is made, the capacity of the colon to absorb electrolytes and water is missing. Usually this has no major pathophysiologic consequences, but some important principles should be remembered. A normal colon absorbs 1000 ml of water and 100 mEq of sodium chloride daily.[67] More important, these amounts can be augmented; when overloaded progressively, the healthy colon can absorb more than 5 L per day.[68] Also, the colon responds to salt depletion by conserving NaCl avidly; however, the small intestine lacks the capacity to respond similarly. For example, under conditions of extremely low salt intake, fecal losses of sodium can be reduced to 1 or 2 mEq per day,[69] whereas patients with ileostomies have obligatory losses of sodium of 30 to 40 mEq per day.[70]

Ileostomies that function well discharge 500 to 600 g of material daily; 90% of this is water.[71]

Foods containing much unabsorbable residue increase the total output by increasing the amount of solids discharged. The response to specific foods varies from patient to patient, and changes are usually minimal. Prunes, which contain a chemical cathartic (diphenylisatin), increase the volume of outputs.

Functional Sequelae. When oral intakes of sodium, chloride, and fluid are adequate, patients with ileostomies do not become depleted; however, negative sodium balance may follow periods of diminished oral intake, vomiting, or even excessive losses in perspiration.[71] In addition, chronic oliguria is to be anticipated because normal stools contain approximately 100 ml of water, whereas ileostomies discharge 500 to 600 ml daily. Ileostomists also have lower $Na^+:K^+$ ratios in urine owing to compensatory renal conservation of sodium and water.[71] These changes in the composition of urine presumably contribute to the increased incidence of urolithiasis (about 5%) in these patients. The stones are predominately urate or calcium salts.[71] When ileostomy is accompanied by resection of terminal ileum, abnormalities of bile acid reabsorption and malabsorption of vitamin B_{12} result. Steatorrhea and greater daily losses of fluid (1000 ml per day or more) should also be anticipated.

Lack of a colon also reduces the exposure of bile acids to the metabolic effects of the fecal flora. Following ileostomy, secondary bile acids largely disappear from bile,[72] but no metabolic disturbances of significance have been recognized. The flora of ileostomy effluents has quantitative (10^4 to 10^7 organisms per ml) and qualitative characteristics (ratio of anaerobes-to-aerobes) that are intermediate between those of feces and those of normal ileal contents.[73]

Pathophysiologic sequelae are therefore mainly the potential consequences of a "salt-losing state;" patients should be advised to use salt liberally and to increase their fluid intake, especially at times of stress. Unfortunately, the limited ability of the small intestine to absorb sodium and water means that stomal volumes will also increase when the oral intake is increased.

Complications and Management. Major long-term complications relate to malfunctioning ileostomies, to prestomal ileitis, and to irritation of the peristomal skin. If the ileostomy was improperly constructed (with newer techniques this is now a much less frequent problem), the stoma may become obstructed. Obstruction leads to cramping, abdominal pain, increased ileal discharge, fluid and electrolyte depletion, and small bowel dilatation. Excessive ileal output arises, at least in part, from increased small bowel secretion as the result of small bowel dilatation proximal to the obstructed stoma. Stomal obstruction can usually be demonstrated by examining the stoma with the little finger, by endoscopy with a small sigmoidoscope, or by barium enema through the stoma. Roentgenograms will reveal a dilated ileum proximal to the point of obstruction. Many of these ileostomies require reconstruction. Ulcerations are often found in the resected terminal ileum during surgical treatment; their pathogenesis is unclear but probably relates in some way to the mechanical problem of obstruction.

Prestomal ileitis is a much less common problem.[74] Patients with this syndrome exhibit the features of mechanical obstruction, but they also have signs of systemic toxicity (fever, tachycardia, and anemia). The ileum has numerous punched-out ulcers, sometimes extending to the serosa. It is not clear whether prestomal ileitis has a different pathogenesis from the changes that follow simple mechanical obstruction of the stoma. Both may develop in a segment of ileum that was normal histologically at the time of colectomy. "Backwash ileitis" does not seem to predispose the patient to the development of either problem. On the other hand, in patients who have had colectomy and ileostomy for Crohn's disease, subsequent problems with the ileal stoma may arise from recrudescence of transmural granulomatous disease in the new terminal ileum. In some instances, it may be difficult to determine with certainty whether stomal dysfunction is caused by mechanical obstruction or recurrent Crohn's disease.

Diarrhea in Ileostomy Patients. Diarrhea in patients with conventional or continent ileostomies can best be defined as a fecal volume of greater than 1 L per day. Patients with ileoanal anastomosis may be troubled by increased stool frequency even when fecal volumes are normal, and a small number of these patients also have fecal incontinence.[75,76]*

Although diarrhea after proctocolectomy is usually caused by conditions unique to the par-

---

*Editors' note: see also Pemberton, J. H., et al.: Ann. Surg., 1987, in press; results of study of 390 patients with ileal pouch-anal anastomosis for chronic ulcerative colitis; mean follow-up; 2 to 3 years. Good long-term results.

ticular postoperative anatomy, it can also be secondary to any condition that affects the intact gut. Moreover, lacking a colon, the patient with an ileostomy is more susceptible to the consequences of any diarrhea. Even an otherwise mild condition (lactose intolerance, giardiasis, or gastric hypersecretion) can be "unmasked" or greatly exaggerated after colectomy.

Conventional Ileostomy. Perhaps the most common cause of persistently elevated ileostomy output following conventional ileostomy is ileal resection, particularly if this is accompanied by steatorrhea. This phenomenon can be manifest with resections of less than 20 cm of terminal ileum, and is almost always present when more than 50 cm of terminal ileum has been resected.[71] Chemical analysis of the high volume effluent reveals a greater than normal output of Na^+ and K^+, and often also of nitrogen and fat, when compared to patients who have not had ileal resection.[77] Fat malabsorption is related to impairment of bile salt absorption resulting from loss of the terminal ileum, with a secondary depletion of the bile salt pool.[50] Malabsorption of electrolytes and nutrients can result from the effects of excessive amounts of luminal fat on the small bowel,[78] or may merely reflect rapid small bowel transit or a decreased absorptive surface.[77] Such patients may manifest clinical symptoms of salt and water depletion and B_{12} deficiency, or they may be asymptomatic.

Partial small bowel obstruction is another frequent cause of elevated ileostomy output. This can occur at any point distal to the ligament of Treitz, including the ileostomy stoma. Though approximately 10% of patients with ileostomies will develop small bowel obstruction postoperatively, the risk is greatest soon after colectomy. The most frequent mechanism of extrinsic small bowel obstruction is an adhesive band. Why partial obstruction produces increased effluent is not completely understood. It has been demonstrated that with complete obstruction, not only an impairment of fluid and electrolyte absorption is present, but also an increased secretion of fluid into the bowel proximal to a point of obstruction occurs.[79] Such a phenomenon, if also present in partial obstruction, would result in an increase in the volume of effluent delivered to the distal small bowel, and a resultant increase in ileal effluent.

Recrudescent regional enteritis represents another important cause of chronic ileostomy diarrhea. In this regard, it should be noted that even a pathologic diagnosis of "typical" ulcerative colitis does not completely exclude the subsequent recurrence of "typical" regional enteritis. Recurrence rates of Crohn's disease in the small intestine following colectomy for Crohn's disease vary from 7 to 43%.[80–82] Undoubtedly, such rates depend on the criteria used to distinguish Crohn's colitis from ulcerative colitis, and the length of follow-up. Although recurrent enteritis may be seen at any site in the small bowel after colectomy, frequently it involves the ileum just proximal to the stoma. In the early postoperative period, peritonitis or localized abdominal infection also results in increased ileal effluent. The mechanism causing this is uncertain, but it may be analogous to that of partial obstruction, in which the segment of bowel adjacent to the area of inflammation has abnormal motility and thereby acts as a functional obstruction.

Though gastric hypersecretion is a known sequela to colectomy in experimental animals and man,[83] persistent hypersecretion of acid is a rare complication of simple proctocolectomy. It should be considered more seriously when the small bowel has been extensively resected. Hypersecretion can produce low pH levels in the jejunum, impaired micellar solubilization of fat, steatorrhea, and diarrhea.

Continent Ileostomy (Kock Pouch). Approximately 20% of patients develop a syndrome that has been variously referred to as pouchitis, bacterial overgrowth syndrome, or mucosal enteritis.[84,85] It can manifest at any time after construction of the pouch, but initial episodes usually occur in the first postoperative year. Patients present with a syndrome that includes: high volume, watery, and sometimes bloody ileostomy effluent; peristomal discomfort; and difficulty with intubation of the pouch. Features suggestive of a systemic illness, malaise, fever, arthralgias, uveitis, anorexia, and weight loss are less common manifestations. Occasionally, high ileostomy output with steatorrhea can be the only clinical manifestation.

The etiology of this syndrome is unknown; but certain analogies have been drawn to bacterial overgrowth and the blind loop syndrome. Clinical studies in symptomatic patients have revealed increased numbers of anaerobic bacteria in jejunal aspirates as compared to subjects with conventional ileostomies or to asymptomatic subjects with continent ileostomies.[85] On the other hand, bacteriologic studies of ileal effluent have been contradictory. Some have reported no qualitative or quantitative abnormalities of the effluent flora,[85] whereas others have shown increased bacterial concentrations in the ileal effluent, primarily of Bacteroides.[86,87] Tests of absorptive function in symptomatic patients have revealed abnormal Schilling tests in 30% and steatorrhea in 50% of the patients.[84,85] Most of the symptoms and pathophysiologic abnormalities are reversible by a course of metronidazole, which decreases concentrations of anaerobes in jejunal aspirates and ileal effluent.

ILEAL POUCH-ANAL PROCEDURE.* By conventional definition, all patients with an ileal pouch-anal anastomosis have diarrhea, because the stool frequency will usually range from 4 to 7 movements daily. In these patients, diarrhea is best defined either in terms of daily fecal outputs greater than 1000 ml, or a greater than expected stool frequency.

As in other patients with ileostomies, partial small bowel obstruction, recurrent regional enteritis, and bacterial overgrowth syndromes can produce diarrhea in patients with pouch-anal procedures. In addition, mechanical factors related to the pouch can produce similar, if not identical, symptoms. Following closure of the temporary ileostomy, a period of adaptation lasting approximately 6 months takes place during which stool frequency gradually decreases. Improvement in anorectal function can be expected thereafter; continence is improved, the need for antidiarrheals decreases, and perianal irritation lessens.[75,76]

Bacterial overgrowth syndromes ("pouchitis") after ileal pouch-anal anastomosis produces a syndrome similar to that seen in patients with Kock pouches. It has been reported in 8% of patients with "J" pouches,[75,76] but is more common in patients with lateral internal pelvic reservoirs.[88] Defecatory frequency and urgency, high volume of fecal output, pelvic discomfort, hematochezia, and deterioration in continence with perianal discomfort are the most common complaints. Often, perianal discomfort is the most troublesome symptom, and this can at times be severe.

Ineffective evacuation of the pouch has been proposed as a cause of frequent passage of stools following pouch-anal anastomosis. Patients with pouches who have good results show that the pouch can evacuate 61% of a slurry of artificial stool; this compares to a mean rectal evacuation of 65% of a comparable bolus by normal controls.[89] Ineffective evacuation, which has been demonstrated in some patients with poor postoperative results, may be secondary to mechanical or a functional obstruction distal to the pouch. Minor degrees of narrowing at the pouch-anal anastomosis are common after any of these procedures, and a tight postoperative stricture will probably produce incomplete evacuation, fecal retention, increased stool frequency, impaired continence, and possibly an overgrowth of bacteria.

Another cause of excessive frequency of bowel movements is decreased capacity of the pouch. This can be measured manometrically. Normally, the size of the pouch increases with time, though capacities vary among patients.[75] Total daily fecal volume in such patients is normal, but the number of bowel movements remains in the range of 5 to 10 daily.

RENAL CALCULI AND GALLSTONES. Development of symptoms referable to the urinary tract raises questions concerning the development of the renal complications of IBD. Though some conditions are seen in the patient who has not undergone surgical treatment (such as obstructive uropathy, which is usually on the right side and results from involvement of the ureter in an inflammatory mass of Crohn's disease), or with an enterovesical fistula,[90] the more usual setting is in the postoperative patient.

Renal calculi are more common in all patients with IBD, but are particularly prevalent (3 to 18% in different series) in patients with ileostomy or extensive ileal resection.[91] The subject is discussed elsewhere (see Chap. 16), but a summary of factors thought to contribute to postoperative nephrolithiasis includes: (1) decreased capacity to alkalinize the urine caused by a mild, systemic acidosis; (2) decreased urine volume from excessive intestinal loss of water; (3) effects of drugs (for example, steroids increase urinary excretion of calcium); (4) residual obstruction or infections of the urinary tract; and (5) enteric hyperoxaluria.

The prevalence of cholesterol gallstones is increased in IBD, particularly when the ileum is affected by Crohn's disease or has been resected.[92,93] Figures usually given are that approximately 30% of such patients have gallstones, and some have suggested that the longer the history of ileitis and the more extensive the disease or resection, the more likely gallstones

---

*Editors' note: see also Pemberton, J. H., et al.: Ann. Surg., 1987, in press; results of study of 390 patients with ileal pouch-anal anastomosis for chronic ulcerative colitis; mean follow-up; 2 to 3 years. Good long-term results.

are to develop. Patients who have had ileal resection usually have bile that is abnormally saturated with cholesterol (lithogenic), and Marks also reported lithogenic bile in patients with ileitis prior to resection.[93] In this small group, only 12% of all patients with ileitis had gallstones; the mean length of history was only 5 years in the unresected group, so that patients with lithogenic bile but without cholelithiasis might be expected to develop stones later. It must be recognized, however, that cholesterol saturation of bile, though important, is not the sole determinant of cholesterol cholelithiasis. Marks also studied 7 persons with ulcerative colitis; cholesterol saturation was not significantly different from control subjects.

In summary, it is important to keep in mind that each of the major clinical features of IBD may have more than one mechanism; these may pertain to different patients or may operate concurrently in an individual. Though the theoretic basis for underlying mechanisms is far from complete, enough is known to indicate that one's clinical approach to a particular patient can be improved by an appreciation of the pathophysiologic variants. Thus, Sir Thomas Lewis warned with regard to the etiology of disease that "diagnosis is a series of more or less guesses, in which the end-point achieved is a name. These names, applied to disease, come to assume the importance of specific entities, whereas they are for the most part no more than insecure and temporary conceptions."[94] We should extend this warning to the clinical features of those diseases that have no identifiable etiology. Although the patient with IBD has diarrhea (or pain, or anorexia), this is not in itself a symptomatic or therapeutic end-point. The physician is challenged to ascertain what is the cause of diarrhea in this patient. Better understanding of the clinical features of IBD is the goal to which this chapter is addressed.

References

1. Hawkins, C.: IBD historical review. *In*: Inflammatory Bowel Diseases. Edited by R. N. Allen, M. R. B. Keighley, J. Alexander-Williams, and C. Hawkins. New York, Churchill Livingstone, 1983.
2. Kirschner, B. S., Voinchet, D., and Rosenberg, I. H.: Growth retardation in children with inflammatory bowel disease. Gastroenterology, *75*:504, 1978.
3. Kirschner, B. S., et al.: Reverse of growth retardation in Crohn's disease with therapy emphasizing oral nutritional restitution. Gastroenterology, *80*:10, 1981.
4. Homer, D. R., Grand, R. J., and Colodny, A. H.: Growth, course and prognosis after surgery for Crohn's disease in children and adolescents. Pediatrics, *59*:717, 1977.
5. Henkin, R. I., et al.: Idiopathic hypogeusia with dysgeusia, hyposomia and dysomia. A new syndrome. J. Am. Med. Assoc., *217*:434, 1971.
6. Hambridge, K. M., Hambridge, C., Jacobs, M., and Brum, J. D.: Low levels of zinc in hair, anorexia, poor growth, and hyogeusia in children. Pediatr. Res., *6*:868, 1972.
7. McClain, C. J.: Zinc deficiency: A complication of Crohn's disease. Gastroenterology, *78*:272, 1980.
8. Wolman, S. L., Anderson G. H., Marliss, E. B., and Jeejeebhoy, K. N.: Zinc in total parenteral nutrition: requirements and metabolic effects. Gastroenterology, *76*:458, 1979.
9. Fleming, C. R., et al.: Zinc nutrition in Crohn's disease. Dig. Dis. Sci., *26*:865, 1981.
10. Goldberg, H. I., Caruthers, S. B., Nelson, J. A., and Singleton, J. W.: Radiographic findings of the National Cooperative Crohn's disease study. Gastroenterology, *77*:925, 1979.
11. Taffet, S. L., Das, K. M.: Sulfasalazine: Adverse effects and desensitization. Dig. Dis. Sci., *28*:833, 1983.
12. Goldman, P., and Peppercorn, N. A.: Sulfasalazine. N. Engl. J. Med., *293*:20, 1975.
13. Das, K. M., Eastwood, N. A., McManus, J. P. A., and Sircus, W.: Adverse reactions during salicylazosulfapyridine therapy and the relation with drug metabolism and acetylator phenotype. N. Engl. J. Med., *289*:491, 1973.
14. Spiller, R. C., et al.: The ileal brake—inhibition of jejunal motility after ileal fat perfusion in man. Gut, *25*:365, 1984.
15. McFarlane, A., Kinsman, R., Read, N. W., and Bloom, S. R.: The presence of food in the ileum delays small bowel transit and gastric emptying. Gastroenterology, *84*:1407, 1983.
16. Grill, B. B., et al.: Delayed gastric emptying in children with Crohn's disease. J. Clin. Gastroenterol., *7*:216, 1985.
17. Jones, L. A., Harries, A. D., and Rhodes, J.: Normal energy intake in undernourished patients with Crohn's disease. Br. Med. J., *288*:193, 1984.
18. Barot, L. R., Rambean, J. L., Faurer, I. D., and Mullen, J. L.: Caloric requirements in patients with inflammatory bowel disease. Ann. Surg., *195*:214, 1982.
19. Chan, A. T. H., Fleming, C. R., O'Fallon, W. M., and Huizenga, K. A.: Estimated versus measured basal energy requirements in patients with Crohn's disease. Gastroenterology, *91*:75, 1986.
20. Fleming, C. R., and Phillips, S. F.: Responses of the small intestine to nutritional deficiencies. *In* Small Intestine. Edited by V. S. Chadwick, and S. F. Phillips. Boston, Butterworths, 1982.
21. Peña, A. S., and Truelove, S. C.: Hypolactasia and ulcerative colitis. Gastroenterology, *64*:400, 1973.
22. Kirschner, B. S., DeFavaro, M. V., and Jensen, W.: Lactase malabsorption in children and adolescents with inflammatory bowel disease. Gastroenterology, *81*:829, 1981.
23. Anderson, I. H., Levine, A. S., and Levitt, M. D.: Incomplete absorption of the carbohydrate in all-purpose wheat flour. N. Engl. J. Med., *304*:891, 1981.
24. Levitt, M. D.: Malabsorption of starch: a normal phenomenon. Gastroenterology, *85*:769, 1983.
25. Stephen, A. M., Haddad, A. C., and Phillips, S. F.: Passage of carbohydrate into the colon. Direct measurements in humans. Gastroenterology, *85*:589, 1983.
26. Chapman, R. W., Sillery, J. K., Graham, M. M., and Saunders, D. R.: Absorption of starch by healthy ileostomates: effect of transit time and carbohydrate load. Am. J. Clin. Nutr., *41*:1244, 1985.
27. Salem, S. N., and Truelove, S. C.: Small intestinal and gastric abnormalities in ulcerative colitis. Br. Med. J., *1*:827, 1965.
28. Chakravarti, K. R., Sehgal, A. K., Chakravarti, R. N., and Chhuttani, P. N.: A study of intestinal function and mor-

28. phology in non-specific ulcerative colitis in acute phase and in remission in India. Am. J. Dig. Dis., *18*:191, 1973.
29. Wollaeger, E. E.: Role of the ileum in fat absorption. Mayo Clin. Proc., *48*:836, 1973.
30. Felipsson, S.: Malnutrition and malabsorption in Crohn's disease. Thesis, University of Goteborg, 1977.
31. Hulten, L., et al.: Regional intestinal blood flow in ulcerative colitis and Crohn's disease. Gastroenterology, *72*:388, 1977.
32. Kalser, M. H., Roth, J. L. A., Tumen, H., and Johnson, T. A.: Relation of small bowel resection to nutrition in man. Gastroenterology, *38*:605, 1960.
33. Longstreth, G. F., and Newcomer, A. D.: Drug induced malabsorption. Mayo Clin. Proc., *50*:284, 1975.
34. Smiddy, F. G., Gregory, S. D., Smith, I. B., and Goligher, J. C.: Faecal loss of fluid, electrolytes, and nitrogen in colitis before and after ileostomy. Lancet, *1*:14, 1960.
35. Caprilli, R., et al.: Salt losing diarrhea in idiopathic proctocolitis. Scand. J. Gastroenterol., *13*:331, 1978.
36. Hofmann, A. F.: Unpublished observations.
37. Schilli, R., et al.: A comparison of the composition of fecal fluid in Crohn's disease and ulcerative colitis. Gut, *23*:326, 1982.
38. Lennard-Jones, J. E., et al.: Observations on idiopathic proctitis. Gut, *3*:201, 1962.
39. Lennard-Jones, J. E., Langman, M. J. S., and Jones, F. A.: Faecal stasis in proctocolitis. Gut, *3*:301, 1962.
40. Denis, P., et al.: Elastic properties of the rectal wall in normal adults and in patients with ulcerative colitis. Gastroenterology, *77*:45, 1979.
41. Duthie, H. L., Watts, J. M., DeDombal, F. T., and Goligher, J. C.: Serum electrolytes and colonic transfer of water and electrolytes in chronic ulcerative colitis. Gastroenterology, *47*:525, 1964.
42. Harris, J., and Shields, R.: Absorption and secretion of water and electrolytes by the intact human colon in diffuse untreated procto-colitis. Gut, *11*:27, 1970.
43. Head, L. H., Heaton, J. W., and Kivel, R. M.: Absorption of water and electrolytes in Crohn's disease of the colon. Gastroenterology, *56*:571, 1969.
44. Rask-Madsen, J., Hammersgaard, E. A., and Knudsen, E.: Rectal electrolyte transport and mucosal permeability in ulcerative colitis and Crohn's disease. J. Lab. Clin. Med., *81*:342, 1973.
45. Hawker, P. C., McKay, J. S., and Turnberg, L. A.: Electrolyte transport across colonic mucosa from patients with inflammatory bowel disease. Gastroenterology, *79*:508, 1980.
46. Archampong, E. Q., Harris, J., and Clark, C. G.: The absorption and secretion of water and electrolytes across the healthy and the diseased human colonic mucosa measured in vitro. Gut, *13*:880, 1972.
47. Racusen, L. C., and Binder, H. J.: Effect of prostaglandin on ion transport across isolated colonic mucosa. Dig. Dis. Sci., *25*:900, 1980.
48. Donowitz, M.: Arachidonic acid metabolites and their role in inflammatory bowel disease. Gastroenterology, *88*:580, 1985.
49. Stenson, W. F.: Pharmacology of sulfasalazine. Viewpoints on Dig. Dis., *16*:13, 1984.
50. Hofmann, A. F.: Bile acid malabsorption caused by ileal resection. Arch. Intern. Med., *130*:597, 1972.
51. Phillips, S. F., and Gaginella, T. S.: Intestinal secretion as a mechanism in diarrheal disease. *In* Progress in Gastroenterology. Vol. III. Edited by G. B. Jerzy Glass. New York, Grune and Stratton, 1977.
52. Cummings, J. H., James, W. P. T., and Wiggins, H. S.: Role of the colon in ileal resection diarrhea. Lancet, *1*:344, 1973.
53. Mitchell, J. E., et al.: The colon influences ileal resection diarrhea. Dig. Dis. Sci., *25*:33, 1980.
54. McJunkin, B., Fromm, H., Serva, R. P., and Armin, P.: Factors in the mechanism of diarrhea in bile acid malabsorption: fecal pH—a key determinant. Gastroenterology, *80*:454, 1981.
55. Ruppin, H., et al.: Absorption of short-chain fatty acids by the colon. Gastroenterology, *78*:1500, 1980.
56. Ritchie, J.: Mechanisms of pain in the irritable bowel syndrome. *In* Irritable Bowel Syndrome. Edited by N. W. Read. New York, Grune and Stratton, 1985.
57. Dawson, A. M.: Origin of pain in the irritable bowel syndrome. *In* Irritable Bowel Syndrome. Edited by N. W. Read. New York, Grune and Stratton, 1985.
58. Summers, R. W., Anuras, S., and Green, J.: Jejunal manometry patterns in health, partial intestinal obstruction and pseudo-obstruction. Gastroenterology, *85*:1290, 1983.
59. Quigley, E. M. M., et al.: Motility of the terminal ileum and ileocecal sphincter in healthy humans. Gastroenterology, *87*:856, 1984.
60. Kruis, W., Azpiroz, F., and Phillips, S. F.: Contractile patterns and transit of fluid in canine terminal ileum. Am. J. Physiol., *249*:12:G264, 1985.
61. Spiller, R. C., Brown, M. L., and Phillips, S. F.: Decreased fluid tolerance, accelerated transit, and abnormal motility of the human colon induced by oleic acid. Gastroenterology, *91*:100, 1986.
62. Goulston, S. J. M., and McGovern, V. J.: The nature of benign structures in ulcerative colitis. N. Engl. J. Med., *281*:290, 1969.
63. Morson, B. C.: Pathology of ulcerative colitis. *In* Inflammatory Bowel Disease. 2nd Ed. Edited by J. B. Kirsner, and R. G. Shorter. Philadelphia, Lea & Febiger, 1980.
64. Bond, J. H., Prentiss, R. A., and Levitt, M. D.: The effects of feeding on blood flow to the stomach, small bowel and colon of the conscious dog. J. Lab. Clin. Med., *93*:594, 1979.
65. Bond, J. H., Prentiss, R. A., and Levitt, M. D.: The effects of anesthesia and laparotomy on blood flow to the stomach, small bowel and colon of the dog. Surgery, *87*:313, 1980.
66. Daly, D. W.: Outcome of surgery for ulcerative colitis. Ann. R. Coll. Surg. Engl., *42*:38, 1968.
67. Phillips, S. F., and Giller, J.: Contribution of the colon to electrolyte and water conservation in man. J. Lab. Clin. Med., *81*:733, 1973.
68. Debongnie, J. C., and Phillips, S. F.: Capacity of the human colon to absorb fluid. Gastroenterology, *74*:698, 1978.
69. Dole, V. P., et al.: Dietary treatment of hypertension: Clinical and metabolic studies of patients on the rice-fruit diet. J. Clin. Invest., *29*:1189, 1950.
70. Kramer, P.: The effect of varying sodium loads on the ileal excreta of human ileostomized subjects. J. Clin. Invest., *45*:1710, 1966.
71. Hill, G. L.: Historical introduction. *In* Ileostomy: Surgery, Physiology and Management. Edited by G. Hill. New York, Grune and Stratton, 1976.
72. Gadacz, T. R., Kelly, K. A., and Phillips, S. F.: The continent ileal pouch: Absorptive and motor features. Gastroenterology, *72*:1287, 1977.
73. Gorbach, S. L., Nahas, L., and Weinstein, L.: Studies of intestinal microflora IV. The microbiology of ileostomy effluent: A unique microbial ecology. Gastroenterology, *53*:874, 1967.
74. Knill-Jones, R. P., Morson, B., and Williams, R.: Prestomal ileitis: Clinical and pathological findings in five cases. Q. J. Med., *39*:287, 1970.
75. Taylor, B. M., et al.: A clinicophysiological comparison of ileal pouch-anal and straight ileoanal anastomosis. Ann. Surg., *198*:462, 1983.

76. Metcalf, A. M., et al.: Ileal "J" pouch-anal anastomosis: Clinical outcome. Ann. Surg., 202:735, 1985.
77. Neal, O. E., Williams, N. S., Barker, M. C. J., and King, R. F. G. J.: The effect of resection of the distal ileum on gastric emptying small bowel transit and absorption after proctocolectomy. Br. J. Surg., 71:666, 1984.
78. Ammon, H. V., Thomas, P. J., and Phillips, S. F.: Effects of long-chain fatty acids on solute absorption: perfusion studies in the human ileum. Gut, 18:805, 1977.
79. Shields, R.: The effect of experimental obstruction on the intestinal absorption of water, sodium, and potassium. In Surgical Physiology of the Gastrointestinal Tract. Edited by A. N. Smith. Edinburgh, The Royal College of Surgeons of Edinburgh, 1963.
80. Korelitz, B. I., Present, D. H., and Alpert, L. I.: Recurrent ileitis after ileostomy and colectomy for granulomatous colitis. N. Engl. J. Med., 287:110, 1972.
81. Ritchie, J. K.: Ileostomy and excisional surgery for chronic inflammatory disease of the colon: A survey of one hospital region. Gut, 12:528, 1971.
82. Watts, J., DeDombal, F. T., and Goligher, J. C.: Long term complications and prognosis following major surgery for ulcerative colitis. Br. J. Surg., 53:1014, 1966.
83. Landor, J. H., Alcancia, E. Y., and Fulkerson, C. C.: Effect of colectomy on gastric secretion in dogs. Am. J. Surg., 113:32, 1967.
84. Kelly, D. G., Branon, M. E., Phillips, S. F., and Kelly, K. A.: Diarrhea after continent ileostomy. Gut, 21:771, 1980.
85. Kelly, D. G., et al.: Dysfunction of the continent ileostomy: Clinical features and bacteriology. Gut, 24:193, 1983.
86. Loeschke, K., et al.: Bacterial overgrowth in ileal reservoirs (Kock pouch); extended functional studies. Hepatogastroenterology, 27:310, 1980.
87. Schjonsby, M., Halvorsen, J. F., Hofstad, T., and Hovdenak, N.: Stagnant loop syndrome in patients with continent ileostomy (intra-abdominal reservoir). Gut, 18:795, 1977.
88. Fonkalsrud, E. W.: Endorectal ileo-anal anastomosis with isoperistaltic ileal reservoir after colectomy and mucosal proctectomy. Ann. Surg., 199:151, 1984.
89. O'Connell, P. R., et al.: Enteric bacteriology, absorption, morphology and emptying after ileal pouch-anal anastomosis. Br. J. Surg., 73:909, 1986.
90. Present, D. H., Rabinowitz, J. G., Banks, P. A., and Janowitz, H. D.: Obstructive hydronephrosis. N. Eng. J. Med., 280:523, 1969.
91. Dobbins, J. W., and Binder, H. J.: Derangements of oxalate metabolism in gastrointestinal disease and their mechanisms. In Progress in Gastroenterology III. Edited by J. B. J. Glass. New York, Grune and Stratton, 1977.
92. Baker, A. L., Kaplan, M. M., Norton, R. A., and Patterson, J. F.: Gallstones in inflammatory bowel disease. Am. J. Dig. Dis., 19:109, 1974.
93. Marks, J. W., et al.: Gallstone prevalence and biliary lipid composition in inflammatory bowel disease. Am. J. Dig. Dis., 22:1097, 1977.
94. Lewis, T.: Reflections upon reform in medical education. Lancet, 1:619, 1944.

14 · Gastrointestinal Complications of Ulcerative Colitis and Crohn's Disease

KENNETH A. HUIZENGA, M.D. AND KENNETH W. SCHROEDER, M.D.

The local complications of chronic ulcerative colitis and Crohn's disease to be discussed are summarized in Table 14-1. Malignant degeneration in inflammatory bowel disease is discussed elsewhere (see Chap. 15).

Anorectal Complications

Complications from idiopathic inflammatory bowel disease are usually encountered in the anorectal area. They are more frequent in Crohn's disease and, while not necessarily serious compared to some other complications, they are often a major source of concern to the patient and his or her physician. Perianal complications of inflammatory bowel diseases may be classified as outlined in Table 14-2.[1] Some of these lesions may be nonspecific reactions to chronic diarrhea, some are associated with bowel inflammation, while others occur only with Crohn's disease.

The chance of developing such complications during the course of Crohn's disease is reported to vary from 22 to 80%,[1-4] with equal distribution between males and females. Children and adolescents, aged 9 months to 21 years, experience these complications at about the same rate as adults.[5] Though usually occurring after onset of intestinal disease, these complications may be the first symptom in Crohn's disease, at times preceding other symptoms or manifestations by months or even years.[2-3] Baker and Milton-Thompson observed that 24% of their patients experienced anorectal lesions prior to the onset of intestinal symptoms by 1 month to 22 years, with a mean interval of 4 years.[3] Two-thirds of this group developed signs of the intestinal disease within 5 years of the onset of the anal lesion, and four-fifths of the patients had involvement of the colon with or without ileal involvement. Williams et al. reported a 22% incidence of anal complications in over 1,000 patients with Crohn's disease.[4] Associated colonic involvement (52%) was more common than small bowel involvement (14%). A similar incidence for fissure (29%), fistula (28%), and abscess (23%) was noted, with 20% of patients experiencing multiple manifestations.

In ulcerative colitis, the anal lesions occur in less than 20% of patients and present less of a clinical problem, usually becoming manifest after the onset of diarrhea.[6] de Dombal et al. reported that fissure in ano is more commonly associated with active disease than quiescent symptoms and is more common when the colon is extensively involved.[6] Abscess and fistula in ano were less clearly associated with the severity or extent of disease. Rectovaginal fistulae were not noted in the absence of active colitis. In their group of 465 patients with longstanding chronic ulcerative colitis, de Dombal and colleagues reported an incidence of 6% for perianal

TABLE 14-1. *Relative Frequency of Gastrointestial Complications in Inflammatory Bowel Disease.*

Complication	Chronic Ulcerative Colitis	Crohn's Disease
Anorectal Lesions	< 20%	20-80%
Fissure in ano	< 15%	25-30%
Perianal abscess	< 10%	20-25%
First symptom	Very infrequent	20-25%
Fistula in ano	< 6%	25-30%
Multiple and complex	Never	Common
Multiple anorectal complications	Very infrequent	20%
Massive hemorrhage		
Colon	3%	< 3%
Small bowel	Never	< 2%
Intra-abdominal abscess	Very rare	15-25%
Internal fistulae	Very rare	20-40%
Free perforation	Uncommon	Very uncommon
Toxic megacolon	2-10%	< 8%
Pseudopolyposis	15-30%	Less common
Strictures	11-15%	Very common

abscess, 5.4% for fistula in ano, 3.6% for rectovaginal fistula, and 12.3% for fissure in ano. The incidence of these abnormalities directly relates to the care with which the anal area is examined, because, as in Crohn's disease, the extent of the perianal disease can be determined in some patients only by a thorough examination while the patient is anesthetized. These anorectal complications most commonly are identified during the first year of chronic ulcerative colitis. Thereafter, duration of symptoms has little effect on the incidence of such complications.

Because anorectal complications are less common in ulcerative colitis, the diagnosis of Crohn's disease should be strongly suspected with the finding of spontaneous perineal fistulae, rectovaginal fistulae, indolent ulcers and fissures, and edematous anal tags. This may be more definitive if the rectal mucosa appears macroscopically normal at the time of sigmoidoscopic examination. Alternatively, the presence of isolated ulcers of the rectal mucosa at sigmoidoscopy would support a diagnosis of Crohn's disease.

Skin Lesions

Edematous skin tags are most common with Crohn's disease, and are often confused initially with hemorrhoids. Though perianal hygiene may be aggravated by such tags, they typically cause no pain, bleeding, or other discomfort, and generally no treatment is indicated.[1] Surgical resection in particular may lead to problems with subsequent healing.

TABLE 14-2. *Perianal Complications in Inflammatory Bowel Disease.*

Skin Lesions
  Maceration
  Erosion
  Ulceration
  Abscess
  Skin tags
  External hemorrhoids
Anal Canal Lesions
  Fissure
  Ulcer
  Stenosis with induration
  Abscess
  Internal hemorrhoids
Fistulae
  Low (anal canal to skin)
  High (rectum to skin)
  Rectovaginal

Other skin lesions, such as skin maceration or erosion, are primarily a result of skin irritation from chronic diarrhea and associated scratching.[1] The skin may become edematous, with corrugated, irregular features, making local cleansing a problem.

Deep ulceration of the skin in Crohn's disease ("metastatic ulcers") may occur some distance from the anus, with apparently normal intervening skin (Fig. 14-1).[1] This is rarely painful. Skin abscesses may also form with nonhealing ulceration occurring thereafter.

Rectal bleeding attributed to hemorrhoids must be carefully evaluated to exclude the presence of inflammatory bowel disease, particu-

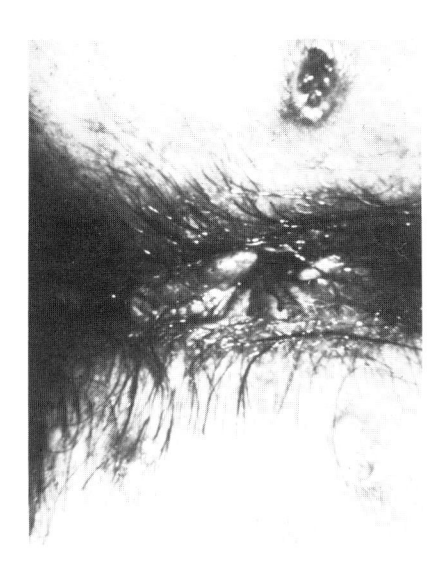

FIG. 14-1. Perianal Crohn's disease with satellite or metastatic ulcers on both buttocks.

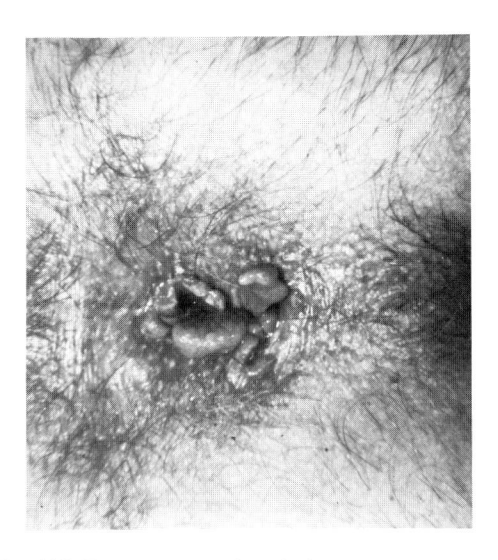

FIG. 14-2. Perianal tags and anal ulcer in a patient with Crohn's disease and delayed healing following hemorrhoidectomy.

larly if surgical treatment is to be considered. Routine careful anal inspection and proctosigmoidoscopy are essential; double contrast barium studies or colonoscopy and small bowel roentgenograms may be helpful if the history or examination suggests the possibility of inflammatory bowel disease. While surgical treatment of hemorrhoids in the presence of ulcerative colitis has a relatively low complication rate, the latter is high in patients with Crohn's disease. In one series, surgery led to perianal abscess and fistula formation or persistent pain, and 6 of 20 patients with Crohn's disease required rectal excision for complications apparently dating from surgical treatment of hemorrhoids (Fig. 14-2).[7] These results suggest that the surgical treatment of symptomatic hemorrhoids is relatively safe in patients with chronic ulcerative colitis, but generally is contraindicated in those with Crohn's disease.

Anal Canal Lesions

FISSURE IN ANO. The most common lesion, found in both Crohn's disease and ulcerative colitis, is fissure in ano and its occurrence is directly related to the severity of the diarrhea that produces ulceration at the anal verge or linear splits in the perianal skin.[1,2,6] Its most common symptom is pain that accompanies or shortly follows defecation, and a burning, constant discomfort may persist for an hour or more before gradually subsiding. The fissure in ano in Crohn's disease may be asymptomatic, however. Multiple fissures may be present and coalesce beneath bridges of skin in patients with Crohn's disease. While fissures may penetrate into the sphincter muscles this rarely leads to incontinence.

ANAL STENOSIS. Narrowing of the anal canal may occur as a sequel of longstanding fissure in ano or anal ulceration.[1] Though the stenosis may be severe, patients will often experience minimal discomfort because the bowel inflammation may lead to soft or liquid stools that pass without difficulty.

PERIANAL ABSCESS. A painful, indurated area may appear during the active phase of inflammatory bowel disease, though sometimes an abscess may present when no clinical sign of activity is apparent. Usually proctosigmoidoscopic or x-ray examination will reveal the presence of active inflammatory bowel disease. Patients with Crohn's disease are apt to develop this lesion (with an incidence of 20 to 25%) at some stage in the course of their disease, particularly in early attacks.[1-4] The complication has been reported in 6% of patients with ulcerative colitis, either in the first attack or in an acute relapse of long-established disease.[6] In ulcerative colitis, the abscess usually is well-localized, but in Crohn's disease of the colon there may be extension into the ischiorectal fossa, or into the submucosal space, producing a more complex lesion (Fig. 14-3). Once the abscess has extended into the ischiorectal fossa, it may involve the anal sphincter musculature medially and the

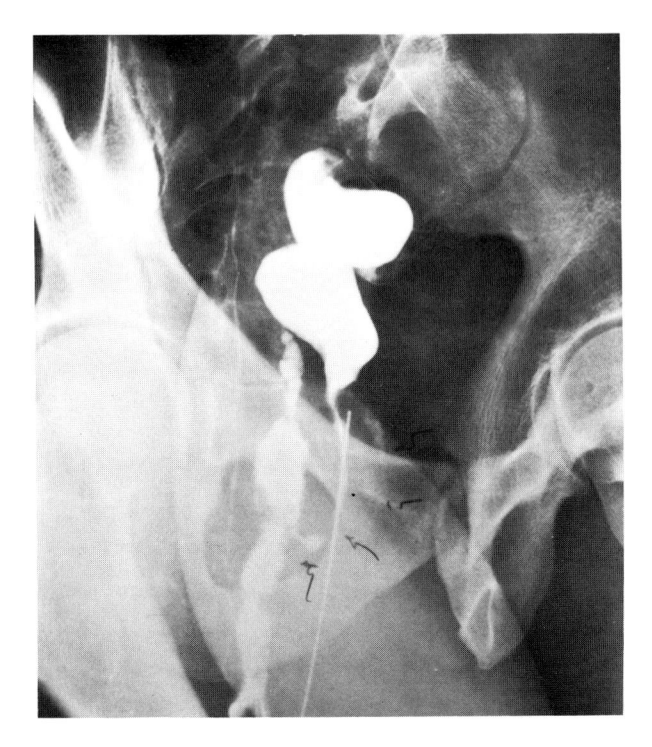

FIG. 14-3. Large complex perianal abscess in a patient with Crohn's disease documented by barium enema.

obturator internus muscle laterally. Anteriorly, the abscess may reach the pubis, and posteriorly it may extend to the sacrotuberal ligament. The reasons for such extensions are poorly understood but probably they are related to the pathogenesis of the granulomatous inflammatory process.

A major and early symptom of perianal abscess is severe pain that is aggravated by walking, sitting, or defecation. Examination usually shows an area of induration, swelling, and redness in close relationship to the anus. Digital examination of the rectum is painful for the patient and commonly reveals induration in the perineum outside the anal canal and below the level of the anorectal ring. If an ischiorectal abscess is present, the patient may feel ill, weak, and febrile. No pain will be present in some instances, but on inspection of the perineum asymmetry of the perineal tissue is found that only later may become indurated and red. Rectal examination reveals a large, tense, tender swelling outside the anal canal, extending above the anorectal ring. Drainage of a perianal abscess, either spontaneously or by incision, will relieve pain but may lead to a fistula or to a nonhealing ulcer.

Fistula in Ano

This problem may arise secondary to a perineal abscess or develop spontaneously without clinical evidence of acute infection.[8,9] The lesion produces a persistent or intermittent discharge from the fistulous opening that irritates the surrounding skin and soils the clothes. On clinical examination, the external opening may consist of a tuft of granulation tissue or, if healed, simply of an area of scar tissue. The external opening usually is located within 5 cm of the anus and the internal opening can be palpated by digital examination or detected by endoscopic examination at about the level of the anal valves. While a probe or fistulogram may demonstrate the extent of the tract produced by the fistula, this is painful and usually unnecessary. With the patient in the prone position, and with comparison of the anus to the dial of a clock, if an external fistula is present between 9 and 3 o'clock the internal opening usually will be found between 11 and 1 o'clock. If the external opening is in the anterior anal section between 3 and 9 o'clock, however the internal opening may be anywhere.

In Crohn's disease, the fistulae tend to become multiple and complex. The external opening may appear at a considerable distance from the perianal area by burrowing through the adjacent tissue to form several tracts that may extend into adjacent structures, the vulva, the groin, the scrotum, and the penile urethra.

Treatment of Anorectal Lesions

The medical treatment of the anal lesions in inflammatory bowel disease begins with therapy of the primary disease process affecting the bowel and will usually use sulphasalazine or corticosteroids, or both, with appropriate symptomatic therapy to the anal area to minimize diarrhea or seepage.[4,6-9]

Minor lesions, such as skin changes, hemorrhoids, and the fissure in ano, usually respond to those forms of treatment aimed to diminish diarrhea, and to local measures such as improved anal hygiene, sitz baths several times a day, and the application of hot compresses. The local application of steroid and analgesic ointments often will provide substantial relief of these perianal symptoms.[1] Caution is required in using analgesic ointments, however, because they tend to induce allergic or hypersensitivity reactions.

Anal stenosis may require no therapy, though in some, gentle dilatation, sometimes under anesthesia, may be required.[1,8,9]

Simple anal fistulae may respond symptomatically to the measures described above, especially if the inflammatory bowel disease is mild or limited to a short segment. In some patients the lesions will heal and become asymptomatic, while in others the lesions do not heal completely, persisting with minor discomfort and a slight discharge of mucus and stool. Nevertheless, commonly these are tolerated by the patients and require no further treatment. It is important to emphasize that it is *not* necessary to treat fistulae just because they are present.

Perianal abscesses should be drained as soon as fluctuance is confirmed. These may then heal but, unfortunately, some become simple or complex fistulae. Local hygiene is an important adjuvant treatment for these abscesses.

Complex perianal fistula or fistulae with extensions to adjacent tissue and organs do not respond readily to medical measures directed at the control of inflammatory bowel disease. Even with extensive fistulae, however, an occasional patient has only mild symptoms and minimal inconvenience and tolerates the situation in the hope of avoiding radical surgical treatment that may involve resection of the rectum and variable amounts of the colon, plus the establishment of a stoma. In such individuals, if the fistulae are complicated by anal stenosis, with or without fecal incontinence, gentle and frequent anal dilatation, usually under anesthesia, may be helpful.

METRONIDAZOLE. Recent experience with metronidazole has shown promise for medical control of symptomatic perineal disease associated with Crohn's disease. Bernstein et al. used metronidazole at a dose of 20 mg/kg/day in divided doses for perineal Crohn's lesions in patients with simple, multiple, or complicated sinuses and fistulae, abscesses, rectovaginal fistulae, rectolabial fistulae, unhealed wounds after excision of hypertrophied anal skin tags, and "metastatic Crohn's ulcers" in the groin.[10] Bowel involvement was also present in one or more sites of the small intestine, colon, or rectum. Complete healing of the perineal disease was noted in 45% of patients, while 23% of the patients improved but with incomplete healing.

In the healing process, the discharge changed from purulent to serous in character. Fistulous openings developed a nipple-like projection that later resolved leaving only a dimple. When large ulcers had been present, large depressed areas with rolled edges were left after healing. Subjective improvement occurred in 91% of the patients while on treatment, with reduction in stool frequency, improved consistency of the stool and stabilization or reversal of weight loss; some individuals also showed improvement in the hematocrit and serum albumin levels.

A follow-up report showed that decreasing the metronidazole dose in one group of patients resulted in worsening of symptoms in all after intervals of 2 weeks to 3 months, the dose at the time of the flare ranging from 20 to 80% of the original dose.[11] Following complete discontinuation of the drug in another group of patients who had experienced complete healing, 72% had recurrent perineal disease within 1 week to 9 months. When the drug was restarted, the perineal disease healed once again and remained healed in 28% of the patients for periods ranging from 7 to 16 months.

Prolonged treatment with metronidazole for 12 to 36 months was used in one group: half of them showed complete healing while the others had advanced but incomplete healing.

Jakobovits and Schuster reported their experience in treating 8 patients with chronic perineal Crohn's disease that had been present for 1 to 14 years.[12] All patients were continued on prednisone, with additional doses of 1000 to

1500 mg/day of metronidazole. The number of draining fistulae was reduced 20-fold, a 50% decrease in the number of detectable fistulous openings was noted, and other bowel symptoms were improved. Symptomatic improvement was maintained for six months after cessation of treatment. Side effects occurred in all patients, but resolved in 88% within 1 to 3 weeks after discontinuation of the drug. Side effects represent the major deterrent to the use of metronidazole. Peripheral neuropathy with numbness and tingling of the lower extremities developed in as many as 75% of these patients after 3 months of treatment.[12] Duffy et al. found an 85% incidence of peripheral neuropathy by formal nerve conduction studies in a group of adolescents with Crohn's disease treated with metronidazole for 4 to 11 months.[13] Only 38% of these patients actually experienced paresthesias or hypoesthesias of the lower extremities. When the dosage was reduced or the drug was stopped, nerve conduction studies improved or resolved in all but one patient. Clinically, a similar effect has been noted, as symptoms usually improve with decreasing the dosage or if the drug is discontinued.[10-12] Other untoward effects of the drug include metallic taste, darkening of the urine, anorexia, nausea, vomiting, and vertigo. A disulfuram-like effect with alcohol ingestion is rare. Though frequently cited, little evidence to date supports a potential concern over mutagenesis and carcinogenesis caused by metronidazole.

Hatoff reported a liver abscess resulting from streptococcus milleri (not sensitive to metronidazole) in a patient with ileal and perianal Crohn's disease treated unsuccessfully with large doses of metronidazole for several months.[14] Because most patients with perineal disease will respond within four months, patients showing no response during this interval probably should not receive further treatment with metronidazole.

The mechanism of action of metronidazole for Crohn's perianal disease may relate to its action against anaerobic organisms. Krook et al. demonstrated reduction in species of Bacteroides in the stools of outpatients treated with metronidazole, while gut flora in healthy individuals changed little.[15]

Though these several reports suggest a benefit for perineal Crohn's disease from relatively high dose metronidazole therapy, no controlled studies have been reported. Virtually all patients treated with the drug have also been on other agents, usually including corticosteroids. The high incidence of its symptomatic side effects often limits the usefulness of the drug.

IMMUNOSUPPRESSIVE THERAPY. The use of 6-mercaptopurine for perianal disease is reviewed in the discussion of intra-abdominal abscesses and fistulae.

NUTRITIONAL MEASURES. Elemental diets have been used in the treatment of Crohn's perianal fistulae. Calam et al. treated 6 patients for 4 weeks or longer, and 4 experienced improvement or healing of the fistulae. Refeeding usually led to recurrent drainage, however.[16] Though promising, elemental diets used as a "medical bypass" remain unproven as therapy for such lesions.

SURGICAL TREATMENT. Surgical therapy for perianal disease associated with chronic ulcerative colitis can be undertaken with little concern about significant sequelae from the surgery.[6] The perianal disease seen with Crohn's disease has been more commonly associated with poor healing, however, and, hence, poor results;[1,17] in particular, surgery for hemorrhoids or edematous skin tags should be avoided.[7] Some reports have suggested that local definitive surgical therapy for perianal abscesses and fistulae in patients with Crohn's disease can be successful.[17-19] When severe Crohn's-associated perianal disease is present, complete resection of the anorectum with a stoma is usually required.

Massive Hemorrhage
Colonic

Bloody stools are a common accompaniment of active ulcerative colitis, often producing a chronic anemia. On occasion, however, bleeding from the rectum may be acute and massive. While many have had experience with this type of colonic bleeding, only a few reports deal with the complication. Truelove reported an incidence of up to 3% in patients with ulcerative colitis, while massive bleeding in Crohn's colitis was considered to be uncommon.[20] A more recent study by Greenstein et al. showed an incidence of 2.5% in a group of 160 patients with Crohn's colitis and ileocolitis,[21] however. In chronic ulcerative colitis, the bleeding may be diffuse from large areas of ulcerated mucosa, but in Crohn's disease the bleeding is often from a localized source and is caused by erosion of a blood vessel within the bowel wall associated with multiple deep ulcerations that extend into the submucosa or deeper layers of the intestinal wall.

Upper Gut

Life-threatening gastrointestinal hemorrhage, manifested by hematemesis and/or melena, in Crohn's disease of the small intestine may be the initial manifestation of the disease or occur in patients with previously documented disease. Crohn and Yarnis noted gross hemorrhage in 25 patients in a series of 542 patients with regional enteritis involving the terminal ileum, an incidence of 4.6%.[22] Peptic ulcers were present concurrently in 20 patients, however, leaving only 5 with regional enteritis as the sole possible source—a revised incidence of 1.1%. While recurrent hemorrhage is considered to be infrequent, Sparberg and Kirsner reported 3 patients who had 5 or more hemorrhages, an incidence of 1.5% in their group of 195 patients.[23] These reports indicate that in Crohn's disease of the upper gut the ileum is the most frequent site of the hemorrhage in patients who manifest bleeding from the rectum. When hematemesis accompanies the massive bleeding, Crohn's disease in the duodenum is the most likely source, but an active duodenal or gastric ulcer first must be excluded.

Treatment

Acute and massive bleeding may complicate an acute severe attack of inflammatory bowel disease involving any segment of the large or small intestine, or may be associated with a toxic megacolon. Such acute bleeding episodes often are associated with varying degrees of shock, manifested by excessive sweating, tachycardia, and hypotension; they require immediate multiple transfusions that ordinarily will support the patient, and the bleeding often subsides spontaneously in this situation. On rare occasions, however, repeated transfusions may not cope with persistent heavy bleeding and emergency surgery is required to control the hemorrhage. In this situation, the possibility of a defect in coagulation should be considered, particularly a prolonged prothrombin time caused by deficiency of vitamin K-dependent clotting factors.[24]

As emphasized previously, in those instances in which upper gastrointestinal bleeding occurs, it is important to localize the site of the bleeding and to determine, if possible, whether the bleeding is directly related to Crohn's disease or some other unrelated cause. Gastric lavage for blood in the stomach and panendoscopy of the esophagus, stomach, and duodenum will frequently identify the site and cause of bleeding. If these studies are nondiagnostic and active bleeding persists at a significant rate (that is, greater than 0.5 ml/min.), however, then selective mesenteric angiography may be helpful in localizing the bleeding site (Fig. 14-4). The localization of the bleeding site is best followed by conservative resection of the involved bowel.[25] A brief trial of selective vasopressin infusion may be employed, however, when the bleeding occurs early in the course of the disease and the angiographic pattern is that of hyperemia with dilata-

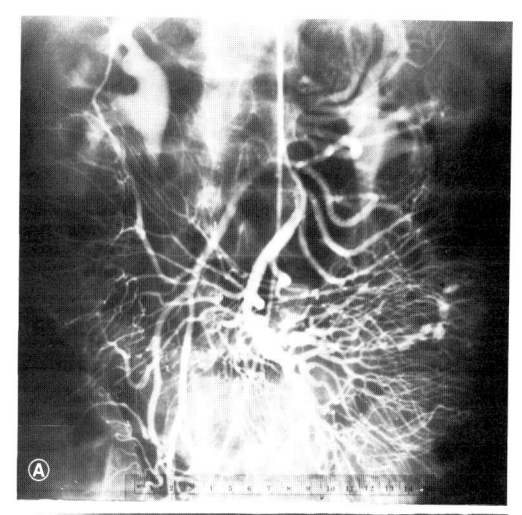

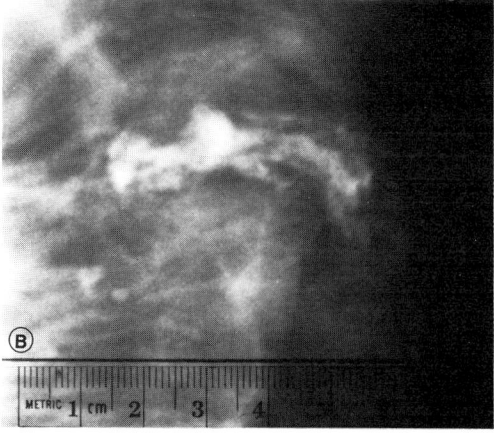

FIG. 14-4. Visceral angiogram: (a) showing active bleeding site in upper ileum; and (b) pooling of contrast material in ileum shows abnormal mucosal pattern consistent with Crohn's disease.

tion of submucosal vessels. In the later stage of the disease, the angiographic and pathologic pattern reveals thickening of vessel walls and narrowing of luminal diameter, and vasopressin infusion in this setting has a potential risk because of diminished blood flow and probable inadequate collateral blood flow. Nevertheless, the successful use of vasopressin infusion has been reported in a few incidences.[26]

Colonoscopic examination, especially after an acute bleeding episode has stopped, may be helpful to identify the region or specific site of the colonic bleeding. The decision to operate when colonic bleeding occurs may be influenced not only by the acute complication itself but also by other coexisting factors. Surgical treatment takes on added significance because total proctocolectomy is the only procedure that can ensure complete control of the hemorrhage and, under these urgent circumstances, the surgical risk is significantly increased. Of course, if the bleeding persists despite multiple transfusions, surgical treatment is the only recourse. In some patients, surgical treatment may be advised when the bleeding is less acute but extends over several days, requiring multiple daily transfusions to maintain a stable hematocrit, and with no indications that the daily loss of blood is diminishing. If this occurs in a patient with other potential indications for colectomy, the decision for surgical treatment is easier. Furthermore, if a massive hemorrhage occurs in those with chronic disabling disease, emergency colectomy may be the treatment of choice, and should be performed early in the course of the bleeding to prevent significant deterioration of the patient's general status.

Intra-abdominal Abscesses and Internal Fistulae

Internal fistulae are characteristic of Crohn's disease and virtually do not occur in ulcerative colitis. In the past, fistulae involving the colon were described in patients with ulcerative colitis; however, when these cases are reviewed in light of the current distinctive characteristics of ulcerative colitis and Crohn's disease of the colon, they are more appropriately placed in the latter category.

Abscesses and fistulae should be considered as part of the same pathologic process, namely, the extramural extension of a fissure ulcer. If the process remains localized, an abscess may be formed in the intraperitoneal space or adjacent organ. If it extends to the skin surface or into adjacent viscera, it becomes a fistula. The incidence of abscess formation varies between 15 and 25%, and that of fistulae between 20 and 40%.[27] Abscesses may occur de novo or following surgical therapy. Postoperative abscesses occurring during the first 1 to 2 months after resective surgical treatment usually result from anastomotic leaks or infected hematomas, while those identified 6 months or later after surgical treatment are probably a result of recurrent disease.[28] Postoperative abscesses are more likely to occur if the original surgical treatment was done for an intra-abdominal abscess. Fistulae are more common when Crohn's disease involves the small bowel than when the colon alone is diseased.[29]

Intra-abdominal Abscesses

Intra-abdominal abscesses associated with Crohn's disease may present either with an onset of a "new" abdominal pain or as a change in the character of established abdominal pain.[29,30] Spiking fever and an abdominal mass may accompany the pain or be the sole manifestation of the lesion. Some abscesses are detected only at surgical therapy performed for other reasons.

Laboratory findings are usually nonspecific and include neutrophil leukocytosis, an elevated serum alkaline phosphatase, hypoalbuminemia, and mild anemia.[28]

Diagnosis may be aided by flat plate and upright abdominal roentgenograms, colon roentgenogram,[32] radionucleotide scanning with Gallium-67,[31] and imaging by computerized tomography (CT).[33] Ultrasonography may be useful,[30] though loops of bowel and previous scars may hinder the examination. Serial ultrasonography at 2 to 3 day intervals also may be helpful in questionable situations.

When detected, abscesses should be drained. Though CT-directed techniques for drainage are available,[34] the patient with Crohn's disease who is drained percutaneously will often have recurrent abscess formation and surgical resection of the involved bowel is usually necessary.[30]

Bacteriologic analysis of abdominal abscesses has shown Escherichia coli (54%), Bacteroides fragilis (44%), enterococci (41%), and viridans streptococci (31%) as the predominant organisms.[28] Broad spectrum antimicrobial antibiotic therapy, including coverage for anaerobes, should be used preoperatively and during the first few days postoperatively.

The potential locations of intra-abdominal

TABLE 14-3. *Location of Intra-abdominal Abscesses in Crohn's Disease.*

Enteroperitoneal
Interloop
Intramesenteric
Retroperitoneal-ileopsoas
Hepatic
Splenic

abscesses are summarized in Table 14-3. Those occurring within the abdominal cavity have been characterized as: (1) enteroperitoneal, with at least one surface in contact with parietal peritoneum and remaining margins bound by viscera and adhesions; (2) interloop, surrounded by loops of diseased bowel; and (3) intramesenteric, enclosed within the leaves of the mesentery of the involved intestinal segment.[30] The terminal ileum and colon (especially sigmoid) are the primary areas of intestinal involvement and origin of intra-abdominal abscesses.[28,35]

Intra-abdominal abscesses may also affect solid abdominal organs or tissues. Ileopsoas abscesses may develop from ileal Crohn's disease with symptoms of weakness and pain on flexion of the right hip.[36] Hepatic abscesses may present with right upper abdominal pain and fever in addition to the symptoms of active bowel disease.[37] Splenic abscesses have been reported but are rare, and contiguous spread from adjacent bowel or bacteremic seeding of the spleen are proposed mechanisms.[38] Drainage of these abscesses in conjunction with appropriate antibiotic coverage will usually be effective.[36-38]

Fistulae

The relative incidence of internal fistulae in Crohn's disease is summarized in Table 14-4.

RECTOVAGINAL FISTULAE. Though rectovaginal fistulae occur both in ulcerative proctitis/colitis and Crohn's proctitis/colitis, they are more common in Crohn's disease and may result from ex-

TABLE 14-4. *Incidence of Internal Fistulae in Crohn's Disease.*

Rectovaginal	3-5%
Enterovesical, enterourethral enteroureteral	2-6%
Enterocutaneous	< 20%
Enteroenteral	< 20%

tension of a perirectal abscess;[39] such fistulae are more common during active disease. The symptoms related to the fistulae are dependent upon their size and location. While pain is usually minimal, small fistulae may be associated with a foul, profuse vaginal discharge, and large lesions may lead to the passage of feces and flatus through the vagina. Sigmoidoscopic and/or vaginal speculum examination usually will enable the examiner to detect the site and size of the fistula. In some instances, however, it can be identified *only* by barium enema examination. On other occasions, even radiologic methods fail to demonstrate the communication and the clinician must rely on the injection of a colored marker, such as methylene blue, into the rectum to determine whether it will find entrance into the vagina as detected on a tampon previously inserted into the vagina.

Rectovaginal fistula may require no therapy if the patient finds it a minor inconvenience. Corticosteroids or sulfasalazine typically has little effect on healing of the fistula. If diarrhea is a major aggravating factor for the patient, medical therapy of the inflammatory bowel disease may prove helpful to control symptoms, and metronidazole may facilitate healing in some patients.[10,11] When symptoms fail to respond adequately, surgical intervention may prove beneficial but often this requires an abdominal perineal resection or diverting colostomy.[40] A case of adenocarcinoma within a rectovaginal fistula has been described as a rare complication.[41]

URINARY TRACT FISTULAE. Enterovesical, enterourethral, or enteroureteral fistulae may occur in Crohn's disease, usually arising from the ileum, sigmoid, or rectum.[42] An abscess may form initially, followed by fistula development between involved bowel and adjacent urinary structures. Direct fistulization, usually to the urinary bladder, may also occur without abscess formation. Rarely, malignancy may develop at the site of a chronic entero-urinary tract fistula, especially if this arises from bypassed small bowel.

Enterovesical fistulae occur in 2 to 6% of patients with Crohn's disease, more commonly in males and at an average interval of ten years after the onset of symptoms of bowel disease.[42,43] Symptoms include pneumaturia (which is virtually pathognomonic), recurrent cystitis, or fecaluria. Physical findings are minimal, though a mass of inflamed bowel may be noted. Pyuria and positive cultures of urine may be found. Bowel symptoms may not be particularly severe, though a concomitant abscess may be symptomatic. Bouts of urinary tract infections can be avoided by using chronic antibiotic suppressive therapy, though serious urinary tract sepsis is rare.

Diagnosis may be difficult. Barium contrast studies of the bowel (Fig. 14-5), intravenous pyelogram, voiding cystogram, and cystoscopy have been used to identify such fistulae, though often these techniques fail. Then it may be necessary to identify the fistula at surgery. When surgical treatment is required, the bladder defect may be either closed or, in some instances, resected, and usually the involved bowel also must be resected. After such surgical therapy, recurrence of these fistulae is rare. Spontaneous healing is unusual and medical therapy rarely results in healing of enterovesical fistulae.[42,43]

ENTEROCUTANEOUS FISTULAE. External fistulae occur in up to 15 to 20% of patients with Crohn's disease.[44] Enterocutaneous fistulae most commonly are complications of prior surgical resection.[45] An anastomosis may leak with resulting local abscess formation that then drains externally, often at the incision.[45,46] This situation often arises in the absence of active bowel disease. Enterocutaneous fistulae may also develop either when a loop of involved small intestine develops a deeply penetrating sinus that then opens onto the abdominal wall, or as the result of spontaneous drainage through the skin of a subcutaneous abscess that also communicates with a loop of bowel.

The identification of bowel contents at the skin makes recognition of this entity easy. Localizing the exact anatomic connection and classification as simple (with involvement of a single loop of bowel) or complex (multiple loops of bowel or abscess) is possible by obtaining a fistulogram and may be supplemented by CT scanning.[47] Standard barium contrast studies can be performed to establish the associated bowel inflammation.

Management of the enterocutaneous fistula will involve replacement of fluid, electrolytes, protein, and calories as the initial stage: this can be simplified by the use of total parenteral nutrition (TPN).[48] Local skin care also is important, using standard stomal therapy techniques.[49] Any associated sepsis or abscesses must also be treated. In the postoperative situation, where active disease is unlikely, a trial of TPN for six weeks is reasonable; if improvement is seen, surgical treatment may be avoided. The fistulae associated with active bowel disease are unlikely to heal unless surgical resection of the inflamed region is performed, however.[44-46] Total parenteral nutrition will serve to improve readiness for surgical treatment in such cases. The prognosis for enterocutaneous fistulae is good with modern nutritional support, infection control, and surgical techniques (see also Chap. 27).[48]

ENTEROENTERAL FISTULAE. Enteroenteral fistulae may develop in Crohn's disease. Such fistulae involve a loop of diseased bowel, especially terminal ileum, and an adjacent loop of small bowel or colon, especially the sigmoid; the adjacent bowel may or may not be primarily involved by

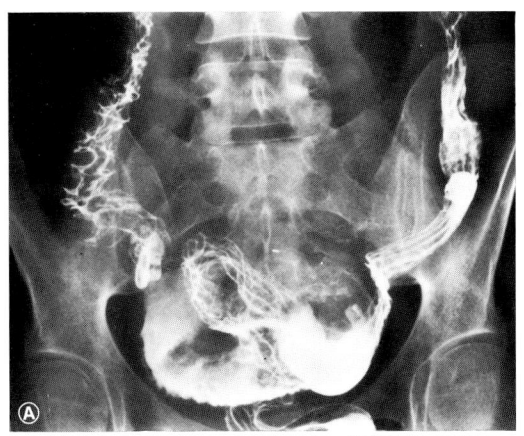

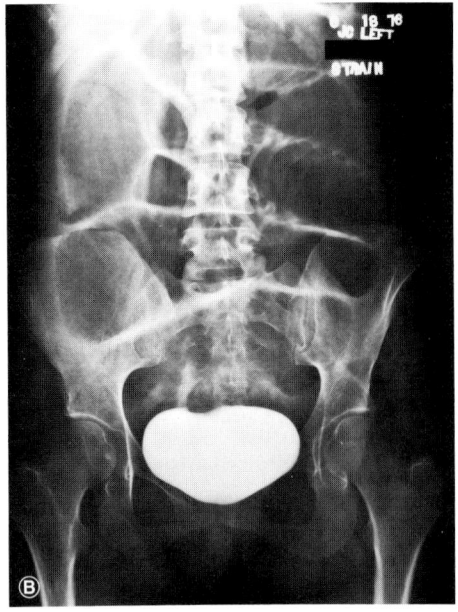

FIG. 14-5. Enterovesical fistula in Crohn's disease seen at barium enema (a) and retrograde cystogram (b).

Crohn's disease. These fistulae appear to develop as a result of deep ulceration penetrating directly from the involved bowel through the wall of the adjacent bowel wall. Abscess cavities may also be involved. Broe et al. reported an incidence of 18.5% or enteroenteral fistulae in a group of 348 patients.[50] Active Crohn's disease in such individuals is most commonly located in the ileum and colon (58%), terminal ileum (20%), colon (11%), and jejunoileal area (11%). Perianal disease may be present also.

Symptoms in patients with such fistulae are usually those caused by the associated pathology, i.e., obstruction or abscess, including abdominal pain, fever, weight loss, diarrhea, abdominal mass, or bleeding. Symptoms attributable to the fistulae per se are rare, and in the absence of associated active Crohn's disease, commonly such patients are asymptomatic. When relatively large tracts are present between stomach or duodenum and the distal small bowel or colon (Fig. 14-6), diarrhea and weight loss are usually noted.

Enteroenteral fistulae are most commonly identified incidentally as other symptoms are being investigated. Barium contrast studies will diagnose about 75% of the fistulae, while others are detected at surgery.[50]

Symptoms of the Crohn's disease accompanying such fistulae should be treated in the usual manner because control of the active inflammatory response will often be sufficient therapy, even though the fistulae do not heal. If fistulae are felt to be responsible for significant symptoms, then elemental diets, total parenteral nutrition, or immunosuppressive therapy may allow healing in some patients. Such improvement will often be transient, however, as fistulae commonly recur once therapy is discontinued. Hence, surgical therapy will often be necessary, with resection of the primary area of involvement.[51-53] When the adjacent loop of bowel does not have primary evidence of Crohn's disease, the fistula may be resected with oversewing of the defect. If the other loop is also involved by Crohn's disease, however, resection of active disease from this portion is necessary as well. In the study by Broe et al. of 64 patients, 48 were diagnosed by barium contrast studies and the remainder were found only during surgical treatment.[50] Twenty-four underwent surgical treatment within two weeks of diagnosis. Twenty-four patients were treated conservatively: of these, 10 required surgical treatment within one year (for intestinal obstruction, enterovesical fistula, increasing ileostomy output, and hemorrhage), and fourteen patients were managed nonoperatively for periods of 15 months to 9 years (mean 3.5 years). Eight of these fourteen required surgical treatment for intestinal obstruction, perforation, enterocutaneous fistula, or further control of symptoms. Of the total of 64 patients, 6 did not require surgical treatment during the study period, with 4 being controlled well medically and 2 showing disappearance of the fistulae on serial barium studies.

If an abscess is detected in conjunction with an enteroenteral fistula, surgical therapy is required typically (see also Chap. 27).

IMMUNOSUPPRESSIVE THERAPY FOR FISTULAE IN CROHN'S DISEASE. As noted, medical therapy to induce healing of fistulae using corticosteroids and sulfasalazine in Crohn's disease commonly fails. Recent experience with immunosuppressive therapy suggests that this may offer one alternative to surgical therapy, however. Present et al. performed a two-year, randomized, double-

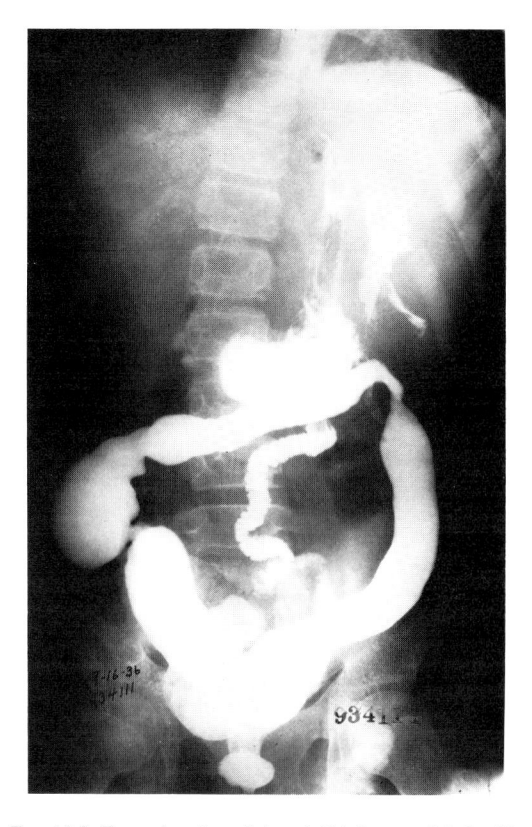

FIG. 14-6. Example of an internal fistula associated with Crohn's disease of the colon. Radiograph shows presence of gastrojejunocolic fistula demonstrated by barium enema. Note the disease in the splenic flexure at the site of the fistula. Radiographs of the stomach and small intestine showed no evidence of the fistula.

blind, placebo-controlled, crossover study of the introduction of 6-mercaptopurine (6-MP) into the treatment of Crohn's patients, while maintaining their previous treatment with corticosteroid and/or sulfasalazine. Thirty-six patients with 40 fistulae were involved, and the dosages of 6-MP averaged 1.5 mg/kg/day. Fistulae were present in perirectal, abdominal wall, enteroenteric, rectovaginal, and vulvar locations. In the 29 patients who received 6-MP, 9 (31%) completely healed while 7 (24%) partially improved; the placebo group of 17 patients experienced complete healing in 1 (6%) and partial healing in 3 (18%). A follow-up report, which included 27 of the original patients treated with 6-MP and a total of 34 patients, showed complete closure in 13 (39%), while improvement was noted in 9 (26%). The mean time to full response was 3.1 months, with almost a quarter of the patients requiring over 4 months of therapy. The site of intestinal involvement was not significant in influencing the outcome, but individuals with prior surgical therapy generally did less well than those without such therapy. Chronic therapy at full dosage was required to maintain healing, but in many instances the dose of corticosteroids was discontinued or continued at a lower level.

Side effects of 6-MP therapy include bone marrow suppression, acute pancreatitis, drug hepatitis, or "allergic" reactions. Furthermore, a potential risk of the development of neoplasia is a concern in chronic therapy with 6-MP.

The relative roles of immunosuppressive therapy and surgical treatment for Crohn's fistulae has not been clearly established. In patients with limited Crohn's disease, in whom resection may have little effect on the physiologic bowel function, surgical therapy may be preferred. Patients with extensive disease or prior extensive surgical resections may be appropriate candidates for a trial of 6-MP therapy, as long as they are willing to accept the careful monitoring involved.

Free Perforation

Colon

Acute free perforation of the colon is potentially the most dangerous complication of inflammatory bowel disease and occurs almost exclusively in patients with ulcerative colitis,[20] only a few cases having been reported in Crohn's colitis.[56-58] Free perforation often complicates toxic megacolon but, on occasion, it is seen in the absence of this condition. Most perforations occur in patients with severe attacks of ulcerative colitis, a few occur in moderately severe attacks, but none has been recorded in attacks that are mild. First episodes of colitis are especially likely to lead to free perforation, possibly because of a lack of fibrosis and scarring from previous attacks that might provide a barrier to the perforation of the intestinal wall by the acute inflammatory process. Furthermore, it is speculated that the absence of serosal involvement and adhesions to adjacent organs facilitates the occurrence of acute free perforation. In Edwards and Truelove's series,[20] 13 of 20 patients suffering perforations developed them during the first attack. Most perforations occur in the left colon, the sigmoid being the most vulnerable. Steroid therapy has been implicated as a contributing factor in the development of colonic perforation, but this was not substantiated by Edwards and Truelove who found no increase in its frequency when they compared a group of patients under treatment with steroids with a similar group who were seen before the introduction of this form of therapy.[20] By confining themselves to patients with the first attack, and by including only those with severe or moderately severe activity, these authors found that the incidences of perforation in the presteroid and steroid eras were essentially the same: 13.6% in the presteroid era and 9.1% in the steroid era.

In Crohn's disease of the colon, free perforation may result from the tendency of the fissure ulcers to penetrate deeply into, and sometimes through, the bowel wall. As noted previously, this penetration commonly leads to the formation of a fistula or abscess because of the attachment of inflamed loops of intestine that become attached to adjacent organs. Free perforation into the peritoneal cavity sometimes occurs, however. On other occasions, free perforation may be noted in the bowel proximal to an obstructed segment. In this instance, the perforation may result either from penetration of the bowel wall by the inflammation in a diseased area, or from changes secondary to obstruction that result in local ischemia, necrosis, and perforation in normal bowel proximal to the obstructive lesion. The latter most often occurs in the cecum.

Small Intestine

Free perforation of the small intestine is being reported in Crohn's disease with increasing frequency.[59,60] While the terminal ileum is most frequently the site of the perforation, probably this reflects the fact that this is the most common site of gross involvement by Crohn's disease because perforation also may occur with disease in the proximal ileum or in the jejunum. Again, as in the colon, perforation may occur with or without the presence of associated intestinal obstruction. When stenosis occurs in the distal small intestine, stasis of the intestinal content is conducive to the formation of calcified enteroliths, and, rarely, such an enterolith may perforate the ileum.[61]

Diagnosis of intestinal perforation is not difficult when the patient shows the classic signs of an "acute abdomen." In view of the fact that many patients already are acutely ill and have varying degrees of abdominal pain and tenderness associated with the IBD, notoriously few local signs of perforation may be present and the only suggestion of the presence of a surgical emergency may be an abrupt clinical deterioration of the patient associated with varying degrees of abdominal pain, often mild to moderate. The diagnosis is best established by prompt x-ray examination of the abdomen to detect the presence of free air. Most clinicians have recommended the use of three exposures—upright, flat, and lateral decubitus, the latter often demonstrating the presence of gas between the area of liver dullness and the right lateral thoracoabdominal wall where perforation has occurred.

A good prognosis for this complication depends upon its prompt recognition and early surgical treatment. The attending physician must always be alert for its occurrence and consider it in the differential diagnosis in patients with severe attacks of IBD in whom a sudden worsening occurs in their clinical status. This was emphasized by Edwards and Truelove who noted that three-fourths of their patients with this complication died, and that half of the instances of perforation were diagnosed only at postmortem examination.[20] While surgical treatment carries a significant risk, it offers the best chance for survival.

Acute Toxic Megacolon

This potentially lethal complication usually occurs in a severe attack of inflammatory bowel disease and is characterized by total or segmental colonic dilation. The colon becomes widely distended, losing its ability to contract, and commonly is associated with deterioration in the patient's clinical state, producing "a toxic condition."[62]

A formal definition of toxic megacolon has proven difficult because no pathognomonic histologic findings are available. Criteria for the clinical diagnosis have been outlined by Jalan, however, and include radiographic evidence of colon distension in addition to at least three of these four conditions: (1) fever over 101.5° F (38.6° C), (2) tachycardia over 120 beats per minute, (3) neutrophil leukocytosis greater than 10,500, or (4) anemia.[63] At least one sign of toxicity, that is, dehydration, mental changes, electrolyte disturbance, or hypotension also must be present. Physical examination of the abdomen may show distension or signs of peritoneal irritation.

This complication has an overall reported incidence of 1.6 to 8% in all patients with chronic ulcerative colitis.[64,65] It may achieve an incidence of 10% in patients hospitalized for ulcerative colitis who are ill enough to require transfusions or have a temperature of 102° F (38.9° C) or higher during the hospital stay, however.[66] Although its occurrence is more likely in those with universal colonic involvement, it has been seen in patients with disease limited to the left colon.[67]

The risk of developing toxic dilation seems to be directly related to the severity of the attack, and it may even occur during the first episode of the disease. In a series of 55 patients, 23 developed the toxic dilation within 3 months of the first onset of symptoms of colitis.[63] Thirty-two patients were in relapse with a wide variation in the duration of the disease, but the majority had had colitis for less than 5 years.

At one time this complication was considered to occur only in patients with ulcerative colitis, but it is being observed with increasing frequency in Crohn's disease of the colon.[68] Farmer et al. reported that 38 of 592 (6.4%) patients with Crohn's disease developed toxic megacolon.[69] In patients requiring surgical treatment for Crohn's disease, toxic megacolon was the indication in 5% of those with ileocolitis, 26.6% of those with colonic or anorectal disease, and 2.1% of patients with small intestinal disease.

Toxic megacolon has also been recognized as a complication of pseudomembranous, bacterial or amebic colitis, and cholera.

Pathophysiology

While the cause of the substantial colonic dilation occurring during the course of inflammatory bowel disease remains obscure, several factors may combine to produce the complete clinical picture. The disturbed motility, with loss of the colon's ability to contract, seems to relate to the extension of the inflammation to involve the muscularis, serosa, and visceral peritoneum. The resulting severe muscular destruction, and perhaps, damage to the myenteric plexus, results in an atonic bowel that loses its ability to contract and thus becomes dilated.[62,64] Depending upon the extent of the inflammation, a segment or the entire colon may be so affected. Hypokalemia may aggravate the already weakened peristalsis, and hypoproteinemia may augment the edema of the bowel wall. Gross pathologic examination of the colon reveals severe and extensive mucosal ulcerations or, in some instances, complete denudation. When the ulcerations are severe, they may be extremely friable and perforations, which are common, usually occur through such areas. The muscularis may be grossly affected by deep ulcerations while the remaining wall of the colon is correspondingly thin. The serosa may show signs of peritonitis and, at times, the peritoneal fat is edematous. Microscopic examination in the areas of ulceration shows denudation of the mucosa with replacement by highly vascular granulation tissue heavily infiltrated with histiocytes, plasma cells, lymphocytes, and polymorphonuclear leukocytes.[70] This inflammatory process extends into the inner and outer muscular coats with varying degrees of degeneration and necrosis of muscle fibers. In many instances, the individual muscle fibers in both layers are peculiarly shortened and rounded with aggregates of eosinophilic-staining cytoplasm present in the myofibrils. The myenteric plexuses may be distorted and edematous, especially in areas adjacent to extensive mucosal ulceration. The serosa shows, in contrast to the colon in ulcerative colitis without colonic dilatation, evidence of acute and chronic inflammation with leukocytic infiltration and formation of new capillaries. The transmural involvement of the colon seen in toxic megacolon may make the distinction between CUC and Crohn's colitis difficult (see also Chap. 18).[71]

Limited studies of absorption and secretion of water and electrolytes in ulcerative colitis show differences from those in the normal human colon. These studies indicate that the colonic absorption of water and sodium is impaired and the secretion of potassium is increased. Harris and Shields found that the reserve capacity for the colon to absorb sodium and water was lost in patients with ulcerative colitis, so that the mean rate of absorption of sodium was reduced to one-third of that observed in healthy adults and the mean rate of water absorption was reduced to one-seventh.[72] They also found that potassium was secreted into the gut four times more rapidly than in the healthy subject. Additional potassium losses may result from desquamation of the intestinal mucosa, hemorrhage, and pus formation. For these reasons, significant depletion of water and electrolytes may occur, particularly in toxic megacolon. Hypoalbuminemia is frequently present but the serum globulins are rarely affected. This probably results from protein loss secondary to an exudative enteropathy associated with the ulcerative mucosa, and from the decreased synthesis of protein caused by the presence of chronic infection.

Risk Factors

Possible risk factors for toxic megacolon development are summarized in Table 14-5.

In some instances the development of toxic dilation seems to be related to the therapeutic use of anticholinergic drugs or narcotics that adversely affect the disturbed motility. Motility studies of the colon in different stages of active ulcerative colitis have shown a diminution or absence of phasic activity and an abnormal incidence of mass peristaltic waves.[73] The dilated colon is adynamic and loses its normal contractility, tone, and propulsive movement. Thus, it is unable to empty, leading to further distension or, alternatively, to an "overflow" type of diarrhea resulting from the continuous flow of small intestinal contents through the ileocecal valve. Furthermore, the absorptive function of the colonic mucosa is probably impaired and may become secretory in character. Anticholinergic drugs in therapeutic doses inhibit colonic tone

TABLE 14-5. *Possible Risk Factors for the Development of Toxic Megacolon.*

Pharmacologic
   Narcotic analgesia
   Anticholinergics
   Antidiarrheals
      Diphenoxylate hydrochloride with atropine sulphate
      Loperamide
   Psyllium seed products
Diagnostic
   Barium enema
   Proctosigmoidoscopy
   Colonoscopy
Metabolic Derangements
   Electrolyte abnormalities, especially hypokalemia
   Hypoproteinemia

and motility, while narcotics produce a loss of propulsive activity accompanied by an increase in tone. Thus, when these drugs are used in treatment of inflammatory bowel disease as a part of the therapy to control diarrhea or pain, they do so by impairing the ability of the colon to empty, thus accentuating the colon's existing inability to empty itself. A temporal relationship between the initiation of opiate treatment, or increased doses, and the development of toxic dilation has been noted. Seventeen of 18 patients who received either tincture of opium or an increased dose of opiate developed toxic megacolon within 1 to 3 days.[73] Loperamide therapy has also been associated temporally with the development of toxic megacolon.[74]

The onset of toxic megacolon may follow barium enema examination of the colon in patients with acute exacerbations of ulcerative colitis,[66,75] particularly in those who at the time of x-ray examination have abdominal pain with tenderness and fever. It is speculated that the rapid distension of the colon may aggravate the mucosal ulceration by forcing, under pressure, bacteria and intestinal contents into the bowel wall and into the open capillary plexuses. Furthermore, the impaired blood supply to the bowel wall, which results from edema and vascular thromboses, may be further reduced by the increased intraluminal pressure that accompanies the barium enema. In one series, 43% of 37 patients with toxic dilation developed their symptoms within 9 days of barium enema examinations.[66] Because the diagnosis of inflammatory bowel disease usually can be made on the basis of history and sigmoidoscopic examination, the barium x-ray examination usually should be deferred in acutely ill patients, especially in those with established disease in an acute flare-up, who are febrile, anemic, and have abdominal pain and tenderness. In rare situations, however, a carefully performed barium roentgenogram may be possible.[76] Care must be taken in doing proctoscopic examinations so that air insufflation is minimized because this procedure also may be followed by toxic dilatation,[77] and colonoscopy also has been followed by onset of toxic megacolon.[78] Factors that have been suggested as potential risks in the development of toxic megacolon include hypokalemia, hypoproteinemia, the use of hydrophilic agents (such as psyllium seed products), and corticosteroids, but none of these has been proven to be a cause of toxic megacolon. Caution in ordering barium enema or colonoscopic examinations, recognition and correction of metabolic derangements, and avoidance of antidiarrheal drugs, narcotics, and psyllium seed products in the ill patient with inflammatory bowel disease are judicious, however.[64]

Diagnostic Features

CLINICAL FINDINGS. The development of toxic dilation of the colon during an episode of acute fulminating colitis may be suspected by an acute change in abdominal pain from a cramping intermittent type to a steady diffuse pain that is not relieved by bowel movements.[64-66] Fever, with spikes to over 101° F (38.3° C), and tachycardia often accompany this clinical situation. Bowel habits show no consistent pattern but, frequently, diarrhea persists without change in severity. In other patients, however, the number of stools may decrease, which may initially give a false impression of clinical improvement, while a few may have an increased stool frequency and an occasional patient will have fecal incontinence. General examination of the abdomen commonly reveals visible distension, diffuse tenderness to palpation, rebound tenderness, and diminished bowel sounds. This combination of findings suggests impending perforation or the possibility of peritonitis. Patients appear acutely and profoundly ill, and may show some alteration of the sensorium or mental balance as manifested by anxiety, hysterical behavior, lethargy, depression, or extreme listlessness. Clinical toxicity may be further manifested by the presence of systemic complications such as thrombophlebitis, which is sometimes complicated by pulmonary embolism and liver disease. Other extraintestinal manifestations of active inflammatory bowel disease that are sometimes present include pyoderma gangrenosum, urticaria, arthritis, uveitis, erythema nodosum, jaundice, and perianal complications such as fissure in ano.[64] Pneumomediastinum with subcutaneous air about the neck also may occur from retroperitoneal air tracking into the mediastinum, even without colon perforation.[79] It should be noted as a caveat, however, that not infrequently a significant discrepancy exists between the paucity of physical findings and the degree of colonic dilatation found in an x-ray film of the abdomen.

RADIOLOGIC FINDINGS.* The judicious use of x-ray examination of the abdomen will alert the attending physician to this complication of IBD early in its course and is the only reliable means

---
*See also Chapter 20.

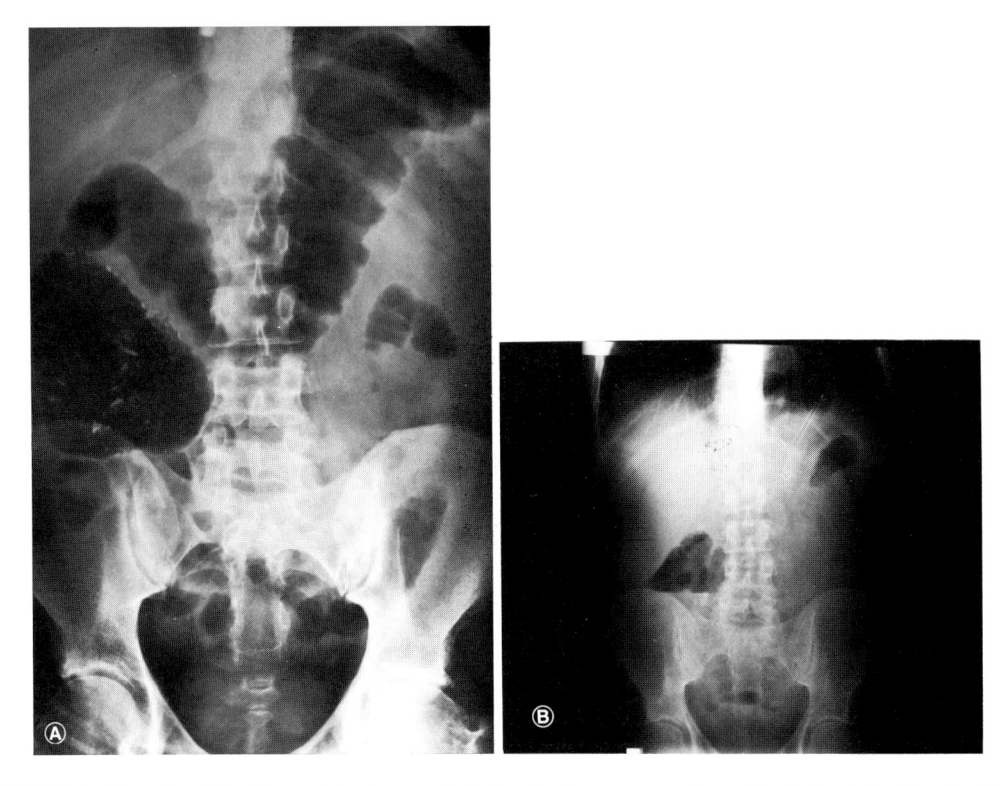

FIG. 14-7. Toxic Megacolon. This 37-year-old male presented after a barium enema performed by his local physician for bloody diarrhea. (A) Note prominent dilatation of the cecum and transverse colon. (B) Flecks of retained barium are present in the cecum. Three days after institution of medical therapy, the dilatation has improved substantially. The patient was successfully managed medically.

of establishing the diagnosis. For this reason, flat films of the abdomen should be obtained in all acutely ill patients with colitis. A striking feature of the abdominal x-ray picture is extreme colonic dilation, which is usually maximal in the transverse colon (Fig. 14-7).[80-82] The entire colon may be involved or segments of the right and left colon may be included with the transverse colon. It is uncommon to find distension of the rectum, even though it is involved in the ulcerative process. The dilated transverse colon usually exceeds 6 cm in diameter and is the most distended segment of the colon if abdominal films are obtained supine.[83] When patients are placed in the prone position, dilatation will probably affect the ascending and descending colon, as the bowel gas is redistributed. Hence, the distribution of bowel gas in the patient with toxic megacolon is primarily affected by gravity. At times, a subserosal radiolucent line is present in the wall of the colon. Other features include: (1) the loss of the normal haustral pattern, (2) a scalloped or wavy contour of the bowel lumen with an occasional "deep-tooth" projection, and (3) numerous broad-based polypoid projections that extend into the lumen from the bowel wall. Frequently some gas is in the small intestine, but this usually presents the appearance associated with aerophagia rather than that of small bowel obstruction. Serial flat plate films of the abdomen at 12 to 24 hour intervals can be useful in determining the clinical course of the patient (see also Chap. 20).

LABORATORY FINDINGS. Neutrophil leukocytosis of 10,000 to 20,000/mm^3 is usually present in patients with toxic megacolon, and the peripheral blood smear may show toxic changes in the neutrophilic leukocytes and rouleaux formation of the erythrocytes. Anemia is common and is secondary to blood loss and infection. Colonic losses of water, protein, and electrolytes are usually excessive in toxic megacolon, and lead to depletion of total body stores. Hence, hypokalemia, hypocalcemia, and hypoalbuminemia are common. Prothrombin time may be prolonged but usually responds to vitamin K administration.

Treatment

MEDICAL THERAPY. In view of the potentially lethal nature of this complication, it should be regarded as an acute medical and surgical emergency requiring constant and close observation. The goal of medical management should be to provide, as quickly as possible, optimal conditions for remission while at the same time achieving the best possible preoperative status of the patient should surgical treatment become necessary. This is best accomplished by early consultation with a gastrointestinal surgeon. Careful monitoring of the vital signs and fluid and electrolyte balance is mandatory, frequently necessitating the nursing care that can be provided only in an intensive care unit. A summary of the management of toxic megacolon is presented in Table 14-6.

Stool samples for culture of enteric pathogens, for parasites, especially ameba, and assay for C. difficile toxin should be taken early in order to establish the presence of treatable infectious causes for toxic megacolon.

Once the diagnosis is established, the bowel should be put to rest by the omission of oral feedings and by the institution of continuous suction applied to a nasointestinal tube (Fig. 14-3). A long tube, such as a Miller-Abbott or Cantor tube, with its tip placed in the distal ileum to produce decompression of the bowel may be used rather than a nasogastric tube. In passing the tip of the tube into the duodenum, fluoroscopy is helpful and avoids the delays associated with reliance on spontaneous passage into the small intestine. Continuous aspiration reduces the amount of small-bowel content that enters the dilated, atonic colon, thus diminishing the contribution of this factor to the pathophysiology of toxic megacolon. Some advocate the use of rectal tubes as well.[84] Frequent radiographs of the abdomen are necessary, not only to check the position of the suction tube but also to follow the progress of the colonic dilatation and for the early detection of a free perforation. Frequent auscultation of the abdomen is a useful clinical guide in this circumstance as a simple but informative approach to the peristaltic activity of the bowel. Opiates and narcotics should be avoided because of their adverse effects on colonic motility.

Intravenous replacement and maintenance of water and electrolytes should be carefully monitored, based on estimates of the pretreatment losses and subsequent measurements of daily losses in urine, stool, and gastrointestinal aspiration. Because Caprilli et al.[85] have suggested that severe electrolyte and metabolic disorders increase the risk in toxic megacolon, intensive fluid and electrolyte replacement are critical to the overall support of the patient. Total parenteral nutrition often is helpful, because many patients are malnourished and some may need surgical intervention. Blood transfusions frequently are required to replace losses from bleeding and to maintain a hemoglobin of 10 g % or a hematocrit of approximately 35%. Hypoalbuminemia not corrected by blood transfusion or parenteral nutrition may require the intravenous administration of salt-free albumin in daily amounts of 25 to 37.5 g to raise the serum concentration to at least 3 g/100 ml. Vitamins B, C, and K should be added to the intravenous fluid because deficiencies are not uncommon. Antibiotics are often given because of concern for impending perforation and/or peritonitis that may exist in this situation. Ideally, the antibiotics used should cover the broad spectrum of both anaerobic and aerobic organisms commonly present in the lumen of the colon. Before initiating antibiotic treatment, blood and stool cultures should be obtained to detect the presence of specific organisms that might influence the choice of antibiotics.

The value of adrenocorticotropin (ACTH) and parenteral steroids in treating toxic megacolon has not been firmly established,[86,87] though many authors strongly recommend their use. Because corticosteroids became widely used at about the same time as the general intensive medical and surgical approach (described previously), it is not known what benefit has been solely caused by the corticosteroids. Concerns about the possible harmful effects of these drugs in toxic megacolon and the surgical therapy thereof include the risk of masking clinical

TABLE 14-6. *Management of Toxic Megacolon.*

Supportive
    Correction of anemia, hypoproteinemia,
        electrolyte imbalance
    Vitamin supplements
    Total parenteral nutrition
    Nasogastric or nasojejunal suction
    Rectal tube
Pharmacologic
    Broad spectrum antibiotics
    Corticosteroids
    Adrenocorticotropin (ACTH)
Surgical
    Colectomy or proctocolectomy

signs of perforation, impairing wound healing, promoting wound sepsis or general sepsis, wound dehiscence, initiating paralytic ileus, peptic ulceration, and psychosis. It is generally accepted, however, that when given in the short term with careful, regular scrutiny of the patient, they are a helpful, albeit unproven, therapy for the initial treatment of toxic megacolon.

Patients with symptomatically active inflammatory bowel disease will usually be receiving corticosteroids for treatment, and if toxic megacolon develops, these patients require continued therapy to avoid adrenal insufficiency.[87] If toxic dilatation, with or without perforation, develops in a patient who discontinued steroid therapy within six months of the attack, such therapy should be reinstituted in full therapeutic doses. On the other hand, if a patient develops toxic dilatation associated with clinical evidence of free perforation or sealed-off perforation, and has not recently received steroids, they should be avoided.

When steroid therapy is indicated in a patient with toxic megacolon, parenteral administration is most frequently used.[86,87] Corticosteroids, such as prednisolone acetate, at a dosage of 60 to 80 mg daily, or similar steroids in equivalent doses are commonly used either alone or simultaneously with ACTH. The drug is continued in lower doses and eventually tapered if a remission occurs without surgical intervention. If the patient requires surgical treatment the dosage can be gradually reduced postoperatively, following the usual recommendations, and then discontinued. Some prefer ACTH alone, which may be given in doses of 80 units intravenously over the first 24-hour period, and then diminished by 10 units daily until the patient requires surgical treatment or until it is discontinued on the eighth or ninth day.[80,87]

SURGICAL THERAPY.* Many patients who develop toxic megacolon will require surgical intervention for definitive treatment; however, its timing during the acute phase of this complication is one of the most difficult decisions encountered in its management. This decision must take into consideration not only the acute problem but also the previous history of the disease and its other manifestations, complications, disability, and response to previous treatment.

In the acute situation, medical management should be continued only in patients who show definite signs of clinical improvement within the first 24 to 48 hours.[78] This improvement should be manifested by both decreasing signs of distension and clinical toxicity. During this interval, the colon may diminish in diameter, and the depleted electrolytes, fluids, albumin, and red cell mass may be replenished. Surgical treatment of toxic megacolon usually should be undertaken for the following reasons: (1) persistent or progressive increase in dilatation and clinical toxicity despite supportive measures beyond 24 to 48 hours; (2) colonic perforation, as demonstrated by clinical examination and/or radiography of the abdomen; or (3) massive bleeding requiring immediate transfusions.

The nature of the surgical treatment will be individualized by the surgeon. Commonly performed procedures include proctocolectomy with ileostomy,[78] subtotal colectomy and ileostomy with mucous fistula, the Hartman procedure, or an ileorectostomy.[88] Rectal removal usually follows at a later date. Turnbull described a diverting loop ileostomy and skin level decompressive colostomy ("blow-hole" procedure), which may occasionally be used.[89]

RESULTS. The relative merits of medical and surgical therapy have been debated in the literature since the condition was recognized in the early 1950's. Early reports generally favored medical therapy because the surgical mortality was high. In the report by McInerney et al., 23 of 28 treated medically survived while 3 of 8 who underwent surgical therapy survived.[70] Some later studies, however, have favored early surgical therapy, suggesting that it was delayed too long in the earlier series resulting in unnecessarily high mortality figures.[90,91]

Katzka et al. emphasized early recognition as critical to successful medical management.[92] Medical therapy in patients in whom toxic megacolon was recognized early was successful in 13 of 19, while only 2 of 8 were successfully managed by this method after full-blown symptoms had developed. Current literature suggests successful medical management is possible in 30 to 70% of patients, while the remainder require surgical intervention during the same hospitalization. Greenstein et al. identified three factors affecting outcome of therapy: (1) age—those under 40 years of age did better (5% mortality) than those 40 years or older (30% mortality); (2) timing of surgical therapy—elective surgical treatment had better results (6% mortality) than when surgical procedure was performed in those critically ill, requiring an operation within 5 days of onset of megacolon (30% mortality) or

*See also Chapters 26 and 27.

when delayed over a month for other medical reasons (40% mortality); (3) perforation—those with perforation did less well (44% mortality) than those without perforation (2% mortality).[93] The mortality related to perforation or sepsis is reported to be approximately 30% for medical therapy and 20% for surgical therapy.[94]

Grant and Dozois reviewed the clinical course and ultimate outcome in 38 patients successfully treated medically, 32 of whom had ulcerative colitis, while 6 had Crohn's disease.[95] Eighteen patients (47%) ultimately came to colon resection (15 as urgent procedures). Functional assessment suggested that many of the patients who received medical but not surgical treatment remained significantly symptomatic.

In summary, it appears that many patients will ultimately require surgical intervention for toxic megacolon. Medical therapy should be effective in some, however, while for those whose colitis continues to be symptomatic despite such treatment, elective surgical treatment can then be performed with less risk to the patient. Those not initially responding to medical management should undergo surgical therapy early in the course of their disease.

Pseudopolyposis

This is essentially a mucosal lesion and generally is regarded as a more common complication of ulcerative colitis than of Crohn's disease of the colon. Dukes described three types of inflammatory pseudopolyps: (1) the polypoid, edematous mucosal type; (2) polyps composed of granulation tissue covered by mucous membrane; and (3) polyps composed of connective tissue covered by a layer of glandular epithelium.[96] Goldgraber, while reviewing surgical and postmortem specimens, identified an additional type of inflammatory pseudopolyp that shows evidence of adenomatous hyperplasia and may achieve a rather significant size—up to 20 times the average thickness of the colonic mucosa.[97] Pseudopolyps usually occur as discrete lesions or in clusters, but on occasion the mucosa may be diffusely studded by them.

The incidence of pseudopolyps is higher in patients with severe disease and extensive colonic involvement. Disease limited to the rectosigmoid is seldom complicated by pseudopolyps. The methods used for diagnosis also influence the reported incidences of this complication. On clinical examination by sigmoidoscopy and barium enema, pseudopolyps are present in 15 to 30% of patients with CUC, most commonly in the rectum and descending colon. When proctocolectomy specimens are examined,[98] however, the frequency of the pseudopolyps is found to be even greater, approaching 80 to 90%. This probably reflects the severity of the colitis in the patients requiring surgical treatment, plus the advantage of direct examination of the resected colon and rectum. In these specimens, pseudopolyps are most common in the transverse and descending colon and least common in the rectum, particularly its lower two-thirds. Pseudopolyps may form during the initial attack, and they become more common with chronic continuous symptoms. On occasion, the pseudopolyps disappear as the disease becomes chronic. Rarely, diffuse pseudopolyposis may present as the only manifestation of quiescent ulcerative colitis.[99] No specific symptoms suggest the presence of pseudopolyps; their presence is established only by sigmoidoscopic, colonoscopic, and x-ray examination.

Most evidence supports the concept that pseudopolyposis per se is not a precancerous change in CUC, but some workers have attempted to show a transition from pseudopolyps to adenoma and, subsequently, to malignancy.[100] Contrary to this concept, however, is the fact that carcinoma is not more common in patients with IBD with pseudopolyposis than in those without.

In view of the previously mentioned evidence, the findings of pseudopolyposis in itself does not require any specific treatment nor is it an indication for colectomy. In contradistinction to adenomatous polyps, pseudopolyps occasionally disappear spontaneously. This was demonstrated by Sloan et al., who noted a regression in 90% of the patients with this complication.[101]

Occasionally pseudopolyps reach "giant" size in a localized area of the colon, thus mimicking a neoplasm and suggesting the presence of a villous adenoma or a polypoid carcinoma. In one instance, the giant pseudopolyp was the only residual evidence of healed Crohn's disease of the colon.[102] In this circumstance surgical treatment may be indicated, but it should be possible to establish the diagnosis by using biopsy at colonoscopy. Occasionally, these large polyps cause intestinal obstruction by virtue of their size or by producing intussusception and hence require colonoscopic or surgical resection.[103,104]

In contrast to giant pseudopolyps, filiform polyposis (Fig. 14-8) of the colon has been de-

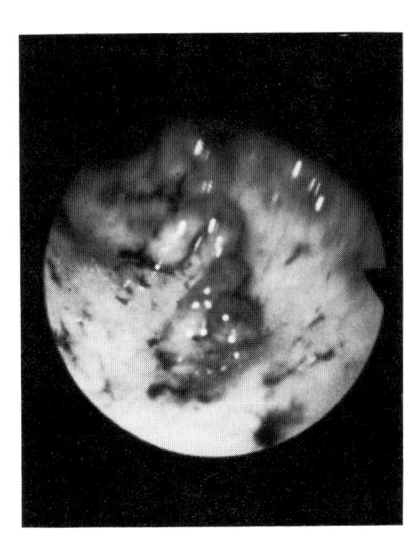

FIG. 14-8. Colonoscopically demonstrated filiform pseudopolyposis seen in longstanding ulcerative colitis.

scribed in ulcerative colitis and in Crohn's disease.[105] These polyps are characterized by multitudinous, worm-like projections of mucosa and submucosa associated with a moderate degree of edema and inflammation. Occasionally arborescence and diameter uniformity are striking features. Although only a few cases are available for review, filiform polyposis has not been associated with cancer and does not represent an indication for colectomy. In a few instances, however, it has presented as massive hemorrhage or mimicking toxic megacolon.[106,107]

Pseudopolyps of the small intestine in Crohn's disease have been described. These occurred in a patient with ileocolitis and showed microscopic features resembling either colonic pseudopolyps or localized nodular lymphangiectasia.[108]

Strictures

Ulcerative Colitis

Some disagreement exists regarding both the frequency of this complication in ulcerative colitis and the nature of its pathology. The underlying concern with strictures is the possibility of a malignancy. While some workers consider strictures to be a rare complication, it is probable that they are found in 11 to 12% of cases of ulcerative colitis.[98,107] Goulston and McGovern found areas in which the diameter of the lumen was reduced by two-thirds or more in 12% of their surgical specimens.[109] These workers, by careful histologic examination, showed that stricture resulted from hypertrophy and thickening of the muscularis mucosa, and that fibrosis, when present, usually was minimal. Generally, strictures occurred in patients with extensive disease and chronic and continuous symptoms, though they may become apparent at any time during the course of the disease. In Truelove's series, one-third occurred within 5 years of the onset of colitis, but the majority appeared in disease with a duration of between 5 and 25 years.[20] Strictures may be seen in any segment of the large bowel, but are most common in the sigmoid and rectum and generally are not found in the right side of the colon. Grossly, most strictures are well localized and the narrowing is restricted to 2 to 3 cm in length. Some, however, are diffuse, achieving lengths up to 15 to 30 cm.

Clinically, it is most difficult to assess the effect of a stricture on the symptoms of colitis because it, in itself, may cause diarrhea indistinguishable from the underlying disease. On occasion, however, it may produce symptoms of partial colonic obstruction in patients whose disease is quiescent. Strictures in the rectum may give the patient a sense of incomplete evacuation of a formed stool or difficulty with continence when the stool is liquid or semiformed.

Radiologically, benign strictures appear to be smooth and fusiform with tapered margins, and pliable, with the mucosa showing either the abnormalities of acute colitis or a smooth, "burned-out" mucosal pattern. Malignancy may mimic a benign stricture, but typically can be expected to present irregular margins in the constricted area, destruction of the mucosal pattern, and rigid tapered extremities with some dilation of the proximal bowel (see also Chap. 20). Biopsies of strictures within reach of the sigmoidoscope or colonoscope should be done to assess the nature of the lesion. Unfortunately, such biopsies may have diagnostic limitations and then the question of benignancy must be based on a clinical assessment of the patient's situation. If the stricture develops within the first few years of the disease, the chance of malignancy is less likely. On the other hand, if a stricture appears for the first time in the second decade of the disease, malignancy must be considered despite the apparent benignancy suggested by radiologic, proctoscopic, and mucosal biopsy examinations.

Considerable differences of opinion are held regarding the use of medical treatment for strictures developing during the course of ulcerative colitis. One widely held view is that the finding of the stricture per se is a strong indication for surgical treatment because of the difficulty of distinguishing a benign from a malignant stricture. Of course, if the stricture is associated with symptoms of partial or complete obstruction, medical treatment is contraindicated. Furthermore, if the strictured area radiologically or colonoscopically shows any indication of malignancy, surgical treatment would be the only course of action.

In view of the features described by Goulston and McGovern, however, the simple stricture in ulcerative colitis is potentially reversible.[109] For this reason, the potential exists for a limited trial of medical treatment with careful observation to determine if the stricture is reversible. Medical treatment should be restricted to those lesions that develop during the first few years of the disease, in the absence of other indications for surgical treatment, and at a stage of the disease when the risk of malignancy is minimal. No specific forms of medical therapy for strictures are available, apart from those used for uncomplicated disease. Such an approach to the treatment of a stricture has limitations and, if adopted, careful follow-up examinations, including colonoscopic evaluation and the use of biopsies, are essential to be certain that improvement occurs both from the standpoint of the symptoms and from the gross appearance of the stricture. If no improvement is apparent in the degree of stricturing within a matter of a few months, even in the absence of evidence of malignancy on biopsy, the question of surgical intervention should seriously be reconsidered.

When the stricture is found late in the course of the disease, particularly as a new development by comparison with previous roentgenograms, it is almost impossible to exclude the possibility of malignancy even with a negative biopsy obtained at colonoscopy. Thus, surgical treatment is strongly indicated.

Crohn's Disease

COLON. These strictures are generally considered to be a part of the disease, rather than a complication, resulting from the transmural nature of the inflammation associated with fibrosis and scarring. The existence of a stricture in this form of colitis, in contrast to chronic ulcerative colitis, is not as suggestive of an underlying malignancy but this possibility should not be ignored. The strictures in Crohn's disease tend to be longer than those seen in ulcerative colitis, and examples of such strictures are shown in Figure 14-9. As pointed out, the possibility of malignancy should not be dismissed casually in Crohn's disease, however, in view of evidence to suggest an increased risk of colorectal cancer in patients with long-standing disease.[110]

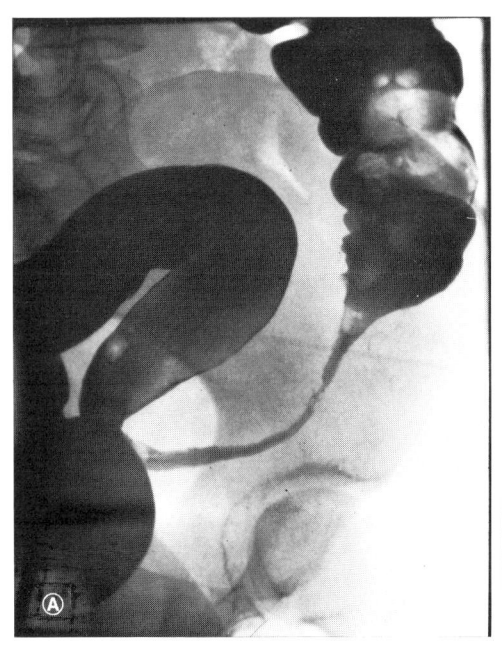

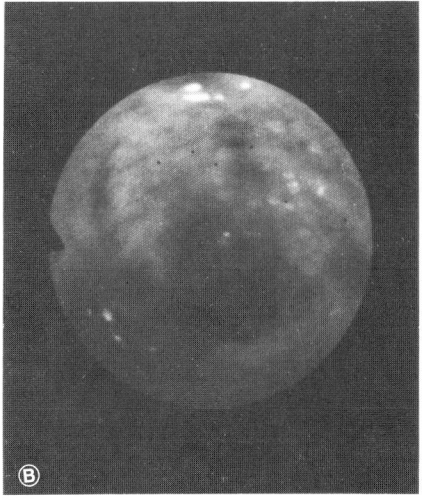

FIG. 14-9. A. Radiograph of Crohn's disease of the colon with a long, benign stricture in the sigmoid area. B. Colonoscopic view of a similar benign, inflammatory stricture in the sigmoid colon.

SMALL INTESTINE. Stricturing is a rather common complication of Crohn's disease involving the small intestine, and approximately 25% of patients hospitalized with the disease will be affected. The most common result is the occurrence of small bowel obstruction secondary to the narrowing of the diseased segment of the bowel that results from scarring and/or inflammation and edema. These pathologic changes usually lead to symptoms, initially of partial, intermittent obstruction that then may slowly become complete. The nature of the obstructive symptoms and signs depends upon the level of the stricture in the small intestine. Distal obstruction is more common, because the ileum is the most frequent site of intestinal involvement and symptomatically is characterized by intermittent cramping, abdominal pain, associated with varying degrees of abdominal distention. Vomiting is infrequent or occurs late in the course of the obstruction, and at times may be feculent. More proximal obstruction is usually associated with frequent vomiting without significant abdominal distension. Gastric outlet obstruction is common when Crohn's disease involves the antrum or duodenum.[111]

Surgical management is usually required to relieve the symptoms of gastrointestinal obstruction secondary to scarring and fibrosis. If it is suggested that the obstruction is secondary to inflammation and edema, however, a short trial of medical therapy with steroids is justified. In some patients with extensive Crohn's disease of the small bowel, surgical management may not be feasible except at the risk of extensive resections that would leave the patient with insufficient small intestine to maintain a normal state of nutrition. In this circumstance, Alexander-Williams has found it possible to simply overcome the stenotic segment(s) by longitudinal incision and transverse suture in the gut, as in a pyloroplasty for duodenal ulcer disease.[112] As a last resort, a combination of nutritional therapy, either an elemental diet administered through a nasogastric tube or total parenteral nutrition, with or without steroid therapy, has given significant palliation to avoid surgical treatment (see also Chaps. 22 and 24).[113,114]

References

1. Buchmann, P., and Alexander-Williams, J.: Classification of Perianal Crohn's Disease. Clin. Gastroenterol., 9:323, 1980.
2. Homan, W. P., Tang, C., and Thorbjarnarson, B.: Anal lesions complicating Crohn's disease. Arch. Surg., 111:1333, 1976.
3. Baker, W. N. W., and Milton-Thompson, G. J.: The anal lesion as the sole presenting symptom of intestinal Crohn's disease. Gut, 12:865, 1971.
4. Williams, D. R., et al.: Anal complications in Crohn's disease. Dis. Colon Rectum, 24:22, 1981.
5. Markowitz, J., et al.: Perianal disease in children and adolescents with Crohn's disease. Gastroenterology, 86:829, 1984.
6. de Dombal, F. T., et al.: Incidence and management of anorectal abscess, fistula and fissure, in patients with ulcerative colitis. Dis. Colon Rectum, 9:201, 1966.
7. Jeffery, P. J., Ritchie, J. K., and Parks, A. G.: Treatment of hemorrhoids in patients with inflammatory bowel disease. Lancet, 1:1084, 1977.
8. Alexander-Williams, J.: Fistula-in-ano: Management of Crohn's fistula. Dis. Colon Rectum, 19:518, 1976.
9. Jackman, R. J.: Management of anorectal complications of chronic ulcerative colitis. Arch. Intern. Med., 94:420, 1954.
10. Bernstein, L. H., Frank, M. S., Brandt, L. J., and Boley, S. J.: Healing of perineal Crohn's disease with metronidazole. Gastroenterology, 79:357, 1980.
11. Brandt, L. J., Bernstein, L. H., Boley, S. J., and Frank, M. S.: Metronidazole therapy for perineal Crohn's disease: A follow-up study. Gastroenterology, 83:383, 1982.
12. Jakobovits, J., and Schuster, M. M.: Metronidazole therapy for Crohn's disease and associated fistulae. Am. J. Gastroenterol. 79:533, 1984.
13. Duffy, L. F., et al.: Peripheral neuropathy in Crohn's disease patients treated with metronidazole. Gastroenterology, 88:681, 1985.
14. Hatoff, D. E.: Perineal Crohn's disease complicated by pyogenic liver abscess during metronidazole therapy. Gastroenterology, 85:194, 1983.
15. Krook, A., et al.: Relation between concentrations of metronidazole and bacteroides spp in faeces of patients with Crohn's disease and healthy individuals. J. Clin. Pathol., 34:645, 1981.
16. Calam, J., Crooks, P. E., and Walker, R. J.: Elemental diets in the management of Crohn's perianal fistulae. JPEN, 4:4, 1980.
17. Williams, N. S., Macfie, J., and Celestin, L. R.: Anorectal Crohn's disease. Br. J. Surg., 66:743, 1979.
18. Hobbiss, J. H., and Schofield, P. F.: Management of perianal Crohn's disease. J. R. Soc. Med., 75:414, 1982.
19. Sohn, N., Korelitz, B. I., and Weinstein, M. A.: Anorectal Crohn's disease: Definitive surgery for fistulas and recurrent abscesses. Am. J. Surg., 139:394, 1980.
20. Edwards, F. C., and Truelove, S. C.: The course and prognosis of ulcerative colitis. Part III. Complications. Gut, 5:15, 1964.
21. Greenstein, A. J., Kark, A. E., and Dreiling, D. A.: Crohn's disease of the colon. Controversial aspects of hemorrhage, anemia and rectal involvement in granulomatous disease involving the colon. Am. J. Gastroenterol., 63:40, 1975.
22. Crohn, B. B., and Yarnis, H.: Regional Ileitis. 2nd Ed. New York, Grune and Stratton, 1958.
23. Sparberg, M., and Kirsner, J. B.: Recurrent hemorrhage in regional enteritis. Am. J. Dig. Dis., 11:652, 1966.
24. Lee, J. C. L., et al.: Hypercoagulability associated with chronic ulcerative colitis: Changes in blood coagulation factors. Gastroenterology, 55:251, 1968.
25. Harvey, J. C., et al.: Massive lower gastrointestinal bleeding: An unusual complication of Crohn's disease. Can. J. Surg., 21:444, 1978.
26. Mellor, J. A., Chandler, G. N., Chapman, A. H., and Irving, H. C.: Massive gastrointestinal bleeding in Crohn's dis-

27. ease: Successful control by intra-arterial vasopressin infusion. Gut, 23:872, 1982.
27. Steinberg, D. M., Cooke, W. T., and Alexander-Wiliams, J.: Abscess and fistulae in Crohn's disease. Gut, 14:865, 1973.
28. Keighley, M. R. B.: Incidence and microbiology of abdominal and pelvic abscess in Crohn's disease. Gastroenterology, 83:1271, 1982.
29. Greenstein, A. J., Kark, A. E., and Dreiling, D. A.: Crohn's disease of the colon. Fistula in Crohn's disease of the colon, classification, presenting features and management in 63 patients. Am. J. Gastroenterol. 62:419, 1974.
30. Nagler, S. M., and Poticha, S. M.: Intra-abdominal abscess in regional enteritis. Am. J. Surg., 137:350, 1979.
31. Chennells, P. M., and Simpkins, K. C.: The barium enema diagnosis of paracolic abscess. Clin. Radiol., 32:73, 1981.
32. Holdstock, G., Ligorria, J. E., and Krawitt, E. L.: Gallium-67 scanning in patients with Crohn's disease: An aid to the diagnosis of abdominal abscess. Br. J. Surg., 69:277, 1982.
33. Chintapalli, K., Thorsen, M. K., Foley, W. D., and Unger, G. F.: Abdominal abscesses with enteric communications: CT findings. AJR, 141:27, 1983.
34. Gerzof, S. G., et al.: Percutaneous catheter drainage of abdominal abscesses. N. Engl. J. Med., 305:653, 1981.
35. Rankin, G. B., Watts, H. O., Melnyk, C. S., and Kelley, M. L.: National Cooperative Crohn's Disease Study: Extraintestinal manifestations and perianal complications. Gastroenterology, 77:914, 1979.
36. Van Dongen, L. M., and Lubbers, E. J. C.: Psoas abscess in Crohn's disease. Br. J. Surg., 69:589, 1982.
37. Nelson, A., Frank, H. D., and Taubin, H. L.: Liver abscess. A complication of regional enteritis. Am. J. Gastroenterol. 72:282, 1979.
38. Wechter, D. G., and Willson, R. A.: Splenic abscess: A rare complication of Crohn's colitis. Dig. Dis. Sci., 30:802, 1985.
39. Rothenberger, D. A., and Goldberg, S. M.: The management of rectovaginal fistulae. Surg. Clin. North Am., 63:61, 1983.
40. Tuxen, P. A., and Castro, A. F.: Rectovaginal fistula in Crohn's disease. Dis. Colon Rectum, 22:58, 1979.
41. Buchmann, P., Allan, R. N., Thompson, H., and Alexander-Williams, J.: Carcinoma in a rectovaginal fistula in a patient with Crohn's disease. Am. J. Surg., 140:462, 1980.
42. Greenstein, A. J., et al.: Course of enterovesical fistulas in Crohn's disease. Am. J. Surg., 147:788, 1984.
43. Talamini, M. A., Broe, P. J., and Cameron, J. L.: Urinary fistulas in Crohn's disease. Surg. Gynecol. Obstet., 154:553, 1982.
44. Irving, M.: Assessment and management of external fistulas in Crohn's disease. Br. J. Surg., 70:233, 1983.
45. McIntyre, J. K., et al.: Management of enterocutaneous fistulas: A review of 132 cases. Br. J. Surg., 71:293, 1984.
46. Hawker, P. C., et al.: Management of enterocutaneous fistulae in Crohn's disease. Gut, 24:284, 1983.
47. Alexander, E. S., Weinberg, S., Clark, R. A., and Belkin, R. D.: Fistulas and sinus tracts: Radiographic evaluation, management, and outcome. Gastrointest. Radiol., 7:135, 1982.
48. Fischer, J. E.: The pathophysiology of enterocutaneous fistulas. World J. Surg., 7:446, 1983.
49. Devlin, H. B., and Elcoat, C.: Alimentary tract fistula: Stomatherapy techniques of management. World J. Surg., 7:489, 1983.
50. Broe, P. J., Bayless, T. M., and Cameron, J L.: Crohn's disease: Are enteroenteral fistulas an indication for surgery? Surgery, 91:249, 1982.
51. Broe, P. J., and Cameron, J. L.: Surgical management of ileosigmoid fistulas in Crohn's disease. Am. J. Surg., 143:611, 1982.
52. Block, G. E., and Schraut, W. H.: The operative treatment of Crohn's enteritis complicated by ileosigmoid fistula. Ann. Surg., 196:356, 1982.
53. Heimann, T., Greenstein, A. J., and Aufses, A. H.: Surgical management of ileosigmoid fistula in Crohn's disease. Am. J. Gastroenterol., 72:21, 1979.
54. Present, D. H., et al.: Treatment of Crohn's disease with 6-mercaptopurine. N. Engl. J. Med., 302:981, 1980.
55. Korelitz, B. I., and Present, D. H.: Favorable effect of 6-mercaptopurine on fistulae of Crohn's disease. Dig. Dis. Sci., 30:58, 1985.
56. Javett, S. L., and Brooke, B. N.: Acute dilatation of colon in Crohn's disease. Lancet, 2:126, 1970.
57. Tugwell, P., Southcott, D., and Walmesley, P.: Free perforation of the colon in Crohn's disease. Br. J. Clin. Pract., 26:44, 1972.
58. Suk, C. H., Posner, G. L., and Bopaiah, V.: Colonic perforation in Crohn's disease. Am. J. Gastroenterol., 79:695, 1984.
59. Ferraro, V., and Hunt, P. S.: Perforation in Crohn's disease of the small bowel. Med. J. Aust., 140:101, 1984.
60. Janevicius, R. V., Bartolome, J. S., and Schmitz, R. L.: Acute free perforation as a presenting sign of regional enteritis. Am. J. Gastroenterol., 74:143, 1980.
61. Zeit, R. M.: Enterolithiasis associated with ileal perforation in Crohn's disease. Am. J. Gastroenterol., 72:662, 1979.
62. Roth, J. L. A., Valdes-Dapena, A., Stein, G. N., and Bockus, H. L.: Toxic megacolon in ulcerative colitis. Gastroenterology, 37:239, 1959.
63. Jalan, K. N., et al.: An experience of ulcerative colitis. I. Toxic dilation in 55 cases. Gastroenterology, 57:68, 1969.
64. Thomford, N. R.: Toxic megacolon. Surg. Annu., 12:341, 1980.
65. Truelove, S. C., and Marks, C. G.: Toxic megacolon. Part I: Pathogenesis, diagnosis and treatment. Clin. Gastroenterol. 10:107, 1981.
66. Odyniec, N. A., Judd, E. S., and Sauer, W. G.: Toxic megacolon. Significant improvement in surgical management. Arch. Surg., 94:638, 1967.
67. Kisloff, B., and Adkins, J. C.: Toxic megacolon developing in a patient with long-standing distal ulcerative colitis. Am. J. Gastroenterol. 75:451, 1981.
68. Whorwell, P. J., and Isaacson, P.: Toxic dilatation of colon in Crohn's disease. Lancet, 2:1334, 1981.
69. Farmer, R. G., Whelan, G., and Fazio, V. W.: Long-term follow-up of patients with Crohn's disease. Gastroenterology, 88:1818, 1985.
70. McInerney, G. T., Sauer, W. G., Baggenstoss, A. H., and Hodgson, J. R.: Fulminating ulcerative colitis with marked colonic dilation: A clinicopathologic study. Gastroenterology, 42:244, 1962.
71. Carman, R., Jannuccilli, E. A., and Thayer, W. R.: Toxic megacolon in inflammatory bowel disease: A new perspective. RI Med. J., 61:342, 1978.
72. Harris, J., and Shields, R.: Absorption and secretion of water and electrolytes by the intact human colon in diffuse untreated proctocolitis. Gut, 11:27, 1970.
73. Garret, J. M., Sauer, W. G., and Moertel, C. G.: Colonic motility in ulcerative colitis after opiate administration. Gastroenterology, 53:93, 1967.
74. Brown, J. W.: Toxic megacolon associated with Loperamide therapy. J. Am. Med. Assoc., 241:501, 1979.

75. Marshak, R. H., et al.: Toxic dilation of the colon in the course of ulcerative colitis. Gastroenterology, 38:165, 1960.
76. Thomas, B. M.: The instant enema in inflammatory disease of the colon. Clin. Radiol., 30:165, 1979.
77. Reddy, K. R., and Thomas, E.: Toxic megacolon after proctosigmoidoscopy in ulcerative colitis. South. Med. J., 76:1072, 1983.
78. Hartong, W. A., Arvanitakis, C., Skibba, R. M., and Klotz, A. P.: Treatment of toxic megacolon. A comparative review of 29 patients. Dig. Dis. Sci., 22:195, 1977.
79. Mogan, G. R., et al.: Toxic megacolon in ulcerative colitis complicated by pneumomediastinum: report of two cases. Gastroenterology, 79:559, 1980.
80. Neschis, M., Siegelman, S. S., and Parker, J. G.: Diagnosis and management of the megacolon of ulcerative colitis. Gastroenterology, 55:251, 1968.
81. McConnell, F., Hanelin, J., and Robbins, L. L: Plain film diagnosis of fulminating ulcerative colitis. Radiology, 71:674, 1958.
82. Wolf, B. S., and Marshak, R. H.: "Toxic" segmental dilatation of the colon during the course of fulminating ulcerative colitis: Roentgen findings. Am. J. Roentgenol., 82:985, 1959.
83. Kramer, P., and Wittenberg, J.: Colonic gas distribution in toxic megacolon. Gastroenterology, 80:433, 1981.
84. Present, D. H., et al.: The medical management of toxic megacolon: Technique of decompression with favorable long-term follow-up. Gastroenterology, 80:1255, 1981.
85. Caprilli, R., Colaneri, V. O., and Frieri, G.: Risk factors in toxic megacolon. Dig. Dis. Sci., 25:817, 1980.
86. Binder, H. J.: Steroids and toxic megacolon. Gastroenterology, 76:888, 1979.
87. Meyers, S., and Janowitz, H. D.: The place of steroids in the therapy of toxic megacolon. Gastroenterology, 75:729, 1978.
88. Jamart, J., Boissel, P., Debs, A., and Grosdidier, J.: Total colectomy with ileorectal anastomosis in surgical management of toxic megacolon. Langenbecks Arch. Chir., 360:159, 1983.
89. Turnbull, R. B., Hawk, W. A., and Weakley, F. L.: Surgical treatment of toxic megacolon: Ileostomy and colostomy to prepare patients for colectomy. Gastroenterology, 122:325, 1971.
90. Chare, M. J. B., and Aubrey, D. A.: Management of toxic megacolon. Br. J. Clin. Pract., 36:175, 1982.
91. Muscroft, T. J., Warren, P. M., Asquith, P., and Montgomery, R. D.: Toxic megacolon in ulcerative colitis: A continuing challenge. Postgrad. Med. J., 57:223, 1981.
92. Katzka, I., Katz, S., and Morris, E.: Management of toxic megacolon: The significance of early recognition in medical management. J. Clin. Gastroenterol. 1:307, 1979.
93. Greenstein, A. J., et al.: Outcome of toxic dilatation in ulcerative and Crohn's colitis. J. Clin. Gastroenterol., 7:137, 1985.
94. Strauss, R. J., et al.: The surgical management of toxic dilatation of the colon: A report of 28 cases and review of the literature. Ann. Surg., 184:682, 1976.
95. Grant, C. S., and Dozois, R. R.: Toxic megacolon: Ultimate fate of patients after successful medical management. Am. J. Surg., 147:106, 1984.
96. Dukes, C. E.: The surgical pathology of ulcerative colitis. Ann. R. Coll. Surg. Engl., 14:389, 1954.
97. Goldgraber, M. B.: Pseudopolyps in ulcerative colitis. Dis. Colon Rectum, 8:355, 1965.
98. de Dombal, F. T., et al.: Local complications of ulcerative colitis: Strictures, pseudopolyposis and carcinoma of colon and rectum. Br. Med. J., 1:1442, 1966.
99. Lesher, D. T., Phillips, J. C., and Rabinowitz, J. G.: Pseudopolyposis as the only manifestation of ulcerative colitis. Am. J. Gastroenterol., 70:670, 1978.
100. Dawson, I. M. P., and Pryse-Davies, J.: The development of carcinoma of the large intestine in ulcerative colitis. Br. J. Surg., 47:113, 1959.
101. Sloan, W. P., Bargen, J. A., and Baggenstoss, A. H.: Local complications of chronic ulcerative colitis based on the study of 2000 cases. Proc. Staff Mtg. Mayo Clin., 25:240, 1950.
102. Schneider, R., Dickersin, G. R., and Patterson, F. J.: Localized giant pseudopolyposis: A complication of granulomatous colitis. Am. J. Dig. Dis., 18:265, 1973.
103. Forde, K. A., Gold, R. P., and Weber, C.: Giant pseudopolyposis and antegrade colonic obstruction: Report a case. Dis. Colon Rectum, 23:583, 1980.
104. Forde, K. A., et al.: Giant pseudopolyposis in colitis with colonic intussusception. Gastroenterology, 75:1142, 1978.
105. Spark, R. P.: Filiform polyposis of the colon. Am. J. Dig. Dis., 21:809, 1976.
106. Renison, D. M., Forouhar, F. A., Levine, J. B., and Breiter, J. R.: Filiform polyposis of the colon presenting as massive hemorrhage: An uncommon complication of Crohn's disease. Am. J. Gastroenterol., 78:413, 1983.
107. Antonow, D. R., Gebhard, R. L., Dykoski, R. K., and Sumner, H. W.: Filiform polyposis in Crohn's colitis mimicking toxic megacolon. Dig. Dis. Sci., 26:1051, 1981.
108. Kahn, E., and Daum, F.: Pseudopolyps of the small intestine in Crohn's disease. Hum. Pathol., 15:84, 1984.
109. Goulston, S. J. M., and McGovern, V. J.: The nature of benign strictures in ulcerative colitis. N. Engl. J. Med., 281:290, 1969.
110. Weedon, D. D., et al.: Crohn's disease and cancer. N. Engl. J. Med., 289:1099, 1973.
111. Fielding, J., et al.: Crohn's disease of the stomach and duodenum. Gut, 11:1001, 1970.
112. Alexander-Williams, J.: Conservative nonresection operations for Crohn's disease. In Advances in Gastrointestinal Surgery. Edited by J. S. Najarian, and J. P. Delaney, Chicago, Year Book Medical Publishers, 1984.
113. Navarro, J., et al.: Prolonged constant rate elemental enteral nutrition in Crohn's disease. J. Pediatr. Gastroenterol. Nutr., 1:541, 1982.
114. Priebe, W. M., and Simon, J. B.: Crohn's disease of the stomach with outlet obstruction: A case report and review of therapy. J. Clin. Gastroenterol., 5:441, 1983.

15 · Neoplasia and Gastrointestinal Malignancy in Inflammatory Bowel Disease

CHARLES J. LIGHTDALE, M.D. AND PAUL SHERLOCK, M.D.[*]

For patients with inflammatory bowel disease the increased risk of cancer is a specter that increases with time. A nearly asymptomatic colitic patient presenting with metastatic cancer in the prime of life is a frightening and widespread scenario. Patients with ulcerative colitis have been thought to be most susceptible, but there is growing evidence of increased risk in Crohn's disease. Pathologic identification of dysplasia in the bowel mucosa of patients with inflammatory bowel disease has provided a new focus for cancer surveillance. While barium enema remains important, colonoscopy has assumed the major role in diagnosis, facilitating detection of cancer at an early stage when surgical cure is still possible.

Ulcerative Colitis

Extent of Risk

Patients with ulcerative colitis are at greater than average risk of developing adenocarcinoma of the colon, but the extent of the risk has been difficult to quantify.[1] Many reports have expressed the risk of cancer as the percentage of a given population of patients with ulcerative colitis who develop cancer. Prevalence rates have varied widely, from 0 to 17%.[2-21] In several large series, however, prevalence has been 3 to 5%, a range often taken to be the approximate lifetime risk of cancer in ulcerative colitis.[3-11]

The statistical parameter of relative risk is also based on prevalence. It compares the observed number of patients with ulcerative colitis who develop cancer to the expected number of cancers in the general population. The risk of cancer in ulcerative colitis has been calculated to be 3 to 30 times that of the general population.[2,4,8,11,12]

The variation in prevalence rates might be explained by biologic, genetic, or environmental factors, but they are more likely related to methodology. Virtually all reports fail key statistical standards, allowing major biases that might affect results. Most series are from hospital based centers with wide areas of referral. This implies unavoidable selection bias from larger groups of patients of unknown size and fate. Some patients are included who were referred primarily because of the diagnosis of cancer.[22-25]

Prevalence does not take into account the duration of the colitis and the extent of disease in the colon; these are major factors influencing the risk of cancer.[2,26] Early age of onset of colitis, a severe first attack, and continuous activity

---

[*]Internationally esteemed as a skilled physician, superb teacher, and wise administrator, Dr. Sherlock was a prime mover in gastrointestinal oncology. His research efforts focused on the early detection of gastrointestinal cancer and the recognition of premalignant disease. His untimely death at the age of 56 was on May 6, 1985.

of disease are possibly additional risk factors, but they do not seem to independently influence cancer risk.[1]

DURATION OF DISEASE. The mixture of patients with recent onset and longstanding ulcerative colitis will have a major influence on the percentage developing cancer. The development of cancer is rare for the first seven years after the onset of disease, and the incidence is low until ten years, when a precipitous and continuous increase in the number of cases occurs.[8,15,18,26-28]

The expression of risk of cancer with duration of ulcerative colitis has been presented most successfully as the cumulative incidence of cancer (%) per years of disease (Fig. 15-1). Actuarial methods that employ project risk with duration of disease have been used, but what is the best statistical approach remains controversial.[24,29] In studies from major referral centers, about 2% of patients develop cancer during the first ten years of ulcerative colitis, after which the risk increases to 10 to 20% per decade.[15,18,26,28] Estimates are based on progressively fewer patients, but the risk may approach 30% after 25 years of disease, and 50% by the fourth decade.[18,26] Although reports from several referral centers are in agreement, the risk may be overestimated because of selection biases. A report analyzing a large office-based practice determined the risk to be lower.[29,30] Further prospective studies designed to minimize statistical compromises have been proposed.[23]

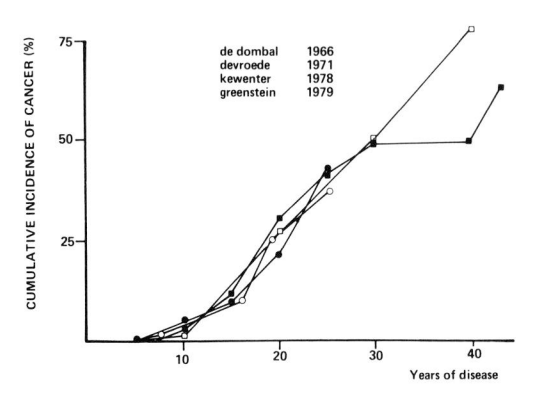

FIG.15-1. Cancer risk with time in extensive ulcerative colitis. (Used with permission from Devroede, G.: In Colorectal Cancer: Prevention, Epidemiology and Screening. Edited by S. Winawer, D. Schottenfeld, and P. Sherlock. Raven Press, New York, 1980.)

EXTENT OF DISEASE. Patients with left-sided colitis have a lower risk of cancer than those with disease involving the total colon.[8,18,26] In left-sided colitis, cancer tends to occur about 10 years slower than in pancolitis; the first cancers usually don't present until about 20 years after the onset of the disease.[2,26] The increased risk is minimal in those patients with ulcerative proctitis, where the inflammatory process is limited to the rectum and most distal sigmoid.[31-35] If proctitis progresses proximally, however, the risk of cancer rises.[26]

Published studies estimating the risk of cancer according to extent of disease began before the era of colonoscopy, and are largely based on rigid sigmoidoscopy and barium enema examinations. It has been established that even double contrast barium studies might not detect right-sided inflammatory changes in ulcerative colitis that can be diagnosed by the use of colonoscopy and biopsy.[36,37] Defining the extent of disease by colonoscopic and histologic criteria may alter current concepts established by roentgenologic methods.

Patients with pancolitis who have a subtotal colectomy and ileorectal anastomosis maintain a high risk of developing rectal cancer.[7,38-41] In one study of patients with ileorectal anastomosis, the risk of rectal cancer was estimated to be nil at 10 years, 6% at 20 years, 15% at 30 years, and 32% at 43 years.[42]

ONSET AND ACTIVITY OF DISEASE. The age at the onset of ulcerative colitis seems to have little effect on the risk of cancer.[1,2,26] Studies that found childhood onset increased the risk of cancer did not take into account the longer duration of disease and follow-up possible when ulcerative colitis begins at an early age.[7,8] Childhood onset of colitis is also more likely to involve the total colon than adult onset of disease.[18,28] When patient-years of follow-up and age-specific incidences are calculated, no tendency for a greater risk of cancer was found associated with childhood onset.[26] Although one analysis did conclude a greater risk existed with onset below the age of 30, and another only with an onset between the ages of 5 and 9, these were of minimal magnitude.[11,18]

Cancer complicating ulcerative colitis occurs at a younger average age, 40 to 50 years, than colon cancer in the general population, where the mean age ranges two decades older.[4,8,14,32,43-45] This is reflected in the high relative risk of children and young adults with ulcerative colitis to develop colon cancer, which is uncommon before age 50 in the general population.[2,11] The risk of cancer in ulcerative colitis is the same for both sexes.[43]

A severe first attack of colitis has been suggested to be associated with an increased cancer risk, along with continuous activity of the disease. Severity and activity are more difficult to standardize among groups of patients and institutions, and no actuarial analysis of these factors has been performed. Patients with relatively mild, intermittent colitic symptoms have been reported to be as prone to cancer as those with more sustained activity.[18,24,26] Periods of prolonged remission are not protective. Patients with severe symptoms are more likely to undergo colectomy, thus eliminating the risk of cancer. It has been speculated that improved medical therapy has allowed more patients with ulcerative colitis to live with an intact colon, providing a larger population at risk.[23]

Pathologic Features

Cancers complicating universal ulcerative colitis are distributed in a nearly even manner throughout the large bowel. A trend toward a more proximal distribution for colon cancer has been found in the general population, but cancer in ulcerative colitis is much more likely to involve the ascending and transverse colon than the de novo adenocarcinoma.[14,43-46] Patients with ulcerative colitis limited to the left colon develop cancer in the area of the affected bowel.[43]

Multiple synchronous colon cancers are a characteristic feature of malignant degeneration in ulcerative colitis. In the general population, synchronous cancers of the colon occur in the 2 to 3% range.[46] Multicentric cancer has been reported in 4 to 26% of ulcerative colitis.[4,8,14,43]

Colon cancer generally assumes one of four predominant gross shapes: annular, exophytic, ulcerating, or infiltrating.[46] Although adenocarcinoma complicating ulcerative colitis may appear as any of these formations, usually it is infiltrating, with ill-defined margins. The appearance is typically a flat, plaque-like mass. Infiltrating cancer may produce a narrowed lumen that may mimic the benign strictures that occur in ulcerative colitis.[43,47-49] In one series, 18 of 26 cancers in patients with ulcerative colitis appeared as plaques or strictures.[50]

Adenocarcinoma cells in ulcerative colitis are more likely to be poorly differentiated than in de novo cancer. Colloid cancer and exuberant mucous production are other striking features

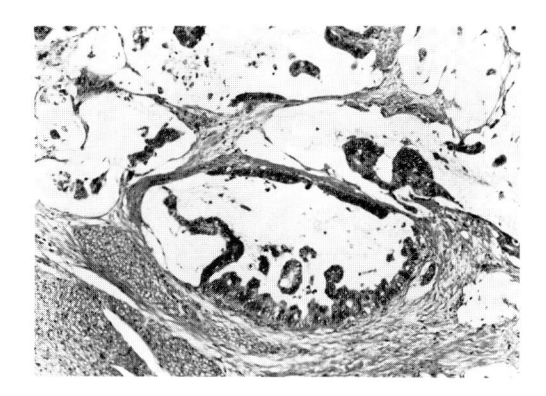

FIG.15-2. Colloid (mucinous) carcinoma that developed in the sigmoid colon in a patient with universal ulcerative colitis (Dukes' stage B). Neoplastic glands are seen in a mucinous stroma separated by fibrous septae (H&E × 250). (Courtesy of Dr. C. Urmacher, Memorial Sloan-Kettering Cancer Center, Department of Pathology.)

of malignancy in ulcerative colitis (Fig. 15-2), occuring in 15 to 50% of patients.[43,48]

As indicated elsewhere in this book (see Chap. 14), inflammatory polyps or pseudopolyps are common in ulcerative colitis, but they do not seem to have an increased potential to evolve into adenomas or carcinomas.[48,52-54] Most, if not all, colon cancer in the general population evolves from adenomatous polyps.[46] This is not the case in ulcerative colitis, where precancerous changes or dysplasia, typically seen in large polyps, have been described in flat or nearly flat mucosa.[53] Dysplasia may not always be in areas that can be histologically described as adenomatous.[54] Like the cancers that develop in ulcerative colitis, dysplastic changes tend to be multifocal and spread throughout the colon.[53-58]

Diagnosis

Even with awareness of the risk, it is difficult to diagnose cancer in ulcerative colitis on the basis of symptoms.[10,14,47] Rectal bleeding, the key symptom in the diagnosis of colorectal cancer, is a common feature in ulcerative colitis. In a study by Greenstein et al. that compared clinical characteristics of cancer in ulcerative colitis with a control group of ulcerative colitis patients, rectal bleeding was present in nearly all patients in both groups.[43]

Diarrhea was usually present in colitis patients both with and without cancer. Abdominal pain was common, although the pain tended to be more severe in metastatic carcinoma.[43] In general, cancer-related symptoms imply that the cancer is advanced. Two statistically significant ($p < 0.001$) features of cancer compared to controls were intestinal obstruction and abdominal mass. Constitutional symptoms of advanced cancer, anorexia, weight loss, and fatigue, were also present to the same extent in the ulcerative colitis controls.[43]

Advanced colonic cancers in ulcerative colitis tend to follow the usual pattern according to location. Cancers of the cecum and ascending colon grow large and ulcerate, presenting with anemia, fatigue, and weight loss. Beyond the hepatic flexure, the cancers primarily obstruct, sometimes causing proximal dilation. Rectal lesions typically cause bloody diarrhea, fistulas, perineal pain, and tenesmus.[43,46]

The timing of symptoms may help alert the clinician to the possibility of cancer. A long asymptomatic period prior to a recrudescence has been noted in up to 50% of ulcerative colitis patients developing cancer.[10,43] Physical examination is not usually of help in diagnosis unless a rectal mass or palpable abdominal mass is present. Abdominal tenderness does not differentiate carcinoma from uncomplicated ulcerative colitis.[43] Evidence of metastatic disease such as an enlarged supraclavicular lymph node or nodular liver is ominous.

Symptoms are usually investigated first by barium enema. The double contrast air-barium examination is strongly preferred.[59-61] This method allows identification of suspicious masses, ulcerations, and contour defects. The location of an obstruction can be documented, and strictures can be defined. About one-fourth of carcinomas complicating ulcerative colitis are found as strictures on barium enema.[4,43,52] While 80 to 90% are benign, a stricture on barium enema in ulcerative colitis is always regarded as suspicious for carcinoma (see also Chap. 20).[8,61,62]

While barium enema suggests the diagnosis of cancer in ulcerative colitis about 90% of the time, preoperative diagnosis is usually confirmed by doing a biopsy at colonoscopy. Benign lesions that are suspicious on barium enema, such as large pseudopolyps, can be assessed at colonoscopy.[62] Barium enema and colonoscopy together are synergistic in providing the most accurate diagnosis. Although infiltrating cancer is difficult to target, a tissue diagnosis can be achieved by doing a biopsy or brush cytology at colonoscopy in more than 90% of patients with symptomatic cancer.[62,64]

Barium enema is helpful to the colonoscopist as a guide to suspicious areas. For example, strictures evident on barium enema may be difficult for the colonoscopist to visualize. Some clinicians, however, defer barium enema and use colonoscopy as the primary examination in an effort to decrease expense, time, and the need for repeat preparation (see also Chap. 19). It is not clear whether this approach will have an important effect on diagnostic accuracy. Colonoscopy is usually completed to the cecum with ease in the patients with chronic ulcerative colitis who often have a shortened colon, but when this is not possible an air-contrast barium examination can provide an excellent view of the right colonic mucosa.[61]

Treatment and Prognosis

The treatment of choice for carcinoma complicating ulcerative colitis is total proctocolectomy.[65] Segmental resection should not be considered because of the high incidence of multiple synchronous cancers, and the widely distributed precancerous changes in the mucosa. Operations that leave the rectum intact usually leave the patient with poor quality function and exposed to an increasing risk of rectal cancer.[7,38-42] This is true whether or not an immediate ileorectal anastomosis is performed.[66] Ileoanal anastomosis following complete stripping of the rectal mucosa is theoretically a safe procedure, but this has not been proven.[67] The principles of modern surgical oncology that govern the resection of colon cancer with wide en bloc lymphatic resection apply to cancers developing in ulcerative colitis.

The prognosis of colitis-cancer after surgical resection is stage-dependent, just as in de novo cancer.[14,32,43,46] Most patients with ulcerative colitis and symptomatic cancer present at an advanced stage, usually with lymph node metastases (Dukes' C) or distant metastases.[4,48,51] This probably relates to two factors: aggressive tumor biology and delay in diagnosis because of nonspecific symptoms.

Primarily infiltrating cancers, as usually occur in ulcerative colitis, tend to invade and metastasize rapidly.[46,50] The cancer develops in flat mucosa and progresses in a submucosal manner, as opposed to beginning in a large polyp. The tendency of colitis-cancers to be poorly differentiated histologically correlates with more aggressive tumor biology.[51] Copious mucous production frequently seen in colitis-cancer also has been linked to rapid progression and metastasis.[46]

The nonspecificity of symptoms related to the development of cancer in patients with ulcerative colitis has commonly led to delays in diagnoses. Patients who have had periods of rectal bleeding, diarrhea, and abdominal pain for years are often not alarmed when these symptoms recur, and may often self-medicate with past regimens rather than seek medical attention. Physicians may similarly institute a trial of therapy rather than submit the patient to diagnostic procedures that might exacerbate an active inflammatory state.

Following surgical treatment for colon cancer in ulcerative colitis, five-year survival (equated with cure) has been reported in the range of 18 to 40%.[4,14,32,43,52] Survival curves after surgical therapy in colitis-cancer patients have been similar to those in de novo cancer controls, where the five-year postsurgical survival rate is about 50%. An initial rapid drop in postsurgical survival may occur in patients with colitis-cancer (Fig. 15-3), probably reflecting the advanced disease often found in these patients.[43] No survival benefit has been established from postsurgical adjuvant treatment, including radiation, chemotherapy, and immunotherapy.[46]

The best treatment for colonic cancer complicating ulcerative colitis is to prevent its occurrence, and the most direct way is total proctocolectomy. This procedure has been advocated for cancer prophylaxis in patients with universal ulcerative colitis of greater than 10 years.[20,27] Supporting this recommendation is the operative mortality of less than 2% for proctocolectomy and ileostomy versus the serious and increasing risk of cancer. A contraindication to prophylactic surgical therapy is the knowledge that many patients will never develop cancer, but they face an immediate risk of operative death and postoperative sexual dysfunction, and also some degree of permanent disability associated with ileostomy.[69] If ulcerative colitis is inactive or controlled medically, most patients are reluctant to undergo proctocolectomy. It is easier to consider the risk of cancer as an additional factor favoring surgical intervention for the patient whose medical management is unsuccessful.

For the majority of patients with ulcerative colitis in the high risk category of 10 years disease duration and total colon involvement, the alternatives of prophylactic surgical treatment and hoping blindly against disaster are equally untenable. A third choice, a program of active surveillance for cancer, seems preferable.

Surveillance

The concept of screening high risk groups for colon cancer is rooted in the belief that cancers discovered and removed before they cause symptoms are more likely to be cured. Ample evidence is available from screening programs for colon cancer not caused by colitis that cancers diagnosed in asymptomatic individuals tend to fall into the more favorable Dukes' A and B pathologic stages.[46] Because the prognosis

SURVIVAL RATES OF PATIENTS WITH COLORECTAL CANCER

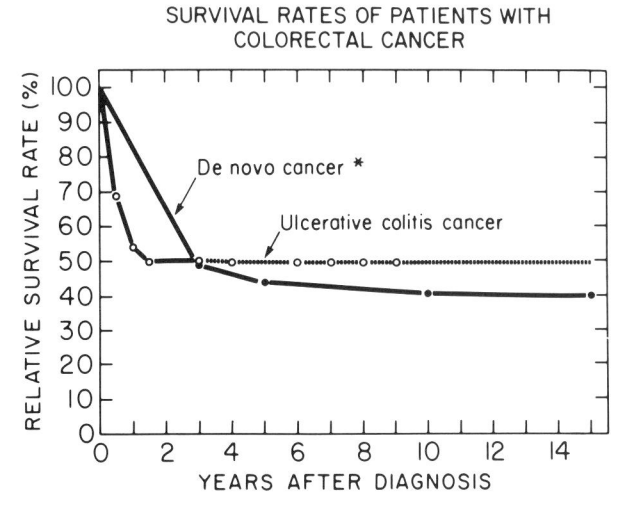

*Modified from "End results in cancer", report no.4, DHEW, 1972

FIG.15-3. Postoperative survival curve in patients with ulcerative colitis and colorectal cancer (open circles) compared with colorectal cancer patients in the general population (closed circles). (Used with permission from Greenstein, A. J., et al.:. Mt. Sinai J. Med., 46:25, 1979.)

after surgical treatment in colon cancer complicating ulcerative colitis is Dukes' stage dependent, it is likely that if colitis-cancer could be diagnosed earlier, survival would be improved.[67]

Some screening methods used for other high risk groups are not applicable for patients with ulcerative colitis. Tests for occult blood in the stool are useless because blood is commonly present in the stool of ulcerative colitis patients.[46] Serum levels of carcinoembryonic antigen are also often elevated in patients with ulcerative colitis in the absence of colon cancer.[70,71] Barium enema is not suitable for surveillance because the meticulous technique needed to detect small abnormalities generally is not available.[60] Another concern is the possible deleterious effects of cumulative x-ray exposure.[72]

In a key paper in 1967, Morson and Pang suggested dysplasia on rectal biopsy as a marker to identify patients with ulcerative colitis at highest risk.[53] In this report, nine patients were found to have histologic changes labelled precancer on rectal biopsy, of whom five had one or more foci of invasive cancer in the colon on examination after colectomy. A review of 23 colectomy specimens removed for cancer showed precancer in all, usually scattered throughout the colon in a patchy distribution.[53] Multiple studies have confirmed and expanded these findings. Dysplasia is present in over 80% of colectomy specimens in which a carcinoma is found.[54-58]

Concurrent with the prospect of using dysplasia as an indicator of precancer in ulcerative colitis, colonoscopy developed as a major new technique, providing a magnified view and tissue sampling capability throughout the entire colon.[55,73] Although invasive and expensive, total colonoscopy with multiple biopsy has emerged as the best available cancer surveillance method. Biopsies are smaller and more difficult to interpret for dysplasia than rectal biopsies taken via rigid sigmoidoscope. The ability to identify mucosal abnormalities and to perform biopsies throughout the colon is a critically important advantage for colonoscopy; however, dysplasia may not always be present in the rectum. In a review by Dobbins, dysplasia was found in 88% of 108 colectomy specimens containing cancer, but dysplasia was present in the rectum in only 66%.[74]

A major problem in using dysplasia for surveillance has been the need for a clear histologic definition that can be widely applied. In an effort to resolve this dilemma, an international group of twelve pathologists has developed a classification of dysplasia.[75] Specimens are classified as negative, indefinite, and positive, with positives divided into low grade and high grade, replacing the previous categories of mild, moderate, and severe. High grade dysplasia is clearly defined, and encompasses carcinoma in situ. It can be difficult to distinguish dysplastic changes from those associated with inflammation and repair. Dysplasia appears to be a preneoplastic abnormality, but the timing of its evolution and possible regression remains to be elucidated.[74,75]

In judging the benefits of surveillance, it is important to separate colonoscopies done for diagnosis. For example, colonoscopies performed because of suspicious symptoms or barium enema abnormalities are considered diagnostic.[76] All abnormal areas seen on colonoscopy should be examined with a biopsy. Dysplasia with an associated lesion or mass, labelled with the acronym DALM by the group at the University of Chicago, carries a high probability of carcinoma being present deeper in the area.[77,78]

Waye has emphasized the importance of the colonoscopy with multiple biopsies in detecting carcinoma in addition to dysplasia (see also Chap. 19).[76] Biopsies should be performed on suspicious pseudopolyps. Adenomatous polyps should be totally removed. Small abnormalities should not be overlooked. Morson has described early infiltrating cancers in ulcerative colitis on pathologic examination as sometimes being easier to feel than see.[74] Lavage cytology has not been effective, but brush cytology (Fig. 15-4)

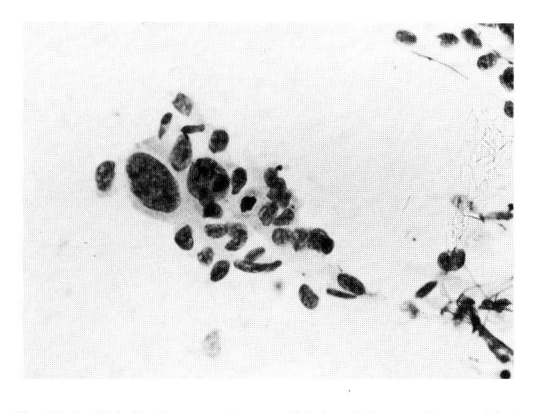

FIG.15-4. Cytologic specimen obtained by using guided brushing of a nodular lesion seen in the ascending colon of a patient with extensive ulcerative colitis. A loosely cohesive cluster of atypical and malignant epithelial cells is seen (Papanicolaou stain × 570). (Courtesy of Dr. S. Hajdu, Memorial Sloan-Kettering Cancer Center, Department of Pathology.)

may be a useful adjunct to performing a biopsy.[79] In seeking dysplasia, which probably is found most often in flat mucosa, about 12 biopsies should be taken systematically through the colon at roughly 10 cm intervals. The most common approach is to take biopsies from the cecum, ascending colon, hepatic flexure, transverse colon, splenic flexure, descending colon, sigmoid colon, and rectum. Biopsies from areas not actively inflamed are more easily interpreted for dysplasia.[75]

Based on multiple studies, about one-third to one-half of patients with high grade dysplasia found on biopsy have a synchronous occult cancer.[80-86] The longest prospective experience using dysplasia as the focus of a surveillance program comes from St. Mark's Hospital in London.[86] Of 186 patients with a history of ulcerative colitis greater than 10 years, carcinoma was detected in 13. Three patients had 2 cancers each. Of the 16 cancers, 11 were Dukes' A, 3 Dukes' B, 1 Dukes' C, and 1 inoperable. Others have noted a similar early stage pattern in patients with carcinomas discovered at the time of surgical treatment done because of dysplasia found on biopsy.[80-85] At St. Mark's, it was assumed that cancer was prevented in 8 additional patients on the basis of the severe dysplastic changes in the colectomy specimens.[86]

Although the efficacy of surveillance strategy centered on endoscopic examination for dysplasia is not fully proven, these encouraging results make it seem reasonable to offer patients such a follow-up program in lieu of automatic proctocolectomy. In this way those at highest risk can be identified for surgical treatment to prevent cancer. The risk of cancer is not eliminated by this surveillance, but cancers that develop are largely amenable to surgical cure. Attention to the personal needs and idiosyncrasies of each patient is critical in maintaining the surveillance effort. Diagnostic intervention is interjected as dictated by clinical events.[86] A cost benefit analysis of a surveillance program for cancer in ulcerative colitis has not been accomplished.

The design of most surveillance programs is basically the same, with variation in the frequency of colonoscopy and sigmoidoscopy with mucosal biopsies. Air-contrast barium enema is an important means of following individuals in whom complete colonoscopy cannot be satisfactorily completed. Surveillance need not be instituted before 7 to 8 years in pancolitis, or 15 to 20 years in disease limited to the left colon. Patients with proctitis need not be screened, but patients who have had ileoproctostomy for severe pancolitis should be included in a surveillance program. The availability of a surgical pathologist who has experience in the interpretation of biopsies for dysplasia is essential.

Optimal procedures and timing are far from established (Fig. 15-5). In many programs, colonoscopy every 2 to 3 years, with annual sigmoidoscopy, is recommended, although others prefer annual colonoscopy. High grade dysplasia or any dysplasia associated with a lesion, such as a mass or stricture, is a strong indication for colectomy, and should be confirmed by repeat biopsy.[76,80] The greatest difficulty is to decide how to follow low-grade dysplasia in flat mucosa.[80] This finding may be used as an indication for more frequent examinations, or may tip the scale toward recommending colectomy in an otherwise borderline clinical situation.[81,82] Long-term prospective studies are in progress that should define the natural history of low-grade dysplasia.

Better clinically applicable markers of premalignancy in ulcerative colitis have not been identified. Areas of active investigation include analysis of mucosal biopsies by flow cytometry, electron microscopy, thymidine labelling, biochemical measurements, and immunologic tests for tumor-associated antigens.[87-90]

Crohn's Disease

Extent of Risk

Crohn, Ginzburg, and Oppenheimer described granulomatous involvement of the small bowel in 1932.[91] In 1956, Ginzburg reported the first case of adenocarcinoma in what had come to be

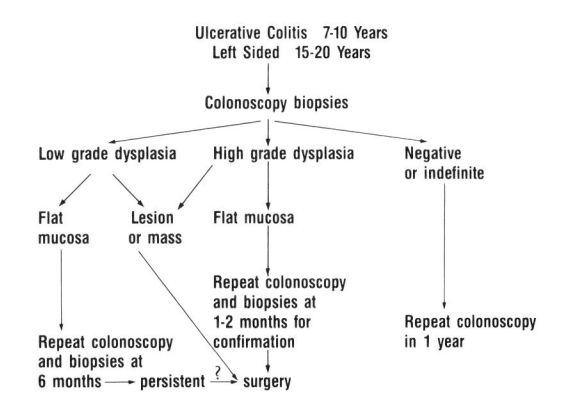

FIG.15-5. A proposed system of surveillance for cancer in ulcerative colitis using colonoscopy and biopsy. (Adapted from Lennard-Jones, J., Ritchie, J., Morson, B., and Williams, C.: Lancet., 2:149, 1983)

called Crohn's disease.[92] Crohn's disease of the colon has been accepted as a separate entity from ulcerative colitis for only about 25 years.[93] Unlike ulcerative colitis, it was assumed that Crohn's disease of the colon was not premalignant.[94,95] In cases of atypical inflammatory bowel disease, the occurrence of a carcinoma was sometimes considered to be diagnostic of ulcerative colitis.[96] A steady trickle, and a recent flood, of more than 100 case reports of adenocarcinoma in Crohn's disease involving both the small and large intestine have erased all doubt.[97-178] The opinion, however, runs the gamut from the belief that the risk of cancer in Crohn's disease is minimal to suggestions that the risk is equivalent to ulcerative colitis.[179-182]

In epidemiologic studies from the United States and the United Kingdom, the risk of developing colon cancer in Crohn's disease has been estimated at 4 to 20 times greater than in the general population.[183-187] These reports are subject to the same biases as studies in ulcerative colitis.[23-25] The report showing a 4-fold increased risk from the Cancer Epidemiology Research Unit in Birmingham, England, is actually a reversal of previous findings from the same group indicating no association between Crohn's disease and cancer.[95,184] Given the relatively recent recognition of Crohn's colitis, it is likely that some cases diagnosed as carcinoma in ulcerative colitis were actually in Crohn's colitis.[181,188] The group from the Radcliffe Infirmary at Oxford reported in 1968 an incidence of colon carcinoma in patients with Crohn's colitis in the same range as patients studied with ulcerative colitis.[154] The report from the Mayo Clinic showing a 20-fold increased risk is comparable to the relative risk estimates in universal ulcerative colitis.[183] Studies from the Mount Sinai Hospital in New York have calculated the absolute incidence rate of gastrointestinal cancer in Crohn's disease to be about one-third that of ulcerative colitis.[185] For colorectal cancer, the observed-to-expected ratio in Crohn's disease was 6:9, compared to 8:6 in left-sided ulcerative colits, and 26:5 in universal ulcerative colitis.[186]

SMALL INTESTINE. Adenocarcinoma of the small bowel is an uncommon disease in the United States and the United Kingdom with an incidence of 0.1 to 0.3 per 100,000 population per year.[120,189] Crohn's disease may be increasing in frequency but it is still not common. Using a prevalence for Crohn's disease of 9 per 100,000 population, Darke and colleagues estimated the likelihood of the two diseases occurring independently in the same patient to be more than one in a billion. Analyzing groups with Crohn's disease, they reported one case of small bowel adenocarcinoma per 354 patients, much greater than expected by chance.[120] In patients with regional enteritis and ileocolitis, at the Mount Sinai hospital in New York, the observed (O)-to-expected (E) ratio for small bowel cancer was 85:8. In the regional enteritis group alone, the O/E ratio was 114:5.[186] Reviews of the literature in 1983 and 1985 identified 64 cases of adenocarcinoma of the small intestine complicating Crohn's disease.[132,190] An association of the two diseases seems likely. With the incidence of small intestinal adenocarcinoma so low in general, however, larger series than are now available will be needed to demonstrate the association in a statistically significant manner.

Other factors indicating an association between small intestinal Crohn's disease and adenocarcinoma are cancers developing at a younger age and in different locations than usual. In Crohn's disease, cancer has been detected in patients ranging in age from 20 to 80 years, with a mean of 47.9 years.[190] The average age of onset of de novo adenocarcinoma of the small intestine is 61 years.[120,189] In patients with Crohn's disease, more than 30% of the small bowel cancers have developed in patients younger than 40 years. Most carcinomas have occurred in areas of the small intestine grossly involved with Crohn's disease. Thus, 70% of cancers in Crohn's disease have been reported in the ileum, where clinically evident Crohn's disease is most common.[132,190] This is in sharp contrast to de novo small bowel adenocarcinoma, which predominates in the proximal small bowel, usually within 20 cm of the ligament of Treitz.[189] Primary adenocarcinoma of the ileum is a rare disease.

COLORECTUM. Because adenocarcinoma of the colon and rectum is a much more common disease than small intestinal adenocarcinoma, the possibility of a chance occurrence of colon cancer in Crohn's disease is a greater consideration. Epidemiologic reports show a consistently greater observed compared to expected risk, however.[183-187] Again, the cancers tend to occur at a younger age on average than de novo colon cancer, at least a decade earlier. Nearly 30% of reported cases occurred before the age of 40, the age at which de novo cancer first begins to increase in frequency.[191] The distribution of cancers occurring in Crohn's disease seemed to be more proximal and more evenly distributed throughout the colon than in de novo cancer, but a recent review of 84 cases showed the differences to be insignificant.[120,145,165,191]

DURATION OF DISEASE. The onset of ulcerative colitis is usually distinguished by bloody diarrhea, a dramatic symptom that allows a reasonably accurate assessment of disease duration. Crohn's disease, on the other hand, is more often characterized by smoldering, indolent symptoms of abdominal pain and diarrhea. Symptoms may be initially subclinical, or well tolerated for long periods. Thus, it is more difficult to quantify the duration of Crohn's disease.[191] Several reviews describe an increased risk of carcinoma in Crohn's disease of long duration. In the small intestine, the interval between the diagnosis of Crohn's disease and intestinal cancer is 18 years, and in the colon the interval is greater than 20 years.[190,191] On the other hand, 20 to 30% of patients with carcinoma complicating Crohn's disease present initially at the time the carcinoma is diagnosed.[191] Even when these patients are excluded from analysis, no initial period free of cancer risk in Crohn's disease exists (Fig. 15-6). This is in sharp contrast to ulcerative colitis, where a 7 to 10 year delay between onset of disease and risk of cancer is solidly established.[18,27,81]

EXTENT OF DISEASE. In Crohn's disease, several studies have shown that gastrointestinal mucosa outside grossly involved areas may be abnormal.[192,193] Although the disease may appear to be segmental, it may more often be subclinically diffuse.[194] Most carcinomas complicating Crohn's disease have been reported in bowel clinically involved by the inflammatory process.[145,190,191] The epidemiologic study from Birmingham pointed to a higher cancer risk in the colon with more clinically extensive Crohn's colitis.[184] The question remains unresolved, but no direct correlation between extent of Crohn's disease and cancer risk has been established, again in contrast to ulcerative colitis.[26,195]

SURGICALLY BYPASSED BOWEL. A striking number of reports describe adenocarcinoma occurring in surgically bypassed segments of bowel involved with Crohn's disease. Almost a third of reported cases of carcinoma complicating Crohn's disease of the small intestine developed in bypassed loops of ileum or jejunum.[190] In a review of 132 patients who had surgical bypass for Crohn's disease, 7 carcinomas (5.3%) developed in excluded intestine.[129] About 20% of the reported cases of large bowel carcinomas occurring in Crohn's disease developed in bypassed segments of the colorectum.[195] Most of these cancers occurred many years following diversionary surgical therapy.[129,142,165,169,190] It is not clear whether the apparently increased risk results from an undefined effect of the bypass or reflects the long duration of the disease.[195]

ONSET AND ACTIVITY OF DISEASE. The study by Weedon et al. from the Mayo Clinic shows a 20-fold increase in the risk of colon cancer in Crohn's disease and was based on 356 patients with Crohn's colitis diagnosed before the age of 21 years.[183] The average age of onset was 15 years. The reports from Birmingham and from Mount Sinai showing 4-fold and 7-fold increased risks were based largely on patients with adult onset of Crohn's disease.[184,185] The mean age of onset was 23 and 26 years, respectively. The significance of age of onset remains unclear, because duration of Crohn's disease may be the more important factor.

The effect of activity of the inflammatory process on the risk of cancer in Crohn's disease is not established. It is well documented that cancer has developed in areas of the bowel not clinically active.[185] On the other hand, several reports emphasize the occurrence of cancers in areas of intense Crohn's disease activity, particularly in strictures and fistulas.[145,195-198]

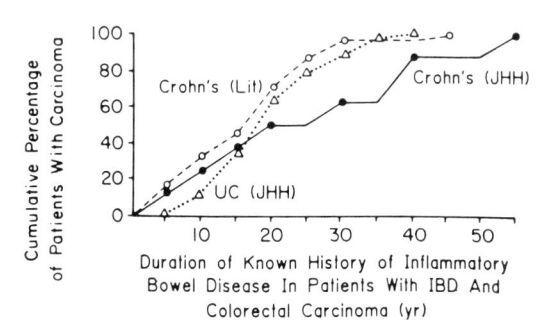

FIG.15-6. Cumulative graph showing duration of known history of inflammatory bowel disease (IBD) in patients with IBD and colorectal carcinoma. Patients not known to have Crohn's disease until they presented with colorectal carcinoma are excluded from both the Johns Hopkins Hospital (JHH) group and the literature group. No clear delay between onset of symptoms of Crohn's disease and diagnosis of colorectal carcinoma is evident in either the JHH series or the literature (Lit) series. This finding contrasts with the usual 7 to 10 year delay reported in patients with colorectal carcinoma and ulcerative colitis, as illustrated by the JHH patients, all of whom had an antecedent history of IBD. (Reprinted with permission from Hamilton, S.R.: Gastroenterology, 89:398, 1985.)

Pathologic Features

Histopathologically, adenocarcinomas associated with Crohn's disease fill the spectrum from well-differentiated to anaplastic.[162] Like cancer in ulcerative colitis, mucinous or colloid carcinoma appears more frequently in Crohn's disease than in de novo cancer.[43,48,191] In a report from Johns Hopkins, 5 out of 10 (50%) "Crohn's-carcinomas" of the colon were mucinous, compared to 11 out of 118 (9%) de novo colon cancers.[191] "Crohn's-carcinomas" tend to be infiltrative in type, and a desmoplastic reaction may occur, particularly in the small intestine.[150] Multifocal cancers seem to be more common in Crohn's disease than in de novo cancer of the colon.[198]

Dysplasia, with features resembling the changes in ulcerative colitis, has been described both in proximity and distant to cancers developing in Crohn's disease.[75,116,165,191] Focal and diffuse dysplastic changes have been found in the small intestine.[162] In the Johns Hopkins study, high-grade dysplasia was contiguous with invasive adenocarcinoma in all 10 colectomy specimens, and high-grade dysplasia was present at a distant colonic site in 6 out of 10 patients. Low-grade dysplasia was present in a seventh patient.[191]

Diagnosis

Preoperative diagnosis of carcinoma in Crohn's disease is even more difficult than in ulcerative colitis. The signs and symptoms of carcinoma, such as anorexia, weight loss, abdominal mass, pain, obstruction, bleeding, and fistulization, can all be produced by Crohn's disease. Barium-contrast roentgenograms of the small bowel usually cannot definitively distinguish changes caused by Crohn's disease from those caused by a carcinoma. Most carcinomas of the small bowel present with obstruction in any case, and surgical treatment is usually performed. Even at laparotomy, a cancer complicating Crohn's disease of the small bowel is recognized grossly in only about one-third of cases, with the diagnosis being established in the majority of cases by histopathologic examination.[132]

Barium enema studies of the colon are equally difficult to interpret for carcinoma in the presence of Crohn's disease. Double contrast technique is limited in the presence of the strictures and deep linear ulcerations typical of Crohn's colitis. Colonoscopy used with biopsy and cytology is the best way to achieve a preoperative diagnosis.[191] Endoscopy is also made difficult by strictures, fistulas, and adhesions that may be present. Strictures and fistulas may harbor a carcinoma, and at colonoscopy should be evaluated with directed forceps and brush biopsy.[145] Again, tests for occult blood in the stool, and serum or tissue analyses for CEA are not helpful in detecting early cancer superimposed on the inflammatory process.[70,71,190]

Treatment and Prognosis

Wide surgical resection with en bloc lymph node dissection is the best treatment for carcinoma in Crohn's disease. The usual principles of oncologic gastrointestinal surgical therapy apply. It is important to preserve sufficient small intestine for adequate absorption. If the colon is involved in a segmental fashion, for example as in ileocolitis, there is no clear indication for total colectomy. Prophylactic colectomies should not be performed in patients with Crohn's disease. In patients with surgically bypassed segments, however, several groups advocate prophylactic resection of those areas not planned for future use.[129,146,190,195] The surgical risks and morbidity in each patient must be weighed against the risk of developing cancer. Those advocating prophylactic removal of bypassed segments emphasize that complicating cancers in excluded bowel usually are advanced when diagnosed, with initial symptoms from metastases.[129] Certainly, in patients with bypassed loops being operated on for other reasons, prophylactic removal of the excluded bowel is recommended. After subtotal colectomy and ileostomy for severe Crohn's disease, Glotzer has proposed resecting even permanently defunctioned rectums that appear normal.[195] The possibility of cancer in Crohn's disease can be used as an additional reason to resect any severely abnormal area of bowel. Resection rather than bypass is the operation of choice in Crohn's disease (see also Chap. 27).

The prognosis of "Crohn's-cancer" after resection appears to be Dukes' stage dependent.[185] Small bowel cancers tend to present at an advanced stage, particularly in bypassed loops.[129,190] Hamilton found no difference in Dukes' stage in 39 patients with Crohn's disease and colon carcinoma compared to 118 usual cancers.[191] Surgical adjuvant therapies have not improved survival.[46]

Surveillance

Attempts have been made only recently to define the magnitude of risk of cancer of the colon in Crohn's disease in the presence of associated dysplasia. Surveillance with the use of colonoscopy and biopsy has not been widely applied. A major problem is the uncertainty of specific characteristics that can identify the patients at highest risk. Patients with Crohn's colitis are currently being entered into established surveillance programs for patients with ulcerative colitis.[190,198] Data should be forthcoming to indicate whether the finding of dysplasia in Crohn's disease can be used as a marker to detect a premalignant state and early stage cancers. The cost of such programs will also need to be addressed.[191,195]

Other Malignancies
Intestinal Cancers

SQUAMOUS CARCINOMA. An unusual cancer in the intestinal tract, squamous-cell carcinoma, has been described in the colorectum of patients with inflammatory bowel disease.[199-201] Squamous-cell cancer of the anus has been reported in Crohn's disease, usually superimposed on chronic perianal inflammation.[202-205] Mixed cloacogenic cancer, adenosquamous or adenoacanthoma, of the upper rectum has occurred both in Crohn's colitis and ulcerative colitis, and such tumors have been described in the colon, including the cecum.[191,199-201] Such instances appear to be uncommon, but are notable considering the rarity of this type of colorectal cancer.

LYMPHOMA. Although the number of patients is small and statistical significance is hard to prove, the occurrence of primary intestinal lymphoma in inflammatory bowel disease has been reported by several groups.[206-225] At least 26 cases of primary colonic lymphoma have been reported in patients with ulcerative colitis.[206-214] Lymphoma of the small intestine and colon has been described in Crohn's disease in at least 13 patients.[214-223] Most of the lymphomas have developed in areas of active inflammation, and most were diagnosed at surgical treatment. The majority of reported lymphomas in inflammatory bowel disease seem to be diffuse histiocytic (high-grade) types. Surprisingly, 4 cases of Hodgkin's disease of the small intestine and colon have been documented as complicating Crohn's disease.[217-220] Primary intestinal Hodgkin's disease is rare, accounting for less than 1% of all gastrointestinal lymphomas.[46,224]

CARCINOID. Five cases of carcinoid tumors involving the ileum in patients with regional enteritis have been reported.[225-228] Although both diseases are uncommon, their propensity to involve the distal ileum makes a chance association seem likely.[224,228] One case of regional enteritis and appendiceal carcinoid has been noted.[229]

Extraintestinal Cancer

In the reports by Greenstein et al., 30 of 267 patients with ulcerative colitis developed malignancies, of which 12% were extraintestinal, and 28 of 579 patients with Crohn's disease developed malignancies, of which 43% were extraintestinal. This did not represent a significant difference between ulcerative colitis and Crohn's disease in the incidence of extraintestinal malignancy.[185,186] A variety of neoplasms have been described in patients with inflammatory bowel disease, including cancers of the urinary bladder, breast, brain, larynx, lung, ovary, skin, thyroid, and uterus. For the most part, extraintestinal malignancy in inflammatory bowel disease has not been found to occur more frequently than expected in the general population.[183-187] Exceptions are biliary tract cancer and, possibly, acute leukemia.

BILIARY TRACT CANCER. Cancer of the biliary tract is an uncommon disease, estimated at 2 cases per 100,000 population per year.[230] At least 70 cases of cancer of the biliary tree have been reported in association with ulcerative colitis, more than half involving extrahepatic bile ducts.[231-242] The remaining cases involved intrahepatic bile ducts or gallbladder. The lifetime risk of developing carcinoma of the biliary tract in ulcerative colitis has been estimated at 0.4 to 1.4%.[231-237] Ritchie et al., reporting 15 well-documented cases, estimated the risk of biliary tract carcinoma to be 10 times greater in ulcerative colitis than in the general population of the United Kingdom.[231]

Bile duct carcinoma associated with ulcerative colitis occurs at a much younger age, on average 30 to 40-years-old, compared with the usual 60 to 70-years-old.[230-232] Bile duct carcinoma largely occurs after long duration of ulcerative colitis (average 15 years), and most often in patients with total colon involvement.[231] No definite relation exists between disease activity and severity of symptoms. The development of bile duct carcinoma many years after proctocolectomy for ulcerative colitis is well documented.[232] Biliary tract carcinomas in ulcerative colitis are not associated with the presence of gallstones.[231]

In contrast, only one patient with Crohn's disease has been reported to develop biliary tract cancer.[243] The incidence of pancreatic cancer does not seem to be increased in either form of idiopathic inflammatory bowel disease. Primary hepatocellular carcinoma has been reported in ulcerative colitis and Crohn's disease, but these appear to be isolated incidents.[244,245]

In patients with ulcerative colitis who develop cholestasis or jaundice, carcinoma of the biliary tract is an important consideration, along with sclerosing cholangitis. The relationship of biliary tract cancer to sclerosing cholangitis in ulcerative colitis is not clear. The cancers are often scirrhous and associated with distinct desmoplastic reaction. Sclerosing cholangitis is also more frequent in ulcerative colitis than Crohn's disease, and may present long after colectomy.[246,247]

ACUTE LEUKEMIA. Inflammatory bowel disease has been reported in at least 15 patients who subsequently developed acute leukemia.[248-252] Patients have had left-sided or universal ulcerative colitis, regional enteritis, or Crohn's colitis. The acute leukemias have been of several types, but in a report from Mount Sinai Hospital in New York, 5 of 6 patients with ulcerative colitis and leukemia had acute promyelocytic (M-3) leukemia.[249] This is a rare type, accounting for only about 5% of all acute myelocytic leukemias. The 5 patients with ulcerative colitis represented one-third of all promyelocytic leukemias seen at Mount Sinai over a 7-year-period.[249]

Etiology

The most widely held theory for the etiology of large bowel cancer is that dietary influences (high fat and low fiber) affect the composition of the fecal stream (bile salt metabolites) and colonic bacteria (high anaerobes), producing carcinogens.[46,253] Carcinogenic compounds are most likely to instigate a malignant process in genetically susceptible individuals. Specific oncogenes may be important.[87]

Abnormalities in inflammatory bowel disease may facilitate or accelerate such mechanisms in a variety of ways. Narrowed and inflamed areas may allow increased proliferation of anaerobic bacteria.[189] The inflamed mucosa may be more vulnerable to carcinogenic agents, either chemical or infectious.[254,255] A defective immune system in inflammatory bowel disease may fail to eliminate malignant cells at an early stage or fail to repel oncogenic viruses.[256,257] The colon mucosa in ulcerative colitis seems to be more susceptible to invasion by cytomegalovirus.[258] The fecal excretion of cholesterol and its bacterial metabolites, coprostanol and cholestane, has been found to be higher in patients with ulcerative colitis than in controls.[259] Such agents have acted as carcinogens and tumor promoters in laboratory models.

Diagnostic radiation has been proposed but not proven to contribute to carcinogenesis in inflammatory bowel disease, particularly to the occurrence of leukemia.[250] No carcinogenic effect has been definitely linked to drugs commonly used to treat inflammatory bowel disease, such as sulfasalazine or metronidazole. Prednisone, azathioprine, and 6-mercaptopurine have immunosuppressive effects, but any role for these agents in the development of malignancy in inflammatory bowel disease has not been established.[190]

In the normal intestine, cell proliferation takes place at the bottom of the mucosal crypts. As cells move up the crypts toward the lumen, maturing cells cease to synthesize DNA.[253] In inflammatory bowel disease, studies using tritiated thymidine have shown DNA synthesis taking place at the top of crypts at the mucosal surface.[260,261] This is similar to the effect of treatment with carcinogens in laboratory animals, and is seen in the colon of individuals at high genetic risk of colon cancer.[254,262] The relationship of mucosal kinetic and biochemical changes to histologic dysplasia in inflammatory bowel disease is not yet defined.[89,255,261]

In summary, malignancies complicating inflammatory bowel disease account for a small fraction of patients with cancer. Adenocarcinoma of the colon in inflammatory bowel disease represents only about 1% of all patients with this common malignancy.[46] The importance of cancer in inflammatory bowel disease transcends the absolute number of patients affected, mainly because of the ability to identify a high risk group for possible intervention. The association offers a great opportunity for investigations in carcinogenesis.[88,263] Current clinical, epidemiologic, and laboratory observations suggest numerous hypotheses that can be tested by further research.

References

1. Sales, D. J.: The prognosis of inflammatory bowel disease. Arch. Intern. Med., *143*:294, 1983.
2. Devroede, R.: Risk of cancer in inflammatory bowel disease. *In* Colorectal Cancer: Prevention, Epidemiology and Screening. Edited by S. J. Winawer, D. Schottenfeld, and P. Sherlock. New York, Raven Press, 1980.

3. Dawson, I. M. P., and Pryse-Davies, J.: The development of carcinoma of the large intestine in ulcerative colitis. Br. J. Surg., 47:113, 1959.
4. Slaney, G., and Brooke, B. N.: Cancer in ulcerative colitis. Lancet, 2:694, 1959.
5. Bargen, J. A., and Gage, R. P.: Carcinoma and ulcerative colitis: Prognosis. Gastroenterology, 39:385, 1960.
6. Nefzger, M. D., and Acheson, E. D.: Ulcerative colitis in the United States Army in 1944. Follow-up with particular reference to mortality in cases and controls. Gut, 4:183, 1963.
7. MacDougal, J. P. M.: The cancer risk in ulcerative colitis. Lancet, 2:655, 1964.
8. Edwards, F. C., and Truelove, S. C.: The course and prognosis of ulcerative colitis. Part IV. Carcinoma of the colon. Gut, 5:15, 1964.
9. Fennessy, J. J., Sparberg, M. B., and Kirsner, J. B.: Radiological findings in carcinoma of the colon complicating chronic ulcerative colitis. Gut, 9:388, 1968.
10. Johnson, W. R., et al.: Carcinoma of the colon and rectum in inflammatory bowel disease of the intestine. Surg. Gynecol. Obstet., 156:193, 1983.
11. Thompson, H., Waterhouse, J. A. H., and Allan, R. N.: Cancer morbidity in ulcerative colitis. Gut, 23:490, 1982.
12. Gilat, T., and Rozen, P.: Risk of colon cancer in ulcerative colitis in low incidence areas—A review. In Colorectal Cancer: Prevention, Epidemiology and Screening. Edited by S. J. Winawer, D. Schottenfeld, and P. Sherlock. New York, Raven Press, 1980.
13. Rosenquist, H., et al.: Ulcerative colitis and carcinoma coli. Lancet, 1:906, 1959.
14. Goldgraber, M. B., and Kirsner J. B.: Carcinoma of the colon in ulcerative colitis. Cancer, 17:657, 1964.
15. de Dombal, F. T., Watts, J. McK., Watkinson, G., and Goligher, J. C.: Local complications of ulcerative colitis: Stricture, pseudopoliposis and carcinoma of colon and rectum. Br. Med. J., 1:1442, 1966.
16. Nedbal, J., and Maratka, Z.: Ulcerative colitis in Czechoslovakia. Am. J. Proctol., 19:106, 1968.
17. Aktan, H., Paykoc, Z., and Erian, A.: Ulcerative colitis in Turkey. Dis. Colon Rectum, 13:62, 1970.
18. Devroede, G. J., et al.: Cancer risk and life expectancy of children with ulcerative colitis. N. Engl. J. Med., 285:17, 1971.
19. Sedlack, R. E., et al.: Inflammatory colon disease in Rochester, Minnesota, 1935-1964. Gastroenterology, 62:935, 1972.
20. Bonnevie, O., Vibeke B., Anthonisen, P., and Riis, P.: The prognosis of ulcerative colitis. Scand. J. Gastroenterol., 9:81, 1974.
21. Gilat, T., Zemishlany, Z., Ribak, J., Benaroya, Y., and Lilos, P.: Ulcerative colitis in the Jewish population of Tel-Aviv Yafo. II. The rarity of malignant degeneration. Gastroenterology, 67:933, 1974.
22. Melton, L. J.: Selection bias in the referral of patients and the natural history of surgical conditions. Mayo Clin. Proc., 60:880, 1985.
23. Sackett, D. L., and Whelan, G.: Cancer risk in ulcerative colitis: scientific requirements for the study of prognosis. Gastroenterology, 78:1632, 1980.
24. Devroede, G. J., and Taylor, W. F.: On calculating cancer risk and survival of ulcerative colitis patients with the life table method. Gastroenterology, 71:505, 1976.
25. Whelan, G.: Cancer risk in ulcerative colitis. Why are results in the literature so varied? Clin. Gastroenterol., 9:469, 1980.
26. Greenstein, A. J., et al.: Cancer in universal and left-sided ulcerative colitis: Factors determining risk. Gastroenterology, 77:290, 1979.
27. Kewenter, J., Ahlman, H., and Hulten, L.: Cancer risk in extensive ulcerative colitis. Ann. Surg., 188:824, 1978.
28. Michener, W. M., Farmer, R. G., and Mortimer, E. A.: Long-term prognosis of ulcerative colitis with onset in childhood or adolescence. J. Clin. Gastroenterol., 1:301, 1979.
29. Katzka, I., Brody, R. S., and Katz, S.: An assessment of colorectal cancer risk in patients with ulcerative colitis: experience from a private practice. Gastroenterology, 85:22, 1983.
30. Yardley, J., Ransohoff, D., Riddell, R., and Goldman, H.: Cancer in inflammatory bowel disease: How serious is the problem and what should be done about it? Gastroenterology, 85:197, 1983.
31. Farmer, R. G., Hawk, W. A., and Turnbull, R. B., Jr.: Carcinoma associated with mucosal ulcerative colitis and with transmural colitis and enteritis (Crohn's disease). Cancer, 28:289, 1971.
32. Cook, M. G., and Goligher, J. C.: Carcinoma and epithelial dysplasia complicating ulcerative colitis. Gastroenterology, 6:1127, 1975.
33. Sparberg, M., Fennessy, J., and Kirsner, J. B.: Ulcerative proctitis and mild ulcerative colitis: A study of 220 patients. Medicine, 45:391, 1966.
34. Farmer, R. G., and Brown, C. H.: Ulcerative colitis confined to the rectum and sigmoid flexure: Report of 124 cases. Dis. Colon Rectum, 10:177, 1967.
35. Nugent, F. W., Haggit, R. C., Colcher, H., and Kutterhuf, G. E.: Malignant potential of chronic ulcerative colitis. Preliminary report. Gastroenterology, 76:1, 1979.
36. Teague, R. H., Salmon, P. R., and Read, A. E.: Fiberoptic examination of the colon—a review of 255 cases. Gut, 14:139, 1973.
37. Elliott, P. R., et al.: Colonoscopic diagnosis of minimal change colitis in patients with a normal sigmoidoscopy and normal air-contrast barium enema. Lancet, 1:650, 1982.
38. Binder, S. C., Miller, H. H., and Deterling, R., Jr.: Fate of the retained rectum after subtotal colectomy for inflammatory disease of the colon. Am. J. Surg., 131:201, 1976.
39. Tompkins, R., et al.: Reappraisal of rectum-retaining operations for ulcerative and granulomatous colitis. Am. J. Surg., 125:159, 1973.
40. Adson, M., Cooperman, A., and Farrow, G.: Ileorectostomy for ulcerative disease of the colon. Arch. Surg., 104:424, 1972.
41. Moss, G. S., and Kiddie, N.: Fate of rectal stump in ulcerative colitis. Arch. Surg., 91:967, 1965.
42. Baker, W. N. W., Glass, R. E., Ritchie, J. K., and Aylett, S. O.: Cancer of the rectum following colectomy and ileorectal anastomosis for ulcerative colitis. Br. J. Surg., 65:862, 1978.
43. Greenstein, A. J., et al.: Cancer in universal and left sided ulcerative colitis: Clinical and pathological features. Mt. Sinai J. Med., 46:25, 1979.
44. Edling, N. P. G., and Eklof, O.: Distribution of malignancy in ulcerative colitis. Gastroenterology, 41:465, 1961.
45. American Cancer Society, Inc. Cancer Facts and Figures. New York, American Cancer Society, 1985.
46. Winawer, S. J., Enker, W. E., and Lightdale, C. J.: Malignant tumors of the colon and rectum. In Bockus—Gastroenterology. Edited by J. E. Berk. Philadephia, W. B. Saunders, 1985.
47. Counsell, P. B., and Dukes, C. E.: The association of chronic ulcerative colitis and carcinoma of the rectum and colon. Br. J. Surg., 39:485, 1952.
48. Morson, B. C., and Bussey, H. J. R.: Predisposing causes of intestinal cancer. Curr. Probl. Surg., 1970.
49. Goulstown, S. J. M., and McGovern, V. J.: The nature of

benign strictures in ulcerative colitis. N. Engl. J. Med., *281*:290, 1969.
50. Welch, C. E., and Hedberg, S. E.: Colonic carcinoma in ulcerative colitis and idiopathic colonic cancer. J. Am. Med. Assoc., *191*:815, 1965.
51. Dukes, C. E.: The surgical pathology of ulcerative colitis. Ann. R. Coll. Surg., *14*:389, 1954.
52. Gyde, S., Prior, P., Thompson, H., Waterhouse, J., and Allan, R.: Survival of patients with colorectal cancer complicating ulcerative colitis. Gut, *25*:228, 1984.
53. Morson, B. C., and Pang, L. S. C.: Rectal biopsy as an aid to cancer control. Gut, *8*:423, 1967.
54. Hulten, L., Kerwenter, J. and Ahern, C.: Precancer and carcinoma in chronic ulcerative colitis: A histopathological and clinical investigation. Scand. J. Gastroenterol., *7*:663, 1972.
55. Dobbins, W. O.: Current status of the precancer lesion in ulcerative colitis. Gastroenterology, *73*:1431, 1977.
56. Lennard-Jones, J. E., et al.: Cancer in colitis: Assessment of the individual risk by clinical and histological criteria. Gastroenterology, *73*:1280, 1977.
57. Yardley, J. H., and Keren, D. F.: "Precancer" lesions in ulcerative colitis: A retrospective study of rectal biopsy and colectomy specimens. Cancer, *34*:835, 1974.
58. Riddell, R. H.: The precarcinomatous phase of ulcerative colitis. Curr. Top. Pathol., *63*:179, 1976.
59. Fraser, G., and Findlay, J.: The double contrast enema in ulcerative and Crohn's colitis. Clin. Radiol., *27*:103, 1976.
60. Frank, R., Riddell, R., Feczko, P., and Levin, B.: Radiological detection of colonic dysplasia (pre-carcinoma) in chronic ulcerative colitis. Gastrointest. Radiol., *3*:209, 1978.
61. Goldberg, H. I., and Jeffrey, R. B.: Recent advances in the radiographic evaluation of inflammatory bowel disease. Med. Clin. North Am., *64*:1059, 1980.
62. Teague, R. H., and Waye, J. D.: Inflammatory bowel disease. *In* Colonoscopy. Edited by R. H. Hunt, and J. D. Waye. England, Chapman and Hall, 1981.
63. Hunt, R. H., Teague, R. H., Swarbrick, E. T., and Williams, C. B.: Colonoscopy in the management of colonic strictures. Br. Med. J., *2*:360, 1975.
64. Crowson, T. D., Ferrante, W. F., and Cathright, J. B., Jr.: Colonoscopy: inefficacy for early carcinoma detection in patients with ulcerative colitis. J. Am. Med. Assoc., *236*:2651, 1976.
65. Glotzer, D. J.: The surgical management of inflammatory bowel disease. Surg. Annu., *14*:221, 1982.
66. Beauregard, G., and Devroede, G. J.: Cancer risk in ulcerative colitis: its independence of luminal factors. Can. J. Surg., *17*:313, 1974.
67. Parks, A. G., Nicholls, R. J., and Belliveau, P.: Proctocolectomy with ileal reservoir and anal anastomosis. Br. J. Surg., *67*:533, 1980.
68. Hughes, P. G., et al.: The prognosis of carcinoma of the colon and rectum complicating ulcerative colitis. Surg. Gynecol. Obstet., *146*:46, 1978.
69. Bauer, J. J., Gelernt, I. M., Salky, B., and Kreel, I.: Sexual dysfunction after proctectomy for inflammatory bowel disease. Gastroenterology, *78*:1138, 1980.
70. Rule, A. H., et al.: Circulating carcinoembryonic antigen (CEA): relationship to clinical status in patients with inflammatory bowel disease. Gut, *14*:880, 1973.
71. Loewenstein, M. S., and Zamcheck, N.: CEA levels in benign gastrointestinal disease states. Cancer, *42*:1412, 1978.
72. Rogers, A. G., and Kirkpatrick, J. R.: The need for a radiation history in patients with gastrointestinal disease: case reports. Gastroenterology, *76*:1228, 1979.
73. Waye, J. D.: Colitis, cancer and colonoscopy. Med. Clin. North Am., *62*:211, 1978.
74. Dobbins, W. O., III: Current status of the precancer lesion in ulcerative colitis. Gastroenterology, *73*:1431, 1977.
75. Riddell, R., et al.: Dysplasia in inflammatory bowel disease: standardized classification with provisional clinical applications. Hum. Pathol., *14*:931, 1983.
76. Waye, J.: Dysplasia and ulcerative colitis—a colonoscopic study. Scand. J. Gastroenterol. (Suppl.), *18*:44, 1983.
77. Blackstone, M., Riddell, R., Rogers, B., and Levin, B.: Dysplasia-associated lesion or mass (DALM) detected by colonoscopy in longstanding ulcerative colitis: an indication for colectomy. Gastroenterology, *80*:366, 1981.
78. Butt, J., Konishi, F., Morson, B. C., Lennard-Jones, J., and Ritchie, J.: Macroscopic lesions in dysplasia and carcinoma complicating ulcerative colitis. Dig. Dis. Sci., *28*:18, 1983.
79. Festa, V. I., Hajdu, S. I., and Winawer, S. J.: Colorectal Cytology in Chronic Ulcerative Colitis. Acta Cytol., *29*:62, 1985.
80. Dobbins, W.: Dysplasia and malignancy in inflammatory bowel disease. Annu. Rev. Med., *35*:33, 1984.
81. Nugent, F. W., and Haggitt, R. C.: Long-term follow-up, including cancer surveillance, for patients with ulcerative colitis. Clin. Gastroenterol., *9*:459, 1980.
82. Rosenstock, E., et al.: Surveillance for colonic carcinoma in ulcerative colitis. Gastroenterology, *89*:1342, 1985.
83. Granqvist, S., Gabrielsson, N., Sundelin, P., and Thorgeirsson, T.: Precancerous lesions in the mucosa in ulcerative colitis. Scand. J. Gastroenterol., *15*:289, 1980.
84. Dickinson, R. J., Dixon, F. M., and Axon, A. T. R.: Colonoscopy and the detection of dysplasia in patients with longstanding ulcerative colitis. Lancet, *2*:620, 1980.
85. Kewenter, J., Hulten, L., and Ahren, C. H. R.: The occurrence of severe epithelial dysplasia and its bearing on treatment of longstanding ulcerative colitis. Ann. Surg., *195*:209, 1982.
86. Lennard-Jones, J., Ritchie, J., Morson, B. C., and Williams, C.: Cancer surveillance in ulcerative colitis. Lancet, *2*:149, 1983.
87. Thor, A., et al.: Monoclonal antibodies define differential ras gene expression in malignant and benign colonic disease. Nature, *311*:562, 1984.
88. Sherlock, P., and Winawer, S. J.: Cancer in inflammatory bowel disease: risk factors and prospects for early detection. *In* Gastrointestinal Cancer. Edited by M. Lipkin, and R. A. Good. New York, Plenum Press. 1978.
89. Hammarberg, C., Slezak, P., and Tribukait, B.: Early detection of malignancy in ulcerative colitis. A flow-cytometric DNA study. Cancer, *53*:291, 1984.
90. Shields, H. M., Best, C. J., and Goldman, H.: Morphometric analysis by scanning electron microscopy of dysplasia in ulcerative colitis. Gastroenterology, *86*:1248, 1984.
91. Crohn, B. B., Ginzburg, L., and Oppenheimer, G. D.: Regional ileitis: a pathologic and clinical entity. J. Am. Med. Assoc., *99*:1323, 1932.
92. Ginzburg, L., Schneider, K. M., Dreizin, D. H., and Levinson, C.: Carcinoma of the jejunum occurring in a case of regional enteritis. Surgery, *39*:347, 1956.
93. Lockhart-Mummery, H. E., and Morson, B. C.: Crohn's disease (regional enteritis) of the large intestine and its distinction from ulcerative colitis. Gut, *2*:189, 1961.
94. Farmer, R. G., Hawk, W. A., and Turnbull, R. B., Jr.: Carcinoma associated with mucosal ulcerative colitis, and

with transmural colitis and enteritis (Crohn's disease). Cancer, 28:289, 1971.
95. Fielding, J. F., Prior, P., Waterhouse, J. A., and Cooke, W. T.: Malignancy in Crohn's disease. Scand. J. Gastroenterol., 7:3, 1972.
96. Thayer, W. R., Jr.: Crohn's disease (regional enteritis): a look at the last four years. Scand. J. Gastroenterol. (Suppl.), 6:165, 1970.
97. Almond, C. H., Neal, M. P, and Moedl, K. R.: Regional ileitis with coincidental ileal carcinoma. Missouri Med., 57:452, 1960.
98. Atwell, J. D., Duthie, H. L., and Goligher, J. C.: The outcome of Crohn's disease. Br. J. Surg., 52:966, 1965.
99. Aufses, A. H., Jr., and Kreel, I.: Ileostomy for granulomatous ileocolitis. Ann. Surg., 173:91, 1971.
100. Beachley, M. C., et al.: Carcinoma of the small intestine in chronic regional enteritis. Am. J. Dig. Dis., 18:1095, 1973.
101. Bearzi, I., and Ranaldi, R.: Small bowel adenocarcinoma and Crohn's disease: report of a case with differing histogenetic patterns. Histopathology, 9:345, 1985.
102. Ben Asher, H.: Adenocarcinoma of the ileum complicating regional enteritis. Am. J. Gastroenterol., 55:391, 1971.
103. Berman, L. G., and Prior, J. T.: Adenocarcinoma of the small intestine occurring in a case of regional enteritis. J. Mt. Sinai Hosp., 31:30, 1964.
104. Bersack, S. R., Howe, J. S., and Rehak, E. N.: A unique case with roentgenological evidence of regional enteritis of long duration with histological evidence of diffuse adenocarcinoma. Gastroenterology, 34:703, 1958.
105. Brill, C. B., Klein, S. F., and Kart, A. E.: Regional enteritis and enterocolitis: a study of 75 patients over 15 years. Ann. Surg., 170:766, 1969.
106. Brown N., Weinstein, V. A., and Janowitz, HD.: Carcinoma of the ileum twenty-five years after bypass for regional enteritis: a case report. Mt. Sinai J. Med., 37:675, 1970.
107. Bruni, H., Lilly, J., Newman, W., and McHardy, G.: Small bowel carcinoma a complication of regional enteritis. South. Med. J., 64:577, 1971.
108. Buchanan, D. P., et al.: Carcinoma of the ileum occurring in an area of regional enteritis. Am. J. Surg., 97:336, 1959.
109. Burbige, E. J., Bedine, M. S., and Handelsman, J. C.: Adenocarcinoma of the small intestine in Crohn's disease involving the small bowel. West. J. Med., 127:43, 1977.
110. Cantwell, J. D., Kettering, R. F., Carney, J. A., and Ludwig, J.: Adenocarcinoma complicating regional enteritis: report of a case and review of the literature. Gastroenterology, 54:599, 1968.
111. Castellano, T. J., Frank, M. S., Brandt, L. J., and Mahadevia, P: Metachronous carcinoma complicating Crohn's disease. Arch. Intern. Med., 141:1074, 1981.
112. Church, J. M., et al.: The relationship between fistulas in Crohn's disease and associated carcinoma. Report of four cases and review of the literature. Dis. Colon Rectum, 28:361, 1985.
113. Clemmensen T., and Johansen, A.: A case of Crohn's disease of the colon associated with adenocarcinoma extending from cardia to the anus. Acta Pathol. Microbiol. Scand., 80:5, 1972.
114. Collier, P. E., Turowski, P., and Diamond, D. L.: Small intestinal adenocarcinoma complicating regional enteritis. Cancer, 55:516, 1985.
115. Cornes, J. S., and Stecher, M.: Primary Crohn's disease of the colon and rectum. Gut, 2:189, 1961.
116. Craft, C. F., Mendelsohn, G., Cooper, H. S., and Yardley, J. H.: Colonic "precancer" in Crohn's disease. Gastroenterology, 80:578, 1981.
117. Crohn, B. B., and Yarnis, H.: Regional Ileitis. 2nd Ed. New York, Grune and Stratton, 1958.
118. Crohn, B. B., and Yarnis, H.: Granulomatous colitis: an attempt at clarification. J. Mt. Sinai Hosp., 33:503, 1966.
119. Crystal, R. D.: Development of carcinoma in regional enteritis. Arch. Surg., 109:124, 1974.
120. Darke, S. G., Parks, A. G., Grogano, S. L., and Pollock, D. N.: Adenocarcinoma and Crohn's disease. A report of two cases and analysis of the literature. Br. J. Surg., 60:169, 1973.
121. Davis, A., and Caley, J. P.: Crohn's disease with carcinoma of the colon. Postgrad. Med. J., 36:380, 1960.
122. Farmer, R. G., Hawk, W. A., and Turnbull, R. B.: Carcinoma associated with regional enteritis: a report of two cases. Am. J. Dig. Dis., 15:365, 1970.
123. Fleming, K. A., and Pollack, A. C.: A case of Crohn's carcinoma. Gut, 16:533, 1975.
124. Floch, H. F., Slattery, L. R., and Hazzi, C. G.: Carcinoma of the small intestine in regional enteritis: presentation of a case and review of the literature. Am. J. Gastroenterol., 70:520, 1978.
125. Frank, J. D., and Shorey, B. A.: Adenocarcinoma of the small bowel as a complication of Crohn's disease. Gut, 14:120, 1973.
126. Fresko, D., Lazarus, S. S., Dotan, J., and Reingold, M.: Early presentation of carcinoma of the small bowel in Crohn's disease ("Crohn's carcinoma"). Case reports and review of the literature. Gastroenterology, 82:783. 1982.
127. Gerwertz, B. L., Dent, T. L., and Appelman, H. D.: Implications of precancerous rectal biopsy in patients with inflammatory bowel disease. Arch. Surg., 111:326, 1976.
128. Goldman, L. I., Bralow, S. P., Cox, W., and Peal, A. R.: Adenocarcinoma of the small bowel complicating Crohn's disease. Cancer, 26:1119, 1970.
129. Greenstein, A. J., et al.: Cancer in Crohn's disease after diversionary surgery. A report of seven carcinomas occurring in excluded bowel. Am. J. Surg., 135:86, 1978.
130. Hamilton, S. R.: Colorectal carcinoma in patients with Crohn's disease. Gastroenterology, 89:398, 1985.
131. Hardy, D. G., and Youngs, G. R.: Crohn's disease and carcinoma of the rectum. Int. Surg., 57:504, 1972.
132. Hawker, P. C., et al.: Adenocarcinoma of the small intestine complicating Crohn's disease. Gut, 23:188, 1982.
133. Heathcote, J., Knauer, C. M., Oakes, D., and Archibald, R. W.: Perforation of an adenocarcinoma of the small bowel affected by regional enteritis. Gut, 21:1093, 1980.
134. Hoffert, P. W., Weingarten, B., Friedman, L. D., and Morecki, R.: Adenocarcinoma of the terminal ileum in a segment of bowel with coexisting active ileitis. NY State J. Med., 63:1567, 1963.
135. Holter, A., and Fischer, J. E.: Adenocarcinoma of the small bowel associated with Crohn's disease. Arch. Surg., 113:991, 1978.
136. Honore, L. H.: Early Crohn's distal ileitis, acute appendicitis and carcinoma of the proximal transverse colon in a 39-year-old woman: a case report. Am. J. Proctol. Gastroenterol. Colon Rectal Surg., 33:6, 1982.
137. Hywel-Jones, J.: Colonic cancer and Crohn's disease. Gut, 10:651, 1969.
138. Keighley, M. R. B., Thompson, H., and Alexander-Williams, J.: Multifocal colonic carcinoma and Crohn's disease. Surgery, 78:534, 1975.
139. Kim, U., Aufses, A. H., and Kreela, I.: Malignant tumors associated with granulomatous enterocolitis. Am. J. Gastroenterol., 63:66, 1975.

140. Kipping, T. A., and Rowntree, T.: Crohn's disease of the colon with carcinoma of the rectum. Proc. R. Soc. Med., 63:753, 1970.
141. Kornfeld, P., Ginzburg, L., and Adlersberg, D.: Adenocarcinoma occurring in regional jejunitis. Am. J. Med., 23:493, 1957.
142. Lavery, I. C., and Jagelman, D. G.: Cancer in the excluded rectum following surgery for inflammatory bowel disease. Dis. Colon Rectum, 25:522, 1982.
143. Lear, P. E.: The physiological basis for the surgical management of regional enteritis. Surg. Clin. North Am., 38:545, 1958.
144. Lennard-Jones, J. E., and Stadler, G. A.: Prognosis after resection of chronic regional ileitis. Gut, 8:332, 1967.
145. Lightdale, C. J., Sternberg, S. S., Posner, G., and Sherlock, P.: Carcinoma complicating Crohn's disease. Report of 7 cases and review of the literature. Am. J. Med., 59:262, 1975.
146. Magnes, M., and DeBell, P.: Carcinoma associated with terminal ileitis. J. Med. Soc. NJ, 66:573, 1969.
147. Martinelli, V., and Bellucci, M.: Ileite terminale e cancero del colon destro. Ann. Ital. Chir., 36:557, 1959.
148. Moesgaard, F., Knudsen, J. T., and Christensen, N.: Adenocarcinoma of the small intestine associated with Crohn's disease. Acta Chir. Scand., 145:577, 1979.
149. Morowitz, D. A., Block, G. E., and Kirsner, J. B.: Adenocarcinoma of the ileum complicating chronic regional enteritis. Gastroenterology, 55:397, 1968.
150. Nesbit, R. R., et al.: Carcinoma of the small bowel. Cancer, 37:2948, 1976.
151. Newman, R. D., Bennett, S. J., and Pascall, R. R.: Adenocarcinoma of the small intestine arising in Crohn's disease. Demonstration of a tumor-associated antigen in invasion and intra-epithelial components. Cancer, 36:2016, 1975.
152. Papp, J. P., and Pollard, H. M.: Adenocarcinoma occurring in Crohn's disease of the small intestine. Am. J. Gastroenterol., 56:149, 1971.
153. Parrish, R. A., Kansten, M. B., McRae, A. T., and Moritz, W. H.: Segmental Crohn's colitis associated with adenocarcinoma. Am. J. Surg., 115:371, 1968.
154. Perrett, A. D., Truelove, S. C., and Massarella, G. R.: Crohn's disease and carcinoma of the colon. Br. Med. J., 2:466, 1968.
155. Perzin, K. H., et al.: Intramucosal carcinoma of the small intestine arising in regional enteritis (Crohn's disease). Report of a case studied for carcinoembryonic antigen and review of the literature. Cancer, 54:151, 1984.
156. Radi, M. F., Gray, G. F., Jr., and Scott, H. W., Jr.: Carcinosarcoma of ileum in regional enteritis. Hum. Pathol., 15:385, 1984.
157. Rha, C. K., Wilson, J. M., Jr., and Klein, N. C.: Adenocarcinoma of the ileum with coexisting regional enteritis. Arch. Surg., 102:630, 1971.
158. Saeed, M., Sims, S., and Burch, B. W.,: Development of carcinoma in regional enteritis. Arch. Surg., 1208:376, 1974.
159. Schofield, P. F.: Intestinal malignancy and Crohn's disease. Proc. R. Soc. Med., 65:783, 1972.
160. Schuman, B. M.: Adenocarcinoma arising in an excluded loop of ileum. N. Engl. J. Med., 283:135, 1970.
161. Sheil, F. O., Clark, C. G., Goligher, J. C.: Adenocarcinoma associated with Crohn's disease. Br. J. Surg., 55:53, 1968.
162. Simpson, S., Traube, J., and Riddell, R. H.: The histologic appearance of dysplasia (precarcinomatous change) in Crohn's disease of the small and large intestine. Gastroenterology, 81:492, 1981.
163. Smith, T. R., Conradi, H., Bernstein, R., and Grewel-dinger, J.: Adenocarcinoma arising in Crohn's disease: report of 2 cases. Dis. Colon Rectum, 23:498, 1980.
164. Steele, D. C., and McNeely, D. T.: Adenocarcinoma arising in a site of chronic regional enteritis. Can. Med. Assoc. J., 83:379, 1960.
165. Traube, J., et al.: Crohn's disease and adenocarcinoma of the bowel. Dig. Dis. Sci., 25:939, 1980.
166. Tyers, G. F. O., Steiger, E., and Dudrick, S. J.: Adenocarcinoma of the small intestine and other malignant tumors complicating regional enteritis. Ann. Surg., 169:510, 1969.
167. Valdes-Dapena, D., et al.: Adenocarcinoma of the small bowel in association with regional enteritis. Cancer, 37:2938, 1976.
168. Van Patter, W. N., et al.: Regional enteritis. Gastroenterology, 26:347, 1954.
169. Victor, D. W., Jr., Thompson, H., Allan, R. N., and Alexander-Williams, J.: Cancer complicating defunctioned Crohn's disease. Clin. Oncol., 8:163, 1982.
170. Warren, S., and Sommers, S. C.: Cicatrizing enteritis (regional ileitis) as a pathological entity. Analysis of one hundred and twenty cases. Am. J. Pathol., 24:475, 1948.
171. Warren, R., and Barwick, K. W.: Crohn's colitis with carcinoma and dysplasia. Report of a case and review of 100 small and large bowel resections for Crohn's disease to detect incidence of dysplasia. Am. J. Surg. Pathol., 7:151, 1983.
172. Wein, M. A., Spector, N., and Robinson, H. M.: Regional ileitis complicated by adenocarcinoma. Am. J. Gastroenterol., 41:58, 1964.
173. Weingarten, B., Parker, J. G., Chazen, E. M., and Jacobson, H. G.: Adenocarcinoma of the jejunum in nonspecific granulomatous enteritis. Arch. Surg., 78:483, 1959.
174. Weingarten, B., and Weiss, J.: Malignant degeneration in chronic inflammatory disease of the colon and small intestine. Am. J. Gastroenterol., 33:203, 1960.
175. Westaby, S., Everett, W. G., and Dick, A. P.: Adenocarcinoma of the small bowel complicating Crohn's disease in a patient treated with azathioprine. Clin. Oncol., 3:377, 1977.
176. Wyatt, A. P.: Regional enteritis leading to carcinoma of the small bowel. Gut, 10:924, 1969.
177. Zinkin, L. D., and Brandwein, C.: Adenocarcinoma in Crohn's colitis. Dis. Colon Rectum, 23:115, 1980.
178. Zisk, J., Shore, J. M., Rosoff, L., and Friedman, N. B.: Regional ileitis complicated by adenocarcinoma of the ileum. A report of two cases. Surgery, 47:970, 1960.
179. Butt, J. H., and Morson, B. C.: Dysplasia and cancer in inflammatory bowel disease (editorial). Gastroenterology, 80:865, 1981.
180. Butt, J. H., Lennard-Jones, J. E., and Ritchie, J. K.: A practical approach to the risk of cancer in inflammatory bowel disease. Med. Clin. North Am., 64:1203, 1980.
181. Kirsner, J. B., and Shorter, R. G.: Recent developments in "nonspecific" inflammatory bowel disease (first of two parts). N. Engl. J. Med., 306:775, 1982.
182. Sachar, D. B.: New concepts of cancer. Mt. Sinai J. Med., 50:133, 1983.
183. Weedon, D. D., et al.: Crohn's disease and cancer. N. Engl. J. Med., 289:1099, 1973.
184. Gyde, S. N., et al.: Malignancy in Crohn's disease. Gut, 21:1024, 1980.
185. Greenstein, A. J., et al.: Patterns of neoplasia in Crohn's disease and ulcerative colitis. Cancer, 46:403, 1980.
186. Greenstein, A. J., et al: Comparison of cancer risk in Crohn's disease and ulcerative colitis. Cancer, 48:2742, 1981.

187. Shorter, R. G.: Risks of intestinal cancer in Crohn's disease. Dis. Colon Rectum, 26:686, 1983.
188. Lindner, A. E., Marshak, R. H., Wolf, B. S., and Janowitz, H. D.: Granulomatous colitis: a clinical study. N. Engl. J. Med., 269:379, 1963.
189. Lightdale, C. J., and Sherlock, P.: Small intestinal tumors (other than lymphoma and carcinoid). In Bockus—Gastroenterology. Edited by J. E. Berk. Philadelphia, W.B. Saunders, 1985.
190. Faintuch, J., Levin, B., and Kirsner, J. B.: Inflammatory bowel diseases and their relationship to malignancy. Crit. Rev. Oncol. Hematol., 2:323, 1985.
191. Hamilton, S. R.: Colorectal carcinoma in patients with Crohn's disease. Gastroenterology, 89:398, 1985.
192. Hamilton, S. R., Bussey, H. J. R., Boitnott, J. K., and Morson, B. C.: Active inflammation and granulomas in grossly uninvolved colonic mucosa of Crohn's disease resection specimens studied with en face histologic technique (abstract). Gastroenterology, 80:1167, 1981.
193. Dvorak, A. M., Connell, A. B., and Dickerson, G. R.: Crohn's disease: a scanning electron microscopic study. Hum. Pathol., 10:165, 1979.
194. Dunne, W. T., Cooke, W. T., and Allan, R. N.: Enzymatic and morphometric evidence for Crohn's disease as a diffuse lesion of the gastrointestinal tract. Gut, 18:290, 1977.
195. Glotzer, D. J.: The risk of cancer in Crohn's disease. Gastroenterology, 89:438, 1985.
196. Chaikhouni, A., Requerya, F. I., and Steven, J. R.: Adenocarcinoma in perianal fistulas of Crohn's disease. Dis. Colon Rectum, 24:639, 1981.
197. Buchman, P., et al.: Cancer in a recto-vaginal fistula in a patient with Crohn's disease. Am. J. Surg., 140:462, 1980.
198. Korelitz, B. I.: Carcinoma of the intestinal tract in Crohn's disease: results of a survey conducted by the National Foundation for Ileitis and Colitis (editorial). Am. J. Gastroenterol., 78:44, 1983.
199. Zirkin, R. M., and McCord, D. L.: Squamous cell carcinoma of the rectum: report of a case complicating chronic ulcerative colitis. Dis. Colon Rectum., 6:370, 1963.
200. Comer, T. P., Beahrs, O. H., and Dockerty, M. B.: Primary squamous cell carcinoma and adenocanthoma of the colon. Cancer, 28:1111, 1971.
201. Crissman, J. D.: Adenosquamous and squamous cell carcinoma of the colon. Am. J. Surg. Pathol., 2:47, 1978.
202. Slater, G., Greenstein, A., and Aufses, A. H., Jr.: Anal Crohn's disease with carcinoma in situ. Dig. Dis. Sci., 25:464, 1980.
203. Preston, D. M., Fowler, E. F., Lennard-Jones, J. E., and Hawley, P. R.: Carcinoma of the anus in Crohn's disease. Br. J. Surg., 70:346, 1983.
204. Daly, J. J., and Madrazo, A.: Anal Crohn's disease with carcinoma in situ. Dig. Dis. Sci., 25:464, 1980.
205. Sommerville, K. W., et al.: Malignant transformation of anal skin tags in Crohn's disease. Gut, 25:1124, 1984.
206. Nugent, F. N., et al.: Colonic lymphoma in ulcerative colitis: report of four cases. Lahey Clin. Med. Bull., 21:104, 1972.
207. Cornes, J. S., Smith, J. C., and Somlinod, N. F.: Lymphosarcoma in chronic ulcerative colitis with report of two cases. Br. J. Surg., 49:50, 1961.
208. Cattell, R. B., and Boehme, E. S.: The importance of malignant degeneration as a complication of chronic ulcerative colitis. Gastroenterology, 8:695, 1947.
209. Renton, P., and Blackshaw, A. J.: Colonic lymphoma complicating ulcerative colitis. Br. J. Surg., 63:542, 1976.
210. Bashiti, H. O., and Kraus, F. T.: Histiocytic lymphoma in chronic ulcerative colitis. Cancer, 46:1695, 1980.
211. Vieta, J. O., and Delgado, G. E.: Chronic ulcerative colitis complicated by colonic lymphoma: report of a case. Dis. Colon Rectum, 19:56, 1976.
212. Bartolo, D., Goepel, J. R., and Parsons, M. A.: Rectal malignant lymphoma in chronic ulcerative colitis. Gut, 23:164, 1982.
213. Barki, Y., and Boult, I.: Two uncommon malignancies complicating chronic ulcerative colitis. J. Can. Assoc. Radiol., 32:136, 1981.
214. Glick, S. N., et al.: Development of lymphoma in patients with Crohn's disease. Radiology, 153:337, 1984.
215. Lee, G. B., Smith, P. M., and Seal, R. M. E.: Lymphosarcoma in Crohn's disease: report of a case. Dis. Colon Rectum, 20:351, 1977.
216. Collins, W. J.: Malignant lymphoma complicating regional enteritis. Case report and review of the literature. Am. J. Gastroenterol., 68:177, 1977.
217. Codling, B. W., Keighley, M. R. B., and Slaney, G.: Hodgkin's disease complicating Crohn's colitis. Surgery, 82:625, 1977.
218. Hecker, R., Sheers, R., and Thomas, D.: Hodgkin's lymphoma: a complication of small bowel Crohn's disease. Aust. NZ J. Surg., 2:603, 1978.
219. Shaw, J. H., and Mulvaney, N.: Hodgkin's lymphoma: a complication of small bowel Crohn's disease. Aust. NZ J. Surg., 52:34, 1982.
220. Morrison, P. D., and Whitaker, M.: A case of Hodgkin's disease complicating Crohn's disease. Clin. Oncol., 8:271, 1982.
221. Case records of the Massachusetts General Hospital. Case 43292. N. Engl. J. Med., 257:135, 1957.
222. Hughes, R. K.: Reticulum cell sarcoma: a case possibly originating in regional enteritis. Am. Surg., 21:770, 1955.
223. Schofield, P. F.: Intestinal malignancy and Crohn's disease. Proc. R. Soc. Med., 65:783, 1972.
224. Lightdale, C. J., Koepsell, T. D., and Sherlock, P.: Small intestine. In Cancer Epidemiology and Prevention. Edited by D. Schottenfeld, and J. Fraumeni Jr. Philadelphia, W.B. Saunders, 1982.
225. Wood, W. S., et al.: Coexistence of regional enteritis and carcinoid tumor. Gastroenterology, 59:265, 1970.
226. Villotte, J., et al.: Crohn's disease revealed by a vesicointestinal fistula and associated with a carcinoid tumor of the small intestine. Sem. Hop. Paris, 45:1620, 1969.
227. Tehrani, M. A., and Carfrae, D. C.: Carcinoid tumor and Crohn's disease. Br. J. Clin. Prac., 29:123, 1975.
228. Van Landingham, S. B., Kluppel, S., Symmonds, R., and Snyder, S. K.: Coexisting carcinoid tumor and Crohn's disease. J. Surg. Oncol., 24:310, 1983.
229. Janin, Y., et al: Crohn's disease and carcinoid tumor of the appendix in a child. Z. Kinderchir., 4:376, 1981.
230. Moertel, C. G.: Extrahepatic bile ducts. In Cancer Medicine. Edited by J. F. Holland, and E. Frei, III. Philadelphia, Lea & Febiger, 1982.
231. Ritchie, J. K., et al.: Biliary tract carcinoma associated with ulcerative colitis. Q. J. Med., 43:263, 1974.
232. Converse, C. F., Reagan, J. W., and DeCosse, J. J.: Ulcerative colitis and carcinoma of the bile ducts. Am. J. Surg., 121:39, 1971.
233. Joffe, N. and Antonioli, D. A.: Primary carcinoma of the gallbladder associated with chronic inflammatory bowel disease. Clin. Radiol., 32:319, 1981.
234. Greenstein, A. J., Janowitz, H. D., and Sachar, D. B.: The extra-intestinal complications of Crohn's disease and ulcerative colitis; a study of 700 patients. Medicine, 55:401, 1976.

235. Morowitz, D. A., Glagov, S., Dordal, E., and Kirsner, J. B.: Carcinoma of the biliary tract complicating chronic ulcerative colitis. Cancer, 27:356, 1971.
236. Ross, A. P., and Braasch, J. W.: Ulcerative colitis and carcinoma of the proximal bile ducts. Gut, 14:94, 1973.
237. Akwari, O. E., van Heerden, J. A., Foulk, W. T., and Baggenstoss, A. H.: Cancer of the bile ducts associated with ulcerative colitis. Ann. Surg., 181:303, 1975.
238. Roberts-Thomson, I. C., Strickland, R. G., and Mackay, I. R.: Bile duct carcinoma in chronic ulcerative colitis. Aust. NZ J. Med., 3:264, 1973.
239. Parker, R. G. F., and Kendall, E. J. C.: The liver in ulcerative colitis. Br. Med. J., 2:1030, 1954.
240. Rankin, J. G., Skyring, A. P., and Goulston, S. J. M.: Liver in ulcerative colitis: Obstructive jaundice due to bile duct carcinoma. Gut, 7:433, 1966.
241. Ham, J. M.: Tumours of the biliary epithelium and ulcerative colitis. Ann. Surg., 168:1088, 1968.
242. Babb, R. R., Lee, R. H., and Peck, O. C.: Cancer of the bile duct and chronic ulcerative colitis. Am. J. Surg., 119:337, 1970.
243. Berman, M. D., Falchuk, K. R., and Trey, C.: Carcinoma of the biliary tree complicating Crohn's disease. Dig. Dis. Sci., 25:795, 1980.
244. Smith, P. M.: Hepatoma associated with ulcerative colitis. Dis. Colon Rectum, 17:554, 1974.
245. Lee, F. L., Murrary, S. M., Prior, J., and Shreeve, D. R.: Primary liver cell cancer occurring in association with Crohn's disease treated with prednisolone and azathioprine. Hepatogastroenterology, 30:188, 1983.
246. Sivak, M. V., Jr., Farmer, R. G., and Lalli, A. F.: Sclerosing cholangitis. Increasing frequency of recognition and association with ulcerative colitis. J. Clin. Gastroenterol., 3:261, 1981.
247. Warren, G. H., and Kern, F., Jr.: The biliary tract in inflammatory bowel disease. Clin. Gastroenterol., 12:255, 1983.
248. Fabry, T. L., Sachar, D. B., and Janowitz, H. D.: Acute myelogenous leukemia in patients with ulcerative colitis. J. Clin. Gastroenterol., 2:225, 1980.
249. Cuttner, J.: Increased incidence of acute promyelocytic leukemia in patients with ulcerative colitis. Ann. Intern. Med., 97:864, 1982.
250. Hanauer, S., et al.: Acute leukemia following inflammatory bowel disease. Dig. Dis. Sci., 6:545, 1983.
251. Cohn, E. M., and Pearlstine, B.: Inflammatory bowel disease and leukemia. J. Clin. Gastroenterol., 6:33, 1984.
252. Giron, J. A., et al.: Crohn's disease and leukemia (letter). Dig. Dis. Sci., 30:410, 1985.
253. Lipkin, M., and Newmark, H.: Effect of added dietary calcium on colonic epithelial-cell proliferation in subjects at high risk for familial colonic cancer. N. Engl. J. Med., 313:1381, 1985.
254. Earnshaw, P., Busuttil, A., and Ferguson, A.: Colorectal cancer. Relevance of colonic mucosal inflammation to aetiology. Recent Results Cancer Res., 83:31, 1982.
255. Boland, C. R., et al.: Abnormal goblet cell glycoconjugates in rectal biopsies associated with an increased risk of neoplasia in patients with ulcerative colitis: early results—a prospective study. Gut, 25:1364, 1984.
256. Asquith, P., Kraft, S. C., and Rothberg, R. M.: Lymphocyte responses to nonspecific mitogens in inflammatory bowel disease. Gastroenterology, 65:1, 1973.
257. Beeken, W. L., St. Andre-Ukena, S., and Gundel, R. M.: Comparative studies of mononuclear phagocyte function in patients with Crohn's disease and colon neoplasms. Gut, 24:1034, 1983.
258. Farmer, G. W., et al.: Dual investigations in ulcerative colitis and regional enteritis. Gastroenterology, 65:8, 1973.
259. Reddy, B. S., Martin, C. W., and Wynder, E. L.: Fecal bile acids and cholesterol metabolites of patients with ulcerative colitis, a high risk group for development of colon cancer. Cancer Res., 37:1697, 1977.
260. Eastwood, G. L., and Trier, J. S.: Epithelial cell renewal in cultured rectal biopsies in ulcerative colitis. Gastroenterology, 64:383, 1973.
261. Biasco, G., et al.: Proliferative and antigenic properties of rectal cells in patients with chronic ulcerative colitis. Cancer Res., 44:5450, 1984.
262. Thurnherr, N., Deschner, E. E., Stonehill, E. H., and Lipkin, M.: Induction of adenocarcinomas of the colon in mice by weekly injections of 1, 2-dimethylhydrazine. Cancer Res., 33:940, 1973.
263. Kirsner, J. B.: Inflammatory bowel disease—consideration of etiology and pathogenesis. In Colorectal Cancer: Prevention, Epidemiology and Screening. Edited by S. J. Winawer, D. Schottenfeld, and P. Sherlock. New York, Raven Press, 1980.

Suggested Readings

1. Brostram, O., Lafberg, R., Ost, A., and Reichard, H.: Cancer surveillance of patients with long-standing ulcerative colitis: A clinical, endoscopical and histological study. Gut, 27:1408, 1986.
2. Krist, N., et al.: Malignancy in Crohn's disease. Scand. J. Gastroenterol., 21:82, 1986.
3. Maratka, Z., et al.: Incidence of colorectal cancer in proctocolitis: A retrospective study of 959 cases over 40 years. Gut, 26:43, 1985.

16 · Extraintestinal Manifestations of Inflammatory Bowel Disease

LLOYD MAYER, M.D. AND HENRY JANOWITZ, M.D.

Although this textbook is devoted to manifestations and complications of inflammatory bowel disease (IBD) affecting the bowel, a significant degree of morbidity in IBD occurs outside the gastrointestinal (GI) tract, i.e., extraintestinal manifestations. Complaints of arthritis, uveitis, or skin eruptions may be the presenting symptom in a patient with IBD, preceding or overshadowing the bowel symptoms. Even when the bowel disease has already been established, some of the symptoms of these extraintestinal disorders may be more difficult to control or more prominent than the GI tract disease itself. In earlier reports, the associated manifestations described were limited in terms of organ involvement (liver, skin, eyes, or joints); however, as we have become more aware of these diseases, newer complications have been described. Extraintestinal manifestations can be divided into three categories: (1) those intimately related to the activity or extent of disease and responsive to therapy directed at the bowel disease; (2) those whose course is independent of the underlying bowel disease, preceding the onset of bowel symptoms or occurring postcolectomy; and (3) those that are direct sequelae of the underlying bowel disease, that is, fistulae, mechanical obstruction of ureters, anemia from GI blood loss, and renal stones. It is possible that the pathogenesis of manifestations in each of the subgroups is distinct, but that within each subgroup similar pathogenetic mechanisms may be involved.

The finding of extraintestinal disorders underscores the fact that IBD is a systemic illness. It should be emphasized, however, that extraintestinal manifestations are not limited to IBD and some have been described in other bowel diseases as well.[1-4] In this chapter we shall examine, by organ system, the various extraintestinal manifestations and their relationship to the bowel disease, therapy, and potential pathogenetic mechanisms.

SKIN AND MUCOUS MEMBRANES

The incidence of skin involvement in IBD is variable from series to series, largely dependent on what is defined as truly associated skin disease. If one considers only erythema nodosum and pyoderma gangrenosum as the major skin disorders, then the incidence ranges from 4 to 10%.[5,6] Increased recognition of vasculitis and aphthous stomatitis in IBD may augment these percentages, but, in general, the incidence of these latter two manifestations is low.

Skin involvement in IBD has been subdivided into four categories by McCallum and Kinmont: (1) involvement by direct extension (fistula in ano or perirectal abscess); (2) vascular reactions such as erythema nodosum, pyoderma,

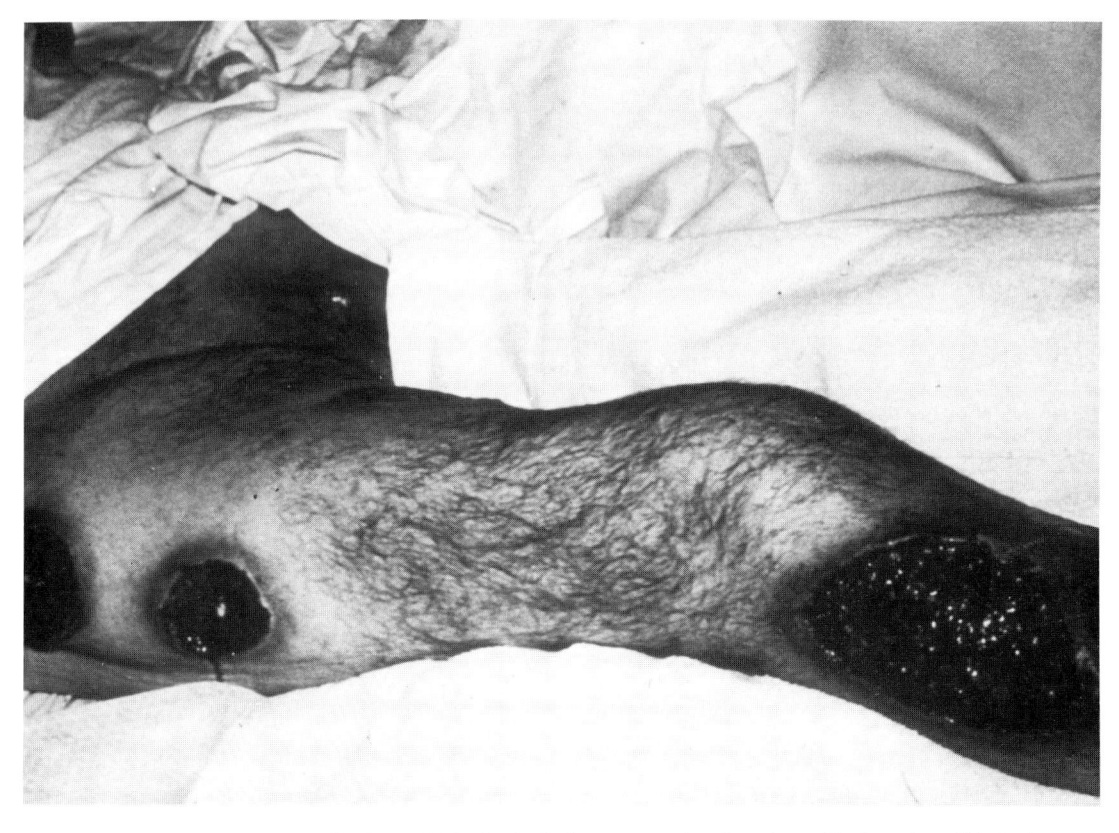

FIG. 16-1. Pyoderma gangrenosum affecting multiple sites in the lower extremity of a patient with ulcerative colitis. Lesions are typical discrete deep ulcers. (Courtesy of Dr. David Sachar.)

and vasculitis; (3) skin lesions secondary to malabsorption; and (4) metastatic Crohn's lesions.[7]

Pyoderma Gangrenosum

Pyoderma gangrenosum (PG) is one of the more interesting complications of IBD. While its actual incidence in ulcerative colitis is low (1 to 5%),[8,11] and it is rarer in Crohn's disease,[12,13] studies of patients with diagnosed PG reveal that the incidence of IBD, predominantly ulcerative colitis (UC), in this disorder is between 36 and 50%.[14–17] Other systemic diseases associated with PG (arthritis, monoclonal gammopathy, carcinoma, and multiple myeloma) are usually found in an older age group, so that younger patients with PG should be evaluated for the presence of subclinical bowel inflammation.[14] These patients with IBD and PG tend to be in the second to third decades, and, especially in UC, the disease is usually present for at least 10 years before the onset of PG.

Pyoderma gangrenosum is more common in patients with colitis and ileocolitis, and is associated more so with extensive and active disease. This is not a hard and fast rule, however. Numerous reports of PG preceding the onset of bowel disease are available, as well as those occurring years after surgical resection.[18] Pyoderma gangrenosum has a predilection for lower extremities, pretibial (Fig. 16-1), but can occur anywhere in the body, including the abdominal wall, face, and arms. A relationship is apparent between the onset of this skin disorder and sites of trauma and needle punctures.* The typical lesion is a discrete undermined ulcer with a necrotic base (Fig. 16-2). Commonly, the lesion starts as multiple nodules that coalesce and ulcerate (Fig. 16-2). The border is surrounded by a violaceous hue, and usually is tender on palpation. Biopsy of these lesions reveals a nonspecific inflammatory response with perivascular mononuclear inflammation, which is thought to induce local ischemia leading to ulceration. Immunofluorescent staining has been variably reported as positive for immunoglobulin and

---

*Editors' note—see also Hickman, J. G. and Lazarus, G. S.: Br. J. Dermatol., 102:235, 1980; and Rees, R. S., et al.: South. Med. J., 78:283, 1985.

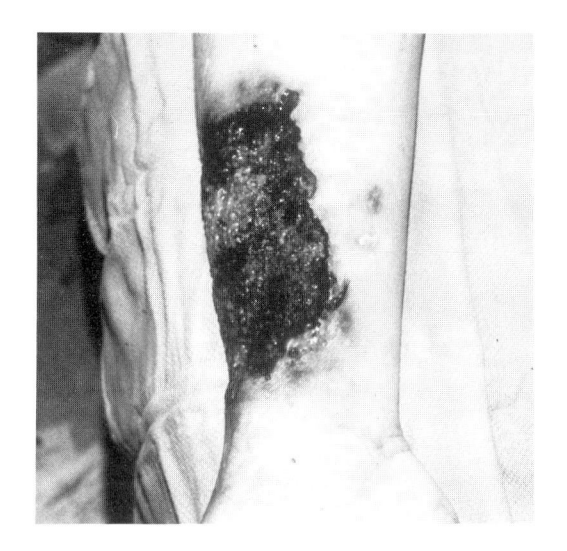

FIG. 16-2. Earlier lesions of pyoderma gangrenosum. This lesion has a more nodular appearance. Nodules coalesce and ulcerate, leaving a discrete undermined ulcer. (Courtesy of Dr. David Sachar.)

complement components, to reports of completely negative results.[17] The major rationale for using biopsy is to rule out a cutaneous vasculitis.

Therapy of PG in IBD is mandated by disease activity. Colectomy is only contemplated if medical therapy fails. Several approaches have been used, such as oral, infralesional, topical, or pulse intravenous steroids, topical antibiotics and debridement, azathioprine, cyclophosphamide, or treatment with dapsone.[19]* Also, a report of a dramatic response to periactin is available.[20]† Response to surgical treatment depends largely on the nature of the underlying disease process. Talansky et al. reported that remission was prompt when resection of moderately to severe disease was performed, but slow when the disease was mild.[21] Patients with a subtotal colectomy leaving an inflamed rectum in place may have a recurrence of PG that responds to proctectomy.[9]

Several other pustular lesions have been described in UC that may be variants of PG or represent distinct entities.[23,24] The differential diagnosis includes pustular psoriasis, dermatitis herpetiformis, bullous pemphigus, or erythema multiforme.

The entity of pyostomatitis vegetans (PV), consisting of vesicles, pustules, and vegetating plaques, was reviewed by Forman, and of 12 cases, 9 also had ulcerative colitis.[25]

Erythema Nodosum

As with pyoderma gangrenosum, erythema nodosum (EN) is associated with several systemic illnesses (such as sarcoidosis, tuberculosis, and streptococcal infections); however, the only overlap between these two skin diseases is in IBD. Erythema nodosum, in contrast to pyoderma, occurs more frequently in patients with Crohn's disease (CD) and is the most common extraintestinal manifestation in children with IBD.[26] The lesions appear to parallel disease activity more closely than those of pyoderma, and are readily treated by directing therapy towards the bowel disease itself. The lesions usually appear when, or shortly after, the diagnosis of bowel disease is made, and tend to recur with "flares." Isolated reports have shown EN occurring prior to the onset of IBD, however.[27]

The lesions characteristically occur on the anterior tibial surface as raised, erythematous, tender nodules (Fig. 16-3). They range in size

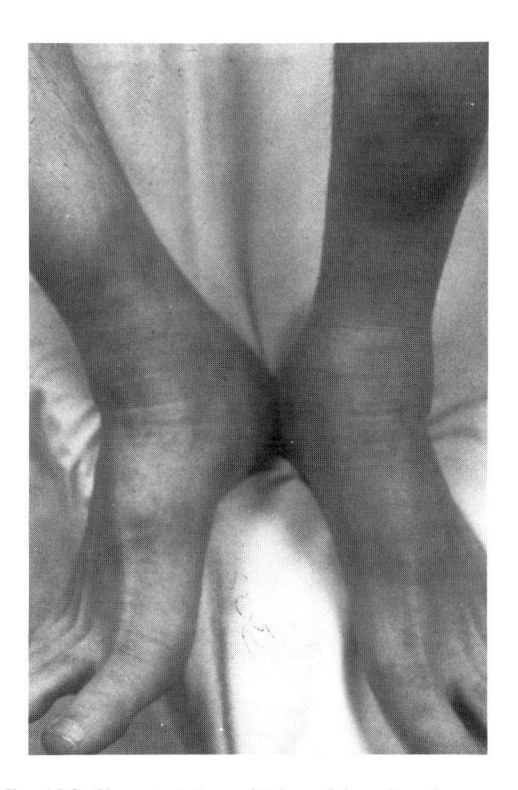

FIG. 16-3. Characteristic, multiple nodules of erythema nodosum on the anterior tibial aspect of the lower extremity. Crops of such lesions are not uncommon during periods of "flare" of the underlying bowel disease. (Courtesy of Dr. Mark Lebwohl.)

*Editors' note—see also Saffouri, B., et al.: Dig. Dis. Sci., 29:183, 1984; Jennings, J. L.: J. Am. Acad. Dermatol., 9:575, 1983; Read, A. E.: Q. J. Med., 55:173, 1985; and Walling, A. D., and Sweet, D.: Am. Fam. Physician, p. 159, January, 1987.
†Merck Sharp & Dohme, West Point, PA 19486

from 1 to 5 cm in diameter. Histologically, there is evidence of a vasculitis or panniculitis, indistinguishable from EN associated with other systemic disorders.

One association of note is the common finding of EN in conjunction with peripheral arthritis and uveitis.[28] In fact, EN or uveitis has been documented in roughly 50% of IBD patients with peripheral arthritis.

As mentioned previously, therapy for EN is not dissociated from therapy of the bowel disease. Steroids or sulfasalazine therapy will induce remission of EN as well. Colectomy, although not indicated for EN alone, is also effective in curing EN.

Vasculitis

Although a rare occurrence, cutaneous vasculitis has been described in IBD.[29–33] The clinical picture may be one of peripheral gangrene or skin necrosis.[29–33] Although treatment for the underlying bowel disease has been reportedly successful in abating the vasculitis, these manifestations do not appear to correlate with disease activity or severity. Steroid or anticoagulant therapy has also been used, presumably directed at circulating cryoglobulins or cryofibrinogens, with reasonable success.[29]

Cutaneous polyarteritis nodosa has been reported in 13 cases of Crohn's disease.[31] No correlation has been found with disease extent or activity, and in some cases the vasculitis is resistant to steroid therapy.[31] Circulating immune complexes have been noted in some of these patients, but are not a consistent finding. Whether these are coincidental diseases or a true extraintestinal association of IBD is unclear at present.

Granulomatous rather than leucocytoclastic vasculitis has been described in some patients with Crohn's disease and may reflect a subgroup of metastatic Crohn's (see the following.)[32] Attempts to associate these lesions with the presence of circulating immune complexes have not been successful.

Oral Mucosa

Poorly recognized but frequently reported is the finding of aphthous stomatitis in Crohn's disease (more so than in UC). The incidence of aphthous stomatitis has been reported to be as high as 10% (Fig. 16-4).[34] In contrast to idiopathic aphthous stomatitis, these ulcers often are pain-

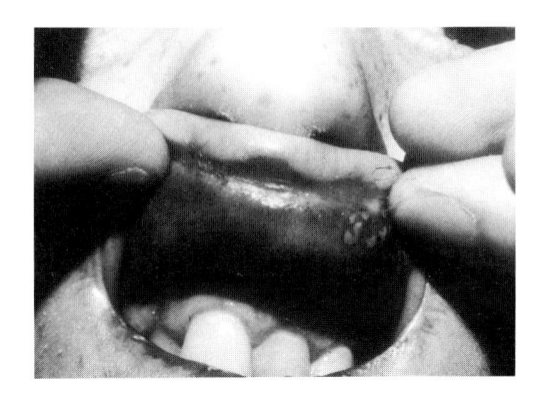

FIG. 16-4. Aphthous stomatitis.

less. They appear to parallel intestinal disease activity and remit after bowel directed therapy is initiated.

Other oral features include cobblestone lesions of the buccal mucosa indistinguishable from CD on biopsy. In older patients, these must be differentiated from denture granulomata.

Glossitis, pharyngeal ulceration or ulceration of the labia may occur secondary to malnutrition, and these are seen mostly in Crohn's disease.

Metastatic Crohn's Disease

Several groups have reported nodular ulcerating skin lesions in patients with CD that, on biopsy, reveal noncaseating granulomas (Fig. 16-5A, B, C).[35–38] As suggested by the name, metastatic Crohn's disease can occur in several sites, including bone, muscle,[35] and the skin of vulva,[36] submammary areas, or arms and thighs. Treatment is that for the underlying bowel disease, with either sulfasalazine or steroids.

Musculoskeleton

Arthritis is the most common extraintestinal manifestation of IBD, occuring in 2 to 23% of patients.[37,38,38a,b] The arthritis may take one of two forms: "colitic arthritis," a nondeforming arthritis affecting the joints of the extremities; or ankylosing spondylitis/sacroiliitis, a progressive destructive arthritis causing extreme debility. Interestingly, even though both forms of arthritis are associated with IBD, one closely parallels disease activity (colitic arthritis) whereas the other runs an independent course (ankylosing spondylitis). Other forms of musculoskeletal disease are not as prominent but include, most notably, clubbing and hypertrophic osteoarthropathy. Myalgias, osteoporosis, and

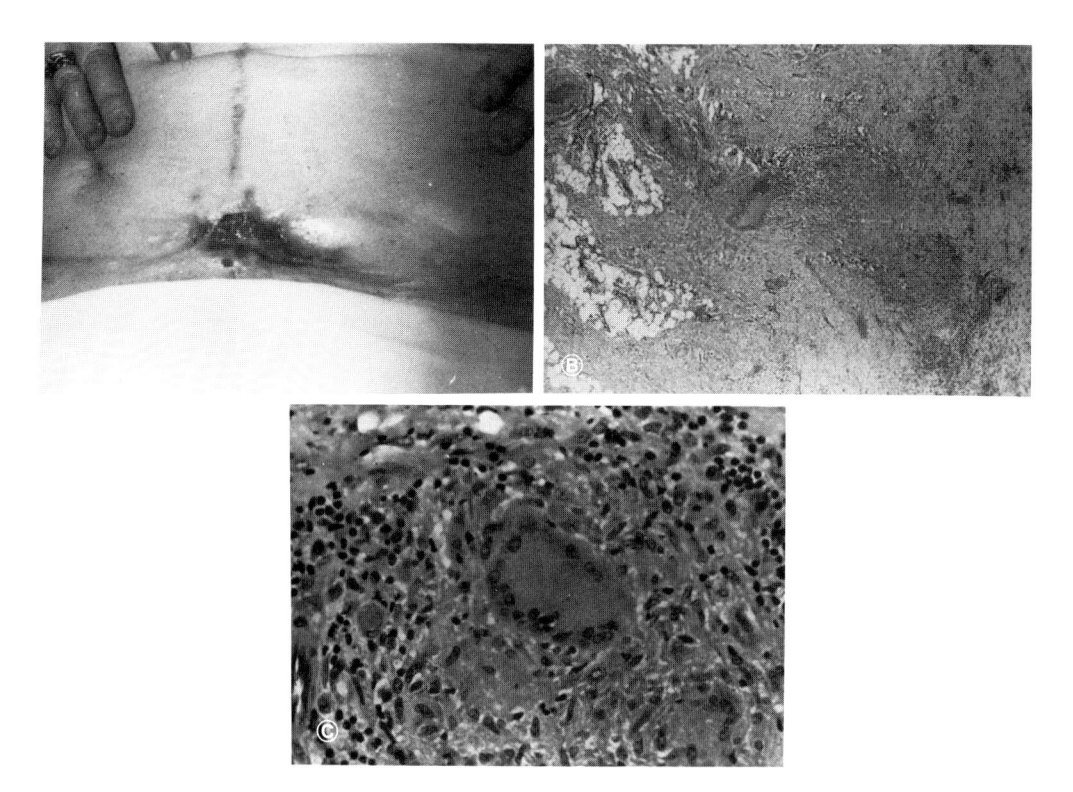

FIG. 16-5 A. Crusted, ulcerating lesion of the skin; metastatic Crohn's disease. B. Histology of the lesion described in Part A demonstrating the presence of a granuloma. C. Higher magnification of a granuloma in metastatic Crohn's disease.

similar disorders do not occur significantly more often in IBD than in other chronic debilitating diseases.

Colitic Arthritis

A frequent presentation of patients with either UC or Crohn's disease (colon > small bowel) is asymmetric, painful swelling and erythema of the knees and ankles. In fact, this association has been so well recognized that the name "colitic" or "intestinal" arthritis has become firmly established.[39–41] The arthritis is migratory and affects knees, hips, ankles, wrists, and elbows, in order of frequency.[42,43] Asymmetric swelling of the proximal interphalangeal joints of the toes was reportedly specific to IBD but it has been seen in Reiter's syndrome as well.[39] Symptoms can mimic rheumatoid arthritis but the lack of bony destruction on roentgenogram and serologic indicators of rheumatoid arthritis (although around 10 to 15% of patients with IBD may have positive rheumatoid factors) can usually rule this out.[44] The arthritis is "pauciarticular," usually affecting less than six joints,[45] and appears to parallel the course of the underlying bowel disease. Frequently, patients can predict a "flare" of their bowel disease by aching of the joints, even when the bowel symptoms are mild. As with erythema nodosum, therapy directed towards the bowel rapidly affects the arthritis as well. Despite this commonality, there have been scattered reports of arthritis bearing no relationship to the colitis and even some cases of arthritis that preceded the colitis by years.[46]

The objective criteria are helpful more for ruling out other etiologies than for aiding in the diagnosis of colitic arthritis. As already indicated, anti-nuclear antibodies (ANA), rheumatoid factors, and elevated blood uric acids are usually absent.[47] Those patients with positive rheumatoid factors probably represent either true rheumatoid arthritis occurring coincidentally, or false-positive tests.[48] The sedimentation rate is invariably elevated. Arthrocentesis reveals a turbid fluid with an inflammatory cellular component (1000 to 50,000 white blood cells, mostly neutrophils) and poor mucin clot. Sugar and protein are normal, and bacteria and rheumatoid factors are absent.[49] A biopsy of the synovium shows only a nonspecific mononuclear cell inflammatory response without significant destruction.[50]

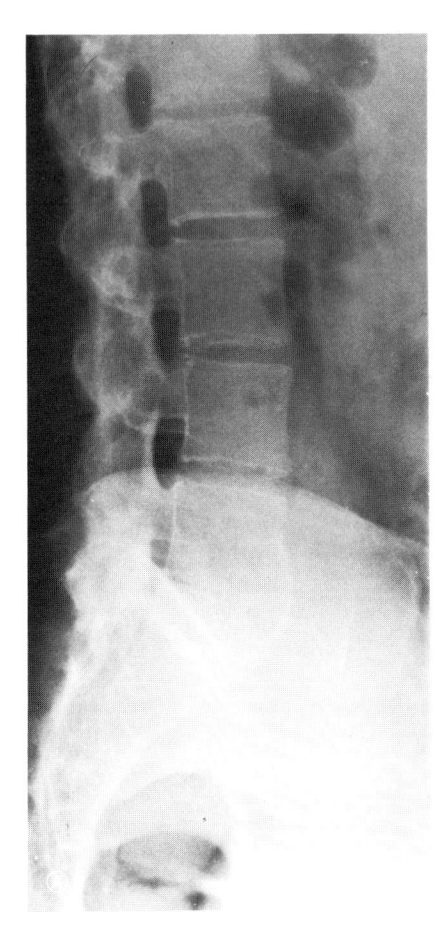

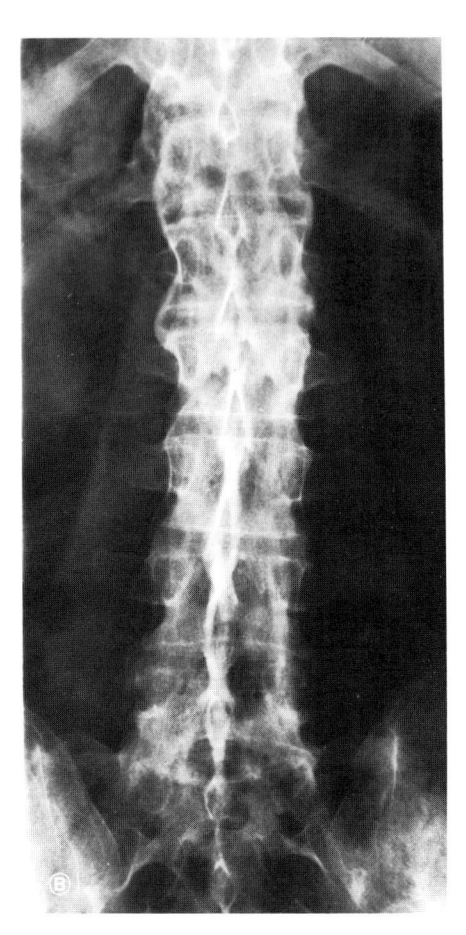

FIG. 16-6. Ankylosing spondylitis in association with sacroiliitis; sclerosis of sacroiliac joints characterized by increased bone density.

As mentioned previously, a striking association exists between colitic arthritis and erythema nodosum and iritis. One or both of these occurs in up to 50% of IBD patients with peripheral arthritis.[28] Therapy directed towards the bowel is usually sufficient for treating the arthritis. Salicylates can be used as a temporary measure, with steroids reserved for the most severe cases. Although the arthritis is cured after colectomy, it should never be the single indicator for such a course of action.

Ankylosing Spondylitis

Like pyoderma gangrenosum, ankylosing spondylitis has a significant association with UC. While patients with UC have a 30-fold greater (2 to 6%) incidence for ankylosing spondylitis than the normal population,[51-52] a significant number of patients with ankylosing spondylitis (10 to 20%) also have UC.[53-54] Several differences exist, however, between the ankylosing spondylitis associated with UC and either the idiopathic variety or that associated with Reiter's syndrome or psoriasis. The ratio of male-to-female is roughly 8 or 9:1 in the idiopathic form,[51] whereas it approaches 40% in UC. In addition, the disease appears to be less severe in UC, usually ceasing before full ankylosis occurs. In addition, the upper vertebrae (cervical and thoracic) are spared in UC (Fig. 16-6). Similarities include the symptom complex of morning stiffness, low back pain, stooped posturing, and the increased risk of aortic valve disease and conduction defects.[55] An association also appears to exist with peripheral arthropathy (20%).[53]

Sacroiliitis (Fig. 16-7) is more common, occurring in roughly 15% of patients with IBD as determined by roentgenogram.[45] The incidence increases to 68% if more sensitive techniques for diagnosis (that is, bone scans) are used.[56] It should be noted, however, despite radiologic evidence of the disease, the majority of these patients are asymptomatic.

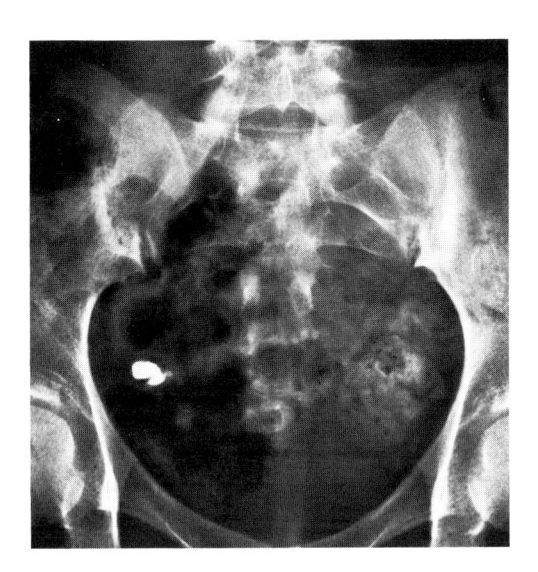

FIG. 16-7. Sacroiliitis.

Laboratory diagnosis of ankylosing spondylitis/sacroiliitis, other than by roentgenogram is partly dependent on HLA typing. Patients with ankylosing spondylitis are almost invariably HLA-B27 positive (90%),[51,52] 5 to 10% of B27 positive individuals develop ankylosing spondylitis (200 times greater than the normal population).[51,52] Although no increased incidence of HLA B27 occurs in patients with IBD, the presence of HLA-B27 greatly increases their risk of developing ankylosing spondylitis. Despite this, about 20% of IBD patients with ankylosing spondylitis are B27 negative.[51] These patients are clinically indistinguishable from those who are B27 positive but it is hoped, by determining the pathogenesis of the arthritis in such patients, that one will be able further to understand the idiopathic variety as well.

The treatment of ankylosing spondylitis is notoriously poor in IBD. Salicylates and associated anti-inflammatory medications help relieve pain and stiffness but do not arrest the disease process. Physical rehabilitation is usually the best approach. Even steroids and irradiation, which have had success in treating the idiopathic variety, are not successful in IBD. In contrast to peripheral arthritis, colectomy is not associated with resolution of symptoms of ankylosing spondylitis and, in fact, may be associated with progression of the disease.

Pelvic Osteomyelitis

Pelvic osteomyelitis occurs as a direct extension of enteric fistulae in patients with Crohn's disease. To our knowledge, nine cases have been reported to date,[57-60] usually associated with psoas abscesses and extension into the hip joint. Anaerobic organisms, such as B. fragilis, peptostreptococcus, and C. perfringens, are usually responsible. Aggressive antibiotic therapy accompanied by adequate surgical drainage is required.

Hypertrophic Osteoarthropathy (Clubbing)

Clubbing is only one form of hypertrophic osteoarthropathy, the others being synovitis and painful periostosis with new bone formation and autonomic dysfunction (sweating of palms and soles).[61-63] Clubbing, although usually not painful or associated with morbidity, is common in Crohn's disease (32 to 58%),[61,62] with a lower incidence in ulcerative colitis (14.5%) and proctitis.[63] The incidence of the other forms of hypertrophic osteoarthropathy is significantly lower, relegated to case reports.[64,65]

A study by Kitis et al. documented a strong correlation of clubbing with disease activity, and evidence exists that clubbing may regress after surgical treatment.[63] Clubbing is more prominent in Crohn's disease affecting the proximal bowel and appears to correlate with the degree of fibrosis in the area.

Renal and Genitourinary Tract

In patients with ulcerative colitis or Crohn's disease, diarrhea, water and electrolyte losses, and malabsorption can all lead to changes in the composition of the urine. Therefore it is not surprising to see renal complications in these diseases. It should be stressed that the lesions (other than amyloidosis) are really *direct complications* of the disease, rather than true extraintestinal manifestations. Structural complications, such as hydronephrosis secondary to trapping a ureter in an inflammatory mass, or pneumaturia secondary to fistulae to the urinary bladder, should also be viewed as complications demanding different therapeutic approaches than one would consider for true extraintestinal manifestations.

Nephrolithiasis*

The incidence of nephrolithiasis in IBD ranges from 2 to 10%,[66-69] the higher percentages being found in Crohn's disease patients. These num-

*See also Chapter 13.

bers are dramatically greater than the incidence in the general population.[67,70] Several "risk factors" have been described for the development of kidney stones in these patients: (1) post-ileostomy, (2) significant ileal disease, and (3) extensive ileal resection. Depending on the risk factor, the patient may develop different stones, urate and oxalate being the most common. In patients with ulcerative colitis, urate stones predominate (59% of stones compared to 5 to 15% of stones in patients without IBD). Surgical intervention is important in this finding. Large ileostomy output leading to dehydration and metabolic acidosis from loss of bicarbonate in the stool can lead to supersaturation of urate in the urine. This is best demonstrated by the finding that at pH 7.0, 158 mg of urate is soluble in 100 ml of urine; however, at pH 5.0, this drops to 8 mg/100 ml.[67] Other factors can increase urate secretion (such as steroids and fever), further complicating matters.

Several series have served to underscore the role of surgical therapy in these patients. Grossman reviewed 544 patients with ileostomy and found that 2.9% had urinary stones.[67] Deren followed this up with a series demonstrating that of 163 patients with ileostomy, 7.4% had stones;[66] in contrast only 2.1% of IBD patients without such treatment had stones. Maratka described 10 patients with kidney stones, 9 of whom had ileostomies.[68] Besides fluid loss, sodium, magnesium, and citric acid losses through the ileostomy increase the insolubility of calcium.[71] The combination of these events all result in calcium urate and calcium phosphate precipitation and stone formation.

Although urate stones are frequently seen in Crohn's disease, oxalate stones appear to be more common, with good pathophysiologic correlations. Earlier studies had claimed that hyperoxaluria was common in Crohn's disease and accounted for the increased incidence of such stones. Subsequent studies have been unable to support this conclusion, however.[72] In 123 patients with IBD, 9 out of 62 hyperoxaluric patients had stones, but 14 out of 61 patients with normal oxalate levels also had stones. A more plausible explanation has been put forth by Dobbins and Binder.[73] Extensive ileal resections or significant ileal disease leads to fat malabsorption that binds calcium. The decrease in available free calcium allows free oxalate to enter the colon and be absorbed systemically. Patients with an ileostomy (no colonic oxalate absorption) never get oxalate stones, a finding that supports this model. Other urinary stones noted in IBD include pyrophosphate stones that are secondary to infections from indwelling catheters.

Initial medical therapy of renal calculi complicating IBD is similar to the approach in "normal" patients with kidney stones, that is, I. V. hydration, pain control, and alkalinization of urine (especially with urate stones). The control of ostomy losses is imperative.

Because nephrolithiasis is relatively common in IBD, it should always be suspected in a patient who complains of severe abdominal pain that is not characteristic of their usual ileitis or colitis pain. Frequently this pain is out of proportion to the abdominal findings, bowel sounds are hypoactive, and the number of bowel movements is decreased.

Amyloid

The incidence of amyloid in IBD varies according to whether premortem (1%) or postmortem studies (25%) are quoted.[38,74] Amyloid is more frequently associated with Crohn's disease, with only rare documentation of this disorder in ulcerative colitis. Amyloid has a strong predilection for the kidney in this association and is listed as one of the causes of death in Crohn's disease.[75] Patients with severe hypoalbuminemia but without sufficient bowel inflammation and malabsorption to account for this, should undergo renal biopsy for amyloid after establishing the degrees of renal protein loss and renal insufficiency. Amyloid itself may affect the bowel causing mucosal ulceration, but it is usually not confused with Crohn's disease.[76] Amyloid was noted to remit in one patient with Crohn's disease after surgical resection of the grossly diseased bowel.[77]

Obstructive Hydronephrosis in Crohn's Disease

A review of this entity was published by Present et al. and described an incidence of 10 in a series of 150 patients.[78] The hydronephrosis is usually right-sided and results from a retroperitoneal inflammatory mass caused by a localization of Crohn's ileitis. The hydronephrosis is easily demonstrated by ultrasonography and is potentially reversible after surgical resection of the affected bowel and the associated mass. Rarely the lesion may be left-sided or bilateral, and result from underlying Crohn's colitis.

Ocular

Ocular manifestations occur in roughly 10% (ranging from 1 to 12%) of patients with IBD,[79] and consist of uveitis, episcleritis, or conjunctivitis. These lesions are frequently independent of disease activity, and may be the cause of significant morbidity. As mentioned earlier, these eye lesions are associated with other extraintestinal manifestations, particularly arthritis and erythema nodosum.

Uveitis and Iritis

Although the incidence of this complication (0.5 to 3%) is lower than that of episcleritis, its potential sequelae are more serious.[80,81] Patients present with the acute onset of blurred vision, headaches, and eye pain.[80,81] Recurrent episodes are common.[82] The onset of uveitis can occur prior to, during, or after the diagnosis of IBD has been made,[83] although some groups have claimed a correlation with severe disease activity.[84]

Diagnosis is achieved by slit lamp examination. Perilimbic edema, cells, and "flare" in the anterior chamber, plus conjunctival injection are uniform findings (Fig.16-8), and are bilateral in approximately 50% of instances. Therapy must be instituted rapidly to prevent the complications of scarring and blindness, local therapy being the treatment of choice.[85] Pupillary dilatation, using atropine or mydriasil, relieves the iridospasm. Topical steroids reduce the inflammatory cellular component, oral steroids being reserved for the most severe cases.[86] Although the evidence is not clear regarding any correlation with disease activity, these ocular lesions have improved following colectomy. In fact, in a study by Billson, just under 50% of affected patients had a complete remission postoperatively.[84] As already discussed, however, colectomy is rarely a treatment of choice for any extraintestinal manifestation.

An interesting observation was made in one series in which slit lamp studies were performed on 26 children with IBD (19 with CD, 7 with UC) who were asymptomatic of any ocular problems.[87] Six of them had cells and "flares" in the anterior chamber that resolved without therapy. It should be stressed that these children were asymptomatic so that any therapeutic extrapolation to symptomatic cases is impossible. Others have claimed, however, that some instances of symptomatic uveitis in patients with UC have remitted within 6 to 8 weeks, regardless of local therapy.[88]

Episcleritis

This is a more benign form of ocular disease, occurring in 3 to 4% of IBD patients, predominantly those with Crohn's colitis.[89] Its occurrence correlates with the presence of disease activity in the gut, but is not related either to its degree or to the extent of disease. Clinically, the patients commonly present with mild symptoms of scleral injection/irritation (Fig. 16-9), burning, and increased secretions, but the lesion may be asymptomatic thus causing its reported incidence to be lower than the true incidence. Topical steroids are an effective treatment, as is therapy directed at the underlying bowel disease.

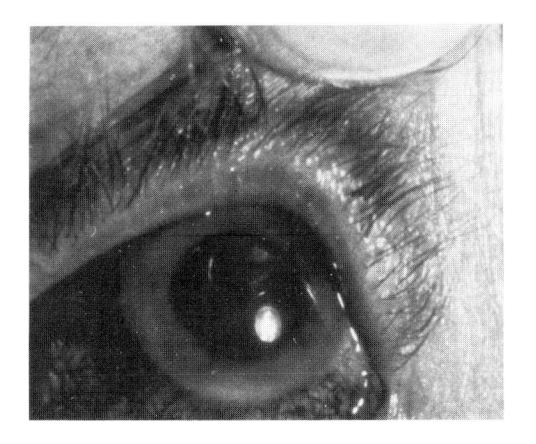

FIG. 16-8. Perilimbic edema, conjunctival injection and corneal cloudiness in a patient with uveitis and IBD.

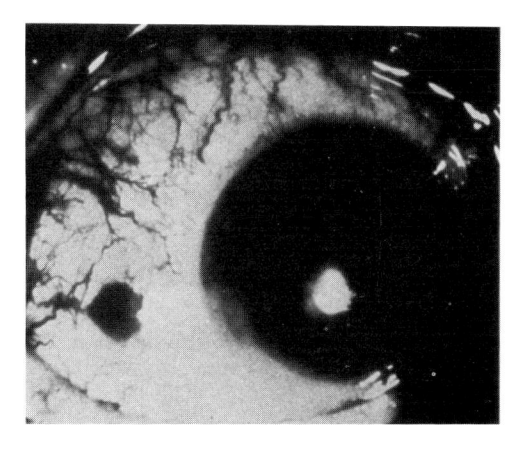

FIG. 16-9. Scleral injection caused by episcleritis. Such patients respond well to topical steroids.

Miscellaneous Ocular Lesions

Conjunctivitis is a frequent, albeit nonspecific, finding in IBD,[90] but whether it is a true association with IBD has yet to be demonstrated. Keratitis is an unusual complication, and may result in corneal ulceration.[91] Topical steroids and an eye patch are usually effective treatments.

Fortunately, retrobulbar neuritis is rare in IBD, because it is a serious lesion. It affects the optic nerve and may cause scarring and loss of vision. For treatment, systemic steroids are used. Cataract formation may complicate prolonged steroid therapy for IBD.

Hematologic and Vascular Complications

Although anemia secondary to GI blood loss is the most consistent hematologic abnormality seen in IBD, nutritional anemias and anemias secondary to autoantibody production have been reported. Hematologic complications affecting the coagulation pathway can result in an increased incidence of deep vein thrombosis, occurring in 6 to 39% of patients in various series.[92,93] This manifestation is of particular importance as it is the third leading cause of death in ulcerative colitis, after peritonitis and cancer. Less commonly, vasculitides have been noted (see earlier and the following), occurring either de novo or in association with cryoglobulins.

Anemia

As stated previously, the most common form of anemia in IBD is a result of chronic blood loss with associated iron deficiency. The anemia of chronic disease, and nutritional anemias (for example B_{12} deficiency caused by resection of ileum, significant ileal disease, or folate deficiency with more proximal disease, or resulting from sulfazaline therapy) also occur but with much less frequency.[94]

Autoimmune hemolytic anemias have been reported in approximately 25 cases of UC.[95–99] These anemias were all Coombs positive by direct assay.[95] No correlation of these with disease activity or duration was apparent,[99–102] although most patients had universal colitis.[95] Some patients with IBD have had documented hemolytic anemias prior to the onset of the intestinal disease,[99] or the anemia has presented after colectomy.[102] The confounding factor in many of these cases has been the use of sulfasalazine, known to cause hemolysis in G6PD deficient individuals,[103] as well as Coombs positive anemias.[104] In addition, several patients with IBD and hemolysis have been septic, disseminated intravascular coagulation accounting for their hemolytic picture.

Therapy of the autoimmune anemia complicating IBD involves a stepwise approach. Initially, high doses of steroids are used, followed by splenectomy in those patients who do not respond to steroids. Total proctocolectomy is reserved for severe cases, where both the colitis and hemolytic anemias are poorly controlled.

Coagulopathy and Deep Vein Thrombosis

Several abnormalities of coagulation have been described in IBD that lead to a hypercoagulable state; for example increase of factors V and VIII, thrombocytosis, and accelerated thromboplastin III levels.[105–108] This background, in association with the fact that patients with IBD are frequently bedridden, septic, or in the perioperative period, can result in an increased incidence of deep vein thrombosis. Autopsy series have described an incidence of thrombosis as high as 39%,[93] although figures in clinical series are generally lower (1 to 7%).[92,108a] Bargen and Barker reported both a clinical and an autopsy series in ulcerative colitis.[92] The incidence in live patients was 18 out of 1500, whereas 14 out of 43 autopsy cases had evidence of deep vein thrombosis. The affected sites are commonly the lower extremities and pelvic veins, but other great veins and organs have been affected including the portal vein,[108b] cerebral veins,[108c] and veins in the lungs, kidneys, and spleen.[92,93] Arterial thromboses are rare.[109]

Vasculitis*

Arteritis of great vessels (aorta, and subclavian) has been described in patients with Crohn's disease or ulcerative colitis.[110–112] As in Takayasu's disease, neurologic symptoms are prominent. Pulmonary vasculitis also has been reported by two groups, the diagnosis being established by transbronchial biopsy;[113] this process was responsive to steroid therapy. As mentioned earlier, cutaneous vasculitis and peripheral gangrene, on the basis of idiopathic vasculitis, polyarteritis nodosa,[31] or cryoglobulins/cryofibrinogens, have been noted in scattered

---

*Editors' note—see also Talbot, R. W., et al.: Mayo Clin. Proc., *61*:140, 1986.

case reports,[29] but any relationship of these syndromes to extent, severity, or duration of disease is, as yet, unestablished.

Bronchopulmonary Abnormalities

Of interest is the description of abnormal pulmonary function in patients with IBD. A study by Eade et al. reported significant reduction in diffusing capacity without other abnormalities, using a correction for anemia.[114,115] Similar, previous studies had shown no significant differences from normal on averaging the calculated values of pulmonary function.[116] Five patients in the latter series had lowered DLco (lung transfer factor) values, however, suggesting that ongoing alveolitis, pulmonary vasculitis, or recurrent pulmonary emboli might have been present. Although the lowered values did not correlate with the IBD activity, a positive correlation appeared with its extent and duration. No relationship existed with sulfasalazine therapy.

Despite these reports, the actual incidence of pulmonary disease is low in IBD.* A report by Kraft et al. described 6 patients (5 with UC, 1 with CD) with chronic bronchiectasis and bronchitis.[117] No relation to disease activity was noted. Other pulmonary complications include a report of fibrosing alveolitis in two patients.[118] It should be noted, however, that this entity has also been described as a complication of sulfasalazine use.[119-120] Pulmonary vasculitis, mentioned previously in IBD,[113] may be similar to other idiopathic pulmonary vasculitides and only occurs by chance in patients with IBD, because there is no relation to the activity or extent of the intestinal disease.

Pleuropericarditis

Like pulmonary disease, the incidence of pleuropericarditis in IBD is low. In fact, in the review of 700 patients by Greenstein et al., no case of pleuropericardial disease was found.[6] Twenty cases have been described in the literature, however, occurring mainly in patients with colonic disease.[121-126] In general, the condition did not correlate well with disease activity or extent. Aspirin and nonsteroidal anti-inflammatory agents were effective in some of these patients,[121] but the majority required steroid therapy to resolve the syndrome;[122-124] in 2 cases pericardial drainage was necessary.[125,126] Although some of these examples may have been a result of intercurrent viral illnesses, a few paralleled "flares" of the bowel disease, suggesting a relationship.

Metabolic and Endocrine Manifestations

IBD, particularly Crohn's disease, may be associated with malnutrition and, in the younger age group, short stature and failure to thrive. Appropriate nutritional therapy can reverse many of these problems, as detailed in Chapters 12, 23, and 24.[127-129]

No endocrinologic abnormality has been defined in IBD, although several studies by Janerot have detected patients with UC and a history of hyperthyroidism (11 out of 300, or 3.7%, compared to a control incidence of 0.8%).[130-132] Follow-up studies revealed minor abnormalities in I[131] uptake and thyroid binding globulin, but these were not associated with overt thyroid disease.[132]

Hepatobiliary Tract

The most frequent and serious extraintestinal manifestations in IBD occur in the liver and biliary tract. These complications do not appear to correlate with disease activity, duration, or severity, with the exception of fatty infiltration of the liver that occurs, as in other chronic illnesses, in the sicker, more debilitated, and malnourished patients. The incidence of hepatobiliary complications ranges from 5 to 95% in various series,[133-136] depending on whether the studies were performed on autopsy, biopsy, or clinical/laboratory series. Because of the patchy nature of some of the hepatic lesions, wedge biopsies at laparotomy offer a better indication of the true incidence. The hepatic complications include fatty liver, "pericholangitis," chronic active hepatitis, granulomatous hepatitis, and cirrhosis. Those affecting the biliary tract include sclerosing cholangitis, cholangiocarcinoma, and gallstones.

Fatty Liver

Fatty infiltration of the liver appears to be more a direct complication of the underlying bowel disease than a true extraintestinal manifestation. Fat malabsorption, sepsis, protein-losing enteropathy, malnutrition, and steroids are all associated with fatty liver, although some reports suggest that other factors also may play a

---

*Editors' note—see also Bonniere, P., et al.: Gut, 27:919, 1986; Walleart, E., et al.: Chest, 87:313, 1985; and Pasquis, P., et al.: Respiration, 41:56, 1981.

role in IBD.[137] The incidence of fatty liver ranges from 15 to 90%, with relatively equal frequencies in Crohn's disease and ulcerative colitis. The overwhelming majority of patients are asymptomatic, with only incidental hepatomegaly on examination. "Liver" enzymes and serum bilirubin are usually within the normal range, although elevations of serum alkaline phosphatase have been reported. In these cases, associated "pericholangitis" may have been present to account for this finding.

"Pericholangitis"

Considerable debate is still going on about whether "pericholangitis" is a distinct entity or is always part of the syndrome of sclerosing cholangitis. The fact that it is the most common hepatic manifestation of IBD, with incidences approaching 50 to 80%, suggests that the latter probably is not so.[138,139] Sclerosing cholangitis is still rare and is associated with significant prognostic implications (see the following). Patients with "pericholangitis" are usually asymptomatic, although there have been reports of acute cholestasis mimicking acute viral hepatitis as well as recurrent cholangitis. Once again, the overlap with intrahepatic sclerosing cholangitis makes it difficult to define the cases of symptomatic "pericholangitis" with concomitant hepatic lesions.* In general, "pericholangitis" runs an independent course from the underlying bowel disease.

Histologically, "pericholangitis" is a portal triaditis with acute inflammation surrounding the portal venules, bile ductules, and lymphatics (Fig. 16–10).[138] Centrilobular hepatic cholestasis may also be present.[138] With chronicity of disease, progressive fibrosis may develop periportally that then extends into the hepatic parenchyma and eventuates in cirrhosis and portal hypertension.[138] Because the earlier lesions may be patchy, random percutaneous liver biopsies may not be sufficient to make the diagnosis. Laboratory abnormalities in the early stages are minor, with only elevations in serum alkaline phosphatase. Bilirubin elevations may be seen in the cholestatic phase but these are uncommon.

Despite the high incidence of "pericholangitis" in IBD, several groups have recommended that if its presence is suspected, a liver biopsy and ERCP should be performed to rule out concomitant sclerosing cholangitis.[140–141] An association exists between the two entities in that 30 to 50% of patients with sclerosing cholangitis

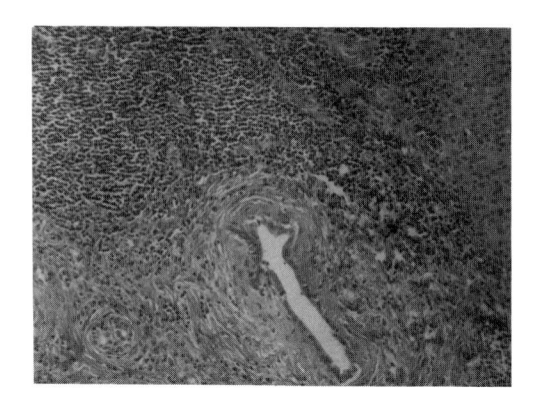

FIG. 16-10. "Pericholangitis" (intrahepatic sclerosing cholangitis) is present in biopsy specimen, with a significant portal and periportal inflammatory reaction that partially occludes the duct. (Courtesy of Dr. Fenton Schaffner.)

have intrahepatic pericholangitis.[140] Because no specific therapies exist for either of these disorders, however, and the prognostic implications of asymptomatic sclerosing cholangitis are not yet appreciated, arguments can be made against such an approach. Therapy for pericholangitis is usually not indicated, but steroids and tetracycline have been used without reproducible success.[142,143]

Chronic Active Hepatitis

An association with chronic active hepatitis has been well documented in ulcerative colitis, occurring in up to 1% of cases, but not in Crohn's disease. In series of patients with chronic active hepatitis, between 4 to 30% had concomitant UC.[144] Although there may be some associated immunologic aberration accounting for both diseases, some of the overlap may relate to chronic active hepatitis from non-A non-B, transfusion-induced viral hepatitis. No good correlation is apparent between disease activity and progression of the liver disease. Unfortunately, a significant number of these patients go on to develop cirrhosis, portal hypertension, and varices with the associated increased mortality.

Cirrhosis

Cirrhosis in IBD has a reported incidence of 1.5%.[145] As noted above, several potential pathways for the development of cirrhosis in these patients exist, namely chronic active hepatitis,

---

*Editors' note—see also Wee, A., and Ludwig, J.: Ann. Intern. Med., *102*:581, 1985; and Ludwig, J., et al.: Hepatology, *6*:560, 1986.

sclerosing cholangitis, and "pericholangitis." Many patients remain asymptomatic from their underlying liver disease until they have developed cirrhosis and its associated complications, portal hypertension, varices, and ascites. Obviously, the diagnosis of cirrhosis carries significant prognostic implications and, in fact, survival rates for patients with both IBD and cirrhosis are lower than for cirrhosis alone.[146]

Granulomatous Hepatitis

Granulomatous hepatitis may exist as an independent idiopathic entity or be associated with other granulomatous diseases (such as sarcoid and tuberculosis), with drugs, or toxins.[147] Granulomatous hepatitis has rarely been reported in Crohn's disease and is usually a benign complication responsive to steroid therapy.[148] Hepatomegaly, fevers and, occasionally, cholestasis may be the presenting symptom, with minor elevation of the alkaline phosphatase. Sequelae are rarely seen from this disorder.

Sclerosing cholangitis

This is one of the most serious complications of IBD occurring in 1 to 4% of patients,[149–150] with a predilection for patients with UC, although it may occur in Crohn's disease.[150] While a primary idiopathic form of sclerosing cholangitis has been found, in studies of patients with SC up to 70% have concomitant IBD. The finding of sclerosing cholangitis has a poor prognosis, with progression to hepatic failure and death within 5 to 10 years.[151] Laparotomy is important in cases where a solitary biliary stricture is seen, to rule out the presence of cholangiocarcinoma, which can have a similar cholangiographic appearance.[152] No strong association exists between sclerosing cholangitis and cholangiocarcinoma.

Sclerosing cholangitis has extrahepatic (Fig. 16–11) and intrahepatic forms, and these two forms may coexist, as discussed previously. Patients present with the classic symptoms of cholangitis: fever, jaundice, and right upper quadrant pain, plus abnormalities of transaminases, bilirubin, and alkaline phosphatase values. Progression to cirrhosis is common. Unfortunately, no adequate medical therapeutic regimen has been described, as both steroids and antibiotics have had limited success. Hepatic allografting is being used in patients with advanced disease.

Two groups have described unusual courses in certain patients with either sclerosing cholangitis or "pericholangitis." Schrumpf et al. evaluated 15 patients with pericholangitis proven by a biopsy using ERCP.[153] None of the 15 had sclerosing cholangitis, but 2 out of 9 went on to develop cirrhosis over a 5 year period. The remainder showed no signs of progression, however. Freese et al. described 2 cases in whom sclerosing cholangitis was diagnosed early and aggressively treated with a combination of steroids and 6-mercaptopurine.[154] Clinical and laboratory improvement was noted in both patients.

The pathogenesis of sclerosing cholangitis is poorly understood. The initial hypotheses of portal bacteremia or toxins have not been proven. An immune mediated injury is more at-

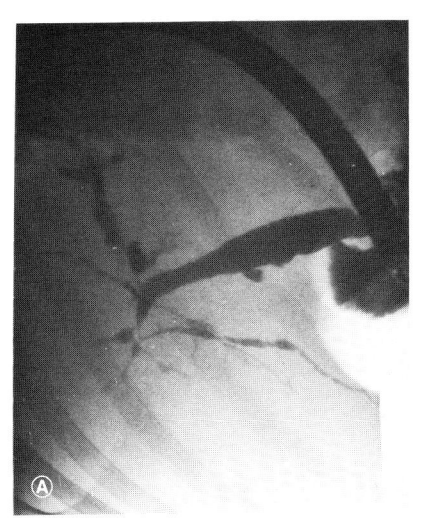

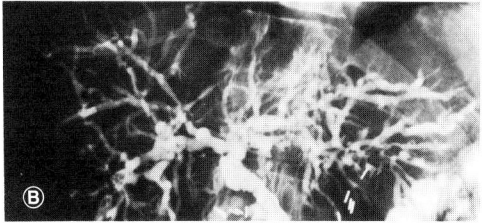

Fig. 16.11 A and B: Cholangiographic findings of sclerosing cholangitis; multiple strictures and areas of dilatation. (Courtesy of Dr. J. B. Kirsner.)

tractive because it may be associated with other "autoimmune" disorders (such as thyroiditis), but no direct evidence for this is available.

Cholangiocarcinoma

Adenocarcinoma of the gallbladder or bile ducts has been recorded by some to occur in 0.4 to 1.4% of patients with IBD,[155] which is a 10 to 20 times greater incidence than the normal population. As with sclerosing cholangitis there is a predilection for these tumors to occur in UC, but they have been found in Crohn's disease as well. Unlike gallbladder cancer in the normal population, those that occur in association with IBD are not associated with chronic cholelithiasis (see also Chap. 15 for greater detail).

Symptoms of right upper quadrant pain, jaundice, and weight loss are common, although 25% of these tumors are diagnosed only at autopsy. As mentioned previously, patients with solitary biliary strictures on ERCP should undergo laparotomy to rule out the presence of cholangiocarcinoma.

Gallstones*

In IBD, incidence of cholelithiasis is only increased in patients with terminal ileal disease, or post-ileal resection, in whom bile salt malabsorption is present.[156] The incidence of gallstones in such patients is between 30 to 35%, whereas the incidence in those with colonic disease alone is equivalent to that in a normal matched population; loss of bile salts leads to changes in bile saturation and predisposes these individuals to stone formation.

Therapy Related

Although the therapeutic armamentarium for IBD is limited, the potential and real side effects of these medications are great. Several "extraintestinal" complications have been recognized as drug related rather than disease related, and there is considerable overlap in terms of the organ systems involved. When such complications develop it is imperative that medications be suspect so that appropriate changes in therapy can be instituted before irreversible damage occurs.

*See also chapter 13.

Sulfasalazine*

By itself, sulfasalazine can result in complications in several organ systems including the skin, lung, liver, joints, blood, testes, and the GI tract. In fact, some of the more unusual extraintestinal manifestations described in the preceding text may actually be intimately related to this drug, rather than to the underlying bowel disease. Of note is the finding that most complications occur in slow acetylators and at high dose.[157] Although there is no association of erythema nodosum or pyoderma gangrenosum with sulfasalazine therapy, urticaria, exfoliative dermatitis, and toxic epidermal necrolysis have been associated with this drug.[158] Several cases of interstitial pulmonary fibrosis,[119-120] indistinguishable from that seen in some patients with UC, has been well characterized, as have scattered pulmonary infiltrates with circulating eosinophilia, the so-called "sulfasalazine lung."[119] Hepatotoxicity related to sulfasalazine is rare.[159] It either consists of a granulomatous hepatitis or mild nonspecific reactive changes. This complication is thought to be caused by the sulfapyridine moiety,[160] because it has been described, along with eosinophilia and rash, with other sulfonamides. Hematologic complications include Coombs positive or negative hemolytic anemias (G6PD deficient individuals), agranulocytosis, and leukopenia related to the free sulfapyridine levels in the blood. Inhibition of folate absorption is well recognized but easily rectified by additional oral folate.[161,162] Arthritis was documented in one case of a lupus-like syndrome consisting of Raynaud's phenomenon, digital vasculitis, cryoglobulins, and antinuclear antibodies, that abruptly reversed when the drug was stopped.[163]

Most important is the recognition of GI tract side effects of nausea, fevers, malaise, and diarrhea. The appropriate action in such cases would be to stop the medication, rather than increase the dose thinking that the symptoms were caused by the underlying bowel disease (see Chaps. 21 and 22).

Reversible infertility in males is another common complication of the use of this drug (see Chap. 21).

Steroids

Most steroid side effects are grossly apparent and readily distinguishable from the complications of IBD (see Chap. 21). In some instances,

*See also Chapters 21, 22, and 23.

however, steroids aggravate certain underlying problems of the disease itself. In this regard, the growth-retarding properties of steroids in children and adolescents is probably the most significant related side effect of their use (see Chaps. 12 and 23)[164] Steroids also aggravate nephrolithiasis by increasing calcium secretion into the urine, thus inducing a supersaturated state.

Hyperalimentation

The increasing use of hyperalimentation therapeutically in IBD has raised the issue of whether its documented acute effects on the liver aggravate underlying hepatic pathology associated with IBD. A study of two groups of patients with IBD given TPN was reported by Bengoa et al.[165] The findings were that both groups, namely those with and those without abnormal liver enzymes prior to TPN, had minor increases in the level of these enzymes during hyperalimentation. It was stressed, however, that the changes were reversible; of the patients studied, the four with the greatest enzyme elevations initially were subjected to liver biopsy that showed only mild, nonspecific changes. Thus, the question remains unanswered whether TPN will affect adversely any severe, existing liver pathology associated with IBD.

Immunosuppressives

In IBD, the use of azathioprine or 6-mercaptopurine has been limited to a small population of patients with Crohn's disease.[166-167] The most frequently recognized complication of this therapy, bone marrow suppression, is reversible. Hepatotoxicity, fevers, and arthralgias also have been reported, but the exact incidences are not known. The complication of acute pancreatitis should always be considered with the onset of a new abdominal pain, nausea, and vomiting,[168] and is easily diagnosed clinically and by the laboratory findings of an elevated serum amylase and abnormal amylase/creatinine clearance ratios. Fortunately, its nature is mild and it remits on withdrawal of the drug.

Extraintestinal Manifestations in Patients Without Inflammatory Bowel Disease

Although the complications seen in IBD are rare in other bowel disorders, there is an increasing awareness of some of the manifestations described in this chapter occurring in some infectious bowel diseases. Skin manifestations appear to predominate, as is illustrated by case reports of erythema nodosum in Shigella or Salmonella infections.[1,169] A recent report described three patients with active diverticulitis who presented with pyoderma gangrenosum and seronegative arthritis.[3] Yersinial infections and, more recently, C. difficile toxin-induced diarrhea have been associated with arthritis/arthralgias indistinguishable from those seen in IBD.[170,171] The finding of such extraintestinal lesions in these other bowel diseases has led to speculation on the role of bacterial antigens and toxins and systemic immune responses in the pathogenesis of these complications.

Pathogenesis of Extraintestinal Manifestations

The four possible mechanisms, probably intimately interrelated, that have been proposed to explain the occurrence of extraintestinal manifestations in IBD are: (1) immune complexes, (2) bacterial antigens and/or toxins, (3) cryoproteins, and (4) malabsorption/malnutrition. In some instances such as oxalate stones and fatty liver, nutritional losses are the obvious antecedents. The mechanisms potentially involved in other hepatic lesions, and those involved in the skin, ocular, and joint manifestations are less distinct, however.

Immune complexes appeared to be the logical cause of many of the serum sickness-like reactions. Unfortunately, although early studies did show some correlation between the presence of immune complexes and hepatic and skin manifestations,[172,173] subsequent studies have not supported this. No immune complexes have been found in the joints, liver, or skin (other than those with polyarteritis nodosa) of these patients, suggesting that other mechanisms are involved. Similarly negative results were obtained from studies evaluating the presence of bacteremias or bacterial toxins.[174] In pericholangitis and sclerosing cholangitis, portal bacteremias were thought to be etiologic.[175] Subsequent studies in man and failure to reproduce the syndrome in experimental animal models suggested that other mechanisms must be in play, however.[137] Cryoproteins may be directly responsible for some of the cutaneous vasculitides,[29] but certainly are not common enough to account for the other manifestations.

It is certainly conceivable that T-cell mediated tissue injury could account for several of these complications and for the lack of antibody and complement in the lesions. In sum, we are as ignorant in understanding the pathogenesis of the extraintestinal manifestations as we are in understanding the pathogenesis of the underlying bowel disease. Perhaps as we advance our knowledge in either of these two areas, we will shed some light on the other.

References

1. Grossman, M. E., and Katz, B.: Salmonella enteritidis enterocolitis: another cause of diarrhea and erythema nodosum. Cutis, *34*:402, 1984.
2. Ellis, M. E., Pope, J., Mokashi, A., and Dunbar, E.: Campylobacter colitis associated with erythema nodosum. Br. Med. J., *285*:937, 1982.
3. Klein, S., Mayer, L., Present, D., and Youner, K.: Extraintestinal manifestations of diverticulitis. Unpublished data.
4. McCluskey, J., Riley, T. V., Owen, E. T., and Langlands, D. R.: Reactive arthritis associated with Clostridium difficile. Aust. NZ J. Med., *12*:535, 1982.
5. Basler, R. S. W.: Ulcerative colitis and the skin. Med. Clin. North Am., *64*:941, 1980.
6. Greenstein, A. J., Janowitz, H. D., and Sachar, D. B.: The extra-intestinal complications of Crohn's disease and ulcerative colitis: A study of 700 patients. Medicine, *55*:401, 1976.
7. McCallum, D. I., and Kinmont, P. D. C.: Dermatologic manifestations of Crohn's disease. Br. Med. J., *80*:1, 1968.
8. Sparberg, M., Fennessy, J., and Kirsner, J. B.: Ulcerative proctitis and mild ulcerative colitis: a study of 220 patients. Medicine, *45*:391, 1966.
9. Mir-Madjlessi, S. H., Taylor, J. S., and Farmer, R. G.: Clinical course and evolution of erythema nodosum and pyoderma gangrenosum in chronic ulcerative colitis: A study of 42 patients. Am. J. Gastroenterol., *80*:615, 1985.
10. Marks, J.: The relationship of gastrointestinal disease and the skin. Clin. Gastroenterol. *12*:693, 1983.
11. Vreeken, J., et al.: Inflammatory bowel disease: Cutaneous manifestations. Compr. Ther., *4*:20, 1978.
12. Schoetz, D. J., Jr., Coller, J. A., and Veidenheimer, M. G.: Pyoderma gangrenosum and Crohn's disease. Eight cases and a review of the literature. Dis. Colon. Rectum, *26*:155, 1983.
13. Korelitz, B. I., and Sommers, S. C.: Pyoderma gangrenosum complicating Crohn's disease. Am. J. Gastroenterol., *68*:171, 1977.
14. Thornton, J. R., Teague, R. H., Low-Beer, T. S., and Read, A. E.: Pyoderma gangrenosum and ulcerative colitis. Gut, *21*:247, 1980.
15. Perry, H. O.: Pyoderma gangrenosum. South. Med. J., *62*:899, 1969.
16. Shatin, H.: How I treat pyoderma gangrenosum. Postgrad. Med. J., *49*:251, 1971.
17. Powell, F. C., Schroeter, A. L., Su, W. P. D., and Perry, H. O.: Pyoderma gangrenosum: A review of 86 patients. Q. J. Med., *55*:173, 1985.
18. Johnson, M. L., and Wilson, H. T.: Skin lesions in ulcerative colitis. Gut, *10*:255, 1969.
19. Soto, L. D.: Diaminodiphenylsulfone and steroids in the treatment of pyoderma gangrenosum. Int. J. Dermatol., *9*:293, 1970.
20. Gelernt, I. M., and Kreel, I.: Pyoderma gangrenosum in ulcerative colitis: Prevention of the gangrenous component. Mt. Sinai J. Med., *43*:467, 1976.
21. Talansky, A. L., Meyers, S., Greenstein, A. J., and Janowitz, H. D.: Does intestinal resection heal the pyoderma gangrenosum of inflammatory bowel disease? J. Clin. Gastroenterol., *5*:207, 1983.
22. O'Loughlin, S., and Perry, H. O.: A diffuse pustular eruption associated with ulcerative colitis. Arch. Dermatol., *114*:1061, 1978.
23. Rice-Oxley, J. M., and Truelove, S. C.: Complications of inflammatory bowel disease. Lancet, *1*:607, 1950.
24. Fenske, N. A., Gern, J. E., Pierce, D., and Vasey, F. B.: Vesiculopustular eruption of ulcerative colitis. Arch. Dermatol., *119*:664, 1983.
25. Forman, L.: The skin and the colon. Trans. St. Johns Hosp. Dermatol. Soc., *52*:139, 1966.
26. Samitz, M. H.: Skin complications of ulcerative colitis and Crohn's disease. Cutis, *16*:533, 1973.
27. Jacobs, W. H.: Erythema nodosum in inflammatory diseases of the bowel. Gastroenterology, *37*:286, 1959.
28. Kelley, M. L., Jr.: Skin lesions associated with chronic ulcerative colitis. Am. J. Dig. Dis., *7*:255, 1962.
29. Mayer, L., Meyers, S., and Janowitz, H. D.: Cryoproteins in Crohn's disease—an etiology of extraintestinal manifestations? J. Clin. Gastroenterol. (Suppl.), *3*:17, 1981.
30. Ball, G. V., and Goldman, L. N.: Chronic ulcerative colitis, skin necrosis, and cryofibrinogenemia. Ann. Intern. Med., *85*:464, 1976.
31. Goshen, J. B., Graham, W., and Lazarus, G. S.: Cutaneous polyarteritis nodosa. Report of a case associated with Crohn's disease. Arch. Dermatol., *119*:326, 1983.
32. Chalvardjian, A., and Nethercott, J. R.: Cutaneous granulomatous vasculitis associated with Crohn's disease. Cutis, *30*:645, 1982.
33. Goldgraber, M. B., and Kirsner, J. B.: Gangrenous skin lesions associated with chronic ulcerative colitis. A case study. Gastroenterology, *39*:94, 1969.
34. Mayer, L.: Oral manifestations of inflammatory bowel disease. Intern. Med. Specialist, *4*:83, 1983.
35. Lebwohl, M., et al.: Metastatic Crohn's disease. J. Am. Acad. Dermatol., *10*:33, 1984.
36. Kremer, M., Nussenson, E., Steinfeld, M., and Zuckerman, P.: Crohn's disease of the vulva. Am. J. Gastroenterol., *79*:376, 1984.
37. Tweedie, J. H., and McCann, B. G.: Metastatic Crohn's disease of the thigh and forearm. Gut, *25*:213, 1984.
38. Mountain, J. C.: Cutaneous ulceration in Crohn's disease. Gut, *11*:18, 1970.
38a. Bowen, G. E., and Kirsner, J. B.: The arthritis of ulcerative colitis and regional enteritis ("intestinal arthritis"). Med. Clin. North Am., *49*:17, 1965.
38b. Lukash, W. M., and Johnson, R. B.: The Systemic Manifestations of Inflammatory Bowel Disease. Illinois, Charles C. Thomas Publishers, 1975.
39. Bywaters, E. G. L., and Ansell, B. M.: Arthritis associated with ulcerative colitis—a clinical and pathological study. Ann. Rheum. Dis., *17*:169, 1958.
40. Hench, P. S., et al.: The problem of rheumatism and arthritis. Review of American and English literature for 1935. Ann. Intern. Med., *10*:754, 1936.
41. Wright, V., and Watkinson, G.: The arthritis of ulcerative colitis. Medicine, *38*:243, 1959.
42. Ansell, B. M.: *In* Infection and Immunology of the Rheumatic Diseases. Edited by D. C. Dumonde. Oxford, Blackwell Scientific Publications, 1976.
44. Haslock, I., and Wright, V.: Musculoskeletal complications of Crohn's disease. Medicine, *52*:217, 1973.

45. McEwen, C., Ling, C., and Kirsner, J. B.: Arthritis accompanying ulcerative colitis. Am. J. Med., *33*:923, 1962.
46. Fernandez-Herlihy, L.: The articular manifestations of chronic ulcerative colitis. An analysis of 555 cases. N. Engl. J. Med., *261*:259, 1959.
47. Miller, M. M.: Ankylosing spondylitis, Reiter's syndrome, psoriatic arthritis and arthritis of inflammatory bowel disease. Primary Care, *11*:271, 1984.
48. Allan, R. N.: Extra-intestinal manifestations of inflammatory bowel disease. Clin. Gastroenterol., *12*:617, 1983.
49. McEwen, C., et al.: The relationship of rheumatoid arthritis to its so called variants. Arthritis Rheum., *1*:481, 1958.
50. Hochberg, M. C., Feinstein, R. S., Moser, R. L., and Ryan, M. J.: Colitic arthritis (clinical conference). Johns Hopkins Med. J., *151*:173, 1982.
51. Brewerton, D. A., et al.: HLA-B27 and arthropathies associated with ulcerative colitis and psoriasis. Lancet, *1*:956, 1974.
52. Russell, A. S.: Arthritis, inflammatory bowel disease and histocompatibility antigens. Ann. Intern. Med., *86*:820, 1977.
53. Acheson, E. D.: An association between ulcerative colitis, regional enteritis and ankylosing spondylitis. Q. J. Med., *29*:489, 1960.
54. Jayson, M. I. V., Salmon, P. R., and Harrison, W. J.: Inflammatory bowel disease in ankylosing spondylitis. Gut, *11*:506, 1970.
55. McEwen, C., et al.: Ankylosing spondylitis and spondylitis accompanying ulcerative colitis, regional enteritis, psoriasis and Reiter's disease—A comparative study. Arthritis Rheum., *14*:291, 1971.
56. Wright, R., et al.: Abnormalities of the sacroiliac joints and uveitis in ulcerative colitis. Q. J. Med., *34*:229, 1965.
57. Simpson, M. B., Jr.: Pelvic-femoral osteomyelitis complicating Crohn's disease. Am. J. Gastroenterol., *79*:379, 1984.
58. Meltzer, S. S.: Granulomatous enterocolitis complicated by osteomyelitis. Am. J. Gastroenterol., *59*:77, 1973.
59. London, D., and Fitton, J. M.: Acute septic arthritis complicating Crohn's disease. Br. J. Surg., *57*:536, 1970.
60. Goldstein, M. J., et al.: Osteomyelitis complicating regional enteritis. Gut, *10*:264, 1969.
61. Fielding, J. F., and Cooke, W. T.: Finger clubbing and regional enteritis. Gut, *12*:442, 1971.
62. Perry, P. M., Evans, G. A., and Davies, J. D.: Regional ileitis, ulcerative colitis and clubbed fingers. Dis. Colon Rectum, *15*:278, 1972.
63. Kitis, G., Thompson, H., and Allan, R. N.: Finger clubbing in inflammatory bowel disease: Its prevalence and pathogenesis. Br. Med. J., *2*:825, 1979.
64. Arlart, I. P., Maier, W., Leopold, D., and Wolf, A.: Massive periosteal new bone formation in ulcerative colitis. Radiology, *144*:507, 1982.
65. Farman, J., Twersky, J., and Fierst, S.: Ulcerative colitis associated with hypertrophic osteoarthropathy. Am. J. Dig. Dis., *21*:130, 1976.
66. Deren, J. J., Porush, J. G., Levitt, M. F., and Khilnani, M. T.: Nephrolithiasis as a complication of ulcerative colitis and regional enteritis. Ann. Intern. Med., *56*:843, 1962.
67. Grossman, M. S., and Nugent, F. W.: Urolithiasis as a complication of chronic diarrheal disease. Am. J. Dig. Dis., *12*:491, 1967.
68. Maratka, Z., and Nedbal, J.: Urolithiasis as a complication of the surgical treatment of ulcerative colitis. Gut, *5*:214, 1964.
69. Gelzayd, E. A., Breuer, R. I., and Kirsner, J. B.: Nephrolithiasis in inflammatory bowel disease. Am. J. Dig. Dis., *13*:1027, 1968.
70. Boyce, W. H., Garvey, F. K., and Strawcutter, H. E.: Incidence of urinary calculi among patients in general hospitals. J. Am. Med. Assoc., *161*:1437, 1956.
71. Hockaday, J. D. R., and Smith, L. H., Jr.: Renal calculi. D. M., Chicago, Yearbook Publications, 1963.
72. Hylander, E., Jarnum, S., and Frandsen, J.: Urolithiasis and hyperoxaluria in chronic inflammatory bowel disease. Scand. J. Gastroenterol., *14*:475, 1979.
73. Dobbins, J. W., and Binder, H. J.: Importance of the colon in enteric hyperoxaluria. N. Engl. J. Med., *296*:298, 1977.
74. Werther, J. L., Shapira, A., Rubinstein, O., and Janowitz, H. D.: Amyloidosis in regional enteritis. A report of 5 cases. Am. J. Med., *29*:416, 1960.
75. Verbanck, J., et al.: Renal amyloidosis as complication of Crohn's disease. Acta Clin. Belg., *34*:6, 1979.
76. Casael, D. E., and Bocian, J. J.: Primary systemic amyloidosis simulating acute idiopathic ulcerative colitis. Am. J. Dig. Dis., *10*:63, 1965.
77. Fitchen, J. H.: Amyloidosis and granulomatous ileocolitis. N. Engl. J. Med., *292*:352, 1975.
78. Present, D., et al.: Obstructive hydronephrosis—a frequent but seldom recognized complication of granulomatous disease of the bowel. N. Engl. J. Med., *280*:523, 1969.
79. Baioco, P. J., Gorman, B. D., and Korelitz, B. J.: Uveitis occurring after colectomy and ileal rectal sleeve anastomosis for ulcerative colitis. Dig. Dis. Sci., *29*:570, 1984.
80. Hopkins, D. J., et al.: Ocular disorders in a series of 332 patients with Crohn's disease. Br. J. Ophthalmol., *58*:732, 1974.
81. Ellis, P. P., and Gentry, J. H.: Ocular complications of ulcerative colitis. Am. J. Ophthalmol., *58*:779, 1964.
82. Edwards, F. C., and Truelove, S. C.: The course and prognosis of ulcerative colitis III. Complications. Gut, *5*:1, 1964.
83. Wright, R. K., et al.: Abnormalities of the sacroiliac joints and uveitis in ulcerative colitis. Q. J. Med., *34*:229, 1965.
84. Billson, F. A., de Dombal, F. T., Watkinson, G., and Goligher, J. C.: Ocular complications of ulcerative colitis. Gut, *8*:102, 1967.
85. Korelitz, B. I., and Coles, R. S.: Uveitis (iritis) associated with ulcerative and granulomatous colitis. Gastroenterology, *52*:78, 1967.
86. Marcoul, K. L.: Ocular changes in granulomatous ileocolitis. Arch. Ophthalmol., *84*:95, 1970.
87. Daum, F., et al.: Asymptomatic transient uveitis in children with inflammatory bowel disease. Am. J. Dis. Child., *133*:170, 1979.
88. Kaufman, H.: Personal interview: Uveitis. Highl. Ophthalmol., *6*:205, 1963.
89. Jampol, L. M., West, C., and Goldberg, M. F.: Therapy of scleritis with cytotoxic agents. Am. J. Ophthalmol., *86*:266, 1978.
90. Crohn, B. B.: Ocular lesions complicating ulcerative colitis. Am. J. Med. Sci., *169*:260, 1925.
91. Petrelli, E. A., McKinley, M., and Troncale, F. J.: Ocular manifestations of inflammatory bowel disease. Ann. Ophthalmol., *14*:356, 1982.
92. Bargen, J. A., and Barker, N. W.: Extensive arterial and venous thrombosis complicating chronic ulcerative colitis. Arch. Intern. Med., *58*:17, 1936.
93. Graef, V., Baggenstoss, A. H., Sauer, W. G., and Spittel, J. A.: Venous thrombosis occurring in nonspecific ulcerative colitis. Arch. Intern. Med., *117*:377, 1966.
94. Ormerod, T. P.: Observations on the incidence and cause of anaemia in ulcerative colitis. Gut, *8*:107, 1967.

95. Altman, A. R., Maltz, C. R., and Janowitz, H. D.: Autoimmune hemolytic anemia in ulcerative colitis. Dig. Dis. Sci., 24:282, 1979.
96. Balint, J. A., Hammock, W. J., and Patton, T. B.: Association of ulcerative colitis and red blood cells coated with autoimmune antibody. Am. J. Dig. Dis., 8:537, 1963.
97. Arner, O., et al.: Autoimmune hemolytic anemia in ulcerative colitis cured by colectomy. Acta Med. Scand., 189:275, 1971.
98. Goldstone, A. H.: Autoimmune haemolytic anaemia in ulcerative colitis. Br. Med. J., 2:556, 1974.
99. Gorst, D. W., Leyland, M. J., and Delamore, I. W.: Autoimmune haemolytic anaemia and ulcerative colitis. Postgrad. Med. J., 51:409, 1975.
100. Lorber, M., Schwartz, L. I., and Wasserman, L. R.: Association of antibody-coated red blood cells with ulcerative colitis. Am. J. Med., 10:887, 1955.
101. Shashaty, G. G., Rath, C. E., and Britt, E. J.: Autoimmune hemolytic anemia associated with ulcerative colitis. Am. J. Hematol., 3:199, 1977.
102. Keene, W. R.: Uncommon abnormalities of blood associated with ulcerative colitis. Med. Clin. North Am., 50:535, 1966.
103. Das, K. M., Eastwood, M. A., McManus, J. P., and Sircus, W.: Adverse reactions during salicylazosulfapyridine therapy. N. Engl. J. Med., 289:491, 1973.
104. Bottinger, C. F., Enstedt, C., Langercrantz, R., and Nyberg, A.: The occurrence of Heinz bodies during azulfidine therapy of ulcerative colitis. Gastroenterol., 100:33, 1963.
105. Lam, A. T., Borde, I. T., Inwood, M. J., and Thompson, S.: Coagulation studies in ulcerative colitis and Crohn's disease. Gastroenterology, 68:245, 1975.
106. Lee, J. C., et al.: Hypercoagulability associated with chronic ulcerative colitis. Changes in blood coagulation factors. Gastroenterology, 54:76, 1968.
107. Talstad, I., Rootwelt, K., and Gjone, E.: Thrombocytosis in ulcerative colitis and Crohn's disease. Scand. J. Gastroenterol., 8:135, 1973.
108. Morowitz, D. A., Allen, L., and Kirsner, J. B.: Thrombocytosis in chronic inflammatory bowel disease. Ann. Intern. Med., 68:1013, 1968.
108a. Dennis, C., and Karlson, K. E.: Surgical measures as supplements to the management of idiopathic ulcerative colitis: Cancer, cirrhosis and arthritis as frequent complications. Surgery, 32:892, 1952.
108b. Capron, J. P., et al.: Gastrointestinal bleeding due to chronic portal vein thrombosis in ulcerative colitis. Dig. Dis. Sci., 24:232, 1979.
108c. Borda, I. T., Southern, R. F., and Brown, W. F.: Cerebral venous thrombosis in ulcerative colitis. Gastroenterology, 64:116, 1973.
109. Braverman, D., and Bogoch, A.: Arterial thrombosis in ulcerative colitis. Am. J. Dig. Dis., 23:1148, 1978.
110. Yassinger, S., et al.: Association of inflammatory bowel disease and large vascular lesions. Gastroenterology, 71:844, 1976.
111. Soloway, M., Moir, T. W., and Linton, D. W.: Takayasu's arteritis: Report of a case with unusual findings. Am. J. Cardiol., 25:258, 1970.
112. Chapman, R., Dawe, C., Whorwell, P. J., and Wright, R.: Ulcerative colitis in association with Takayasu's disease. Am. J. Dig. Dis., 23:660, 1978.
113. Forrest, J. A. H., and Shearman, D. J. C.: Pulmonary vasculitis and ulcerative colitis. Am. J. Dig. Dis., 20:482, 1975.
114. Eade, O. E., Smith, C. L., Alexander, J. R., and Whorwell, D. J.: Pulmonary function tests in patients with inflammatory bowel disease. Am. J. Gastroenterol., 73:154, 1980.
115. Dinakara, P., et al.: Effect of anemia on pulmonary diffusing capacity with derivation of a correction equation. Am. Rev. Respir. Dis., 102:965, 1970.
116. Johnson, N. M. I., Mee, A. S., Jewell, D. P., and Clarke, S. W.: Pulmonary function in inflammatory bowel disease. Digestion, 18:416, 1978.
117. Kraft, S. C., Earle, F. H., Roesler, M., and Eaterly, J. R.: Unexplained bronchopulmonary disease with inflammatory bowel disease. Arch. Intern. Med., 136:454, 1976.
118. McKee, A. L., Rajapaksa, A., Kalish, P. E., and Pitchumoni, C. S.: Severe interstitial pulmonary fibrosis in a patient with chronic ulcerative colitis. Am. J. Gastroenterol., 78:86, 1983.
119. Yaffe, B. H., and Korelitz, B. I.: Sulfasalazine pneumonitis. Am. J. Gastroenterol., 78:493, 1983.
120. Davies, D., and MacFarlane, A.: Fibrosing alveolitis and therapy with sulphasalazine. Gut, 15:185, 1974.
121. Patwardhan, R. V., et al.: Pleuropericarditis: An extraintestinal complication of inflammatory bowel disease. Arch. Intern. Med., 143:94, 1983.
122. Christensen, C. F.: Ulcerative colitis and pericarditis. West. J. Med., 130:560, 1979.
123. Thompson, D. G., Lennard-Jones, J. E., Swarbrick, G. F., and Brown, R.: Pericarditis and inflammatory bowel disease. Q. J. Med., 48:93, 1979.
124. Goodman, M. J., Moir, D. J., Holt, J. M., and Truelove, S. C.: Pericarditis associated with ulcerative colitis and Crohn's disease. Dig. Dis. Sci., 21:98, 1976.
125. Breitenstein, R. A., Salel, A. F., and Watson, D. W.: Chronic inflammatory bowel disease: Acute pericarditis and pericardial tamponade. Ann. Intern. Med., 81:406, 1974.
126. Rheingold, O. J.: Inflammatory bowel disease and pericarditis. Ann. Intern. Med., 82:592, 1975.
127. Kirschner, B., Voinchet, O., and Rosenberg, I. H.: Growth retardation in inflammatory bowel disease. Gastroenterology, 75:504, 1978.
128. Layden, T., et al.: Reversal of growth arrest in adolescents with Crohn's disease after parenteral nutrition. Gastroenterology, 70:1017, 1976.
129. Berger, M., Gribetz, D., and Korelitz, B. I.: Growth retardation in children with ulcerative colitis: The effect of medical and surgical therapy. Pediatrics, 55:459, 1975.
130. Jarnerot, G., Khan, A., and Truelove, S. C.: Thyroid enlargement and hyperthyroidism in ulcerative colitis. Acta Med. Scand., 197:83, 1975.
131. Jarnerot, G., Truelove, S. C., and Warner, G. T.: The daily fractional turnover of thyroxine. Acta Med. Scand., 197:89, 1975.
132. Jarnerot, G., Truelove, S. C., and VonSchenk, H.: Thyroid hormone binding proteins. Acta Med. Scand., 197:95, 1975.
133. Eade, M. N.: Liver disease in ulcerative colitis: analysis of operative liver biopsy in 138 patients having colectomy. Ann. Intern. Med., 72:475, 1970.
134. de Dombal, F. T., et al: Hepatic histological changes in ulcerative colitis; a series of 58 consecutive liver biopsies. Scand. J. Gastroenterol., 1:220, 1966.
135. Dew, M. J., Thompson H., and Allan, R. N.: The spectrum of hepatic dysfunction in inflammatory bowel disease. Q. J. Med., 48:113, 1979.
136. Logan, A. H.: Chronic ulcerative colitis; a review of 117 cases. Northwest. Med., 18:1, 1919.
137. Perrett, A. D., et al.: The liver in ulcerative colitis. Q. J. Med., 40:211, 1971.
138. Christophi, C., and Hughes, E. R.: Hepatobiliary dis-

139. Mistilis, S. P.: Pericholangitis and ulcerative colitis 1. Pathology, aetiology and pathogenesis. Ann. Intern. Med., *63*:1, 1965.
140. Schrumpf, E., and Gione, E.: Hepatobiliary disease in ulcerative colitis. Scand. J. Gastroenterol., *17*:961, 1982.
141. Chapman, R. W. G., et al.: Primary sclerosing cholangitis: a review of its clinical features, cholangiography and hepatic histology. Gut, *21*:870, 1980.
142. Rankin, J. G., et al.: The liver in ulcerative colitis. Lancet, *2*:1110, 1959.
143. Mistilis, S. P., Skyring, A. P., and Goulston, S. J. M.: Effect of long term tetracycline therapy, steroid therapy and colectomy in pericholangitis associated with ulcerative colitis. Australas. Ann. Med., *14*:284, 1965.
144. Gray, N., et al.: Hepatitis, colitis and lupus manifestations. Am. J. Dig. Dis., *3*:481, 1938.
145. Perret, A. D., et al.: The liver in Crohn's disease. Q. J. Med., *40*:187, 1971.
146. Scheuer, P. J.: Liver Biopsy Interpretation. London, Baillière and Tindall, 1973.
147. Guckian, J. C., and Perry, J. E.: Granulomatous hepatitis. An analysis of 63 cases and review of the literature. Ann. Intern. Med., *65*:1081, 1966.
148. Maurier, L. H., et al.: Granulomatous hepatitis associated with regional enteritis. Gastroenterology, *53*:301, 1967.
149. Mihas, A. A., Murad, T. M., and Hirshowitz, B. I.: Sclerosing cholangitis associated with ulcerative colitis. Am. J. Gastroenterol., *70*:614, 1978.
150. Cooperman, A. M., and Judd, E. S.: The role of colectomy in hepatic disease accompanying ulcerative and granulomatous colitis. Mayo Clin. Proc., *47*:36, 1972.
151. Cutler, B., and Donaldson, G. A.: Primary sclerosing cholangitis and obliterative cholangitis. Am. J. Surg., *117*:502 1969.
152. Way, L. W.: Surgical management of sclerosing cholangitis. Gastroenterology, *73*:357, 1977.
153. Schrumpf, E. L., et al.: Sclerosing cholangitis in ulcerative colitis. Scand. J. Gastroenterol., *15*:689, 1980.
154. Freese, D., et al.: Sclerosing cholangitis associated with inflammatory bowel disease. Clin. Pediatr., *21*:11, 1982.
155. Rankin, J. G., Skyring, A. P., and Goulston, S. M.: Liver in ulcerative colitis. Gut, *7*:433, 1966.
156. Baker, A. K., et al.: Gallstones in inflammatory bowel disease. Am. J. Dig. Dis., *19*:109, 1974.
157. Fich, A., et al.: Sulfasalazine hepatotoxicity. Am. J. Gastroenterol., *79*:401, 1984.
158. Lennard-Jones, J. E., and Powell-Tuck, J.: Drug therapy of inflammatory bowel disease. Clin. Gastroenterol., *8*:187, 1979.
159. Kanner, R. S., Tedesco, F. J., and Kalser, M. H.: Azulfidine (sulfasalazine)—induced hepatic injury. Am. J. Dig. Dis., *19*:465, 1974.
160. Losek, J. D., and Werlin, S. L.: Sulfasalazine hepatotoxicity. Am. J. Dig. Dis. Child., *135*:1071, 1981.
161. Pounder, R. E., Craven, E. R., Henthorn, J. S., and Bannatyne, J. M.: Red cell abnormalities associated with sulphasalazine maintenance therapy for ulcerative colitis. Gut, *16*:181, 1975.
162. Schneider, R. E., and Beeley, L.: Megaloblastic anemia associated with sulphasalazine treatment. Br. Med. J., *2*:1638, 1977.
163. Griffiths, I. D., and Kane, S. P.: Sulphasalazine induced lupus in ulcerative colitis. Lancet, *2*:1188, 1977.
164. McCaffery, T. D., Nasr, K., Lawrence, A. M., and Kirsner, J. B.: Severe growth retardation in children with inflammatory bowel disease. Pediatrics, *45*:386, 1970.
165. Benogoa, J. M., et al.: Pattern and prognosis of liver function test abnormalities during parental nutrition in inflammatory bowel disease. Hepatology, *5*:79, 1985.
166. Present, D. H., et al.: Treatment of Crohn's disease with 6-Mercaptopurine. A long-term randomized, double blind study. N. Engl. J. Med., *302*:981, 1980.
167. Klein, M., et al.: Treatment of Crohn's disease with azathioprine: a controlled evaluation. Gastroenterology, *66*:916, 1974.
168. Nogueira, J. R., and Freedman, M. A.: Acute pancreatitis as a complication of Imuran therapy in regional enteritis. Gastroenterology, *62*:1040, 1972.
169. Tami, L. F.: Erythema nodosum associated with Shigella colitis. Arch. Dermatol., *12*:590, 1985.
170. Leino, R., and Kalliomaki, J. L.: Yersiniosis as an internal disease. Ann. Intern. Med., *81*:458, 1974.
171. McCluskey, J., Riley, T. V., Owen, E. T., and Langlands, D. R.: Reactive arthritis associated with clostridium difficile. Aust. NZ J. Med., *12*:535, 1982.
172. Nielsen, H., Binder, V., Daugherty, H., and Sevehag, S. E.: Circulating immune complexes in ulcerative colitis. 1. Correlation to disease activity. Clin. Exp. Immunol., *31*:72, 1978.
173. Fiasse, R., et al.: Circulating immune complexes and disease activity in Crohn's disease. Gut, *19*:611, 1978.
174. Aoki, K.: Endotoxins in inflammatory bowel disease. Acta Med. Okayama, *32*:147, 1978.
175. Brooke, B. N., and Slaney, G. Portal bacteremia in ulcerative colitis. Lancet, *1*:1206, 1958.

17 · Fertility and Pregnancy in Inflammatory Bowel Disease

BURTON I. KORELITZ, M.D.

Between one and two million people have idiopathic inflammatory bowel disease (IBD) in the United States, and approximately half are women. Because both Crohn's disease and ulcerative colitis are predominantly illnesses of young people, many considerations arise regarding coincident or anticipated pregnancy. Until recently, most of the available data were based on patients observed during the 1940's and 1950's when few drugs significantly influenced the course of either disease, and experience with corticosteroids was just developing. These observations have been reviewed,[1-4] and studies supplementing the early observations now have provided answers to some important issues regarding the management of the pregnant IBD patient.

Fertility in Women

Many women with IBD wish to know if their condition will interfere with conception. Although earlier studies suggested that women with ulcerative colitis may be subfertile,[5] recent data indicate that fertility is not significantly diminished.[6-8] Similarly, while it had been claimed that Crohn's disease may decrease fertility,[9,10] this is countered by a study indicating that fertility in 54 patients with Crohn's disease was 88%, a figure not appreciably different from that of the general population.[11]

Precise data to support claims for reduced fertility in Crohn's disease patients are not available.* Such patients, of course, are subject to the same psychologic influences as are women without inflammatory bowel disease, because ovulation, libido, timing of intercourse, and nutritional and environmental factors all influence the fertility rate. More specifically, however, is the systemic impact of Crohn's disease itself; this may be manifested by fever, diarrhea, and abdominal pain, or it may be more subtle. Furthermore, the ovaries and the fallopian tubes, because of their proximity to the involved bowel (especially the right ovary and tube to the terminal ileum), may be involved in the inflammatory process, although this is rare.[12] Multiple labial or perineal abscesses and fistulas may, because of pain, interfere with intercourse, and also reduce libido, either in the patient, the husband, or both. Two studies concluded that fertility is less when

---

*Editor's comment: A study by Mayberry and Weterman (see also Mayberry, J. F., and Weterman, I. T.: Gut, 27:821, 1986), however, concluded that Crohn's disease in European women results in subfertility. Medical advice may have been partly responsible, but contraceptive practices were similar in the patients and controls and the investigators concluded that the disease was primarily responsible for the subfertility.

See also, Purrmann, J., et al.: Gut, 27:1517, 1986, who questioned the finding of the European study; and the reply by Mayberry, J. F.: Gut, 28:112, 1987, who reemphasized that fertility may be reduced, and this does not directly relate to contraceptive practices.

the Crohn's disease involves the colon than when it involves the ileum,[9,12] perhaps because of the higher incidence of perirectal and perineal complications in Crohn's colitis than in ileitis. In contrast, reduced fertility in women with ileitis, as opposed to colitis, has been reported.[10] Until recently, however, studies assessing fertility in Crohn's disease patients failed to consider certain important factors affecting fertility, such as the patient's desire for pregnancy, the age, and the marital status. Only Khosla has considered such factors when calculating fertility rates, and when this was done in 54 patients with Crohn's disease, infertility was noted in 12%, a figure that is approximately the same as in the general population.[11]* According to some observers, a possible reason for the apparently lowered fertility rate in some young women with Crohn's disease is fear. The obstetrician or gynecologist may introduce this fear by warning the patient not to become pregnant because the disease might become worse or the fetus might be damaged; such fear also may be induced by similar concerns of the gastroenterologist.* Such fear is unwarranted, however, as the subsequent observations will indicate.

Fertility in Men

Infertility in the male patient with inflammatory bowel disease caused by sulfasalazine has been well-documented.[13,14] Within two months of starting therapy with the drug, the density of the patient's semen becomes less, abnormal forms of spermatozoa develop, and motility is reduced.[15,16] Gross semen abnormalities have been observed in 86% of males taking sulfasalazine.[15] Fortunately, beginning two to three months after withdrawal of the drug, semen quality returns.[15,16] Often, managing the IBD will be difficult if the male patient is to be deprived of sulfasalazine for this reason, and another drug may be substituted if pregnancy is the priority. Because it appears that 5-aminosalicylic acid (5-ASA) does not cause the semen damage, its use, if proven to be as effective as sulfasalazine in treating inflammatory bowel disease, should solve the problem of male infertility. A reversal of male infertility on changing treatment from sulfasalazine to 5-ASA has been reported.[17,18] Folic acid deficiency reportedly has been associated with reduced male fertility, and simple addition of folic acid, 1 mg twice daily, may occasionally prove helpful. The managing gastroenterologist should share the potential problems relating to this sulfasalazine effect with the patient, but also indicate that the problem is manageable (See Table 17-1).

No information is available on the compromise of fertility in male patients directly attributable to the underlying inflammatory bowel disease itself. Diminished erection or ejaculation may occur when the rectal segment is resected for inflammatory bowel disease. Fortunately, total colonic resection rarely causes impotence and the incidence is even lower when the procedure is performed for inflammatory bowel disease and not for cancer. The age of the patient also may be important.[19]

Risk of Inheriting Inflammatory Bowel Disease

Young women, and/or their husbands, with IBD commonly seek information about the risk of inflammatory bowel disease in their offspring. As emphasized elsewhere in this book (see Chap. 1 and 6), 20% of patients have at least one blood relative who has Crohn's disease or, less often, ulcerative colitis.[20] The most common relationships are father-daughter, father-son, brother-sister, cousin-cousin (first cousins). Familial Crohn's disease occurs both in Jews and non-Jews, but many families with Crohn's disease involving more than two generations have been Jewish. In a study of Crohn's disease in New York City, 281 patients had no known relatives with inflammatory bowel disease, 36 had 1, 15 had 2, 3 had 4, and 8 members in 1 family suffered from Crohn's disease. Farmer et al. reported that 35% of Crohn's disease patients and 29% of ulcerative colitis patients had a family history of IBD.[21] The type of inheritance probably is polygenic, with varying degrees of penetration.[22] Despite familial occurrences, when giving advice on the risk of IBD in poten-

TABLE 17-1. *Guidance for the Physician Managing Male Inflammatory Bowel Disease Patients on Sulfasalazine.*

1. Make the male patient taking sulfasalazine aware of its toxic effect on sperm.
2. If the sulfasalazine is to be continued, reassure the patient that any damage to his sperm will be reversed on cessation of drug.
3. Communicate with the infertility expert being consulted by the patient and his wife whether the sulfasalazine is responsible or not.

*Editor's note: see also, Mayberry, J. F.: Gut, 28:112, 1987.

tial offspring, the patients must be reassured that the risk of such an eventuality is low, and that ulcerative colitis and Crohn's disease are *not* classic genetic disorders.

The Influence of Drug Therapy on the Course of Pregnancy

Concern about the pregnancy and its outcome are usually foremost in the mind of the patient with IBD who is pregnant or contemplating pregnancy, and the issue of the influence of the inflammatory bowel disease upon the fetus cannot be separated from the influence of the drug therapy on the IBD. Commonly, the pregnant patient with inflammatory bowel disease is advised by the obstetrician to discontinue sulfasalazine and corticosteroids in the interest of the safety of the patient and the fetus; a position that is often supported by gastroenterologists. Because, about 85% of all patients with ulcerative colitis or Crohn's disease are taking sulfasalazine, steroids, or other medications, this drug issue is a frequent and important problem.

Concerns about the outcome of pregnancy usually include prematurity, low birth weight, stillbirth, spontaneous abortion, and congenital abnormalities. With the advent of drug therapy, more subtle concerns have arisen regarding the offspring, such as mutagenicity, carcinogenicity, and teratogenicity. Previously these issues were studied primarily in experimental animals, and the results cannot be extrapolated to the human situation.*

Historically, sulfonamides have been reported to displace bilirubin from serum albumin, with the potential for the development of kernicterus. Fortunately, studies have shown that sulfasalazine only weakly displaces bilirubin from albumin,[23] and the incidence of kernicterus in offspring of mothers taking sulfasalazine is low.

Sulfasalazine has been used consistently throughout pregnancy without causing harm to the fetus or newborn. In one large series,[24] sulfasalazine did not alter the rate of spontaneous abortion, prematurity, or fetal weight in 174 patients receiving the drug either alone or in combination with corticosteroids. Baiocco and Korelitz showed that the disease activity and not the drug, probably was the determining factor in the higher complication rates seen in patients receiving sulfasalazine than in those who are not treated.[25] As a general principle, however, no drugs, including sulfasalazine, should be given to pregnant women unless the cost-to-benefit ratio clearly favors their use.*

Sulfasalazine interferes with folic acid absorption in the small bowel.[26] Folates are important to fetal development and a deficiency, especially in the early weeks of pregnancy, might cause defective nucleic acid formation, impaired cell growth, and damage to the placenta, which in turn could lead to abortion or congenital abnormalities.[27] As mentioned elsewhere (see Chap. 21), the macrocytic anemia often attributed to sulfasalazine also might be caused by interference with folic acid absorption. This possibility, therefore, should be counteracted by administration of 1mg of folic acid twice daily.

Metronidazole has been shown to be mutagenic for certain strains of salmonella, to be mildly fetotoxic, and also teratogenic in mice. Fortunately, in one study of more than 2500 pregnant women treated with metronidazole for various illnesses, the incidence of congenital abnormalities did not increase.[28] Nevertheless, the effects of this drug on the outcome of pregnancy are not completely known. Therefore, it should be used during pregnancy only if its therapeutic benefits outweigh potential endangerment to the fetus.

Studies of 6-mercaptopurine and azathioprine have indicated that pregnant rats receiving these drugs produce offspring with reduced weights, small litters,[29] and dead fetuses,[9] but fertility is normal and no tumors develop in the offspring. Although a teratogenic role has been reported in other animals,[30] reports of congenital abnormalities in humans are rare. Nevertheless, massive doses of these agents inadvertently given to humans during pregnancy have been well tolerated.[31] Healthy children have been born to patients suffering from acute or chronic leukemia, lupus nephritis, or with renal transplants, who were treated with large doses of these and other immunosuppressive drugs during pregnancy.[32,33] Several instances of successful pregnancies in patients with IBD receiving immunosuppressives also have been reported.[34] Women with inflammatory bowel disease taking 6-mercaptopurine who became pregnant against advice not to do so, and chose not to have a therapeutic abortion, usually delivered normal offspring. Concern about fertility and mutagenic effects on future offspring is frequently expressed, however. The use of cytotoxic drugs

---

*Editor's note: however, see Mackay, J. M., et al.: Gut, *27*:A1271, 1986.

*Editor's note: see also, Mackay, J. M., et al.: Gut *27*:A1271, 1986.

during the second and third trimesters causes less concern than their use during the first trimester.[35] Questions also arise about the possibly deleterious influence of immunosuppressive drugs on DNA in sperm, leading to organ malformation in the developing fetus. Although the available information supports the safety of 6-mercaptopurine in this regard,[33] male patients with inflammatory bowel disease receiving 6-mercaptopurine commonly have been cautioned to discontinue the drug if they are anticipating impregnating their wives. In these litigious times this is a reasonable approach.

Corticosteroids can increase the rate of abortions and stillbirths in mice and rats,[36] reduce litter size, and decrease DNA synthesis. They also may lead to a cleft palate,[36] exophthalmos,[36] impaired glucose homeostasis, reduced brain size, and decreased growth in neonatal animals. In humans, prematurity has been common in the offspring of patients receiving corticosteroids. Stillbirths occurred in 8 out of 34 patients in one report,[37] although this study did not take into account the effect of the underlying disease on the pregnancy. Corticosteroids have been used by pregnant women with inflammatory bowel disease and the data from two studies indicated that such use is safe. Indeed, Mogadam[24] found that patients treated with conventional therapy, including corticosteroids, had a *lower* incidence of fetal complications than the general population.[24] Although a later report suggested that fetal complications may be higher in a medically treated group,[25] this is likely to be caused by the disease activity and not the effects of corticosteroid therapy alone. Nevertheless, as with all drugs, whenever possible it is advisable *not* to give steroids to pregnant women unless this is warranted by disease severity.

Tetracycline taken by pregnant women may cause cataracts in the fetus, retard skeletal growth, and render the fetus vulnerable to fatty necrosis of the liver, pancreatitis, and possible renal damage. In addition, all antibiotic agents have been found in breast milk. Information about the effects of antibiotics on the fetus is insufficient, and the question must be raised as to whether any antimicrobial agents are safe to use during pregnancy. The safest procedure is either not to give or to discontinue the use of the antibiotic in pregnant women unless the situation is life-threatening for the mother.

Complete or partial bowel rest may be indicated in the patient who is unresponsive to conventional therapy, especially in Crohn's disease. In such circumstances, total parenteral nutrition is necessary to provide adequate caloric and nutritional requirements (see Chap. 21 and 24). Total parenteral nutrition has been used safely during pregnancy for a variety of underlying illnesses.[38-43] Because the caloric requirements are estimated on the basis of the patient's ideal weight, adjustments must be made to ensure adequate weight gain during pregnancy. Although fat emulsions are routinely used in the non-pregnant patient receiving total parenteral nutrition, their use in the pregnancy remains controversial because of the possibility of placental hypoxia, which initiates premature labor.[44] Thus, while pregnancy is not a contraindication to the use of total parenteral nutrition, a physician experienced in its use should be involved in the patient's care.

The Influence of Inflammatory Bowel Disease on the Outcome of Pregnancy

The overall outcome of pregnancy in inflammatory bowel disease patients reported by studies in the 1950's and 1960's has been favorable.[1-6,45-50] The study by Baiocco and Korelitz provides data on fetal outcome influenced by inflammatory bowel disease and its medical treatment.[25] A group of 147 pregnant patients, 77 who had Crohn's disease and 70 who had ulcerative colitis, was divided into those in whom therapeutic drugs were taken during pregnancy, the "treated group," and those in whom none was taken, the "untreated." Overall, the incidence of prematurity, stillbirths, and developmental defects was no greater than in the general population.* The incidence of spontaneous abortion, however, was 12.2%, considerably higher than that in the general population, which was 9.9%.* When the treated group was compared with those who received no therapy for inflammatory bowel disease during pregnancy, the number of premature births among the treated patients was considerably higher.

Fetal complications are more frequent in those pregnant patients with active disease, whether they have ulcerative colitis or Crohn's disease, independent of whether the patients received drug treatment (Table 17-2). This unfa-

---

*Editor's comment: see Mayberry, J. F., and Weterman, I. F.: Gut, *27*:821, 1986, who found an increased incidence of prematurity in infants of mothers suffering from Crohn's disease, but no increase in the rate of abortion. No details of treatment were presented.

TABLE 17-2. *Fetal Outcome of Pregnancy in Inflammatory Bowel Disease: Influence on Drug Therapy*

	Percent Treated	Percent Untreated	Percent Disease Activity
Prematurity	13	1.9	37.5
Stillbirth	2	1	50
Developmental defects	4	2	100
Spontaneous abortion	19.5	8.9	38.8

Adapted from Baiocco, P. J., and Korelitz, B. I.: J. Clin. Gastroenterol., 6:211, 1984.

vorable influence of disease activity on fetal complications was more common in Crohn's disease than in ulcerative colitis (Table 17-3).

The need for urgent surgical intervention for treatment of IBD arises less frequently now than it did decades ago, and pregnancy may continue to term without difficulty in those patients who have required previous total proctocolectomy and ileostomy creation for inflammatory bowel disease.[47,49,51-53] As with nonpregnant individuals, when the pregnant woman with inflammatory bowel disease requires urgent surgical intervention, however, the prognosis is guarded. Toxic megacolon has complicated the course of ulcerative colitis, with subsequent death of the mother and fetus, in many instances.[54,55] Nevertheless, survival of both also has been reported following surgical intervention for fulminating ulcerative colitis in the last trimester,[56-58] and following nonoperative management of toxic megacolon complicating ulcerative colitis, treated with ACTH.[55] Despite the additional concerns of pregnancy, enthusiastic medical treatment of the underlying inflammatory bowel disease and complicating megacolon with intravenous ACTH or hydrocortisone, antibiotic coverage, small bowel tubation, and rectal tube decompression, together with frequent turning of the patient, will probably result in a favorable outcome (see also Chap. 14).

The Influence of Pregnancy on the Course of Inflammatory Bowel Disease

The influence of pregnancy on the course of inflammatory bowel disease now can be evaluated by combining data from large studies, carried out in the 1950's and 1960's,[1-5,9,12,45-50] with more recent data.[5,59] The major variables likely to account for differences in the outcome between the two eras are the use of drugs (ACTH, corticosteroids, antibiotics), and more aggressive nonoperative management.

When ulcerative colitis is inactive at the time of conception, it is likely to remain inactive throughout the pregnancy (Table 17-4). If ulcerative colitis is active at the time of conception, it usually remains active or becomes worse during the course of pregnancy. Data from two studies indicate that approximately one-half of the women who have active ulcerative colitis at the time of conception will have a worsening or minimal improvement of symptoms during pregnancy.[8,59]

As with ulcerative colitis, Crohn's disease that is inactive at the time of conception will probably remain so throughout the pregnancy (Table 17-4). If Crohn's disease is active at the time of conception, reports of the course of disease during pregnancy have been conflicting. Data from older studies suggest that pregnancy has a favorable effect on the course of the disease, with many patients achieving remission.[50] More recent studies support a course similar to that of ulcerative colitis for some patients with active Crohn's disease, that is, a worsening of the illness may occur. Nearly two-thirds of women with active Crohn's disease will maintain the same level of disease activity throughout the pregnancy (Tables 17-4 and 17-5). The course of active IBD during pregnancy, therefore, remains variable, if not controversial; perhaps as the result of variable therapeutic approaches.

Previously undetected ulcerative colitis may emerge for the first time during pregnancy. Ear-

TABLE 17-3. *Influence of Active Disease on Fetal Complications.*

	Percent Treated	Percent Untreated	Percent Total
Ulcerative colitis	30	0	18.7
Crohn's disease	75	50	62.5

Adapted from Baiocco, P. J., and Korelitz, B. I.: J. Clin. Gastroenterol., 6:211, 1984.

TABLE 17-4. *Influence of Pregnancy on Course of Inflammatory Bowel Disease.*

	Risk of Exacerbation
Inactive ulcerative colitis	Small
Active Ulcerative colitis	Large
Inactive Crohn's disease	Small
Active Crohn's disease	Controversial

TABLE 17-5. *Changes in Inflammatory Bowel Disease Activity During Pregnancy.*

	Before	During Percent 0 to Mild	During Percent Moderate to Severe
Ulcerative colitis	0 to mild	72	28
	Moderate to severe	56	44
Crohn's disease	0 to mild	78	22
	Moderate to severe	35	65

Adapted from Mogadam, M., et al.: Am. J. Gastroenterol., 75:265, 1981.

lier literature reported a poor prognosis for such an onset.[45,47,48,50] More recently, however, it has been demonstrated that the outcome need not be any worse than in those in whom the ulcerative colitis was previously diagnosed.[8] Although Crohn's disease diagnosed for the first time during pregnancy also has been reported, the incidence is less than that for ulcerative colitis. Allegedly, such an onset of Crohn's disease has carried a poor prognosis.[9,12,50,60] These observations have not been substantiated subsequently, however.

Postpartum Period

Recurrences of IBD in the postpartum period are common and have been attributed to the stress induced by the newborn infant.[1] It has been claimed that in Crohn's disease such postpartum exacerbations occur more frequently; for example, in as many as 40% of women whose disease was inactive during pregnancy.[9,12] Other, more recent studies failed to substantiate this view, however.[11,59]

As a working rule, the prognosis for women with either ulcerative colitis and Crohn's disease is the same whether pregnant or not.

The Effects of Pregnancy on Previously Established Ileostomy

The patient with a conventional ileostomy may have occasional prolapse or obstruction of the ostomy as pregnancy progresses. The most serious complication of ileostomy dysfunction is intestinal obstruction, which had an incidence as high as 10% in one series.[52] More common problems include cracking or bleeding from the stoma. Frequently, ostomy polyposis and nipple valve retraction may be encountered, requiring surgical correction during pregnancy.[61] Avoiding pregnancy for a year after the construction of the stoma has been recommended to avoid complications.[52,62] While active perineal or perirectal disease may contraindicate episiotomy, its use is appropriate in the majority of pregnant women with IBD. Vaginal delivery in a woman with a previous colectomy can be safely accomplished without risk to the fetus.[49,51,52,53] The ileal pouch-anal anastomosis offers an attractive alternative to the conventional ileostomy in the young patient (see Chap. 29). The limited experience of pregnancy in women with such anastomoses has been favorable, with continence being only mildly affected.[63]

Concern also arises as to diagnostic procedures performed during pregnancy. In general, x-ray procedures should be avoided throughout pregnancy, even though theoretically the risk to the fetus is present only during the first trimester. Actually, there is evidence that the low-dose radiation used for a barium enema examination is not detrimental to the fetus even then.[64] Sigmoidoscopies and rectal biopsies or limited colonoscopies can be performed at any time during pregnancy. As a rule, because the colonoscopy requires air insufflation to distend the colon it should be postponed, but each patient must have individual consideration. Gastroscopy is not contraindicated in the pregnant woman.

Medical Management of Inflammatory Bowel Disease in Regard to Fertility and Pregnancy

Table 17-6 summarizes the observations on the influence of IBD upon the outcome of pregnancy. On the basis of the available data and general principles, the following observations seem appropriate:

1. Although nonspecific antidiarrheal agents such as deodorized tincture of opium should be used with caution in the management of inflammatory bowel disease at any time, an additional concern for narcotic addiction is present in the infant after delivery.
2. Oral therapy with sulfasalazine may be used during pregnancy if the disease activity war-

TABLE 17-6. *Influence of Inflammatory Bowel Disease on Outcome of Pregnancy.*

1. No unfavorable effect.
2. Incidence of complications same as general population.
3. Patients who receive drugs during pregnancy may have increased risk of fetal complications, although drug therapy may represent an innocent bystander compared to disease activity in causing these complications.
4. Risk of fetal complications greater in Crohn's disease than in ulcerative colitis.
5. Rate of fetal complications higher with active Crohn's disease.

rants, but it is a good working rule to give no drugs to pregnant women if such therapy can be avoided without serious hazard to the patient.

3. If oral steroid therapy is established the dose should be gradually reduced and discontinued during pregnancy, as guided by the clinical course. Oral steroids should be introduced or reintroduced only to control active IBD.
4. Immunosuppressive medication and metronidazole should *not* be given during pregnancy since many questions regarding fetal damage cannot be answered at the present time. For the same reason, a plan for pregnancy should be postponed in patients receiving these drugs. If pregnancy occurs inadvertently or otherwise, therapeutic abortion may be considered. However, the incidence of fetal damage seems to be low in those patients receiving 6-mercaptopurine or azathioprine who choose to continue with pregnancy despite this advice.
5. Active inflammatory bowel disease should be treated and brought into remission prior to planning a pregnancy.
6. Therapeutic abortion cannot be depended upon consistently to ameliorate the course of idiopathic inflammatory bowel disease.

References

1. Zetzel, L.: Fertility, pregnancy and idiopathic inflammatory bowel disease. *In* Inflammatory Bowel Disease. 2nd Edition. Edited by J. B. Kirsner, and R. G. Shorter. Philadelphia, Lea & Febiger, 1980.
2. Fielding, J. F.: Pregnancy and inflammatory bowel disease. Ir. J. Med. Sci., *151*:194, 1982.
3. Korelitz, B. I.: Pregnancy and inflammatory bowel disease. Compr. Ther., *8*:67, 1982.
4. Vender, R. J., and Spiro, H. M.: Inflammatory bowel disease and pregnancy. J. Clin. Gastroenterol., *4*:231, 1982.
5. De Dombal, F. T., et al.: Ulcerative colitis and pregnancy. Lancet, *2*:599, 1965.
6. Webb, M. J., and Sedlack, R. F.: Ulcerative colitis in pregnancy. Med. Clin. North Am. *55*:823, 1974.
7. Ganchrow, M. I., and Benjamin, H.: Inflammatory colorectal disease and pregnancy. Dis. Colon Rectum,, *18*:706, 1975.
8. Willoughby, C. P., and Truelove, S. C.: Ulcerative colitis and pregnancy. Gut, *21*:469, 1980.
9. de Dombal, E. T., Burton, I. L., and Goligher, J. C.: Crohn's disease and pregnancy. Br. Med. J., *3*:550, 1972.
10. Homan, W. P., and Thorbjarnarson, B.: Crohn's disease and pregnancy. Arch. Surg. *111*:545, 1976.
11. Khosla, R., Willoughby, C. P., and Jewell, D. P.: Crohn's disease and pregnancy. Gut, *25*:52, 1984.
12. Fielding, J. F., and Cooke, W. T.: Pregnancy and Crohn's disease. Br. Med. J., *2*:76, 1970.
13. Levi, A. J., Fisher, A. M., Hughes, L., and Hendry, W. F.: Male infertility due to sulphasalazine. Lancet, *2*:276, 1979.
14. Birnie, G. C., McLeod, T. I. F., and Watkinson, G.: Incidence of sulphasalazine induced male infertility. Gut, *22*:452, 1981.
15. Toovey, S., Hudson, E., Hendry, W. F., and Levi, A. J.: Sulphasalazine and male infertility: reversibility and possible mechanism. Gut, *22*:445, 1981.
16. Toth, A.: Reversible toxic effect of salicylazosulfapyridine on semen quality. Fertil. Steril., *31*:538, 1979.
17. Cann, P. A., and Holdsworth, C. D.: Reversal of male infertility on changing treatment from sulphasalazine to 5-aminosalicyclic acid. Lancet, *1*:119, 1984.
18. Shaffer, J. L., Kershaw, A., and Berrisford, M. H.: Sulphasalazine-induced infertility reversed on transfer to 5-aminosalicylic acid. Lancet, *1*:1240, 1984.
19. Lee, E. C. G., and Dowling, B. L.: Perimuscular excision of the rectum for Crohn's disease and ulcerative colitis. Br. J. Surg., *59*:29, 1972.
20. Korelitz, B. I.: From Crohn to Crohn's disease—Observations in New York City. Crohn's Workshop. A Global Assessment of Crohn's Disease. Edited by E. C. G. Lee. London, Heyden HM&M Publishers, 1981.
21. Farmer, R. G., Michener, W. M., and Mortimer, E. A.: Studies of family history among patients with inflammatory bowel disease. Clin. Gastroenterol., *9*:271, 1980.
22. Kirsner, J. B., and Spencer, J. A.: Familial occurrence of ulcerative colitis, regional enteritis and ileocolitis. Ann. Intern. Med., *51*:133, 1963.
23. Hensleigh, P. A., and Kauffman, R. E.: Maternal absorption and placental transfer of sulfasalazine. Am. J. Obstet. Gynecol., *127*:443, 1977.
24. Mogadam, M., Dobbins, W. O., III, Korelitz, B. I., and Ahmed, S. W.: Pregnancy in inflammatory bowel disease: The effect of sulfasalazine and corticosteroids on fetal outcome. Gastroenterology, *80*:72, 1981.
25. Baiocco, P. J., and Korelitz, B. I.: The influence of inflammatory bowel disease and its treatment on pregnancy and fetal outcome. J. Clin. Gastroenterol., *6*:211, 1984.
26. Halstead, C. H., Gandhi, G., and Tamura, T.: Sulfasalazine inhibits the absorption of folates in ulcerative colitis. N. Engl. J. Med., *305*:1513, 1984.
27. Hibbard, B. M., and Hibbard, E. D.: Folate metabolism and reproduction. Br. Med. Bull., *24*:10, 1968.
28. Sutherland, J. M., and Light, I. J.: The effect of drugs upon developing fetus. Pediatr. Clin. North Am., *12*:781, 1965.
29. Reimers, T. J., and Sluss, P. M.: 6-Mercaptopurine treatment of pregnant mice: effects on second and third generations. Science, *201*:65, 1978.
30. Scott, J. R.: Fetal growth retardation associated with ma-

ternal administration immunosuppressive drugs. Am. J. Obstet. Gynecol., *128*:668, 1976.
31. Hendrick, D., and Mirkin, B.L.: Metabolic disposition and toxicity of 6-mercaptopurine after massive overdose. Lancet, *1*:277, 1984.
32. Sokal, J. E., and Lessmann, E. M.: Effects of cancer chemotherapeutic agents on the human fetus. J. Am. Med. Assoc., *172*:1765, 1969.
33. Blatt, J., et al.: Pregnancy outcome following cancer chemotherapy. Am. J. Med., *69*:828, 1980.
34. Levy, N., Roisman, I., and Teodor, I.: Ulcerative colitis in pregnancy in Israel. Dis. Colon Rectum, *24*:351, 1981.
35. Nicholson, H. O.: Cytotoxic drugs in pregnancy. Br. J. Obstet. Gynecol., *75*:307, 1968.
36. Fraser, F. C., and Fainstat, T. D.: Production of congenital defects in offspring of pregnant mice treated with cortisone: Progress note. Pediatrics, *1*:527, 1951.
37. Warrel, D. W., and Taylor, R.: Outcome for the fetus of mothers receiving Prednisone during pregnancy. Lancet, *1*:117, 1968.
38. Lolucide, T. A., and Chandrakaar, C.: Pregnancy and jejunoileal bypass: Treatment of complications with total parenteral nutrition. South. Med. J., *73*:256, 1980.
39. Main, A. N. H., et al.: Intravenous feedings to sustain pregnancy in a patient with Crohn's disease. Br. Med. J., *283*:1221, 1981.
40. Gineston, J. L., et al.: Prolonged total parenteral nutrition in a pregnant woman with acute pancreatitis. J. Clin. Gastroenterol., *6*:249, 1984.
41. Hew, L. R., and Deitel, M. L.: Total parenteral nutrition in gynecology and obstetrics. Obstet. Gynecol., *55*:464, 1980.
42. Webb, G. A.: The use of hyperalimentation and chemotherapy in pregnancy: A case report. Am. J. Obstet. Gynecol., *137*:263, 1980.
43. Weinberg, R. B., et al.: Treatment of hyperlipidemic pancreatitis in pregnancy with total parenteral nutrition. Gastroenterology, *83*:1300, 1982.
44. Heller, L.: Parenteral nutrition in obstetrics and gynecology. *In* Current Concepts in Parenteral Nutrition. Edited by J. Greep. The Hague, Hyoff Medical Division, 1977.
45. Crohn, B. B., et al: Ulcerative colitis and pregnancy. Gastroenterology, *30*:391, 1956.
46. Banks, B. M., Korelitz, B. I., and Zetzel, L.: The course of nonspecific ulcerative colitis: review of twenty years' experience and late results. Gastroenterology, *32*:983, 1957.
47. Macdougall, I.: Ulcerative colitis and pregnancy. Lancet, *2*:641, 1956.
48. Abramson, D, Jankelson, I. R., and Milner, L. R.: Pregnancy and colitis. Am. J. Obstet. Gynecol., *61*:121, 1951.
49. McEwan, M. P.: Ulcerative colitis in pregnancy. Proc. R. Soc. Med., *65*:279, 1972.
50. Crohn, B. B., Yarnis, H., and Korelitz, B. I.: Regional ileitis and pregnancy. Gastroenterology, *31*:615, 1956.
51. Barwin, B. N., Harley, J. M. G., and Wilson, W.: Ileostomy and pregnancy. Br. J. Clin. Pract., *28*:256, 1974.
52. Hudson, C. N.: Ileostomy in pregnancy. Proc. R. Soc. Med., *65*:281, 1972.
53. Priest, F. O., Gilchrist, R. K., and Long, J. S.: Pregnancy in the patient with ileostomy and colectomy. J. Am. Med. Assoc., *169*:213, 1959.
54. Holzbach, R. T.: Toxic megacolon in pregnancy. Am. J. Dig. Dis., *14*:908, 1969.
55. Becker, I. M.: Pregnancy and toxic dilations of the colon. Dig. Dis. Sci., *17*:79, 1972.
56. Flatmark, A. L., Nordoy, A., and Gjone, E.: Radical surgery for ulcerative colitis during pregnancy. Scand. J. Gastroenterol., *6*:45, 1971.
57. Bohe, M. G., et al.: Surgery for fulminating colitis during pregnancy. Dis. Colon Rectum, *26*:119, 1983.
58. Nielsen, O. H., et al.: Pregnancy in ulcerative colitis. Scand. J. Gastroenterol., *18*:735, 1983.
59. Mogadam, M., et al.: The course of inflammatory bowel disease during pregnancy and postpartum. Am. J. Gastroenterol., *75*:265, 1983.
60. Martinbeau, P. N., Welch, J. S., and Weiland, L. H.: Crohn's disease and pregnancy. Am. J. Obstet. Gynecol., *122*:746, 1975.
61. Gopal, K. A., et al.: Ostomy and pregnancy. Dis. Colon Rectum, *28*:912, 1985.
62. Scudamore, H. H., Rogers, A. G., Bargen, J. A., and Banner, E. A.: Pregnancy after ileostomy for chronic ulcerative colitis. Gastroenterology, *32*:295, 1957.
63. Metcalf, A., Dozois, R. R., Beart, R. W., and Wolff, B. G.: Pregnancy following ileal pouch-anal anastomosis. Dis. Colon Rectum, *28*:859, 1985.
64. Kohn, H. L., and Fry, R. J. M.: Radiation carcinogenesis. N. Engl. J. Med., *310*:504, 1984.

Section 4 · *Pathology*

18 · Pathology of Idiopathic Inflammatory Bowel Disease

ROBERT H. RIDDELL, M.D.

Idiopathic inflammatory bowel disease essentially includes ulcerative colitis (UC) and Crohn's disease (CD), but these frequently must be distinguished not only from each other, but also from other diseases such as self-limited (infectious) colitis, the solitary rectal ulcer syndrome, and collagenous colitis.

Some overlap is present in the gross and histopathologic features of many colonic inflammatory conditions, and few specific features alone are diagnostic. Patterns sufficiently characteristic to permit a diagnosis that is both accurate and clinically useful only follow careful consideration of a constellation of features, including clinical and radiologic findings. Specific infections must be excluded and many of these are considered in other chapters; although biopsies may suggest an infectious etiology, culture and stool examinations for ova, parasites, and toxins are still essential diagnostic tools. In most western countries, the differentiation of UC from CD is the most common diagnostic dilemma in the histopathologic diagnosis of inflammatory bowel disease.

In this chapter, the pathology of ulcerative colitis and Crohn's disease and their local complications will be considered. Also, those features that are useful in differentiating them from each other and from other forms of inflammatory bowel disease will be examined, and the entity of indeterminate colitis, if it exists, will be discussed. Throughout, an attempt will be made to determine the pathologic features that are strong indicators of the underlying disease. Consideration will also be given to the serious local complications of hemorrhage, toxic dilatation, and perforation that develop as a consequence of severe or fulminant activity; inflammatory polyps and fibromuscular strictures are benign complications, and their importance is mainly in relation to their differentiation from malignancy. The important topics of precancer and cancer in ulcerative colitis as well as extraintestinal manifestations of ulcerative colitis are discussed elsewhere.

Ulcerative Colitis

Ulcerative colitis is characteristically a mucosal disease, usually beginning in the rectum and extending proximally to involve all or part of the remaining colon. In some patients, particularly the young, it may be extensive and involve the entire colon from the beginning. In many patients the disease begins in the rectum and remains limited to that site for its entire course. Most patients with acute ulcerative colitis have only mild to moderately severe disease and do not require colectomy. Macroscopic examination of the colon is now usually performed by the endoscopist, and the material submitted to the pathologist is limited to small mucosal biop sies. Except for the risk of carcinoma, elective resection in disease that is quiescent or only mildly active is now uncommon.

DISTRIBUTION OF THE DISEASE. This is a useful diagnostic feature both for the endoscopist and pathologist, especially when the pathologist has to study multiple, separately identified biopsies. The rectum is usually involved, but the extent of the proximal spread is variable. Some patients have disease that appears to involve much or all of the colon. Others have proctoscopically and histologically indistinguishable disease limited to the rectum that never extends proximally.[1] A small group of patients have an unresponsive and apparently intractable proctosigmoiditis, but nothing is remarkable about its histology. In cases with limited colonic involvement, the transition from diseased to normal mucosa is usually gradual, but occasionally it is abrupt. Proximal spread is in continuity without intervening areas of uninvolved mucosa. This is an important feature of ulcerative colitis that contrasts with the discontinuous pattern of gross involvement often seen in Crohn's colitis. Variation in macroscopic activity and severity may falsely suggest the existence of skip areas. Unless fulminant disease is present, however, biopsies from such apparent "skip" areas always confirm that there is involvement. Likewise, sigmoidoscopically uninvolved rectal mucosa is occasionally observed but invariably is found to be diseased when examined histologically. This emphasises the importance of always obtaining a biopsy from apparently uninvolved mucosa, whether proximal or distal. Endoscopists should remember that, occasionally, normal-appearing mucosa may show obvious disease histologically.

HISTOLOGIC FINDINGS. In ulcerative colitis, they represent a spectrum of changes that often parallel the clinical course of the disease. Active, resolving, and quiescent stages can be recognized histologically in biopsy specimens and reflect corresponding clinical patterns in patients with alternating periods of activity and remission.[2] Some patients, however, have disease that clinically is chronically active; fulminant colitis is less frequent.

Active Ulcerative Colitis

The histopathologic findings in biopsies taken from patients with active ulcerative colitis correlate reasonably well with the endoscopic appearance. Endoscopically, there is variable mucosal hyperemia, granularity, friability, ulceration, and bleeding, depending on the severity of the disease. Histologically, active ulcerative colitis is characterized by features of chronicity, namely alterations of the architecture with features of regeneration; in particular, multiple basal lymphoid aggregates or basal plasma cells are present. Paneth cell metaplasia is frequently found distal to the ascending colon but is a nonspecific feature of mucosal regeneration. Hyperplasia of enteroendocrine cells may also be seen, particularly argentaffin cells. Superimposed are features of activity, including intense mucosal inflammation with crypt abscesses and depletion of goblet cell mucin, erosions, or superficial, but rarely deep, ulcers (Fig. 18-1). Mucosal vascular congestion, with edema and focal hemorrhage, is often present and tends to be more prominent in severe cases. Sometimes this predominates. Shallow ulcers are common in active disease, but deeper ulcers penetrating the

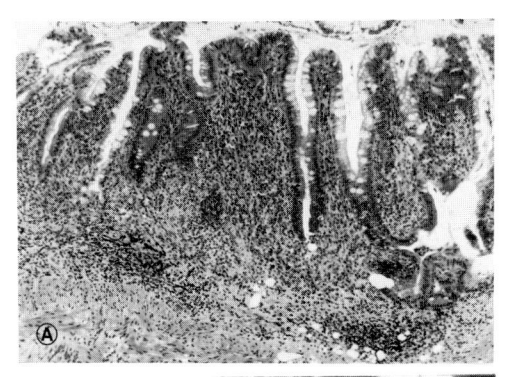

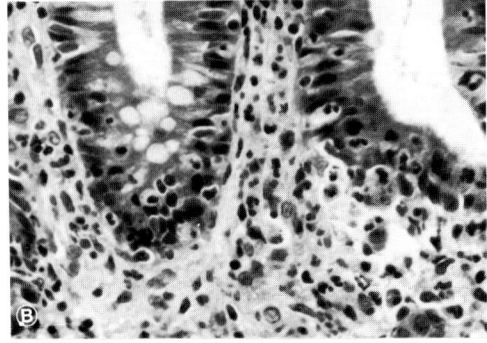

FIG. 18-1A. Active ulcerative colitis. The normal mucosal architecture is distorted, with a reduced number of irregular crypts that also fail to reach the muscularis mucosae. Small basal lymphoid aggregates are present immediately above the muscularis mucosae. Increased numbers of inflammatory cells are seen in the lamina propria. Note the uniformity of the inflammatory infiltrate.
B. Detail of active ulcerative colitis showing polymorphs in the lamina propria that attack the adjacent crypts.

muscularis mucosa into the superficial submucosa occur less often, and are seen principally in severe cases. Most of the histopathologic findings in ulcerative colitis are limited to the mucosa and superficial submucosa with the deeper layers being unaffected, except in fulminant disease.

The mucosal inflammatory infiltrate in active colitis includes an *acute* component associated with crypt abscesses, and a *chronic* component involving the lamina propria more diffusely. Aggregates of neutrophils near and invading the crypt epithelium form crypt abscesses that, when numerous, are characteristic and reliable indicators of activity (Fig. 18-1B). Neutrophilic infiltration ranges from small accumulations of neutrophils within crypt epithelium (cryptitis), to invasion of crypt lumina (crypt abscess), and, ultimately, if crypt ulceration occurs, to large intramucosal abscesses that completely destroy the crypt epithelium and extend into the lamina propria and submucosa. Most crypts in a diseased segment show similar degrees of involvement, with the worst usually occurring in the mid and deeper parts of the crypts. This contrasts with the appearances in infectious acute self-limited colitis (ASLC), which has a distinct tendency for the acute inflammation to affect primarily the luminal epithelium and the superficial portion of the crypts. The presence of chronic disease in the presence of isolated crypt abscesses, intermixed with completely uninvolved crypts, is more typical of Crohn's disease than of ulcerative colitis, however. Polymorphonuclear infiltrate with crypt abscesses is an important characteristic of ulcerative colitis, although it is not specific. It is unlike ulcerative colitis for a polymorphonuclear infiltrate to be present without epithelial invasion. It is important to realize that crypt abscesses are also a feature of acute colitis resulting from numerous other causes; they indicate the *activity* of the acute inflammatory process rather than the underlying etiology.

Depletion of goblet cell mucin is a characteristic and fairly consistent finding in active ulcerative colitis, and, except where dysplasia is present, is another reliable indicator of activity. It is not specific, however, and is found also in CD and ASLC. Mucin depletion tends to affect all crypts and to be pronounced when an intense inflammatory infiltrate is present. Restoration of normal mucin content, usually beginning in the most superficial portion of the crypts, occurs with resolution, and a return to normal levels occurs in the state of quiescence. An increased rate of epithelial cell proliferation may be reflected by increased numbers of mitotic figures, from the average of about one per three crypts to one or more per crypt. Epithelial regeneration may also be seen in active disease. When the acute attack is resolving and the patient's symptoms have diminished, epithelial regeneration becomes a prominent histologic feature.

Typically, in active ulcerative colitis, a chronic inflammatory infiltrate, mostly of lymphocytes and plasma cells accompanied by variable numbers of eosinophils and mast cells, extends diffusely throughout the lamina propria. Indeed, the presence of basal lymphoid or plasma cell aggregates (Fig. 18-1) is useful in distinguishing IIBD from ASLC, in which it is not seen.* In the normal colonic mucosa occasional lymphoid follicles are present adjacent to or straddling the muscularis mucosae. In some diseases, the follicles may become especially large and numerous in the rectum, and, less commonly so, in the colon. They are invariably superficial to the muscularis mucosae, however. This finding has been termed by some "follicular proctitis or colitis," and is often accompanied by epithelium showing regenerative features. Usually it is a variant of active ulcerative colitis and invariably resolves with therapy; rarely it may be seen in Crohn's disease or lymphogranuloma venereum.[3]

Variability in the intensity of the inflammation in ulcerative colitis does occur, particularly during the resolving phase of the disease, and may result in a somewhat patchy distribution, but a clearly focal distribution is more suggestive of Crohn's disease.[4,5] Some studies have reported an increase both in the numbers and proportions of IgG-producing plasma cells,[6,7] but this has not been a universal conclusion.[8] Increased numbers of IgE-containing cells have been reported in the rectal mucosa in some patients with proctitis. One group of workers have suggested that this is a favourable prognostic feature for which they have proposed the term "allergic proctitis."[9] Others, however, have reported increased IgE-cells in patients who have proximal extension, and have found a correlation with duration of the disease.[8]

Eosinophil counts are reported to be higher in the mucosa in patients with long-standing ulcerative colitis and in colitis responding to medical therapy than in patients with a first attack of colitis,[10] especially those who are unresponsive

---

*Editor's footnote: See also, Nostrant, T. T., et al.: Gastroenterology, *92*:318, 1987.

to medical therapy.[11] Eosinophils may form such a large part of the infiltrate, particularly when the disease is quiescent, that the possibility of an eosinophilic colitis may be entertained. However, eosinophilic colitis remains a poorly described entity,[12] and is far less common than ulcerative colitis that has numerous eosinophils in the infiltrate. Assuming that eosinophilic colitis has either an allergic or parasitic basis, the architectural changes seen in UC should be absent.[13]

Resolving Ulcerative Colitis

As patients recover from an acute attack of UC, the signs of clinical resolution often precede those of histologic resolution. In biopsies, activity begins to subside, regenerative features become prominent and epithelial continuity is restored. The epithelium is at first attenuated as it "stretches" over recently ulcerated surfaces, then it gradually becomes columnar. It is important to distinguish the nuclear changes characteristic of regenerating epithelia from those of true dysplasia.[14] Nuclei may be large with prominent nucleoli and an open chromatin pattern, but are widely separated. As the cells become cuboidal to low columnar, the nuclei appear closer together, sometimes overlapping, but may not have their usual polarity. Basal polarity appears after the epithelium has become columnar, but variable degrees of stratification may be seen while columnar differentiation is in progress.

Neutrophils disappear as the acute inflammation subsides but may still be seen in and around the crypts in the early stages of resolution. As the epithelium matures, the goblet cell population is restored and mitotic figures decrease. The final features of the resolution are the gradual decline in the diffuse infiltrate of lymphocytes and plasma cells. Uneven resolution of the chronic inflammation may produce a patchy infiltrate that could be misinterpreted as Crohn's disease. In ulcerative colitis it is uncommon to see distinct focal changes, however, with parts of the mucosa being heavily inflamed while the adjacent mucosa appears virtually normal, which are so typical of some forms of Crohn's disease. If it occurs at all, complete histologic resolution may take several months to occur after the symptoms have resolved and the endoscopic appearances have returned to normal; in some patients, a persistent state of low grade inflammatory activity ensues.

Quiescent Ulcerative Colitis

MACROSCOPIC APPEARANCE. The mucosa may appear normal or be smooth and atrophic. Small nodules, villous foci, or flat plaque-like areas should raise suspicion that either a small carcinoma or dysplasia could be present.[15]

Some shortening and reduction in the diameter of the bowel, usually most apparent distally, is often present and may be severe (Fig. 18-2); such shortening in ulcerative colitis is attributed to muscular contraction and thickening and is not accompanied by fibrosis. This feature is more pronounced in long-standing colitis and is an indicator of prolonged disease. Radiologic manifestations of these muscular changes include loss of haustra, increased sacrorectal distance, and reduction in transverse diameter. A total lack of haustra may ultimately give rise to a tube-like appearance, but these radiologic findings may occasionally revert to normal if the disease remains quiescent for a long period (see Chap. 20).[16]

HISTOLOGY. When the disease is quiescent, an intact but architecturally abnormal mucosa usually persists as an indication of previous mucosal injury. The degree of architectural change varies from slight abnormalities to distinct mucosal atrophy; it seems to be related to the severity, duration, and frequency of attacks of the previous active disease. The normal parallel arrangement of closely packed crypts is lost, crypts being reduced in number, more widely separated, and often branched (Fig. 18-3). Shortening of crypts may leave a prominent gap between the crypt bases and the muscularis muco-

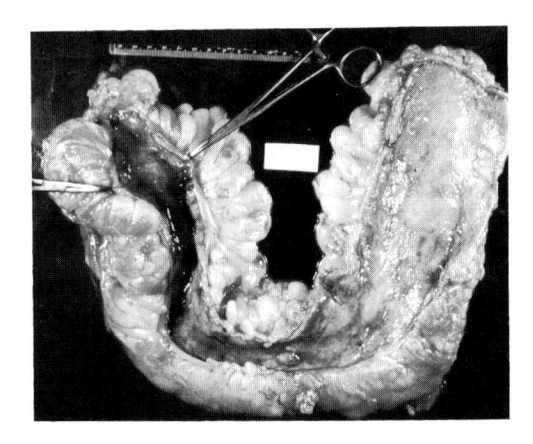

FIG. 18-2. Chronic ulcerative colitis showing a typical "haustra-less" bowel with significant shortening.

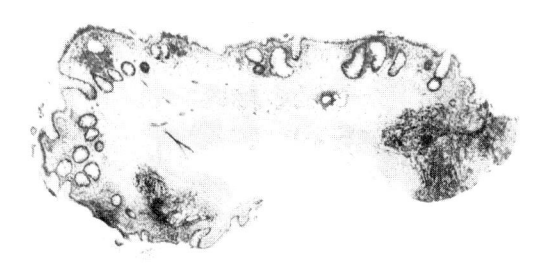

FIG. 18-3. Rectal biopsy in quiescent ulcerative colitis. The biopsy shows a pronounced reduction in the number of crypts that are distorted and fall short of the muscularis mucosae. Note also the presence of several lymphoid aggregates immediately above the muscularis mucosae. These changes are indicative of chronic inflammatory diseases that have caused full thickness mucosal ulceration. The vast majority of these will be on the basis of ulcerative colitis, but occasionally similar changes can be found in patients with Crohn's disease, ischemia, or following irradiation.

sae. Shortening and branching of crypts can be useful in differential diagnosis as it is frequent in ulcerative colitis, less common in Crohn's disease, and rare in other diseases. Some patients may show only minimal loss of parallelism, slightly increased separation, and occasional branching of crypts. Rarely, the mucosa in ulcerative colitis may regenerate so well that it is virtually indistinguishable from normal.

In the quiescent state, the goblet cell population is restored to normal. Inflammatory cell infiltrates are less than in active disease but the degree is variable; other features of active disease usually are absent. An occasional crypt abscess may be present, however, but this is of no significance; in pathology reports it should not be mentioned as being indicative of active disease. Paneth cells, almost never found in the normal colon except in the vicinity of the ileocecal valve, may appear in any region of the colon or rectum. They are usually located at the base of crypts and, occasionally, are numerous. Argentaffin cells also may be increased in number.

Characteristically, hypertrophy of the muscularis mucosae occurs, accompanied by some separation of fibers. It is generally most prominent in the rectum, where the muscularis mucosae normally is thickest (Fig. 18-3). Repeated episodes of activity may cause a multilayered muscularis mucosae, which may be a major factor in the benign strictures sometimes observed in ulcerative colitis.[17] Similar thickening of the muscularis mucosae also is observed in chronic colitides of other etiologies, so it is a nonspecific feature of chronic inflammation of the colon

Chronically active ulcerative colitis

Some patients have disease with persistent clinical symptoms, and the term "chronically active ulcerative colitis" seems appropriate for this group. The mucosa, whether examined endoscopically or grossly in resected specimens, varies in appearance from almost normal to severely inflamed. Histologically, the mucosa in such patients may fall into any of the three stages of active, resolving, or quiescent colitis. Generally the mucosa shows features of resolving disease plus a variable amount of acute inflammation. Crypt distortion and atrophy are usually present.

Severely active ulcerative colitis

About 15% of patients with ulcerative colitis experience a particularly severe or fulminant episode that is unresponsive to intensive medical therapy or accompanied by massive uncontrollable hemorrhage or toxic dilatation requiring urgent colectomy (see Chap. 14). These fulminant attacks tend to occur early in the course of the disease but may be seen in those with longstanding disease. Such cases have formed the basis of most of the macroscopic descriptions of ulcerative colitis. The distribution of lesions in these severe cases usually shows rectosigmoid involvement with variable degrees of proximal extension in continuity. External examination of such specimens commonly reveals only minimal external changes, as might be expected in a disease predominantly affecting the mucosa. In contrast to the minimal change observed on the serosal surface, the mucosal changes usually are dramatic (Fig. 18-4). The most severely involved mucosa is dark red or purple, hemorrhagic, and friable, with extensive ulceration. It is covered by a mixture of blood, mucus, pus, necrotic debris, and liquid stool. Extensive and deep ulceration, which exposes the underlying submucosa or muscularis propria, is common; disease entirely confined to the mucosa rarely, if ever, causes illness sufficiently severe to require urgent colectomy.[18]

Confluence of ulcers may produce longitudinal furrows and often leaves isolated polypoid islands of mucosa (Fig. 18-5). This is possibly the only time when the term "pseudopolyp" is appropriate. Because of the ambiguity of the term "polyp," however, the term "mucosal islands" is preferred. Deep fissuring, which is more characteristic of Crohn's disease, is seen rarely, except in toxic dilatation.

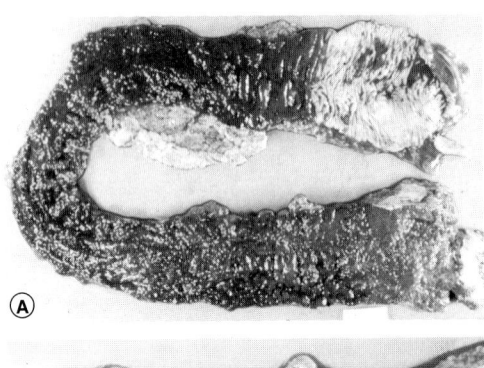

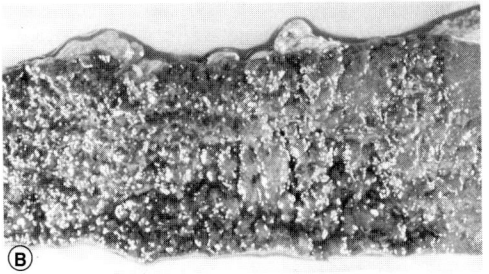

FIG. 18-4A. Fulimant ulcerative colitis. The mucosa is diffusely involved down to the anorectal junction (bottom right). Note that although the proximal extension of disease appears abrupt (top right) in the ascending colon, small patches of active disease are apparent within the "spared" colon. These changes should not be misinterpreted as the focal changes of Crohn's disease and are usual at the proximal extent of severe ulcerative colitis. Similar changes can sometimes be seen in the rectosigmoid in patients with a severe initial attack of the disease.
B. Detail of sigmoid colon with diffuse hemorrhage and ulceration. It should be appreciated that the deep ulcers may perforate in the absence of toxic dilatation.

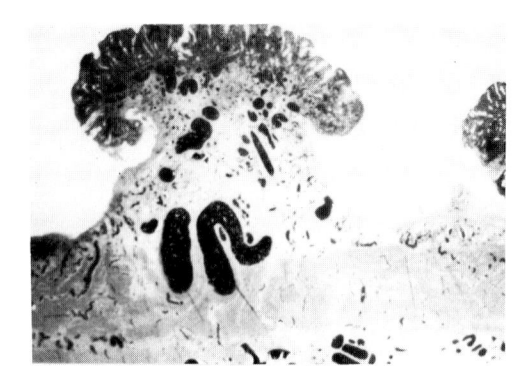

FIG. 18-5. Fulminant ulcerative colitis with mucosal islands. The deep ulcers extend down to the muscularis propria leaving islands of residual mucosa with a polypoid configuration—"true" pseudopolyps.

Histologically, the inflammatory infiltrate is restricted to the immediate vicinity of the ulcer, even in severe cases where ulcers extend into the submucosa or muscularis propria. Occasionally, patients with severe active ulcerative colitis, without toxic dilatation, are unresponsive to medical therapy; they may also have complications because of colonic perforation. These cases show focal cleft-like extension of the mucosal ulcers into the muscularis propria that create potential sites of perforation. The penetration of the muscularis propria is usually less extensive than that in toxic megacolon, and myocytolysis and muscular inflammation are more closely confined to the immediate vicinity of the deep ulcers. They also differ from patients with toxic megacolon in that the inflammatory infiltrate tends to be more prominent relative to the degree of vascular dilatation.

Changes in the remainder of the submucosa are usually limited to vascular dilatation and edema. Fibrosis, granulomas in the subserosa or uninvolved mucosa, lymphocytic aggregates in the submucosa, muscularis, or serosal layers away from areas of ulceration are absent, or, if present, should suggest that the underlying disease is Crohn's disease. Occasional foreign-body granulomas rarely may be found adjacent to deep ulcers that extend into the submucosa, perhaps one of the few occasions when granulomas may be seen in UC. These should not be confused with the sarcoid-like granulomas seen in Crohn's disease, which are independent of overlying ulcers. The foreign body granulomas that occur in ulcerative colitis are usually associated with foreign material, the identification of which may be facilitated by the use of polarized light. Occasionally, a diffuse submucosal "periarteritis-like" vasculitis is present, but this is rare.[19,20] More frequently, involvement of vessels occurs in the base of an ulcer, with ischemic necrosis of the walls.

Toxic Dilatation and Perforation*

The most serious complication of acute ulcerative colitis is colonic perforation, which may occur either in toxic megacolon or in severe colitis without dilatation. The incidence of toxic megacolon is reported to be 2 to 4% of all patients with ulcerative colitis,[21,22] and in up to 13% of hospitalized patients.[22,23] It may develop at any time, but is most commonly seen early in the course of the disease; indeed, it may be the presenting manifestation. Dilatation is most often greatest in the transverse colon or flexures, but it may involve other parts of the colon (Fig. 18-6); occasionally it affects almost the entire colon. In some areas, and sometimes over

*See also Chapter 14

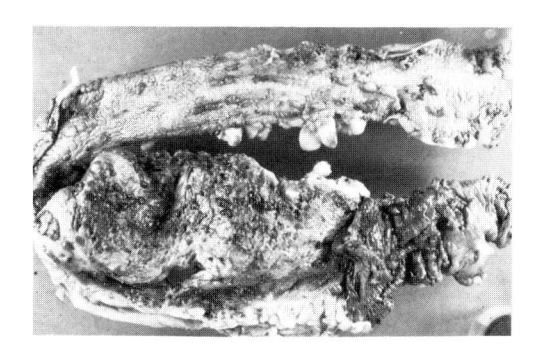

FIG. 18-6. Longstanding ulcerative colitis with dilatation limited to the descending and sigmoid colon with perforation at approximately their junction. The rectum (bottom right) is actively involved but the right colon shows only healed disease.

long segments of bowel, it involves all layers, including the muscularis propria and serosa. The serosa is congested, dull, opaque, and often covered by a fibrinous or fibrinopurulent exudate. The thin friable wall, which has been likened to wet tissue paper, is easily ruptured, and perforation may occur spontaneously or with even the most gentle surgical handling. In the affected area, mucosal ulceration is severe, with cleft-like extensions into the muscularis propria accompanied by extensive myocytolysis. Vascular dilatation and engorgement are often present and may be a more prominent feature than the inflammatory cell infiltrate.

Although no definite explanation is yet available for the state of toxic megacolon, of the specific factors studied, the extent and depth of ulceration has the strongest correlation with the area of dilatation.[18,24] In colectomy, specimens from patients who are successfully brought through an episode of toxic dilatation but in whom colectomy is performed subsequently, regenerated mucosa may be seen to extend into the muscularis propria, presumably representing re-epithelialization of prior deep ulcers. Interestingly, no consistent neurologic abnormality has been reported and obvious obstructive lesions are absent. Hypokalemia and drugs that decrease motility, such as narcotics and anticholinergics, are recognized as aggravating factors but not as primary etiologic agents.[24] Overall mortality is about 15%, but the presence of perforation is the single most important determinant of prognosis, with a mortality of about 50%.[23,24] Patients treated conservatively for several weeks may regenerate the mucosa deep in the muscularis propria (colitis cystica profunda).

Benign Strictures*

Benign strictures are local sequelae of ulcerative colitis that are usually of little consequence to the patient and not an indication for colectomy. Colectomy is sometimes considered if doubt exists concerning their underlying pathology or they prevent the colonoscopist from reaching the proximal colon in cancer-surveillance programs, however. They are usually smooth, may be multiple, are sometimes reversible, and are rarely sufficiently narrow to cause obstruction. Benign strictures have been attributed to hypertrophy of the muscularis mucosae.[17] Strictures that are not reversible are frequently malignant but may include some caused by fibrosis of the submucosa or muscularis propria as a result of previously severe ulcerative disease. Benign strictures are most commonly seen in patients with long-standing disease, although they are occasionally found at the time of presentation.[17,25]

Backwash Ileitis

Total colonic involvement is accompanied by extension of mucosal inflammation into the distal terminal ileum in between 10 and 20% of patients. It is usually associated with a dilated, patulous ileocecal valve. Whether this lesion represents a reaction to regurgitation of colonic content into the terminal ileum or primary ileal involvement is not yet established;[2] morphologically, the ileitis looks almost identical to the colonic disease.[26] The commonly used term "backwash ileitis" should, therefore, not be given too much pathologic significance, nor does it have any prognostic significance; it invariably resolves following colectomy. Despite rare reported cases of ileal perforation in ulcerative colitis,[27] the affected ileum can even be used for anastomosis or ileostomy formation without appreciable hazard.

Inflammatory Polyps*

Polypoid mucosal tags are relatively common sequelae of active ulcerative colitis. The term "pseudopolyp" also is used commonly for these mucosal projections to avoid confusion with adenomas. This is a poor choice of available terms because they are true polyps. These mucosal tags, unlike those seen as "mucosal is-

*See also Chapter 14.

lands" in acute disease, clearly fit the definition of "polyp" and so the alternative term "inflammatory polyp" is preferred.[2] In active disease they consist of isolated, edematous, and congested mucosal remnants resulting from ulcers undermining them, thus producing mucosal tags rising above the surrounding ulcerated surface.

Inflammatory polyps are generally distributed in a diffuse or irregular fashion throughout the colon but are relatively uncommon in the rectum, especially close to the anal verge.[25] They are not exclusive to ulcerative colitis and may be found following ulceration in inflammatory bowel disease of other etiologies. True adenomatous polyps may occur as a coincidental finding in patients with ulcerative colitis,[15] although their incidence is low.

Inflammatory polyps assume many shapes and occasionally form mucosal bridges, and although they may be bifid or trifid, usually they lack the distinct, lobulated "head" typical of predunculated adenomas. Most inflammatory polyps are less than 1.5 cm long, although they show considerable variation in size and occasionally may reach several centimeters in length or diameter. They persist in the quiescent stage after re-epithelialization and often remain as a constant monument to the severity of the preceding ulceration. When especially numerous they can form a forest of polyps for which the term "colitis polyposa" has been used.

The histologic appearance of these inflammatory polyps shows some variability, depending on whether the mucosa originated from a mucosal island, in which case their mucosa may be virtually normal, or from regenerated mucosa that has the typical features of regeneration. Another mechanism of inflammatory polyp formation is the exuberant proliferation of granulation tissue to form polypoid nodules that are later covered with regenerated mucosa. When covered and invaginated by epithelium, these tend to have cystic dilatation, and the crypts may closely resemble juvenile polyps histologically.

Although in the past there has been controversy concerning the precancerous potential of inflammatory polyps,[28] the majority of current opinion considers them benign.[25,29,30] Nevertheless, there is no reason why they should not become dysplastic. Some inflammatory polyps become large and create a suspicion of carcinoma or even cause obstruction.[29,31] Most commonly these occur in patients with severe disease, especially those with total colonic involvement. This is the probable basis for the reported positive association of inflammatory polyps with toxic megacolon and the arthropathy of ulcerative colitis,[30] for both tend to occur with severe total colitis. Patients with mild disease, as judged by clinical criteria, rarely have inflammatory polyposis.

Anal lesions*

Anal lesions occur in a small minority of patients with ulcerative colitis and are thought to be secondary to the diarrhea. These include anal fissure, rectal prolapse, hemorrhoids, perianal excoriations, and perirectal abscesses. In ulcerative colitis the anal complications are considerably less frequent and less severe than in Crohn's disease. Rectovaginal fistulas are rare in ulcerative colitis and should always raise the suspicion of Crohn's disease.

Unusual Biopsy Appearances in Ulcerative Colitis

While the previously described patterns are classical, exceptions occur. Further, these exceptions have clinical significance and must be appreciated. These are as follows:

Specificity of Atrophic or Regenerative Changes

When these changes are present, they undoubtably are indicative of previous full mucosal ulceration. While idiopathic ulcerative colitis is by far the most frequent cause, identical changes may be seen in many other diseases. The most common of these are Crohn's disease (in which such changes are frequently focal), chronic ischemia, irradiation damage, and the solitary rectal ulcer syndrome; rarely, they are seen as a sequel to infections, particularly pseudomembranous colitis or severe Shigellosis.[32]

Lack of Atrophic or Regenerative Changes

The finding of an atrophic mucosa with typical regenerative features in patients with known long-standing ulcerative colitis is always of comfort when reviewing their histology, as it tends to confirm that diagnosis. Further, in patients who are being investigated for bloody diarrhea, the presence of these features, plus acute inflammatory changes involving the crypts, is

*See also Chapter 14.

strong evidence that the patient has UC.[33,34] Nevertheless, such changes are not always found in patients with known UC, particularly under certain well-defined clinical circumstances.

The first of these circumstances is in proximal biopsies from patients with known extensive or total disease with previous exacerbations and either radiologic or endoscopic evidence of activity; in these patients, only distal biopsies may show the typical changes.

The second is in patients who have been quiescent for long periods of time, often a decade or more. In these patients, biopsies from all parts of the large bowel may fail to show regenerative changes.

The third is in patients developing carcinoma in UC, when not only may no regenerative changes occur but also the crypts may be packed tightly together. The implication is that the regenerative changes so typical of UC either never develop in some patients or, more likely, that the mucosa has the ability over time to revert to a more normal pattern. Surprisingly, virtually nothing has been reported in the literature regarding this point, but most pathologists have seen what appear to be bona fide examples of this reversion. Persistent Paneth cell metaplasia may be the only marker of previous disease, but even this may be absent.

The importance of recognizing that this occurs is to alert the clinician that in long-standing quiescent colitis, biopsies may fail to show regenerative changes. Conversely, pathologists must not over-interpret this lack of microscopic involvement and suggest that the patient never had UC. Nevertheless, patients who are undergoing periodic surveillance colonoscopy who change their clinician clearly need some evidence of their former colitis to be passed on to their new gastroenterologist. Prior biopsy documentation is clearly valuable in this respect.

Active Disease Superimposed on Mucosa Lacking Regenerative Changes

Histologic appearances under these circumstances can vary considerably, and in severe attacks can cause the typical crypt-destructive disease, as illustrated in Figure 18-1. Patients with a less severe recrudescence may retain a relatively normal architecture, but show an acute inflammatory reaction that is centered on the epithelium. It is worth remembering that patients with long-standing UC frequently retain either several small lymphoid or plasma cell aggregates immediately above, or involving, the muscularis mucosae, which is a useful indicator of prior long-standing disease. In some patients the typical crypt-centered neutrophil infiltrate may be present, although mucin may not be depleted.

Acute Exacerbation of Ulcerative Colitis by Superimposed Infection

Some apparent exacerbations of UC are accompanied by the finding of a pathogen in the stool.[35-39] Patients with UC seem to be more prone to develop infectious forms of diarrhea, although evidence for this is almost entirely anecdotal. The finding that C. difficile toxins could also be part of this spectrum begged the question of what proportion of apparent exacerbations were in fact caused by pathogens that are not easy to demonstrate. Surprisingly, although the histologic appearances of both active UC and acute infectious (self-limited) colitis are well-documented,[33,34,40] the appearances of acute exacerbations of UC associated with the isolation of a pathogen or toxin have yet to be documented. We have seen occasional biopsies in this setting. Some have an appearance suggesting an infectious process although a pathogen was not isolated. Although such biopsies always raise the question of underlying infection, in the absence of a demonstrable pathogen no specific therapy can be instituted. Conversely, we have seen examples of dramatic clinical responses to steroids by what appeared histologically to be typical UC, but in which Campylobacter was cultured. The exact part that infections play in acute exacerbations of UC is still far from clear, a major problem being that most pathogens can exist in the bowel in a carrier state.

Granulomas in Ulcerative Colitis

A recurring question is that of whether granulomas can be present in ulcerative colitis. Our rule of thumb is that well-formed, sarcoid-like granulomas are not part of the spectrum of UC and that if these are present, an alternative explanation must be found. It should, however, be recognized that crypt abscesses may rupture, causing extravasation of mucin into the lamina propria, and that this can excite foreign-body giant cells and a few histiocytes.[5] Sarcoid-like granulomas are rare in this situation, however, although some might argue that a mucin stain, such as an alcian-blue at pH 2.5, or PAS, or a combination of the two, is worth carrying out if it is thought that a "granuloma" may have resulted on this basis. The finding of granulomas therefore demands that other diseases known to result in granuloma formation be excluded. Granulomas immediately adjacent to foci of acute inflammation, usually ulcers, should also be viewed with caution as these may represent a response to foreign material.

Rectal sparing and irregular transition to active disease in fulminant colitis

A further confusing change that is not uncommon in patients with severely active disease is the presence of relative rectal sparing, particularly in a first attack, with an irregular and patchy transition to active disease, thus suggesting that the underlying disease is Crohn's disease. These changes may cause diagnostic concern if gentle, fiberoptic proctosigmoidoscopy is being carried out when it may be difficult to avoid the conclusion that the underlying disease is Crohn's disease. Multiple biopsies also may confirm this patchy tendency. Nevertheless, if these colons are resected, similar changes are often present at the proximal limit of disease (Fig. 18-4A). In most of such patients, nothing else indicates that the underlying disease is anything other than ulcerative colitis.

Preclinical Ulcerative Colitis

It is not surprising to learn that little is known about the pathophysiology of a first attack of UC, for this would require accidental or incidental biopsies in the preclinical phase of the disease. Yet it is well-documented, even in a first attack of UC, that not only the architectural distortion, but also the excess of basal lymphoid or plasma cell aggregates are present.[33,34] Because the inflammatory features take longer to develop temporally, it is suggested that the preclinical phase of UC is considerably longer than that of ASLC and may be measured in weeks or months.

Our only real experience of this phase of the disease has been with that group of patients with colitis whose disease seems to date from an episode of ASLC that never completely resolved. Exactly when these patients cease being thought of as having post-infectious diarrhea and are considered to have UC usually coincides with an exacerbation in which no pathogen is isolated. Only anecdotal data are available regarding the clinical and histologic appearances in these patients.

In those with established UC, repeated biopsies indicate an increased chronic inflammatory component in the lamina propria, often over a period of weeks or months, before the appearance of polymorphs in large numbers that correlate best with clinical activity.

Crohn's Disease

This disease can affect any part of the gastrointestinal tract and is characterized in its active phase by aphthoid ulceration with adjacent cobblestoning, by a chronic inflammatory process characterized by lymphoid aggregates that may be transmural, by fissures and fistulous tracts, in the resolving phase by fibrosis that may result in strictures, and by focal or multifocal disease radiologically, endoscopically, and pathologically. Noncaseating granulomas occur in some patients. As in ulcerative colitis, a variety of accompanying extraintestinal diseases may be present, but, unlike UC, evidence exists that CD, as manifest by granulomatous disease, may sometimes affect other tissues or organs.

The diagnosis of CD rests upon the demonstration of the microscopic features referred to previously; commonly, the gross appearances will strongly suggest the diagnosis. In its differential diagnosis from other forms of inflammatory bowel disease, the gross appearances may be worth any number of histologic sections in demonstrating focality, cobblestoning, or aphthoid ulcers, all of which can be difficult to be certain about when reviewing a series of slides.* To this end the importance of taking gross photographs cannot be overemphasized, particularly when dealing with disease of the large intestine.

Because resections are only carried out for complications of the disease, the range of changes encountered grossly by the pathologist is now relatively limited. These include resections for strictures causing obstructive symptoms, fistula, or, less frequently, active disease usually with bleeding that is unresponsive to treatment, fulminant colitis, or carcinoma. Conversely, endoscopists are familiar with the cobblestone/aphthoid ulcer phase of the disease.

---

*Editor's note: see also, Dvorak, A. M., and Silen, W.: Ann. Surg., 201:53, 1985.

Active Crohn's Disease

The characteristic lesion of active Crohn's disease is the aphthoid ulcer, which can be found anywhere along the GI tract. In the smallest lesions identifiable by light microscopy, it is apparent that while they can occur anywhere in the gastrointestinal tract, even towards the tips of small intestinal villi, these have a real predilection for the epithelium overlying lymphoid aggregates; in the small intestine these cells are the M-cells.[41] The lymphoepithelial complex, which contains the M-cell in the small intestine, has a counterpart in the large intestine that also is predisposed to the development of aphthoid ulcers.[42] This offers at least a partial explanation for the frequent association of aphthoid ulcers with underlying lymphoid tissue. Because any epithelium may be affected, however, some aphthoid ulcers need not be associated with underlying lymphoid tissue or may incite the development of underlying lymphoid aggregates as a secondary phenomenon.

Development and Resolution of Cobblestone Mucosa and Linear Ulceration

In examining multiple biopsies or resected specimens from patients with CD, one can invariably find in the least affected areas simple, aphthoid ulcers that are well-circumscribed. In more severely affected mucosa, however, aphthoid ulcers often are larger and have a more stellate appearance (Fig. 18-7). Although these stellate ulcers tend to fuse primarily in a longitudinal direction, they also fuse transversely to form islands of spared mucosa surrounded on all sides by aphthoid ulceration. The mucosa only is slightly edematous, but the underlying submucosa is very edematous with significant lymphangiectasia. It is the submucosal disease that results in the cobblestone appearance. It is unclear why the mucosa and submucosa should show these changes in the absence of demonstrable lymphatic obstruction. It can be argued that the large ulcers impede lymphatic flow, although one could argue equally that loss of fluid into the lumen would be the more likely result. The background mucosa is frequently normal, although a whole spectrum of changes from architecturally normal to atrophic mucosa can be found in which the inflammatory component varies from normal to an excess of either acute or chronic inflammatory cells, often both. Mast cells are present in large numbers in this phase of the disease, both in the submucosa and in the muscle.[43]

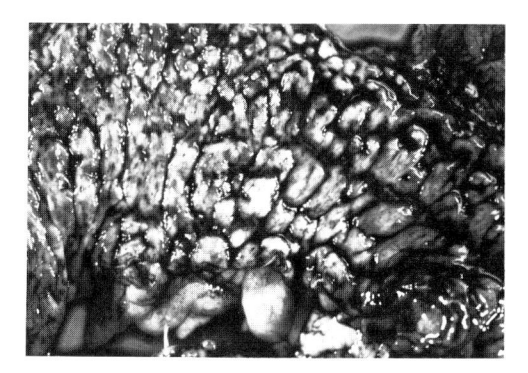

FIG. 18-7. Crohn's disease. To the left, numerous aphthoid ulcers are visible, some of which have enlarged and fused with formation of transverse and longitudinal ulcers, giving a typical "cobblestone" appearance.

How do such changes resolve? Mucosal ulceration ultimately resolves by the development of typical regenerative changes, as described above in UC. In the small intestine, metaplasia to pyloric-type glands is a frequent but nonspecific finding, while regenerative changes may also be found. In addition, patients who have undergone ileal resection frequently show adaptive changes in the neoterminal ileal mucosa that develops the invaginations and numbers of absorptive cells similar to those seen in jejunal rather than ileal villi.

Edema can either be reabsorbed or undergo gradual fibrosis. The latter would certainly explain at least some of the tight strictures (Fig. 18-8) that primarily seem to involve the submucosa rather than the full thickness of the bowel wall.

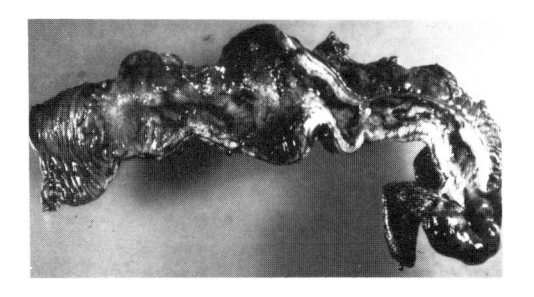

FIG. 18-8. Typical terminal ileal stricture from Crohn's disease causing obstructive symptoms. Note that ulcerations are present not only within the stricture but also within the diseased mucosa proximally.

Development of Fissures and Fistula

While these are a characteristic of Crohn's disease, remarkably little is known of their formation. Nevertheless, in random histologic sections the earliest phase of this process can sometimes be observed. Fissures are always seen to arise from the bases of aphthoid ulcers, invariably the lateral edges. It is presumed that fistulous tracts represent extensions from these, although the time frame over which such tracts develop is not clear. Because free perforation in the absence of toxic dilatation occurs but is rare in Crohn's disease, it seems unlikely that fistulae develop quickly; instead, sufficient time is probably available for a serositis to develop on the external surface of the bowel, allowing adhesion to an adjacent loop(s) of bowel into which these fissures may pass. Occasionally, large inflammatory masses are encountered that are the result of adherent loops of bowel with fistulae and abscesses in between (Fig. 18-9).

Fissures are invariably lined by neutrophils with a surrounding infiltrate of histiocytes and other mononuclear cells. Yet, with time it is not uncommon to observe attempts to reepithelialize these tracts, at least in part. This has important clinical connotations, for it is reasonable to suppose that if the driving force causing tracts to form is removed, whether by diversion of intestinal contents, parenteral nutrition, antibiotics, or combinations of these, the fissures and fistulae might undergo some degree of healing. Yet if they were to become completely epithelialized, it is almost inconceivable that they could close down permanently, any more than a loop of defunctioned bowel might become resorbed.

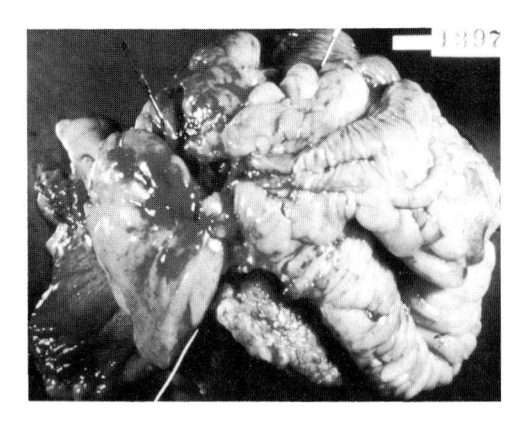

FIG. 18-9. Inflammatory mass in Crohn's disease caused by matted loops of small bowel with abscess formation and numerous fistulae, some of which are demarcated by probes.

Transmural Inflammation

This is characterized by lymphoid tissue and/or aggregates that are most dense in an expanded submucosa, with a second row immediately external to the muscularis propria. When both are well-developed, the diagnosis of CD can be made with confidence, the two rows of lymphoid "beads" being apparent. Occasional lymphoid aggregates within the muscularis propria complete the transmural inflammatory changes. Noncaseating granulomas may accompany the lymphoid aggregates, but when present are often situated adjacent to dilated lymphatics; indeed, the same also applies to the lymphoid aggregates. Interestingly, transmural inflammation is uncommon in surgical specimens resected during the acute or active phase of Crohn's disease, namely when fulminant disease (toxic dilatation) is present, or in resections for uncontrollable bleeding during the cobblestone/aphthoid ulcer phase of the disease; it is also relatively uncommon when rectal stumps are excised for persistent anorectal disease. Even in resections for otherwise unremarkable Crohn's disease, a considerable search is sometimes required to find transmural disease. These findings suggest that lymphoid aggregates develop in long-standing disease and are markers of chronicity.

Granulomas

Great variations exist between series concerning the likelihood of finding noncaseating granulomas either in biopsies or resected specimens. Even if granulomas are present, the chance of finding them in biopsies depends on their frequency and size, the number of slides examined, and the number of sections on each slide. Finally, the diligence of the examiner and the criteria used to call something a granuloma are important.[44] My preference is for a localized, well-formed aggregate of epithelioid histiocytes; the presence of giant cells or a surrounding cuff of lymphocytes is *not* required; solitary giant cells and indefinite aggregates of histiocytes are excluded, but prompt a search in adjacent sections or further slides from the same block for better formed granulomas.

Central necrosis can occasionally be seen in granulomas in Crohn's disease, but true caseation should raise the question of an alternative diagnosis, particularly tuberculosis. I regard granulomas that are less than about 4 cells in diameter to be dubious; in practice, this is rarely a problem as multiple sections usually resolve questions regarding whether a lesion is really a granuloma. If any doubts are voiced, my reports usually state that it is possible that a poorly-formed granuloma is present. Depending on the clinical circumstances I may, if multiple levels through the block are unrevealing, request a repeat biopsy or simply inquire whether any other clinical evidence suggests underlying granulomatous disease, particularly Crohn's disease. Some have found that biopsies from the edges of aphthoid ulcers have a high yield of granulomas, but I have been less fortunate in this regard.

It has been suggested that granulomas can be found in patients with Crohn's disease at some time in about 66% of instances, while careful examination of two rectal biopsies may reveal granulomas in 25%, if carefully sought.[45] It is a fact that in countries where Crohn's disease is rare, the diagnosis depends on the demonstration of granulomas, but with increasing experience this criterion is less important.

Of interest is the evolution of Crohn's disease within a country or society. Initially, the disease seems to be confined to atypical small intestinal lesions such as a single longitudinal ulcer that is often mesenteric and contains granulomas. As further cases come to light, more typical disease becomes endemic and the proportion of large bowel disease increases. We are becoming increasingly impressed by the recent dearth of granulomas in biopsies and resected specimens in North America, and also by the increased incidence (or detection) of gastroduodenal disease.

Significance of a Solitary Granuloma

The incidental finding of a granuloma in an otherwise normal biopsy in a patient with Crohn's disease poses a problem of interpretation. First, it may represent a completely different pathologic process, especially if one is practicing in an area where other granulomatous diseases are a consideration. For example, Tuberculosis, Yersinia, or Chlamydia must be excluded by using histologic, culture, and clinical methods. In areas where these diseases only need to be considered rarely, there is usually a clinical or pathologic suspicion that the lesion cannot be attributed to Crohn's disease. If no other cause can be involved, the temptation to consider this active involvement by Crohn's disease should be avoided, and that area of the bowel should not be treated topically in the absence of other local indications of Crohn's disease. Whether this part of the bowel will later become the seat of active disease has yet to be determined.

Granulomatous Crohn's disease may be less aggressive than its nongranulomatous counterpart,[45] thereby resembling other diseases such as leprosy and primary biliary cirrhosis in which patients with the granulomatous forms of the diseases do better than those with the nongranulomatous types.

Histologic Features in Resected Bowel

In long-standing disease, the "double row of beads" effect is by far the most comforting feature, particularly if accompanied by occasional granulomas and with a relatively intact mucosa. This combination is well-recognized and virtually diagnostic of Crohn's disease. Even in the absence of granulomas, other histologic pointers are adequate evidence on which to base a firm diagnosis. However, it must be stressed again that because granulomatous and other features may be focal, multiple additional sections are sometimes required to establish the diagnosis. In the absence of noncaseating granulomas, numerous submucosal lymphoid aggregates in the submucosa in the absence of transmural disease are probably the minimal change on which a confident diagnosis of Crohn's disease can be made; all other diagnoses are more presumptive. The finding of neuronal hyperplasia,[46] sometimes extending into the mucosa, may help confirm the diagnosis. Ulceration within tight strictures is the rule, irrespective of the underlying disease, and therefore is not helpful. Focal ulceration outside the strictured segment of bowel is also a useful pointer (Fig. 18-8), because it is an indicator of multifocal disease.

In active disease, the presence of cobblestoning can be seen better by visualizing the slide with the naked eye. Aphthoid ulcers appear within what is often unremarkable mucosa; indeed, the presence of a nonspecific superficial ulcer with adjacent normal mucosa is typical of such lesions.

Histologic Traps in Diagnosis

V-SHAPED ULCERS IN FULMINANT COLITIS. Perhaps the easiest mistake is to interpret the V-shaped ulcers in fulminant ulcerative colitis that may penetrate into, although rarely through, the muscularis propria, as being indicative of the transmural inflammation of Crohn's disease. These ulcers can be found in the active or fulminant phase of any of the inflammatory diseases including infections, and, therefore, are not specific. They may be accompanied by a surrounding chronic inflammatory infiltrate that, if it extends through the muscularis propria, generally can be incorporated into the term "transmural inflammation" even though the aggregates so characteristic of Crohn's disease are absent.

GRANULOMAS. The possibility that these might be caused by something other than Crohn's disease, including mucin-leak into the lamina propria, has been discussed previously. The possibility of a reaction to foreign material should always be considered, especially if the granuloma is in close proximity to an area of ulceration.

DIFFERENTIAL DIAGNOSIS OF UNUSUAL DISEASE. Occasionally Crohn's disease may present with unusual clinical or pathologic features, such as single or multiple large, but otherwise nonspecific, serpiginous or longitudinal ulcers of the large or small bowel. Even in the presence of granulomas the diagnosis may be difficult because of this unusual appearance; in their absence the differential diagnosis is that of nonspecific ulceration and includes ischemia, infections such as amebiasis or resolving (nongranulomatous) tuberculosis, involvement by Behçet's disease, or drug-induced disease such as that caused by potassium chloride or digoxin (especially in the ileum, which probably is also ischemic), ulcerative jejunoileitis, ulcers in celiac sprue, lymphoma, and sometimes ulcers that are "idiopathic." Those associated with other diseases depend on the demonstration that such disease is present, or that ingestion of the appropriate drug has occurred.

Biopsy Diagnosis of Crohn's Disease

Single biopsy

Features suggesting that the underlying disease is Crohn's disease are the following:

GRANULOMAS. In North America, Crohn's disease is probably the most common underlying disease, but the presence of granulomas in biopsies remains relatively uncommon unless serial sections are carried out, as indicated earlier. The differential diagnosis depends to a large extent on which part of the gastrointestinal tract is being examined by using a biopsy. As stressed previously, however, a variety of infections causing granulomas are known occasionally to involve the gastrointestinal tract, and these include tuberculosis, fungi, Yersinia, Chlamydia, or, rarely, syphilis. Sarcoid is similarly uncommon. In the stomach, food granulomas, idiopathic granulomatous gastritis, and reactions to tumors are all rare causes of granulomas. In a patient with known Crohn's disease, granulomas can be found in any part of the gastrointestinal tract including minor salivary glands, and are perhaps least common in the esophagus.

APHTHOID ULCERS. These produce a characteristic biopsy appearance with an ulcer on one edge of the biopsy (Fig. 18-10). Because superficial ulceration can occur in a variety of diseases, a useful pointer is that in Crohn's disease the adjacent mucosa is frequently either normal or only minimally inflamed, and often the crypts contain more mucus. In the large bowel this is in direct contrast to ulcerative colitis where ulceration or erosion invariably occurs against a

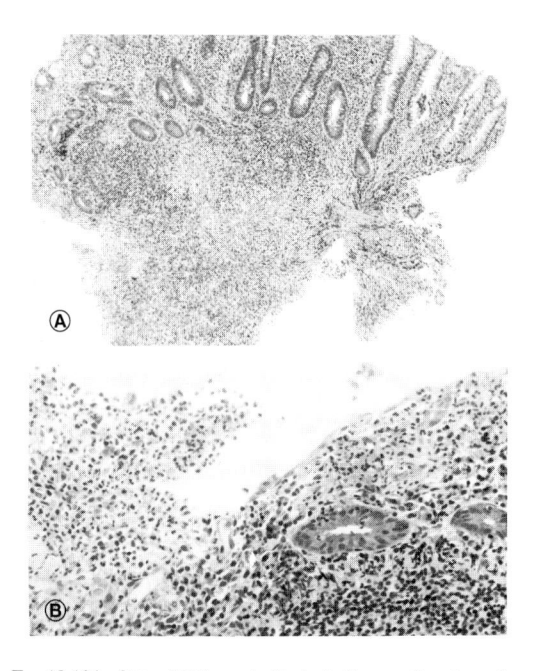

FIG. 18-10A. Sigmoid biopsy in Crohn's disease. Crypts on the right are relatively preserved with normal architecture and mucous production; on the left, both are abnormal. Multiple basal lymphoid aggregates confirm chronic disease.
B. Detail from left edge of Part A shows the edge of an ulcer (left). The combination of an ulcer in one part of the biopsy with relatively preserved mucosa in another is characteristic of tissue from an aphthoid ulcer.

background of heavy inflammation, with diffuse mucin depletion and a neutrophil infiltrate that shows a real propensity to attack the crypts. In biopsies of aphthoid ulcers a large part of the biopsy may fail to show even mucin-depletion.

In the large bowel, given an appropriate clinical and endoscopic setting, such biopsies are virtually diagnostic of CD; however, in the upper gastrointestinal tract localized ulcer disease, particularly that associated with aspirin or nonsteroidal anti-inflammatory drugs, can produce virtually identical biopsy findings. The endoscopic finding of cobblestoning, in the distal duodenum, or combined gastroduodenal disease all increase the index of suspicion of Crohn's disease. Because upper gastrointestinal CD invariably occurs in patients with documented CD elsewhere in the gastrointestinal tract, we are cautious about making a *primary* diagnosis of Crohn's disease in the upper part of the gastrointestinal tract.

DISPROPORTIONATE SUBMUCOSAL INFLAMMATION. This applies only to large bowel biopsies and consists of a heavy submucosal infiltrate with a relatively normal overlying mucosa. The clinical correlation of this is a biopsy taken from what appeared to be inflamed mucosa. If only normal appearing mucosa is obtained, the possibility of disproportionate submucosal disease, indicative of Crohn's disease, should always be considered. Note that this does not include either a large solitary lymphoid nodule, which may be normal but always either straddles or is immediately below the muscularis mucosae, or multiple small lymphoid aggregates on either side of the muscularis mucosae, which rather are markers of any form of chronic inflammatory bowel disease.

FOCAL MUCOSAL DISEASE. This is the least specific variant of aphthoid ulcers and disproportionate submucosal inflammation and it consists of a great variability in the quantity of inflammation in different parts of the same biopsy or between biopsies. In the upper gastrointestinal tract similar changes can also be seen in a variety of inflammatory conditions, including peptic ulcer disease. It is, therefore, most useful when present in the more distal duodenum where peptic ulcer and drug-induced disease are less common. In the large bowel, similar changes can be seen in active or resolving infections, and in ulcerative proctitis or colitis near the transition with more normal mucosa. As a finding in a single biopsy, this change is relatively unhelpful other than to pinpoint that part of the bowel as having inflammatory disease, although significant focality is uncommon in UC.

TERMINAL ILEITIS. The presence of an acute terminal ileitis in an appropriate clinical setting strongly favors Crohn's disease (Fig. 18-11). Adaptive changes are effectively limited to biopsies of neoterminal ileum following prior ileocecal resection, and consist of relative "jejunalization" of terminal ileal villi. If extensive small bowel resection has been carried out, some may argue that this merely indicates normal mid-ileal villi. We have noted it in patients with relatively extensive small bowel disease who have had limited resections, however, and therefore consider it a genuine finding.

PYLORIC METAPLASIA. Although of no diagnostic value in the upper gastrointestinal tract, this may also be found in biopsies from the terminal ileum. While merely an indicator of preexisting

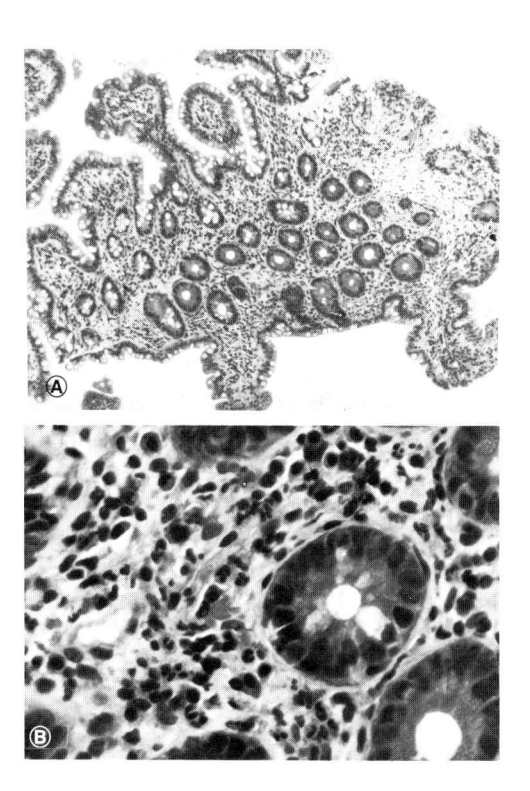

FIG. 18-11A. Terminal ileal biopsy with relatively normal initial appearance. Crypts in the lower half are depleted of goblet cells, however.
B. Detail shows numerous polymorphs in the lamina propria but little evidence of crypts. These features are those of acute terminal ileitis and suggest the presence of CD in a patient with other evidence of the disease.

chronic inflammatory disease, in North America this effectively indicates Crohn's disease and it is useful in the distinction from UC. In other parts of the world, however, it is a less specific diagnostic finding.

Multiple Biopsies from the Same Level

These can be used to advantage to demonstrate the focal nature of Crohn's disease on light microscopy. Thus, while architecturally some biopsies may have a normal crypt structure, others may show atrophic and regenerative changes. Focality of inflammation may be apparent in some biopsies that are heavily inflamed, while others are only focally so, and some have no excess of inflammatory cells. Possible exceptions are considered in the "Focal Mucosal Disease" section. It should be noted, however, that in the large bowel, infections only rarely cause atrophic changes.[32]

Multiple Biopsies from a Variety of Levels

In the upper gastrointestinal tract, this can be useful in demonstrating the focal nature of distal duodenal CD with sparing of the proximal duodenum, features that are uncommon in peptic ulcer disease. However, these biopsies really come into their own in the large bowel where the diagnosis of Crohn's disease can be strongly suggested not only because of the presence of many of the features already described, but also because they can add the dimension of the light microscopic distribution of disease. In ulcerative colitis, if architectural changes are present they always occur in the most distal biopsies but may be present in continuity proximally. Similarly, if active disease is present it invariably follows the same distribution, with the most active disease being distal. Crohn's disease is, however, invariably focal on light microscopy so that in a series of biopsies from cecum to rectum neither the architectural damage nor, most importantly, the severity of the inflammatory infiltrate present is predictable, and this haphazard pattern is helpful in establishing a positive diagnosis of CD.

"Indeterminate Colitis"

The term "indeterminate colitis" has been proposed as an appropriate appellation for those cases that show maximal overlap of the pathologic features of ulcerative colitis and Crohn's disease.[47,48] In these a firm diagnosis either of ulcerative colitis or Crohn's disease may depend on the review of previous material or have to await the evidence from resection or subsequent follow-up. In resected specimens this essentially comes down to estimating the number of features that are unlike ulcerative colitis and thus raise the odds that CD is the underlying disease, despite the absence of bona fide evidence for CD.

Clearly, a range of degrees of certainty exists with which a diagnosis of Crohn's disease can be made, that is, definite, probable, possible, and no evidence. The first and last of these pose no problems; however, the others, "possible" and "probable" Crohn's disease, can be handled in one of two ways. Either or both can be referred to as "indeterminate colitis;" alternatively, "possible" and "probable" Crohn's disease can be designated as "inflammatory bowel disease". The real question is what criteria should be used for either of these categories, and how sensitive are these for prognosticating the development of more specific features of Crohn's disease.

Perhaps the simplest example is a colectomy specimen in which a solitary granuloma is present for which no apparent cause is found in 20 sections of bowel (see earlier). Assuming that this is not a reaction to mucin, other demonstrable foreign material, or another definable cause, is this sufficient grounds for a diagnosis of Crohn's disease? Most pathologists would be hesitant, even if this were present only in the serosa and away from all other inflammation. Similarly, most would also hesitate to make an unequivocal diagnosis of ulcerative colitis. This problem can be handled either by using "indeterminate colitis" or "inflammatory bowel disease," or "possible" or "probable" (depending on one's own degree of uncertainty) Crohn's disease, but its clinical value in predicting subsequent more florid CD remains largely undefined. Similarly, the number of granulomas required for "possible CD" to become "probable CD" or "definite CD" has never been defined; some might feel that a single granuloma is adequate for an unequivocal diagnosis. The clinical significance relates little to medical therapy, but becomes important prognostically, especially if the patient is being considered for a reservoir/pouch procedure.

In my practice the term "indeterminate colitis" is used relatively rarely, with ulcerative colitis being used unless features exist that raise the question of underlying Crohn's disease. If these are present, the thought is expressed in terms of "possible" or "probable" disease. If Crohn's disease has been considered because a single feature of that disease is present I tend to use "possible;" if two features such as a granuloma and serosal lymphoid tissue are present in an area of mucosal ulceration, I tend to use "probable." If more than this evidence is present, it is usually possible to make a definitive diagnosis of CD. It is currently unwise to proceed to pouch or reservoir procedures without serious consideration of the potential disadvantages, when there is even a suggestion of underlying Crohn's disease. Importantly, in instances where patients with apparent ulcerative colitis underwent resection and subsequently developed features of Crohn's disease, in most (but not all) "soft" evidence of Crohn's disease could be found retrospectively in the resected colonic specimen.

As implied earlier, a variety of traps exist into which the unwary may fall in the presence of fulminant disease that question whether it is possible in this situation to make the diagnosis of Crohn's disease. It is certainly possible, but with the following provisos:

GRANULOMAS. In the presence of granulomas, particularly in the submucosa and/or subserosa away from areas of ulceration or in lymph nodes, in the absence of any other cause, the diagnosis of CD is relatively simple.

LYMPHOID TISSUE. The presence of lymphoid aggregates or nodules in an expanded submucosa or, better, in the subserosa, in a segment of bowel that is not ulcerated, is strong evidence that the underlying disease is in fact Crohn's disease. If they are present, plus they have superficial mucosal erosions, the diagnosis of CD is invariably correct. As ulceration extends to involve the full mucosa or superficial mucosa, lymphoid aggregates in the submucosa should probably be interpreted as a reaction to the local ulceration. Under these circumstances, a row of lymphoid nodules in the subserosa may be taken as evidence of Crohn's disease. Once ulceration extends into the muscularis propria, it is unwise to regard this as evidence of the transmural inflammation of CD, as it is nonspecific.

RECTAL SPARING. As already emphasized, in a few patients with ulcerative colitis the characteristic features of the disease are obscured or absent during fulminant attacks.[47,48] The rectum, although usually involved, may be spared, particularly in a severe first attack, with the brunt of the disease falling on the mucosa proximal to the rectum. The role of steroid enemas as a cause of apparent rectal sparing is unclear but it is sometimes evoked as an explanation. Before the advent of steroid therapy, rectal sparing was often attributed to the effect of cod liver oil or other enemas popular at the time (Kirsner, J.B., personal communication). In such cases careful sigmoidoscopy often reveals relatively normal appearing rectum and, above that, scattered ulcers, before the more proximal diffusely affected mucosa is seen. Multiple biopsies therefore may show focal disease and can easily be misinterpreted as Crohn's disease because of the focality. A normal rectal mucosa is probably acceptable in UC in a first attack of the disease; this feature itself should not negate a diagnosis of UC under these circumstances. Nevertheless, this reflects my personal experience and has never been critically evaluated.

FISSURING ULCERS. In severely diseased areas fissuring ulcers, extending into the muscularis propria as V-shaped clefts, are frequently accompanied by some degree of dilatation of the colon (see previous section). In ulcerative colitis these are always found in areas of extensive ulceration and are accompanied by signs of myocytolysis and vascular dilatation in the adjacent tissue. They differ from the typical fissures of Crohn's disease that have a more prominent inflammatory cell component, show less myocytolysis in adjacent muscle, and are not limited to areas of extensive overlying mucosal ulceration. This is not useful as a distinguishing criterion, however. Such cases represent some of the 10% of colectomy specimens that cannot be confidently identified as either ulcerative colitis or Crohn's disease.[47,48]

NEURONAL PROLIFERATION. The neuronal proliferation seen in CD may extend into the submucosa where it may be detected immunocytochemically using neuron-specific enolase.[49] Although only a preliminary finding at the time of writing, if present this would support a diagnosis of CD. If this change is dependent on longstanding disease, however, a negative finding is probably not indicative that the underlying disease is UC, particularly in a first attack.

Coexistent Ulcerative Colitis and Crohn's Disease

A question asked with increasing frequency is whether ulcerative colitis can coexist with Crohn's disease in the same patient. Suggestions that this might occur have appeared in the literature.[50-52] Clearly, if both diseases ultimately prove to have different etiologies there is no reason, statistically, why this should not happen. Indeed, because the prevalence of ulcerative colitis is approximately 40 to 80/100,000 and that of Crohn's disease is approximately 15/100,000, coexistence of the two would be expected to occur in 6 to 12/100,000,000 of the population, or 15 to 30 cases in the United States. Conversely, if they prove to be different manifestations of the same etiologic agent it should not happen at all, unless it represents changes in the nature of the etiologic agent and/or the host responses to it. The underlying bias of trying to make most diseases fit one category or another might prevent the recognition of such cases when they occur. Thus, any patient with typical ulcerative colitis in whom a biopsy or resected material shows typical granulomas or other features of Crohn's disease is usually classified as having Crohn's disease. This approach is, of course, pragmatic because most of such patients ultimately appear to behave like Crohn's disease patients, with the risk of any or all of its complications, and, if follow-up is sufficiently long, most are not cured by proctocolectomy.

In a few patients the evolution of the disease may necessitate a change in diagnosis; this is invariably from ulcerative colitis to Crohn's disease rather than the other way round. In some of these patients a careful review of previous material may reveal either pronounced focality or "missed" granulomas. It should be remembered that Crohn's colitis passed unrecognized as a clinical entity until the early 1960's; patients undergoing proctocolectomy and ileostomy before that time were virtually all diagnosed as having ulcerative colitis; some returned later with "ileostomy dysfunction" or further disease in the small bowel that was clearly the result of CD. In a few patients, however, such recrudescences may indicate the coexistence of both diseases rather than a failure to differentially diagnose them.

Differential Diagnosis

Ischemia

In the elderly or arteriopathic patient it may be difficult to differentiate histologically between acute ulcerative colitis and low-grade ischemic colitis. The subsequent clinical course provides better differentiation than does the evolution of the histologic changes. Although hemosiderin deposition is said to distinguish ischemic colitis, it is, in fact, a nonspecific finding.[53]

Infection (Acute Self-limited Colitis)

As mentioned previously, some forms of infective colitis may resemble ulcerative colitis clinically. For example, bacillary dysentery and gonococcal proctitis produce mucosal inflammation with a macroscopic distribution similar to that of ulcerative colitis or proctitis. The clinical picture and microbiologic studies of the stool or mucus usually establish the correct diagnosis, however. Several points are worth remembering. Standard microbiologic methods may be inadequate and special methods are necessary to isolate some organisms such as Campylobacter or Yersinia. Furthermore, a predisposition for salmonella infection has been reported in patients with ulcerative colitis and Crohn's disease,[35,36] and, in some patients, exacerbations of ulcerative colitis occur with stools that contain Campylobacter or the C. difficile toxin.[37-39] It is not clear whether the apparent predisposition to infection by these organisms is peculiar to ulcerative colitis, a consequence of antibiotics or steroid therapy, or simply represents a carrier state.

The histologic features of acute self-limited colitis (ASLC) may differ from those that are typical of ulcerative colitis (Fig. 18-12).[33,34]* In infective colitis the architecture is preserved and the active inflammation tends to be superficial with epithelial destruction, in contrast to ulcerative colitis in which the acute inflammation and crypt abscesses are usually basal. In infective colitis mucin depletion and accompanying chronic inflammatory cell infiltration are less than is expected in ulcerative colitis. Basal lymphoid or plasma cell aggregates are conspicuously absent. Unfortunately, such differences may be difficult to detect. Recovery from infective colitis is usually followed by restoration of histologically normal mucosa. The diffuse mucosal atrophy and crypt distortion indicative of previous active disease, which typify quiescent ulcerative colitis, are notably absent, unless infection is superimposed on underlying ulcerative colitis. Gram stains are rarely successful in demonstrating the infecting organisms and, therefore, are usually of little value in differential diagnosis.

---

*Editor's note: see also Nostrant, T. T., et al.: Gastroenterology 92:318, 1987.

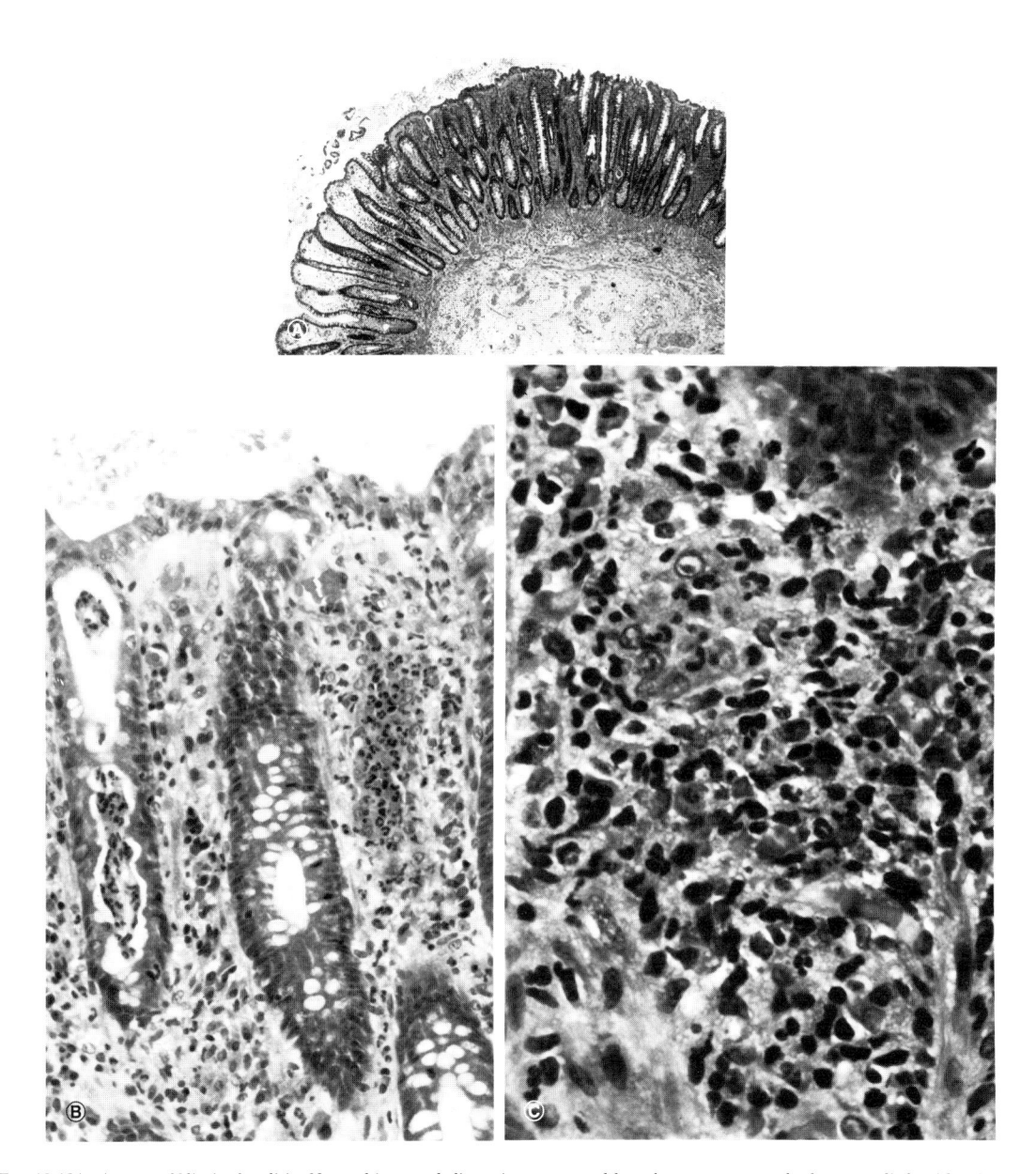

FIG. 18-12A. Acute self-limited colitis. No architectural distortion occurs although crypts are pushed apart a little either by edema (left) or the inflammatory infiltrate. No basal lymphoid infiltrates that indicate longstanding inflammatory bowel disease are present.
B. Detail showing a superficial crypt abscess; although polymorphs in the lamina propria are plentiful they show little tendency to infiltrate crypts.
C. Higher power with numerous neutrophils.

Solitary Rectal Ulcer Syndrome

The clinicopathologic "spectrum" of this disease is well-described and has characteristic histology (Fig. 18-13).[55,56] Nevertheless, it may escape diagnosis if the pathologist or clinician is not familiar with the typical appearances or if the biopsy is taken from an area of mucosa that is minimally involved. Solitary rectal ulcer syndrome (SRUS) is only a factor in the differential diagnosis of IBD limited to the rectum and distal sigmoid colon, and not in the differential diagnosis of more proximal disease.

Collagenous Colitis

Since its description in 1976,[56] it has become apparent either that this disease is more com-

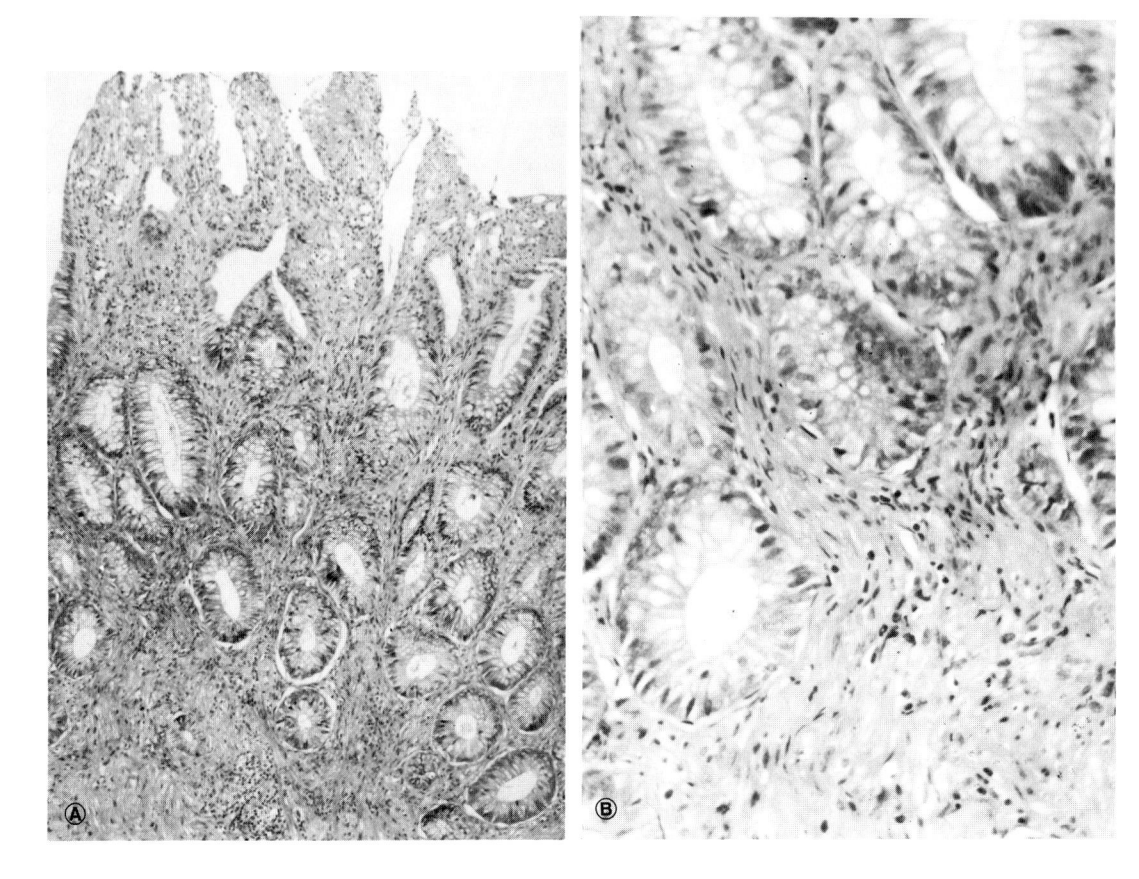

FIG. 18-13A. Solitary rectal ulcer syndrome. The lamina propria is obliterated by fibromuscular tissue derived from the hyperplastic muscularis mucosae. Note the early superficial ulceration.
B. Detail of Part A, showing fibromuscular tissue in the lamina propria.

mon than was originally thought or it is increasing rapidly in incidence; most large centers for intestinal diseases have seen many cases.[57-59*] It has been shown that normally the subepithelial basement membrane does not exceed 10μ, and that in symptomatic patients with collagenous colitis it is always greater than 15μ.[60] Because collagenous colitis is now so well-recognized it is unlikely to be missed on biopsy. Clinically, it is the most likely diagnosis in middle aged to elderly women presenting with watery diarrhea. While some resolve dramatically, others persist or recur. We have seen examples that seem almost certainly to be ischemic in etiology, but others where this seemed most unlikely.**

Drug-induced Proctitis and Colitis

Enemas and laxatives can cause mucin depletion, superficial epithelial damage, and even a superficial polymorph infiltrate;[61] however, the use of GoLytely lavage has largely overcome these effects.[62†] A variety of other drugs given either topically or systemically can cause colitis or proctitis; these include local NSAID's, penicillamine, sulfasalazine, methyldopa, and gold.[63] A correct drug history is indispensible in the investigation of all patients with diarrhea. Finally, it should be remembered that ingestion of laxatives remains a relatively common cause of diarrhea, and one of the best reasons for advocating routine biopsies for patients with diarrhea who are undergoing colonoscopy is that evidence of anthraquinone ingestion, as manifest by melanosis coli, remains relatively common, but this may not be obvious endoscopically and the patient may deny the ingestion.

Diversion Colitis and "Pouchitis"

These sequelae of surgical therapy are currently the subject of considerable controversy. Both

*Editor's note: see also Rams, H., et al: Ann. Intern. Med., 106:108, 1987.
**Editor's note: see also Nostrant, T. T., et al.: Gastroenterology 92:318, 1987.

†Braintree Laboratories, Inc.; 285 Washington St., Braintree, MA 02184

may cause symptoms and show inflammation, and in both the question is always whether the symptoms and pathology are caused by organisms or their toxins or represent recurrent disease, especially CD. Since the description of diversion colitis it appears that whatever its morphology, this disease can largely be ignored as all features disappear when rejoined to proximal bowel.[64] While the endoscopic appearances may be patchy and even aphthous ulcers can develop,[65] these resolve following reanastomosis. The situation with inflammation in Koch, "J," or "S" pouches may be similar, but some of these are more likely to be caused by recurrent CD. Perhaps the most frustrating aspect is that there seems little correlation between the patient's symptoms and either the endoscopic or histologic appearances. It is hoped that current work in this field will help resolve these problems.

References

1. Farmer, R. G.: Long-term prognosis for patients with ulcerative proctosigmoiditis (ulcerative colitis confined to the rectum and sigmoid colon). J. Clin. Gastroenterol., 1:47, 1979.
2. Morson, B. C., and Dawson, I. M. P.: Gastrointestinal Pathology. London, Blackwell, 1979.
3. de la Monte, S., and Hutchins, G.: Follicular proctocolitis and neuromatous hyperplasia with lymphogranuloma venereum. Hum. Pathol., 16:1025, 1985.
4. Yardley, J. H., and Donowitz, M.: Colo-rectal biopsy in inflammatory bowel disease. In The Gastrointestinal Tract. Edited by J. H. Yardley and B. C. Morson. Monograph of the International Academy of Pathology. Baltimore, Williams & Wilkins, 1977.
5. Haggitt, R. C.: The differential diagnosis of idiopathic inflammatory bowel disease. In Pathology of the Colon, Small Intestine and Anus. Edited by H. T. Norris. New York, Churchill Livingstone, 1983.
6. Bookman, M. A., and Bull, D. M.: Characteristics of isolated intestinal mucosal lymphoid cells in inflammatory bowel disease. Gastroenterology, 77:503, 1979.
7. Brandtzaeg, P., Baklien, K., Fausa, O., and Hoel, P. S.: Immunohistochemical characterization of local immunoglobulin formation in ulcerative colitis. Gastroenterology, 66:1123, 1974.
8. O'Donoghue, D. P., and Kumar, P.: Rectal IgE cells in inflammatory bowel disease. Gut, 20:149, 1979.
9. Rosekrans, P. C. M., Meijer, C. J. L. M., Van Der Wal., A. M., and Lindeman, J.: Allergic proctitis: a clinical and immunopathological entity. Gut, 21:1017, 1980.
10. Willoughby, C. P., Piris, J., and Truelove, S. C.: Tissue eosinophils in ulcerative colitis. Scand. J. Gastroenterol., 14:395, 1979.
11. Heatley, R. V., and James, P. D.: Eosinophils in the rectal mucosa. A simple method of predicting the outcome of ulcerative proctitis? Gut, 20:787, 1978.
12. Naylor, A. R., and Pollet, J. E.: Eosinophilic colitis. Dis. Colon Rectum, 28:615, 1985.
13. Goldman, H., and Proujansky, R.: Allergic proctitis and gastroenteritis in children. Clinical and mucosal biopsy features in 53 cases. J. Surg. Pathol., 10:75, 1986.
14. Riddell, R. H., et al.: Dysplasia in inflammatory bowel disease. Standardized classification with provisional clinical implications. Hum. Pathol., 9:931, 1983.
15. Riddell, R. H.: The precancerous lesions of ulcerative colitis. In The Gastrointestinal Tract. Edited by J. H. Yardley and B. C. Morson. Monograph of the International Academy of Pathology. Baltimore, Williams & Wilkins, 1977.
16. Kirsner, J. B., Palmer, W. L., and Klotz, A. P.: Reversibility in ulcerative colitis: clinical and roentgenologic observations. Radiology, 57:1, 1951.
17. Goulston, S. J. M., and McGovern, V. J.: The nature of benign strictures in ulcerative colitis. N. Engl. J. Med., 281:290, 1969.
18. Buckwell, N. A., Williams, G. T., Bartram, C. I., and Lennard-Jones, J. E.: Depth of ulceration in acute colitis. Gastroenterology, 79:19, 1980.
19. Warren, S., and Sommers, S. C.: Pathogenesis of ulcerative colitis. Am. J. Pathol., 25:657, 1949.
20. Lumb, G., and Protheroe, R. H. B.: Biopsy of the rectum in ulcerative colitis. Lancet, 2:1208, 1955.
21. Edwards, F. C., and Truelove, S. C.: The course and prognosis of ulcerative colitis. Gut, 5:1, 1964.
22. Jalan, K. N., et al.: An experience of ulcerative colitis. I. Toxic dilatation in 55 cases. Gastroenterology, 57:68, 1969.
23. Greenstein, A. J., et al.: Outcome of toxic dilatation in ulcerative and Crohn's colitis. J. Clin. Gastroenterol., 7:137, 1985.
24. Norland, C. C., and Kirsner, J. B.: Toxic dilatation of colon (toxic megacolon): etiology, treatment and prognosis in 42 patients. Medicine, 48:229, 1969.
25. deDombal, F. T., and Watts, J. McK., Watkinson, G., and Goligher, J. C.: Local complications of ulcerative colitis: stricture, pseudopolyposis, and carcinoma of colon and rectum. Br. Med. J., 2:1442, 1966.
26. Saltzstein, S. L., and Rosenberg, B. F.: Ulcerative colitis of the ileum and regional enteritis of the colon, a comparative histopathologic study. Am. J. Clin. Pathol., 40:610, 1963.
27. Markowitz, A. M.: The less common perforations of the small bowel. Ann. Surg., 152:240, 1960.
28. Dawson, I. M. P., and Pryse-Davies, J.: The development of carcinomas of the large intestine in ulcerative colitis. Br. J. Surg., 47:113, 1959.
29. Hinrichs, R. H., and Goldman, H.: Localized giant pseudopolyposis of the colon. J. Am. Med. Assoc., 205:108, 1968.
30. Jalan, K. N., et al.: Pseudopolyposis in ulcerative colitis. Lancet, 2:555, 1969.
31. Kelly, J. K., et al.: Giant and symptomatic inflammatory polyps of the colon in idiopathic inflammatory bowel disease. Am. J. Surg. Pathol., 10:420, 1986.
32. Anand, B. S., et al.: Rectal histology in acute bacillary dysentery. Gastroenterology, 90:654, 1986.
33. Surawicz, C. M., and Belic, L.: Rectal biopsy helps to distinguish acute self-limited colitis from idiopathic inflammatory bowel disease. Gastroenterology, 86:104, 1984.
34. Kumar, N. B., Nostrant, T. T., and Appelman, H. D.: This histopathologic spectrum of acute self-limited colitis (acute infectious-type colitis). Am. J. Surg. Pathol., 6:523, 1982.
35. Dronfield, M. W., Fletcher, J., and Langman, M. J. S.: Coincident salmonella infections and ulcerative colitis: problems of recognition and management. Br. Med. J., 1:99, 1974.
36. Lindeman, R. J., Weinstein, L., Levitan, R., and Patterson, J. F.: Ulcerative colitis and intestinal salmonellosis. Am. J. Med. Sci., 106:856, 1967.
37. Newman, A., and Lambert, J. R.: Campylobacter jejuni

causing flare-up in inflammatory bowel disease. Lancet, 2:919, 1980.
38. Bolton, R. P., Sheriff, R. J., and Read, A. D.: Clostridium difficile associated diarrhoea: a role in inflammatory bowel disease. Lancet, 1:383, 1980.
39. LaMont, J. T., and Trnka, Y. M.: Therapeutic implications of clostridium difficile toxin during relapse of chronic inflammatory bowel disease. Lancet, 1:381, 1980.
40. Dickinson, R. J., Gilmour, H. M., and McClelland, D. B. L.: Rectal biopsy in patients presenting to an infectious disease unit with diarrhoeal disease. Gut, 20:141, 1979.
41. Owen, R. L.: And now pathophysiology of M-cells—good news and bad news from Peyer's patches. Gastroenterology, 85:468, 1983.
42. O'Leary, A. D., and Sweeney, E. C.: Lymphoglandular complexes of the colon: structure and distribution. Histopathology, 10:267, 1986.
43. Dvorak, A. M., Monahan, R. A., Osage, J. E., and Dickerson, G. R.: Crohn's disease: Transmission electron microscopic studies. II. Immunologic inflammatory response. Alteration of mast cells, basophils, eosinophils and the microvasculotase. Hum. Pathol., 11:606, 1980.
44. Surawicz, C. M., et al.: Rectal biopsy in the diagnosis of Crohn's disease: value of multiple biopsies and serial sectioning. Gastroenterology, 81:66, 1981.
45. Chambers, T. J., and Morson, B. C.: The histopathological evolution of Crohn's disease. *In* Recent Advances in Crohn's Disease. Edited by A. S. Peña, I. T. Weterman, C. C. Booth, and W. Strober. The Hague, Martinus Nijhoff, 1981.
46. Dvorak, A. M., Monahan, R. A., Osage, J. E., and Dickerson, G. R.: Crohn's disease: Transmission electron microscopic studies. III. Target tissues. Proliferation of and injury to smooth muscle and the autonomic nervous system. Hum. Pathol., 11:620, 1980.
47. Lee, K. S., Medline, A., and Shockey, S.: Indeterminate colitis in the spectrum of inflammatory bowel disease. Arch. Pathol. Lab. Med., 193:173, 1979.
48. Price, A. B.: Overlap in the spectrum of non-specific inflammatory bowel disease—'colitis indeterminate'. J. Clin. Pathol., 31:567, 1978.
49. Troster, M., and Grignon, D.: Enteric nerve fibres, ganglion cells and Schwann cells in Crohn's disease and ulcerative colitis: an immunohistochemical study using S-100 protein and neuron-specific enolase. Lab. Invest., 54:64, 1986.
50. Voitk, A. J., Owen, D. R., and Lough, J.: Coexistent regional enteritis and ulcerative colitis. Int. Surg., 61:535, 1976.
51. Eyer, S., et al.: Simultaneous ulcerative colitis and Crohn's disease. Am. J. Gastroenterol., 73:345, 1980.
52. Jones, B. J. M., Gould, S. S., and Pollock, D. J.: Coexistent ulcerative colitis and Crohn's disease. Postgrad. Med. J., 61:647, 1985.
53. Mitros, F., and Johlin, F.: Relative nonspecificity of hemosiderin deposition in colon as a marker for ischemia. Lab. Invest., 54:44, 1986.
54. Rutter, K. R. P., and Riddell, R. H.: The solitary ulcer syndrome of the rectum. Clin. Gastroenterol., 4:505, 1975.
55. Ford, M. J., et al.: Clinical spectrum of "solitary ulcer" of the spectrum. Gastroenterology, 85:1533, 1983.
56. Lindstrom, C. S.: Collagenous colitis with watery diarrhoea—a new entity? Pathol. Europe; 11:87, 1979.
57. Kingham, J. G. C., et al.: Collagenous colitis. Gut, 27:570, 1986.
58. Palmer, K. R., et al.: Collagenous colitis—a relapsing and remitting disease. Gut, 27:578, 1986.
59. Fausa, O., Foerster, A., and Hovig, T.: Collagenous colitis. A clinical, histological and ultrastructural study. Scand. J. Gastroenterol. (Suppl.), 107:8, 1985.
60. Gledhill, A., and Cole, F. M.: Significance of basement membrane thickening in the human colon. Gut, 25:1085, 1984.
61. Meisel, J. L., et al.: Human rectal mucosa: proctoscopic and morphological changes caused by laxatives. Gastroenterology, 72:1274, 1977.
62. Pockros, P. J., and Foroozan, P.: GoLytely lavage versus a standard colonoscopy preparation. Effect on normal colonic mucosal histology. Gastroenterology, 88:545, 1985.
63. Riddell, R. H.: The gastrointestinal tract. *In* Pathology of Drug-Induced and Toxic Diseases. Edited by R. H. Riddell. New York, Churchill-Livingstone, 1982.
64. Glotzer, D. J., Glick, M. E., and Goldman, H.: Proctitis and colitis following diversion of the fecal stream. Gastroenterology, 80:438, 1981.
65. Lusk, L. B., Reichen, J., and Levine, J. S.: Aphthous ulcerations in diversion colitis. Clinical implications. Gastroenterology, 87:1171, 1984.

Acknowledgements. I would like to thank Janice Butera and Lydia Wilson for their secretarial expertise and kind assistance.

Section 5 · *Endoscopy and Radiology*

19 · Endoscopy in Idiopathic Inflammatory Bowel Disease

JEROME D. WAYE, M.D.

Endoscopy plays a well-defined role in the diagnosis and management of patients with inflammatory bowel disease, particularly when the large bowel is involved.[1] In most instances colonoscopy is the last step in a succession of diagnostic examinations carried out during the evaluation of a problem arising in the course of disease in the patient with colitis. When colonoscopy is performed for specific indications the information obtained may be valuable. Colonoscopy is an invasive procedure requiring a rigorous preparation, however, and should follow the barium enema x-ray examination except in a few selected situations, such as post-operative evaluation and during screening for premalignant conditions. Colonoscopy is complementary to the roentgenographic examination that is a standardized procedure, can be performed rapidly, and provides a permanent record with x-ray films available for later review and comparison (see Chap. 20).[2,3]

One current problem with colonoscopy is that the clinician must rely upon the endoscopist's interpretation of intracolonic events that, to a large extent, is subjective and depends upon the experience of the colonoscopist in dealing with inflammatory bowel disease. The new electronic video endoscopes provide the possibility for permanent electronic imaging but problems are created by the need both to store videocasettes from every endoscopic procedure and to retrieve a specific segment of any desired videotape.

Although colonoscopy does not provide a permanent record of the examination (in the absence of a multitude of photographs), it offers two particular advantages:

1. It has the ability to detect changes in color and to visualize bleeding (erythema, vascular engorgement, and friability).
2. It permits the collection of biopsy specimens for interpretation by the histopathologist and samples for microbiologic studies.

The diagnosis and management of idiopathic inflammatory bowel disease (IBD) is usually established by clinical "parameters" along with information obtained from radiology, sigmoidoscopy, and colorectal biopsy; most patients do not require colonoscopy. When the interpretation of a barium enema is difficult, colonoscopy may be a valuable aid for the diagnosis of the patient with inflammatory bowel disease. Indications for colonoscopy in inflammatory bowel disease are shown in Table 19-1.

Other than for finding cancer or precancer in patients with IBD, colonoscopy rarely helps determine the need for surgical intervention in any individual instance.[4] Dealing with an acutely ill patient requires careful clinical observation with ongoing assessment, frequently necessitat-

TABLE 19-1. *Indications for Colonoscopy in Inflammatory Bowel Disease.*

Differential diagnosis
Determination of extent of disease
Investigation of radiographic abnormalities
    Mass lesions
    Stricture
Perioperative endoscopy
Screening for premalignant and malignant features
Evaluation of unexplained diarrhea

---

ing hourly reevaluation and continuous monitoring by members of the medical/surgical team; colonoscopy does not have a role in the evaluation and therapy of such patients, nor does it contribute to the decision for surgical treatment in those whose disease progresses inexorably despite the judicious use of intensive medical treatment. In the majority of instances the decision for surgical intervention is based on the sudden onset of clinical features that arise as complications of the disease, such as uncontrolled hemorrhage, free or confined perforation of the bowel, or toxic megacolon. In the nonemergency patient with IBD, the decision for surgical therapy is a clinical judgment based on a complex integration of several "parameters," most of which are poorly measured but include response to therapy and the rate of progress of the total disease process. Other complications of colitis, such as growth retardation and other extra-intestinal manifestations including ocular involvement, arthritis, pyoderma gangrenosum, and hepatic abnormalities, must be handled by a multidisciplinary approach in which colonoscopy plays only a minor role (see Chaps. 12, 16, and 23). In only a few of the total number of colitis patients requiring surgical treatment does colonoscopy offer definitive assistance in reaching a surgical decision.

Whenever colonoscopy is indicated during the course of inflammatory bowel disease, complete intubation of the entire large bowel is desirable. If the predetermined goal of colonoscopy can be achieved by partial examination, however, it may be wise in some instances to discontinue the procedure rather than risk a perforation in a noticeably inflamed bowel during vigorous but misguided attempts to perform total colonoscopy. The endoscopist-clinician must be aware, however, that when the indication for an examination is the determination of precancer or cancer, total endoscopy should be achieved, whereas a complete colonic inspection may not be necessary to evaluate a stricture or other radiographic abnormality.

In a series of 289 consecutive examinations of patients with inflammatory bowel disease,[4] endoscopy to the cecum was accomplished in 94% of those with ulcerative colitis and in 74% of patients with Crohn's disease. A similarly high success rate for total colonic intubation was reported previously in 92% of ulcerative colitis patients by Grandqvist et al.[5] The usual reason for incomplete colonoscopy in those with ulcerative colitis is either a stricture or poor bowel preparation. Termination of the examination in Crohn's disease is usually a result of the severity of the inflammatory process with large, deep ulcerations and the increased risk of colonic perforation.

When the colorectal mucosa is examined with a flexible fiberoptic endoscope, the glistening surface and progressive branching of the vascular network can be immediately identified and be seen throughout the entire extent of the normal colon.[6] The visible vasculature is at the surface of the submucosa, immediately beneath the mucosal layer. Normally, the mucosal lining of the colon is transparent, and the surface is uniformly salmon pink throughout. Arborization of the superficial vascular pattern is a characteristic of the surface topography, and must be present for the endoscopist to accept the normality of that mucous membrane. Vascularity is typically more prominent in the rectum than in any other area of the colon; there, large blood vessels are present whose caliber increases in diameter distally. One characteristic that never varies in health is the smoothness of the colorectal mucosal surface. No nodulations or irregular projections should be seen except in the occasional pediatric patient or young adult with lymphoid hyperplasia. Throughout the entire colon, the various interhaustral septa are ordinarily "paper-crease" sharp in their semicircular or triangular configuration; no bleeding is seen nor is pus or mucus present on the bowel wall. Only rarely does the bowel preparation for endoscopic examination give rise to visible alterations in the surface mucosa, such changes consisting only of mild erythema or slight edema, recognized as loss of the normal bright, glistening appearance of the mucosal surface. Contact bleeding, or friability, *never* develops as a result of preparation with cathartics and enemas.[2]

Endoscopy to Evaluate the Extent of Inflammatory Bowel Disease

Although easily performed, it is unusual to require colonoscopy simply to evaluate the extent of idiopathic colitis because that information rarely is vital in determining the clinical approach to the patient. When "proctitis" does not respond to a course of topical therapy, however, the physician should consider that the disease might extend more proximally than the rectosigmoid region; under these circumstances, colonoscopy and multiple proximal biopsies can provide the desired information.[7,8] Such biopsies may double the "yield of pathology" when compared to the endoscopically visible amount of inflammation,[9] and can be three times more informative than the barium enema x-ray examination.[10] Fifty percent of patients with treatment resistant proctitis and a negative proximal roentgenogram will be shown to have more proximal inflammation in colonoscopic biopsies in the absence of gross mucosal abnormalities. Radioactive scanning methods using indium-111 or gallium-67 may help to delineate the extent of colon involvement if colonoscopy is not desirable or available.[11,12]

All of the current studies on the surveillance for precancer in ulcerative colitis are based on the extent of disease as determined radiographically.[13] No data are available that evaluate the clinical significance of finding total colonic involvement by endoscopy and biopsy when the barium enema x-ray examination shows only left-sided involvement.

Endoscopy, Strictures, and Mass Lesions in Inflammatory Bowel Disease

Two major problems that may not be resolved by the barium enema examination are the precise identification of the nature of mass lesions and strictures in patients with IBD. Strictures occur with equal frequency in those with ulcerative or Crohn's colitis and may be the result of muscular hypertrophy and spasm, fibrosis, or carcinoma (see Chap. 14).[14] Any stricture occurring in a patient with ulcerative colitis should raise the suspicion of carcinoma and must be further evaluated. The best method for investigating such strictures is colonoscopy, which permits direct inspection of the segment and also allows collection of biopsies and cytologic samples.[15] Many strictures in patients with ulcerative colitis are benign, but carcinoma still must be ruled out even though malignancy accounts for less than 20% of these narrowed segments.[16] Hunt et al. demonstrated via colonoscopy that only 12.5% of the strictures in 24 patients with ulcerative colitis were associated with malignancy,[15] while Grandqvist et al. reported that no cancer was found on similar evaluations of 14 colitic patients.[5]

To investigate a stricture, the colonoscope should be passed through the area to determine its extent and nature. If intubation is not possible with standard size instruments, it should be repeated with a narrower endoscope, such as a pediatric colonoscope or a small caliber upper intestinal gastroscope.[17] Many strictures found on barium enema examination can be successfully negotiated with the standard-size colonoscope because air insufflation during endoscopy may distend the narrow lumen, especially when the cause is muscle hypertrophy or spasm.[10] Some radiographically identifiable strictures may not be seen endoscopically because of spherical aberrations related to the wide angle (fish-eye) lens systems of modern fiberendoscopes. Narrowing of the barium column may be obvious on the x-ray film but if the stricture is wide enough to allow passage of the endoscope, it may be barely detectable by the examiner only as a minor change in lumenal caliber.

When evaluating a stricture endoscopically, a visual impression is insufficient to provide an accurate diagnosis so it must be supplemented by biopsies at the edge of and within the strictured segment, as well as by brush cytology. Fibrotic strictures are usually short and web-like (Plate I-1), while inflammatory strictures are usually concentric and notable for the presence of ulcers, friability, and mucosal erythema within them (Plate I-2). Carcinoma causing a stricture is usually identified endoscopically as an eccentric, friable, plaque-like mass within the narrow segment (Plate I-3). Endoscopic features that may signal the presence of malignancy within a stricture are rigidity of the edge, an eccentric lumen, an abrupt shelf-like margin, nodularity within or at the stricture margins, and difficulty in intubation (Plate I-4).[17] Although carcinoma originates from the mucosal surface of the colon, there has been a report of a carcinoma in colitis spreading submucosally, associated with negative mucosal biopsies.[18] Thus, a biopsy that does not reveal a cancer in a stricture that appears suspicious should not be interpreted as proving the absence of malignancy because sampling error may occur. Conversely, a biopsy from a stricture that appears malignant may demonstrate it to be benign, as reported in a case of colitis cystica profunda.[19] To prevent the possibility of overlooking a cancer, strictures that appear endoscopically to be malignant should raise considerations for surgical intervention rather than be repeatedly monitored by colonoscopic evaluations.[20] Strictures too narrow to be intubated with the standard or pediatric endoscope also should be referred for surgical treatment because adequate colonoscopic inspection is not possible.

The endoscopist must be prepared to terminate the examination if a stricture resists gentle attempts at intubation. No role exists for the use of the tip of the colonoscope as a dilating probe in strictures occurring in ulcerative colitis. The colonic wall in ulcerative colitis usually is thinned and the mucosa friable, which does not permit the longitudinal stretching tolerated by the normal, noncolitic bowel. Because of this, the endoscopist should exert only minimal pressure when attempting to pass through strictures in patients with ulcerative colitis, lest the bowel wall be traumatized and perforation result. Although strictures can be dilated by balloons that are passed through the colonoscope's channel, the risks and benefits of such a procedure have not been determined in inflammatory bowel disease.

Mass lesions found at barium enema examination in IBD may range in importance from carcinoma to the nonneoplastic pseudopolyp. Pseudopolyps are usually small, glistening, and multiple throughout the colon, and they are found in both ulcerative colitis and Crohn's disease.[4,21] (Plate I-5) They may consist of regenerative epithelial islands that have not been involved in the surrounding destructive ulcerations in colitis, or, alternatively, they may be composed of granulation tissue or inflammatory nodules (see also Chap. 14).[22] Whatever their etiology, they have no malignant potential and any mass lesion definitely identified as a pseudopolyp can be safely ignored.[23,24] Although pseudopolyps are usually small (less than 7mm in size) and multiple, some not only may be solitary but also may grow to several cm in diameter.[25] A large pseudopolyp or a collection of small pseudopolyps may obstruct the lumen,[26-28] or act as a nidus for intussusception of the colon,[29] and they can be mistaken for an irregularly shaped carcinoma.[28,30-32] Biopsies from a suspicious mass will usually establish the correct diagnosis, however. A tissue sample from a pseudopolyp may or may not show inflammation, but will definitely reveal the mass not to be a neoplasm. Whether sessile or pedunculated (Plate I-6), pseudopolyps may be removed endoscopically but resection is not usually required unless they are causing symptoms of partial obstruction or bleeding (see also Chap. 14). In the presence of surrounding inflammation, healing of the polypectomy site may be delayed following endoscopic excision of a pseudopolyp,[33] and interference with healing may lead to immediate or delayed hemorrhage from the site. When multiple pseudopolyps are encountered, it is not possible, or necessary, to biopsy them all. Histologic sampling should be reserved for those with features that may be possessed by a carcinoma or an adenoma; thus biopsies should be taken when a polyp exceeds 1 cm in diameter, has spontaneous surface bleeding, is different in color from other pseudopolyps, or has an irregular surface configuration.

Adenomatous polyps may be present in as many as 5% of patients with idiopathic colitis, but rarely are identified as such by the colonoscope. The typical appearance of an adenoma, so commonly encountered in the noncolitic colon, is infrequently seen in colitis, with most adenomas resembling pseudopolyps (Plate I-7), and only biopsy may sort out the true nature of a colonic mass lesion.[33,34] In some instances, when a diagnosis of adenoma is made from a biopsy specimen, the endoscopist may be surprised because grossly the lesion resembled a pseudopolyp. Adenomas may be removed endoscopically by the same technique used for colon polypectomy in the normal bowel. Once a polyp in the colitic colon is discovered to be an adenoma, the bowel does not need to be resected subsequently if no malignant change is present.

Endoscopy and the Differential Diagnosis of Colorectal Inflammatory Bowel Disease

The differential diagnosis between ulcerative and granulomatous colitis (Crohn's disease) is usually made with the aid of the history, sigmoidoscopy, rectal biopsy, and barium enema x-ray examination (see Chap. 20). In every case, the correct diagnosis requires that a clinician familiar with the diseases should review the information obtained from a number of different sources, the most important being a careful and detailed history of all pertinent events leading up to the onset of illness, including travel information, diet, antibiotic usage, and sexual preference. Because the presentation of several varieties of diarrheal illness may be similar, even the most skilled gastroenterologist may have difficulty in differentiating between infectious colitis and idiopathic inflammatory bowel disease because many of their features overlap (see Chaps. 8, 9, 10, and 18).[35] The clinician must always consider the possibility of a treatable, infectious etiology for any diarrheal illness, even in those patients in whom the diagnosis of idiopathic inflammatory bowel disease has been established over a considerable period of time, because the possibility always exists that an acute exacerbation of such a chronic illness may be provoked by a superimposed infectious event (see Chaps. 8, 9, and 10).

Most patients with diarrhea of acute onset respond to symptomatic therapy, but those who do not respond rapidly or develop debility require more intensive medical attention to ascertain whether a treatable etiologic agent is responsible for the illness. Although diarrhea is the hallmark of infectious colitis, the presence of rectal bleeding is relatively common but is not voluminous in amount. Unfortunately for the endoscopist the gross visual examination of the mucosal lining both in infectious and inflammatory colitis may be indistinguishable, as is also true of many histologic features in tissue specimens obtained during endoscopy (see Chap. 18). Because of the multiple similarities presented by many conditions affecting the large bowel, the astute endoscopist must always keep diagnostic options open even when "typical" evidence of nonspecific inflammatory bowel disease is encountered because this excludes an infectious etiology and emphasizes the need for microbiologic studies in all cases.[36] The probability of an infectious process decreases with the duration of diarrhea, while the probability of idiopathic inflammatory disease increases with the length of symptoms. If the diarrheal syndrome progresses to the subacute stage (longer than 4 weeks), however, the differential diagnosis continues to be complex because some infectious agents may be responsible for long-standing diarrheal illness;[37,38] these include colitis secondary to campylobacter, tuberculosis, schistosomiasis, and amebiasis (see Chap. 10).

Approximately one-third of all patients with a diarrheal illness of 6 weeks' duration considered clinically by history and sigmoidoscopy to have idiopathic inflammatory bowel disease actually prove to have an infectious etiology when extensive laboratory investigations are performed.[38]

The reason why endoscopy and biopsy alone may fail to render a correct diagnosis in colitis is that the intestinal lining has a limited number of responses to any process that affects its integrity. The initial response to any inflammatory process is an increase in local blood supply, seen endoscopically as erythema. If the mucosal surface is ulcerated, spontaneous or "contact" bleeding may occur. Any type of inflammatory condition of the colon may cause a change in the smoothness of the surface lining, alter its color, or affect the delicate branching vascular pattern. Not only may gross visible patterns of disease be indistinguishable regardless of the underlying inflammatory process, but also biopsies may be remarkably similar and therefore of limited assistance in further differentiation between these various entities. The responses evoked are rarely specific for any etiologic factors.

Even when a specific infectious etiology has been excluded and a diagnosis of colonic IBD is made, considerable difficulty still may exist in differentiating between CUC and Crohn's colitis. Because endoscopy allows total colonic visualization and can provide tissue specimens for histologic study, the endoscopist will frequently be requested to assist in this differentiation.

Because ulcerative and granulomatous colitis affect the bowel differently, the gross appearance of the two colitides often is sufficiently distinct to enable the endoscopist to distinguish between them (Table 19-2). Therefore, a detailed description of the endoscopic findings in these two types of idiopathic inflammatory bowel disease will be presented.

Ulcerative colitis mainly affects the mucosal layer while Crohn's disease involves the full thickness of bowel wall, including the mucosa and the submucosa (see Chap. 18). Because mucosal involvement is not prominent early in the course of Crohn's disease, the surface vascular pattern tends to remain intact because the endoscopically visualized blood vessel network lies between the mucosa and the submucosal layers. Scanning electron microscopy studies have demonstrated that the aphthous ulcer in granulomatous colitis originates in the submucosal lymphatic follicles and an inflammatory eruption penetrates through the superficial layers (see Chap. 18).[39] The pathogenesis of these tiny ulcers makes them among the earliest lesions of Crohn's disease, a tiny ulcer in an otherwise completely normal mucosal surface, including normal vascularity.[40,41] The earliest phases of colonic involvement in ulcerative colitis, on the other hand, are manifested by an increase in surface blood flow creating an endoscopic picture of diffuse erythema (Plate I-8). The mucosal inflammation is frequently associated with concomitant edema, resulting in an inability to visualize the mucosal vascular architecture. Mucosal edema is colonoscopically recognized as "granularity," with the finely "granular" surface resulting from multiple reflections of light (highlights) from individual mounds of edema punctuated by the colon crypts (Plate

TABLE 19-2. *The Colonoscopic Visual Differential Diagnosis of Inflammatory Bowel Disease.*

Visible Feature	Ulcerative Colitis	Granulomatous (Crohn's) Colitis
Mucosal granularity	+	±
Mucosal friability	+	±
Cobblestoning	−	+
Thick interhaustral septum	+	+
Pseudopolyps	+	+
Narrowing of lumen	+	+
Strictures	+	+
Mucosal bridge	+	+
Ulcers	In abnormal mucosa	In grossly normal mucosa
Mucosal involvement	Contiguous	Discontinuous
Rectum	Involved	Commonly not involved
Vascular pattern	Distorted	Normal

I-9), a pattern that resembles wet sandpaper. The engorged mucosa in ulcerative colitis is friable and bleeds readily when traumatized by the endoscope or a cotton swab (contact bleeding). As the inflammation progresses in ulcerative colitis, minute surface ulcerations occur that, in combination with the mucosal hyperemia, cause the spontaneous bleeding so characteristic of the disease. The nature of the inflammatory response in ulcerative colitis, with its progression from vascular engorgement to mucosal edema is the reason why the small ulcers in this disease occur in a bed of surrounding colon inflammation (Plate I-10). Multiple linear ulcers of several centimeters in length, the so-called "bear claw" ulcers, may occur representing coalescence of smaller surface erosions, but large surface ulcers are more common in Crohn's disease. The small aphthous inflammatory erosions (Plate I-11) in granulomatous colitis tend to enlarge concentrically and encroach upon areas of apparently normal surface mucosa as they increase in diameter. Unless the disease has spread to involve a broad segment of the colon, even large ulcers in Crohn's disease typically appeared to be surrounded by normal mucosa (Plate I-12).

Tables 19-3 and 19-4 list certain endoscopic features that may serve to distinguish between ulcerative colitis and Crohn's disease.[1] The distributions of the inflammatory processes in the colon may give some help in their differential diagnosis; it is uncommon for ulcerative colitis to show endoscopic and histologic rectal sparing unless topical steroids have been used. Similarly, isolated, right-sided ulcerative colitis is unusual. Endoscopically it is also uncommon to see total Crohn's disease of the colon ending abruptly at the ileocecal valve with a normal terminal ileum. More typically the valve itself is involved, becoming stenosed and rigid with changes of Crohn's disease in the terminal ileum. Nodular lymphoid hyperplasia, common in young people, should not be confused with granulomatous ileitis because the coloration of the bumpy lymphoid nodules is the same as that of surrounding ileal mucosa, and the overlying mucosa is not friable. An abrupt change to normality at the ileocecal valve is more suggestive of ulcerative colitis in which the valve is often incompetent and easily intubated. The most important endoscopic criteria to distinguish between the two major types of idiopathic inflammatory bowel disease are as follows:[22]*

1. Aphthous ulcers are pathognomonic of Crohn's colitis, although they may be seen in many of the other types of inflammatory bowel disease.
2. Cobblestoning is pathognomonic of Crohn's colitis.
3. Ulcers may occur in segments of diffusely abnormal mucosa in both forms of colitis, but if they are seen in an area of otherwise apparently normal mucosa the diagnosis is *never* ulcerative colitis.
4. Granularity and friability are both common in early ulcerative colitis, but may be late findings in Crohn's colitis.

Additional distinguishing points are the tendency for Crohn's disease to spare the rectum, an area almost always involved in ulcerative colitis, and the contiguous nature of the inflammatory response in the latter disease. The gross involvement in granulomatous colitis is patchy

*Editor's note: See also Pera, A., et al.: Gastroenterology, *92*:181, 1987.

TABLE 19-3. *Colonoscopy in Ulcerative Colitis.*

Rectum usually involved
Diffuse erythema replaces usual vascular pattern
Mucosal granularity frequent
Mucosal friability occurs
If present, ulcerations always are seen in areas of mucosal inflammation

and asymmetric, often with one wall showing evidence of inflammation that is not grossly evident on the opposite wall of the same segment.

In most instances of relatively early disease, endoscopic differences help in the differential diagnosis but the late stages of both types of colitis may resemble each other so closely that correct differentiation may not be possible endoscopically.

The clinical severity of colitis tends to correlate with the endoscopic estimation of the mucosal reaction. Characteristically in ulcerative colitis, ulcerations are a manifestation of severe disease and do not occur in mild colitis. On the other hand, loss of vascular pattern and friability are features of relatively mild disease. Tiny aphthous ulcers are seen early in Crohn's colitis; progression of the disease produces larger ulcers that coalesce, become longitudinal, and may extend for several centimeters with deep fissuring. Rarely, Crohn's ulcers may be "punched-out." This particular appearance is associated with easy bleeding and perforation.

Cobblestoning is caused by submucosal involvement by Crohn's disease and may be described differently by pathologists and endoscopists (see Chap. 18). Endoscopists consider cobblestoning to be uniform nodulations caused by submucosal edema. Although ulcerations may be present in the area recognized as cobblestoning, they do not define this entity endoscopically. Characteristically, the endoscopic type of cobblestoning is low in height with a broad base, and bears little relation to ulcers (Plate II-1). These nodulations are easily recognized and will never be mistaken for the small, "nubbly" mucosal surface irregularities indicative of dysplasia in patients with ulcerative colitis. Cobblestoning must be distinguished from multiple pseudopolyps projecting into the lumen; a pseudopolyp is characteristically taller than its base is broad, and areas of flat mucosa may be immediately adjacent, whereas the low nodulations of cobblestoning are contiguous although they may be asymmetric.

Many of the mucosal features at endoscopy are common to both diseases, and therefore may not be helpful in differentiating ulcerative from granulomatous colitis. Pseudopolyps occur in both forms of colitis and their presence does not favor the diagnosis of one or the other (see Chap. 14). Mucosal bridges share a common pathogenesis with pseudopolyps, and are created when two adjacent ulcerations meet by burrowing beneath an area of inflamed mucosa instead of destroying it; as healing occurs, re-epithelialization of the ulcers and the under surface of the mucosal strip occurs, thereby producing a mucosally covered tube connected at both ends. Mucosal bridges are seen in either type of colitis (Plate II-2) and may (although rarely) cause obstruction to passage of the colonoscope. Another similarity between the two types of idiopathic inflammatory colonic disease is that the healing phase of chronic disease may be associated with loss of haustral folds, while fibrotic strictures and linear scars may be seen on the mucosal surface.

It might appear that the differential diagnosis between CUC and Crohn's colitis would be greatly enhanced by the ability to obtain unlimited biopsies throughout the colon in every case in which endoscopy is performed. Because the mucosa of the large bowel has limited reactions to a wide variety of insults, however, only a few specific diagnostic features are available that permit the pathologist to recognize patterns of injury. The histopathologist often provides little assistance to the endoscopist's ability to differentiate between ulcerative and granulomatous colitis. Granulomas are the hallmark of Crohn's colitis but, according to some studies, these are seen in less than 10% of mucosal biopsies from granulomatous colitis,[13,42,43] although others report their presence in the majority of patients.[44,45] The discrepancies in the reported incidence of granuloma identification on endoscopic biopsy may be a result of the type of patients referred for colonoscopy, because early cases with small aphthous ulcers tend to yield the highest incidence of granulomas. The yield

TABLE 19-4. *Colonoscopy in Granulomatous (Crohn's) Colitis.*

Rectum often grossly normal
Asymmetric and discontinuous disease common
Discrete ulcers may occur in otherwise grossly normal mucosa
Linear ulcers common
Mucosal friability unusual
"Cobblestoning" often occurs in severe cases

of granulomas is greatest when biopsies are taken from the center of small ulcers; as ulcers enlarge, they tend to engulf and destroy the original epithelioid cluster of cells, causing a low incidence of granulomas in mucosal biopsies from patients with long-standing disease. A study of rectal biopsies from normal appearing mucosa in patients with Crohn's colitis demonstrated granulomas in 6% of patients and minute collections of macrophages termed "microgranulomas" in 14% (see also Chap. 18).[46]

Whenever endoscopy is used to assist in the differential diagnosis between the idiopathic inflammatory bowel diseases, multiple biopsies should be provided for histopathologic study. Each specimen must be labelled as to its location in the colon because the mapping of inflammation provides additional information to assist in unravelling the diagnostic dilemma. A pattern of progressively increasing distal inflammation on multiple biopsies is consistent with ulcerative colitis, whereas patchy inflammation throughout the colon or even variations of distribution of inflammatory cells within one of the tiny tissue specimens is more characteristic of Crohn's disease.[47] A common feature of Crohn's disease is "disproportionate" inflammation, a term that refers to the tendency for the cellular infiltrate to be more prominent in the submucosa than in the mucosa (see also Chap. 18).[48,49]

In some cases of long-standing Crohn's disease amyloid may be found in vessel walls on endoscopic biopsy of the mucosa;[1] this has not been reported in ulcerative colitis.

Ileoscopy and biopsy of the distal small bowel mucosa are possible by inserting the colonoscope through the ileocecal valve. This can be accomplished in 80 to 97% of patients in whom total colonic intubation is achieved.[50,51] The gross visualization of small ulcerations on the valve or in the small bowel has a high predictive value in establishing the diagnosis of Crohn's disease (Plate II-3).[52] Biopsies of the terminal ileum may reveal a pattern of inflammation "compatible with Crohn's disease" but there is a low yield of granulomas in the presence of known regional enteritis.

As stressed previously, however, many of the endoscopic and biopsy abnormalities described as characteristic for the two major types of idiopathic inflammatory bowel disease may also be seen in patients with infectious colitis. Some infections of the colon appear to be ulcerative colitis while others affect deeper portions of the colon wall and appear identical to Crohn's disease. In many circumstances, the endoscopist's intraluminal view is not diagnostic, and the etiology of the colitis is determined by integrating all the data from multiple sources, with the history from the patient as a primary informational factor aided by the results of stool cultures and/or biopsy specimens.[53-55] The results of stool cultures may not be available at the time of an endoscopic examination and, as emphasized earlier, the suspicion of an infectious etiology should always be in the forefront of the differential diagnosis when dealing with any patient having diarrhea. Fortunately, most of the infective diarrheas are self-limiting and for this reason colonoscopy is rarely performed in these patients. It is not uncommon, however, to examine the rectum and sigmoid colon with a sigmoidoscope during an acute phase of diarrheal illness. Any physician who looks at the colonic mucosa using any instrument, either rigid or flexible, must therefore be familiar with the gross characteristics of the various types of inflammatory bowel disease, both specific and nonspecific.

Some endoscopic features that may be more common in infections of the colon than in idiopathic inflammatory bowel disease include the fact that infectious diarrhea may have a yellowish tenacious exudate that partially or completely covers the mucosal surface. Free pus, identified by its thick consistency and creamy color, may be seen with infection but is unusual with either of the idiopathic inflammatory bowel diseases. Visible ulcerations that are common in Crohn's disease are not usually seen in most of the infectious colitides. Many infections cause the surface mucosa to become intensely reddened, almost magenta-colored in contrast to the deeper red of idiopathic inflammatory bowel disease. One of the most characteristic patterns in the endoscopic appearance of infectious colitis is patchy involvement within the same colon segment where multiple small areas in the same visual field may be obviously inflamed with normal mucosa intervening.[38] In ulcerative colitis the pattern of involvement is contiguous, whereas small aphthous ulcerations would be expected in some of the areas of patchy redness in granulomatous colitis. Because mucosal edema is responsible for the granularity so characteristic of inflammatory bowel disease, it is not surprising that granularity may also be present in colonic infections.

Confusion concerning the endoscopic differentiation between the specific and nonspecific inflammatory bowel diseases has arisen because various authors attribute different endoscopic appearances to the same infectious agent. For example, some observers have reported one agent to cause a picture resembling Crohn's disease while others state that the same organism causes the endoscopic appearance of ulcerative colitis. The variation in mucosal response to the same infection is undoubtedly related to several factors, including the degree of aggressiveness of that particular organism in each specific patient, the duration of infection when endoscopy is performed, and the host's response to inflammation.

An interesting histopathologic study on a blind evaluation of rectal biopsy specimens taken at endoscopy from a series of patients with acute self-limited (infectious) colitis and patients with idiopathic inflammatory bowel disease demonstrated a number of histologic criteria that were highly discriminant because they occurred often in idiopathic inflammatory bowel disease and rarely, if at all, in acute self-limited colitis.[56] Five features with a high predictive probability (100% in this study) for the diagnosis of idiopathic inflammatory bowel disease were as follows:

1. Crypt architecture distortion
2. Mixed lamina proprial cellularity
3. Villous surface
4. Crypt atrophy
5. Basal lymphoid aggregates

It should be noted that in this study granulomas were present in 25% of the patients with idiopathic inflammatory bowel disease. Almost half of all idiopathic inflammatory bowel disease biopsy specimens showed distorted crypt architecture, but this was not present in acute self-limited colitis. Crypt architecture was deemed to be distorted if two or more branched crypts were present in the well-oriented central core of an adequate size biopsy. The type of inflammatory cells seen in the lamina propria was also helpful in the differential diagnosis, with an increase in both round cells and neutrophils in idiopathic inflammatory bowel disease. An increase in polymorphonuclear cells alone was not characteristic for either the self-limited colitis or idiopathic inflammatory bowel disease. An endoscopic biopsy showing a "villous surface structure" resulting from a separation of the crypts yielding broad villous-like projections was seen only in idiopathic inflammatory bowel disease, as was the finding of crypt atrophy. Collections of lymphocytes, without reactive centers, located between the muscularis mucosa and the crypts were termed "basal lymphoid aggregates." Like crypt atrophy, these crypts were present in about 20% of patients with idiopathic inflammatory bowel disease but not in any patients with acute self-limited colitis.*

Common Infections of the Colon

Table 19-5 lists the most common infections of the colon and indicates whether they are likely grossly to resemble ulcerative or granulomatous colitis; in some instances the same infectious condition at different stages may resemble either form of IBD. A description of the endoscopic findings in each of many colon infections is presented (see also Chap. 10).

Amebiasis

A protozoal infection primarily affecting the large bowel, amebiasis may resemble Crohn's disease.[57,58] Symptoms may vary from none to an acute fulminating course with explosive bloody diarrhea, abdominal cramps, tenesmus, and fever. Endoscopy during the acute phase may demonstrate diffuse edema, granularity, and friability resembling ulcerative colitis. Patients with chronic amebiasis have cecal involvement in 80 to 90% of cases. The most characteristic appearance of chronic amebiasis is discrete ulcers with undermined edges in a bed of normal mucosa. The ulcers may be covered with a yellowish-white exudate (Plate II-4). Biopsies should be taken from the ulcer margins because this area provides the best yield for demonstration of trophozoites. The amebic ulcer is often associated with a reddened rim, a finding that may assist the astute observer in a visual differentiation between amebiasis and Crohn's disease.

Antibiotic-associated Colitis

Antibiotic-associated colitis may resemble ulcerative colitis,[59-64] and is a specific type of colitis caused by clostridium difficile that is frequently identifiable endoscopically because an easily recognizable pattern of disease exists. Although the rectum is usually involved, the distribution is not always uniform and may be confined to the right colon or to the sigmoid area. A yellowish membrane is often present covering much of the mucosal surface (Plate II-5). Frequently, small (2 to 5 mm in diameter) elevated creamy yellowish plaques dot the surface of the

---

*Editors' note: See also Nostrant, T.T., et al.: Gastroenterology 92:318, 1987.

TABLE 19-5. *Infectious Colitis Resembling Idiopathic Inflammatory Bowel Disease.*

Infectious Agent	Resembles Ulcerative Colitis	Resembles Crohn's Disease
Amebiasis		+
Antibiotic associated colitis	+	
Balantidium Coli		+
Campylobacter	+	+
Cytomegalovirus	+	+
Histoplasmosis		+
Salmonella		+
Schistosomiasis	+	
Shigella	+	
Tuberculosis		+
Yersinia	+	+

moderately inflamed bowel wall. The mucosa between these plaques is not ulcerated but may vary from being edematous and friable to having hemorrhagic features similar to ulcerative colitis. The plaques may occur diffusely without a sharply demarcated border of involvement, and their biopsy may induce bleeding. Histology demonstrates a polymorphonuclear exudate with the typical "volcano" lesions associated with this condition. Not all cases of pseudomembranous colitis are associated with the prior ingestion of antibiotics, but even then the endoscopic findings are typical for the disease and the histopathologic diagnosis of the pseudomembrane is characteristic.

Balantidium coli

Possibly resembling Crohn's disease, Balantidium coli is an unusual infection that resembles amebiasis in all its characteristics.[65] The trophozoites may be distinguished from amebiasis by their histologic characteristics in biopsy samples.

Campylobacter Fetus Subspecies Jejuni

Campylobacter fetus subspecies jejuni colitis may resemble ulcerative colitis or Crohn's disease.[66,67] This organism has been recognized to have the capability of producing an acute colitis indistinguishable from ulcerative colitis, with erythema and friability in the early stages, as well as granularity, spontaneous bleeding, and diffuse exudate over the mucosal surface. In addition to the usual endoscopic findings of inflammation, inflammatory mass lesions have been described. Commonly, the rectum is involved, while the right colon is only rarely affected. Not all patients infected by campylobacter present these "typical" features, and in some instances an endoscopic picture closely resembling Crohn's disease occurs with segmental patchy involvement showing hyperemia, friability, edema, and occasional small ulcers. In most patients the disease is of short duration, but organisms may persist up to seven weeks after the onset of symptoms.

Cytomegalovirus

Cytomegalovirus colitis may resemble ulcerative colitis or Crohn's disease (Plate II-6).[68] This is an opportunistic infection that occurs in immunosuppressed patients, most commonly those with malignant disease receiving cytotoxic drugs or steroids. Infection by this organism has also been identified in homosexual males with the acquired immunodeficiency syndrome (AIDS), however. Patients either may be asymptomatic or complain of abdominal pain and intermittent diarrhea containing occult or gross blood. The proctosigmoidoscopic appearance may resemble ulcerative colitis with granularity and mucosal friability. The presence of discrete, "punched-out", shallow ulcers can resemble Crohn's disease, however, because these may occur in the cecum with normal appearing surrounding mucosa. In contrast to granulomatous colitis, however, the cytomegalovirus ulcers are usually single and vary in size from 2 to 6 mm. Biopsies from the edges of the ulcerations will reveal the CMV inclusions in cells on sections stained with hematoxylin and eosin.

Histoplasmosis

Although it may resemble Crohn's disease endoscopically, histoplasmosis rarely affects the colon.[69] If colitis develops, the rectum is usually spared while the ileocecal area is the area most involved, showing ulcers, pseudopolyps, hyperemia, and friability. When the rectum is involved, discrete, granular plaque-like lesions may be seen and biopsies of these usually demonstrate the organism. The patchy nature of inflammation and the predominantly right-sided distribution of this mycotic infection may cause it to be mistaken for granulomatous colitis.

Salmonellosis

Salmonellosis may resemble Crohn's disease, and is a bacterial infection that primarily involves the small intestine but may affect the colon.[70] If so, a segmental involvement of the entire colon exists with rectal sparing. Early endoscopic findings include edema, hyperemia, and granularity, while progressive disease may result in mucosal friability with petechial hemorrhages. Deep ulcerations and concomitant strictures have been reported but are distinctly rare.

Schistosomiasis

Schistosomiasis, which may resemble ulcerative colitis, is a parasitic infection of the colon that is rarely encountered in temperate climates.[71] The colonoscopist should be alerted, however, to the possibility of this infestation by the finding of large inflammatory polypoid lesions that have a whitish exudate on their surfaces. These polyps, which may involve the entire colon, are produced by the inflammatory response to degenerating ova. More commonly, these mucosal changes occur only in the proximal colon, while the rectum and sigmoid are completely normal. The histologic finding of encysted schistosomes in a resected polyp or biopsy specimen is the unique feature of this disease. If the rectum is involved, the appearances are similar to ulcerative colitis with hyperemia, friability, edema, and granularity of the mucosa with shallow ulcerations.

Shigellosis

Possibly resembling ulcerative colitis, shigellosis is commonly known as bacillary dysentery.[36] This disease is caused by infection with shigella dysenteriae, a gram negative bacterium that primarily affects the large intestine. The onset of disease is sudden, with fever, crampy abdominal pain, tenesmus, and mucoid diarrhea often containing gross blood. The endoscopic appearances range from erythema and mild granularity to multiple ulcers with considerable exudate. The involvement is characteristically patchy, but otherwise may closely resemble the endoscopic findings in ulcerative colitis. Crypt abscesses may be found on biopsy in addition to the cellular infiltration of acute inflammation. In this infection, the bowel wall erythema is particularly intense and often magenta-colored, a clue to the astute endoscopist that an infectious etiology is present instead of idiopathic inflammatory bowel disease.

Tuberculosis

An infection that can affect any part of the large bowel or the terminal ileum, tuberculosis produces appearances indistinguishable from Crohn's disease (Plate II-7).[72,73] Commonly the rectum is spared so the sigmoidoscopic examination may be normal. The right side of the colon and ileocecal area are most often affected, with deformity of the ileocecal valve and lumenal narrowing. Colonoscopy may demonstrate diffuse nodules, linear ulcerations, and strictures. The ulcerations usually have surrounding edema and erythema; like Crohn's disease they are often located in an area of otherwise normal-appearing mucosa. In this chronic infection, mass lesions or tuberculomas can be present, and fistularization may occur between loops of bowel. Cobblestoning has been reported resulting from submucosal involvement with thickening of the bowel wall, and inflammatory pseudopolyps may be present throughout the colon. The differentiation between Crohn's disease and tuberculosis can be difficult even for the most experienced endoscopist because the two illnesses so closely resemble each other. Some points that may assist in the correct visual diagnosis are that the "skip areas" are shorter in the colon affected by M. Tuberculosis, and the ulcers may have rolled edges and lack the sharp definition usually associated with ulcerations in Crohn's disease. Appropriate microbiologic studies of tissue samples will resolve the problem if those involved are alert to the possibility of the presence of a specific infection.

Yersinia Enterocolitica

Yersinia enterocolitica is an infection that produces diffuse edema, erythema, and friability throughout the entire colon, resembling ulcerative colitis in about 50% of the patients affected.[74] Others may have patchy or right-sided distribution (including involvement of the terminal ileum), however, with aphthous ulcers adjacent to areas of normal mucosa, a combination strongly suggestive of Crohn's disease. A normal rectum is often encountered because 40% of affected patients have endoscopically identifiable disease only proximal to the rectosigmoid area. Symptoms of Yersinia colitis may persist for months, and cultures of tissue can take several weeks to demonstrate growth of the organism. If the disease is suspected, the laboratory must be specifically requested to inoculate the appropriate growth media to increase the chance of obtaining a positive culture.

The Gay Bowel Syndrome

A number of colon infections are related to anal intercourse and are most commonly associated with homosexual activity between males.[75-80] A variety of infectious agents are responsible for the mucosal changes seen in the gay bowel syndromes, and whenever a nonspecific proctitis is diagnosed in any patient, a history of sexual activity and its nature should be obtained because anal intercourse may transmit easily overlooked specific rectal infections. Homosexual males have been found to be particularly susceptible to unusual diseases affecting the large bowel, and even to illnesses that have not yet been proven to be infectious in etiology. Some of the infectious colonic diseases described earlier may occur as a part of the gay bowel syndrome, with amebiasis and shigellosis as frequent infections, and cytomegalovirus is a fairly common opportunistic invader in the immunologically deficient host. In addition, infections by Gonococci, anorectal herpes simplex infection, syphilis, and lymphogranuloma venereum may produce proctitis. The last of these, which is caused by chlamydia trachomatis, may be associated with rectal stricturing close to the anal margin that may cause difficulty in visually differentiating this infection from Crohn's disease. This distinction is made more difficult by the tendency of the organism to provoke a tissue reaction similar to granulomatous proctitis, with crypt abscesses and granulomas containing giant cells.

Involvement by Kaposi's sarcoma in the colon is recognized by the presence of dark magenta-colored nodules that are only slightly elevated (Plate II-8); biopsies are positive in only half of the instances because the lesion is in the submucosa and may be beyond the reach of the endoscopic forceps. This disease may be patchy in distribution, with infrequent nodules occurring in the midst of otherwise normal appearing mucosa.

Other Inflammatory Conditions of the Colon

Diverticular disease of the colon represents a wide spectrum of pathology,[81] with only a few responses that may be directly germane to the topic of this chapter. The known muscular hypertrophy in this disorder is usually not associated with any true inflammatory reaction, but the sequela of the hypercontractile state may closely resemble inflammatory bowel disease endoscopically and will, therefore, be described. It is not difficult to recognize the individual orifices of diverticula and the commonly associated muscular hypertrophy. Uncomplicated diverticulosis, even with severe luminal narrowing, is *not* associated with any grossly visible mucosal inflammatory response. Strictures encountered during colonoscopy in diverticular disease are not at all similar to the areas of mucosal narrowing in strictures of idiopathic inflammatory bowel disease. The term "stricture" when used by the endoscopist who cannot advance the colonoscope beyond the sigmoid colon in a patient with diverticular disease may have either of two meanings: one is impedance of instrument passage caused by pronounced tortuosity of the colon, while the other is the presence of a true, fibrotic narrowed segment resulting from recurrent infection with scarring. Whenever fixation or fibrosis cause difficulty during colonoscopy, the safest course is discontinuation of the procedure.

The endoscopist may recognize a peculiar color pattern in diverticular disease that must be differentiated from idiopathic inflammatory bowel disease. Patchy, red areas may be seen at the tips of several adjacent hypertrophied folds in the sigmoid colon in diverticulosis; these areas do not bleed spontaneously and are not friable when touched by the tip of the endoscope or by the biopsy forceps. The redness is characteristically uniform and confluent on the edge of folds, but becomes discontinuous over a distance of a few millimeters toward the haustral pouches. When viewed closely, the redness consists of myriads of tiny red dots, each of which resembles a petechia. The contractile pressure generated by muscular activity in the narrowed and hypertrophic sigmoid colon may actually cause capillary rupture, or diapedesis of red cells across intact capillary walls. Biopsies of the reddened mucosa do not demonstrate any inflammation, but red cells may be seen or hemosiderin found in the extravascular tissues. If a broad segment is involved, friability may develop and, rarely, spontaneous bleeding may occur. In the presence of bleeding, the endoscopic appearance may be consistent with an isolated segment involved by inflammatory bowel disease, but biopsy samples are characteristic for their hemorrhagic infiltration and lack of inflammatory cell response.

Colonoscopy is *not* indicated in acute diverticulitis, but because this is usually a clinical diagnosis, occasionally endoscopists may be requested to evaluate a sigmoid segment noted on roentgenograms to be the site of a mass lesion, or may be called upon to investigate complete obstruction to the retrograde flow of barium during an x-ray examination. A variety of responses are seen in the endoscopic examination of patients with acute diverticulitis, the most localized being pus issuing from the diverticular orifice. In the presence of acute diverticulitis, there is invariably rather prominent severe spasm in the diseased segment, with the presence of pus in the narrowed irregular lumen (Plate II-9). Only rarely can the actual site of infection be identified, and the infected segment is usually devoid of the expected signs of inflammation such as redness, granularity, and friability. When complete retrograde obstruction of the barium enema is caused by diverticular disease, the tip of the colonoscope can be passed up to an area of progressive irregular luminal narrowing that cannot be intubated. In spite of the tiny caliber, often neither change in coloration nor friability of the narrowed segment occurs; this is an important point in distinguishing it from a carcinoma causing such a radiographic blockage because, when a tumor is present, it is always seen as a typical bleeding lesion, impeding progress of the colonoscope.

Ischemic Colitis

Ischemic colitis has variable appearances according to the severity of the ischemia.[82-84] The type of damage seen endoscopically is related to the various categories of ischemic injury that may occur and include the following:

1. Transient mucosal necrosis followed by complete resolution.
2. Partial resolution, often with transmural scarring and subsequent stricture formation.
3. Full thickness necrosis (gangrene).

Although easily recognized on the barium enema, the spectrum of changes seen endoscopically are being increasingly well-described. The most common site for ischemic colitis is the descending colon just distal to the splenic flexure, although it may occur in the sigmoid colon and rectum.

Endoscopists must take special care when ischemic bowel disease is suspected, and be wary of excessive air insufflation as well as the amount of pressure exerted during passage of the flexible fiberoptic endoscope because the compromised bowel has an increased liability to damage during instrumentation and can even perforate spontaneously. In mild cases only slight edema may occur with loss of vascular pattern, but the blue-black coloration of incipient gangrene is present in severe cases. A segment of acutely ischemic mucosa may be hemorrhagic, friable, and ulcerated, with a sharp demarcation from normal mucosa at each end. Ulcerations in ischemia may resemble aphthous ulcerations or be linear and irregular (Plate II-10). Ischemic episodes with overt rectal bleeding may occur with or without abdominal pain; colonoscopy performed within hours of the onset of ischemia may reveal fresh blood in the lumen, serpiginous superficial ulcers, and reduced colonic motility. The healing phase of ischemia may be manifested by patchy ulcerations in an area of otherwise normal-appearing mucosa. When this is seen, a short history of clinical disease accompanied by rectal bleeding may be the only clue that the underlying disease is not Crohn's colitis. The development of a stricture may accompany the healing process and cause pronounced luminal constriction. A pseudomembrane may overlie the ischemic area that, when removed, reveals a reddened, friable mucosa with contact bleeding. A syndrome of induced bowel ischemia, mimicking Crohn's colitis, has been described in women taking oral contraceptives, estrogens, or progesterones.[85] The clinical course in these women resembles ischemic bowel disease, and endoscopy either may reveal discrete ulcers in areas of mucosa that are otherwise completely normal, or confluent friability and edema in the involved segment. The clinical occurrence of colonic ischemia in a young woman is the clue to this diagnosis and a history of hormone ingestion must be sought. On biopsy, acute ischemic injury is characterized by mucosal necrosis with epithelial cells sloughing into empty "ghost" tubules.[49,82] Microthrombi are commonly noted in the mucosa and submucosa. The submucosa frequently shows edema and hemorrhagic changes, with dilated capillaries that present radiographically as filling defects known as "thumb-printing." Acute damage may resolve quickly leaving only nonspecific sequelae. Biopsy of healed ischemic strictures may be fairly characteristic, the histology usually showing hemosiderin deposition within macrophages, a finding of considerable diagnostic importance.[8]

Solitary Ulcer of The Rectum

This is a well-recognized syndrome, often of unknown cause, which may be confused endoscopically with Crohn's disease.[86-90] The ulcers occur primarily in young women with symptoms of rectal bleeding associated with rectal discomfort and mucous discharge, but they also have been reported in men. A flat, irregularly shaped ulcer, covered with slough and rimmed by erythema, is typically seen on the anterior wall of the rectum, approximately 5 to 10 cm from the anal verge (Plate II-11). The histologic features consist of fibrous replacement of the normal lamina propria, with thickening of the muscularis mucosal fibers.[49] Nonspecific solitary ulcers also may occur more proximally in the colon, usually in the cecum, and may present with rectal bleeding; the pathogenesis of these proximal lesions is unknown but it is probably an ischemic episode. Ischemia may be a pathogenic factor in rectal ulceration in elderly patients,[91] but in the younger patient, self-induced trauma may be causative. When an isolated shallow ulcer is discovered within reach of a fully inserted index finger, the patient should be queried as to the habit of digital extraction of stool, or other invasive practices.

Radiation Colitis

The mucosa of the large bowel may be damaged during radiation therapy.[92] The most common condition for which such treatment is prescribed is malignant pelvic disease in women. The proximal rectum and distal sigmoid are the areas most commonly affected, although the mid- and upper sigmoid may become involved when adhesions of previous surgical treatment cause a fixed loop to lie within the radiated area. The mid-ascending and descending colon also may be damaged during irradiation of the kidneys. The mucosa bears the brunt of injury from x-ray treatment, while the deeper layers survive the insult relatively intact. A colitic response of short duration frequently follows radiotherapy of the pelvic organs, and may include diarrhea and tenesmus with the passage of mucus and occasional blood. The endoscopist will rarely be called upon to examine this well-recognized and self-limited phenomenon in which an edematous, inflamed mucosa is seen with granularity, loss of vascular pattern, and multiple small bleeding sites. This acute reaction usually heals spontaneously, but even in the absence of immediate damage, long lasting tissue destruction may occur that does not become recognized until a considerable time after the radiotherapy has been completed; symptoms of bleeding may be evident within six months but may also be reported as long as 20 years following treatment.

The endoscopic appearance of long-standing irradiation damage is characteristically one of mucosal friability, spontaneous bleeding, and granularity with multiple telangiectases (Plate II-12). These are not to be confused with spontaneous telangiectases, which usually are discrete and occur in the right colon. It is important to differentiate the bleeding in radiation colitis from that caused by ulcerative colitis or idiopathic proctitis, because a considerable amount of blood may bathe the mucosal surface, thus obscuring the true nature of the bleeding sites following irradiation injury.

Perioperative Endoscopy in Crohn's Disease

Colonoscopy is of limited benefit in the preoperative evaluation of Crohn's disease.[93] The endoscopic discovery of patches of inflammation either near to or far from the area of contemplated resection is not important to the surgeon because the anastomosis may be made in an area of diseased bowel and the presence of inflammation elsewhere does not seem to be a factor in the tendency for recrudescence of Crohn's disease.[94-96]

One reason for performing colonoscopy in the preoperative phase in a patient with an ileocolonic fistula, however, is to determine whether the colon is primarily involved by Crohn's disease or is only a passive participant in the inflammatory process, being affected from the small bowel.[97] This distinction may be made by observing the area around the fistula in the colon and noting whether the segment of inflammation extends beyond the immediate area around the orifice of the fistula. When the adjacent colonic segment is inflamed and ulcerated, a diagnosis may be made of primary colonic Crohn's disease.[14] Usually, however, the segments of colon around a fistula are normal and surgical therapy can be planned accordingly.

Endoscopy and the Ileostomy

Several operative procedures are currently available for CUC patients who require surgical intervention. When the entire colon is removed and an ileostomy is required, such patients may have either a standard Brooke ileostomy or some form of continent ileostomy. Both of these types of ileostomies may be associated with obstruction to outflow, bleeding, pain in the area of the stoma, and increased ileostomy output, and the clinician occasionally may be concerned about the presence of inflammatory disease.

Continent ileostomies have additional problems that may require resolution, including incontinence, difficulty in intubating the pouch, and foreign bodies retained within the pouch (see Chaps. 29 and 30).[98] In contrast to CUC, no "pouch" procedures should be performed in patients with Crohn's disease for fear of recrudescence in the pouch, although some pouches were created in the past.

Roentgenograms of the small bowel may be followed through, possibly permitting localization of the site of a particular problem within an ileostomy stoma.[99] Frequently, the presence of inflammation in the most distal portion of a Brooke's ileostomy stoma may be associated with such severe spasm and contractility of the bowel that adequate roentgenographic examination of that segment is not possible. In these circumstances endoscopy may permit visualization of the distal 10 or 20 cm of the ileostomy stoma, a distance usually adequate to allow the correct diagnosis to be made, including recrudescence of Crohn's disease. For x-ray evaluation of the continent ileostomy, a specially trained radiologist must interpret the radiographic findings, because seeking the presence of a nipple within a nonperistaltic pouch may be a difficult task.

An upper intestinal endoscope is commonly used for examination of stomas and may be placed into the stomal orifice under direct vision. A circumferential view of the lumen of a pouch ileostomy may be obtained with the endoscope. The endoscopist should be aware of the normal pattern of the valvulae conniventes in the small bowel, and should seek the presence of aphthous ulcerations, diffuse erosions, linear ulcerations, and tumors. The continent ileostomy requires some experience in intubation, because the outflow tract to the skin is not straight.

In the continent ileostomy pouch, the ileal inflow tract is located adjacent to the nipple.[98] The ileal inflow tract can usually be intubated for several centimeters, and an assessment of the integrity of this portion of the bowel may be accomplished endoscopically. Normally, the mucosal lining is glistening pink, and linear suture lines can be easily identified. A small amount of fluid is normally present within the ileal pouch after the patient has emptied it by catheter intubation. A U-turn maneuver can be easily accomplished by the endoscopist by retroflexing the tip of the instrument within the pouch while advancing the endoscope shaft. The normal anatomy reveals a nipple standing away from the pouch walls and arising in a column-like projection (Plate III-1). By torquing the instrument to the right or the left, a circumferential view of the base of the nipple can be accomplished so that the most frequent site of a fistula can be inspected and any small fistulous orifices can be identified (Plate III-2). If the nipple is sitting in a slight depression, this usually indicates partial intussusception of the nipple into the outflow tract. If only a portion of the nipple is seen during retroflexion with the instrument pressed against the colon wall, a rather severe degree of nipple intussusception into the outflow tract exists, a condition requiring surgical repair (Plate III-3). Any degree of intussusception causes the patient to have difficulty in intubating the pouch, and is the most common cause of this problem. Occasionally, an adhesive band is seen extending from the nipple to one wall of the pouch, causing tethering of the nipple and partial incontinence. This can be severed using a wire snare and diathermy current. A shortened nipple may be associated with incontinence and occasionally a total absence of the nipple (because of postoperative slough) may be seen upon instrument retroflexion (Plate III-4).

"Pouchitis" can be identified when the lining becomes reddened, friable, and nodular (Plate III-5). Small aphthous-type ulcerations may be seen scattered over the surface of the pouch, closely resembling Crohn's disease. "Pouchitis" is an inflammatory response of unknown etiology, but it has been postulated that it may be caused by stasis of intestinal contents within the ileal reservoir (see Chaps. 29, 30, and 31).

Occasionally, a patient with a continent ileostomy is completely unable to intubate with the drainage catheter. This may become a gastroenterologic emergency, and every effort must be made to drain the pouch or an emergency surgical procedure may be required. The usual cause for inability to intubate is severe intussusception of the nipple with concomitant angulation of the outflow tract. During endoscopy, considerable "torquing" of the instrument shaft may be necessary to find the lumen because the tip cannot be angulated enough to permit full visualization of the entire tortuous tract. Once the pouch is entered, no attempt should be made to totally examine the pouch because patients who cannot intubate have a considerable amount of retained ileal contents in the ileostomy reservoir. It is rarely possible to suction out the pouch via the endoscope channel because the solid matter plugs its orifice. A large caliber catheter should be placed into the pouch for continuous drainage of the ileal contents. This can be accomplished by using the Seldinger technique of passing the catheter over a wire inserted through the endoscope channel.

Most ileoscopies are performed with the patient recumbent and unsedated. The patient should ingest only a full liquid diet for 24 hours prior to the examination; in the case of continent ileostomies the patient should drain the pouch (if possible) within a half hour of the endoscopy.

Ileoanal anastomoses also may be associated with problems of evacuation, continence, and bleeding. The ileoanal pouch may be intubated in a fashion similar to the continent ileostomy, always maintaining direct visual control of intubation.

The mucous fistula, or retained rectal segment, can be directly intubated with the endoscope. No preparation is necessary for this examination, and because a significant incidence of carcinoma has been found within retained rectal segments, they should be examined on a regular basis. If strictures occur, a pediatric endoscope (upper gastrointestinal type) may be successfully employed. The endoscope should be placed through the entire extent of the retained rectal segment, and biopsies taken. Most rectal segments appear to have considerable inflammation within them, and are friable, with grossly irregular surface markings. It should be noted, however, that this may be a manifestation of "bypass" colitis, and multiple biopsies should be obtained within these segments for any evidence of dysplasia.

Endoscopy and the Evaluation of Unexplained Diarrhea

There are certain patients with diarrhea whose diagnostic investigations, including sigmoidoscopy and roentgenograms, are entirely normal but in whom endoscopy *with biopsy* demonstrates the presence of colitis.[23,100-103] Although the radiographic examination is usually important in the diagnosis of inflammatory bowel disease, it may not be sensitive enough to detect those minor abnormalities of the mucosa that may be found by using colonoscopy and biopsy.[104] As mentioned earlier the rectum is usually involved in ulcerative colitis, while Crohn's disease often spares the distal bowel; however, in 5% of patients with ulcerative colitis, the rectum appear normal on sigmoidoscopy,[100] and the correct diagnosis may be made only on biopsy. Rectal biopsy features may also permit a diagnosis of Crohn's Disease in the presence of normal, gross appearances.

Preparation for Colonoscopy in Patients with Diarrhea

Cathartics should not be given to any patient during an acute exacerbation of colitis activity, nor for several weeks thereafter.[17,105] Colitis patients with chronic diarrhea need not receive cathartics, but a liquid diet prior to the procedure (28 to 48 hours) will insure the absence of large particulate matter within the colon. If the patient's symptoms are stable, but consist of less than three bowel movements daily, a mild cathartic such as 150 to 300 ml of citrate of magnesia may be given on the night prior to colonoscopy following one day of a clear liquid diet. To insure visualization during colonoscopy, all patients, even those with liquid bloody diarrhea, must receive mechanical cleansing of the colon by enemas. Two enemas are preferred, but this may be modified according to the clinical condition of each patient. Unless the patient receives adequate preparation, colonoscopy should not be performed. Oral osmotic, whole gut irrigation with a balanced electrolyte solution may be used for some patients with inflammatory bowel disease.

Screening for Premalignant and Malignant Features*

Each patient with CUC or Crohn's colitis presents a unique challenge to the physician and surgeon because that person belongs to an identifiable population subgroup in whom malignancy develops with a greater frequency than in the general population.[106-119] Long-term management decisions would be straightforward if colonic IBD behaved like familial polyposis, invariably resulting in the development of colon cancer, but fortunately the incidence of malignancy in colonic IBD patients is not inevitable. This section will review the role of endoscopy in cancer surveillance programs in CUC and Crohn's colitis.

Cancer in the bowel in ulcerative colitis patients has a different pathogenesis to that occurring in patients without colitis. According to some, in non-colitis patients, most large bowel carcinomas develop via a mechanism of malignant change in an adenoma.[120,121] Colitic cancer, in contrast, develops diffusely along the colonic mucosal surface that has been the site of previous (or continuous) inflammation. The preneoplastic changes that may occur in the colitis mucosa can be recognized by the patholo-

---

*See also Chapter 15.

Color Plates

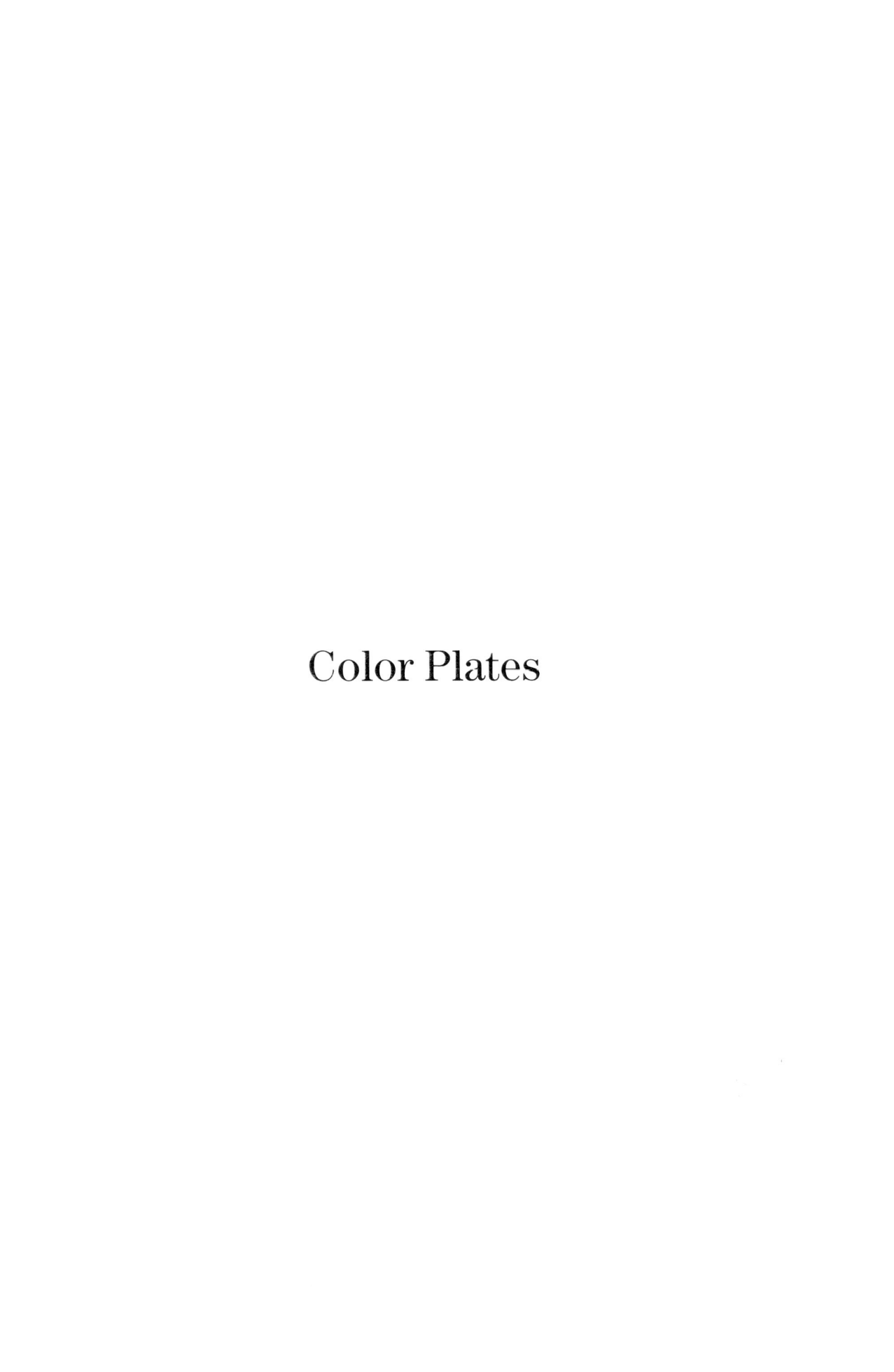

PLATE I-1. Fibrotic stricture in ulcerative colitis. Pseudopolyps are present at the edge of the stricture. Friability resulted from an attempt to pass the endoscope through the stricture.

PLATE I-2. Inflammatory stricture with concentric narrowing and pronounced inflammatory response.

PLATE I-3. Colonic stricture with carcinoma causing flattening of the left wall with eccentricity of the lumen. Biopsies were positive for carcinoma.

PLATE I-4. This large irregular adenocarcinoma caused significant lumenal narrowing and eccentricity. It was located at the hepatic flexure in a patient who had ulcerative colitis for 30 years with no evidence of colitic activity for two decades.

PLATE I-5. Multiple small pseudopolyps in a patient with inactive ulcerative colitis. Note the abnormal vasculature on the colonic wall.

PLATE I-6. A pedunculated pseudopolyp in a patient with ulcerative colitis. This polyp was resected because it was a source of continued bleeding.

PLATE I-7. A group of broad-based polyps that, on resection, proved to be tubular adenomas. They were completely removed endoscopically.

PLATE I-8. Diffuse erythema in a patient with early ulcerative colitis. The vascular pattern is completely absent.

PLATE I-9. Granularity of the colon in ulcerative colitis. The surface resembles wet sandpaper, and the multiple reflections of light are caused by edema surrounding colon crypts.

PLATE I-10. A large irregular ulcer (ulcerative colitis) in an area of diffuse colonic inflammation, as evidenced by spontaneous bleeding, erythema, loss of vascular pattern, and granularity.

PLATE I-11. A tiny aphthous ulcer in Crohn's disease of the colon. Note the red border and the normality of the surrounding mucosa.

PLATE I-12. A large irregular ulcer in granulomatous colitis. Note the absence of inflammation in the surrounding nonulcerated mucosa.

I-1　　　　　　　　　　　　　I-2　　　　　　　　　　　　　I-3

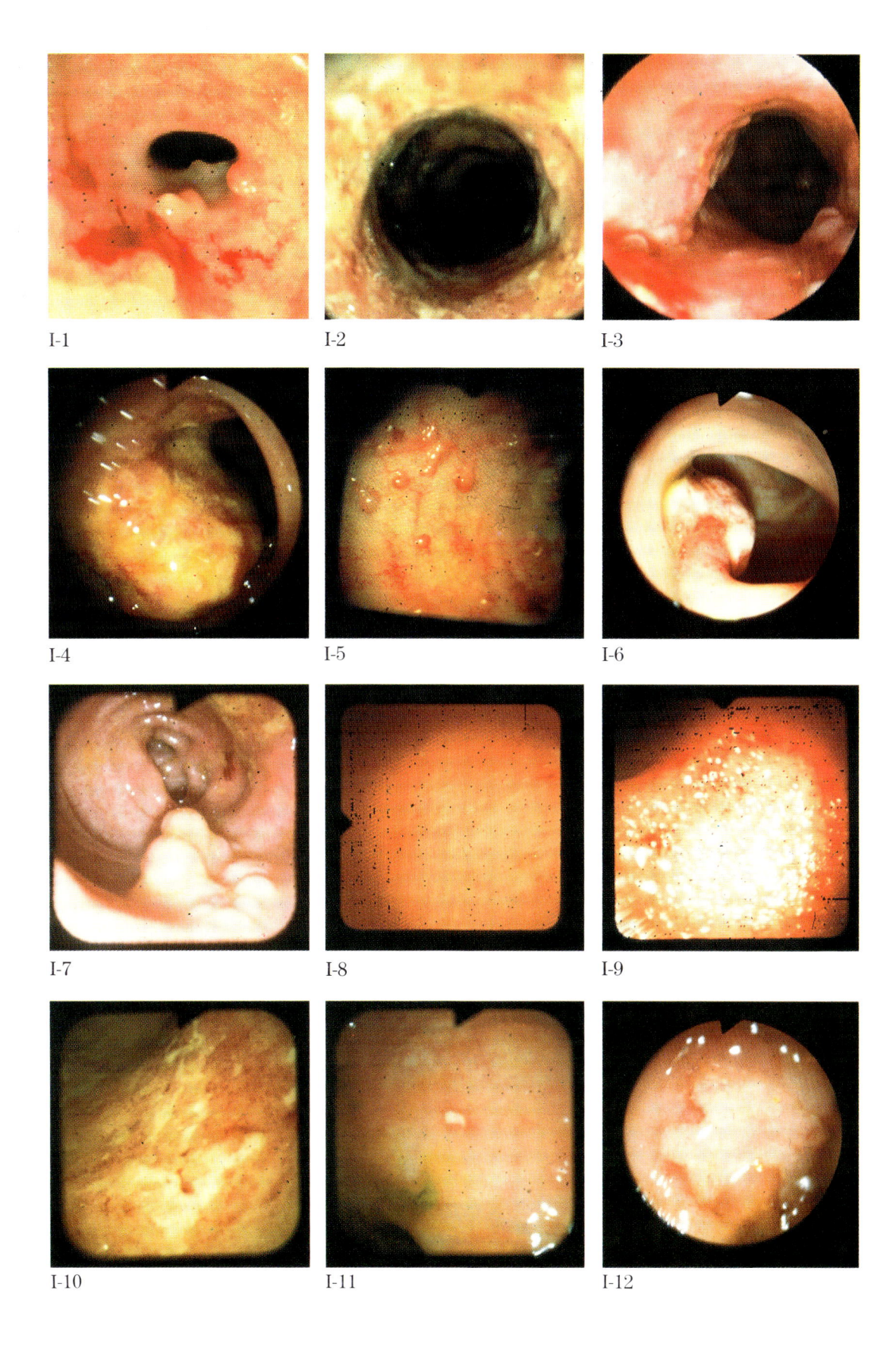

I-4　　　　　　　　　　　　　I-5　　　　　　　　　　　　　I-6

I-7　　　　　　　　　　　　　I-8　　　　　　　　　　　　　I-9

I-10　　　　　　　　　　　　 I-11　　　　　　　　　　　　　I-12

PLATE II-1. Cobblestoning in granulomatous colitis. This is caused by submucosal involvement with Crohn's disease. Ulcerations are present in the upper portion of the involved wall, but are not present in the area on the lower right.

PLATE II-2. A mucosal "bridge" in Crohn's disease. Activity of disease is no longer present, having healed completely.

PLATE II-3. The small bowel in a patient with active Crohn's disease. Multiple ulcerations are present in the terminal ileum, intubated following total colonoscopic evaluation of the large bowel.

PLATE II-4. Irregular rectal ulcers in amebiasis. The ulcerations have a red rim, and although undermining of the mucosa is common it has not occurred in this case.

PLATE II-5. Antibiotic-associated colitis can be diagnosed visually by the multiple creamy plaques on the mucosal surface.

PLATE II-6. Discrete ulcers in a surrounding zone of normal right colon mucosa in cytomegalovirus complicating chemotherapy-induced immunodeficiency disease.

PLATE II-7. Caseating granulomas were found in the cecum of this patient who presented with colonic bleeding. Cultures proved this to be an atypical Mycobacterium.

PLATE II-8. Kaposi sarcoma of the colon typically presents as a slightly elevated, purplish, well-demarcated lesion.

PLATE II-9. In acute diverticulitis, free pus may be seen in the lumen. The actual infected orifice is rarely identified.

PLATE II-10. A linear ulceration may be seen in the subacute phase of ischemic colitis. This stage closely resembles Crohn's disease.

PLATE II-11. Solitary rectal ulcer usually presents as an irregular, superficial-appearing ulceration in the mid to upper rectum.

PLATE II-12. Telangiectasias of the rectum are commonly found in radiotherapy-induced rectal injury. Bleeding may occur from these telangiectasias many years after radiation.

II-1

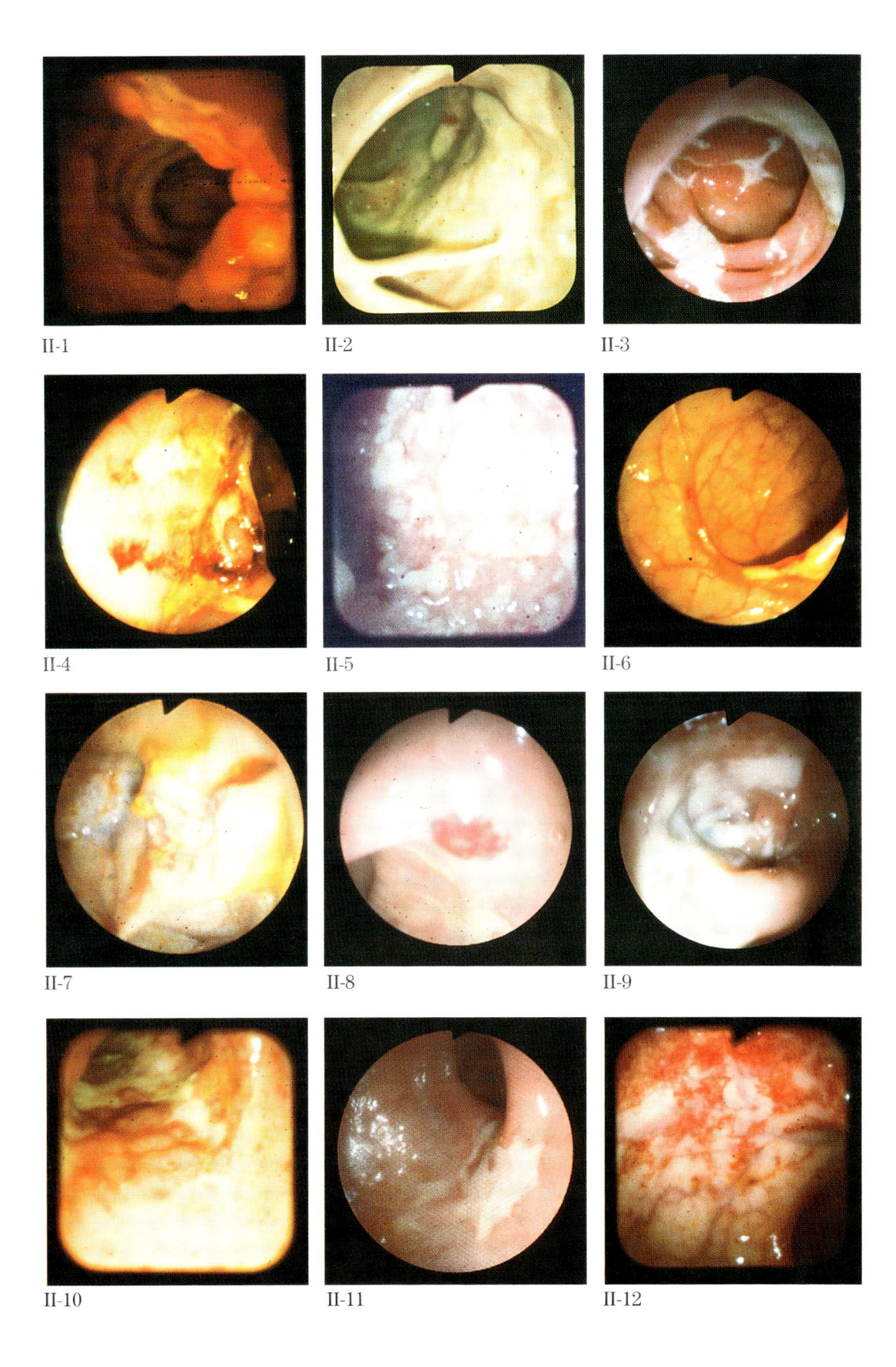

II-2

II-3

II-4

II-5

II-6

II-7

II-8

II-9

II-10

II-11

II-12

Plate III-1. The endoscope has been passed into a continent ileostomy, and is seen at the 2 o'clock position. The nipple arises smoothly from the pouch wall and surrounds the instrument in a column-like fashion. The pouch walls are smooth and glistening.

Plate III-2. A small fistula can be identified at the base of the nipple. Part of the nipple is present in the left upper portion of this picture, and the fistula, the slit-like orifice, communicates with the outflow tract.

Plate III-3. This nipple is partially intussuscepted, and only a portion of it can be seen. Most of the nipple lies within the outflow tract. This is a common cause for difficulty with intubation. Note the multiple small erosions/ulcerations in the pouch. This patient also has a moderate severe "pouchitis."

Plate III-4. A "U-turn" maneuver within the continent ileostomy demonstrates almost complete loss of the nipple caused by slough following surgical treatment. This patient was totally incontinent.

Plate III-5. This patient's abdominal pain and fever was caused by inflammation within the continent ileostomy. "Pouchitis" is frequently associated with spontaneous bleeding.

Plate III-6. Dysplasia in ulcerative colitis usually presents no particular visual abnormality. These small mucosal nodulations were proven to be dysplastic on biopsy.

Plate III-7. Dysplasia was present in this segment of the ascending colon in a 21-year-old patient with inactive ulcerative colitis for 15 years.

Plate III-8. Dysplasia was found over the surface of this mass lesion that, at surgical treatment, proved to be carcinoma of the right colon.

Plate III-9. Crohn's disease of the stomach. The antrum is nodular and lacks distensibility. A small ulcer is seen in the right mid-portion. The pylorus is concentric.

III-1

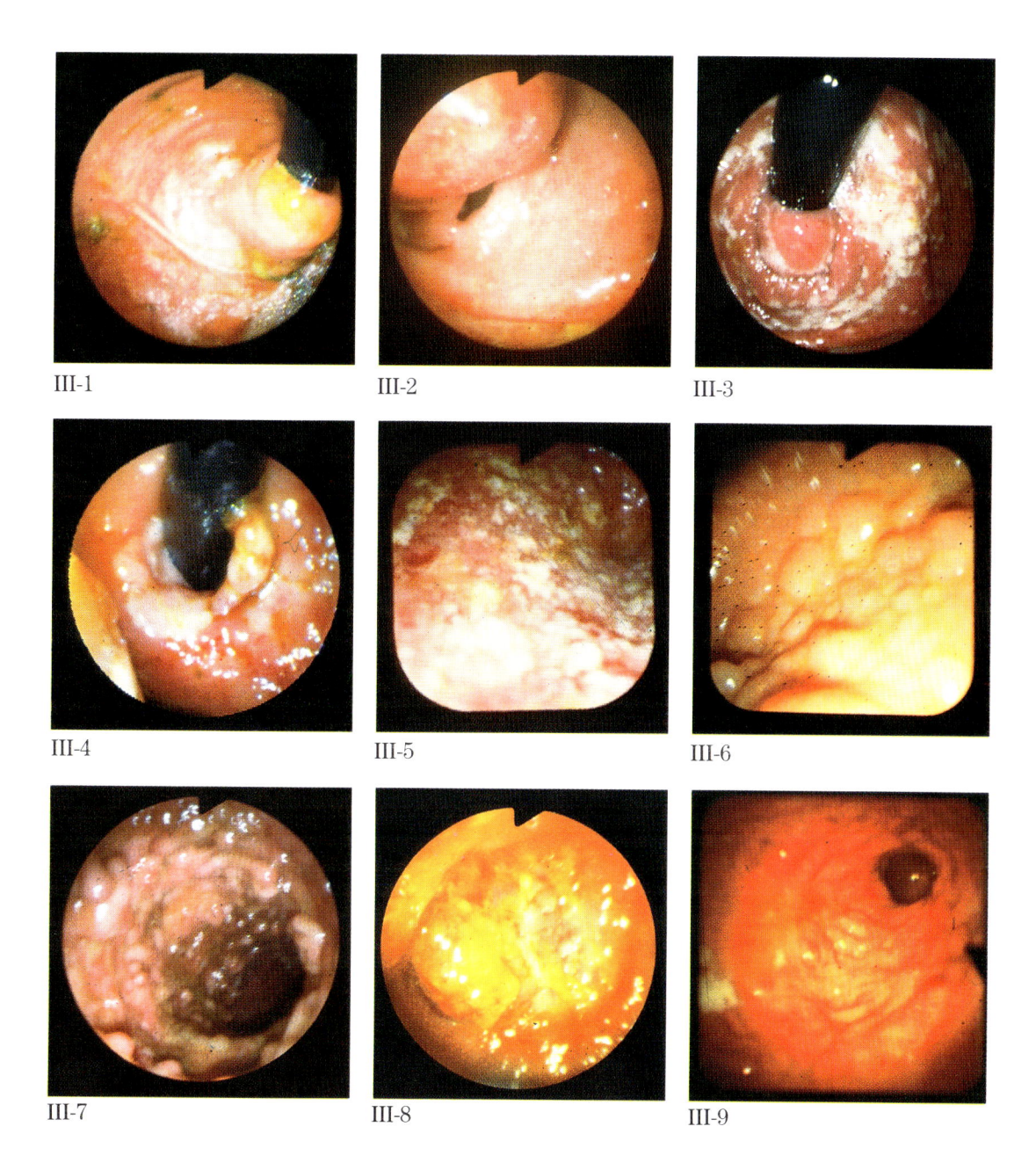

III-2

III-3

III-4

III-5

III-6

III-7

III-8

III-9

gist,[122] and they consist of architectural alterations as well as the cytologic abnormalities of cellular pleomorphism and stratification of hyperchromatic nuclei that have lost their normal polarity. Such histopathologic abnormalities are seen in some patients with ulcerative colitis and are termed dysplasia. The areas of dysplasia that may develop in the patient with chronic ulcerative colitis are focal, but such foci may occur throughout the length of the bowel. The propensity for dysplastic changes to affect any part of the colon that had been the site of inflammatory activity means that the entire colonic surface in patients with universal disease is potentially at risk for the development of cancer.[110]

The tendency for the direct development of neoplastic mucosal changes without passing through a precursor mass lesion, such as an adenoma, accounts for the reason that the carcinoma in patients with ulcerative colitis is characteristically flat and may be difficult to recognize on endoscopy or on the barium enema x-ray examination. The likelihood of carcinoma in a dysplastic proliferative lesion rises with the number and size of such areas throughout the colon.[123-125]

Data concerning dysplasia in the colorectal cancer occurring in Crohn's disease have been conflicting, with one study of endoscopy and surgical resection specimens reporting the absence of any dysplastic changes in several patients,[126] while others have described dysplasia, both nearby and remote from the Crohn's colitic cancer.[112,113,127-129] The latter findings indicate that a "working approach" to Crohn's colitis and cancer is that such patients should be managed similarly to those with CUC whenever possible.

Dysplasia*

As mentioned earlier, dysplasia is a histopathologic finding that is identified by submitting samples of colonic tissue for microscopic identification (Table 19-6). Mucosal specimens may be obtained either by sigmoidoscopic biopsies or through the use of the flexible fiberoptic colonoscope.

Rectal Biopsies and the Detection of Dysplasia

Until recently, rectal biopsies were considered to reflect the presence of dysplasia in the proximal intestinal tract.[130] The initial claims of a high correlation between dysplasia in rectal biopsy tissue and that occurring in the proximal portion of the colon have failed to be confirmed, however, and a significant proportion of patients with colonic dysplasia (up to 90%) may not have concomitant dysplasia in the rectum.[131-133]

Colonoscopic Biopsies and the Detection of Dysplasia

Because dysplasia occurs in various noncontiguous areas throughout the colon, colonoscopic biopsies provide a method of obtaining tissue specimens from representative areas of the entire colon. A considerable sampling error occurs during the gathering of mucosal specimens on surveillance colonoscopy because the tiny pinch biopsy represents only a fraction of the total mucosal surface at risk. The endoscopist should approach the surveillance examination with the knowledge that dysplasia may be missed because it may occur in patches as small as 1 cm in extent, and dysplasia on one wall of a particular segment may not be detected by a biopsy from the opposite wall of the same segment. The highest yield for dysplasia is achieved when the endoscopist directs the biopsy forceps to an area of visible surface irregularity.[138]

When using colonoscopy for screening in high risk patients with colonic IBD, multiple biopsies should be taken from each area of the colon.[133] The current recommendation is to biopsy at 10 cm intervals,[17,120,134] which implies that one or more biopsies should be taken from the cecum, ascending colon, hepatic flexure, transverse colon, splenic flexure, descending colon, sigmoid colon, and from the rectum. Biopsies should be labeled separately so that the segment from which the tissue was obtained can subsequently be identified to permit directed rebiopsy if dysplastic changes are found in only one of the several areas sampled.

Potentially, dysplastic areas may be extremely difficult to recognize endoscopically because these areas may be flat or only slightly elevated above the level of the atrophic colonic mucosa (Plate III-6).[135,136] Dysplasia is rarely found in the segments of shiny mucosa with an intact vascular pattern, but is most likely to be present in areas of featureless "atrophic" mucosa. The use of a dye-spray technique to enhance the endoscopist's perception of surface irregularity may eventually prove to be useful in the identification of specific sites for directed biopsy, but currently it is tedious and usually nonproductive. Because it is not possible to make a naked-eye diagnosis of dysplasia,[137] the endoscopist is encouraged to take particular in-

*See also Chapter 15.

TABLE 19-6. *Classification of Dysplasia in Ulcerative Colitis and Schema for Patient Management.**

Biopsy Classification	Implications for Patient Management
Negative	
Normal	Follow-up with colonoscopy yearly or colonoscopy every 2–3 years with interval annual rectal biopsies
Inactive colitis	
Active colitis	
Indefinite (probably negative)	
Unknown	
Probably positive	Repeat biopsies in 3 months
Positive	
Low-grade dysplasia	Treat colitis and repeat biopsy in 3 months. Consider colectomy if dysplasia associated with mass or if dysplasia is confirmed.
Positive	
High-grade dysplasia	Consider colectomy if dysplasia confirmed

terest in raised lesions (Plate III-7). If a mass lesion is seen, multiple biopsies should be taken from that area because dysplasia associated with the presence of a mass lesion takes on a much greater significance than when found in a flat area of mucosa. The mass lesion found to have dysplasia on endoscopic biopsy may be termed polypoid dysplasia, and has been noted to have a high incidence of associated carcinoma (Plate III-8).[125,138] Conversely, dysplasia in a flat segment of mucosa is reported to have a lower correlation with the presence of cancer.[138] Scanning electron microscopy may complement light microscopy in the diagnosis of colonic dysplasia.[139]

When the entire colon had been removed and was available for pathologic examination, dysplasia was found to be present in 88% of ulcerative colitis colons containing carcinoma.[140] This figure is not applicable to the clinical situation where the entire colon is not available for microscopic examination and there is a need for cancer surveillance in a patient with ulcerative colitis. The effectiveness of surveillance colonoscopy and biopsy for the detection of dysplasia in the high-risk group of patients with universal ulcerative colitis for over eight years has been addressed by many authors.[132,138,141-148] Random colonoscopic biopsies at 10 cm intervals may demonstrate carcinoma in as many as 3% of patients,[132,145] and dysplasia may be discovered in 7 to 40% of patients in the high-risk group.[132,144] The overall result in a total of 877 patients reported in the literature (Table 19-7) to have had colonoscopic surveillance biopsies is that 20 patients (2%) had carcinoma diagnosed as a result of the discovery of dysplasia, and an additional 11 patients (1%) had carcinoma discovered on direct mucosal biopsies. Not all patients with colitic cancer have concomitant dysplasia, as evidenced by the finding that 10% (3 out of 31) of the patients with cancer did not have dysplasia in any of the colonoscopic biopsies. Thus regular surveillance colonoscopies in the high-risk patient serves two purposes, that of discovering dysplasia, with its possible implications, and the discovery of carcinoma by visual identification of abnormal areas for directed biopsy.[150]

The merits of surveillance colonoscopy in Crohn's colitis have yet to be defined because the realization that the risk of colorectal cancer is increased in this form of IBD is relatively recent.[128] Dysplasia has been found in resection specimens in the immediate vicinity of all colon cancers in Crohn's disease, however, and remote from the cancer in 60% of cases.[112]

Frequency of Colonoscopy and Biopsy for Cancer Surveillance*

The frequency for surveillance colonoscopy and biopsies in colonic IBD is a subject of controversy.[144,151,152] Some authors are concerned about patient compliance for an annual colonoscopic examination, as well as the cost involved, and recommend colonoscopy with multiple biopsies every other year, alternating with sigmoidoscopy and multiple rectal biopsies.[147] However, if it is true that colonoscopy may uncover small carcinomas prior to the time that they are clinically identifiable, then perhaps annual colonoscopy should be the procedure of choice in patients who are at high risk for the development of cancer, with high-risk patients being those with total colonic disease for over

---

*See also Chapter 15. Editor's note: see also Lennard-Jones, J. E.: Gut, *27*:1403, 1986; and Broström, O., et al.: Gut, *27*:1408, 1986.

TABLE 19-7. *Colonoscopic Surveillance in Ulcerative Colitis (877 Patients).*

First Author	Number of Patients	Number of Patients with Dysplasia	Percent with Dysplasia	Number of Patients with Dysplasia Leading to Cancer Diagnosis	Number of Patients with Dysplasia and Cancer Found Simultaneously	Number of Patients with Cancer without Dysplasia
Brostrom[146]	52	8	15	1	0	0
Dickinson[143]	43	9	20	2	0	0
Grandqvist[142]	150	12	8	1	0	0
Hanauer[144]*	107	43	40	4	0	0
Lennard-Jones[104]‡	72‡	7	—	2	0	0
Nugent[149]§	131	34	26	6	0	0
Rosenstock[132]‖	259	18	7	4	7	2
Waye[145]	63	5	8	0	1	1
Total	877	136	16%	20	8	3

*Includes data from Blackstone, et al.: Gastroenterology, *80*:366, 1981.
†Their most recent article does not provide separate colonoscopy data.[147]
‡Patients examined in the colonoscopy era.
§Includes data from Nugent, et al.: Gastroenterology, *76*:1, 1979.
‖Includes data from Fuson, et al.: Am. J. Gastroenterol. *73*:120, 1980.

eight years duration. A practical solution to this frequency problem may be to offer annual colonoscopy and biopsy to patients with a featureless and grossly irregular mucosal pattern, and biennial examinations to those with a completely normal vascular pattern throughout, whose initial biopsies show no suspicious abnormalities.

Risk of the Retained Rectal Segment

Patients who have had a subtotal colectomy with the rectal segment retained are also at risk of developing carcinoma in the mucosa of the rectum, whether the underlying disease was Crohn's disease or ulcerative colitis.[112,153,154] Following eight years of colitis, such patients are at the same high risk for the subsequent development of carcinoma as are patients with an intact large intestine because intestinal discontinuity does not protect against malignant transformation.[155,156]

Complications of Colonoscopy

In the group of infectious and inflammatory conditions affecting the large intestine, the following three areas should be considered as potential causes of complications of colonoscopy:

1. Complications from instrumentation itself.
2. The possibility of transmitting infection via the colonoscope.
3. Infection of endoscopy staff via contaminated materials and equipment.

The endoscopist must remember that the inflamed large bowel is probably more friable and less able than the normal colon to adapt to the stress of stretching and distension imposed by the passage of the colonoscope. Every effort must be made to maintain the shaft as straight as possible, with a minimum of loop formation; the amount of air insufflation should be a constant consideration.[1] Mucosal friability may cause bleeding after an endoscopic examination whether or not biopsies are taken. Fortunately, colonoscopists have been extremely cautious when endoscoping inflammatory bowel disease and reported complications are rare.[157-159]

General standards of cleanliness are required whenever an endoscopic procedure is performed in a patient with potentially infectious colitis, but the technique of "reverse isolation," with gowns, gloves, and masks, is not recommended except for cases of acquired immunodeficiency syndrome (AIDS). When cultures are necessary, colonic secretions can be collected in a bronchoscopic-type suction trap and sent to the microbiology laboratory in the sealed container without the need to inoculate specimens in the endoscopy suite. Although few reports have been made of infections transmitted from patient to patient via the flexible fiberoptic endoscope,[160] it is considered prudent to disinfect the equipment after each case of infectious or inflammatory colitis. In addition to meticulous mechanical cleansing, the instrument and accessories should be soaked in the manufacturer's suggested disinfection solution.[161] The current recommendation in patients with AIDS is gas sterilization of the colonoscope and all ancillary equipment. Gas sterilization is not recommended following endoscopy in any other condition.

Endoscopy in Upper Gastrointestinal Involvement by Crohn's Disease

Crohn's disease can affect the entire gastrointestinal tract from the mouth to the anus, with a variety of presentations in the upper intestine. Ulcers may occur in the oral cavity with or without periodontal disease.[162] The pharynx or esophagus involved rarely is involved. Clinical evidence of gastric and duodenal Crohn's disease is not common, but, if present, almost all patients also will have radiographic and symptomatic Crohn's disease of the small or large bowel.[163,164] The reported incidence of upper gastrointestinal Crohn's disease ranges from 0.5 to 4%.[165,166]

In the stomach, the antrum is most commonly involved. The affected segments may appear tubular, narrowed, and lack distensibility. The mucosa may have multiple large bumpy nodulations similar to cobblestoning of the colon (Plate III-9). Ulcerations are unusual, but when present are linear in configuration and are found in obviously diseased segments of the stomach as opposed to the large bowel where ulcerations often occur in otherwise normal segments.

Duodenal involvement may resemble a classic peptic ulcer but the endoscopist is more likely to visualize diffuse evidence of disease with linear ulcerations and thickening of the mucosal folds. The descending duodenum is often the segment most severely affected. In the presence of diffuse jeunoileitis,[167,168] it may be possible to orally pass a long enteroscope (or a properly sterilized colonoscope) deep into the upper small bowel for purposes of visual identification of small ulcers as well as obtaining tissue for histopathologic evaluation.

Endoscopic biopsy of involved mucosa shows characteristic granulomas only in a minority of cases, causing difficulty in making a definitive diagnosis of Crohn's disease in the upper gastrointestinal tract.[169,170] Despite the low incidence of clinical upper gastrointestinal involvement with Crohn's disease, endoscopic biopsy studies of the upper gastrointestinal tract in patients with only distal bowel involvement have uniformly demonstrated a high prevalence of histologic abnormalities in the stomach and duodenum.[171-173]

References

1. Waye, J.: The role of colonoscopy in the differential diagnosis of inflammatory bowel disease. Gastrointest. Endosc., *23*:150, 1977.
2. Kettlewell, M., and Harper, P.: Colonoscopy in the management of Crohn's disease. In Gastrointestinal Endoscopy. Advances in Diagnosis and Therapy. Edited by P. R. Salmon. London, Chapman and Hall, 1984.
3. Bartram, C.: Radiology in the current assessment of ulcerative colitis. Gastrointest. Radiol., *1*:383, 1977.
4. Waye, J., and Braunfeld, S.: Colonoscopy and the indications for surgery in ulcerative colitis. In Gastrointestinal Endoscopy. Advances in Diagnosis and Therapy. Edited by P. R. Salmon. London, Chapman and Hall, 1984.
5. Grandqvist, S. et al.: Precancerous lesions in the mucosa in ulcerative colitis. A radiographic, endoscopic, and histopathologic study. Scand. J Gastroenterol., *15*:289, 1980.
6. Waye, J.: Colonoscopy intubation technique without fluoroscopy. In Colonoscopy. Techniques, Clinical Practice and Colour Atlas. Edited by R. Hunt, and J. Waye. London, Chapman and Hall, 1981.
7. Hogan, W., Hensley, G., and Geenan, J.: Endoscopic evaluation of inflammatory bowel disease. Med. Clin. North Am., *64*:1083, 1980.
8. Mitros, F.: The biopsy in evaluating patients with inflammatory bowel disease. Med. Clin. North Am., *64*:1037, 1980.
9. Das, K., Farid, T., and Berkowitz, J.: Value of colonoscopy in the investigation of inflammatory bowel disease. Gastroenterology, *66*:681, 1974.
10. Holdstock, G., DuBoulay, C., and Smith, C.: Survey of the use of colonoscopy in inflammatory bowel disease. Dig. Dis. Sci., *29*:731, 1984.
11. Stein, D., et al.: Location and activity of ulcerative and Crohn's colitis by indium 111 leukocyte scan. A prospective comparison study. Gastroenterology, *84*:388, 1983.
12. Jones, B., Abbruzzese, A., Hill, T., and Adelstein, S.: Gallium-67-citrate scintigraphy in ulcerative colitis. Gastrointest. Radiol., *5*:267, 1980.
13. Williams, C., and Waye, J.: Colonoscopy in inflammatory Bowel Disease. Clin. Gastroenterol., *7*:701, 1978.
14. Waye, J.: Endoscopy in inflammatory bowel disease. Clin. Gastroenterol., *9*:279, 1980.
15. Hunt, R., Teague, R., Swarbrick, E., Williams, G.: Colonoscopy in the management of colonic strictures. Br. Med. J., *2*:360, 1975.
16. Greenstein, A., et al.: Cancer in universal and left-sided ulcerative colitis: factors determining risk. Gastroenterology, *77*:290, 1979.
17. Waye, J.: Colitis, cancer and colonoscopy. Med. Clin. North Am., *62*:211, 1978.
18. Crowson, T., Ferrante, W., and Cathright, J.: Colonscopy: Inefficacy for early carcinoma detection in patients with ulcerative colitis. J. Am. Med. Assoc., *236*:2651, 1976.
19. Nielsen, O., Sondergaard, J., and Aru, A.: Colitis cystica profunda lokalisata. Acta Chir. Scand., *150*:191, 1984.
20. Cook, M., and Goligher, J.: Carcinoma and epithelial dysplasia complicating ulcerative colitis. Gastroenterology, *68*:1127, 1975.
21. Margulis, A.: Radiology of ulcerating colitis. Radiology, *105*:251, 1972.
22. Teague, R., and Waye, J.: Endoscopy in inflammatory bowel disease. In Colonoscopy: Techniques, Clinical Practice and Colour Atlas. Edited by R. Hunt, and J. Waye. London, Chapman and Hall, 1981.
23. Edwards, F., and Truelove, S.: The course and prognosis of ulcerative colitis, III and IV. Gut, *5*:1, 1964.
24. Jalan, K., et al.: Pseudopolyposis in ulcerative colitis. Lancet, *2*:555, 1969.
25. Corless, J., Tedesco, F., Griffin, J., and Panish, J.: Giant ileal inflammatory polyps in Crohn's disease. Case Reports. Gastrointest. Endosc., *30*:352, 1984.
26. Shah, S., Rogers, H., and Nagal, N.: Localized giant pseudopolyposis in Crohn's disease: colonoscopic findings. Dis. Colon Rectum, *21*:104, 1978.
27. Jones, B., and Abbruzzese, A.: Obstructing giant pseudopolyps in granulomatous colitis. Gastrointest. Radiol., *3*:437, 1978.
28. Kirks, D., Currarino, G., and Berk, R.: Localized giant pseudopolyposis of the colon. Am. J. Gastroenterol., *69*:609, 1978.
29. Forde, K., et al.: Giant pseudopolyposis in colitis with colonic intussusception. Gastroenterology, *75*:1142, 1978.
30. Martinez, C., et al.: Localized tumor-like lesions in ulcerative colitis and Crohn's disease of the colon. Johns Hopkins Med. J., *140*:249, 1977.
31. Fishman, R., Fleming, C., and Stephens, D.: Roentgenographic simulation of colonic cancer by benign masses in Crohn's colitis. Mayo Clin. Proc., *53*:447, 1978.
32. Levinson, J., Wall, A., and Kirsner, J.: The problems of carcinoma in inflammatory disease of the bowel. South. Med. J., *65*:209, 1972.
33. Waye, J., and Hunt, R.: Colonscopic diagnosis of inflammatory bowel disease. Surg. Clin. North Am., *62*:905, 1982.
34. Teague, R., and Read, A.: Polyposis in ulcerative colitis. Gut, *16*:792, 1975.
35. Rutgeerts, P., et al.: Acute infective colitis caused by endemic pathogens in Western Europe: Endoscopic features. Endoscopy, *14*:212, 1982.
36. Tedesco, J., and Moore, S.: Infectious diseases mimicking inflammatory bowel disease. Am. Surg., *48*:242, 1982.
37. Tedesco, F.: Differential diagnosis of ulcerative colitis

and Crohn's ileo-colitis and other specific inflammatory disease of the bowel. Med. Clin. North Am. *64*:1173, 1980.
38. Tedesco, F., Hardin, R., Harper, R., and Edwards, B.: Infectious colitis endoscopically simulating inflammatory bowel disease: a prospective evaluation. Gastrointest. Endosc., *29*:195, 1983.
39. Rickert, R., and Carter, H.: The "early" ulcerative lesion of Crohn's disease: Correlative light-and scanning electron-microscopic studies. J. Clin. Gastroenterol., *2*:11, 1980.
40. McGovern, V., and Goulston, S.: Crohn's disease of the colon. Gut, *9*:164, 1968.
41. Morson, B.: The early histological lesion of Crohn's disease. Proc. R. Soc. Med., *65*:71, 1972.
42. McGovern, V., and Goulston, S.: Crohn's disease of the colon. Gut, *9*:164, 1968.
43. Geboes, K., Desmet, V., DeWolf-Peters, C., and Van Trappen, G.: The value of endoscopic biopsies in the diagnosis of Crohn's disease. Am. J. Gastroent. Colon Rect. Surg., *29*:21, 1978.
44. Lux, G., Fruhmorgen, P., Philip, J., and Zeus, J.: Diagnosis of inflammatory disease of the colon. Endoscopy, *10*:279, 1978.
45. Hogan, W., Hensley, G., and Geenen, J.: Endoscopic evaluation of inflammatory bowel disease. Med. Clin. North Am., *64*:1083, 1980.
46. Korelitz, B., and Sommers, S.: Rectal biopsy in patients with Crohn's disease. Normal mucosa on sigmoidoscopic examination. J. Am. Med. Assoc., *237*:2742, 1977.
47. Rotterdam, H., and Sommers, S.: Biopsy diagnosis of the digestive tract. New York, Raven Press, 1981.
48. Morson, B.: The technique and interpretation of rectal biopsies in inflammatory bowel disease. Pathol. Annu., *9*:209, 1974.
49. Rickert, R.: The important "impostors" in the differential diagnosis of inflammatory bowel disease. J. Clin. Gastroenterol., *6*:153, 1984.
50. Gaisford, W.: Fiberendoscopy of the cecum and terminal ileum. Gastrointest. Endosc., *21*:13, 1974.
51. Nagasako, K., Yazawa, C., and Takemoto, T.: Biopsy of the terminal ileum. Gastrointest. Endosc., *19*:7, 1972.
52. Coremans, G., et al.: The value of ileoscopy with biopsy in the diagnosis of intestinal Crohn's disease. Gastrointest. Endosc., *30*:167, 1984.
53. Goldgraber, M., and Kirsner, J.: "Specific" diseases simulating "non-specific" ulcerative colitis-lymphopathia venerum, acute vasculitis, scleroderma and secondary amyloidosis. Ann. Int. Med. *47*:939, 1957.
54. Curtis, K., and Sleisenger, M.: Infectious and parasitic diseases. In Gastrointestinal Disease. Edited by Sleisenger MH, Fordtran, J., 2nd Ed. Philadelphia: WB Saunders, 1978.
55. Farman, J., Rabinowitz, J., and Meyers, M.: Roentgenology of infectious colitis. Am. J. Roentgenol. Rad. Ther., *119*:375, 1973.
56. Surawicz, C., and Belic, L.: Rectal biopsy helps to distinguish acute self-limited colitis from idiopathic inflammatory bowel disease. Gastroenterology, *86*:104, 1984.
57. Crowson, T., and Hines, C.: Amebiasis diagnosed by colonoscopy. Gastrointest. Endosc., *24*:254, 1978.
58. Tucker, P., Webster, P., Zachary, M., and Kilpatrick, A.: Amebic colitis mistaken for inflammatory bowel disease. Arch. Int. Med., *135*:681, 1975.
59. Scott, A., Nicholson, G., and Kerr, A.: Lincomycin as a cause of pseudomembranous colitis. Lancet, *1*:1232, 1973.
60. DeFord, J., Molinaro, J., and Daly, J.: Lincomycin—and clindamycin-associated colitis. Gastrointest. Endosc., *21*:19, 1974.
61. Beavis, J., Parsons, R., and Salfield, J.: Colitis and diarrhea—a problem with antibiotic therapy. Br. J. Surg., *63*:299, 1976.
62. Bartlett, J., Chang, T., Gurwith, M., Gorbach, S., and Onderdonk, A.: Antibiotic associated pseudomembranous colitis due to toxin-producing clostridia. N. Engl. J. Med., *298*:531, 1978.
63. Tedesco, F.: Antibiotic associated pseudomembranous colitis with negative proctosigmoidoscopy examination. Gastroenterology, *77*:295, 1979.
64. Peikin, S., Galdibini, J., and Bartlett, J.: Role of clostridium difficile in a case of nonantibiotic-associated pseudomembranous colitis. Gastroenterology, *79*:948, 1980.
65. Knight, R.: Giardiasis, isosporiasis and balantidiasis. Clin. Gastroenterol., *7*:31, 1978.
66. Blaser, M., Parsons, R., and Lou-Wang, W.: Acute colitis caused by Campylobacter fetus ss. jejuni. Gastroenterology, *78*:448, 1980.
67. Loss, R. Jr., Mangla, J., and Pereira, M.: Campylobacter colitis presenting as inflammatory bowel disease with segmental colonic ulcerations. Gastroenterology, *79*:138, 1980.
68. Goodman, Z., Boitnott, J., and Yardley, J.: Perforation of the colon associated with cytomegalovirus infection. Dig. Dis. Sci., *24*:376, 1979.
69. Haws, C., Long, R., Caplan, G.: Histoplasma capsulatum as a cause of ileocolitis. Am. J. Radiol., *128*:692, 1977.
70. Saffouri, B., Bartolomeco, R., Fuchs, B.: Colonic involvement in salmonellosis. Dig. Dis. Sci., *24*:203, 1979.
71. Nebel, O., et al.: Schistosomal colonic polyposis: endoscopic and histological characteristics. Gastrointest. Endosc., *20*:99, 1974.
72. Franklin, G., Mohapatra, M., and Perillo, R.: Colonic tuberculosis diagnosed by colonoscopic biopsy. Gastroenterology, *76*:362, 1979.
73. Bhargava, D. et al.: Diagnosis of ileocecal and colonic tuberculosis by colonoscopy. Gastrointest. Endosc., *31*:68, 1985.
74. Vantrappen, G., et al.: Yersinia enteritis and enterocolitis. Gastroenterology, *72*:220, 1977.
75. Lebedeff, D., and Hochman, E.: Rectal gonorrhea in men: diagnosis and treatment. Ann. Int. Med., *92*:464, 1980.
76. Goldmeier, D.: Proctitis and herpes simplex virus in homosexual men. Br. J. Vener. Dis., *56*:111, 1980.
77. Quinn, T., et al.: Chlamydia trachomatis proctitis. N. Engl. J. Med., *305*:195, 1981.
78. Quinn, T., et al.: Rectal mass caused by Treponema pallidum, Gastroenterology, *82*:135, 1982.
79. Levy, J., and Zeigler, J.: Acquired immonodeficiency syndrome is an opportunistic infection and Kaposi's Sarcoma results from secondary immune stimulation. Lancet, *2*:78, 1983.
80. Petras, R., Carey, W., and Alanis, A.: Cryptosporidial enteritis in a homosexual male with an acquired immunodeficiency syndrome. Clev. Clin. Q., *50*:41, 1983.
81. Williams, C.: Diverticular disease and strictures. In Colonoscopy: Techniques, Clinical Practice and Colour Atlas. Edited by R. Hunt, J. Waye. London, Chapman and Hall, 1981.
82. McNeill, C., Green, G., Bannayan, G., and Weser, E.: Ischemic colitis diagnosed by early colonoscopy, Gastrointest. Endosc., *20*:124, 1974.
83. Hunt, R., and Buchanan, J.: Transient ischemic colitis-colonoscopy and biopsy in diagnosis. J. R. Nav. Med. Serv., *65*:15, 1979.
84. Scowcroft, C., Sanowski, R., and Kozarek, R.: Colonos-

copy in ischemic colitis. Gastrointest. Endosc., *27*:156, 1981.
85. Tedesco, F., Volpicelli, N., and Moore, F.: Estrogen-and progesterone-associated colitis: a disorder with clinical and endoscopic features mimicking Crohn's colitis. Gastrointest. Endosc., *28*:247, 1982.
86. Madigan, M., and Morson, B.: Solitary ulcer of the rectum. Gut, *10*:871, 1969.
87. Rutter, K., and Riddell, R.: The solitary ulcer syndrome of the rectum. Clin. Gastroenterol., *4*:505, 1975.
88. Ford, M., et al.: Clinical spectrum of "solitary ulcer" of the rectum. Gastroenterology, *84*:1533, 1983.
89. Alberti-Flor, J., Halter, S., and Dunn, G.: Solitary rectal ulcer as a cause of massive lower gastrointestinal bleeding. Gastrointest. Endosc., *31*:54, 1985.
90. Devroede, G., Beaudry, R., Haddad, H., and Enriquez, P.: Discrete ulcerations of the rectum and sigmoid. Dig. Dis. Sci., *18*:695, 1973.
91. McNeill, C., Green, G., Bannayan, G., and Weser, E.: Ischemic colitis diagnosed by early colonoscopy. Gastrointest. Endosc., *20*:124, 1964.
92. Moss, W., and Brand, W.: Radiation Oncology. St. Louis, C.V. Mosby, 1979.
93. Block, G.: Current concepts: Surgical management of Crohn's colitis. New Engl. J. Med., *302*:1068, 1980.
94. Whelan, G., Farmer, R., Fazio, V., and Goormastic, M.: Recurrence after surgery in Crohn's disease. Gastroenterology, *88*:1826, 1985.
95. Hamilton, S., et al.: No role for resection margin frozen sections in the surgical management of Crohn's disease. Gastroenterology, *82*:1078, 1982.
96. Lee, E., and Papaioannou, N.: Recurrences following surgery in Crohn's disease. Clin. Gastroenterol., *9*:419, 1980.
97. Yardley, J., and Donowitz, M.: Colo-rectal biopsy in inflammatory bowel disease. *In* The Gastrointestinal Tract. Edited by J. Yardley, B. Morson, and M. Abell. Baltimore, Williams & Wilkins, 1977.
98. Waye, J., Kreel, I., Bauer, J., and Gelernt, I.: The continent ileostomy: Diagnosis and treatment of problems by means of operative fiberoptic endoscopy. Gastrointest. Endosc., *23*:196, 1977.
99. Franchini, A., Cola, B., and Stevens, P.: Atlas of stomal pathology. Verona, Cortina International. New York, Raven Press, 1983.
100. Elliott, P., et al.: Colonoscopic diagnosis of minimal change colitis inpatients with a normal sigmoidoscopy and normal air-contrast barium enema. Lancet, *1*:650, 1982.
101. Shearman, D.: Colonoscopy in ulcerative colitis. Scand. J. Gastroenterol., *8*:289, 1973.
102. Williams, C.: Evaluation of the colonoscopic examination: results of three studies. Dis. Colon Rectum, *18*:365, 1975.
103. Read, N., et al.: Chronic diarrhea of unknown origin. Gastroenterology, *78*:264, 1980.
104. Lennard-Jones, J., et al.: Cancer in colitis: assessment of the individual risk by clinical and histological criteria. Gastroenterology, *73*:1280, 1977.
105. Adler, M., et al.: Whole gut lavage for colonoscopy—a comparison between two solutions. Gastrointest. Endosc., *30*:65, 1984.
106. Weedon, D., et al.: Crohn's disease and cancer. N. Engl. J. Med., *289*:1099, 1973.
107. Greenstein, A., et al.: Patterns of neoplasia in Crohn's disease and ulcerative colitis. Cancer, *46*:403, 1980.
108. Gyde, S., et al.: Malignancy in Crohn's disease. Gut, *21*:1024, 1980.
109. Greenstein, A., et al.: A comparison of cancer risk in Crohn's disease and ulcerative colitis. Cancer, *48*:2742, 1981.
110. Yardley, J., et al.: Cancer in inflammatory bowel disease; how serious is the problem and what should be done about it? Gastroenterology, *85*:197, 1983.
111. Sachar, D.: Crohn's disease in Cleveland: A matter of life and death. Gastroenterology, *88*:1996, 1985.
112. Hamilton, S.: Colorectal carcinoma in patients with Crohn's disease. Gastroenterology, *89*:398, 1985.
113. Korelitz, B.: Carcinoma of the intestinal tract in Crohn's disease. Results of a survey conducted by the National Foundation for Ileitis and Colitis (editorial). Am. J. Gastroenterol., *78*:44, 1983.
114. Glotzer, D.: The risk of cancer in Crohn's disease. Gastroenterology, *89*:438, 1985.
115. Slater, G., Greenstein, A., Aufses, A., Jr.: Anal cancer in patients with Crohn's disease. Ann. Surg., *199*:348, 1984.
116. Devroede, G., et al.: Cancer risk and the life expectancy of children with ulcerative colitis. N. Engl. J. Med., *285*:17, 1971.
117. Rosenqvist, H., et al.: Ulcerative colitis and carcinoma coli. Lancet, *1*:906, 1959.
118. Farmer, R., Hawk, W., Turnbull, R.: Carcinoma associated with mucosal ulcerative colitis and with transmural colitis and enteritis (Crohn's disease). Cancer, *28*:289, 1971.
119. Greenstein, A., et al.: Cancer in Crohn's disease after diversionary surgery. A report of seven carcinomas occurring in excluded bowel. Am. J. Surg., *135*:86, 1978.
120. Riddell, R.: Dysplasia in inflammatory bowel disease. Clin. Gastroenterol., *9*:439, 1980.
121. Morson, B., and Konishi, F.: Dysplasia in the colorectum; *In* Recent Advances in Gastrointestinal Pathology. Edited by R. Wright. London, W.B. Saunders Co., 1980.
122. Riddell, R., et al.: Dysplasia in inflammatory bowel disease: standardized classification with provisional clinical applications. Hum. Pathol. 14:931, 1983.
123. Butt, J., et al.: Macroscopic lesions in dysplasia and carcinoma complicating ulcerative colitis. Dig. Dis. Sci., *28*:18, 1983.
124. Yardley, J., Bayless, T., and Diamond M.: Cancer in ulcerative colitis (editorial). Gastroenterology, *76*:221, 1979.
125. Blackstone, M., Riddell, R., Rogers, B., and Levin, B.: Dysplasia associated lesion or mass (DALM) detected by colonoscopy in long-standing ulcerative colitis: an indication for colectomy. Gastroenterology, *80*:366, 1981.
126. Farmer, R., Whelan, G., and Fazio, V.: Long-term follow-up of patients with Crohn's disease. Relationship between the clinical pattern and prognosis. Gastroenterology, *88*:1818, 1985.
127. Simpson, S., Traube, J., and Riddell, R.: The histologic appearance of dysplasia (precancerous change) in Crohn's disease of the small and large intestine. Gastroenterology, *81*:492, 1981.
128. Shorter, R.: Risk of intestinal cancer in Crohn's disease. Dis. Colon Rectum, *26*:686, 1983.
129. Warren, R., and Barwick, K.: Crohn's colitis with carcinoma and dysplasia. Report of a case and review of 100 small and large bowel resections for Crohn's disease to detect incidence of dysplasia. Am. J. Surg. Pathol., 7:151, 1983.
130. Riddell, R., and Morson, B.: Value of sigmoidoscopy and biopsy in detection of carcinoma and premalignant change in ulcerative colitis. Gut, *20*:575, 1979.
131. Kewenter, J., Hulton, L., and Ahren, C.: The occurrence of severe epithelial dysplasia and its bearing on treat-

ment of longstanding ulcerative colitis. Ann. Surg., 195:209, 1982.
132. Rosenstock, E., et al.: Colonoscopic surveillance for dysplasia and cancer in chronic ulcerative colitis. Gastrointest. Endosc., 30:145, 1984.
133. Vatn, M., Elgjo, K., and Bergan, A.: Distribution of dysplasia in ulcerative colitis. Scand. J. Gastroenterol., 19:893, 1984.
134. Waye, J.: Role of colonoscopy in surveillance for cancer in patients with ulcerative colitis. In Colorectal Cancer: Prevention, Epidemiology, and Screening. New York. Raven Press, 1980.
135. Morson, B., and Pang, L. Edited by S.J. Winawer, D. Schottenfeld, and P. Sherlock. Pang, L.: Rectal biopsy as an aid to cancer control in ulcerative colitis. Gut, 8:423, 1967.
136. Yardley, J., and Keren, D.: "Precancer" lesions in ulcerative colitis. Cancer, 34:835, 1974.
137. Dawson, I., and Pryse-Davies, J.: The development of carcinoma of the large intestine in ulcerative colitis. Br. J. Surg., 47:113, 1959.
138. Stah., D., Tyler, G., Fischer, J.: Inflammatory bowel disease—relationship to carcinoma. Curr. Probl. Cancer, 5:1, 1981.
139. Shields, H., et al.: Scanning electron microscopic appearance of chronic ulcerative colitis with and without dysplasia. Gastroenterology, 89:62, 1985.
140. Dobbins, W.: Current status of the precancer lesion in ulcerative colitis. Gastroenterology, 73:1431, 1977.
141. Fuson, J., Farmer, R., Hawk, W., and Sullivan, B.: Endoscopic surveillance for cancer in chronic ulcerative colitis. Am. J. Gastroenterol., 73:120, 1980.
142. Granqvist, S., Gabrielsson, N., Sundelin, P., and Thorgeirsson, T.: Precancerous lesions in the mucosa in ulcerative colitis. Scand. J. Gastroenterol., 15:289, 1980.
143. Dickinson, R., Dixon, F., and Axon, A.: Colonoscopy and the detection of dysplasia in patients with longstanding ulcerative colitis. Lancet, 2:620, 1980.
144. Hanauer, S., Riddell, R., and Levin, B.: Variability and significance of dysplastic findings in patients with chronic ulcerative colitis (CUC). Gastroenterology (Abstr.), 84:1181, 1983.
145. Waye, J.: Dysplasia and ulcerative colitis—a colonoscopic study. Scand. J. Gastroenterol. (Suppl.), 18:44, 1983.
146. Brostrom, O.: The role of cancer surveillance in long-term prognosis of ulcerative colitis. Scand. J. Gastroenterol. (Suppl.), 18:40, 1983.
147. Lennard-Jones, J., Ritchie, J., Morson, B. C., and Williams, C.: Cancer surveillance in ulcerative colitis. Lancet, 2:149, 1983.
148. Nugent, F., Haggitt, R., Colcher, H., and Kutteruf, G.: Malignant potential of chronic ulcerative colitis: preliminary report. Gastroenterology, 76:1, 1979.
149. Nugent, F., and Haggitt, R.: Long-term follow-up, including cancer surveillance, for patients with ulcerative colitis. In Clinical Medicine. Edited by J.A. Spittell. Philadelphia, Harper & Row, 1984.
150. Riddell, R.: Dysplasia and cancer in ulcerative colitis: a soluble problem? Scand. J. Gastroenterol. (Suppl.), 104:137, 1984.
151. Farmer, R.: Extended management of chronic ulcerative colitis and the problem of carcinoma. Prim. Care, 8:321, 1981.
152. Yardley, J., Ransohoff, D., Riddell, R., and Goldman, H.: Cancer in inflammatory bowel disease: how serious is the problem and what should be done about it? Gastroenterology, 85:197, 1983.
153. Johnson, W., et al.: The risk of rectal carcinoma following colectomy in ulcerative colitis. Dis. Colon Rectum, 26:44, 1983.
154. Johnson, W., McDermott, F., Pihl, E., and Hughes, E.: Mucosal dysplasia: a major predictor of cancer following ileorectal anastomosis. Dis. Colon Rectum, 26:697, 1983.
155. Baker, W., Glass, R., Ritchie, J., and Aylett, S.: Cancer of the rectum following colectomy and ileorectal anastomosis for ulcerative colitis. Br. J. Surg., 65:862, 1978.
156. Khubchandani, I., Stasik, J., and Nedwich, A.: Prospective surveillance by rectal biopsy following ileorectal anastomosis for inflammatory disease. Dis. Colon Rectum, 25:343, 1982.
157. Teague, R., Salmon, P., and Read, A.: Fiberoptic examination of the colon—a review of 255 cases. Gut, 14:139, 1973.
158. Rogers, B., et al.: Complications of flexible fiberoptic colonoscopy and polypectomy. Gastrointest. Endosc., 22:73, 1975.
159. Smith, L.: Complications of colonoscopy and polypectomy. Dis. Colon Rectum, 19: 407, 1976.
160. Dean, A.: Transmission of Salmonella typhi by fiberoptic endoscopy. Lancet, 2:134, 1977.
161. Geenen, J., Pfeifer, M., and Simonsen, L.: Cleaning and disinfection of endoscopic equipment. Gastrointest. Endosc., 24:185, 1978.
162. Scully, C., et al.: Crohn's disease of the mouth—an indicator of intestinal involvement. Gut, 23:198. 1982.
163. Netto, G. M., et al.: Crohn's disease with exclusive gastric involvement: A case report and review of the literature. Rev. Hosp. Clin. Fac. Med. Sao Paulo, 38:259, 1983.
164. Fielding, J. F., Toye, D. K. M., Benton, D. C., and Cooke, W. T.: Crohn's disease of the stomach and duodenum. Gut, 11:1001, 1970.
165. Farman, J., Faegenburg, D., Dallemand, S., and Chen, C. K.: Crohn's disease of the stomach: The "Ram's Horn" sign. A. J. R., 123:242, 1975.
166. Johnson, O. A., Hoskins, D. W., Todd, J., and Thorbjarnarson, B.: Crohn's disease of the stomach. Gastroenterology, 50:571, 1966.
167. Swan, C. H. J., Cooke, W. T.: Treatment and prognosis in diffuse jejuno-ileitis. Gut, 12:864, 1971.
168. Colon, A. R., and Klein, L. H.: "Universal" Crohn's disease. South. Med. J., 72:1476, 1979.
169. Danzi, J., Farmer, R., Sullivan, B., and Rankin, G.: Endoscopic features of gastroduodenal Crohn's disease. Gastroenterology, 70:9, 1976.
170. Hoagland, B., Wieman, T. J., and Shively, E. H.: Gastroduodenal Crohn's disease. J. Ky. Med. Assoc., 82:224, 1984.
171. Korelitz, B. I., et al.: Crohn's disease in endoscopic biopsies of the gastric antrum and duodenum. Am. J. Gastroenterol., 76:103, 1981.
172. Van Spreeuwel, J. P. et al.: Morphological and immunohistochemical findings in upper gastrointestinal biopsies of patients with Crohn's disease of the ileum and colon. J. Clin. Pathol., 35:934, 1982.
173. Schmitz-Moormann, P., Malchow, H., and Pittner, P. M.: Endoscopic and bioptic study of the gastrointestinal tract in Crohn's disease patients. Pathol. Res. Pract., 178:377, 1985.

20 · Radiology of Inflammatory Bowel Disease

HARLEY C. CARLSON, M.D.

The gut is the site of many forms of inflammatory change, including those induced by chemical damage, specific infections and infestations, and ischemia. But the most common and interesting forms of inflammatory disease seen by the radiologist are those in which the underlying cause of the process is unknown, such as chronic ulcerative colitis (CUC) and Crohn's disease (CD). It is true that specific infections of the gut can closely resemble these two diseases, radiologically. But, in reality, by careful history taking, physical examination, and appropriate laboratory tests, the bedside physician identifies these conditions before radiologic examination and extensive endoscopy become necessary. Occasionally, nevertheless, patients with such diseases do present themselves for examination and the radiologist must keep them in mind, especially if the pathologic process seen is in any way unusual.

During the past decade, new radiologic modalities have assumed widespread use in the examination of the abdominal organs, and they have increased the capacity to visualize the pathologic processes of inflammatory bowel disease more completely. Computerized tomography, ultrasound, and retrograde cholangiography have improved our understanding of these conditions. Contrast x-ray examination of the gut, however, is still the most direct, safe, and accurate way to detect, identify, and characterize these entities.

Endoscopy, especially fiberoptic endoscopy, is used more often in the diagnosis and management of CUC and CD during this decade, particularly in patients with colonic involvement (see Chap. 19). Any patient who has needed a barium enema also has needed endoscopic examination of the anal canal, rectum, and low sigmoid. This is at least as true in the study of patients with possible colitis as it is in those suspected of neoplasm. Colonoscopy and barium enema are complementary examinations. Each has its strengths and weaknesses. Endoscopy can assess the nature of the bowel content, color, and vascularity of the mucosa, and efficiently detect small isolated inflammatory lesions as well as remove tissue for microscopic examination and culture. Barium enema almost always results in visualization of the entire colon, is more sensitive to subtle changes in distensibility, can usually see beyond pronounced deformity or partial obstruction, and can visualize deep ulceration and fistulae more graphically. Endoscopy is more sensitive in the detection of minimal disease. Barium enema is probably more effective in the characterization of more severe changes and produces a visual record of them.[1,2]

Methods of Contrast Examination

If the inflammatory disease is acute and severe and involves the colon (acute toxic colitis), barium enema is contraindicated. Radiography of the abdomen in the recumbent and upright or lateral decubitus positions will usually allow characterization of the disease when combined with proctoscopy and history. Severe small bowel disease is rarely a reason to defer contrast examination unless high-grade obstruction is present, in which case contrast is usually unnecessary, immediately, for management.

Colon

The colon is most effectively examined for inflammatory disease by means of careful double contrast radiography, using a viscous suspension of barium sulfate of high density. This is best pumped in under pressure using large bore tubing. Fluoroscopy and palpation by the radiologist help characterize the anatomy, detect fistulae and obstruction of any degree, and allow the examiner to determine when an adequate amount of barium has entered the colon. A moderate amount should be present just beyond the hepatic flexure, then the surplus drained out through the rectal tube. When the appropriate amount remains, air is pumped in under fluoroscopic control until the colon is thoroughly distended. Appropriate films are then made in various positions in order to visualize the entire colon in several projections. This usually requires nine or ten 14 × 17 in. films, at least half of which should be made with a horizontal x-ray beam.[3,4]

Single contrast examination of the colon is also effective, but it does not display the granular appearance of the mucosa in CUC of mild to moderate severity, or the discrete, shallow ulcers of minimal CD as well as does double contrast. Good post evacuation films after single contrast examination can reveal even more subtle mucosal changes than double contrast, however, but such films with the correct amount of residual barium and firm contraction of the colon are not regularly obtainable.

Small Intestine

Two ways exist to effectively examine the small intestine. The patient may drink the barium suspension, usually two to four 12 oz. cups, and, as the stomach empties, the radiologist carries out fluoroscopy with vigorous palpation of the opacified bowel in various projections at frequent intervals until the entire bowel has been visualized. A film is made after each visit. Abnormalities are detected fluoroscopically and recorded on film.

In the other way to examine the small intestine, a tube may be passed through the stomach and into the proximal jejunum. The patient is given a small bowel enema while the radiologist carries out fluoroscopy combined with vigorous manual palpation and appropriate films. Fundamental to both methods is careful fluoroscopy and visualization of segments of opacified bowel with separation by manual palpation or compression and appropriate films. Either method, if properly done, should detect and identify about 95% of CD in the small intestine. The practice of taking periodic films of the small intestine without fluoroscopy after oral ingestion of barium is inadequate and will result in many errors of omission as well as commission.[5,6]

Esophagus, Stomach, and Duodenum

The esophagus, stomach, and duodenum can be satisfactorily examined with either the single contrast or double contrast technique. If single contrast examination is elected, fluoroscopy with careful, vigorous manual compression is essential to detect limited distensibility, so-called aphthous ulcers, and enlarged but pliable folds in the stomach and duodenum. Esophageal involvement manifests itself through ulceration that may penetrate into the submucosa and muscularis just as in the small and large intestines, with localized limited distensibility. Double contrast technique, with highly fluid, high density barium suspension ingested with gas-producing salts, can also graphically show all of the same abnormalities.

Chronic Ulcerative Colitis

Although double contrast study is almost always preferable for the diagnosis of CUC, two situations arise in which single contrast examination using a fluid barium and fluoroscopy and palpation is better. The first is when obstruction or fistula is suspected. Single contrast examination gives better control of distention and better adaptation of barium flow, positioning, and filming to best demonstrate the abnormality. The second instance in which a single contrast study is at least as satisfactory as a double contrast study is when the inflammation is inactive, the diagnosis having been securely made already, and the reason for periodic examination being the detection of cancer. In this situation, the single contrast examination is simpler, faster, less expensive, and just as sensitive as the double

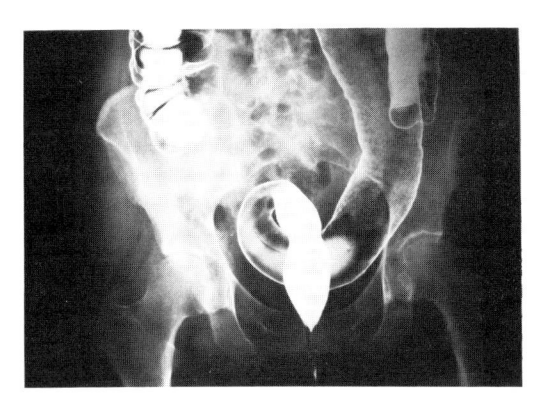

FIG. 20-1. Chronic ulcerative colitis with limited distensibility of the rectum and a smooth mucosal surface. The sigmoid is also devoid of haustral indentation and the mucosa, there and above, is finely granular.

contrast examination in the detection of neoplasms if done with careful fluoroscopy and palpation.[7]

Minimal or mild ulcerative colitis is often confined to the distal bowel, and the most sensitive radiologic finding is limited distensibility of the involved segment. This results in a somewhat shortened, tubular form of the lumen. The haustral indentations disappear, the overall diameter of the bowel lumen is diminished, the normal tortuous configuration is lost and a generalized shortening in the length of the involved portion of the colon occurs (Fig. 20-1). In cases of mild or moderate severity, determined by the appearance of the mucosa, this lack of haustration, narrowing, and shortening can be completely reversible radiologically if the disease enters remission. In more severe disease present for a sustained time, however, narrowing, shortening, and lack of haustration may become fixed and irreversible. (Fig. 20-2). The mucosa in mild disease may look perfectly smooth and normal even though proctoscopy demonstrates minimal CUC.[2] Usually, however, the mucosa has a fine granular appearance face-on, its profile has a finely irregular outline, and the lumen may be either contracted or normally distensible. (Figs. 20-3 to 20-7). In somewhat more severe forms of involvement, the granular appearance is more coarse and might be described better as a finely nodular and reticular pattern. This is sometimes shown most dramatically after evacuation (Figs. 20-8 and 20-9). Scattered over the surface of this finely nodular pattern, one can often see small

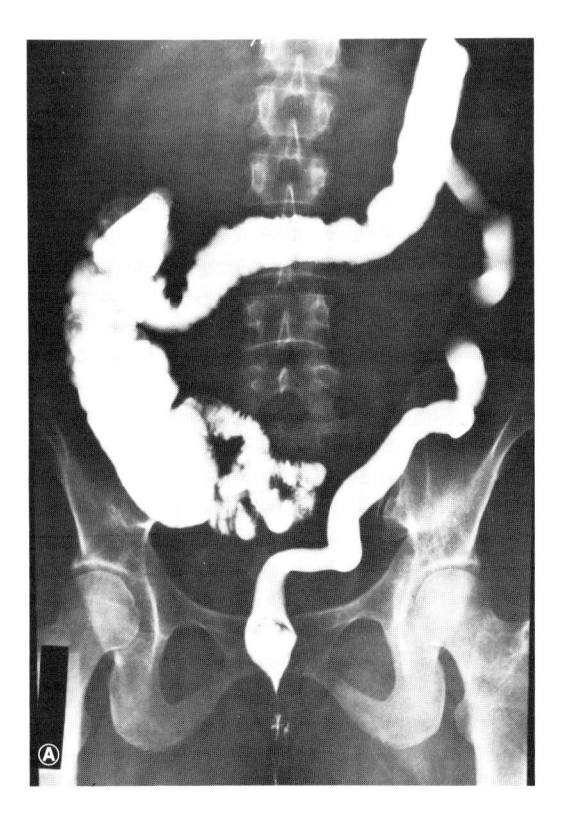

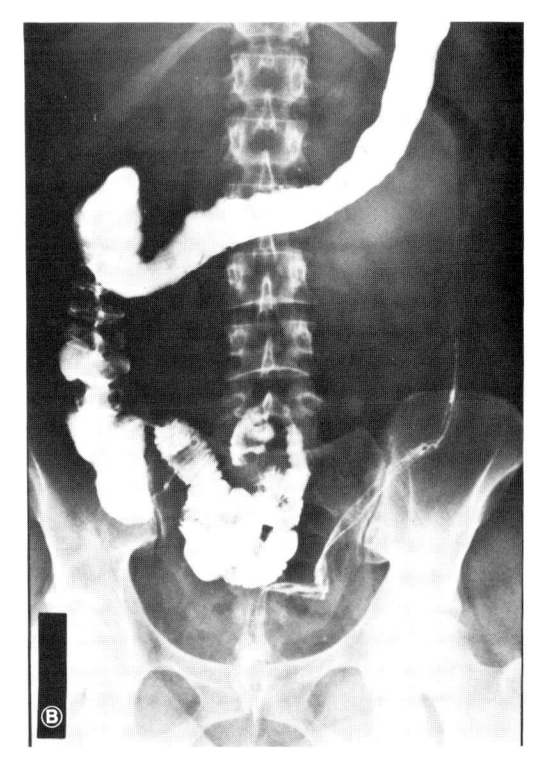

FIG. 20-2. Chronic ulcerative colitis 20 years. Generalized, probably permanent, narrowing of the left colon and rectum with a finely irregular mucosal surface both when filled (A) and after evacuation (B).

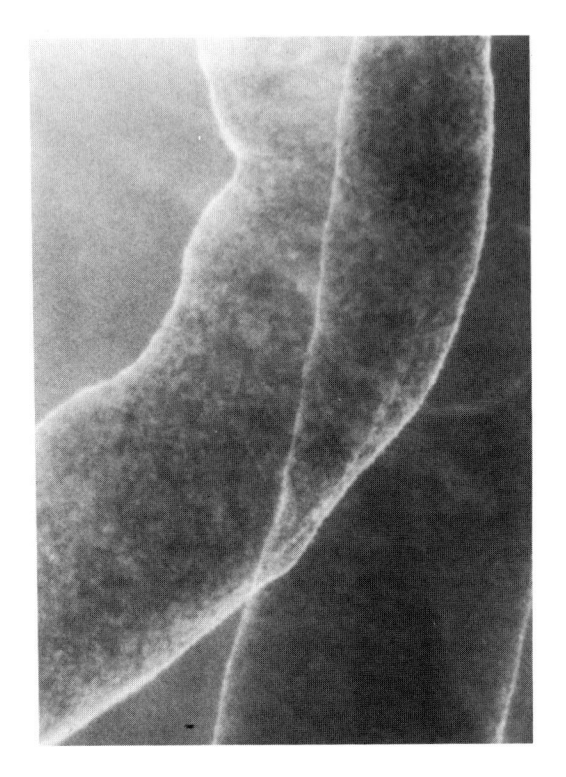

FIG. 20-3. Pancolitis (CUC) with diffuse moderate granularity and loss of haustration.

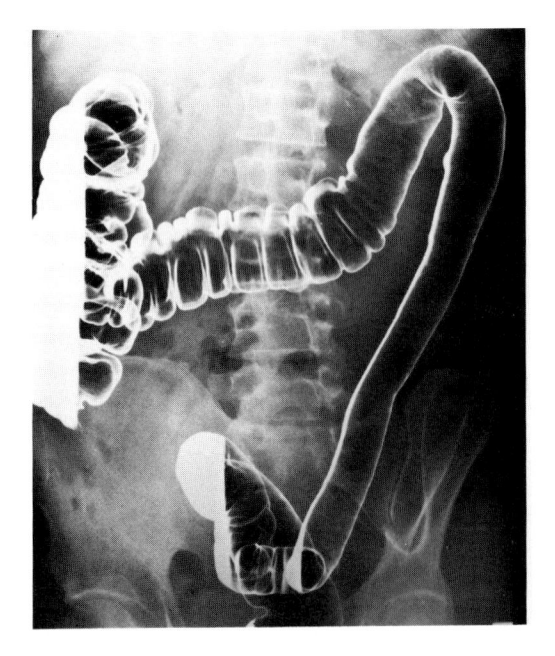

FIG. 20-4. Chronic ulcerative colitis with lack of haustration and finely granular mucosa from the distal transverse colon to the anus.

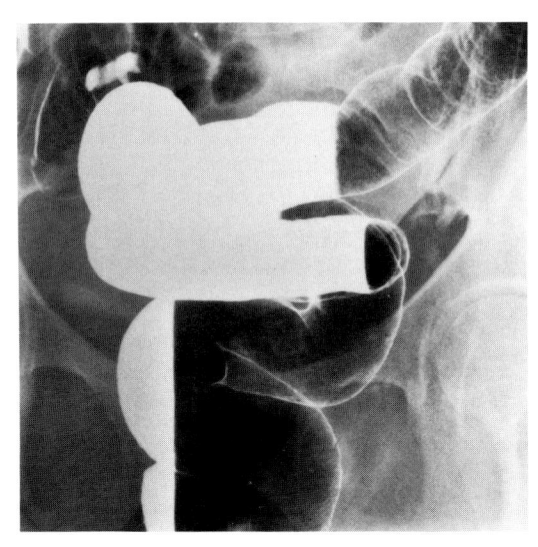

FIG. 20-5. Fine granularity of the rectal and sigmoid mucosa with normal distensibility.

discrete ulcer craters with surrounding mounds of infiltrate. These are best seen face-on but can also be seen if caught precisely in profile (Fig. 20-10).

Even more severe disease is manifested radiologically by penetrating ulcers into the mucosa and submucosa that are seen face-on as small collections of barium, but they are most convincingly visualized in profile where one can see their tendency to dissect a bit in the mucosa along the long axis of the bowel, or become confluent (Figs. 20-11 to 20-15). Permanent shortening and narrowing usually result after a period of time.

Scattered or isolated dominant nodules may form on the surface of the granular or finely nodular mucosa. When small (a few millimeters in diameter), they are spherical in shape and rather smooth. The larger nodules are somewhat more irregular. These nodules may form clusters, or one or two may become very large. Rarely, nodular inflammatory polyps cover almost the entire colonic mucosal surface and resemble severe adenomatous polyposis. They are grossly indistinguishable from neoplastic polyps radiologically, but histologic examination shows them to be composed of inflammatory tissue (Figs. 20-16 to 20-18). Endoscopy and biopsy are usually decisive in the distinction.

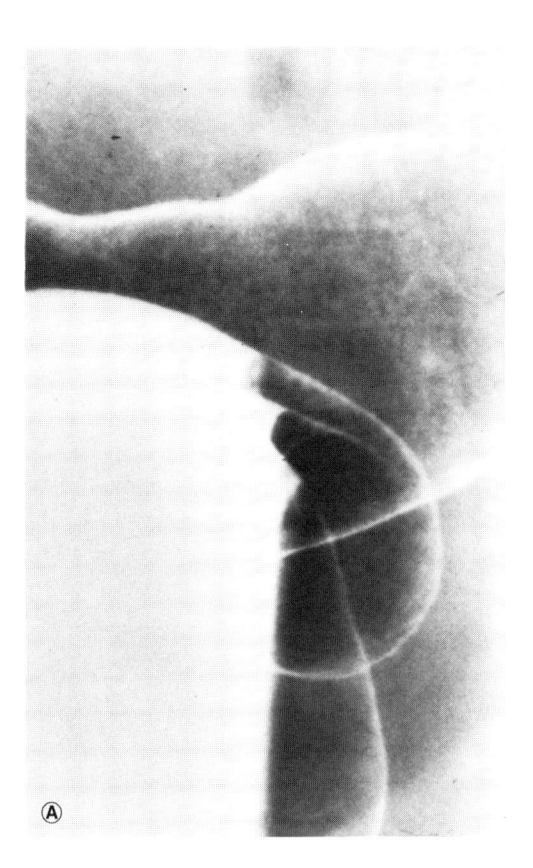

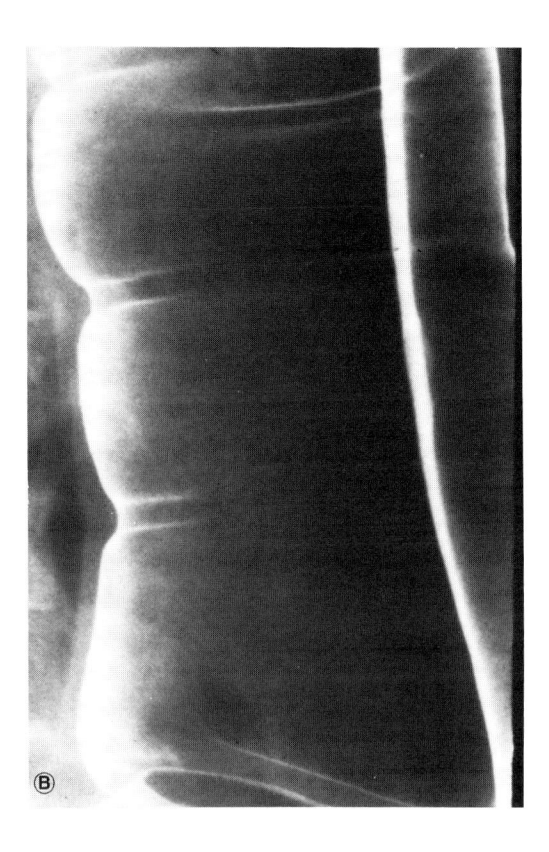

FIG. 20-6. A. Chronic ulcerative colitis limited to rectum and sigmoid showing fine granularity. B. Normal splenic flexure for comparison.

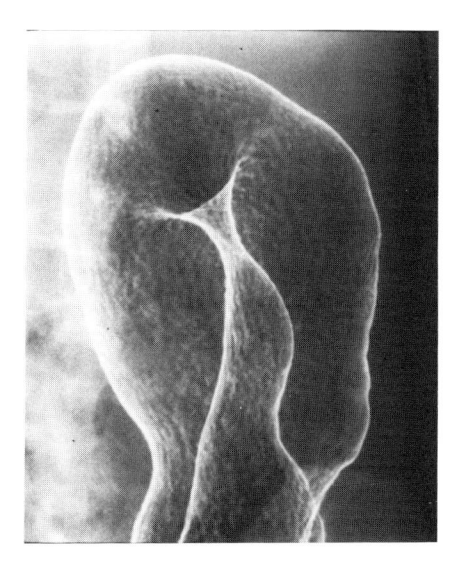

FIG. 20-7. Chronic ulcerative colitis with wavy granularity in the splenic flexure.

Continuity of the Inflammatory Process

Beginning with the rectum, continuity of the inflammatory process is often cited as characteristic of CUC, and this is often true. If the patient is examined soon after the onset of symptoms, the rectum is usually involved, and as the process continues or recurs, it often involves more and more proximal colon in continuity with the rectum. As patients are followed, however, especially those with involvement of the entire colon, remissions occur that may not affect the entire colon uniformly. Some segments may become less severely involved or even normal, while other portions of the same colon may not undergo improvement. In this way the distal colon, including the rectum, may be normal when examined, while more proximal segments are clearly involved with characteristic radio-

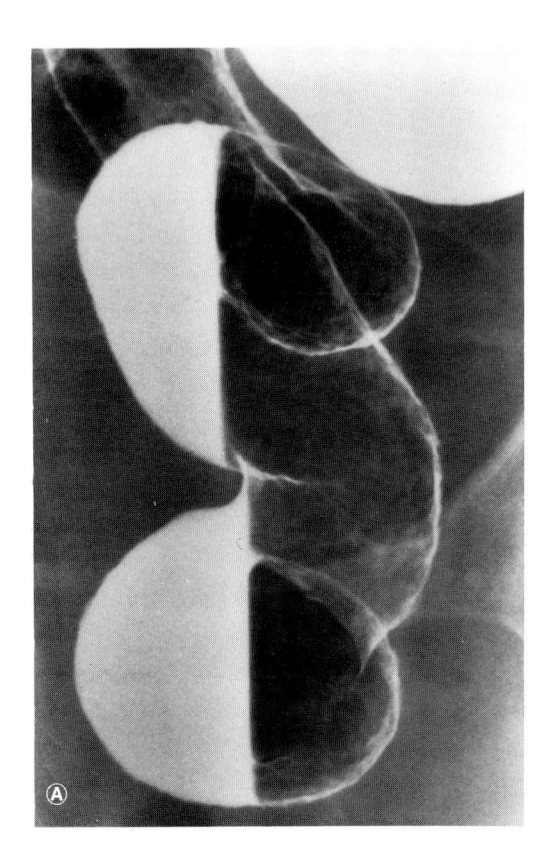

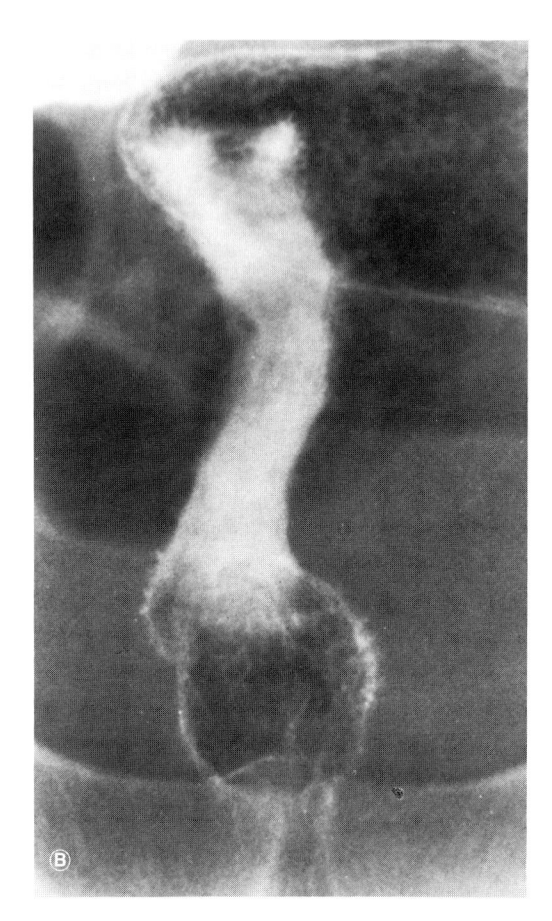

FIG. 20-8. Chronic ulcerative colitis with coarse granularity of the rectum seen when distended (A) and after evacuation (B).

logic findings of CUC. If a patient is first encountered in this situation, it appears that he has segmental, or right-sided, CUC. In this situation the radiologist must rely upon the surface pattern and general form of the involved colon to identify the process as CUC, and, if possible, obtain old films to reconstruct the genesis of the process (Figs. 20-19 to 20-24).

Inflammatory Polyps*

As pointed out previously, inflammatory polyps that form on actively inflamed mucosal surfaces have approximately the same form, radiologically, as adenomatous polyps, and only their association with inflamed mucosa makes them likely to be non-neoplastic (Figs. 20-16 to 20-18).

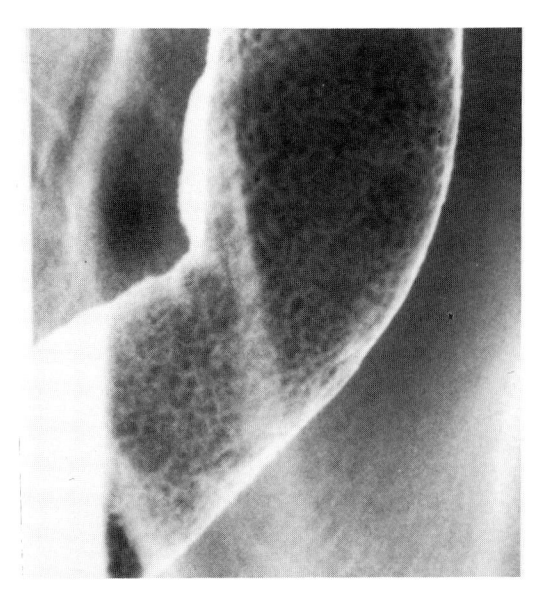

FIG. 20-9. Chronic ulcerative colitis with nodular granularity.

*See also Chapter 14.

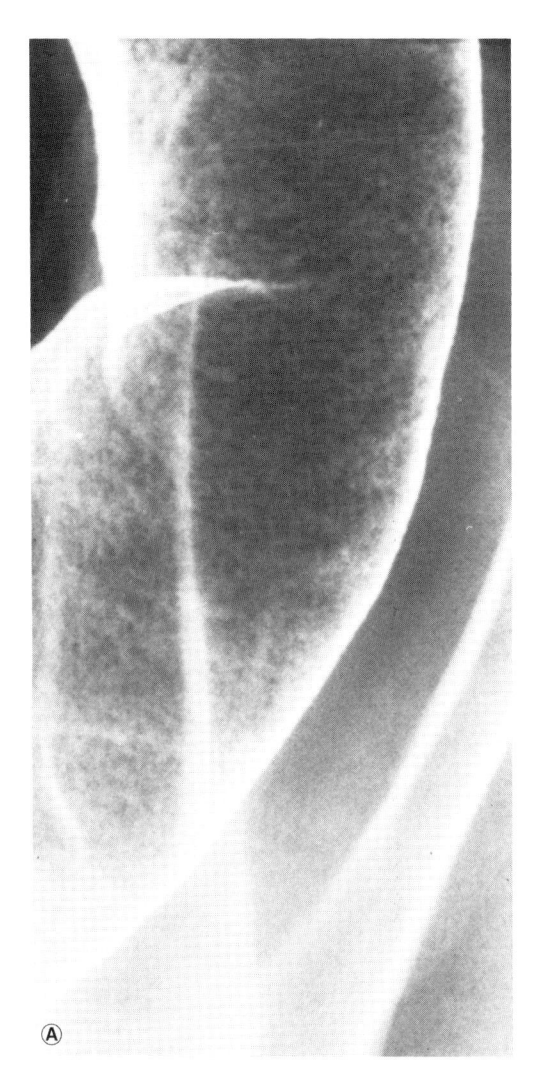

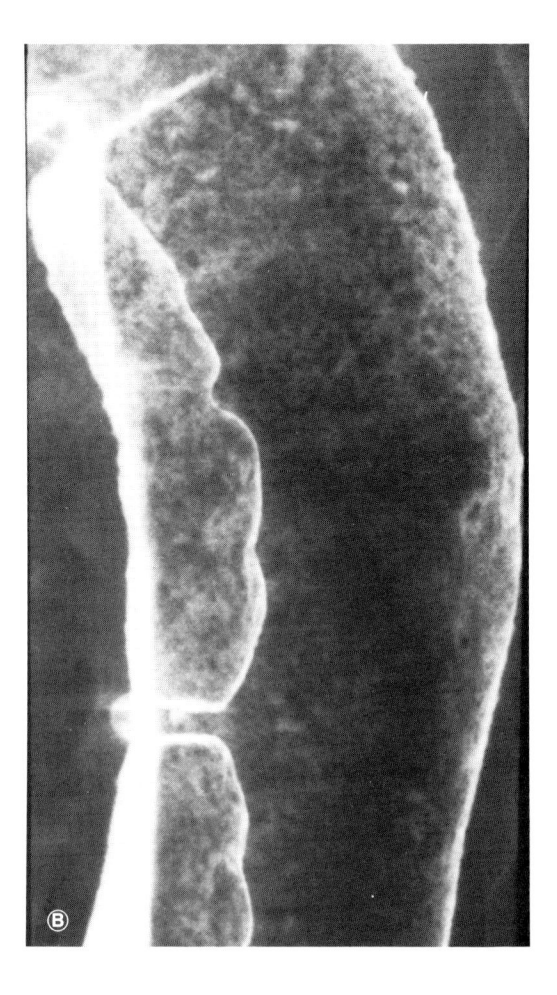

FIG. 20-10. Varying severity in CUC. Moderate granularity in the low descending colon (A) and visible, discrete ulcers in the splenic flexure (B).

Another form of inflammatory polyps may occur, however, as healing of inflamed mucosa takes place. These often have a thread-like appearance of varying length and thickness, hence are called filiform pseudopolyps. They are often found upon relatively normal looking mucosal surfaces, indicating that the area in which they are located was once involved in active inflammatory disease, usually CUC. They may also occur together, with more nodular-shaped inflammatory polyps on actively inflamed mucosa. They do not indicate an increased risk of carcinoma. Such polyps are more rare with CDC (Figs. 20-25 to 20-30).[8]

Strictures

Strictures are common in CUC as time passes (see also Chap. 14). Most of the limited distensibility encountered on x-ray examination, especially in the early, active stage, is caused by muscular contraction that can be variable during the examination (Fig. 20-31), and often reverts to normal during quiet periods of the illness. Occasionally, however, localized narrowing of the bowel actually progresses because of fibrosis in the mucosa and muscularis, and the lumen may become permanently narrow. Clinical obstruction of the colon resulting from such an inflam-

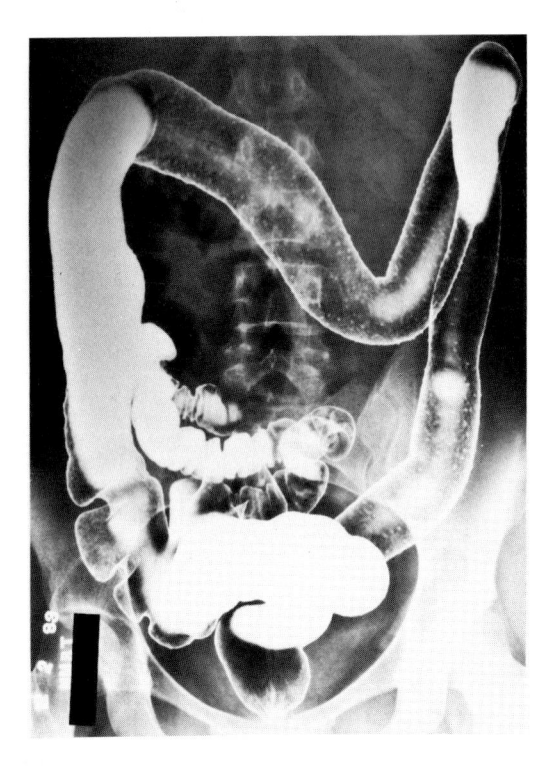

FIG. 20-11. Chronic ulcerative colitis with diffuse penetrating ulcers and lack of haustration.

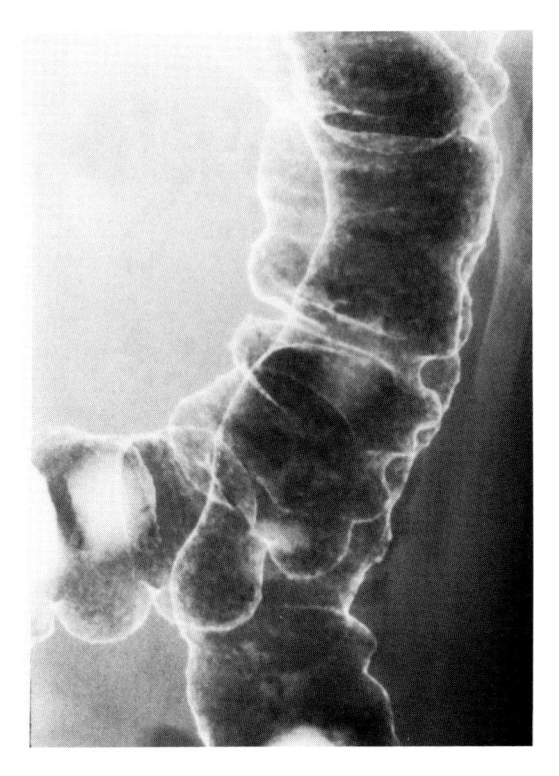

FIG. 20-12. Chronic ulcerative colitis with blunted haustra and diffuse small discrete penetrating ulcers.

matory stricture almost never happens. If such a stricture forms in the rectum, it may make the use of conventional enema tips or endoscopes impossible. A pediatric tip or catheter can be effectively substituted. The significance of a stricture in CUC is its close resemblance to carcinoma that occurs with increased frequency in patients with this disease (Figs. 20-32 to 20-35).

Carcinoma

Carcinoma is probably at least one hundred times as common in patients with CUC, overall, as in the general population (see Chap. 15). About two-thirds of such cancers have an infiltrative, stricturing form and do not prominently protrude into the lumen. When not annular, such infiltration can closely resemble the broad haustral indentation present in relatively inactive inflammatory disease and, thus, elude detection. Even when the infiltration becomes annular, it may be difficult to distinguish from an inflammatory stricture. Irregularity of the lumen, any suggestion of a protruding nodule into the lumen, or the sense of rigidity or mass when compressed with a gloved hand at fluoroscopy should make carcinoma a likely consideration, and resection should be undertaken. Endoscopy with recovery of non-neoplastic tissue from biopsy should not delay surgical treatment in the presence of suspicious radiologic evidence (Figs. 20-36 to 20-43).

Although double contrast barium enema would seem ideal in the search for early cancer in patients with CUC, it is no more sensitive than single contrast barium enema with fluoroscopy and palpation. Both methods fail to diagnose such lesions in about equal proportions. A rather large experience would indicate that radiologic methods fail to detect neoplasm in about 15% of patients with CUC and cancer, and fail to definitely diagnose about 30% of all lesions, because multiplicity is common.[7,10]

Periodic colonoscopy and systematic biopsy may improve this, but it is not clearly established as true, yet.

Dysplasia

Dysplasia (see Chap. 15), or precancer of colonic mucosa, is reportedly increased in longstanding CUC. It may occur in mucosa that has an abnormal, nodular surface appearance, but it can also be found in smooth, grossly normal mucosa. The diagnosis must be made by an experienced pathologist, who usually examines tissue that is removed systematically by an endoscopist for surveillance, or by a directed biopsy of a suspicious area identified by either barium enema or endoscopy. It seems unlikely that barium enema will ever be useful in excluding the presence of dysplasia with confidence, though it is probably useful in directing the efforts of the colonoscopist toward the thorough biopsy of possible dysplasia (Figs. 20-44 and 20-45).[11]

Terminal Ileum

The terminal ileum is often abnormal in CUC if the right colon, including the cecum, is involved in radiologically active disease. The ileocecal valve is deformed and open, the caliber of terminal ileum is greater than normal, and it often

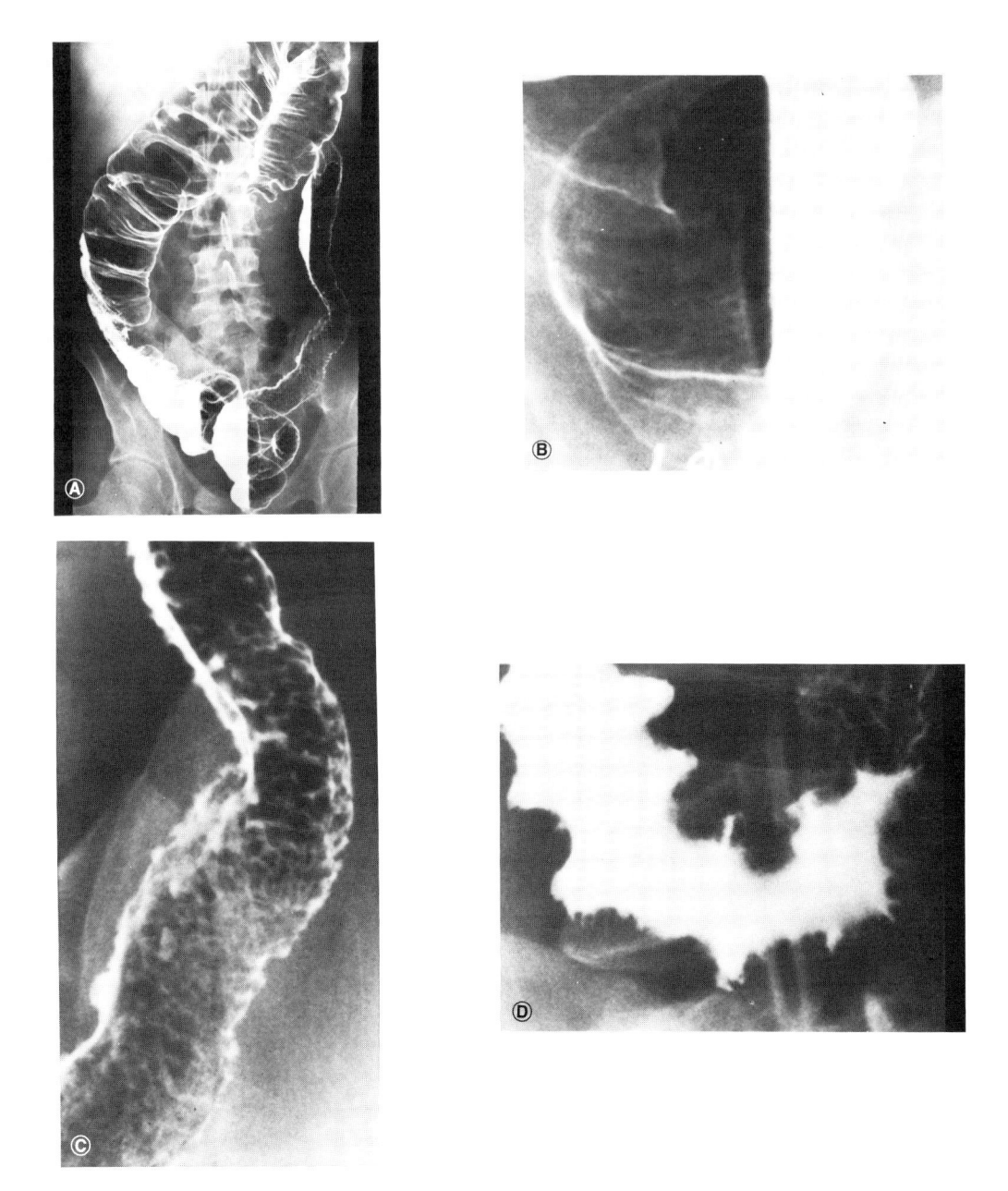

FIG. 20-13. A. Chronic ulcerative colitis with significantly variable severity. B. Fine granularity in the rectum. C. Somewhat penetrating ulcers in the low descending colon. D. Deep ulceration and narrowing in the transverse colon.

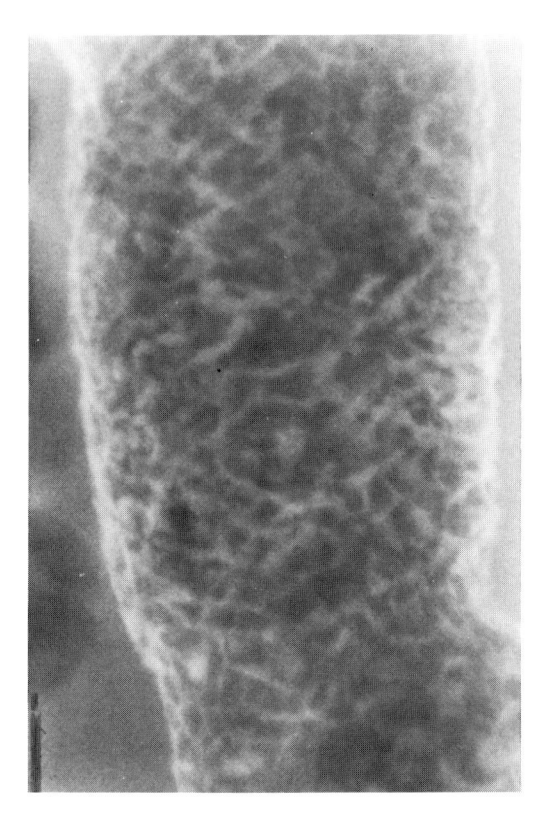

Fig. 20-14. Chronic ulcerative colitis with confluent ulceration.

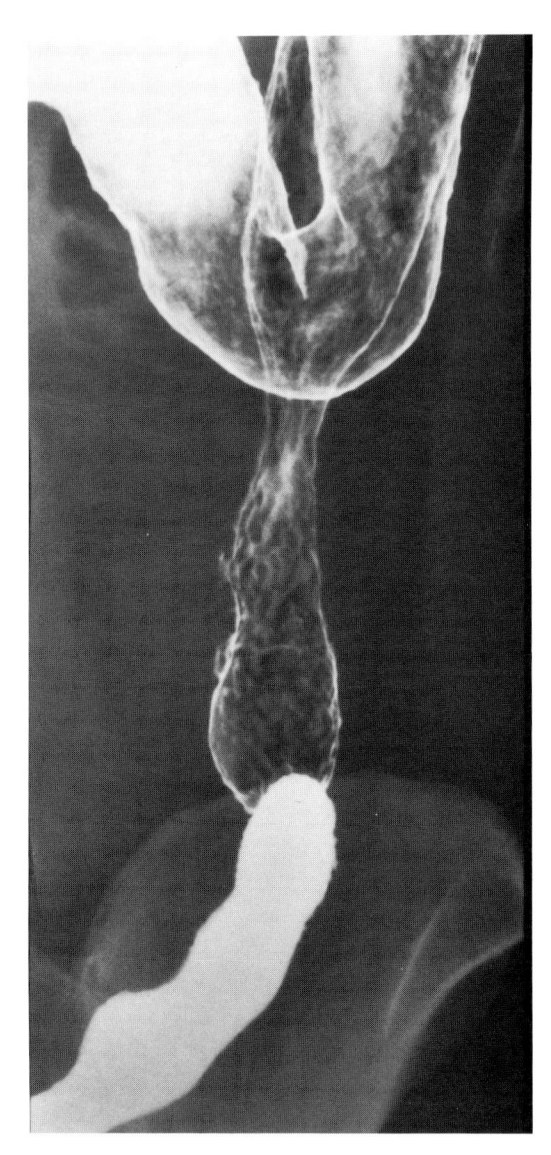

Fig. 20-15. Chronic ulcerative colitis with focal, penetrating, longitudinally dissecting ulcer craters.

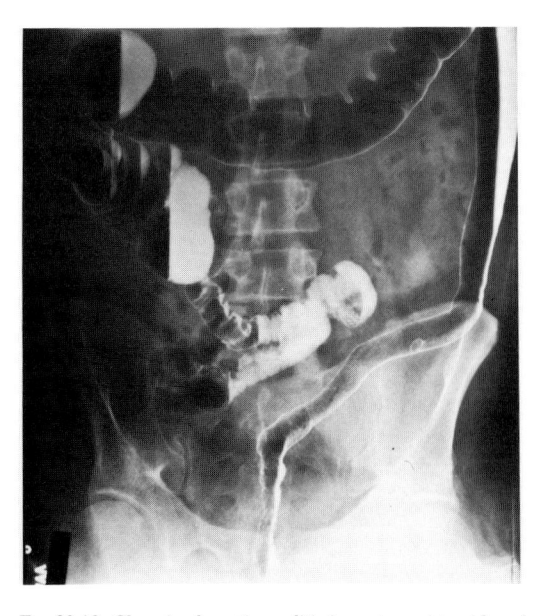

Fig. 20-16. Chronic ulcerative colitis in rectum, sigmoid, and descending colon with solitary inflammatory polyp.

stays distended with barium longer than normal because of a reduction of its usual motor activity. The mucosal folds may be slightly thickened and have a rather fuzzy surface. The bowel wall is not thickened or stiff when palpated at fluoroscopy, and usually no narrowing or visible penetrating ulceration is present. Occasionally, however, the mucosal surface may be involved in a manner similar to that of the colon. Its appearance is in contrast to that of Crohn's disease with its nodularity, ulceration, narrowing of the lumen, thickening of the wall, and fistula formation (Figs 20-19, 20-21 to 20-23, and 20-46).

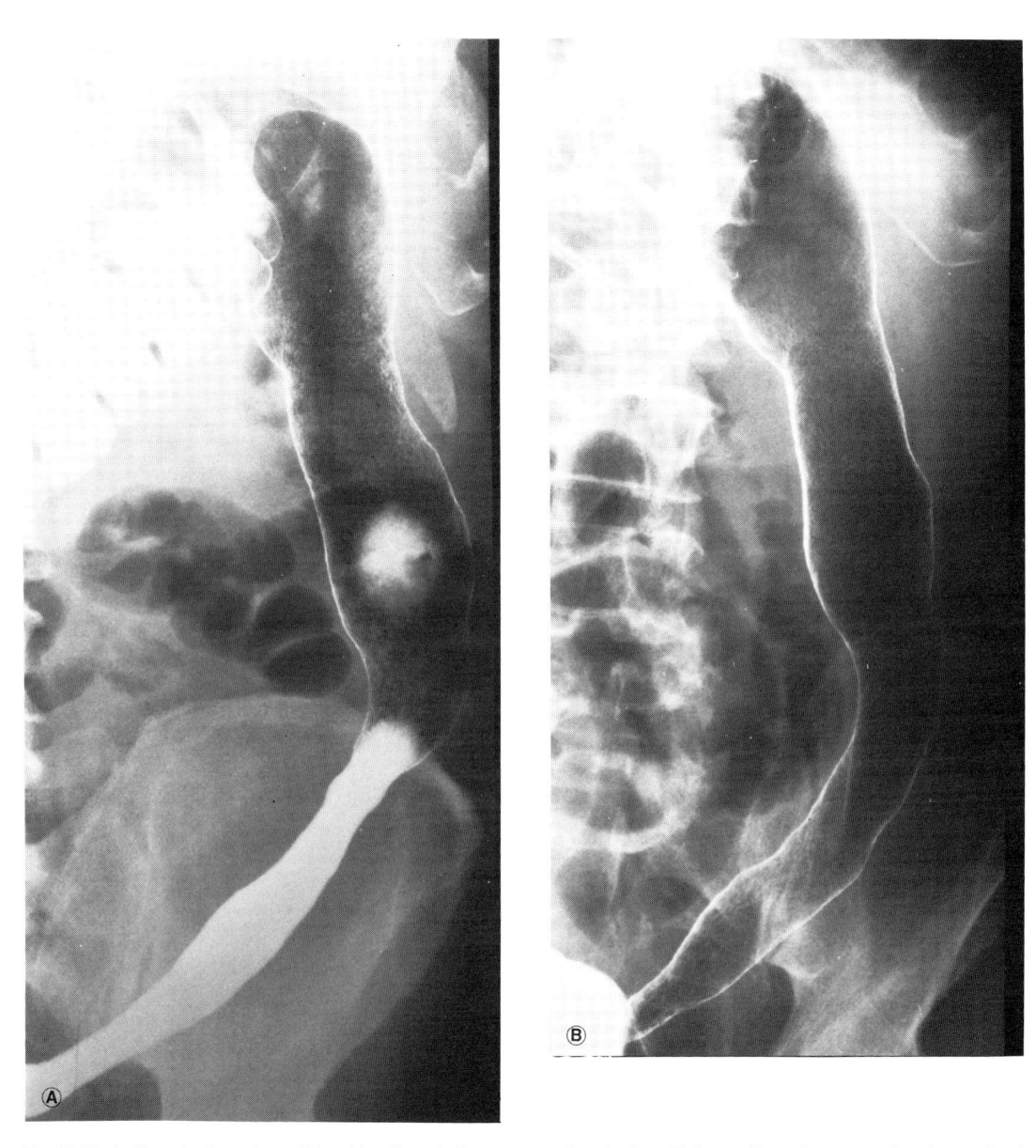

FIG. 20-17. A. Chronic ulcerative colitis with solitary inflammatory polyps in the mid-descending colon, seen only when outlined by barium in the dependent pool. B. Polyps suspended from the superior surface are often not visible on double contrast films.

Distinction from Other Disease of the Colon

Although differentiation of CUC from other disease of the colon is usually straightforward (see Chap. 10), two situations cause occasional difficulty. The first is that of distinguishing severe, longstanding universal CUC from moderately severe Crohn's disease limited to the colon (Fig. 20-47). The second situation arises in the patient with relatively acute but sustained symptoms of colitis, in whom the likelihood of a specific infection is reasonably high. These organisms include Campylobacter fetus and Clostridium difficile, the latter usually following administration of antibiotics and producing pseudomembranous colitis. Both of these infections produce a similar and somewhat characteristic appearance on barium enema. The haustral indentations may be broadened and, occasionally, the

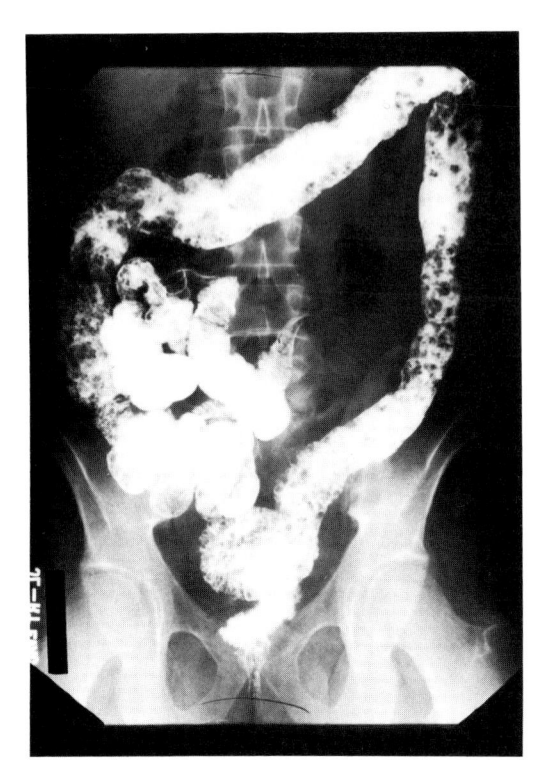

FIG. 20-18. Chronic ulcerative colitis of the entire colon and rectum with profuse inflammatory polyps, several of which are rather large. This closely resembles severe neoplastic polyposis.

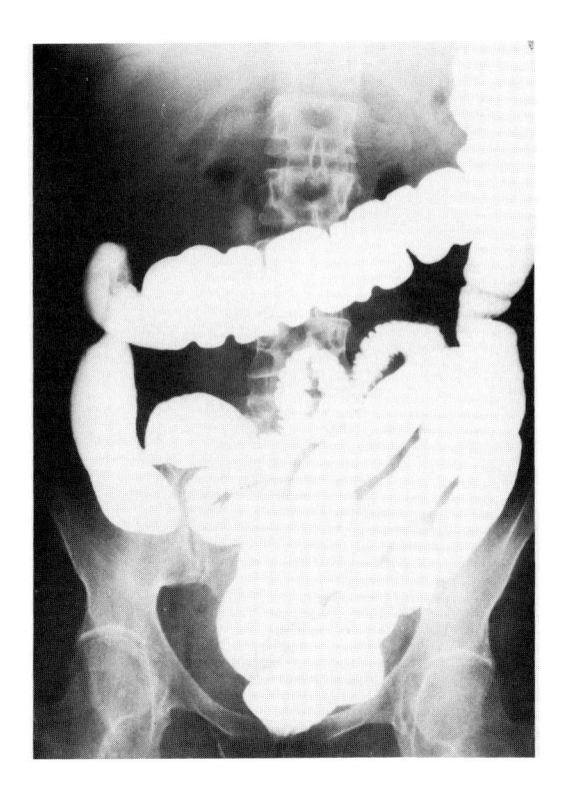

FIG. 20-19. Characteristic CUC involving the cecum and ascending colon with "backwash ileitis" in the terminal ileum. The left colon was normal. Proctoscopy showed minimal changes of CUC up to 14 cm above the anal canal and was normal above this.

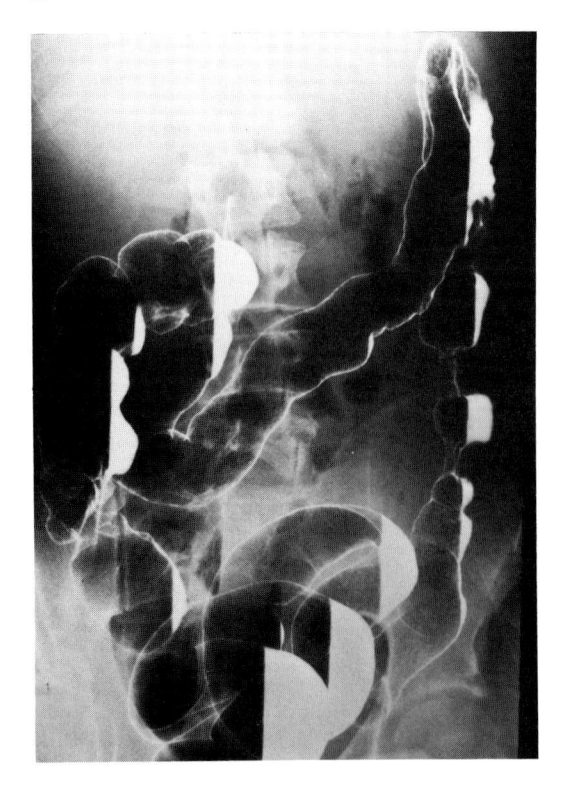

FIG. 20-20. Chronic ulcerative colitis with lack of haustration and granularity above the rectum. The rectum had been involved previously but was now normal radiologically and proctoscopically.

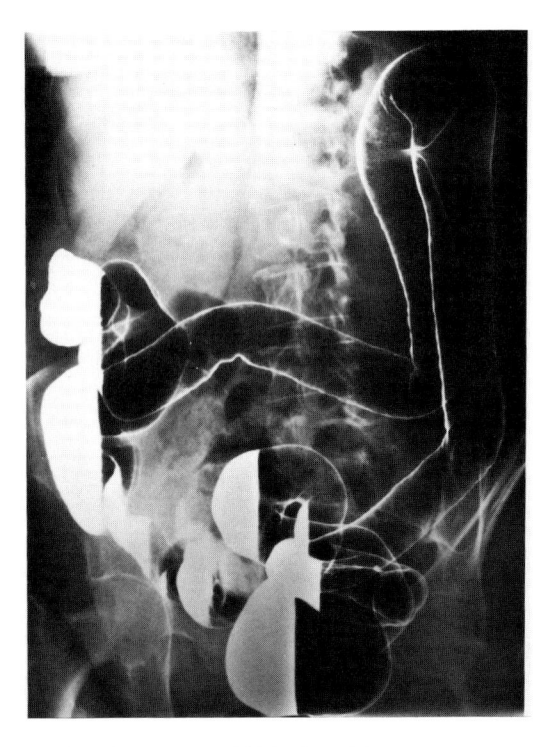

FIG. 20-21. Prior universal CUC. Now CUC above the sigmoid and rectum that were normal radiologically and endoscopically. Moderate "backwash ileitis."

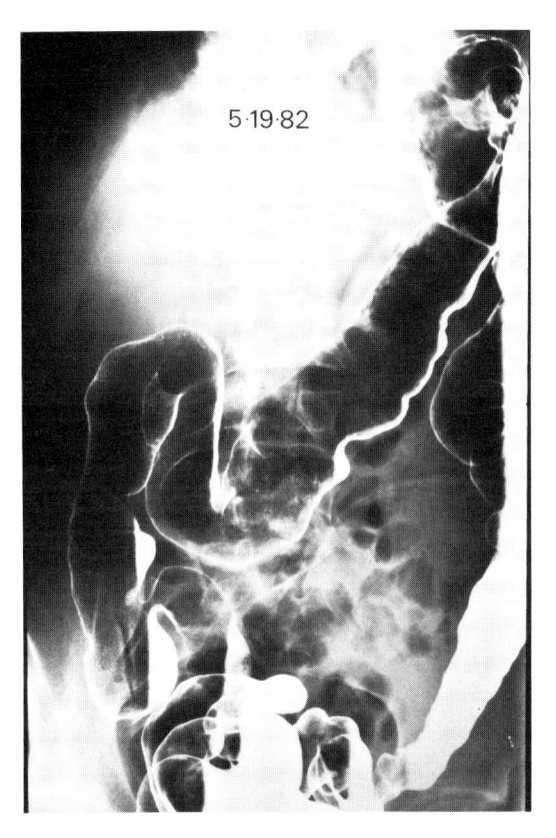

FIG. 20-22. Chronic ulcerative colitis above the sigmoid with "backwash ileitis." The rectum was visually normal at endoscopy, but a biopsy was characteristic of moderately severe IBD.

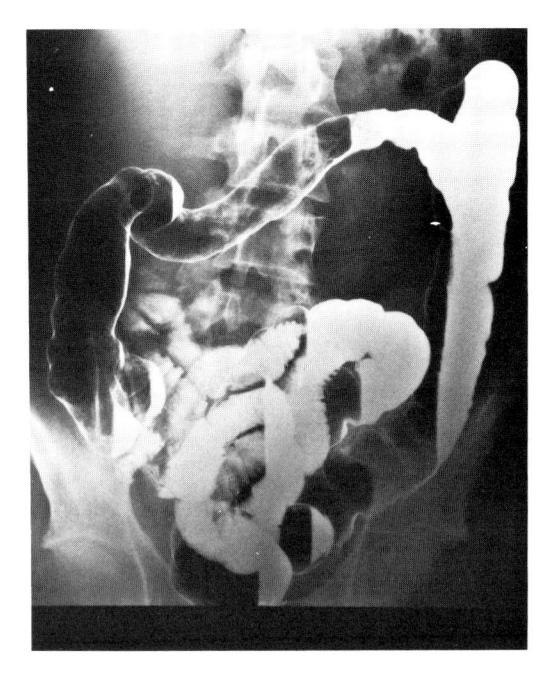

FIG. 20-23. Chronic ulcerative colitis above the splenic flexure. Although proctoscopy showed CUC 6 years previously, it is now normal. Patient also has sclerosing cholangitis.

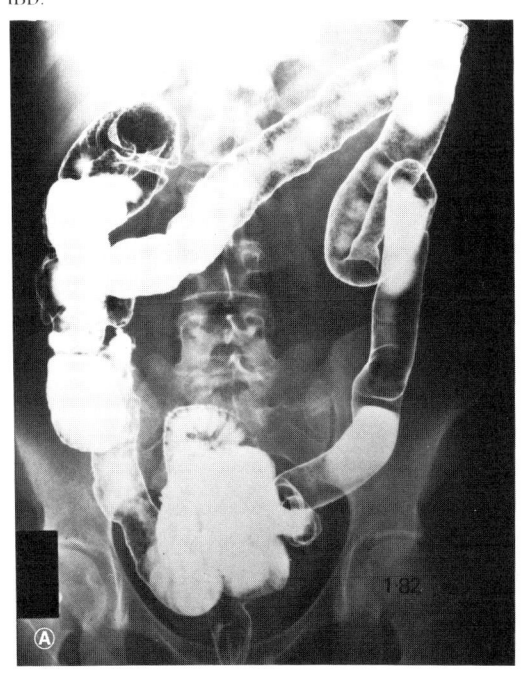

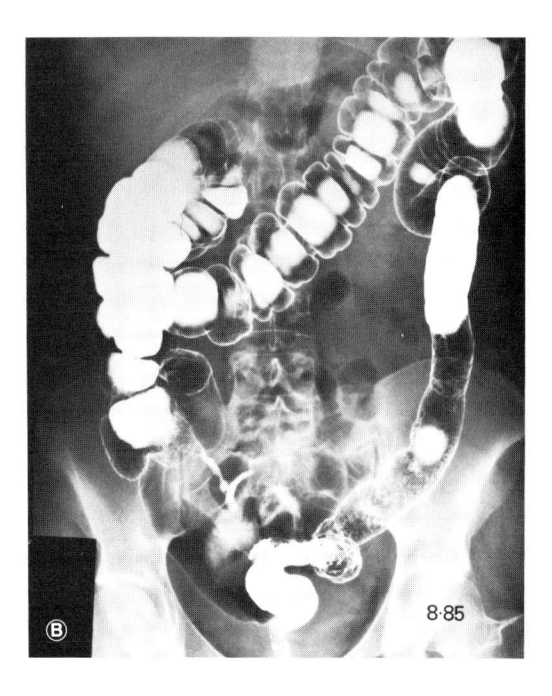

FIG. 20-24. A. and B. Chronic ulcerative colitis with backwash ileitis. Healing of the transverse colon with more severe disease developing in the lower left colon in 3 years.

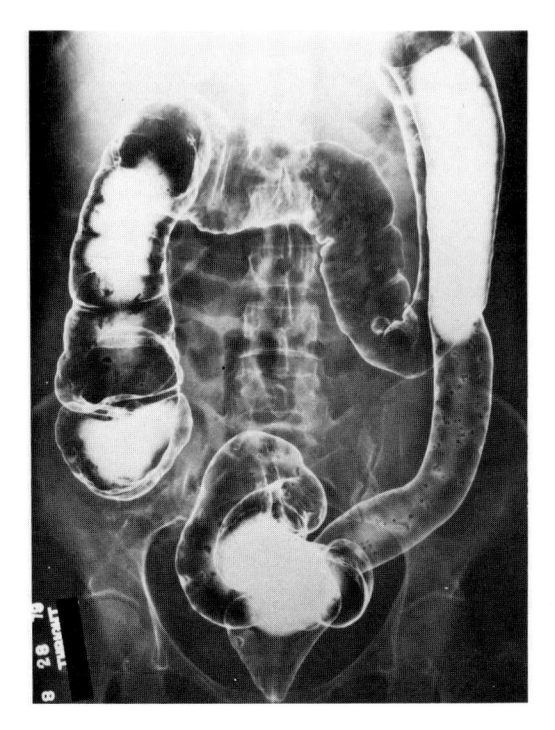

FIG. 20-25. Quiescent chronic ulcerative colitis with filiform and nodular inflammatory polyps scattered throughout the colon and rectum on normal looking mucosa.

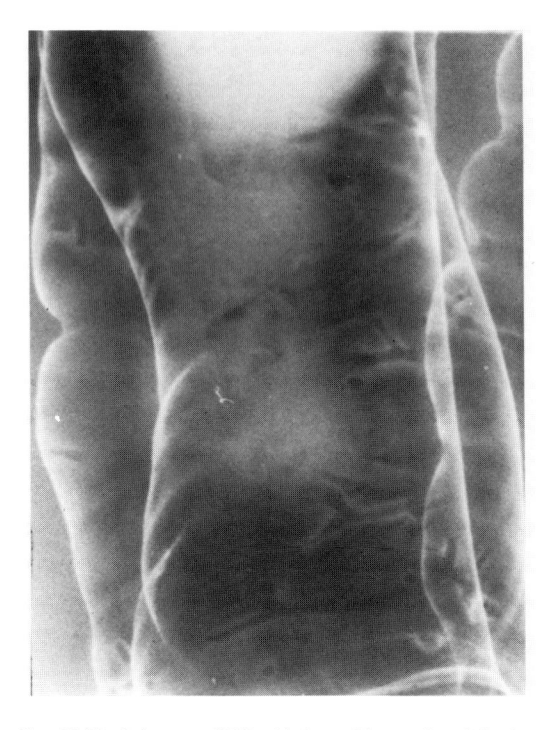

FIG. 20-26. Quiescent CUC with branching and nodular inflammatory polyps upon radiologically normal mucosa.

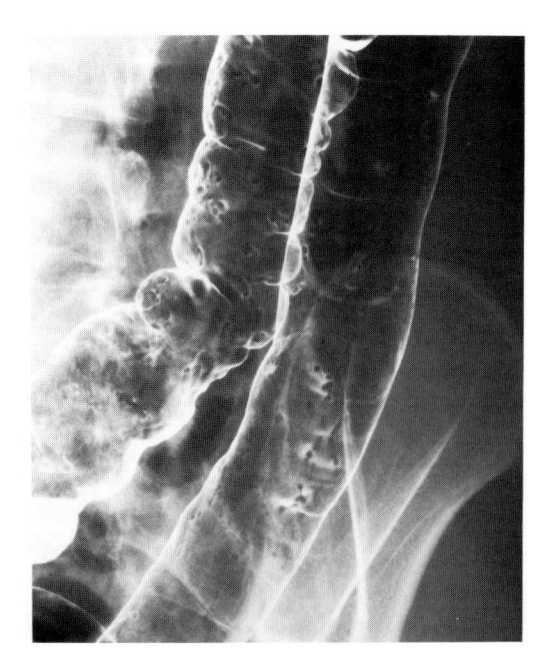

FIG. 20-27. Chronic ulcerative colitis that was asymptomatic for ten years. Filiform and nodular inflammatory polyps on normal mucosa.

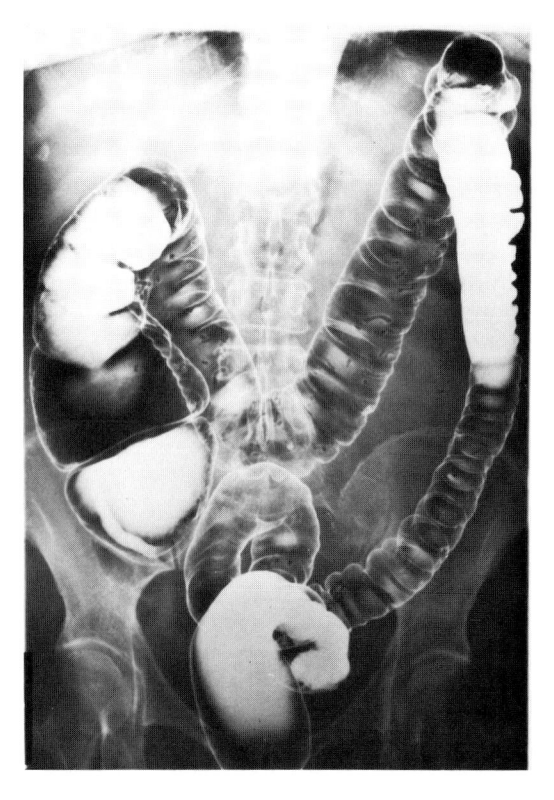

FIG. 20-28. Quiescent CUC. Filiform and nodular inflammatory polyps on normal mucosa.

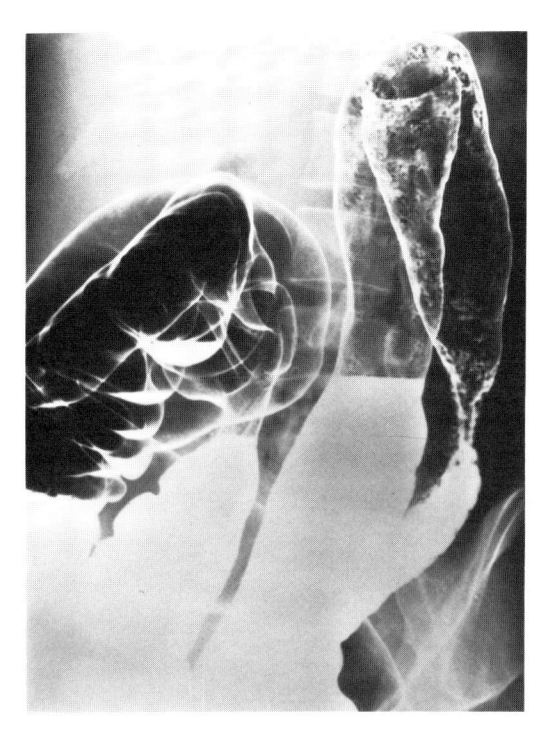

FIG. 20-29. Profuse filiform and nodular inflammatory polyps in the splenic flexure and descending colon. Endoscopy with a 60 cm instrument was reported as normal to the "distal transverse colon," undoubtedly an error in perceived location.

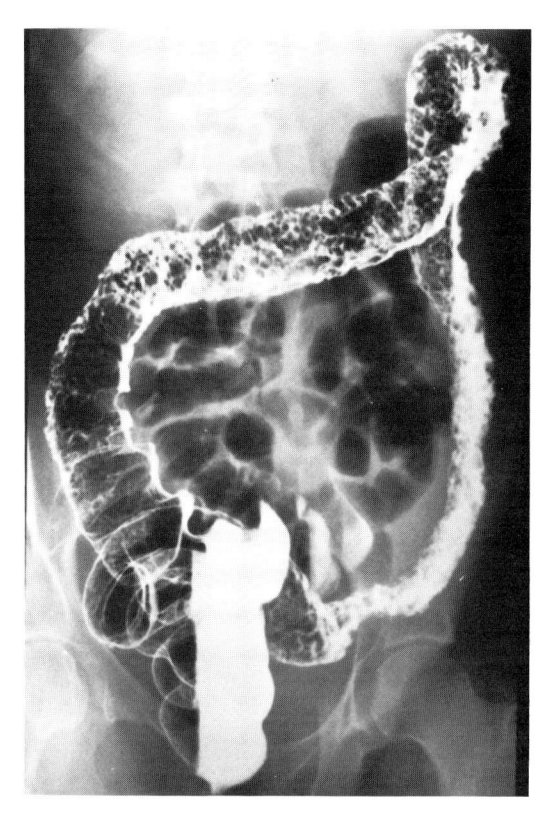

FIG. 20-30. Chronic ulcerative colitis with extremely profuse inflammatory polyps above the rectum with active inflammatory disease.

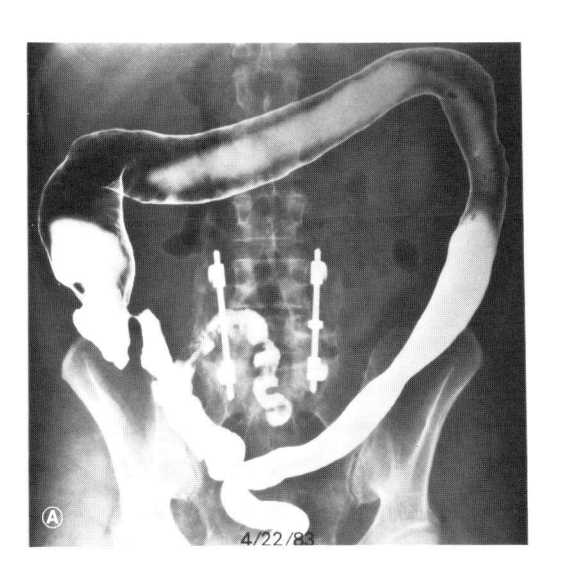

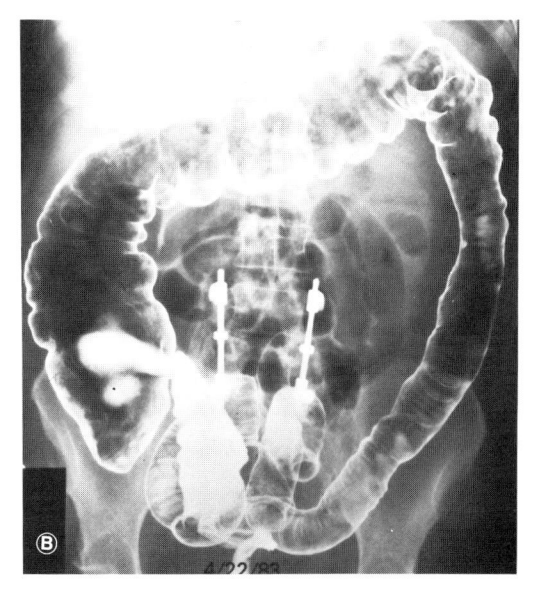

FIG. 20-31. A. and B. Chronic ulcerative colitis showing widely variable overall forms of the colon because of variation in muscular tone during the same examination.

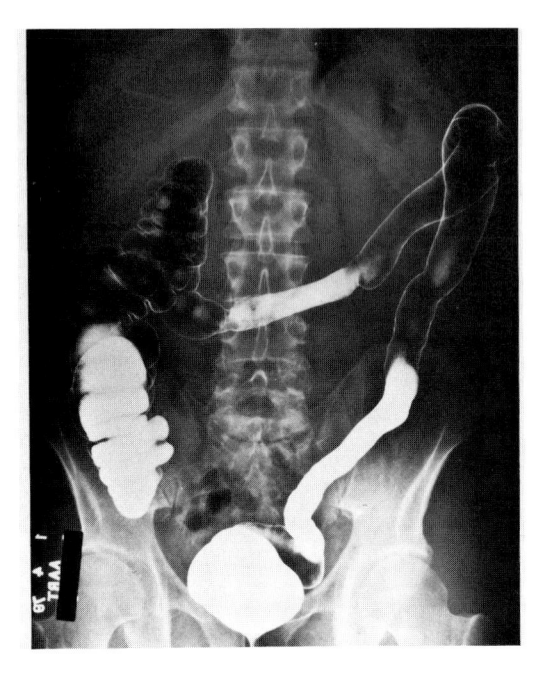

FIG. 20-32. Localized stricture of left transverse colon. Careful biopsy yielded inflammatory tissue. Unchanged from 3 years prior.

nodularity of the mucosal surface may be sharply circumscribed (Fig. 20-48). A majority of patients with such infections, however, will have a normal barium enema. Pseudomembranous

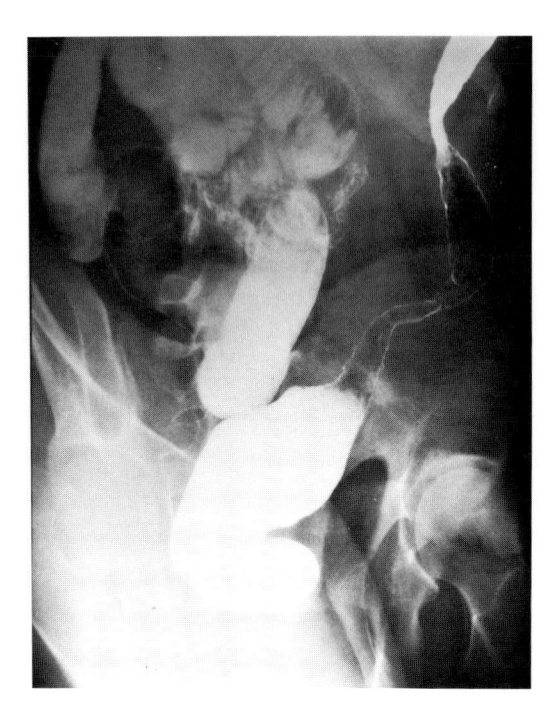

FIG. 20-33. Chronic ulcerative colitis with multiple inflammatory strictures in descending colon. Rectum showed only minimal changes endoscopically. Total proctocolectomy with ileoanal anastomosis.

colitis often has a characteristic appearance on proctoscopy. Acute amebiasis of the colon can be indistinguishable from CUC, but, again, most patients with amebic infestation will have a normal x-ray examination. Proctoscopic examination can also be helpful in this instance.[12-15]

Severe laxative abuse can result in colonic shortening, lack of haustration, and the appearance of backwash ileitis. Careful history will usually identify the condition, but, occasionally, endoscopy and biopsy will be necessary to exclude the possibility of CUC (Fig. 20-49). Finally, normal post evacuation films occasionally suggest CUC because of trapping barium in normal intersecting creases in the mucosal surface. This somewhat alarming appearance disappears completely when the colon is fully distended (Fig. 20-50).

Crohn's Disease

Unlike CUC, Crohn's disease may afflict any or all of the segments of the gut. This tends to lend credibility to the idea that these are different diseases, though their cause(s) are not understood.

Of all cases of Crohn's disease, about 20% are restricted to the colon, about 20% to the small

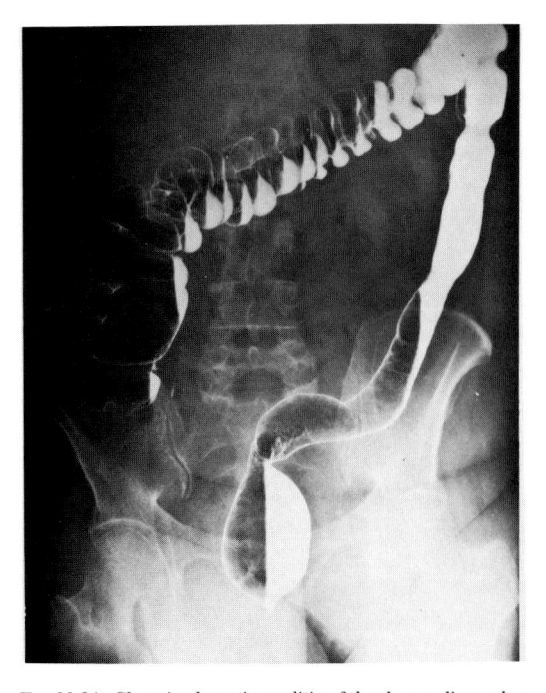

FIG. 20-34. Chronic ulcerative colitis of the descending colon and rectum with benign stricture in upper rectum.

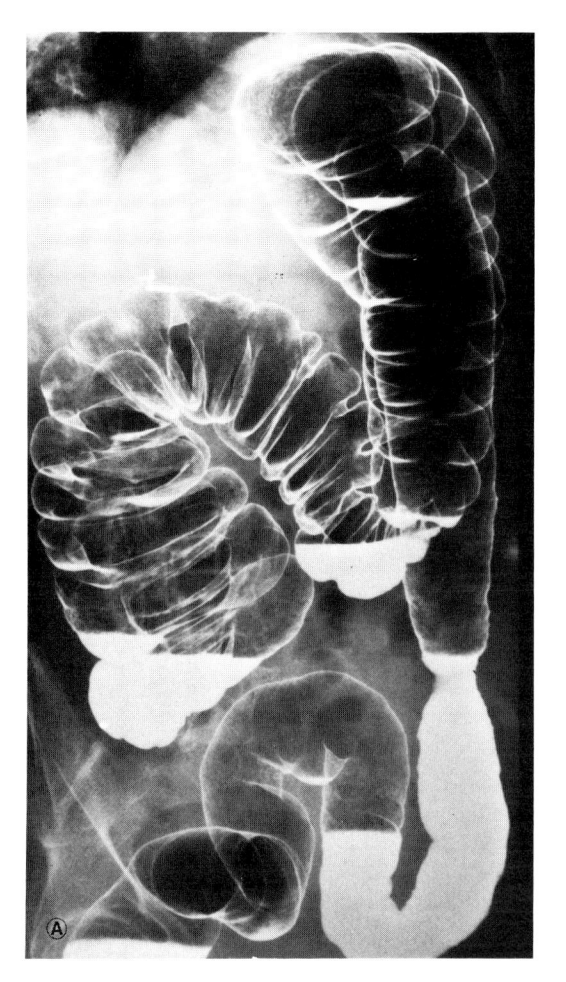

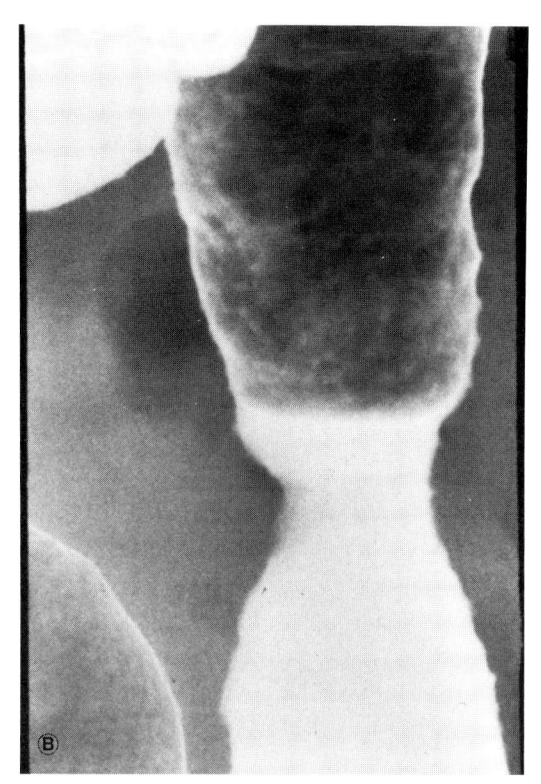

Fig. 20-35. A. and B. Chronic ulcerative colitis for 30 years. Active disease distal to splenic flexure. Stricture descending colon. Colonoscopy did not perceive the stricture but multiple biopsies yielded inflammatory tissue.

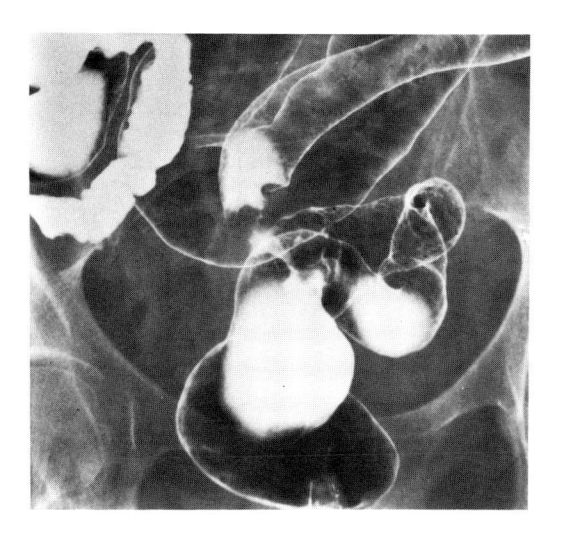

Fig. 20-36. Chronic ulcerative colitis for 40 years. Typical, annular carcinoma of the sigmoid seen on double contrast examination.

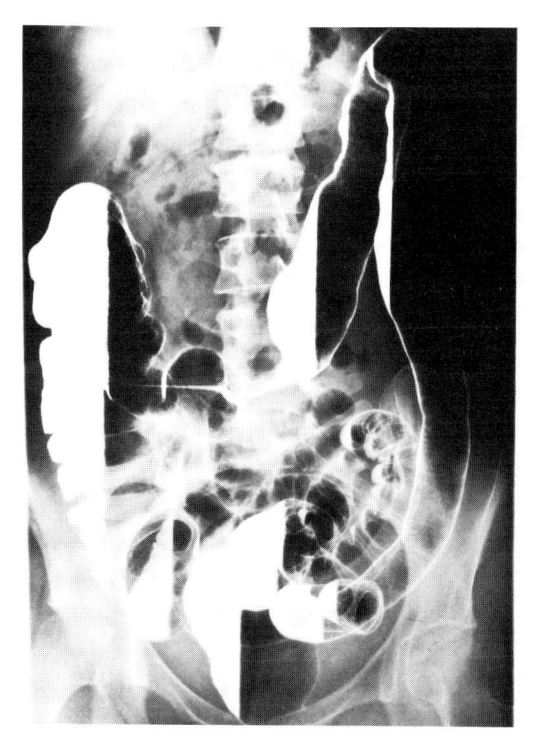

Fig. 20-37. Chronic ulcerative colitis for 15 years. Annular carcinoma, transverse colon with somewhat tapered, infiltrative junction with adjacent gut.

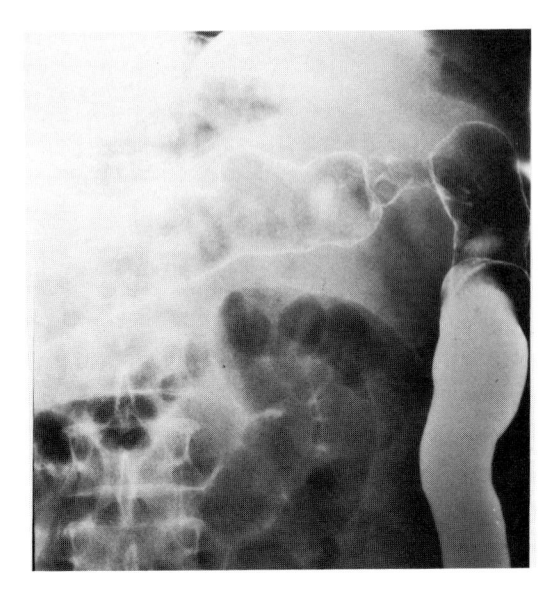

FIG. 20-38. Chronic ulcerative colitis for 14 years. Annular carcinoma near splenic flexure. Irregular surface but no overhanging polypoid mass.

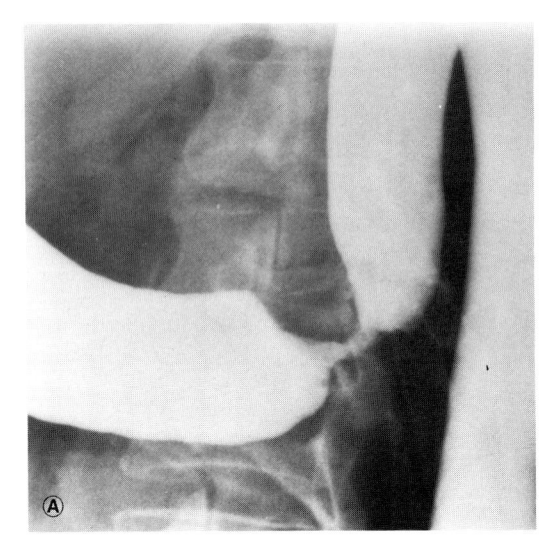

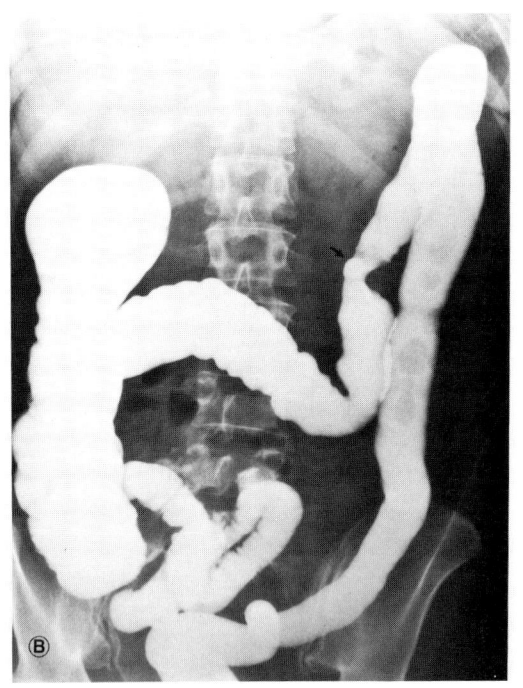

FIG. 20-39. Chronic ulcerative colitis for 33 years. A. Annular tapered carcinoma with irregular surface. B. Barium enema almost 2 years previously shows smooth, sessile indentation not thought to be pathologic, but which, in retrospect, probably was.

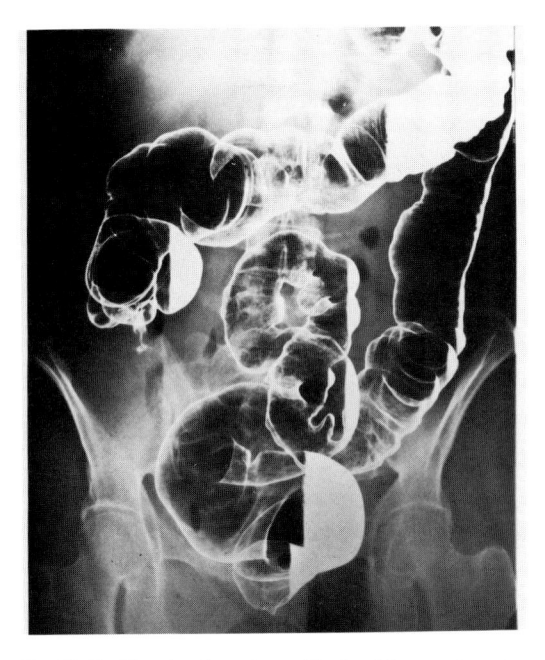

FIG. 20-40. Chronic ulcerative colitis for 18 years. Annular, obstructing carcinoma of the cecum.

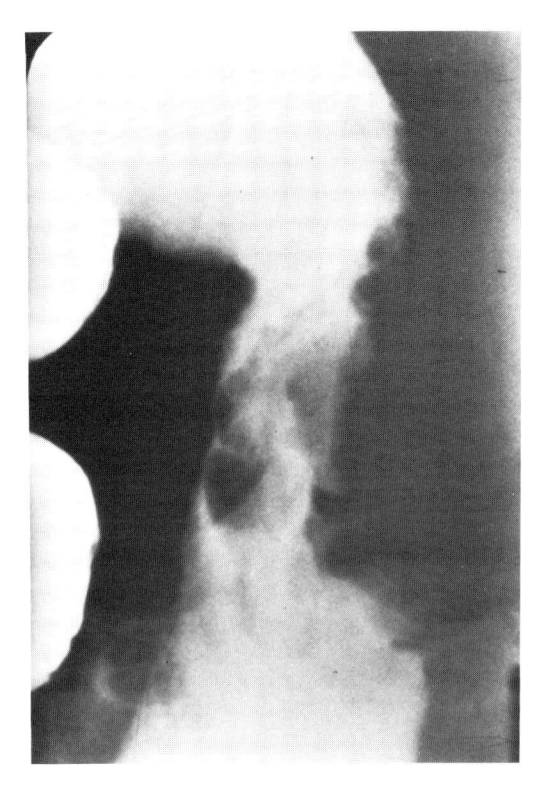

FIG. 20-41. Chronic ulcerative colitis for 13 years. Sessile, nodular carcinoma of the descending colon that is atypical in form.

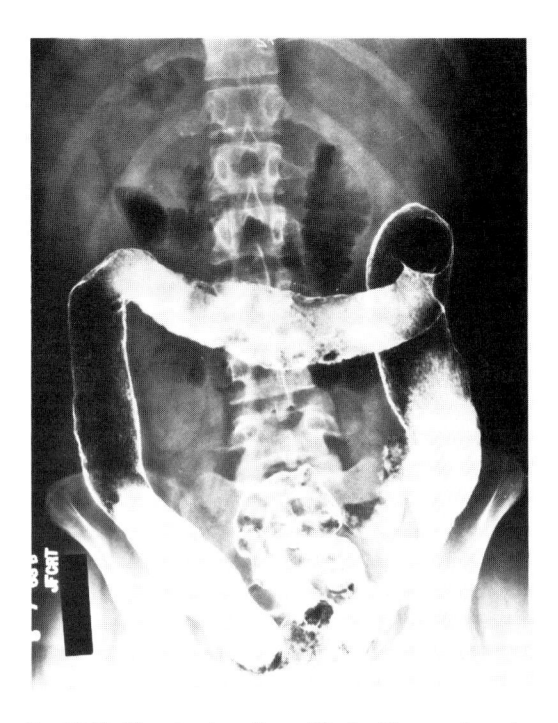

FIG. 20-42. Chronic ulcerative colitis for 12 years. Irregular masses in the transverse colon thought to be large inflammatory polyps. Total colectomy was performed, and multiple carcinomas were found in the resected specimen, with several in the transverse colon.

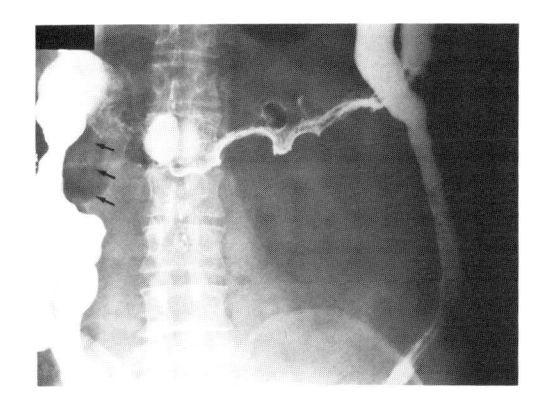

FIG. 20-43. Chronic ulcerative colitis with carcinoma. Colonoscopic examination showed distortion of the right colon. Biopsy revealed mild CUC with no dysplasia. The patient was explored because of high cancer suspicion on roentgenogram, and extensive carcinoma of the ascending colon was found.

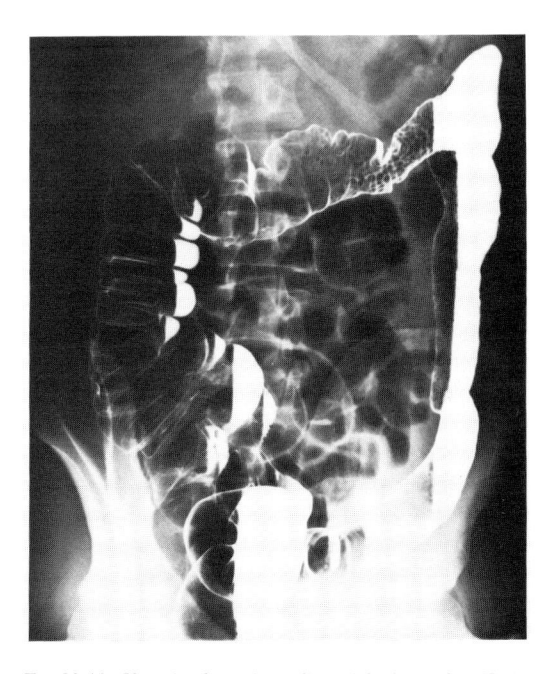

FIG. 20-44. Chronic ulcerative colitis of the left colon. Nodular surface near the splenic flexure thought to be suggestive of dysplasia. Extensive biopsy showed only moderate active colitis. The rectum was normal endoscopically.

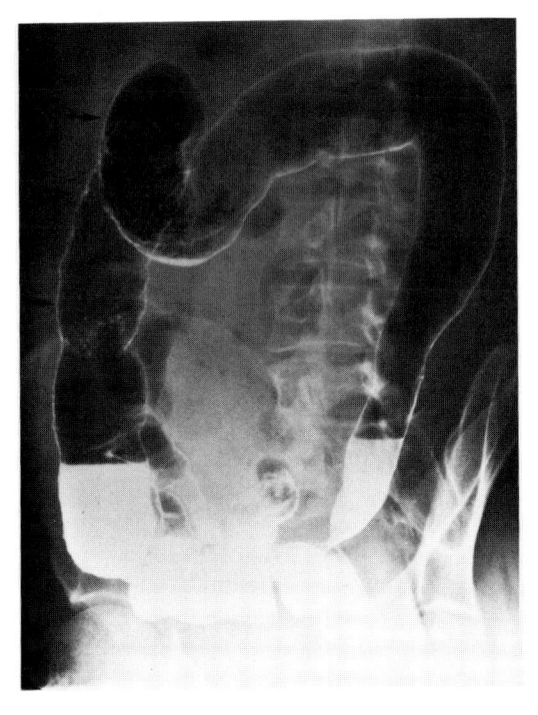

FIG. 20-45. Chronic ulcerative colitis for 14 years. Dysplasia suggested radiologically in upper ascending colon, and mild dysplasia was found there after total colectomy.

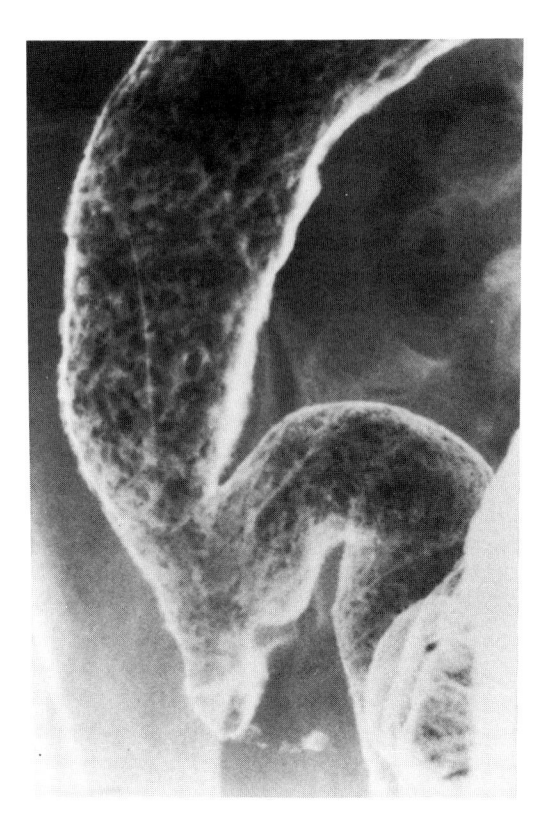

FIG. 20-46. Severe CUC of the entire colon with severe "backwash ileitis." Total colectomy was performed with a Brooke ileostomy fashioned from the terminal ileum, without complication.

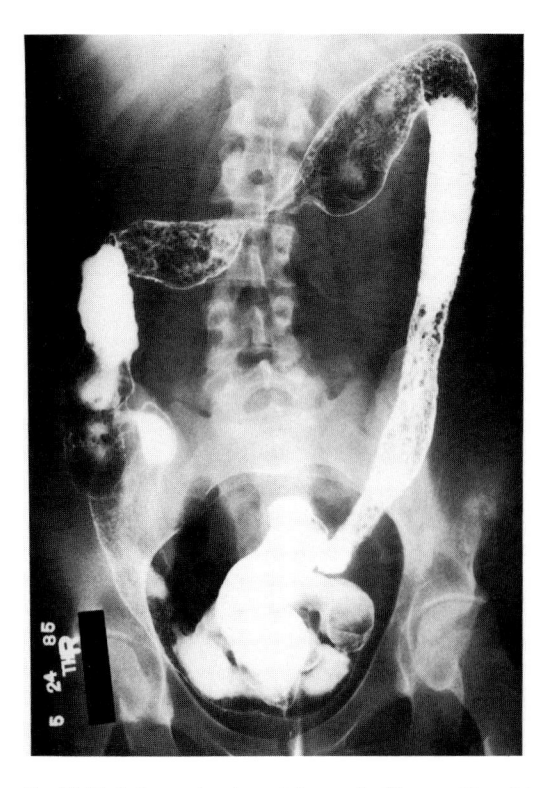

FIG. 20-47. Inflammatory bowel disease for 10 years. Thought to represent moderately severe CUC with backwash ileitis radiologically. The surgeon thought the terminal ileum was not typical of regional enteritis, but the pathologist believed this represented transmural, granulomatous disease in both the colon and resected ileum. A Brooke ileostomy was performed without complication.

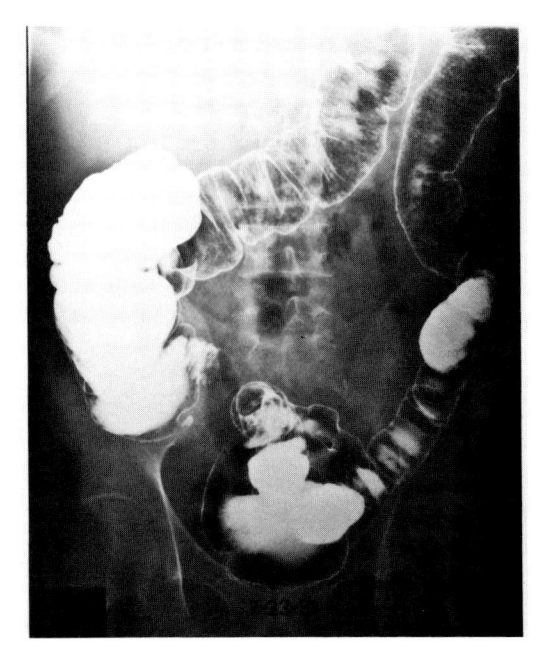

FIG. 20-48. Subacute Campylobacter colitis that cleared slowly but completely over a period of one year.

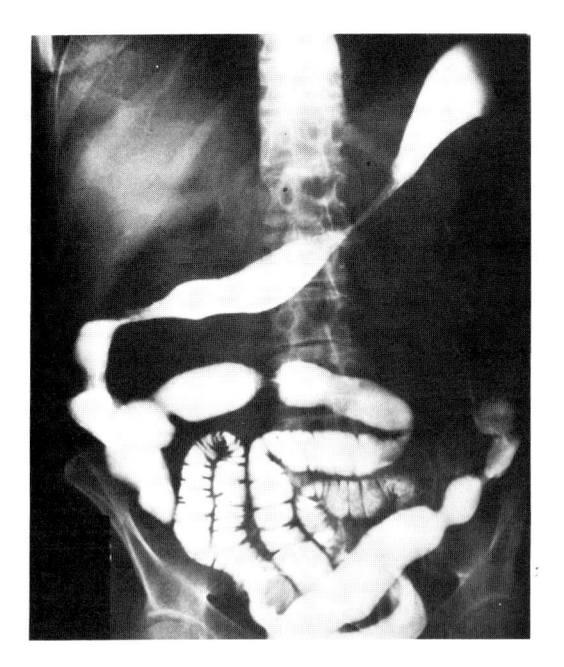

FIG. 20-49. Severe laxative abuse resembling CUC and "backwash ileitis."

intestine, and about 60% involve both organs. The stomach and duodenum rarely manifest the disease in an easily recognizable form, perhaps 1 to 2% of cases, but more subtle abnormalities may be recognized with careful study during endoscopy and radiologic examination in a larger group of patients, perhaps as high as 10 to 20% of all cases. Pathologic changes are rarely seen in the esophagus.[16]

The Colon

TECHNIQUE

The technique of examination is similar to that applied to CUC. Ordinarily, double contrast examination is most useful for the detection and identification of Crohn's disease of the colon (CDC). If obstruction and/or fistula are suspected, single contrast study will probably produce the desired diagnostic information. Fistulous tracts, rather common in this disease, are best seen by barium "undiluted" by gas.

SEGMENTAL INVOLVEMENT

Segmental involvement of the colon is characteristic, with no predilection for any particular segment in disease limited to the colon. If the terminal ileum is diseased, however, the cecum is the most frequent site of colonic pathologic change. Anal canal disease is usually seen in association with severe abnormalities in the colon and rectum, but this may happen with only small intestinal involvement and, rarely, may be the first definite manifestation of Crohn's disease (Fig. 20-51). Inspection of the perianal area, digital examination, and endoscopy are the best ways to examine this segment, but occasionally, barium enema demonstrates unsuspected sinuses (Fig. 20-52).[17]

The mildest form of CDC demonstrated by barium enema is small, discrete ulcers seen as a small collection of barium surrounded by a radiolucent halo of infiltrate. These are usually multiple and are separated by normal intervening mucosa. When these ulcers are small, the colon has normal distensibility and haustral patterns. These so-called aphthous ulcers, however, may also be seen in other conditions such as Behçet's disease, tuberculosis, Shigellosis, and amebiasis, as well as some unidentified afflictions of the colon. The finding of aphthous ulcers alone is not diagnostic of Crohn's disease. These small lesions may disappear or deepen and enlarge and connect to one another, and are then visible radiologically as collections of barium that grow more irregular as they increase in size, leaving a nodular mucosa between them (Figs. 20-53 to 20-58).[18]

DISTENSIBILITY

Distensibility of the colon becomes limited as the ulcers deepen, connect, and form fistulae between the craters in the wall of the colon. This deformity of the lumen may be localized and affect only a portion of the circumference, leaving the opposite wall practically normal, or it may form circumferential strictures that can result in clinical obstruction. These strictures have somewhat tapered ends, an irregular lumen without normal mucosal pattern, and are easily distinguished from primary uncomplicated carcinoma. This severe form of involvement is usually segmental, but the entire colon and rectum may be completely involved, often with considerable variation in severity along the length of the organ (Figs. 20-59 to 20-71).

INFLAMMATORY POLYPS

These can be seen often in CDC and have a wide variety of shapes and sizes. Most are nodules,

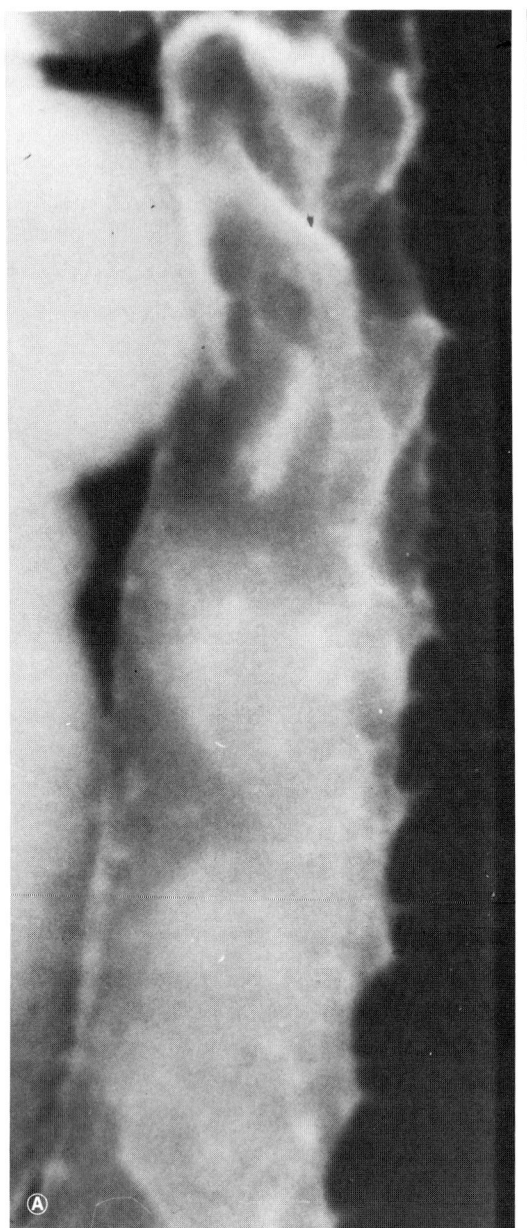

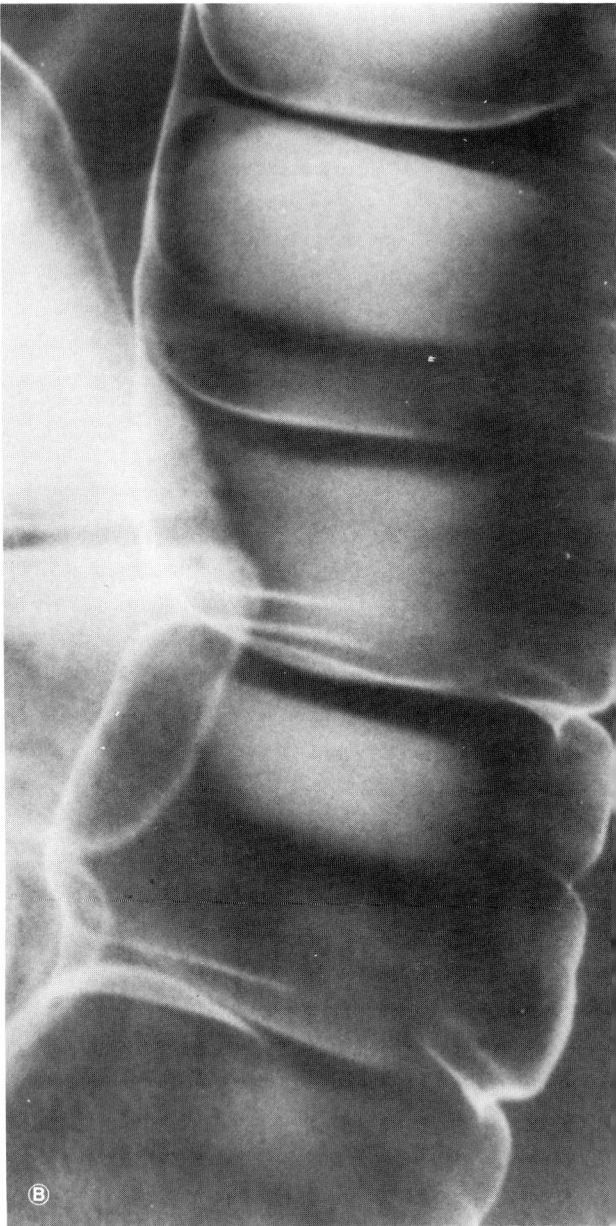

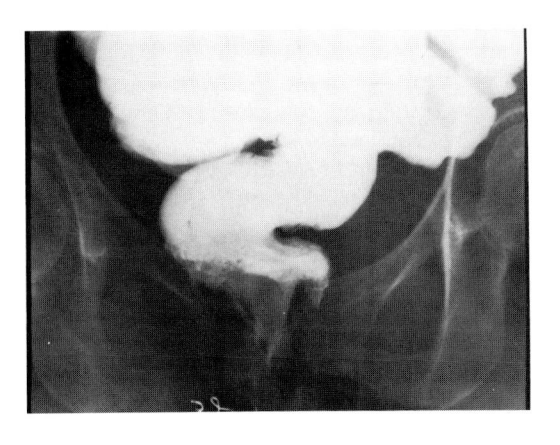

FIG. 20-50. A. Normal postevacuation film resembling moderately severe CUC resulting from prominent intersecting mucosal creases. B. When fully distended, the mucosa is perfectly normal.

FIG. 20-51. Crohn's disease confined to the rectum and anus.

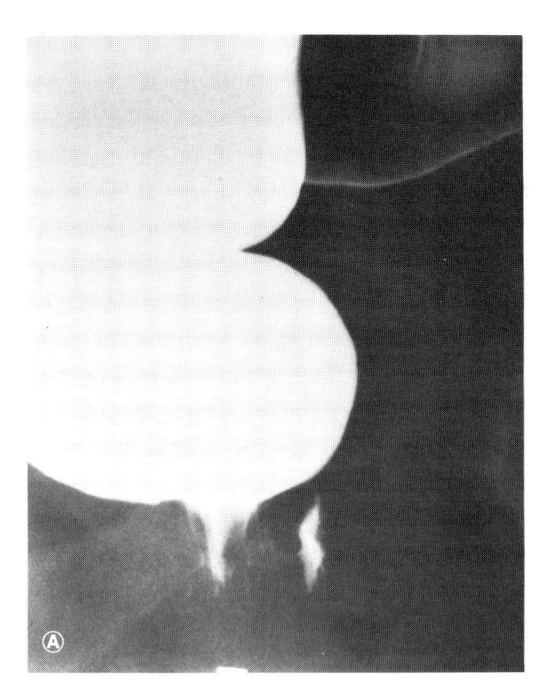

FIG. 20-52. A. Sinus arising from anal canal unobserved endoscopically. B. Crohn's disease in the descending colon.

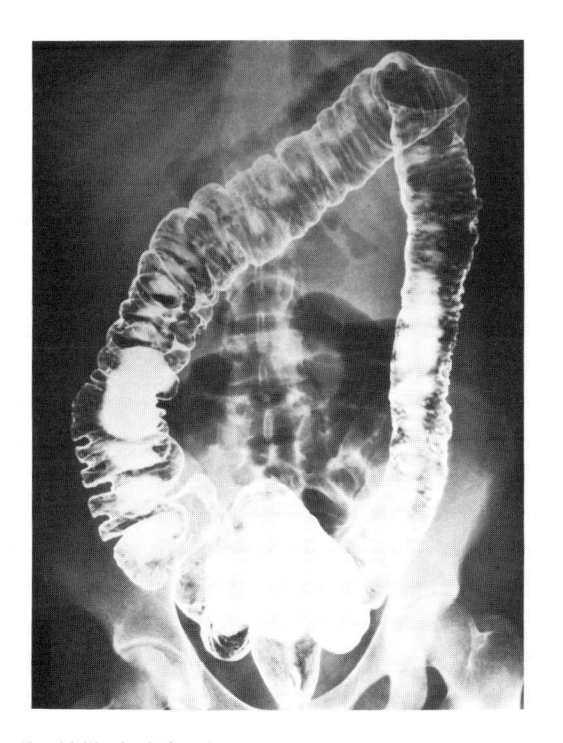

FIG. 20-53. Crohn's colitis with extensive discrete ulceration throughout the colon and similar changes in the terminal ileum. No gross deformity in either organ.

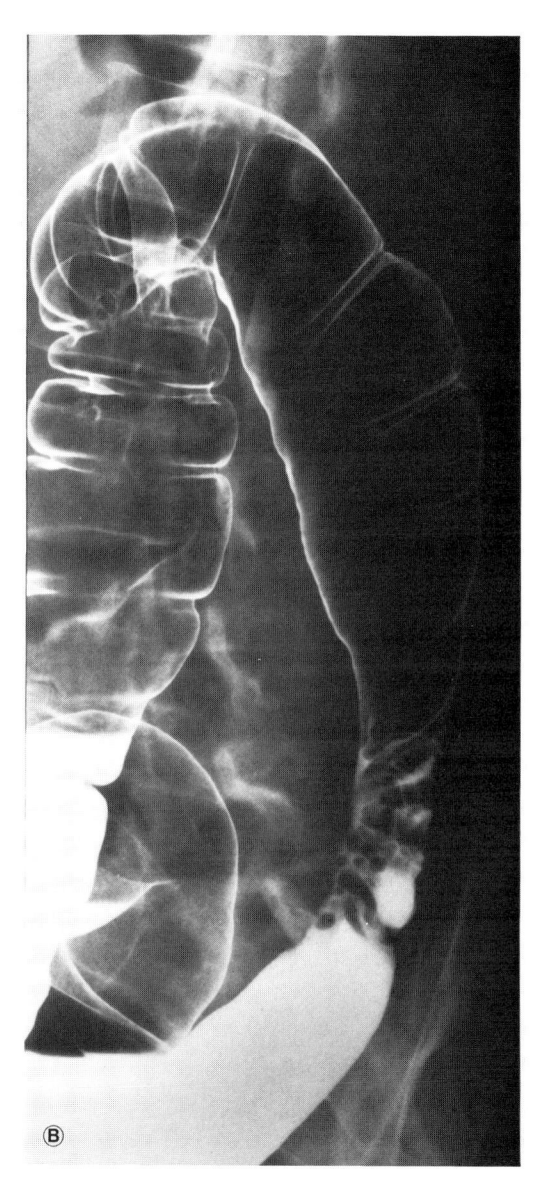

but they may be spherical and irregular, large, or filiform (Figs. 20-61 to 20-63, and 20-72 to 20-74).

FISTULAE

Although these most commonly form between ulcers in the wall of the bowel, fistulae may perforate the wall, form an abscess, and extend to the skin, especially in the perianal region, or to adjacent organs such as the small intestine, urinary bladder, vagina, and urethra (Figs. 20-75 to 20-79).

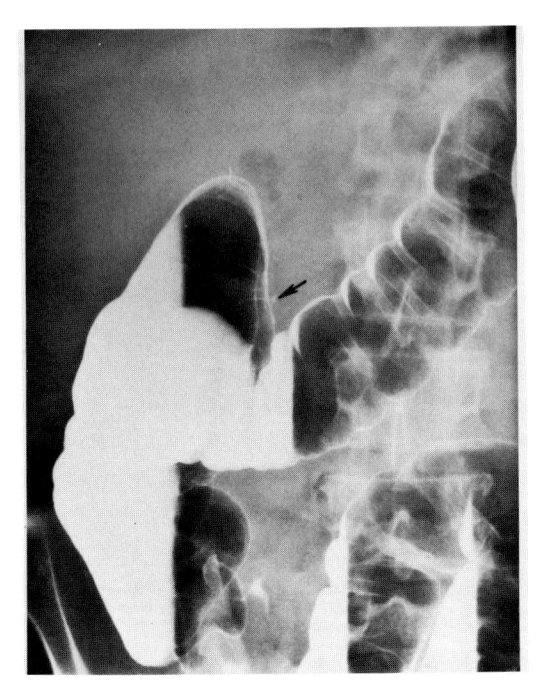

FIG. 20-54. Isolated penetrating ulcer in CDC (arrow). The colon is not deformed. The colonic mucosa has a somewhat granular appearance. Haustration is normal. Biopsy of the ulcer showed granulomas.

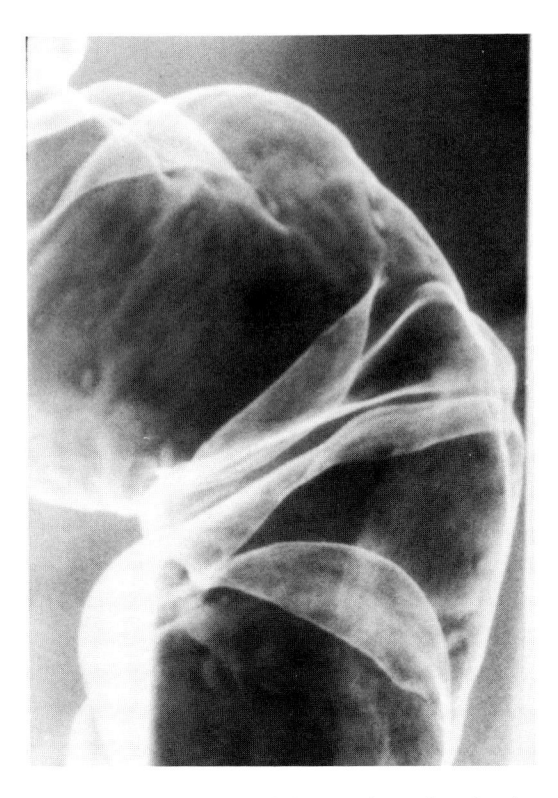

FIG. 20-55. Crohn's colitis with discrete ulcers of varying size with some visible nodules that are not ulcerated.

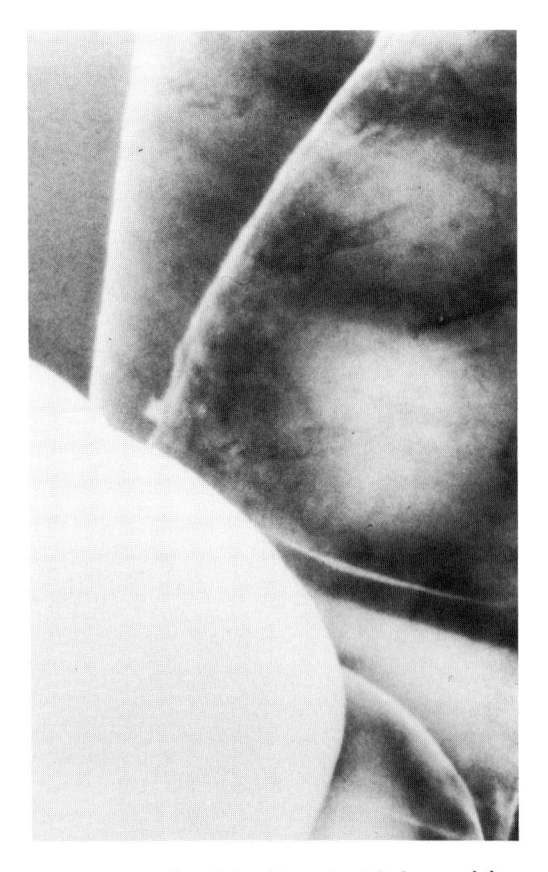

FIG. 20-56. Crohn's colitis with moderately large aphthous ulcer in profile.

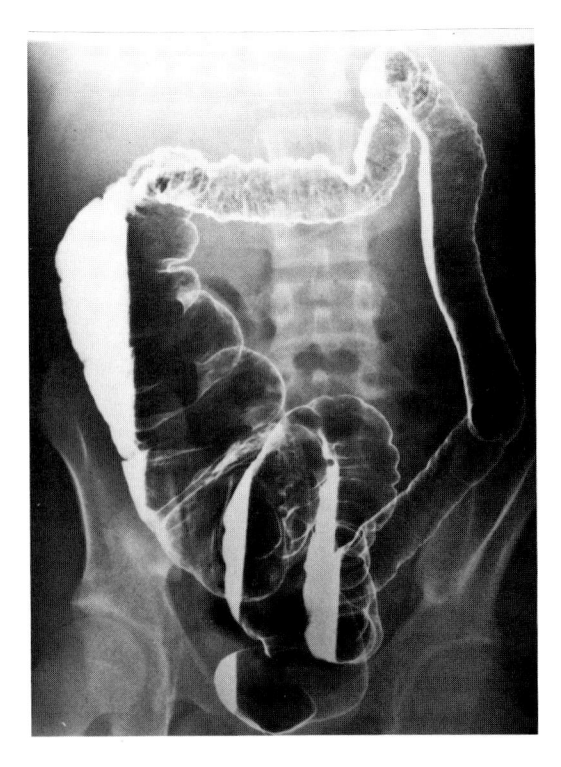

FIG. 20-57. Crohn's colitis with involvement of varying severity. A somewhat granular surface in the descending colon with shallow, small ulcers. The transverse colon is much more deformed with larger discrete ulcers, linear ulcers, and mucosal nodules.

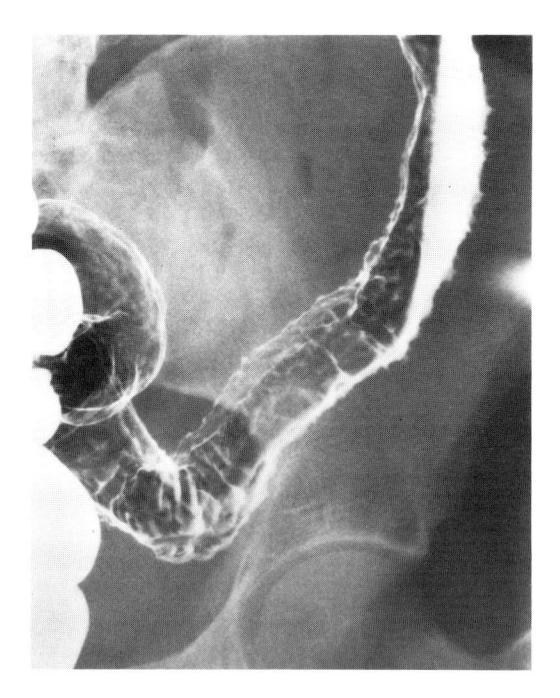

FIG. 20-58. Crohn's colitis with some narrowing of the lumen, deep, rather large discrete ulcers, linear ulcers, and a nodular mucosal surface.

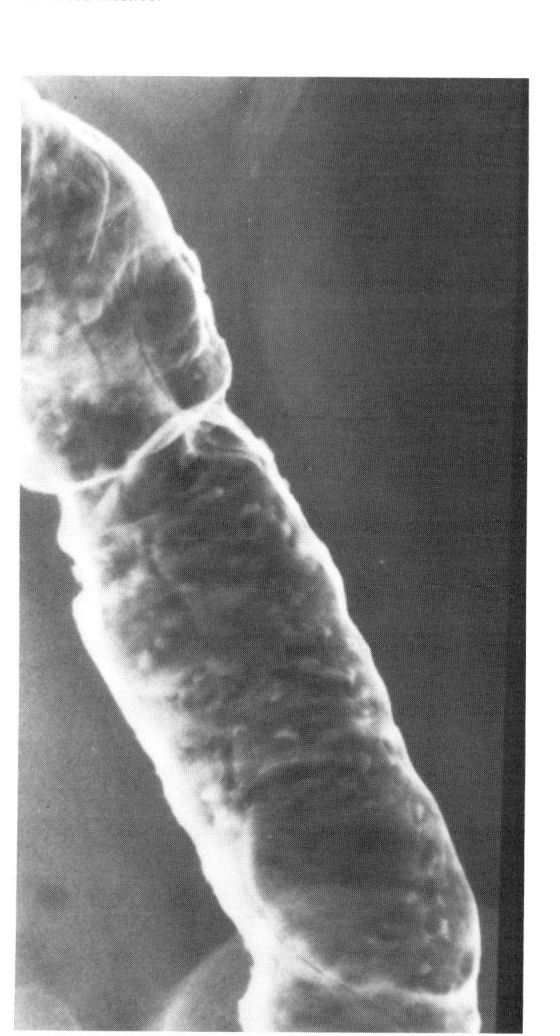

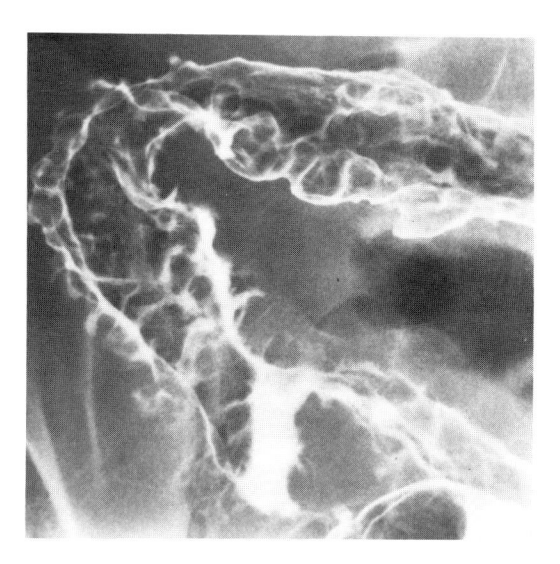

FIG. 20-60. Crohn's disease of the terminal ileum and colon with deep penetrating and linear ulceration, narrowing, and nodular surface.

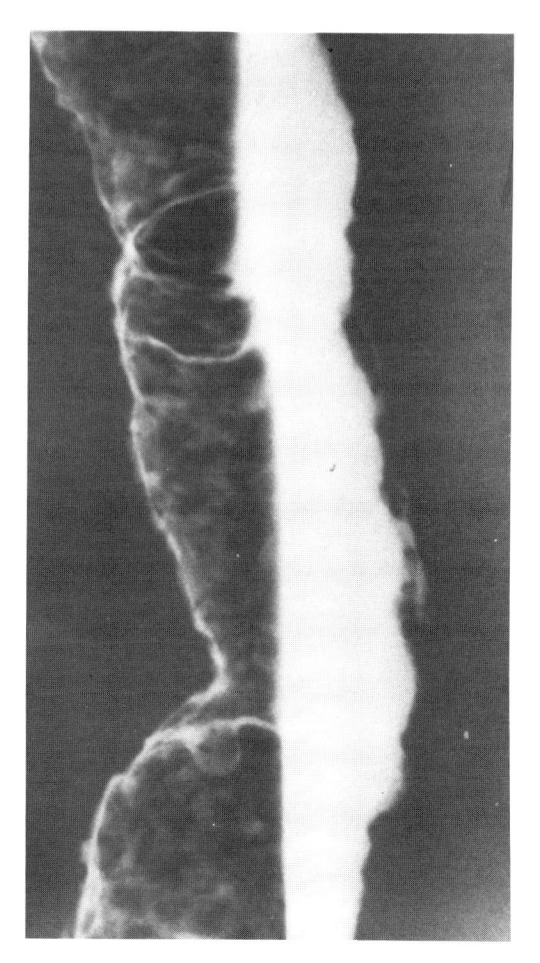

FIG. 20-61. Crohn's colitis with deep ulcers that connect in the wall of the bowel. A small inflammatory polyp also is present.

FIG. 20-59. Discrete ulcers in CDC with early limited distensibility of the lumen.

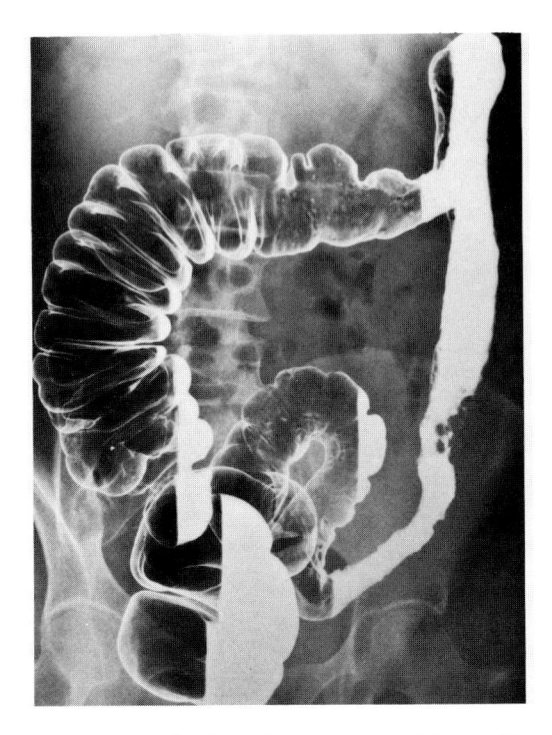

FIG. 20-62. Crohn's colitis with narrowing and intramural fistulae in the descending colon, discrete ulcers in the transverse colon, and residual inflammatory polyps (some filiform) in the sigmoid.

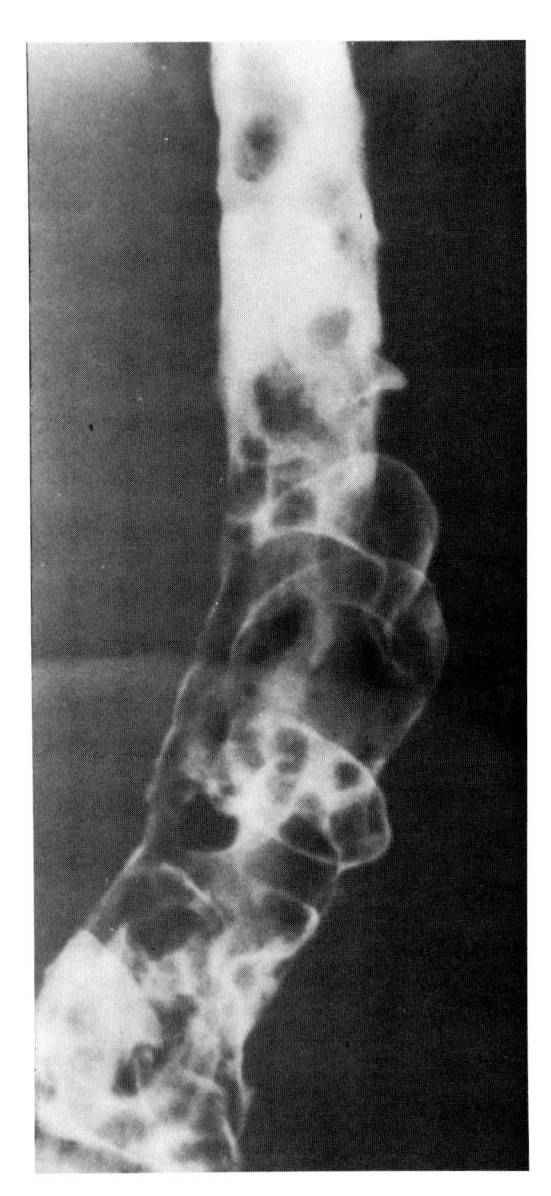

FIG. 20-63. Shortening of the medial wall of the descending colon with normal distensibility of the lateral wall forming pseudodiverticulae. Inflammatory nodules or polyps are present in this segment as well.

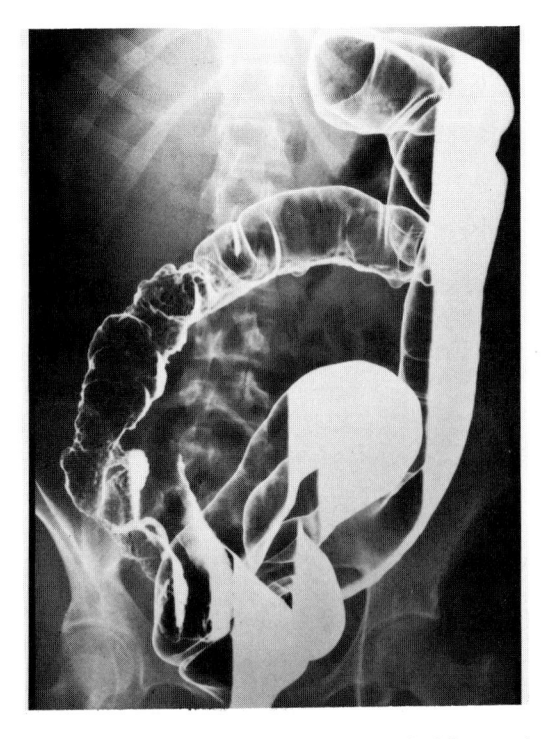

FIG. 20-64. Crohn's disease involving the terminal ileum and right colon with discrete ulcers, nodular surface, and narrowing. Only the caudad aspect of the transverse colon is abnormal.

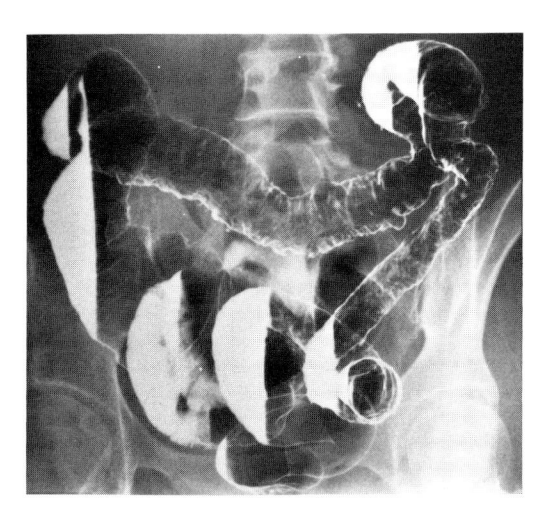

FIG. 20-65. Crohn's colitis with scattered deep ulceration, many small superficial ulcers, scattered normal bowel, and a somewhat nodular surface. The rectum showed only widely scattered discrete ulcers.

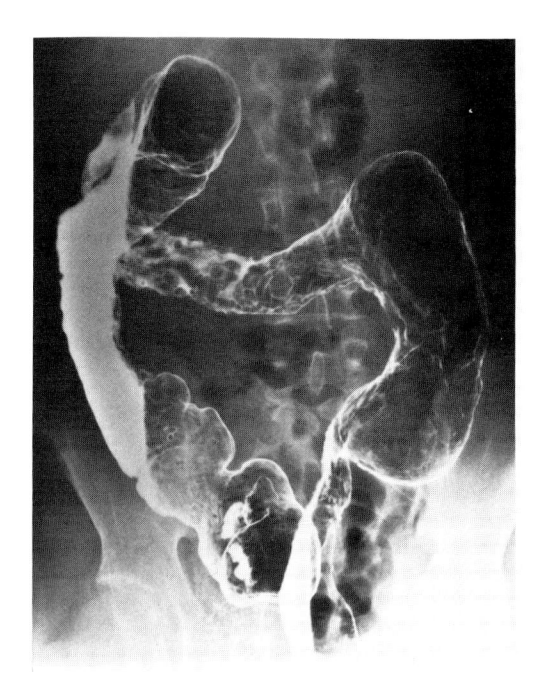

FIG. 20-66. Generalized CDC with slight stricture in the sigmoid.

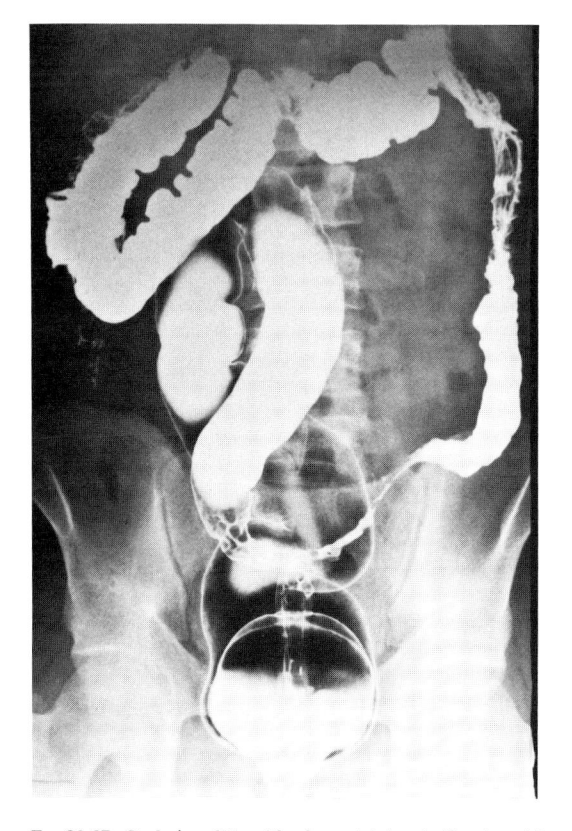

FIG. 20-67. Crohn's colitis with a long stricture in the sigmoid and a characteristic nodular surface.

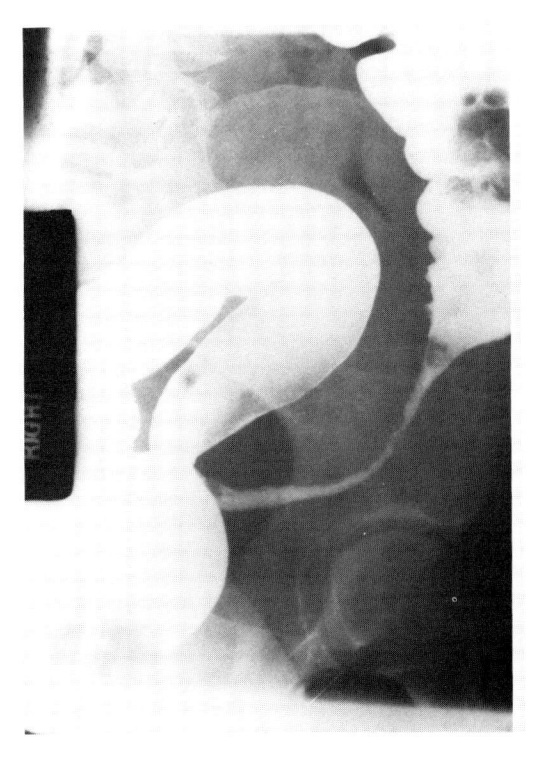

FIG. 20-68. Crohn's colitis with long, smooth stricture in the sigmoid.

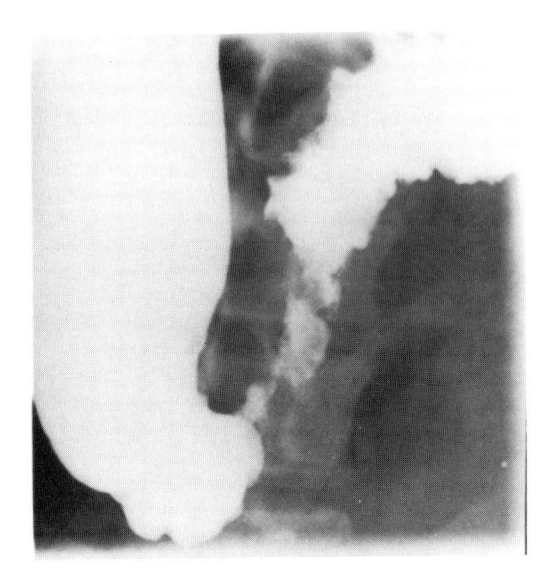

FIG. 20-69. Crohn's colitis with irregular focal stricture in the splenic flexure.

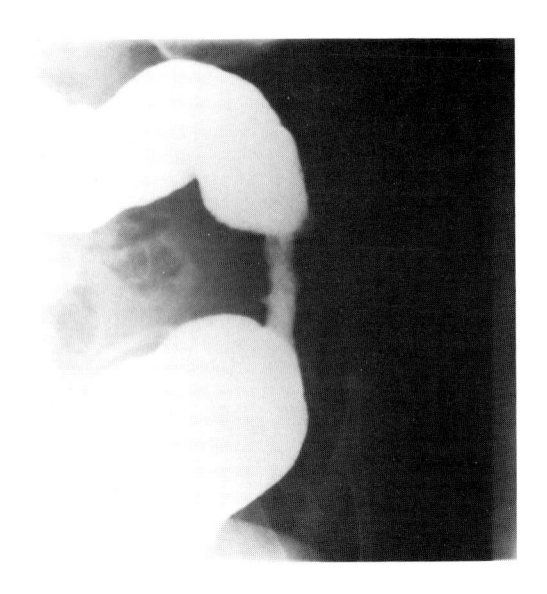

FIG. 20-70. Crohn's colitis with abrupt, irregular, benign stricture in the splenic flexure. Cancer is suspected.

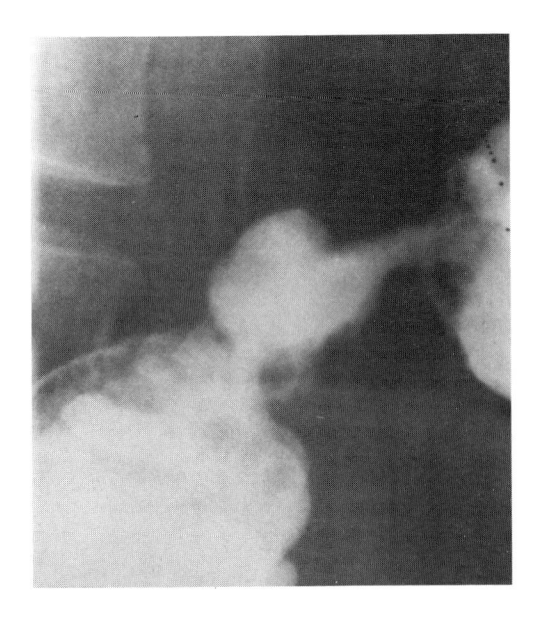

FIG. 20-71. Crohn's colitis with abrupt, irregular, benign stricture in the hepatic flexure that was called "probable cancer" on barium enema.

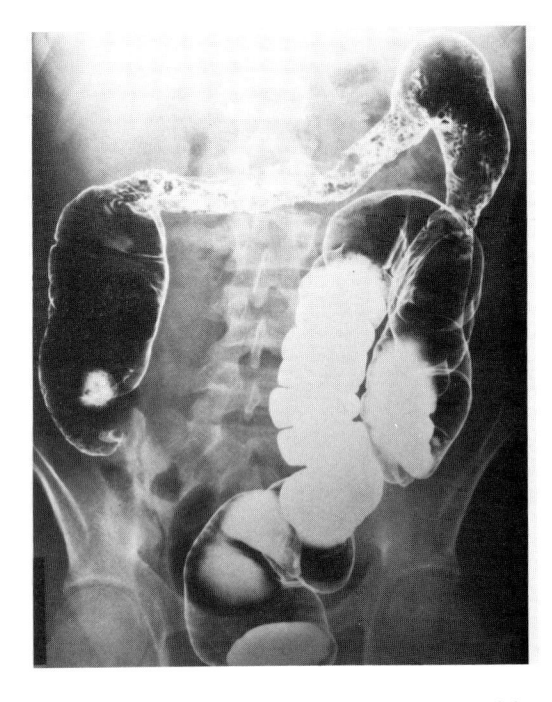

FIG. 20-72. Crohn's colitis with narrow lumen and nodular mucosal surface. Several of these inflammatory polypoid masses are rather large. Filiform inflammatory polyps are present in the splenic flexure.

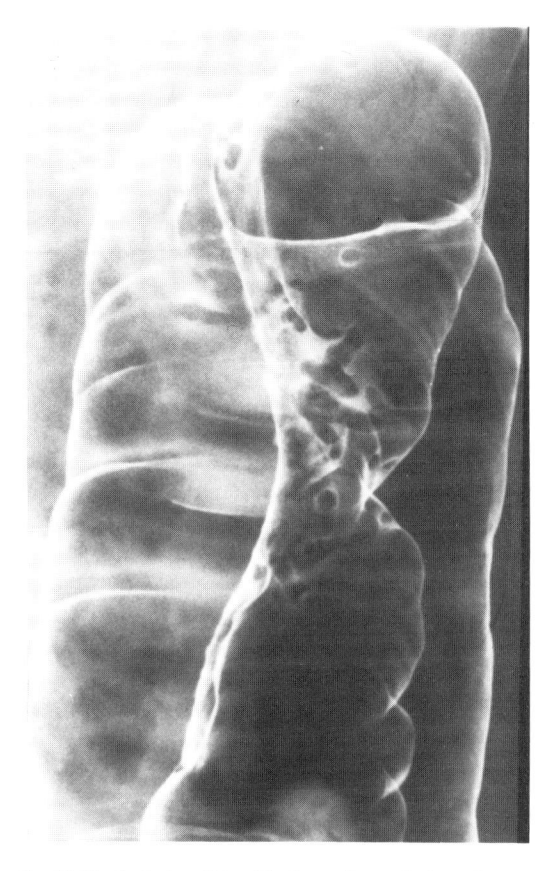

FIG. 20-73. Crohn's colitis with shortening and ulceration on the medial aspect of the descending colon with local inflammatory polyps.

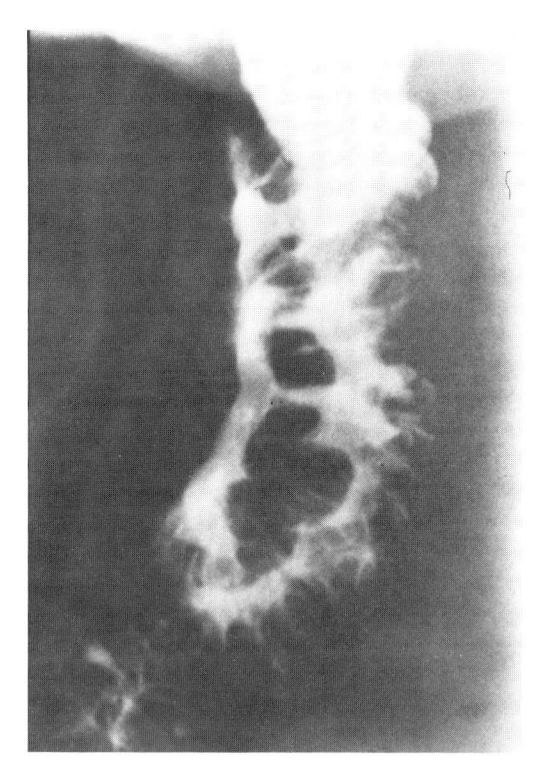

FIG. 20-75. Crohn's colitis with long, wide intramural fistula in the sigmoid.

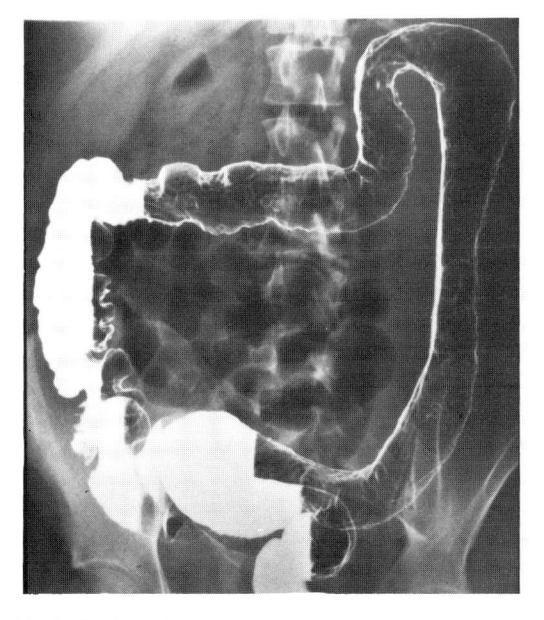

FIG. 20-74. Crohn's colitis with penetrating ulcers in the splenic flexure and inflammatory polyps in the left transverse colon and sigmoid regions.

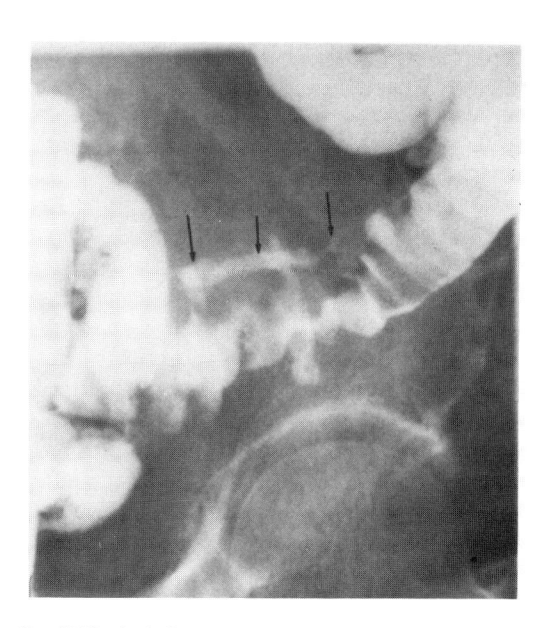

FIG. 20-76. Crohn's colitis with intramural fistula (arrows) connecting diverticulae.

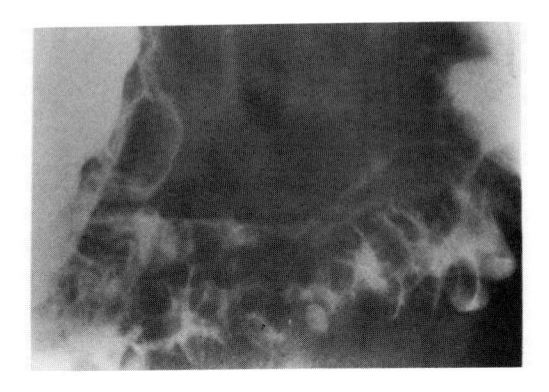

FIG. 20-77. Crohn's colitis involving the transverse colon and sigmoid colon with intramural fistula and nodular surface in the sigmoid.

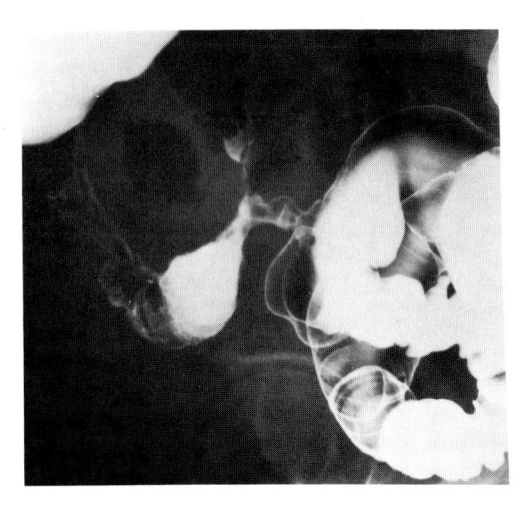

FIG. 20-78. Fistula connecting a relatively normal sigmoid colon with ileum involved with rather severe CD.

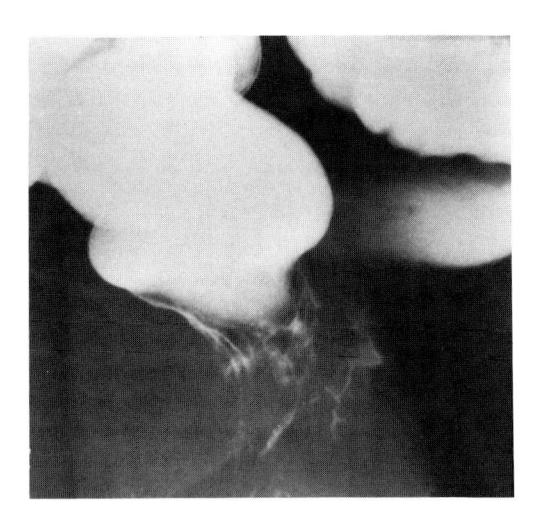

FIG. 20-79. Crohn's colitis with rectovaginal and cecovesical fistulae.

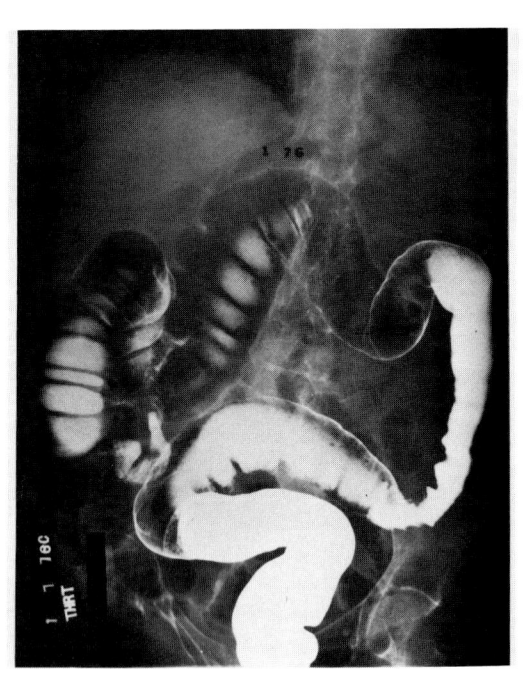

FIG. 20-80. Acute changes of ischemia in the descending colon in a patient with dermatomyositis.

DISTINCTION FROM OTHER DISEASES

It is usually easy to distinguish CDC limited to the colon from other diseases (see Chap. 10). If the involvement is moderately severe and includes the rectum in continuity with more proximal abnormalities, however, differentiation from severe CUC may be difficult and even impossible, and this is especially true if the entire colon is diseased.[19] Segmental ischemia can closely resemble CDC, but its acute onset and transient nature, with frequent prompt reversions to normal, serves to separate them. Occasionally, however, the symptoms are vague and an irregular stricture may form that can be impossible to differentiate from those seen in Crohn's disease (Figs. 20-80 to 20-82). Perforated diverticulitis is a common disease that may result in intramural fistulae and narrowing of the lumen. It can usually be recognized by a

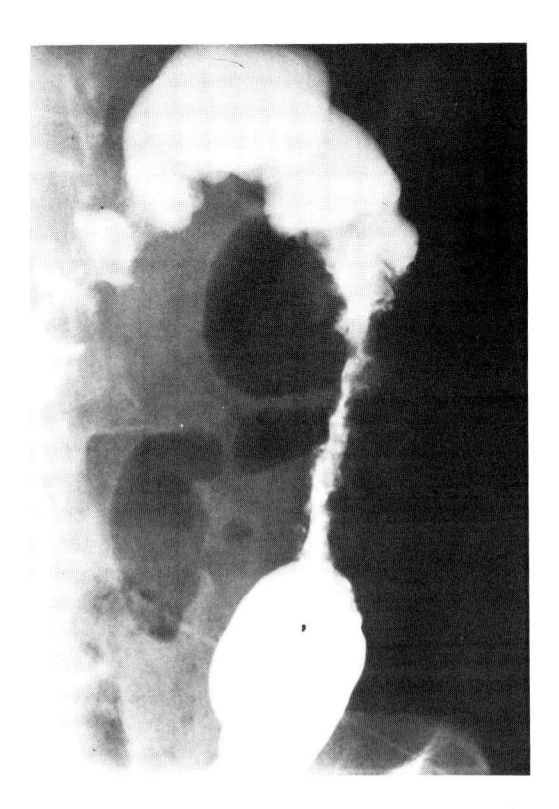

FIG. 20-81. Severe ischemic stricture of the descending colon with mucosal ulceration.

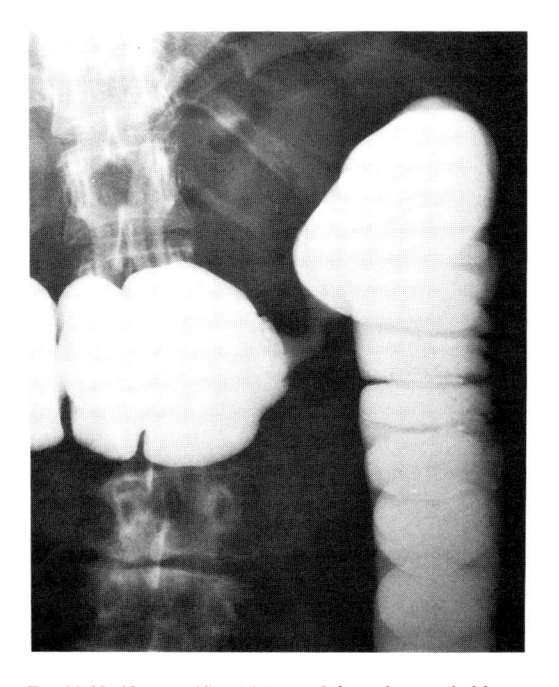

FIG. 20-82. Nonspecific stricture of the colon, probably secondary to prior ischemia. Mucous membrane was covering this stricture but it was smooth and without pattern.

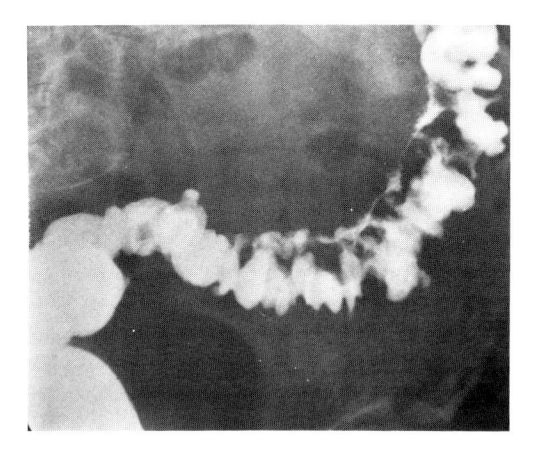

FIG. 20-83. Perforated diverticulitis with pericolonic fistula connecting many diverticulae.

normal mucosal pattern within the narrow segment, the presence of many diverticulae connected by fistulae, and its tendency to occur in the aged; however, the mucosal pattern is often difficult to assess, fistulae may form with adjacent organs, and the distinction between the two conditions may have to await examination of the resected tissue by the surgical pathologist (Fig. 20-83).[20] Perforated appendicitis can also result in fistula formation and closely resemble CD in the ileocecal region (Fig. 20-84). Tuberculosis can completely mimic CDC but its rarity in Western populations almost eliminates it as a realistic consideration.[21] A more urgent consideration today is venereal proctocolitis in homosexual males.[22] This may closely mimic CDC, and only a careful history and culture of pathologic lesions will accurately identify the process (Fig. 20-85). Occasionally, discrete ulcers are identified that are transient and their cause is never deter-

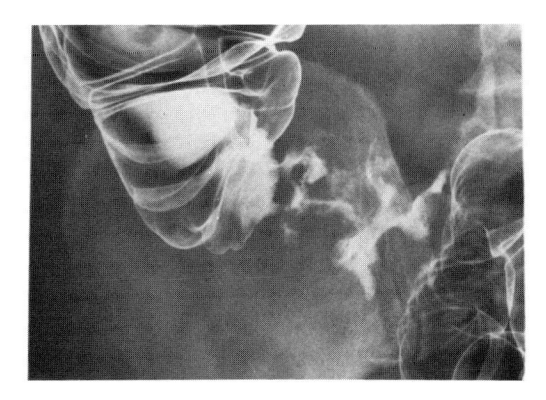

FIG. 20-84. Perforated appendicitis that formed a fistula back into the cecum.

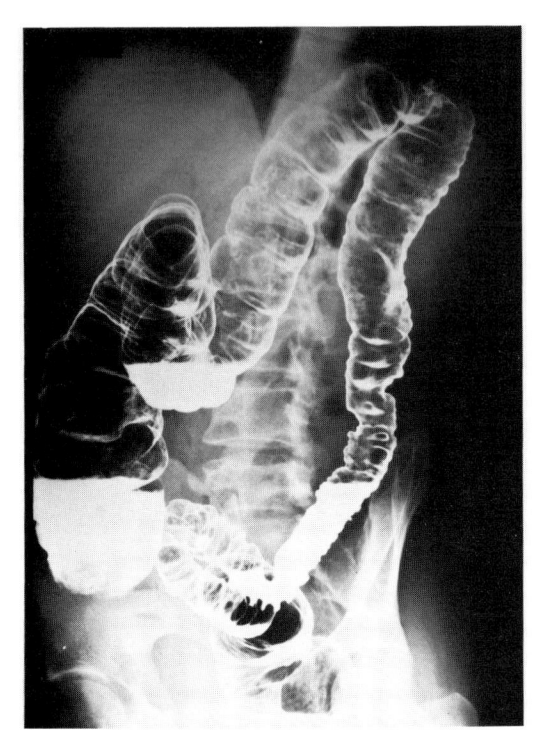

FIG. 20-85. 43-year-old homosexual male with discrete ulcers throughout the descending colon, sigmoid, and rectum. Culture positive for Neisseria variant.

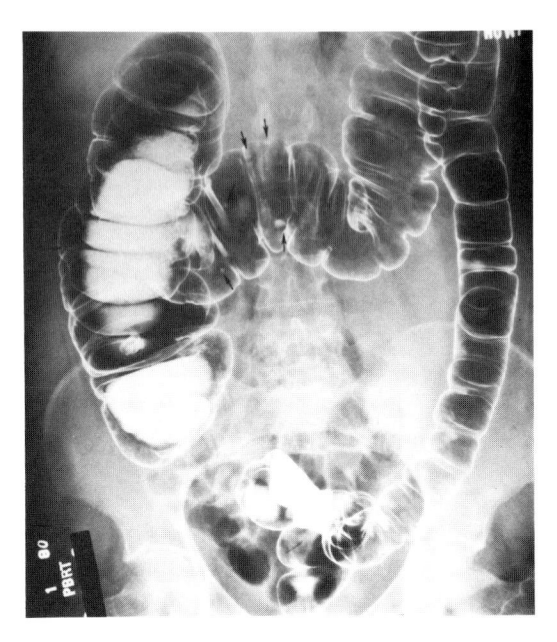

FIG. 20-86. Discrete ulcers in the transverse colon. Proctoscopy was normal. Reexamination one year later was normal, with no definite diagnosis.

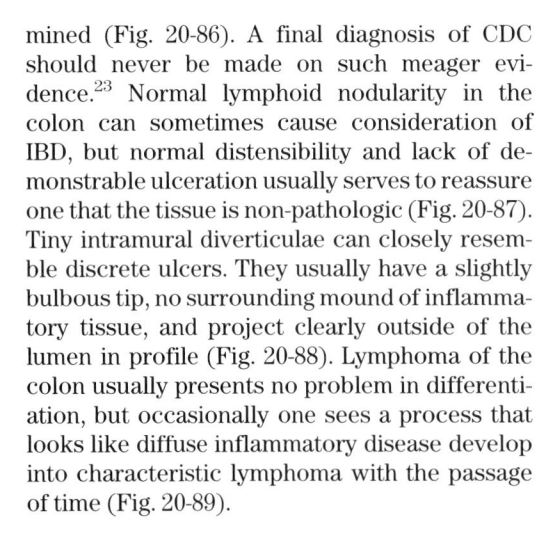

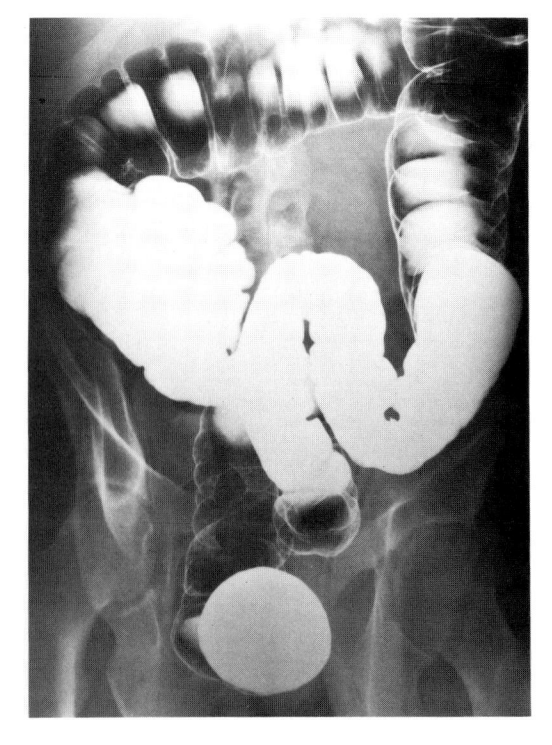

FIG. 20-87. Somewhat prominent lymphoid nodules in the rectum and sigmoid, with normal endoscopy.

mined (Fig. 20-86). A final diagnosis of CDC should never be made on such meager evidence.[23] Normal lymphoid nodularity in the colon can sometimes cause consideration of IBD, but normal distensibility and lack of demonstrable ulceration usually serves to reassure one that the tissue is non-pathologic (Fig. 20-87). Tiny intramural diverticulae can closely resemble discrete ulcers. They usually have a slightly bulbous tip, no surrounding mound of inflammatory tissue, and project clearly outside of the lumen in profile (Fig. 20-88). Lymphoma of the colon usually presents no problem in differentiation, but occasionally one sees a process that looks like diffuse inflammatory disease develop into characteristic lymphoma with the passage of time (Fig. 20-89).

ACUTE TOXIC COLITIS

This can occur in CD, and, as in CUC, barium enema should be withheld until this phase quiets. A plain film of the abdomen often allows identification of an acute, severe pathologic

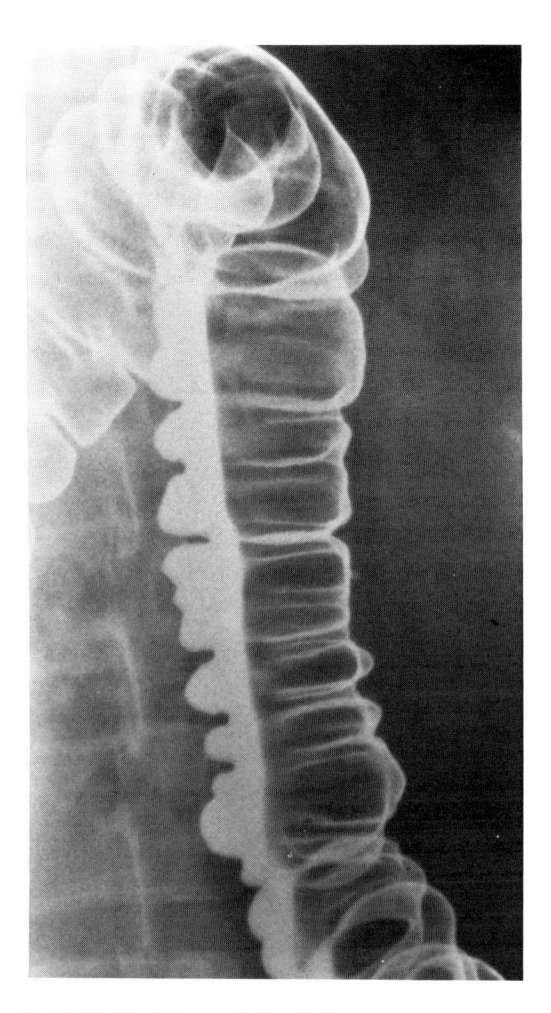

FIG. 20-88. Tiny intramural diverticulum.

process involving the colon by virtue of altered overall configuration and a nodular irregular surface. This information combined with the medical history and proctoscopic examination usually allows a definite diagnosis.

The Small Intestine

Whether oral ingestion or tube injection is used to opacify this segment of the bowel, careful fluoroscopy with palpation and proper positioning of the patient for detailed viewing of the anatomy and physiology are fundamental to the success of the examination. If carefully performed, each method will probably accurately identify about 95% of active CD of the small intestine.[5,6,24]

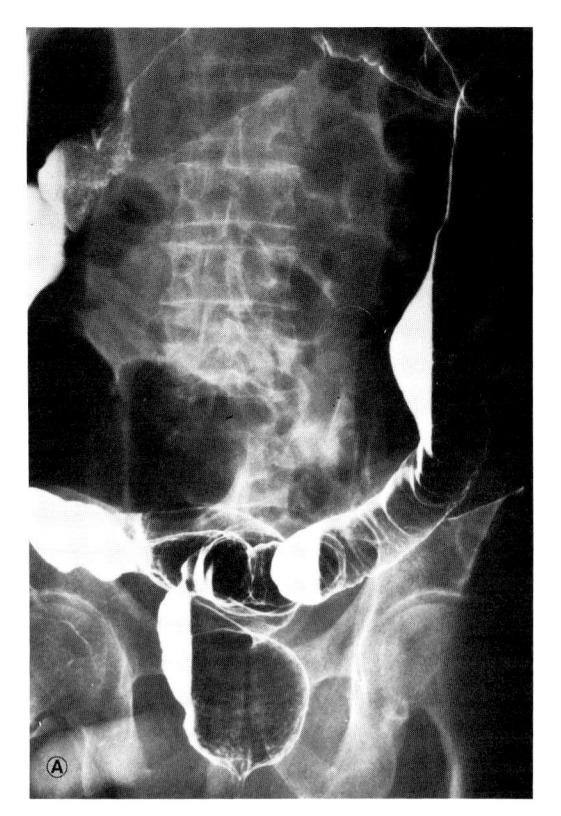

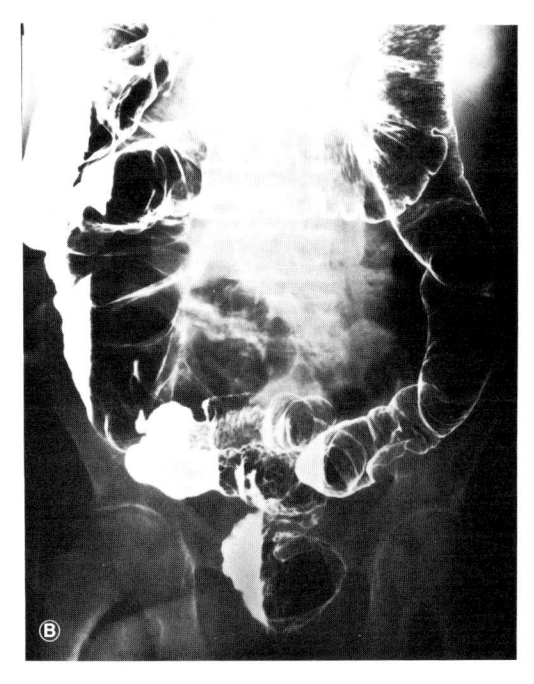

FIG. 20-89. A. Changes of active IBD in the rectum and sigmoid that was confirmed by biopsy. B. Three years later the patient returned with nodular mucosa in the rectum and sigmoid colon and a sessile mass in the upper sigmoid colon. A non-Hodgkin's malignant lymphoma was present.

ORAL INGESTION

Oral ingestion is simple, comfortable, reasonably sparing of time, allows assessment of small bowel motor physiology and bowel content, and allows ready evaluation of the esophagus, stomach, and duodenum at the same time. It has the disadvantages of requiring repeated visits to the fluoroscopic and filming rooms, possibly taking more total time for the patient, and not providing controlled distention of the small bowel lumen.

SMALL BOWEL ENEMA

This probably consumes less fluoroscopic time and may take less total time for the patient, and also provides controlled distention of the intestine via the indwelling tube. Its disadvantages include inability to immediately precede the enema with a radiologic examination of the esophagus, stomach, and duodenum, the professional effort and patient discomfort of intubation, difficulty in assessing the motor physiology of the small bowel during an enema, and limited opportunity to assess the mucosal pattern of the contracting and contracted lumen.

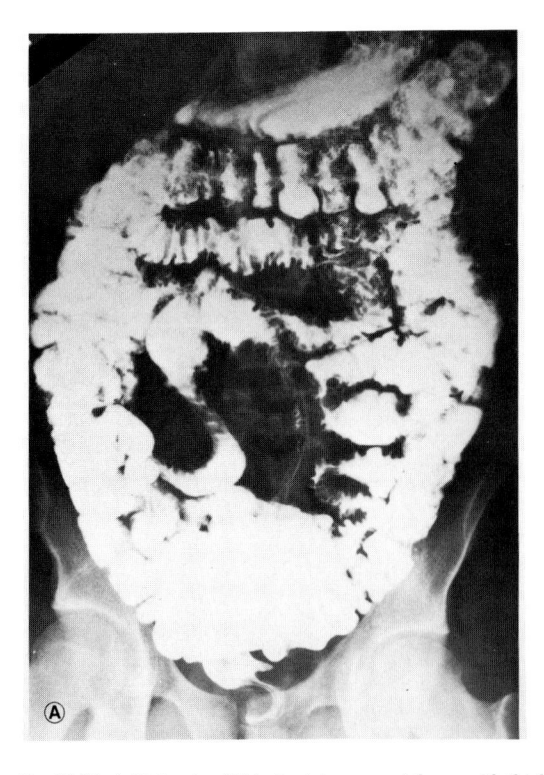

THE TERMINAL ILEUM

The most common segment of the small intestine involved is the terminal ileum, often together with the adjacent colon. This Crohn's ileocolitis is the most common presentation of the disease. As in the colon, involvement of multiple segments with intervening normal bowel is common. The disease occasionally may manifest itself only in the jejunum or proximal ileum, however. Inflammation of the region of the anal canal, with a tendency to form sinuses and fistulae, may accompany small intestinal CD in the presence of an otherwise uninvolved colon and rectum. Rarely, the anal disease may precede recognizable changes in the small intestine and colon (Figs. 20-90 and 20-91).[17]

Small discrete ulcers surrounded by a nodule of inflammatory infiltrate probably constitute the earliest radiologic sign of CD in the small bowel, but they are much less commonly seen than in the colon. As in the colon, they are not diagnostic of CD because they can be seen in Yersinia enteritis and in some unidentified inflammatory processes.[25] The most common and reliable early sign is thickening of the circular mucosal folds accompanied by a sense of stiffness when palpated at fluoroscopy. As severity increases, some folds become much thicker and

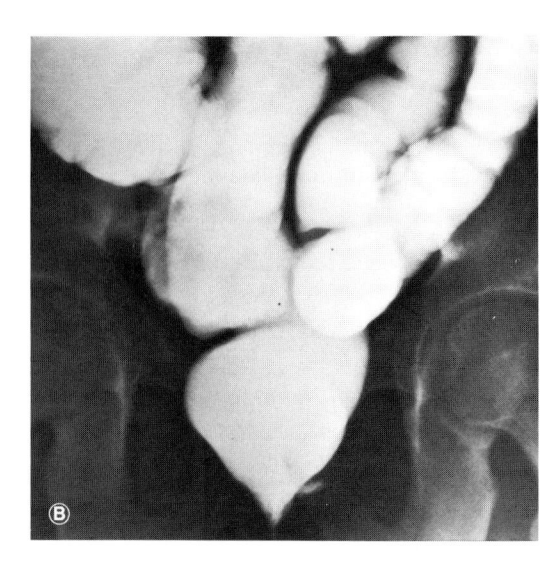

FIG. 20-90. A. Extensive CD in the jejunum and ileum with thickening of the folds, nodularity, and some narrowing of the lumen throughout much of the small intestine. B. The colon was normal except for a small sinus tract arising just proximal to the anal canal.

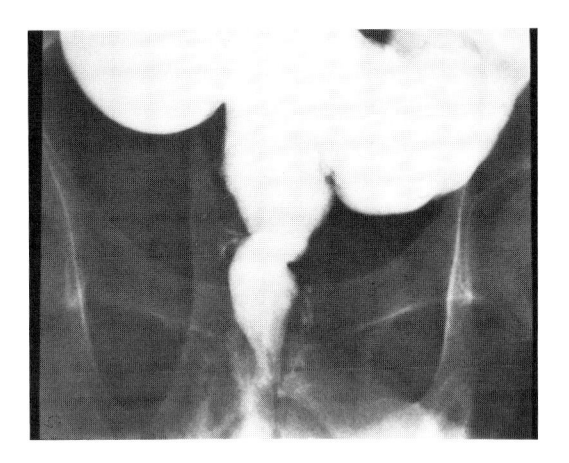

FIG. 20-91. Severe perianal disease associated with severe CD in the ileum.

nodular with the formation of visible ulcers on or adjacent to the nodules. The ulcers may widen and produce areas completely devoid of mucous membrane and mucosal pattern and, if annular, may resemble neoplasm. They also frequently deepen and communicate intramurally forming small fistulous tracts. This penetrating ulceration is always associated with thickening of the wall seen radiologically as separation of

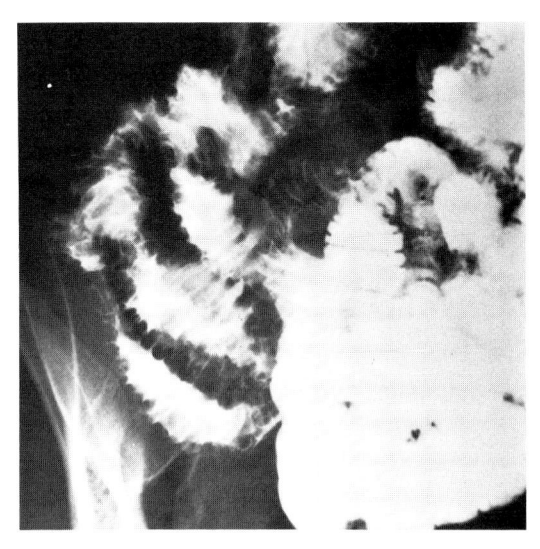

FIG. 20-92. Recurrent CD adjacent to an ileostomy after resection of terminal ileum and colon for severe disease.

the lumens of adjacent segments of opacified gut. The sense of mass involving the bowel wall and its adjacent mesentery is striking when palpating at fluoroscopy (Figs. 20-92 to 20-99).[26]

As in the colon, ulcers may perforate the bowel wall and form an abscess that may then, in turn, extend to adjacent organs such as the colon, other segments of small intestine, the uri-

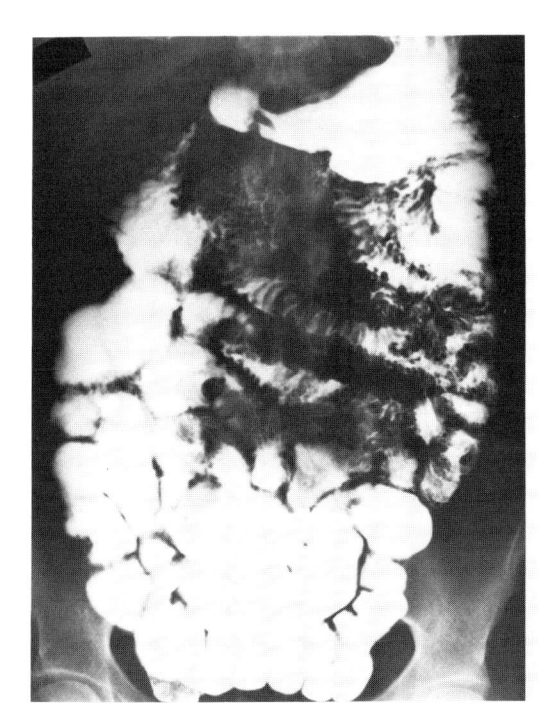

FIG. 20-93. Extensive CD involving almost the entire small intestine with thickening of the folds and scattered nodularity.

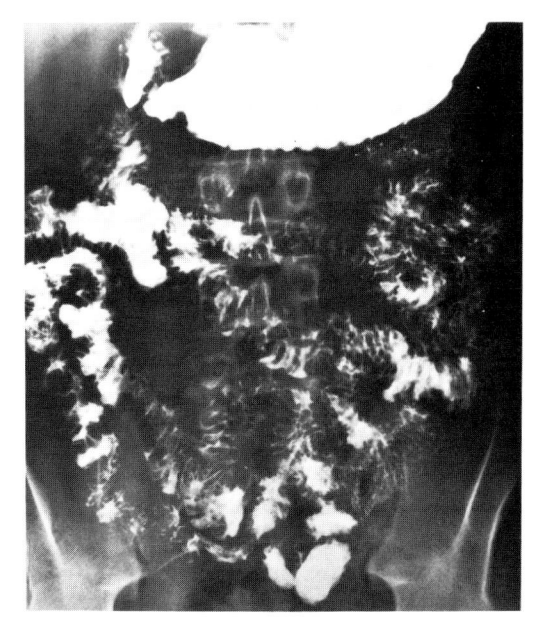

FIG. 20-94. Extensive CD in the jejunum and ileum with nodular mucosa and a few penetrating ulcers. The bowel was pliable with little mesenteric thickening.

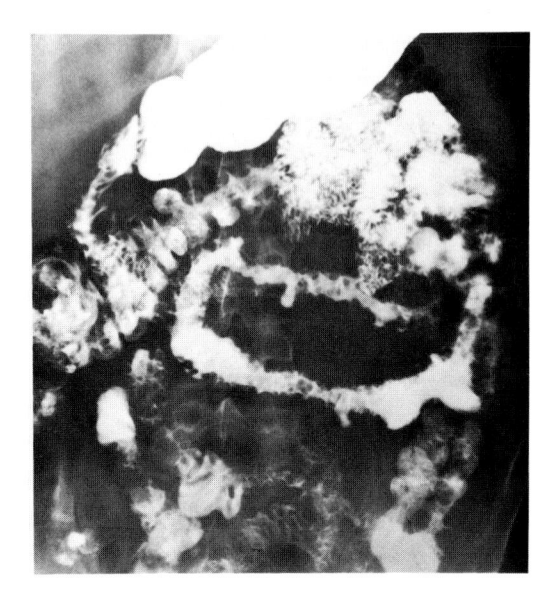

FIG. 20-95. Extensive CD of the jejunum and ileum with nodular mucosal surface, deep ulceration, pseudodiverticulae, strictures, and mesenteric thickening.

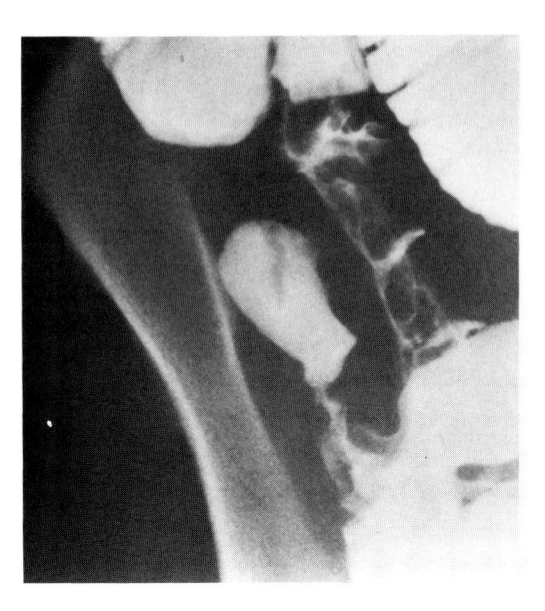

FIG. 20-97. Crohn's disease of the terminal ileum with nodular surface, deep ulceration, and a Meckel's diverticulum, the neck of which is also involved.

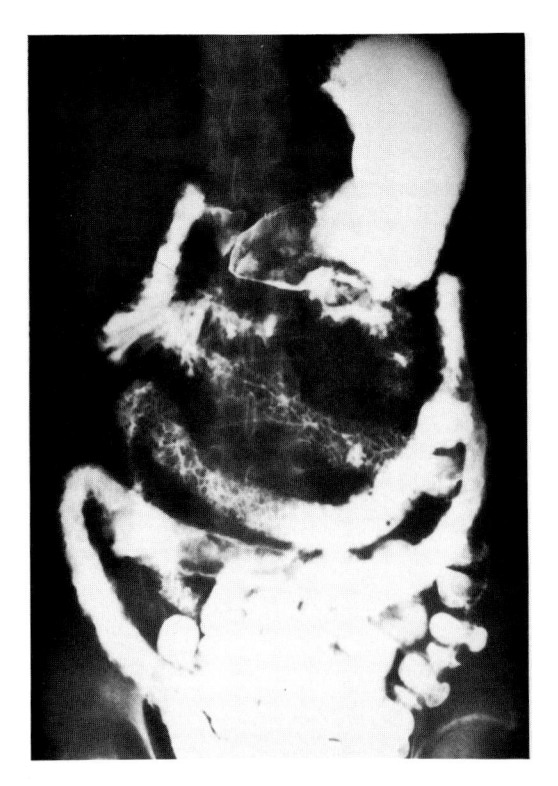

FIG. 20-96. Severe CD of almost the entire small intestine and right colon with extensive nodular mucosa, linear ulceration, and thickened mesentery.

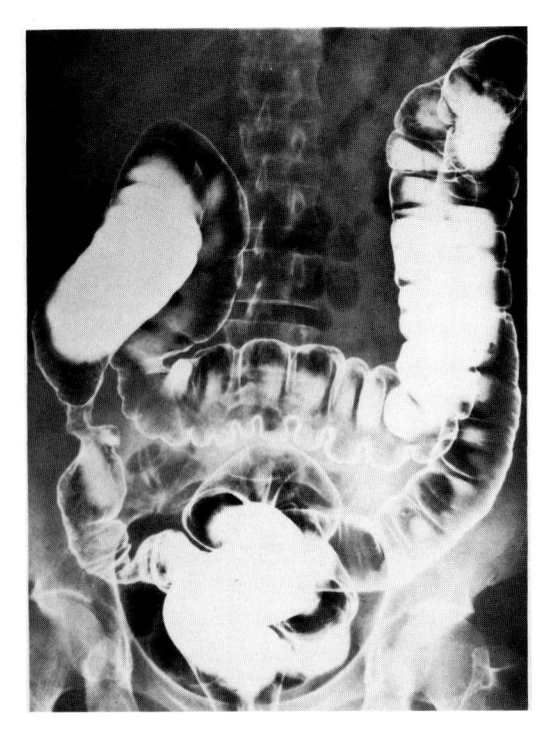

FIG. 20-98. Crohn's disease of the ileocecal region with obliteration of landmarks, stricture and fine, penetrating ulcers laterally, and a thin intramural fistulous tract medially.

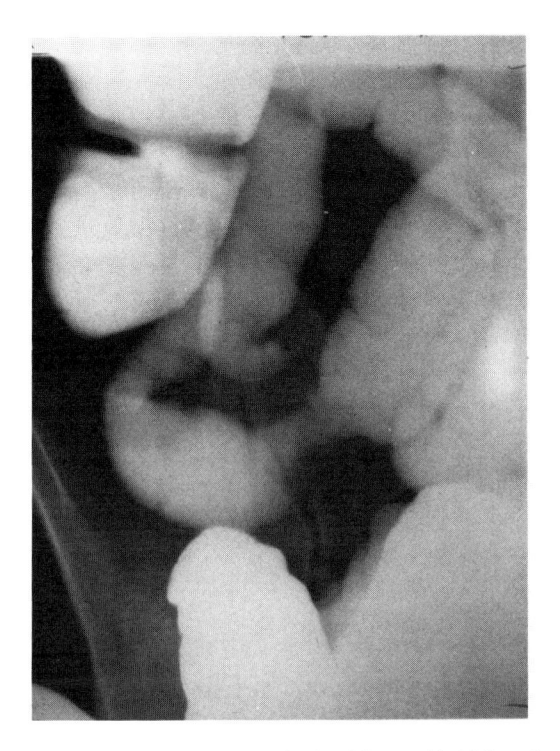

FIG. 20-99. Crohn's disease of the distal ileum with thickened folds and focal annular narrowing and flat ulceration resembling malignant neoplasm.

nary bladder, ureter or urethra, and, rarely, to the skin (Figs. 20-100 to 20-102).

The lumen is usually narrowed by this process, especially if it involves the entire circumference of the bowel wall. This annular narrowing can become severe and result in high-grade obstruction, which is one common indication for surgical intervention (Figs. 20-103 to 20-105). Often, however, the stricturing process is plaque-like and causes localized shortening with compensatory dilatation of the opposite wall, causing it to have the appearance of a broad diverticulum. This appearance, carefully looked for and clearly seen, is virtually pathognomonic of CD (Fig. 20-106). Sometimes symptoms and signs of CD are so vague and seemingly inconsequential that the patient first seeks medical attention because of obstruction.

Mild to moderate forms of CD occasionally return to normal, radiologically, when treated, but more often the changes are relatively stable or slowly progressive.

A fair correlation exists between the clinical estimate of severity of CD and the radiologic abnormalities seen. Those patients with extensive, severe abnormalities, such as obstruction caused by strictures or perforation with fistula or abscess, tend to be quite ill and many must be subjected to surgical treatment. This correlation is far from complete however, and many patients with profound findings on roentgenograms have relatively mild symptoms and maintain normal activity and nutrition (Figs. 20-107

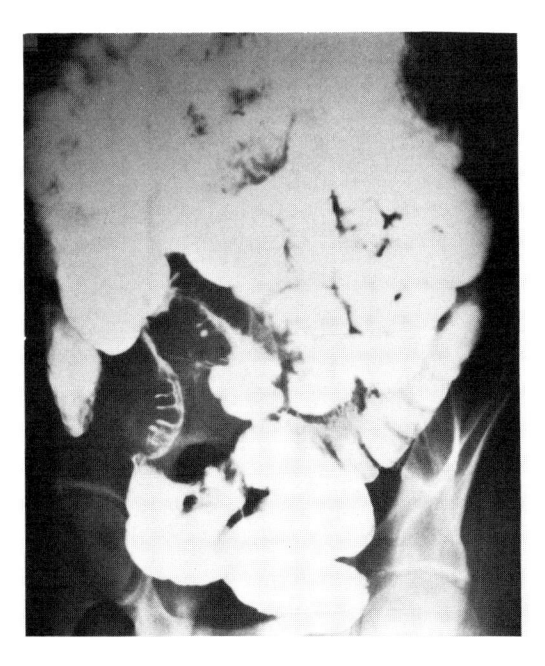

FIG. 20-100. Crohn's disease of the ileum with deep ulceration, and enteroenteric and enterocolic fistulae, as well as strictures and mesenteric thickening.

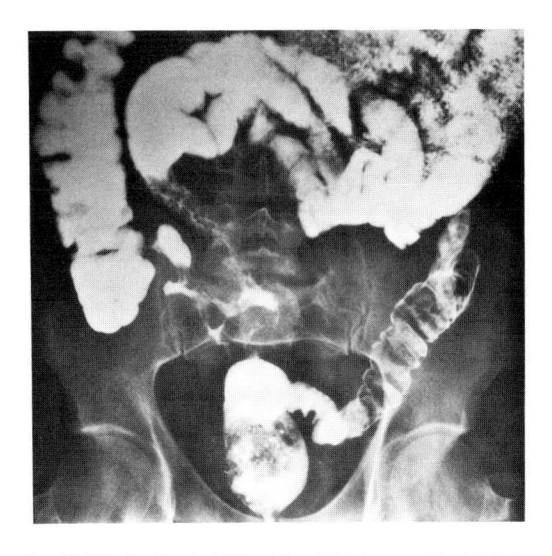

FIG. 20-101. Perforated CD of the distal ileum with fistula to the low sigmoid.

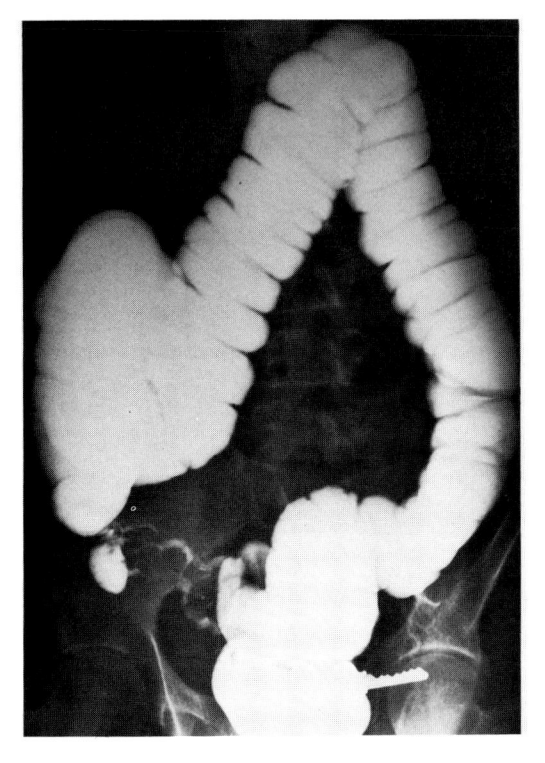

FIG. 20-102. Crohn's disease of the distal ileum and cecum with enteroenteric as well as enterocystic fistulae.

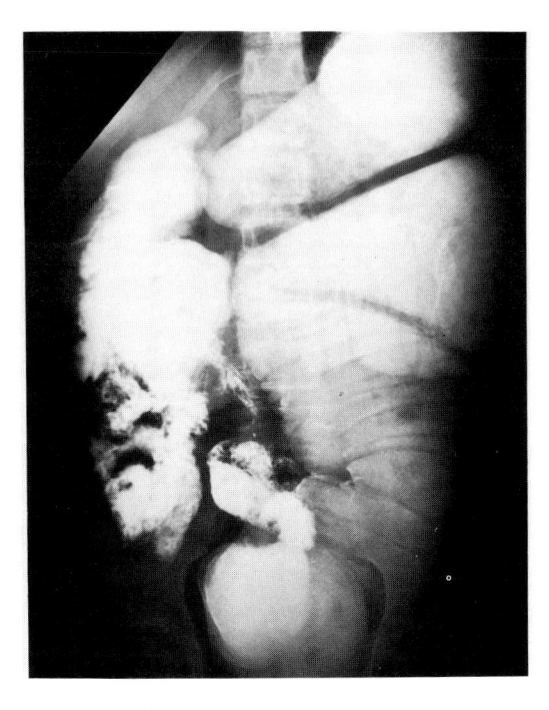

FIG. 20-103. High-grade obstruction of the jejunum caused by CD seen on prior examination.

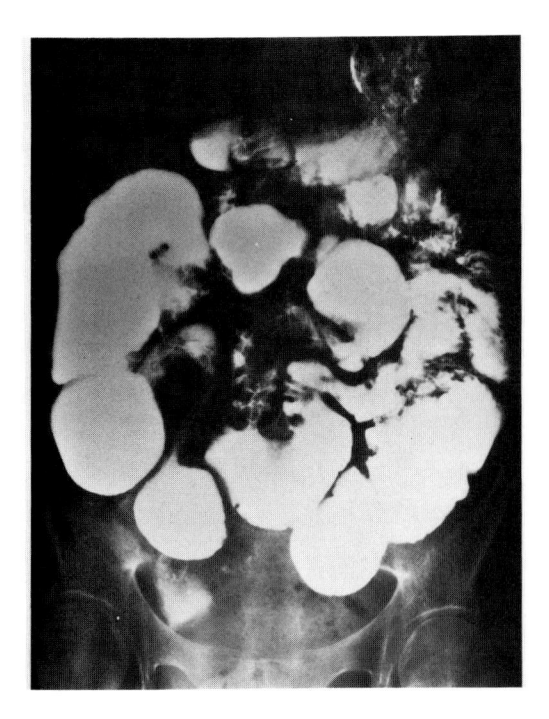

FIG. 20-104. Multiple high-grade strictures caused by CD, with progressive weight loss.

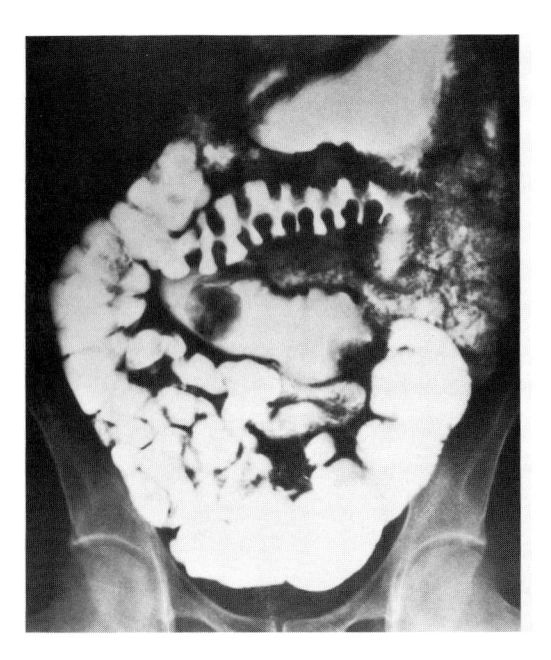

FIG. 20-105. High-grade stricture in the proximal ileum with enterolith caused by CD.

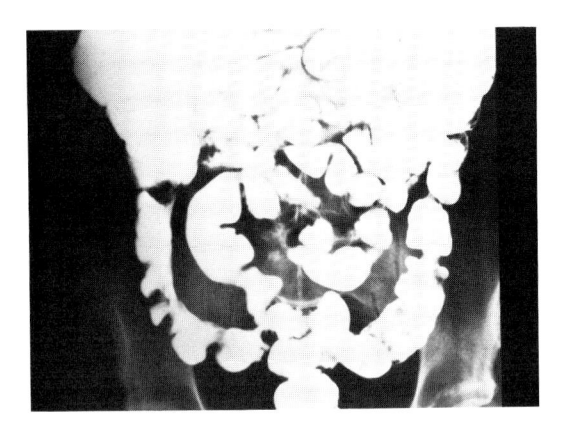

FIG. 20-106. Multiple strictures in the ileum caused by CD. Shortening and flat ulceration of one side of the bowel wall with pseudodiverticulae on the opposite wall.

and 20-108). This is especially true in recurrent CD after surgical resection.[27] It is common to find moderately severe disease in the ileum adjacent to an ileocolonic anastomosis in virtually asymptomatic patients (Figs. 20-109 and 20-110). Periodic x-ray examination of patients with relatively mild and stable clinical situations, in whom the diagnosis is already clear, probably

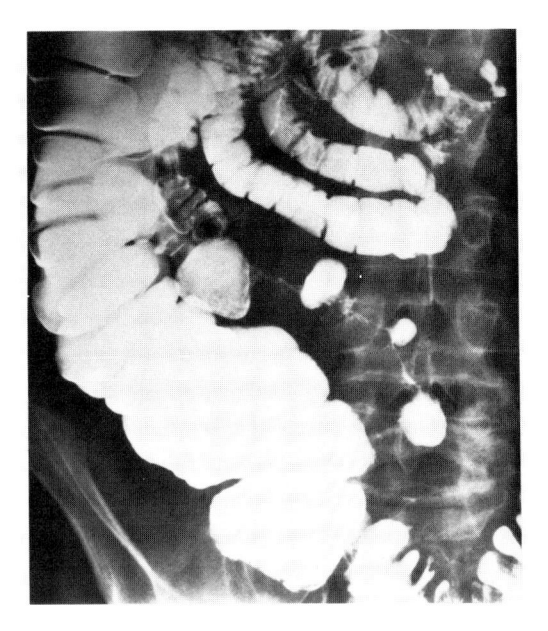

FIG. 20-108. Unsuspected CD involving the terminal ileum in a 75-year-old male who had a barium enema because of change in bowel habit.

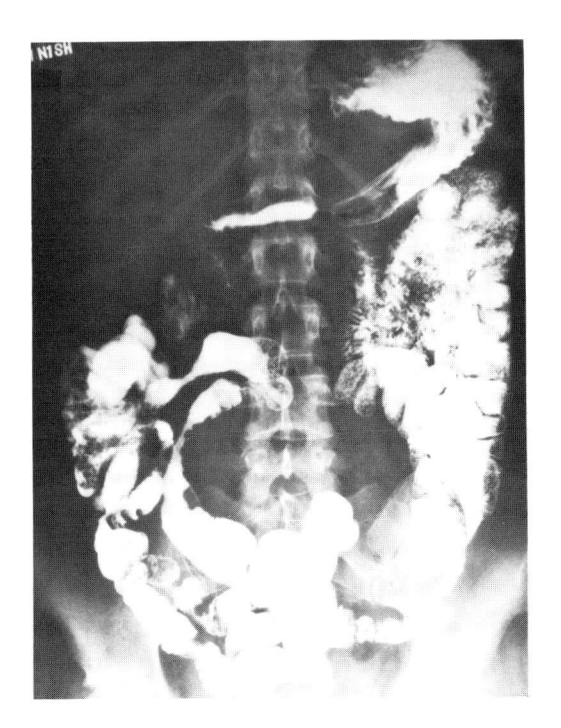

FIG. 20-107. Virtually asymptomatic regional enteritis with multiple strictures discovered during surgical treatment for gallstones and confirmed by roentgenogram.

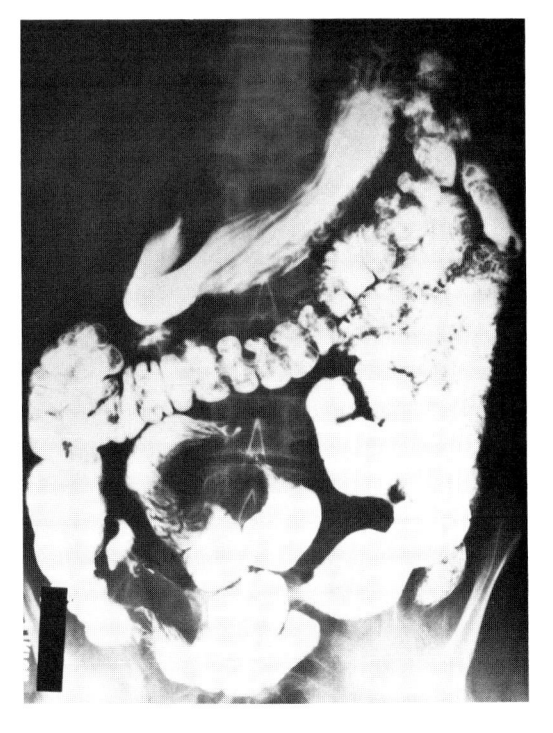

FIG. 20-109. Recurrent CD in the ileum after resection with multiple strictures and moderate obstruction. Few symptoms were present.

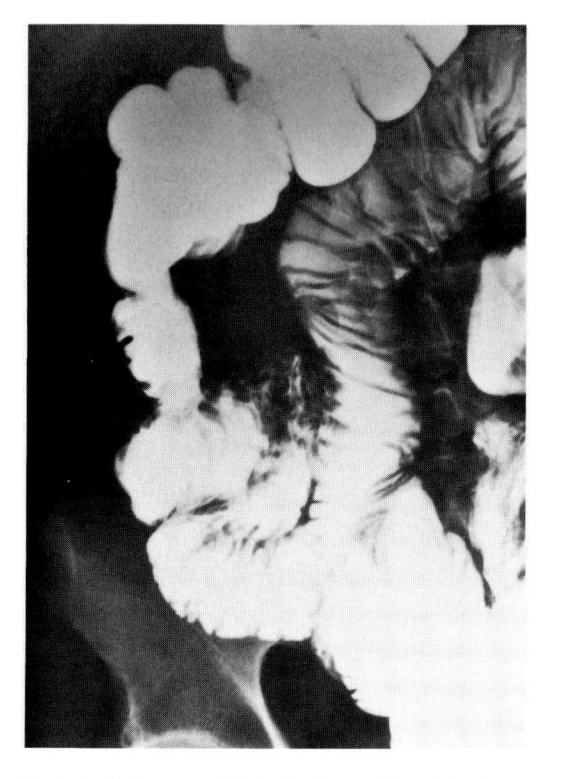

FIG. 20-110. Recurrent CD in the ileum adjacent to ileoascending colostomy with diffuse, flat ulceration and rigidity of the medial wall, and intact mucosa on the opposite wall. Few symptoms of active disease were present.

semble CD of moderate severity with a nodular surface, the sharply circumscribed extramucosal nodules of lymphoma without small area ulceration are usually distinctive. Today, with careful fluoroscopy and with CT available to study the mesentery and the retroperitoneal nodes, it should rarely be necessary to surgically explore the abdomen in order to make a precise and confident diagnosis.[28] Ischemia and other processes that result in irregular necrosis and stricture formation, such as rare cases of sprue or radiation damage, can be difficult to distinguish from CD, and only the examination of the resected specimen by an experienced pathologist may settle the diagnosis (Figs. 20-111 to 20-114). Occasionally, metastatic neoplasm, including carcinoid, may resemble CD (Figs. 20-115 and 20-116). Computerized tomography should be helpful in the distinction of these conditions. Of course, tuberculosis can completely mimic CD, and only bacteriologic studies can distinguish them (Figs. 20-117 and 20-118).

The Esophagus, Stomach, and Duodenum

Severe involvement of the stomach and duodenum is quite uncommon, and that of the esophagus, rare. Either single or double contrast meth-

fulfills no urgent need. One gets the impression that such examinations are often requested to satisfy the curiosity of the patient and referring physician about the state of the disease process. But that, of course, is a valuable function of any physician's consultation.[16]

DISTINCTION FROM OTHER DISEASES

Crohn's disease involving the small intestine is usually readily distinguishable from other diseases. The findings of flat ulceration with contracture and pseudodiverticulum formation, or deep, penetrating ulcers with nodular mucosal surface and fine-tract fistulae, often with a patchy distribution, are virtually pathognomonic of CD. Of course, these changes must be recognized and translated into pathologic terms. The most common question raised is that of lymphoma, sometimes by radiologists who seem to be under the impression that every case of regional enteritis that they encounter could, in reality, be lymphoma. While it is true that diffuse nodular lymphoma of the small bowel can re-

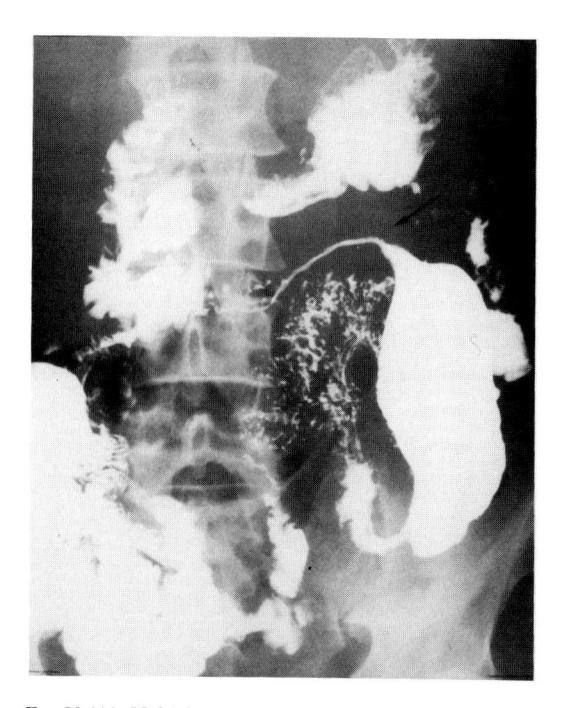

FIG. 20-111. Multiple strictures (arrow) and mucosal ulceration secondary to emboli.

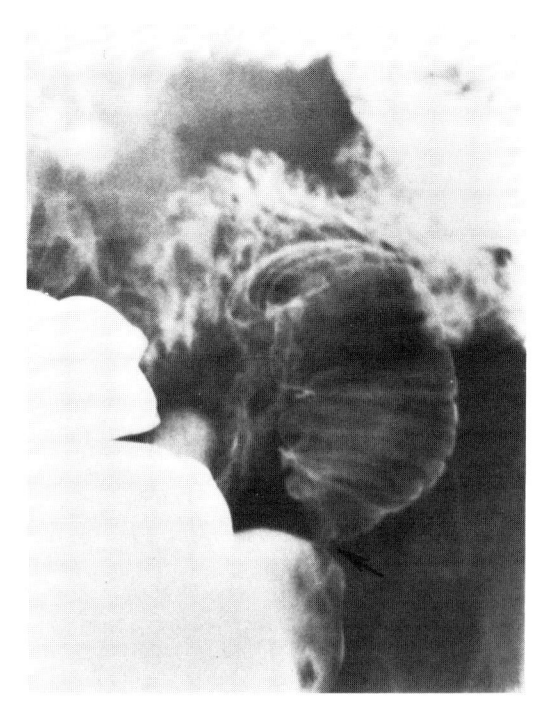

FIG. 20-112. Nonspecific stricture (arrow) and mucosal ulceration, probably caused by ischemia.

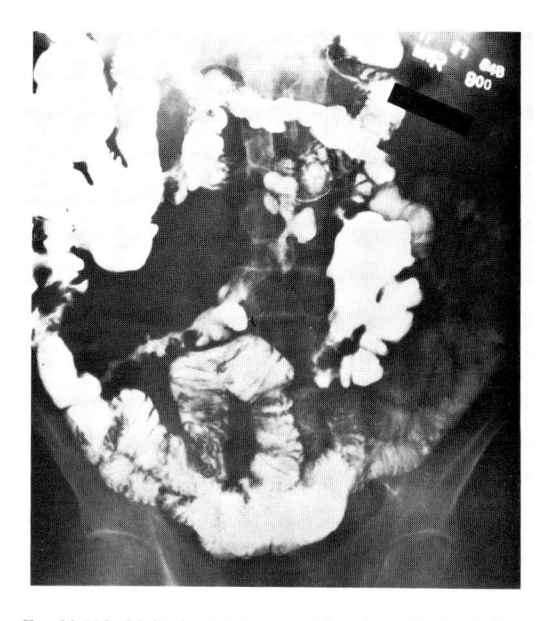

FIG. 20-113. Multiple strictures and flat ulceration in the jejunum with pseudodiverticula associated with long-standing sprue. No evidence of CD existed in resected specimen.

ods can be used to detect and identify the pathologic changes and, if appropriately used, are sensitive.

The least severe changes seen in the stomach and duodenum are thick folds, some stiffening upon palpation at fluoroscopy, and, occasionally, small discrete ulcer craters. These abnormalities are usually confined to the distal stomach, pyloric canal, and duodenum. Larger ulcer craters can be seen in the duodenal bulb especially, and the appearance is that of peptic ulceration. In more severe disease, the lumen of this segment may become generally narrow, and the gross landmarks of the gastric antrum, pyloric canal, and the duodenal bulb disappear. Motor activity also virtually disappears in this area of severe involvement. Diffuse severe involvement of this junctional zone has a distinctive appear-

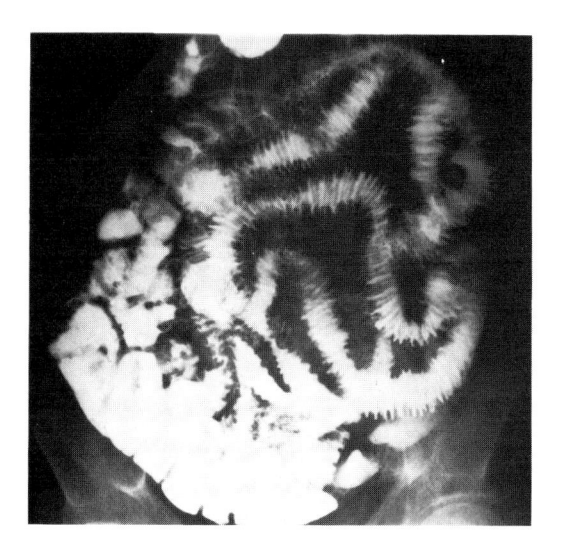

FIG. 20-114. Diffuse thickening of mucosal folds following therapeutic radiation.

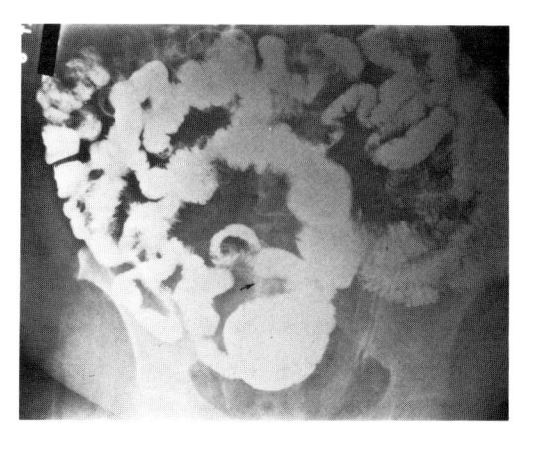

FIG. 20-115. Metastatic carcinoid tumor with extramucosal narrowing and fixation (arrow). The dilated bowel proximal to this has areas of thickened folds suggestive of CD. Thickening of the mesentery occurred in this case because of metastasis.

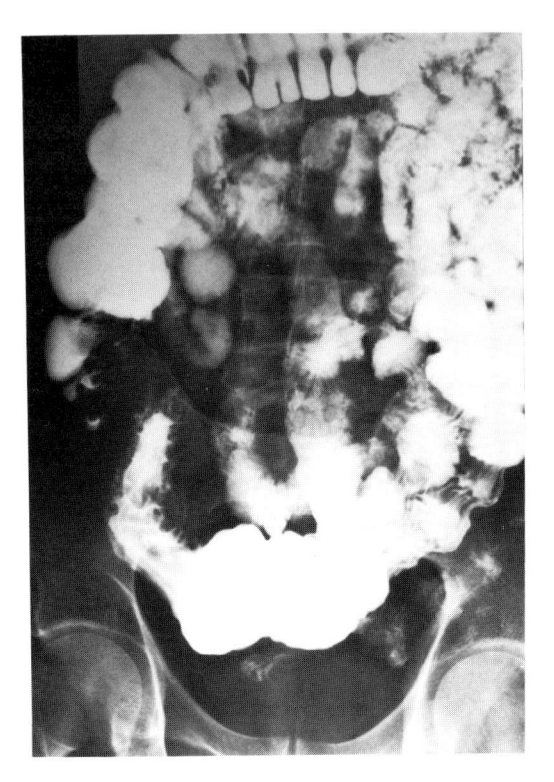

Fig. 20-116. Carcinoid tumor in the distal ileum with mesenteric metastasis causing partial obstruction, and a nodular mucosal surface in the distal ileum resembling CD.

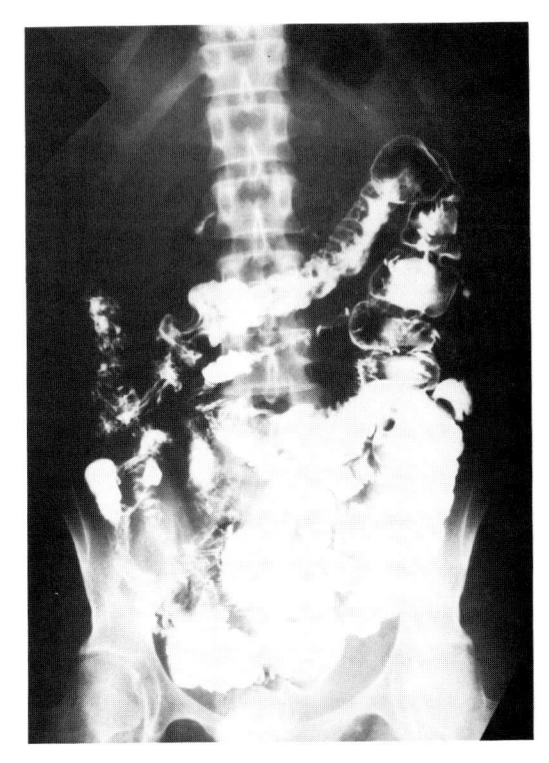

Fig. 20-117. Tuberculosis involving multiple segments of distal ileum with nodular surface, ulceration, and strictures.

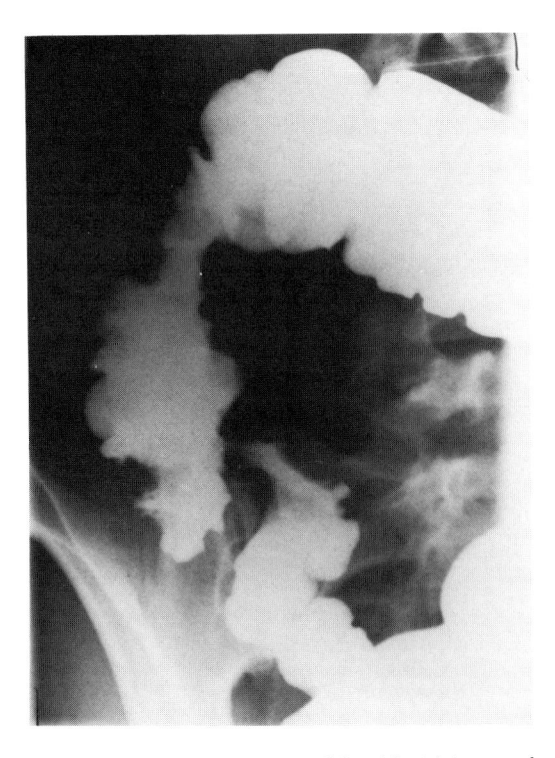

Fig. 20-118. Tuberculous enterocolitis with strictures and nodular mucosal surface.

ance seen in almost no other condition. The duodenum may become narrow and be partially obstructed, sometimes requiring surgical bypass. If the region of the papilla is affected, there may be reflux of barium into the bile duct and pancreatic duct.[29,30] Deep, penetrating ulceration and fistulae do not seem to occur in the stomach and duodenum (Figs. 20-119 to 20-127). In order to make a confident diagnosis of CD of the stomach and duodenum, as well as the esophagus, one must find characteristic disease in the intestine.[31-33] Biopsy of these upper tract lesions is usually not diagnostic. Although metastatic neoplasm and eosinophilic gastroenteritis can closely resemble CD in this region, the lack of characteristic CD distally, together with history and examination of the peripheral blood, promptly resolves the questions (Fig. 20-128).

The findings in the esophagus are somewhat distinctive, either penetrating ulceration with dissection within the wall along the long axis, or thickened folds with linear ulceration between them. Realistically, only when these are found in patients with established CD in the intestine will the diagnosis probably be made radiologically (Figs. 20-129 to 20-131).[34]

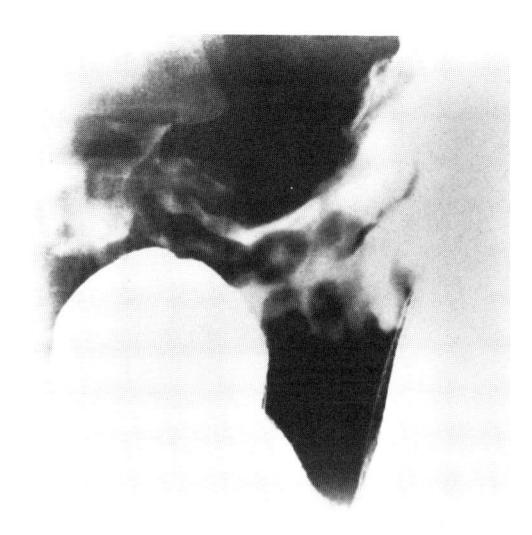

FIG. 20-120. Crohn's disease of the stomach with prominent nodular antral folds and shallow ulcers, and also CD in the colon.

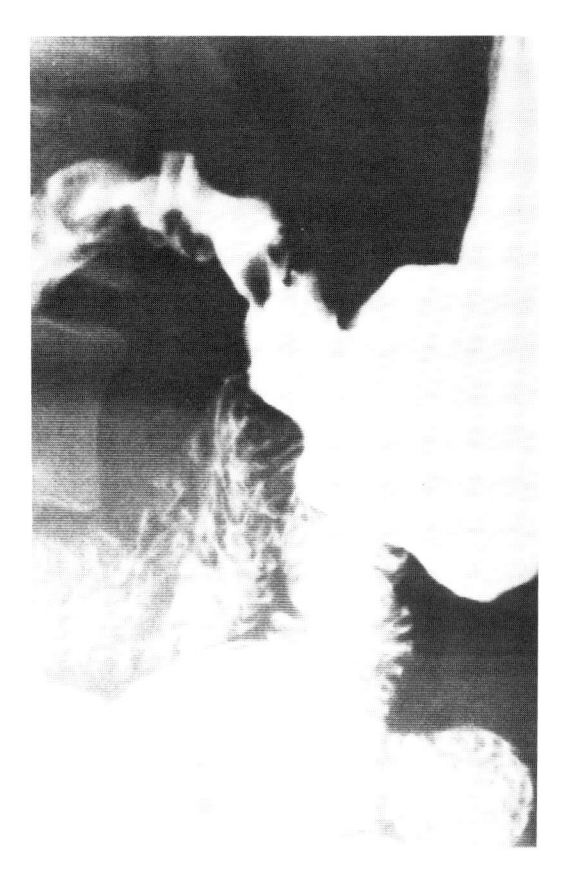

FIG. 20-119. Deformity and somewhat nodular mucosa in the distal antrum, pyloric canal, and proximal duodenum that is probably CD. Prior resection of the ileocecal region had to be done for obstructing regional enteritis.

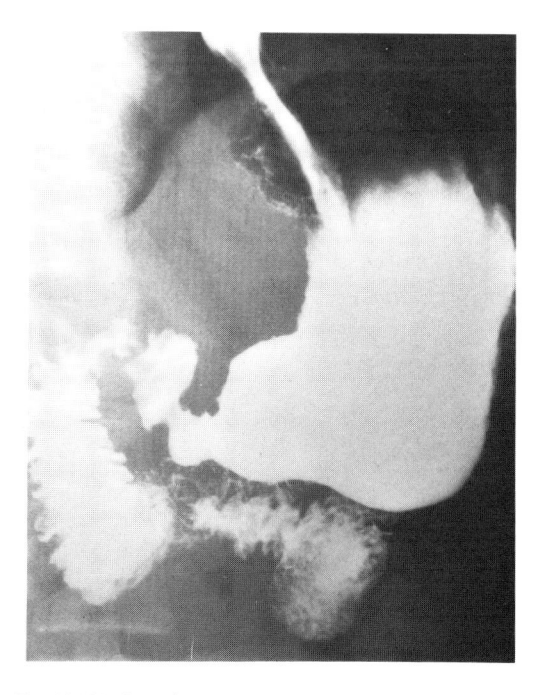

FIG. 20-122. Crohn's disease of the distal stomach with narrowing and finely irregular mucosal surface.

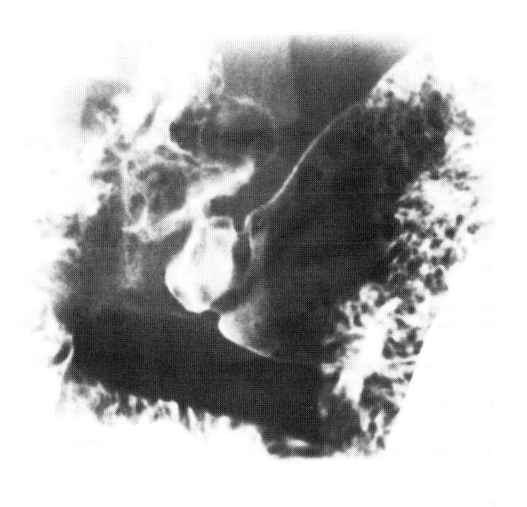

FIG. 20-121. Crohn's disease of the distal stomach with deformity and nodular antral folds and tiny superficial ulcers. CD in the mid-ileum.

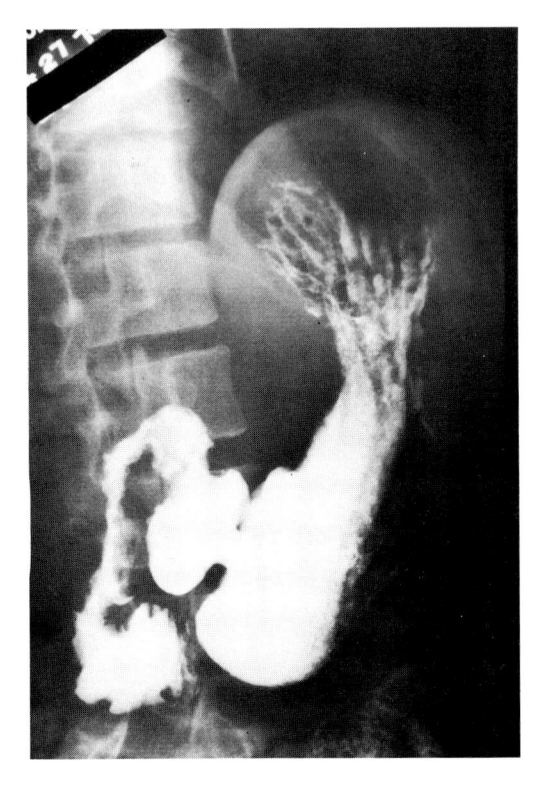

FIG. 20-123. Crohn's disease of the pyloric canal and proximal half of duodenum.

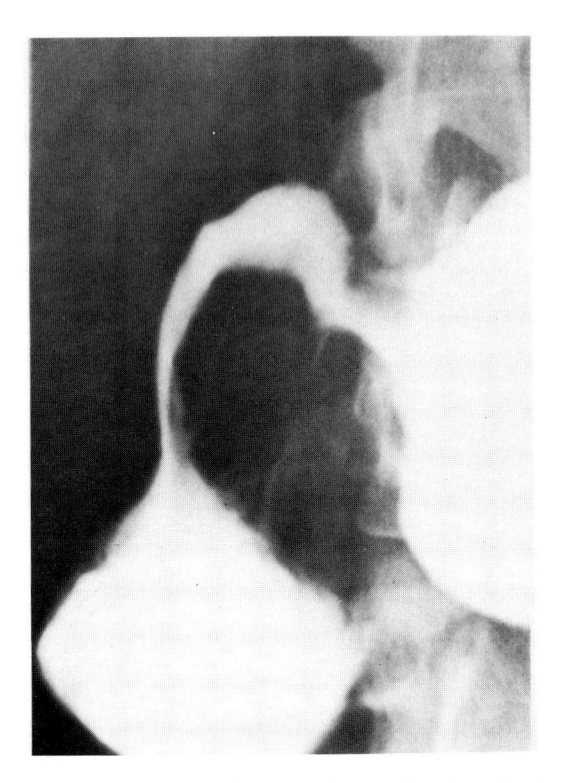

FIG. 20-125. Advanced CD of distal stomach and proximal duodenum with pronounced narrowing and smooth mucosal surface.

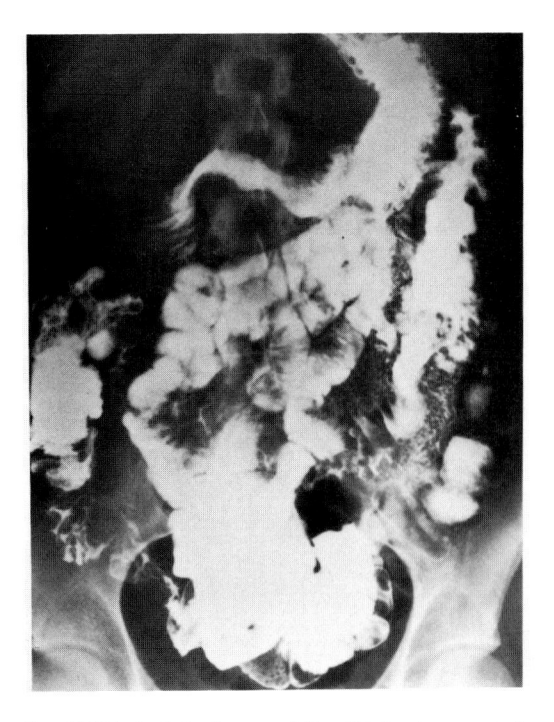

FIG. 20-124. Crohn's disease of the distal antrum, pyloric canal, and proximal duodenum with loss of landmarks and smooth mucosal surface together with extensive, severe disease in the small intestine.

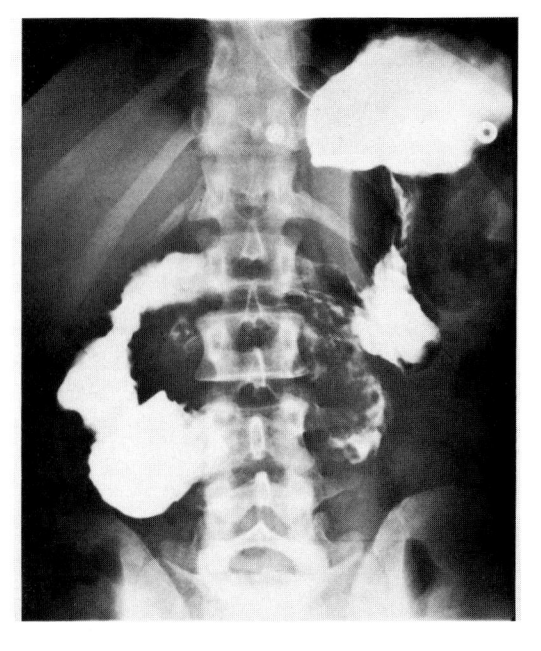

FIG. 20-126. Crohn's disease in the duodenum with thickened, irregular folds and narrowing of the second and third portions.

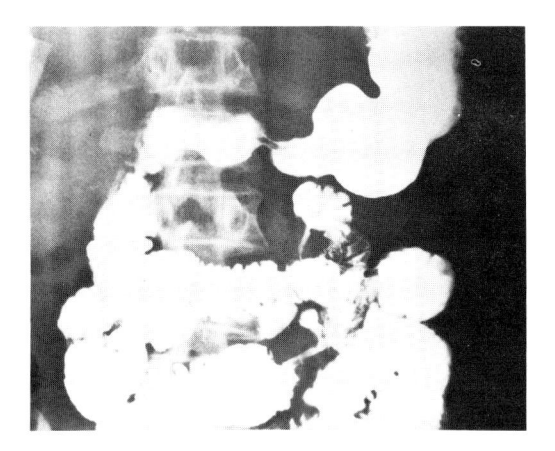

FIG. 20-127. Crohn's disease of the duodenum with focal narrowing of the second portion and more severe narrowing of the distal duodenum and proximal jejunum. Slight irregularity of the lesser curvature of the distal antrum.

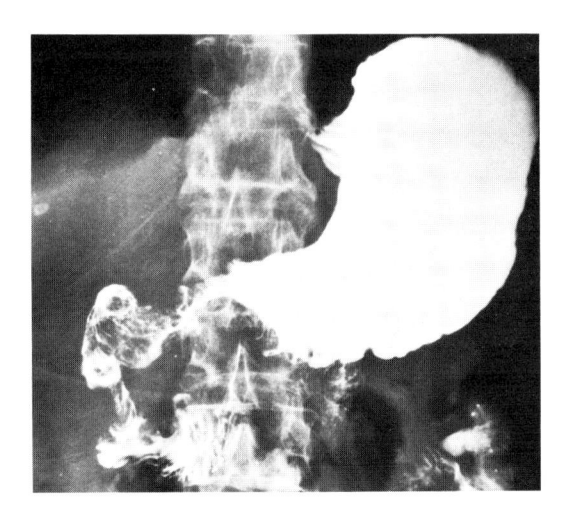

FIG. 20-128. Deformity of the distal antrum and proximal duodenum caused by extramucosal metastatic carcinoma of the breast. This distribution of pathologic change resembles CD.

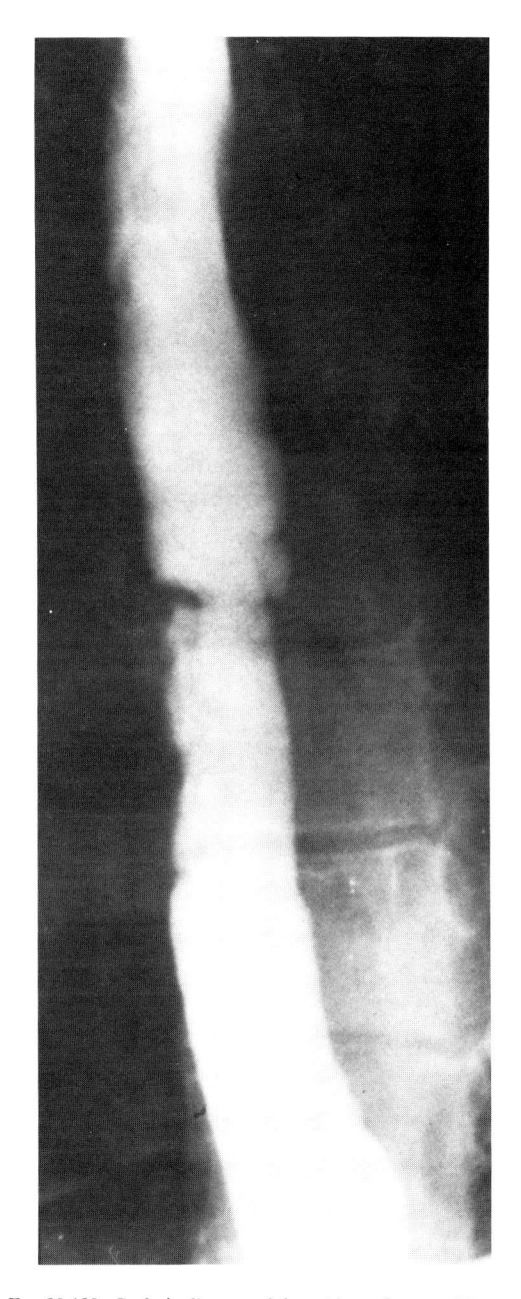

FIG. 20-129. Crohn's disease of the mid-esophagus with narrowing and deep ulceration.

Carcinoma and Crohn's Disease*

The carcinogenic effect of Crohn's disease is definite.[35] Such patients have about twenty times as much intestinal cancer as the general population. It occurs in areas actively involved with inflammatory change. Although it is rarely found at an early stage, the radiologist should be aware of the possibility of cancer if he encounters unusually severe localized deformity. The actual prevalence of this complication is so low, however, that periodic surveillance, radiologically, is not reasonable, nor is prophylactic resection of diseased intestine.

*See Chapter 15.

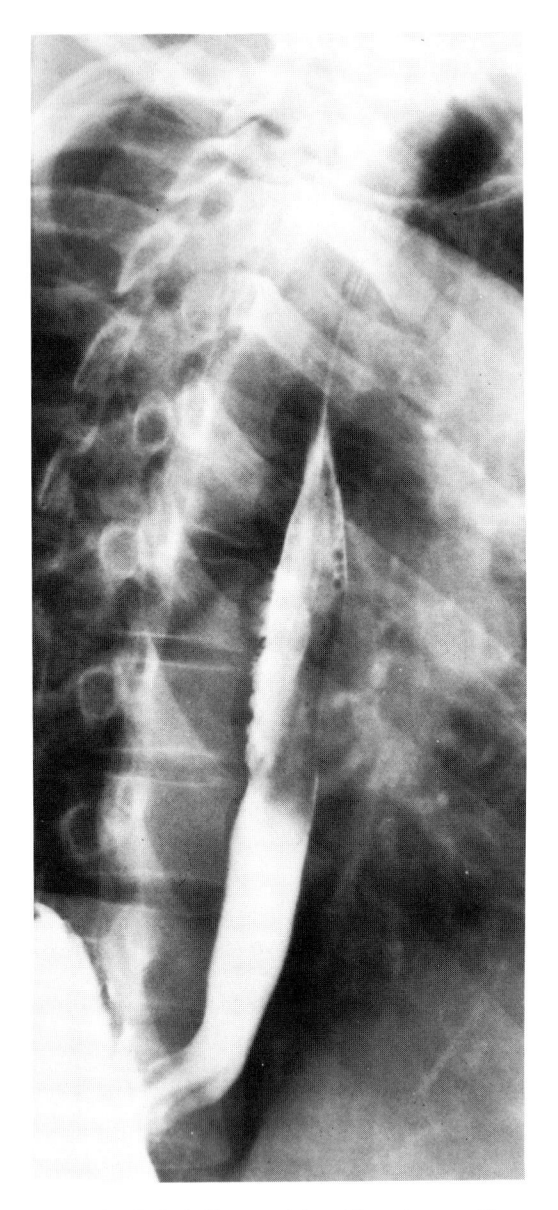

FIG. 20-130. Crohn's disease of the mid-esophagus with extensive irregular ulceration.

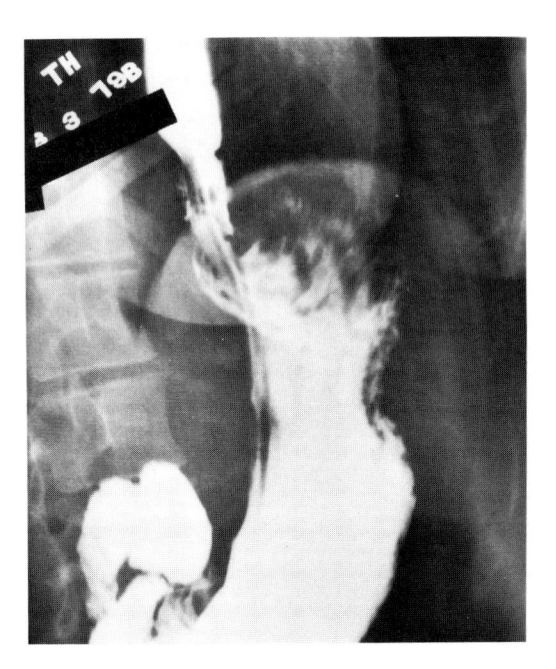

FIG. 20-131. Crohn's disease of the distal esophagus with ulceration and some narrowing.

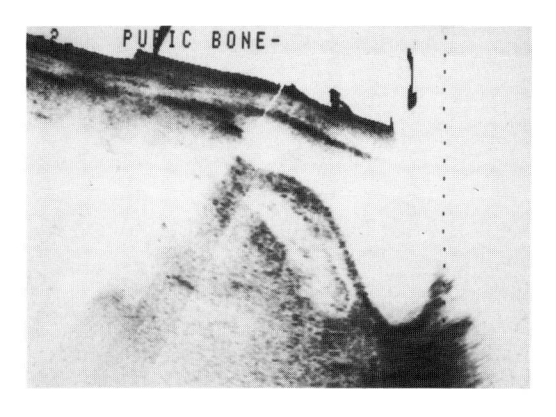

FIG. 20-132. Crohn's disease of the sigmoid colon seen behind the urinary bladder on ultrasound in a young patient with lower abdominal pain.

Methods of Detecting Inflammatory Bowel Disease and Associated Disorders

Ultrasound

This modality is rarely capable of precise identification of IBD, but patients of two varieties are seen with some frequency by the ultrasonographer: 1) the patient with vague, uncharacteristic abdominal complaints in whom ultrasound (US) is used as an extension of the physical examination in an attempt to "rule out" organic disease; and 2) the patient with known IBD in whom perforation and abscess is suspected and US is called upon to detect the presence of such a process and localize it. Involved bowel can be seen in cross section or longitudinal section as a narrow central core of highly echogenic mucous membrane, surrounded by a thick inflamed wall of much lower echogenicity (Fig. 20-132). Often, thickened mesentery of moderate echogenicity separates this segment from other structures. Fluid filled echolucent bowel can be recognized

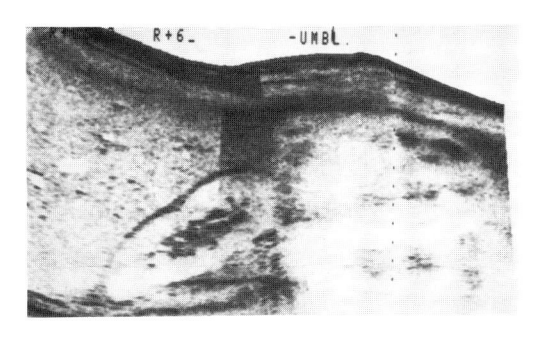

FIG. 20-133. Recurrent CD of the small intestine seen on ultrasound as fluid filled segments of bowel separated by echogenic tissue.

in obstruction (Fig. 20-133), and a matted mass of disorganized variable echogenicity can be seen in the presence of perforation and multiple fistulae. This is similar to the findings in abscess formation.[36-37]

Ultrasound can measure the actual thickness of bowel wall but this is not a particularly useful capacity in the diagnosis and management of IBD at this time.[38]

In patients with jaundice associated with IBD, US can assess the state of liver parenchyma and measure the caliber and configuration of bile ducts in order to exclude focal duct obstruction and proximal dilatation caused by stone or tumor.

Computerized Tomography

As with US, computerized tomography (CT) is usually useful in patients with uncharacteristic abdominal or systemic complaints in undiagnosed Crohn's disease, and in those with possible perforation and abscess as a complication of IBD, especially Crohn's disease. Because these abnormalities can be encountered in undiagnosed patients, the radiologist must be aware of characteristic findings and diagnostic possibilities.

The gut lumen should be opacified by the oral administration of a rather large volume of dilute soluble iodinated contrast medium or by giving it as an enema to visualize the rectum and colon. Computerized tomography produces a more graphic record of cross-sectional pathologic anatomy than does ultrasound, and more precisely determines the relationship of the gut lumen to pathologic processes involving the bowel wall, mesentery, and abdominal spaces. Characteristically, in CD, the lumen is seen as a narrow fluid-filled structure often with proximal dilatation surrounded by a thick bowel wall and an increased amount of tissue surrounding the wall. This tissue has varying density depending upon the relative amount of fat and edema and cellular infiltrate in it. The presence of gas indicates infection with abscess formation (Figs. 20-134 to 20-136).[39-41]

Computerized tomography can be used to perform guided abscess drainage, but this is usually a temporary measure because surgical extirpation of the underlying bowel perforation is often necessary for a satisfactory result. In a pa-

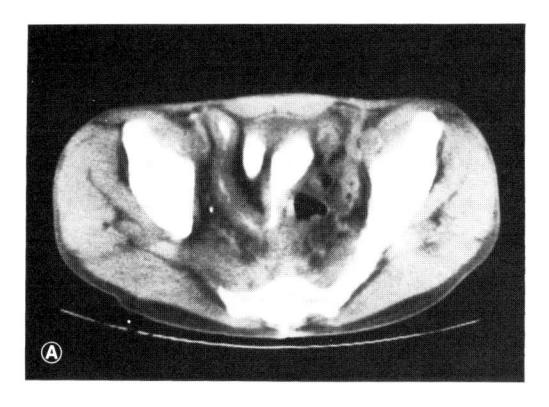

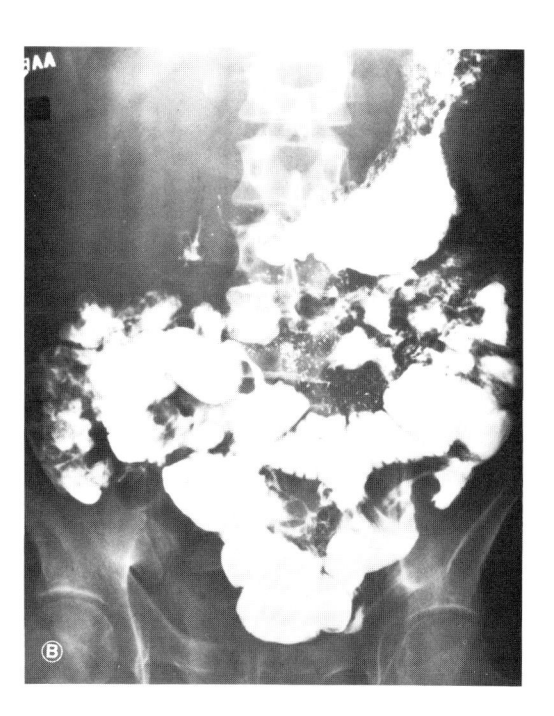

FIG. 20-134. A. Computed tomography showing CD of the ileum with thickened wall and narrowed lumen causing partial obstruction. A presacral mass containing gas is present (abscess). B. Barium examination of the small intestine confirms the CT findings and demonstrates enteroenteric fistulae.

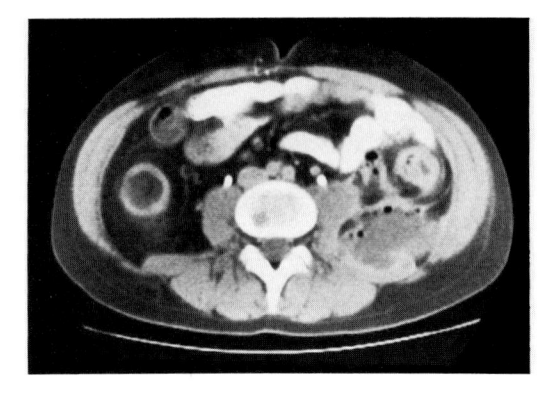

Fig. 20-136. Computed tomography shows CD involving the entire colon with perforation of descending colon and a retroperitoneal abscess.

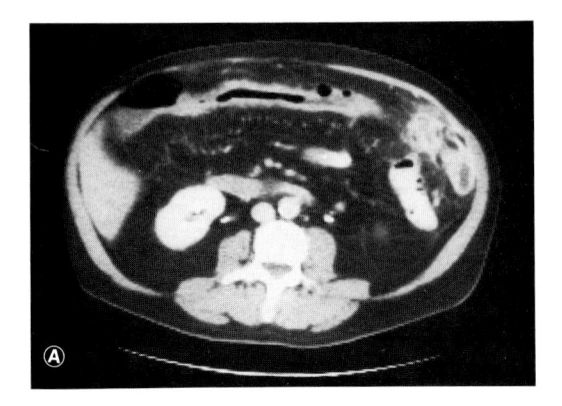

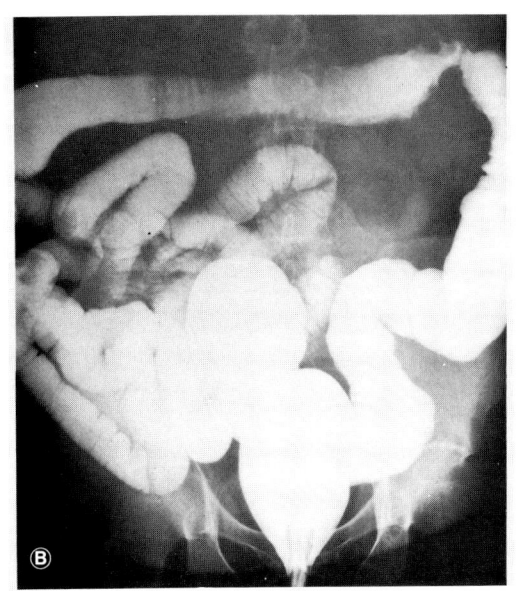

Fig. 20-135. A. Computed tomography showing CD in the transverse colon with thickened walls and lack of haustration. B. Barium enema and subsequent surgical treatment confirmed these findings.

tient with septicemia, however, abscess drainage guided by CT can bring about a prompt and safe resolution of a dangerous circumstance.

Sclerosing Cholangitis*

Sclerosing cholangitis occurs commonly in association with IBD. Rarely, it is the first manifestation of these associated diseases. Such patients commonly have clinical episodes of cholangitis or have abnormal liver function tests indicating bile duct obstruction with or without clinical jaundice. Retrograde cholangiography through an endoscope is the preferred method of study, but if this fails or if the common bile duct has high-grade obstruction, percutaneous transhepatic cholangiography can be used.

Characteristically, the entire bile duct system is irregular with focal narrowing and slight intervening dilatation. The intrahepatic tributaries opacified are reduced in number and the branching takes on an angular pattern rather than a normal smooth flowing together of ducts (Figs. 20-137 and 20-138). Rarely, the common duct is not visibly abnormal and the overall pattern then resembles the cholangiographic findings in severe primary biliary cirrhosis.[42,43]

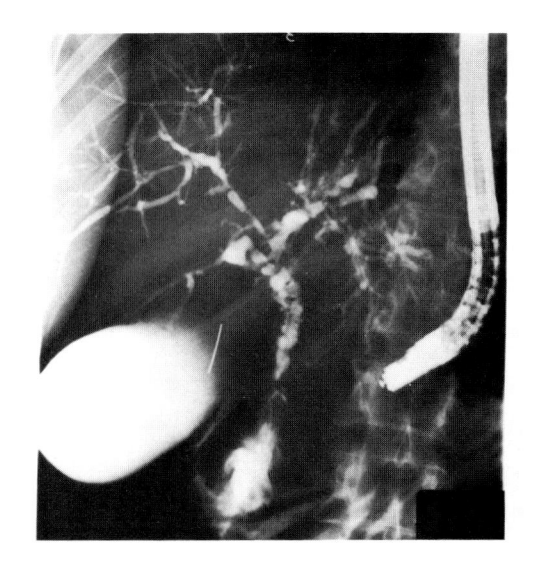

Fig. 20-137. Chronic ulcerative colitis associated with sclerosing cholangitis showing focal band strictures in the common duct and diffuse involvement of the intrahepatic ducts with retrograde cholangiogram.

*See Chapter 16.

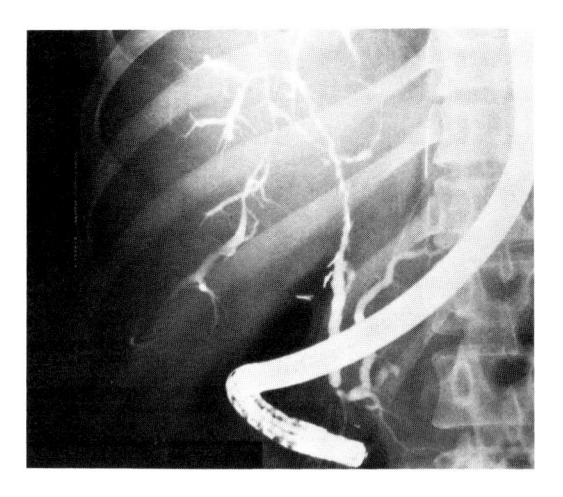

FIG. 20-138. Sclerosing cholangitis associated with CUC shown by retrograde cholangiogram.

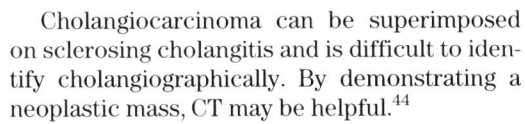

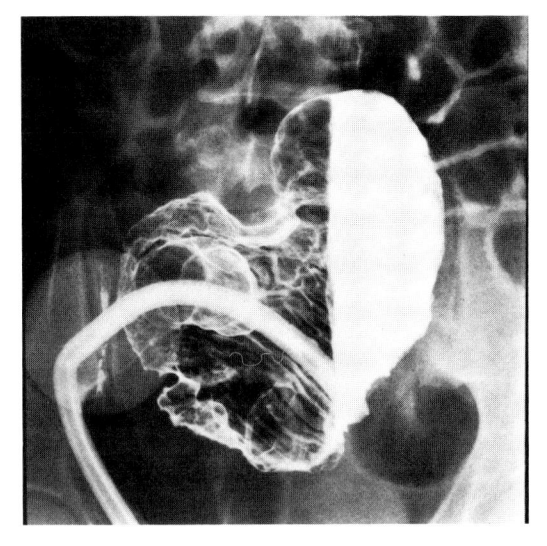

FIG. 20-139. Normal Kock pouch with nipple.

Cholangiocarcinoma can be superimposed on sclerosing cholangitis and is difficult to identify cholangiographically. By demonstrating a neoplastic mass, CT may be helpful.[44]

Because sclerosing cholangitis is so diffuse, relief of obstruction is not successful. Occasionally, however, if there is relatively focal high-grade duct obstruction, transhepatic catheter internal drainage or balloon dilitation can be helpful in the relief of symptoms.

Angiography

Angiography probably has a minor role in the detection and identification of IBD. If, however, a patient is examined for sustained, brisk intestinal hemorrhage to localize the site and possibly treat the hemorrhage with vasoconstricting drugs, the angiographer may see hypervascularity of the bowel wall. Recognition of this pattern as suggestive of IBD may affect the management of the patient including the planning of appropriate surgical intervention.[45]

The Continent Ileostomy*

Total proctocolectomy not only "cures" ulcerative colitis, but obviously it also eliminates the significant threat of colonic cancer.

ILEAL POUCH

With a valve produced by a retrograde intussusception of the efferent loop surgically fixed within its cavity, the ileal pouch has been used for a number of years to improve the quality of life for such patients and make colectomy more acceptable. It may eliminate the necessity for a stomal bag and allow periodic emptying by means of a catheter. Such pouches can become incontinent, develop fistulae or inflammatory disease, or the patient may have difficulty pass-

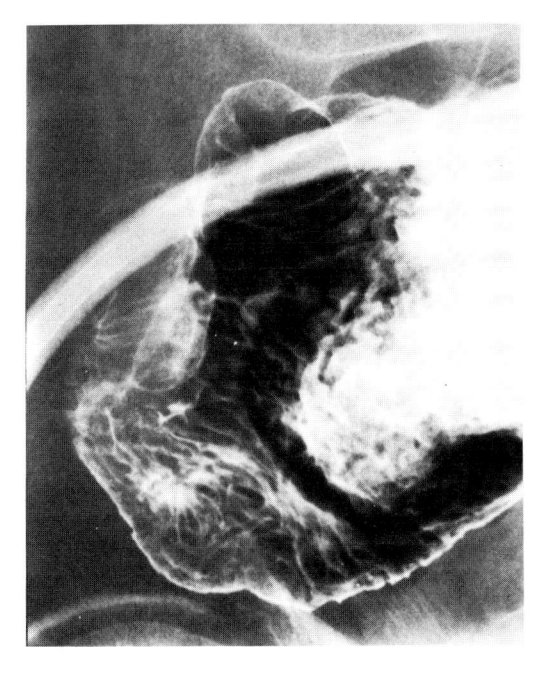

FIG. 20-140. Incontinent Kock pouch with partially reduced nipple.

*See Chapter 29.

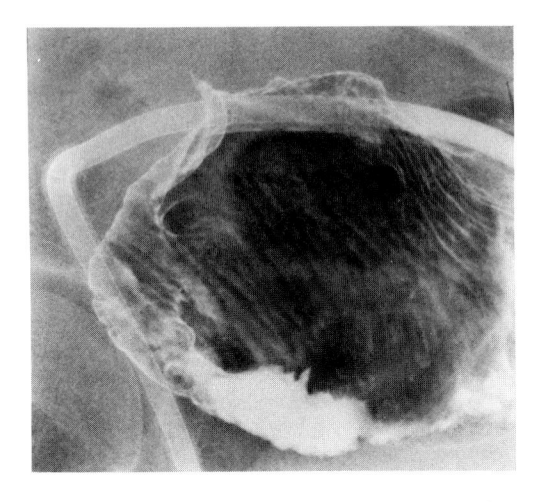

FIG. 20-141. Incontinent Kock pouch caused by completely reduced nipple.

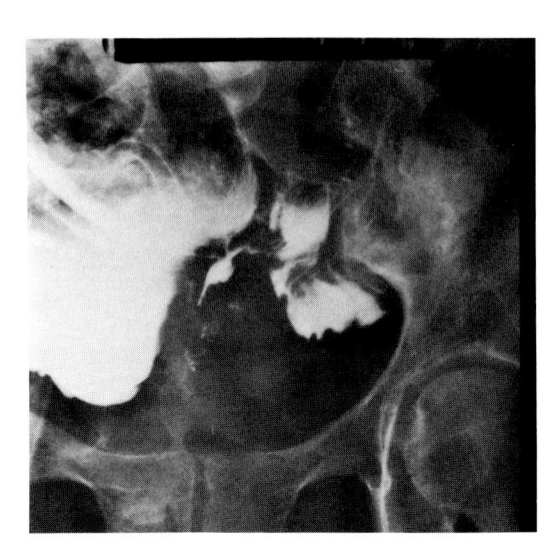

FIG. 20-142. Recurrent CD in a Kock pouch with fistula between the pouch and the afferent loop.

ing a catheter into the pouch. These complications require x-ray examination to detect reduction of the valve, the formation of fistulae, the development of diffuse or focal enteritis, or an abnormal course of the efferent segment. Single contrast injection of the segment between the skin opening and the pouch will identify kinks in this segment that may make catheterization difficult. Then, passage of a catheter followed by injection of dense barium and air allow double contrast examination of the valve nipple, the pouch itself, and the ileum leading into the pouch. The use of horizontal beam films with the patient on his back, sides, and standing usually results in a vivid display of anatomy (Figs. 20-139 to 20-143).[46]

ILEOANAL ANASTOMOSIS

This has become more widely used than the pouch in recent years. In these patients the radiologist is called upon to examine the region of the anastomosis several weeks postoperatively in order to be sure that the anastomosis is firm and that no fistulae or sinuses involving the

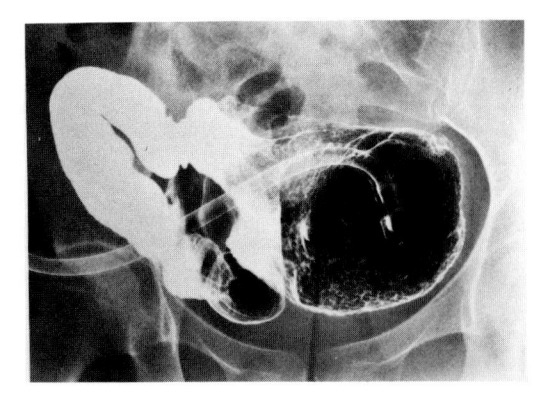

FIG. 20-143. Kock pouch with diffuse inflammatory involvement of the pouch. No evidence of Crohn's disease exists away from the pouch.

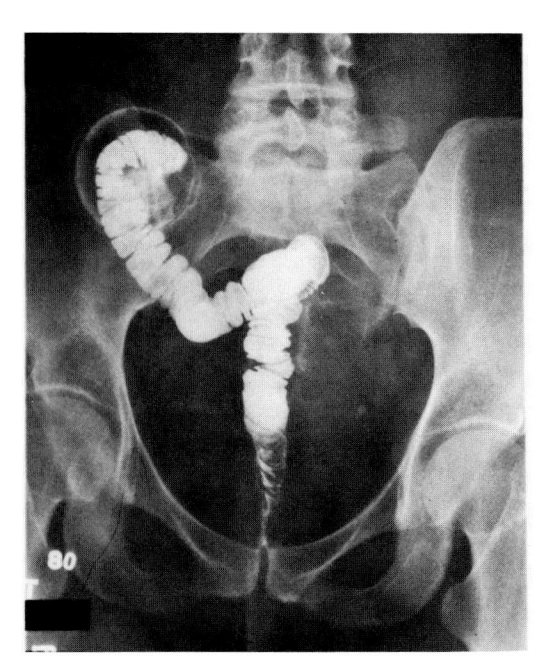

FIG. 20-144. Normal ileoanal anastomosis.

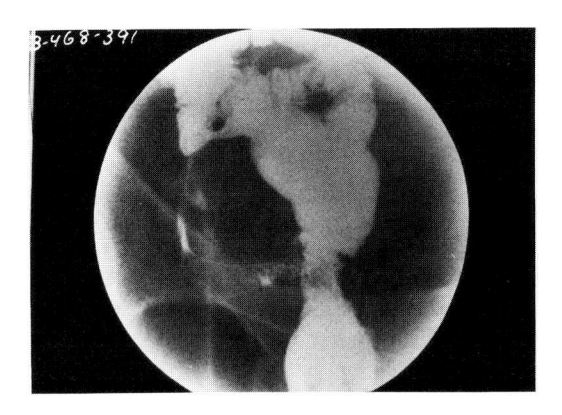

FIG. 20-145. Ileoanal anastomosis nine months after total colectomy for CUC showing persistent sinus tract arising from just above the anastomosis.

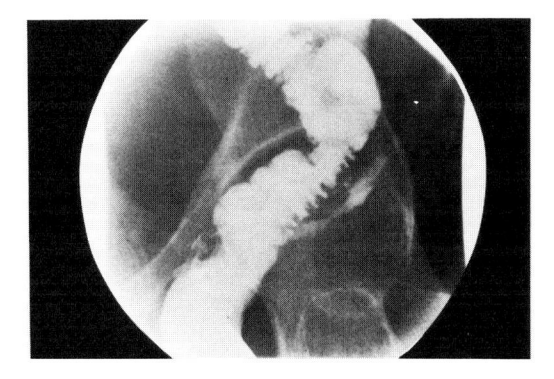

FIG. 20-146. Sinus tract after ileoanal anastomosis for CUC.

anastomosis or pouch are present. Single contrast examination under fluoroscopic control, with films made in the frontal and lateral positions with the bowel filled and also following evacuation, is the most effective procedure. If all is normal, the diverting ileostomy can be closed. If an anastomotic leak or fistula is found, additional time for healing or surgical correction may be necessary (Figs. 20-144 to 20-146).[47,48]

References

1. Gabrielsson, N., Granqvist, S., Sundelin, P., and Thorgeirsson, T.: Extent of inflammatory lesions in ulcerative colitis assessed by radiology, colonoscopy, and endoscopic biopsies. Gastrointest. Radiol., 4:395, 1979.
2. Williams, H. J. Jr., Stephens, D. H., and Carlson, H. C.: Double-contrast radiography: colonic inflammatory disease. Am. J. Radiol., 137:315, 1981.
3. Fork, F. T., Lindstrom, C., and Ekelund, G.: The double contrast examination in inflammatory large bowel disease. Fortschr. Rontgenstr., 137:685, 1982.
4. Winthrop, J. D., et al.: Ulcerative and granulomatous colitis in children. Radiology, 154:657, 1985.
5. Herlinger, H.: The small bowel enema and the diagnosis of Crohn's disease. Radiol. Clin. North. Am., 20:721, 1982.
6. Carlson, H. C.: Perspective: The small bowel examination in the diagnosis of Crohn's disease. Am. J. Radiol., 147:63, 1986.
7. Johnson, C. D., Carlson, H. C., Taylor, W. F., and Weiland, L. P.: Barium enemas of carcinoma of the colon: sensitivity of double- and single-contrast studies. Am. J. Radiol., 140:1143, 1983.
8. Blum, J. C., and Kelvin, F. M.: Radiologic spectrum of polypoid lesions in ulcerative colitis and Crohn's disease. South. Med. J., 74:850, 1981.
9. Deuroede, G. J., et al.: Cancer risk and life expectancy of children with ulcerative colitis. N. Engl. J. Med., 285:17, 1971.
10. James, E. M., and Carlson, H. C.: Chronic ulcerative colitis and colon cancer: can radiographic appearance predict survival patterns? Am. J. Radiol., 130:825, 1978.
11. Kelvin, F. M., et al.: Prospective diagnosis of dysplasia (precancer) in chronic ulcerative colitis. Am. J. Radiol., 138:347, 1982.
12. Kollitz, J. P. M., Davis, G. B., and Berk, R. N.: Campylobacter colitis: a common infectious form of acute colitis. Gastrointest. Radiol., 6:227, 1981.
13. Loughran, C. F., Tappin, J. A., and Whitehouse, G. H.: The plain abdominal radiograph in pseudomembranous colitis due to clostridium difficile. Clin. Radiol., 33:277, 1982.
14. Rimmer, M. J., Freeman, A. H., and Low, F. M.: The barium enema diagnosis of penicillin associated colitis. Clin. Radiol., 33:529, 1982.
15. Strada, M., Meregaglia, D., and Donzelli, R.: Double-contrast enema in antibiotic-related pseudomembranous colitis. Gastrointest. Radiol., 8:67, 1983.
16. Goldberg, H. I., Caruthers, S. B. Jr., Nelson, J. A., and Singleton, J. W.: Radiographic findings of the national cooperative Crohn's disease study. Gastroenterology, 77:925, 1979.
17. DuBrow, R. A., and Frank, P. H.: Barium evaluation of anal canal in patients with inflammatory bowel disease. Am. J. Radiol., 140:1151, 1983.
18. Joffe, N.: Radiographic appearances and course of discrete mucosal ulcers in Crohn's disease of the colon. Gastrointest. Radiol., 5:371, 1980.
19. Joffe, N.: Diffuse mucosal granularity in double-contrast studies of Crohn's disease of the colon. Clin. Radiol., 32:85, 1981.
20. Marshak, R. H., et al.: Longitudinal sinus tracts in granulomatous colitis and diverticulitis. Semin. Roentgenol., 11:101, 1976.
21. Hoshino, M., et al.: A clinical study of tuberculous colitis. Gastroenterol. Jpn., 14:299, 1979.
22. Sider, L., et al.: Radiographic findings of infectious proctitis in homosexual men. Am. J. Radiol., 139:667, 1982.
23. Max, R. J., and Kelvin, F. M.: Nonspecificity of discrete colonic ulceration on double-contrast barium enema study. Am. J. Radiol., 134:1265, 1980.
24. Nolan, D. J., and Gourtsoyiannis, N. C.: Crohn's disease of the small intestine: a review of the radiological appearances in 100 consecutive patients examined by a barium infusion technique. Clin. Radiol., 31: 597, 1980.
25. Ekberg, O., Baath, L., Sjostrom, B., and Lindhagen, T.: Are superficial lesions of the distal part of the ileum early in-

dicators of Crohn's disease in adult patients with abdominal pain? A clinical and radiologic long term investigaion. Gut, 25:341, 1984.
26. Nolan, D. J., and Piris, J.: Crohn's disease of the small intestine: a comparative study of the radiological and pathological appearances. Clin. Radiol., 31:591, 1980.
27. Ekberg, O., Fort, F. T., and Hildell, J.: Predictive value of small bowel radiography for recurrent Crohn disease. Am. J. Radiol., 135:1051, 1980.
28. Sartoris, D. J., Harell, G. S., Anderson, M. F., and Zboralske, F. F.: Small-bowel lymphoma and regional enteritis: radiographic similarities. Radiology, 152:291, 1984.
29. Legge, D. A., Carlson, H. C., and Hoffman, H. N. II: A roentgenologic sign of regional enteritis of the duodenum. Radiology, 100:37, 1971.
30. Barthelemy, C. R.: Crohn's disease of the duodenum with spontaneous reflux into the pancreatic duct. Gastrointest. Radiol., 8:319, 1983.
31. Legge, D. A., Carlson, H. C., and Judd, E. S.: Roentgenologic features of regional enteritis of the upper gastrointestinal tract. Am. J. Radiol., 110:355, 1970.
32. Miller, E. M., Moss, A. A., and Kressel, H. Y.: Duodenal involvement with Crohn's disease: a spectrum of radiographic abnormality. Am. J. Gastroenterol., 71:107, 1979.
33. Gray, R. R., St. Louis, E. L., and Grosman, H.: Crohn's disease involving the proximal stomach. Gastrointest. Radiol., 10:43, 1985.
34. Ghahremani, G. G., Gore, R. M., Breuer, R. I., and Larson, R. H.: Esophageal manifestations of Crohn's disease. Gastrointest. Radiol., 7:199, 1982.
35. Weedon, D. D., et al.: Crohn's disease and cancer. N. Engl. J. Med., 289:1099, 1973.
36. Sonnenberg, A., Erckenbrecht, J., Peter, P., and Niederau, C.: Detection of Crohn's disease by ultrasound. Gastroenterology, 83:430, 1982.
37. Yeh, H. C., and Rabinowitz, J. G.: Granulomatous enterocolitis: findings by ultrasonography and computed tomography. Radiology, 149:253, 1983.
38. Dubbins, P. A.: Ultrasound demonstration of bowel wall thickness in inflammatory bowel disease. Clin. Radiol., 35:227, 1984.
39. Goldberg, H. I., et al.: Computed tomography in the evaluation of Crohn disease. Am. J. Radiol., 140:277, 1983.
40. Frager, D. H., Goldman, M., and Beneventano, T. C.: Computed tomography in Crohn disease. J. Comput. Assist. Tomogr., 7:819, 1983.
41. Frick, M. P., Salomonowitz, E., and Gedgaudas, E.: The value of computed tomography in Crohn's disease. Mt. Sinai. J. Med., 51:368, 1984.
42. MacCarty, R. L., LaRusso, N. F., Wiesner, R. H., and Ludwig, J.: Primary sclerosing cholangitis: findings on cholangiography and pancreatography. Radiology, 149:39, 1983.
43. Kolmannskog, F., et al.: Cholangiographic findings in ulcerative colitis. Acta Radiol. (Diagn.), 22:151, 1981.
44. McCarty, R. L., et al.: Cholangiocarcinoma complicating primary sclerosing cholangitis: cholangiographic appearances. Radiology, 156:43, 1985.
45. Tsuchiya, M., et al.: Angiographic evaluation of vascular changes in ulcerative colitis. Angiology, 31:147, 1980.
46. Stephens, D. H., Mantell, B. E., and Kelly, K. A.: Radiology of the continent ileostomy. Am. J. Radiol., 132:717, 1979.
47. Kremers, P. W., et al.: Radiology of the ileoanal reservoir. Am. J. Radiol., 145:559, 1985.
48. Hillard, A. E., Mann, F. A., Becker, J. M., and Nelson, J. A.: The ileoanal J pouch: radiographic evaluation. Radiology, 155:591, 1985.

Section 6 · *Therapy*

21 · Medical Therapy in Ulcerative Colitis

STEPHEN B. HANAUER, M.D.
JOSEPH B. KIRSNER, M.D., PH.D.

While the cause and the medical cure for ulcerative colitis (UC) continue to elude investigators, the majority of patients with the disease will benefit from prolonged medical therapy. The broad range of clinical patterns and the variable responses to therapy preclude a "routine" approach. Rather, each patient must be assessed individually as to the status of the inflammatory bowel disease, complications, response to prior therapies, and the impact of the illness on lifestyle as a basis for a comprehensive program directed to individual problems and needs.

The physician approaching the medical treatment of UC must recognize the nonspecific nature of the current medical armamentarium. While sulfasalazine and corticosteroids are the mainstays of present therapy, neither deals with a known specific pathogenetic mechanism. Additional elements of treatment also are nonspecific but substantially improve symptoms and therefore, are helpful clinical adjuvants. Furthermore, when confronted with the inability to cure the disease with a potent, yet potentially harmful medical regimen (e.g., steroids), the physician also must consider the option of a surgical approach, especially in patients who fail to respond, suffer significant complications related to therapy, develop intercurrent complications from the disease, or who can no longer cope with the uncertainties and/or limitations upon their lifestyle.

The doctor usually will be working within the extremes of the spectrum (effective therapy versus inability to cure), but must be able to contend with both the frequent and rare contingencies that occur when dealing with a chronic, potentially physically debilitating, or even life-threatening condition such as ulcerative colitis.

Evaluation of the Patient

General Principles

While ulcerative colitis remains a distinct pathophysiologic entity, many of the clinical and pathologic findings are mimicked by other disorders (Table 21-1). In addition to careful review of the diagnosis (see Chap. 8 and 10), potentially exacerbating conditions should be identified. Regular review of the patient's status is important to update the effectiveness of medical therapy, avoid or recognize complications of the disease or its treatment, and assess the impact of the illness on the patient's lifestyle and adaptation to the illness. Patients should be encouraged to maintain regular contact with the physician, allow reconsideration of the medical program, and update the status of clinical effort.

New Cases

In most instances, the chronicity of symptoms (in the absence of identifiable pathogens) associated with typical endoscopic, pathologic, and

TABLE 21-1. *Ulcerative Colitis: Differential Diagnosis.* *

I. Specific Infections
   A. Bacterial:
      Campylobacter
      Salmonella
      Shigella
      E. coli (invasive strains)
      Gonorrhea proctitis
      Clostridium difficile
   B. Fungal:
      Histoplasmosis
   C. Viral:
      Cytomegalovirus
   D. Protozoan:
      Amebic dysentery
      Schistosomiasis
II. Other Diseases
      Acute self-limited colitis
      Crohn's disease
      Radiation proctitis
      Ischemic colitis
      Behçet's disease
      Amyloidosis
      Mercury poisoning
      Hemolytic-uremic syndrome
      Soap colitis
      Irritable bowel syndrome
      Lymphoma

*See also Chapter 10.

FIG. 21-1. Extent of colitis at ation. (Courtesy of Ritchie, J. K., Powell-Tuck, J., and Lennard-Jones, J. E.: Lancet, 1:1140, 1978.)

radiographic features will allow the physician to make a presumptive diagnosis of ulcerative colitis. In uncertain situations continued observation and repeated diagnostic studies often will clarify the diagnosis.[1-3]

Initially, it is important, for both the clinical decision-making process and the prognostic assessment, to determine the anatomic extent of the colitis.[4,5] The choice among therapeutic options will be modified by the extent of the colitis. More distal disease is likely to respond to treatment with locally administered rectal medications, whereas disease of the right colon usually requires oral or systemic therapy. More than half of all patients will have left-sided colitis with involvement of the rectum (100%), sigmoid colon (55%), and descending colon (27%), which is limited proximally to the splenic flexure. Involvement of the transverse colon or the entire colon is noted in approximately 20% of cases categorized as extensive colitis (Fig. 21-1). Radiographic involvement of the hepatic flexure usually signifies mucosal inflammation of the ascending colon as well (see also Chap. 20).*

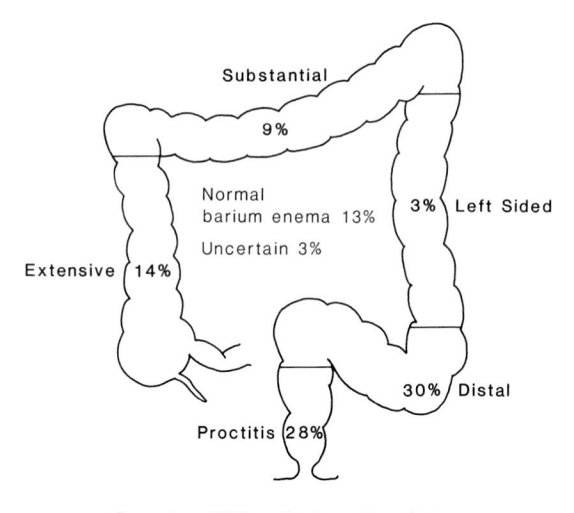

*Frank, P.: Personal communication, 1986.

The anatomic extent of mucosal involvement should be assessed early in the course of disease to determine the most appropriate therapy, preferably by endoscopic and biopsy examinations. Estimating the degree of disease activity by encompassing the clinical features, laboratory findings, and endoscopic and radiographic examinations, is essential for determining optimal therapy.

Clinical Features

Truelove and Witts defined three categories of illness to assess the effectiveness of cortisone therapy in acute ulcerative colitis (Table 21-2).[6] The homogeneous nature of symptoms in patients with UC compared with Crohn's disease has allowed the few clinical criteria of bowel frequency and body temperature to predict the necessity of surgical treatment in acute colitis,[7] while clinical severity, defined by limitation of activities, abdominal pain, bowel frequency, and stool consistency, correlates with a simple scale of sigmoidoscopic appearance.[8] Powell-Tuck's expansion of the profile to a scoring system using ten items (Table 21-3) was used successfully in clinical trials, but the additional features did not significantly improve correlation with the sigmoidoscopic appearance.[8] Additional clinical features, such as rectal urgency, incontinence, nocturnal bowel movements, and ability to work, correlated well with global clinical assessments,[9] but have not improved on the overall assessment made by Truelove and

TABLE 21-2. *Truelove and Witts' Criteria for Disease Activity.*

	Severe	Mild
Bowel movement frequency	≥6 daily	≤4 daily
Blood in stool	++	±
Fever	>37.5	<—>
Pulse rate	>90	nl
Hemoglobin	<75%	nl
ESR	>30 mm/hr	<30 mm/hr

Moderate = "in between"

Witts.[6] This simple index is perhaps too qualitative and subjective for use as a single criterion, however, and can be difficult to interpret when a patient has only some of the characteristics in any category.*

Laboratory Studies

No simple blood test reflects the extent and severity of the inflamed colon. Truelove and Witts used the hemoglobin and erythrocyte sedimentation rate (ESR) in their clinical scale.[6] Data from the Lyon group[10] suggested that the hematocrit has a better correlation with disease activity than does the hemoglobin concentration.[1]

*Singleton, J.: Personal communication, 1986.

Likewise, despite the overall correlation between ESR and disease activity, the wide scatter between categories and the long half-life of the proteins contributing to the ESR preclude its rapid fluctuation, despite clinical improvement.[11] Levels of orosomucoid, an alpha$_1$-glycoprotein that is used more often by European investigators, correlate better than C-reactive protein or the ESR,[12] and have compared favorably with other acute phase reactants in a number of serum protein studies.[10-16]

Additional laboratory studies that more directly reflect the degree of the inflammatory reaction in the colon are currently being evaluated. The usefulness and practicality of Indium-111-labelled autologous leukocytes,[17, 18] or measurement of colonic bicarbonate output,[19] depend upon the cost, difficulty of performing the tests, and exposure to radiation. Serum albumin concentration relates to ongoing protein loss and is a necessary element of the nutritional profile (see the following), but does not reflect rapid clinical change.[9] Neither do serial determinations of prostaglandin metabolites in the stool appear to be of routine, practical clinical use.[9] Stool alpha-1-antitrypsin may be a better indicator of overall inflammatory activity, but this requires further confirmation prior to general acceptance.[20]

TABLE 21-3. *Powell-Tuck Scoring System of Disease Activity.*

Indicant	Score	Guide to scoring
"Well being"	1	Impaired, but able to continue activities.
	2	Activities reduced.
	3	Unable to work.
Abdominal pain	1	With bowel actions.
	2	More continuous.
Bowel frequency	1	3-6/day.
	2	>6/day.
Stool consistency	0	Normal or variably. Normal.
	1	Semi-formed.
	2	Liquid.
Bleeding	1	Trace.
	2	More than a trace.
Anorexia	1	Present.
Nausea or vomiting	1	Present.
Abdominal tenderness	1	Mild.
	2	Prominent.
	3	Rebound.
Eye, joint, mouth, or skin complications	1	1 mild complication.
	2	1 severe complication or at least two mild complications.
Temperature	1	37.1–38°C.
	2	>38°C.

Radiography*

A plain abdominal radiograph can be useful in the assessment of a patient with worsening clinical disease. Colonic dilatation heralds severe colitis, impending toxic megacolon, or perforation. The extent of disease often can be crudely estimated by observing the presence of stool proximally and absent haustrations distal to the border of normal and involved colon. Mucosal islands, "thumbprinting," or pseudopolyps outlined within the gas-filled bowel indicate severe disease. A plain abdominal radiograph taken immediately after a limited proctoscopic examination is also useful. This simple air colonogram can detail the gross extent and severity in sick patients without the risk of more extensive procedures.

Air-contrast barium enemas, useful in determining the extent and severity of an acute episode of colitis, are being replaced by colonoscopy. Endoscopy provides the most reliable indicator of disease activity (see Chap. 19), despite the potential for discrepancies between symptoms and the mucosal appearance; for example, proctoscopic healing may lag behind symptomatic improvement or, conversely, appear paradoxically improved distally subsequent to local steroid therapy, although more severe proximal disease is present. Despite documented variability in sigmoidoscopic interpretation,[21,22] underlying features that are readily classified provide more reliable and reproducible agreement between observers.[8,9,22] Most experienced clinicians can agree upon the presence or absence of bleeding, either spontaneous or induced, whereas descriptions of the vascular pattern, degree of hyperemia, or granularity are more variable, leading Heatly to suggest the four gradations of activity listed in Table 21-4.[22]

Histology†

Similarly, a dissociation often exists between proctoscopic changes and histologic findings.[23]

*See Chapter 20.
†See Chapter 18.

TABLE 21-4. *Heatley's Grade of Mucosal Disease Activity.*

Grade I—Normal mucosa
  II—Hyperemic mucosa with loss of vascular pattern
  III—Bleeding spontaneously or on light contact
  IV—Severe changes with excess mucus, pus, mucosal hemorrhage, or ulceration

(From Heatley, R. V., et al.: Disodium cromoglycate in the treatment of chronic proctitis. Gut, *16*:559, 1975.)

A simplified descriptive scheme consists of three levels of histologic changes and this correlated with the sigmoidoscopic gradation when bleeding was used as the criterion for activity:[8]

1. No acute inflammation; variable chronic inflammatory cell infiltrate without polymorphonuclear leukocytes, intact epithelium with a normal content of mucus.
2. Mild inflammation; variable degree of chronic inflammatory cell infiltrate but with some polymorphonuclear leukocytes; intact epithelium with normal or slightly reduced content of mucus.
3. Moderate or severe inflammation; variable increase in chronic inflammatory cells with numerous polymorphonuclear leukocytes, often with crypt abscesses; reduced mucin content of the epithelium.

Chronicity

While difficult to document, the chronic course of ulcerative colitis will directly influence the expected response to medical treatment. Clinical patterns may vary between acute fulminating colitis to a chronic continuous course (Fig. 21-2). Patients who respond initially to sulfasalazine and/or steroids are likely to continue to respond to a maintenance program. On the other hand, patients with continuous symptoms, despite ongoing or intermittent therapy, experience incomplete remissions that require trials of multiple agents, often with a less than satisfactory outcome.

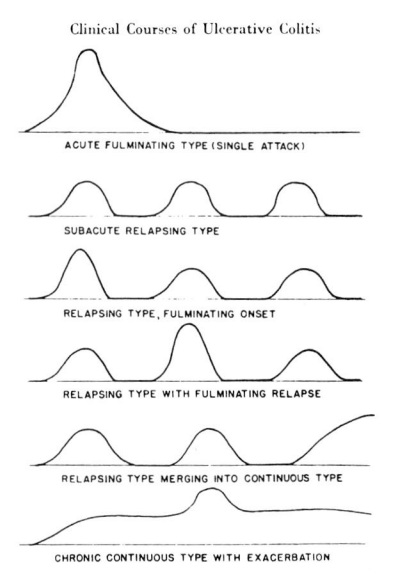

FIG. 21-2. Variable course of ulcerative colitis. (Courtesy of Farmer, R. G.: *In* Bockus Gastroenterology 4th Ed. Edited by J. E. Berk. Philadelphia, W. B. Saunders Co., 1985.)

Complications

The medical complications of UC are detailed within the chapters on gastrointestinal complications, extraintestinal complications and nutritional consequences and therapy (Chaps. 14, 16, and 24).

Medical Management

To define an appropriate program of medical management, several factors must be considered:

Nutrition

The nutritional status of the patient is a critical determinant of the response to medical treatment. In our experience, patients will not respond to such treatment until nutritional deficiencies, often documented by protein deficiency, have been corrected. Mildly ill patients usually are nutritionally replete or may only manifest iron deficiency. Folate deficiency may occur with long-standing sulfasalazine therapy (vide infra). On the other hand, more severely ill patients with protracted diarrhea are likely to be significantly malnourished, often suffering from a combination of protein and calorie malnutrition.

Metabolic Abnormalities

Metabolic abnormalities require attention in severely ill patients. These include losses of bicarbonate, potassium, and sodium in the stool. A negative calcium balance in patients receiving steroids often is aggravated by lactose intolerance and the avoidance of milk and dairy products without adequate supplementation. Similarly, phosphate depletion can exacerbate muscle weakness induced by steroids. Rarely, hypoxia can be caused by hypotension, pulmonary embolization, cardiac decompensation directly (myopericarditis) or indirectly (hypophosphatemia, hypokalemia) related to the inflammatory bowel disease, or respiratory depression secondary to excessive opiate use for the relief of pain. Such cardiopulmonary complications necessitate intensive monitoring in severely ill or toxic patients.

Bowel Hemorrhage

A cardinal sign of ulcerative colitis, bowel hemorrhage, may be aggravated when the IBD is complicated by hepatic disease or severe protein wasting. Vitamin K deficiency may follow prolonged antibiotic treatment and can be replaced by oral or parenteral vitamin K. Occasionally, replacement therapy with fresh frozen plasma is necessary to control active hemorrhage. Likewise, calcium replacement is helpful in preventing the coagulopathy associated with the transfusion of multiple units of citrate-preserved blood products.

Psychosocial Factors*

Assessment of the impact of the ulcerative colitis upon the patient and his family is essential in the overall approach to the patient and a wide spectrum of behavioral adaptations (or maladjustments) can be expected. In most situations, inflammatory bowel disease is a "transfiguring" disease. To use Spiro's terms, "from the patient's perspective it is a life-long transfiguring disease of uncertain cause with inescapable and humiliating symptoms whose therapy has changed little in 30 years. An illness manifest by disability, anxiety, foreboding, and suffering."[24] Spiro urges the physician to view the chronic disease according to the impact of the disability, dependency, depression, the doctor, the diagnostic studies, and the drug therapy upon the individual, while emphasizing the importance of listening to the patient rather than relying solely on the objective findings of the physical, sigmoidoscopic, or laboratory examinations.[24]

Observations of the interaction of the patient with the spouse or other family provide additional insights into the impact of the illness upon the patient's life, and the appropriateness of the adaptive response. Family support is essential for an effective adaptation to the illness.[25] Counterproductive responses from the family occur when the patient becomes a source of guilt for the spouse or parent, or if he is given too much attention at the expense of another family member (e.g., sibling), to the point of excessive dependency.

Insight may also be gained from noting the interactions of the patient with the nursing staff, social workers, and other ancillary care providers. Formal evaluation is helpful in instances when the patient (or family) seems unable to cope. Here, consultation with a psychiatrist or social worker may reveal additional psychologic diagnoses and provide supportive or pharmacologic treatment as an adjunct to medical management.

* See also Chapter 11.

Diet and Nutritional Factors*

Despite the absence of known dietary factors aggravating the inflammatory reaction in ulcerative colitis, the usefulness of diet and nutrition in relieving symptoms should not be ignored. Clearly, adequate provision of macro- and micronutrients is necessary for long-term benefit. It is the manner in which the nutrients are supplied that may affect the general course of the patient's symptoms. Likewise, the overall status of the patient will determine the optimal approach to dietary management.

A "diet history" is necessary to initiate nutritional assessment and planning. In patients with chiefly diarrheal symptoms, factors that aggravate bowel frequency should be explored. Irritants such as highly spiced foods or laxative fruits should be proscribed, and stimulants such as large quantities of caffeinated beverages should be limited. Conversely, patients with proctitis who are troubled by constipation may benefit from additional fiber products or bulk forming agents. The ability to digest lactose should be considered and lactose-tolerance testing should be performed if the history is equivocal. A general reduction in other products that form gas (beans, peas, cabbage) will be helpful in those troubled by bloating or flatus. Roughage such as skins, nuts, and seeds should be avoided by patients who are actively bleeding. A defined outline of dietary advice is necessary and almost always is requested by the patient.

Adequate supplementation with iron is important to compensate for blood loss. Enteral forms of iron, at times, are poorly tolerated, producing either diarrhea or constipation that may necessitate parenteral replacement. In severely active colitis transfusions may be necessary. Folic acid should be prescribed for patients receiving sulfasalazine therapy to compensate for the impaired absorption of folate from the diet. Sufficient calcium intake also should be assured, especially in those on lactose-free diets and for patients on corticosteroids. Additional vitamin and mineral supplementation occasionally is necessary for patients on severely restricted diets or receiving parenteral nutrition. Consultation with an experienced dietician or nutritionist can be helpful.

Although specific approaches to nutrition are described more extensively by Dr. Jeejeebhoy (see Chap. 24), they will be briefly introduced in the approaches to specific clinical situations described in the following section.

*See also Chapter 24.

Therapeutic Agents

Supportive Therapy

Supportive, "steroid sparing therapy," refers to prescribed or proprietary products used to relieve the symptoms of IBD (abdominal cramping, diarrhea, constipation) that would otherwise require higher or maintenance doses of steroids. The potential advantage of such interventions must be balanced against the possible adverse consequences. Again, we emphasize the importance of incorporating the supportive agents into a program of treatment that is fully explained to the patient, whose understanding of the pathophysiology of the symptoms and the mechanisms and purposes of the recommended medications will facilitate reliable and regular conformation to the physician's recommended schedule.

Antispasmodics

Many patients either with active disease or ulcerative colitis in remission have symptoms of intestinal irritability.[26] Anticholinergic medications such as tincture of belladonna, propantheline bromide, dicyclomine hydrochloride, and clidinium bromide may reduce postprandial pain and rectal urgency, and aid in the control of bowel symptoms if given before meals to depress the hyperactive gastrocolic reflex and the increased peristalsis associated with ulcerative colitis. These agents are most effective when taken on a regular (rather than p.r.n.) schedule, beginning with the lowest dose range for each agent, by patients with mild to moderate symptoms. Severely ill patients may overreact pharmacologically to such medications, possibly resulting in excessive inhibition of peristalsis and precipitation of toxic dilatation of the colon. Thus, in moderate to severe attacks these agents either should be taken in small, individually regulated amounts or, preferably, avoided entirely. If given to severely ill individuals, the patient should be closely monitored for the presence of active bowel sounds (by abdominal auscultation), the absence of abdominal distention on physical examination, and colonic dilatation using roentgenograms. The relief of abdominal cramping, urgency, or bloating by antispasmodics often permits continued reduction in steroid dosage.

Antidiarrheal Medication

These preparations can be used by patients with mild to moderate colitis to reduce the frequency of bowel movements and to relieve rectal urgency. A variety of preparations are available (diphenoxylate, loperamide, codeine, paregoric, deodorized tincture of opium) that share properties of opiate-receptor blockade.[27] Few studies have compared individual agents in ulcerative colitis, although loperamide, diphenoxylate, and codeine have been compared in patients with chronic diarrhea and were found to be well-tolerated and to have equal efficacy.[28] Diphenoxylate and loperamide were compared in another group of patients with diarrhea of diverse causes and benefit was shown with each drug, although loperamide seemed to be more effective in those with ileostomies.[29,30] Diphenoxylate, 5mg t.i.d., has been compared to placebo in patients with ulcerative colitis and it resulted in an average reduction in the number of bowel movements of 1.3 per day over six days, at the expense of side effects (nausea, drowsiness, dizziness, fatigue, or pain) in 53% of patients.[31] The absence of adverse effects,[27] and the potential advantage of increased anal sphincter tone,[32] make loperamide a more tolerable, albeit more expensive, option for the relief of diarrhea.

A regular regimen of medication rather than a p.r.n. schedule is preferable for patients with mild inflammatory disease. All of these drugs must be used cautiously in moderately ill individuals, and they are contraindicated in severely ill or potentially toxic patients. Loperamide, codeine, or deodorized tincture of opium also can be used cautiously in patients with tenesmus or inability to retain rectal enemas.

Lidamidine, an aryl substituted amino-urea compound, has both antimotility and antidiarrheal qualities but, as yet, is unavailable in the United States. Clonidine, a derivative that is structurally similar to imidazoline with central and intestinal alpha-adrenergic properties,[33] stimulates intestinal electrolyte absorption and may have additional therapeutic efficacy in ulcerative colitis.[34]

Hydrophilic mucilloids may improve stool consistency and facilitate bowel control for patients (usually those with distal colitis) who experience constipation and diarrhea. Both processed fiber products and bran may be useful in forming a soft, bulky stool, but may be tolerated poorly if bowel activity is intensified or accompanied by excessive flatus or distention. The ultimate advantage of bran or fiber products, however, has not been established in inflammatory bowel disease.

Sedatives and Antidepressants

While emotional disturbances do not cause ulcerative colitis, the chronologic association between significant emotional stresses and the onset, recurrence, and intensification of inflammatory bowel disease is recognized. The central nervous system and the enteric nervous system independently and jointly influence the motor, secretory, and absorptive functions of the gut (as well as its immune response).[35] The adjunctive use of one or more of a variety of sedatives or anxiolytics, together with the supportive care by the sympathetic and interested physician, may be helpful to the patient who has emotional distress. Chronic, recurrent, unpredictable illness tends to induce emotional conflicts, dependency, and a state of regression that may impede the response to medical treatment. Furthermore, medical therapy with steroids and even sulfasalazine may affect mood and induce emotional lability. The introduction of mood altering drugs should be monitored to avoid additional dependency, especially in our "quick-cure," drug-seeking society. Because of the heightened dependency and depressive features of barbiturates, benzodiazepine derivatives are preferable. Occasionally, however, low doses of phenobarbital (or similar short-acting barbiturates), combined with antispasmodics, can be useful. For hospitalized patients, sedation at night may be valuable, especially in the initial phase of treatment.

Antidepressant or antipsychotic medication is reserved for patients with clinically significant psychologic indications. Antidepressants may help patients who have steroid-induced (or unmasked) depression. In this situation, the tricyclic antidepressants, such as amitriptyline, imipramine hydrochloride, or nortriptyline hydrochloride have the advantage of anticholinergic effects that reduce bowel spasms and stool frequency. For schizophrenic patients, antipsychotics should be prescribed under the supervision of a psychiatrist.

Analgesics

Abdominal pain arising from the bowel is treated by suppression of the inflammatory reaction and by the relief of bowel spasms and irritability. Opiates and related analgesics increase bowel spasm and carry the risk of inducing toxic dilatation in the acute patient. Occasionally, patients with severe rectal spasm will benefit from a short course of belladonna and opium suppositories.

Milder analgesics, such as acetaminophen, have minimal value for relieving pain of intestinal origin and have been associated with relapse in ulcerative colitis.[36] Similarly, nonsteroidal anti-inflammatory drugs should be avoided because of their tendency to cause mucosal ulceration and increased colorectal bleeding.[37,38]

A wise precaution in a patient with new or severe abdominal pain not responding to treatment is to exclude extraintestinal causes of abdominal pain, such as renal or biliary colic. Perforation, which may be heralded by diffuse or localized peritoneal signs, should not be overlooked, and it may be difficult to detect initially in a patient receiving steroids.

The supportive therapies described previously can be of great benefit in the management of patients with ulcerative colitis. The use of such agents should not be considered routine and each situation must be managed according to individual requirements. As alluded to earlier, serious adverse consequences have been documented with the use of anticholinergic, antidiarrheal, and analgesic medications. Furthermore, the potential for abuse and/or dependency in young patients with a chronic illness, and the overlying tendency towards regressive or dependent features is significant.[39]

Sulfasalazine Therapy

Currently sulfasalazine (sulphasalazine, salicylazosulfapyradine, salazopyrin, SASP, Azulfidine*) remains the keystone of therapy for ulcerative colitis. This compound of 5-aminosalicylic acid (5-ASA) linked to sulfapyridine (SP) by an azo bond (Fig. 21-3), however, introduced in Sweden by Svartz in the early 1940's,[40,42] will

*Pharmacia Laboratories, Piscataway, NJ 08854.

gradually be replaced by a variety of analogs that deliver the active moiety, 5-ASA, to specific sites along the gastrointestinal tract. The clinical experience, metabolism, mechanism of action, and adverse effects of sulfasalazine will be reviewed before considering the new derivatives.[43]

Clinical Experience

MILD TO MODERATE COLITIS. From an uncontrolled study, Svartz reported an 80 to 90% rate of improvement or recovery in her patients.[42] Subsequent controlled trials also showed beneficial effects. In early studies in the United States, Moertel and Bargen reported "favorable responses" in 64% of patients with a spectrum of severity of disease, compared to 40% in controls.[44] Subsequent British studies found clinical and sigmoidoscopic improvement in 80% of 20 patients with mild ulcerative colitis treated with SASP, compared to 35% of placebo-treated controls.[45] These findings were confirmed by Dick and colleagues, who reported a 77% versus 39% improvement in treated patients compared to controls.[46] These initial controlled studies used doses of 1 to 1.5 g four times daily and demonstrated that clinical improvement might take up to four weeks after initiation of therapy; additional benefit occurred with daily doses above 4 g.

ACUTE OR SEVERE COLITIS. Although sulfasalazine alone has not been studied in patients with severe colitis, when compared to combined ther-

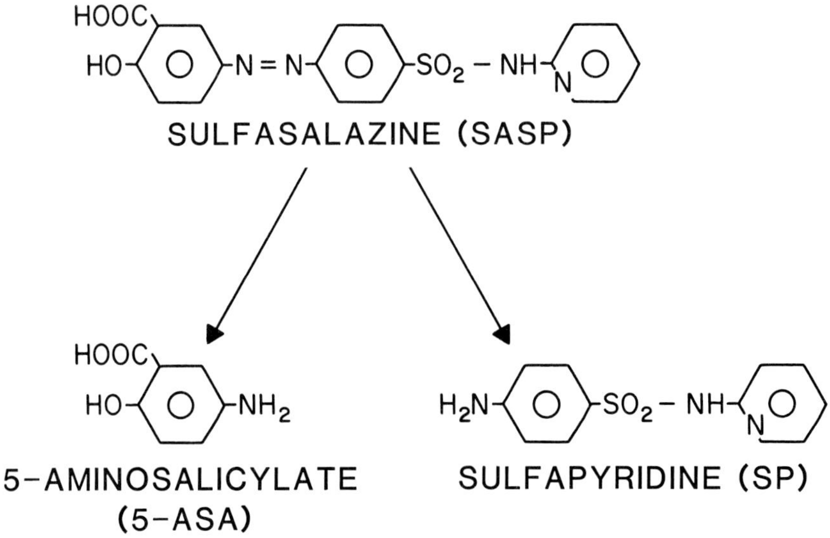

FIG. 21-3. Sulfasalazine. (Courtesy of Stenson, W. F.: Viewpoints on Dig. Dis., 16:13, 1984.)

apy with systemic, low-dose prednisone and hydrocortisone retention enemas, the response to steroids was judged to be superior.[47] These observations led Truelove and colleagues to use sulfasalazine only after a response to steroids and bowel rest had been demonstrated.[48] The response to SASP in patients with severe symptoms may be masked by the similarity of the adverse effects of SASP (fatigue, nausea, abdominal pain) to the acute symptoms of colitis. The use of SASP as adjuvant therapy with steroids in ulcerative colitis also has not been evaluated. Furthermore, the institution of SASP therapy with steroids, while routine practice, may carry the risk of obscuring the few patients whose colitis is aggravated by SASP.

MAINTENANCE THERAPY. The usefulness of SASP as a maintenance therapy to prevent relapse in patients with active disease has been carefully examined in several clinical trials. While Svartz implied that patients responding to therapeutic doses would maintain a remission with smaller doses of 1 to 2 g daily,[42] Misiewicz et al. prospectively followed 67 patients with ulcerative colitis in remission for greater than one year.[49] Seven of 34 patients who were chosen randomly to receive a 2 g daily dose of SASP relapsed during the twelve month observation period compared to 24 out of 33 placebo treated patients. Although a Danish study could not confirm the long-term benefits of SASP maintenance therapy in a smaller group of patients (some of whom received less than 2 g SASP daily),[50] a subsequent British study, which screened patients for sigmoidoscopic remission as well as subsidence of symptoms, documented the benefit of a 2 g daily dose, preventing recurrence in 88% of the patients who were maintained on SASP compared to 45% who were transferred to placebo.[51] Azad Khan et al., in a randomized trial in 172 patients, demonstrated that the likelihood of flare-ups on maintenance SASP is related inversely to the dose.[52] The relapse rates for patients treated with 1, 2, and 4 g daily were 33, 14, and 9% respectively (Fig. 21-4) at one year. A direct correlation was found between dose and side effects such that 13 of 56 patients receiving the higher dose were unable to tolerate continued treatment at a level of 4 g daily. These studies have formed the basis for maintenance therapy with SASP. Most patients will tolerate doses of 2 g daily and have a low risk of recurrence. Those who develop increasing symptoms or a relapse are then treated with doses of 3 to 6 g daily until symptoms and sigmoidoscopic changes resolve, at which point a maintenance dose of 3 to 4 g daily can be attempted. The minimal dose preventing relapse then is maintained for several years in those with a single episode of mild to moderate colitis, or maintained indefinitely for patients with a chronic course or with a frequently relapsing pattern.

Pharmacology

The clinical pharmacokinetics of sulfasalazine (SASP) have been reviewed recently.[53] Sulfasalazine is now considered to be a "prodrug," and is composed of 5-ASA and sulfapyridine (SP) joined by an azo bond. The parent compound was designed to be poorly absorbed and, because of its low water solubility under acid conditions, it is not absorbed from the stomach. The percentage of an oral dose that reaches the systemic circulation varies between 2 to 10% and probably is entirely a result of limited small bowel absorption,[54] because no difference exists between absorption in healthy individuals, patients with colitis, or those with ileostomies.[55,56] In patients with ulcerative colitis, peak serum concentrations after a single dose of 3 or 4 g ranged between 15 and 31 μg/ml after 4 to 8 hours,[57] with an average steady-state serum concentration of 18 μg/ml in those receiving 3 to 6 g daily.[58] Rectal absorption of SASP is low, averaging 13% of an oral dose.[57,59] The bioavailability of tablets (Azulfidine^R) relative to an oral suspension was varied but appeared to be independent of the formula used,[60] and while the systemic availability of enteric-coated tablets averaged only 66% of the uncoated preparation, the total urinary excretion of sulfapyridine was

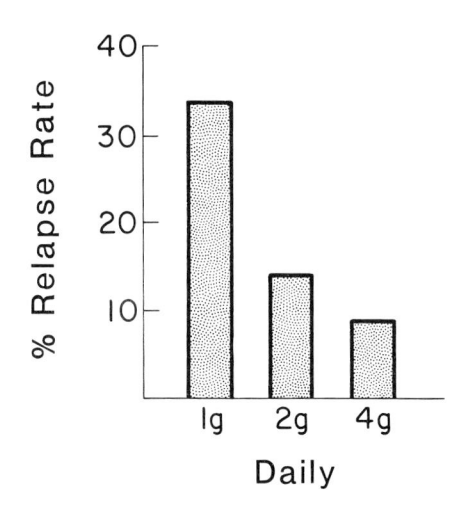

FIG. 21-4. Relapse rate with maintenance sulfasalazine. (Courtesy of Azad Khan, A. K., et al.: Gut, 21:232, 1980.)

similar.[61] Concomitant treatment with corticosteroids has no appreciable effect on the serum concentrations of sulfasalazine or its metabolites.[62]

Once absorbed, SASP is extensively bound to serum proteins, only minimal amounts being available for tissue penetration.[53] The intact molecule is excreted unchanged in the urine with only traces recovered in the feces, although an enterohepatic circulation has been described.[56,57] In pregnant women, SASP crosses the placenta with comparable fetal and maternal blood levels, although only a small amount is excreted in breast milk.[53]

Sulfasalazine is primarily metabolized to SP and 5-ASA within the colon by a wide variety of bacterial species.[63-65] These bacteria possess an intracellular azo reductase enzyme that is inhibited by oxygen. Both accelerated intestinal transit and administration of broad-spectrum antibiotics will impair the splitting of SASP and reduce the amounts of 5-ASA released into the colon.[54,66,67]

Reduction of the azo bond liberates SP and 5-ASA. After oral administration, SP can be detected in the blood in 3 to 6 hours, correlating with intestinal transit to the colonic sites of azo reduction.[58,68] Absorption is almost complete, with peak serum concentrations occurring after 10 to 30 hours,[57,67] and 60 to 80% urinary recovery both in patients with ulcerative colitis and in healthy subjects.[57,68]

The elimination of SP requires hepatic metabolism prior to urinary elimination (Fig. 21-5). The major pathway is via N-acetylation, with genetic phenotypic variation controlling an individual's rate of metabolism.[57,62] Higher serum concentrations of SP are achieved in the 60% of subjects who are slow acetylators. A parallel, and more phenotypically homogeneous, pathway of metabolism involves ring hydroxylation that, by a mechanism similar to that with the N-acetylated SP metabolites, is followed by conjugation with glucuronic acid and/or acetic acid prior to urinary excretion.[53,57,68] As pointed out earlier, sulfapyridine and its metabolites reach similar concentrations in fetal as in maternal serum, although in breast milk the concentration is only about 40% of the maternal serum level.[53]

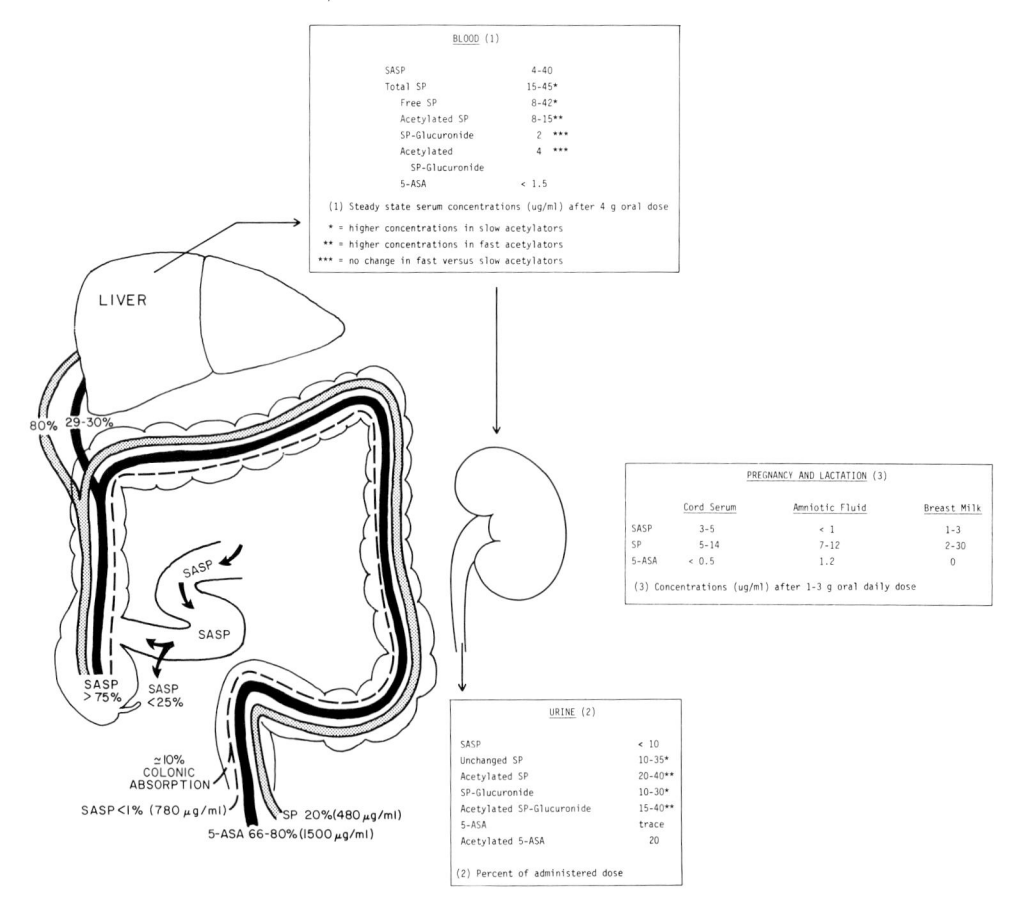

FIG. 21-5. Metabolism of sulfasalazine, sulfapyridine, and 5-ASA.

The 5-ASA liberated from SASP is absorbed much less completely from the colon than is the SP, with about 20 to 30% of the dose being recovered in the urine.[57] Approximately 50% of the administered dose from SASP is recoverable in the feces,[54,68] mostly in the unchanged form, whereas in the urine greater than 80% of 5-ASA appears in the acetylated form (Ac-5-ASA).[57,58] After administration of SASP, plasma concentrations of unchanged 5-ASA are usually less than 1.5 μg/ml with concentrations of Ac-5-ASA being 2 to 5 times higher, suggesting presystemic acetylation. Recently, this has been demonstrated to occur via acetyltransferase activity in the cytosol of human colonic epithelial cells,[69] and as a saturable intestinal and hepatic first-pass system in animals.[70] Approximately 80% of Ac-5-ASA is protein-bound compared to 40% of 5-ASA,[53,71] and the acetylated metabolite has a longer serum half-life, 6 to 9 hours, compared to 0.5 to 1.5 hours for unchanged 5-ASA.[71-73] The acetylation rate for 5-ASA is not genetically controlled and only small amounts of 5-ASA appear in the bile or breast milk,[53] although in one study, concentrations of Ac-5-ASA detected in breast milk were higher than in plasma.[74]

If it is ingested orally without linkage or alternative protection (slow-release forms), 5-ASA is rapidly and extensively absorbed from the upper gastrointestinal tract.[75] Release from slow-release preparations (see the following) depends upon the transit time, the bacterial environment (for azo-bond pro-drugs), and the local pH.[74] Absorption after rectal administration of 5-ASA enema products also is pH dependent, with neutral solutions providing a more rapid rate of absorption and higher serum concentrations of 5-ASA and Ac-5-ASA compared to acidic solutions.[76] Low serum concentrations of 5-ASA and Ac-5-ASA (10 μmol/ml) after continued administration of 5-ASA enemas or suppositories were comparable to equimolar doses of SASP.[53,74] Following rectal installation of 5-ASA the renal excretion, mainly as Ac-5-ASA, averaged 13 to 16% of the administered dose (compared to 17 to 37% urinary recovery of 5-ASA during treatment with SASP), although wide individual variation (4 to 80%) has been reported.[74]

Mechanism of Action

The precise mechanism of action of SASP and its metabolites has yet to be elucidated. Hypotheses and experimentation to clarify potential mechanisms have often paralleled concepts of etiopathogenesis of the underlying disease. Svartz initially reported the drug to be bound to the connective tissue of the bowel and focused on the influence of inflammatory effects on the histologic changes in the connective tissue associated with ulcerative colitis.[76] Subsequently, the antibacterial properties of sulfapyridine were considered, but initial studies were unable to confirm any substantial changes in the fecal flora associated with SASP,[77] and while later investigations using more sophisticated anaerobic techniques have demonstrated changes in the quantity of certain species of clostridia, nonspore forming anaerobes and coliforms, the alterations did not correlate with disease activity.[78] Hence, while efforts continue to search for a bacterial or other infectious etiology of ulcerative colitis, the role of colonic microflora in the pathogenesis of or the CUC response to therapy with SASP remains uncertain.[3]

Some insight into the mechanism of action of SASP can be derived from two studies that attempted to define its active moiety. Azad Khan et al. and, subsequently, Klotz and coworkers demonstrated that suspension enemas composed of SASP or 5-ASA were effective in controlling the symptoms and histologic changes of ulcerative colitis,[79,80] and Crohn's proctitis,[80] whereas SP enemas were of no benefit. The results are in contrast to studies in rheumatoid arthritis where SP appears to be the active component.[81] Efforts since have been directed at attempting to identify how SASP or 5-ASA influence local or systemic mediators of the inflammatory response.

Recently, interest has focused on the arachidonic cascade and its metabolites as potential mediators of the inflammatory response as well as other pathophysiologic processes (electrolyte transport) in inflammatory bowel disease.[3,82,83] Arachidonic acid is metabolized through two separate pathways by means of cyclooxygenase and cyclic endoperoxygenase activity, or via lipoxygenase (Fig. 21-6).[82] The cyclooxygenase metabolites include prostacyclin, thromboxanes, and the prostaglandins. Metabolites of the lipoxygenase pathway include hydroperoxyeicosatetranoic acids (HPETES), hydroeicosatetranoic acids (HETES), and leukotrienes (including the slow-reacting substance of anaphylaxis, SRS-A). The alternative pathways are not equally active in all tissues or cell types.[82] To assess the role of the individual arachidonic acid products, it is necessary to consider the metabolism of arachidonic acid by the intestinal mucosa independently of the inflammatory cell infiltrate, plus the effects

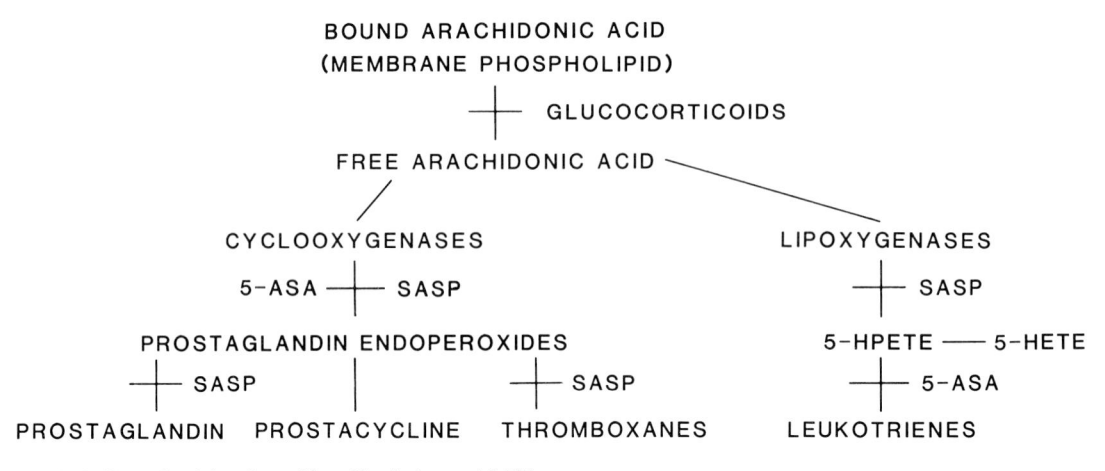

```
BOUND ARACHIDONIC ACID
(MEMBRANE PHOSPHOLIPID)
            ┼──── GLUCOCORTICOIDS
FREE ARACHIDONIC ACID
       /                              \
CYCLOOXYGENASES                    LIPOXYGENASES
5-ASA ─┼─ SASP                        ─┼─ SASP
PROSTAGLANDIN ENDOPEROXIDES         5-HPETE ──── 5-HETE
─┼─ SASP        ─┼─ SASP              ─┼─ 5-ASA
PROSTAGLANDIN  PROSTACYCLINE  THROMBOXANES   LEUKOTRIENES
```

FIG. 21-6. Sites of activity of steroids, sulfasalazine, and 5-ASA.

of local tissue factors (such as kinins) on the arachidonic cascade.[82]

In active ulcerative colitis, the production of the cyclooxygenase derivatives PGE_2, thromboxane and prostacyclin, increases with a return to control values after successful treatment.[83-85] Prostaglandins can induce mucosal dilatation, fever, and colonic secretion.[82,83,86,87] While some cyclooxygenase metabolites are produced by cultured epithelial cells, it has not been clarified whether the elevated mucosal levels in ulcerative colitis are caused by enhanced production by epithelial or mononuclear cells,[88,89] or by reduced degradation.[82] Studies demonstrating PGE_2 accumulation in the rectal lumen or feces using dialysis techniques have identified high levels during active disease with decreases towards control levels during remission.[90,91] Despite the inhibition of prostaglandin biosynthesis by SASP and 5-ASA,[84,85,92,93] some nonsteroidal anti-inflammatory drugs actually appear to worsen ulcerative colitis.[36,37,94-96] Other studies have identified potent inhibition of prostaglandin catabolism by SASP and stimulation of PGI_2 that would elevate levels of endogeneous prostaglandins.[97,98] The latter studies raise the issue as to whether prostaglandins are cytoprotective in ulcerative colitis,[83,93,98,99] despite the following evidence to the contrary: levels of 5-ASA in the colonic lumen are up to 1000 times higher than those resulting in raised prostaglandin levels in vitro;[100] raised PGE_2 levels are normalized with 5-ASA treatment;[91] and, most conclusively, administration of prostaglandin analogue 15-(R)-15 methyl-PGE_2 failed to maintain remission in patients with relapsing ulcerative colitis.[101] While such data only seem to obfuscate the role of local prostaglandins in ulcerative colitis, both SASP and 5-ASA inhibit the cyclooxygenase system at different levels and may produce different profiles of endoperoxide metabolites (Fig. 21-6).[102] Perturbations in the arachidonic acid cascade at alternate levels may shift or redirect precursors into differing pathways.[82]

Redirection of arachidonic acid metabolism away from the cyclooxygenase system may lead to enhanced synthesis of lipoxygenase products.[82,83,102] Normal colonic mucosa does not have an active lipoxygenase system, whereas Stenson and colleagues have demonstrated the formation of leukotriene B_4 and 5-HETE by neutrophils infiltrating the mucosa.[102,103] Leukotrienes may play a role in amplifying the inflammatory response by the chemotactic properties induction of lysosomal enzyme release from neutrophils, and increasing capillary permeability.[82,103,104] Sulfasalazine and, to a lesser degree, 5-ASA are inhibitors of neutrophil lipoxygenase (diminished synthesis of leukotriene B_4 and 5-HETE) at concentrations that are achieved within the stool (but not serum), whereas 5-ASA inhibits the transformation of leukotriene A_4 to leukotriene B_4.[105-107] Benoxaprofen, a relatively weak inhibitor of the lipoxygenase pathway that also inhibits prostaglandin synthesis, was not effective in an open trial in active ulcerative colitis.[108] The current lack of an available nontoxic lipoxygenase inhibitor, however, makes it impossible to evaluate the relevance of enhanced leukotriene B_4 and 5-HETE synthesis in ulcerative colitis, or to assess the differential effects of

SASP, 5-ASA, and the nonsteroidal anti-inflammatory drugs upon the lipoxygenase system.[74,82,109]

The effect of SASP and its metabolites upon the systemic immune system also have been examined. Arachidonic acid derivatives can stimulate (PGE_2) or inhibit (thromboxane, lipoxygenase products) suppressor cell activity,[110] and they may mediate suppression of antigen-dependent cellular cytotoxicity in mucosal lymphocytes.[111] Despite the inhibition of mutagen-induced in vitro lymphocyte cytotoxicity by sulfasalazine,[112] neither SASP, 5-ASA, nor SP altered subpopulations of circulating lymphocytes.[113] Although treatment with SASP reversed changes in circulating lymphocyte populations and function in active disease, incubation of SASP and its metabolites with leukocytes from patients did not alter the immunologic changes or immunoglobulin production by peripheral blood mononuclear cells.[114,115]

SASP also has effects on polymorphonuclear leukocyte function. Molin and Stendahl reported that SASP and SP at concentrations of 0.1 to 0.5 mM inhibited human neutrophil migration, superoxide generation, and lysosomal enzyme release, while neutrophil myeloperoxidase-mediated iodination and cytotoxicity were reduced in the presence of 5-ASA and SP at similar concentrations.[116]* It must be remembered, however, that serum concentrations of SASP and 5-ASA, achieved after oral SASP, are in the range of 0.01 to 0.05 mM,[58] ten times less than required for inhibition. Rhodes et al. also reported that SASP and 5-ASA inhibited neutrophil chemotaxis and random motility, with 50% inhibition at concentrations of 2.5 mM and 33 mM respectively;[117] again, at pharmacologic levels not normally achieved in plasma. Stenson and colleagues have shown, however, that SASP at achievable serum concentrations of 0.01 mM inhibits binding of N-formylmethionylleucyl-phenylalanine (FMLP) to neutrophil receptors.[118] FMLP is thought to be an analog of peptides synthesized by bacteria that, after binding to neutrophils, monocytes, and macrophages, results in lysosomal enzyme release, activation of the respiratory burst, and chemotaxis.[118] 5-ASA also blocks FMLP binding at higher concentrations (5 mM) and, likewise, prevents the chemotactic response, respiratory burst, and enzyme release. These authors have hypothesized that SASP may block the stimulation of the inflammatory response by blocking the binding of bacterial chemotactic factors to neutrophils.[102] Del Soldato et al. have suggested that SASP may exert beneficial actions via the ability of 5-ASA to scavenge oxygen-free radicals,[119] a theory that has been supported by recent in vitro experiments.[120]*

The exact mechanism by which SASP and its metabolites exert a beneficial effect remains uncertain. The influence of the arachidonic acid pathway requires investigation by specific inhibitors of the various pathways. The influence of SASP and metabolites on circulating and intestinal inflammatory cells needs further study at achievable tissue concentrations. Mostly what is required is a better understanding of the etiopathogenesis of inflammatory bowel disease, combined with continued investigation into potential mechanisms of benefit of SASP and its metabolites.

Adverse Reactions

A significant clinical obstacle to the use of sulfasalazine is the frequency of side effects, the incidence of which ranges between 10 and 45% in patients with ulcerative colitis and up to 85% in healthy controls.[121,122] The likelihood of developing side effects is related both to the dose and to the acetylator status.[122,123] Generalized, dose-related side effects occur in approximately 50% of patients receiving doses of 4 g or greater daily; fewer occur with a maintenance dose of 2 g daily.[52] The higher concentrations of SP obtained in patients who are phenotypically slow-acetylators are associated with toxic side effects 2 to 3 times more frequently, with an apparent threshold of approximately 50 μg/ml.[123] Most of the dose-related intolerance develops over the first few weeks of treatment,[124-126] and it will respond to a temporary discontinuation of the drug, with gradual reintroduction and a 50% lowering of the daily dose.[52,121]

Commonly encountered, dose-related side effects include dyspepsia (nausea, pyrosis, vomiting, abdominal pain),[124] headache, anorexia, myalgias, and arthralgias. A bluish discoloration of the skin ("cyanosis"),[123] hair loss, dizziness, anosmia, and palpitations are less frequent.[121,124]

"Hypersensitivity" reactions also are common. A generalized toxic reaction, with fever, skin rash, arthralgias, lymphadenopathy, and

---

*Editors' note: See also Miyachi, Y., et al.: Gut, 28:190, 1987; and Craven, P. A., et al.: Gastroenterology, 92:1998, 1987.

*Editors' note: See also Grisham, M. E., et al.: Gastroenterology, 92:1416, 1987.

hepatitis associated with hypocomplementemia and circulating immune complexes,[126] antinuclear antibodies and antibodies to double-stranded DNA,[127] or systemic granulomata accompanying the Stevens-Johnson syndrome,[127,128] have been reported. These reactions, as well as SASP-induced lupus syndrome or Raynaud's phenomenon, are reversible and also are reproducible with discontinuation and re-challenge.[121]

A variety of cutaneous eruptions ranging from urticaria or maculopapular rashes to toxic epidermal necrolysis or the Stevens-Johnson syndrome have been documented.[43,121] In most instances, the dermatologic reactions are mild and limited so the drug can be continued or temporarily withheld and gradually reintroduced (see the following); however, with more serious or generalized hypersensitivity, as described earlier, the drug should be discontinued.

A spectrum of hepatic reactions has been observed.[43,121] This includes mild to moderate hepatitis with elevations of all liver enzymes,[129] more severe hepatitis and necrosis,[130,131] cholestasis,[132] and granulomatous hepatitis.[133] In one instance, severe hepatotoxicity and a generalized systemic reaction was associated with edema, oliguria, and reduced creatinine clearance with hematuria and pigmented urinary casts, which resolved after withdrawal of the drug.[134] Pancreatitis resulting from SASP therapy also has been described.[135]

Pulmonary hypersensitivity reactions rarely occur with SASP.[43,121] The initial manifestations are dyspnea associated with cough, fever, and/or wheezing, and these are accompanied by a variety of pulmonary functional abnormalities.[136] The onset of symptoms is often delayed by months after initiation of therapy.[137] Chest radiograms may demonstrate a pattern of fibrosing alveolitis and bronchiolitis obliterans,[138] or widespread patchy or nodular infiltrates that are associated with eosinophilia.[139] While pulmonary function tests may be unaltered,[140] withdrawal of the drug is indicated in patients with eosinophilic pneumonia or fibrosing alveolitis.[121]

The spectrum of SASP's effects on the hematopoietic system ranges from metabolic to hypersensitivity reactions.[121] Beginning with the latter, rare idiosyncratic agranulocytosis that occurs independent of dose has been described,[141] and has been seen simultaneously with marrow plasmacytosis and erythroid hyperplasia.[142] Megaloblastic anemia induced by SASP has been reported, associated with selective erythroid and megakaryocytic aplasia.[143] Hemolytic anemia, with or without Heinz bodies, sulfhemoglobin, or methemoglobin, is a well-recognized complication of SASP therapy that is related to slow-acetylator status and higher SP levels.[123,144-146] Daily amounts below 1.5 g appear to be safe maintenance doses that are not associated with red blood cell abnormalities.[144]

Megaloblastic anemia also may be related to folic acid deficiency induced or aggravated by SASP administration.[147-150] While the actual development of anemia is uncommon (less than 5% of patients), low serum folate levels are not infrequent and probably underestimate red blood cell and tissue depletion.[147,149] The mechanisms of folate deficiency appear to relate to interference with a folate recognition site and/or competitive inhibition of folate conjugase in the jejunal brush border.[151,152] Folate conjugase is necessary to hydrolyze dietary, polyglutameal folate into the monoglutamate form for intestinal transport. SASP also behaves as a folate antagonist by inhibiting a variety of folate-dependent systems in lymphocytes,[153] and this has been postulated as a potential mechanism for the inhibition of cytotoxic lymphocyte function previously described.[112]

It has also been speculated that the antifolate action of SASP accounts for some of the observed ("megalo") morphologic changes in spermatozoa.[153,154] Such changes in sperm morphology accompanied reductions in sperm counts in 72% of one series of 21 patients receiving 2 to 4 g SASP daily, and abnormal sperm motility in 86%.[155] Other reports have confirmed the reversible nature of the effects of SASP on sperm size,[156] numbers, and motility.[157] O'Morain et al. studied semen samples from 64 male patients with inflammatory bowel disease who were analyzed according to whether they had never taken SASP,[158] were on the drug for more than three months, or had discontinued SASP for more than three months. Patients who had never taken the drug had normal sperm counts, motility, and morphology. All these observations (on average) were abnormal in those on the drug, but had recovered after three months off SASP. Slow acetylator patients had significantly lower sperm counts than fast acetylators but, despite reduced motility and increased numbers of abnormal sperm in slow versus fast acetylators, the differences were not statistically significant. These investigators also examined semen acid phosphatase, fructose, and PGE_2, all of which were normal, with or without SASP exposure, as were the hormone profiles of luteinizing hormone, follicle stimulating hormone, prolactin, and testosterone after a modified gonadotrophin releasing hormone test. The same report describes studies of male rats treated with SASP, SP, and 5-ASA that demonstrated litter sizes of their pregnant mates to be inversely proportional to the dose of SASP, and also reduced litter sizes from males treated with SP, but not from those given 5-ASA. It has been suggested that SASP and SP may inhibit enzymes in the acrosomal membrane that could be caused by the antifolate effect of SASP, although in an unpublished study, large doses of folate given to patients did not improve sperm counts.[158] Despite the changes in sperm morphology and function related to SASP, the frequency of infertility remains low, does not necessarily correlate with the abnormal semen analysis, and is consistently reversed by discontinuing the drug. Replacement of sulfasalazine by 5-ASA apparently also reverses the abnormal effects upon sperm in patients with ulcerative colitis.[159,160]

Miscellaneous adverse reactions to SASP include tachycardia,[161] hair loss,[162] and two syndromes of reversible neurotoxicity that manifest either as numbness, paresthesias, and ataxia,[163] or confusion, headache, and seizures associated with hepatotoxicity.[164]

Another complication of SASP therapy has been the development of bloody diarrhea with features of acute colitis. This was initially described in two children who had a rapid onset of fever, vomiting, and bloody diarrhea, with recurrent symptoms upon rechallenge.[165] This apparently hypersensitive reaction, with endoscopic and histologic features similar to active ulcerative colitis, has been confirmed in several subsequent reports.[166-169] Schwartz et al. describe a physician who consented to rechallenge with an oral dose and, later, an SASP enema that resulted in nausea, abdominal pain, and bloody diarrhea occurring within 2 or 4 hours after administration by either route.[156] Severe histologic changes were present within 8 hours and the patient developed iridocyclitis a week after each challenge, consistent with systemic consequences of IBD. All of the patients improved after withdrawal of SASP and initial stabilization with corticosteroids.

These few documented case reports differ from pseudomembranous colitis that has been described during SASP therapy for IBD,[170] and raise the possibility that SASP sensitivity may occur more frequently than has been appreciated. Many patients are treated with SASP and steroids concurrently for acute colitis. Perhaps some patients with "steroid dependent" colitis would benefit from a trial period off SASP before abandoning medical therapy (Blackstone, M.O.: Personal communication). Whether a low grade colonic sensitivity to SASP can occur remains to be seen.[166]

Recommendations for Therapy

Sulfasalazine is the initial drug of choice for patients with mild to moderate ulcerative colitis, no matter what the extent of disease. Even for those with distal ulcerative colitis or proctitis in whom 5-ASA or steroid enemas are of equal or greater efficacy, the majority of patients prefer an oral medication to nightly enemas. Most patients are given a gradually increasing dose beginning with 500 mg or 1 g daily with additional increments every few days aiming for 2 to 4 g daily in divided doses. The drug is best tolerated when taken 500 mg to 1 g at a time with food to prevent gastric irritation. Some patients tolerate and prefer 1 to 2 g twice daily to a 500 mg to 1 g q.i.d. schedule. If lower doses are not effective after several weeks of therapy, then trials of up to 6 or 8 g daily may be made, although the frequency of side effects increases significantly with doses above 2 g, as previously discussed. Furthermore, the likelihood of response to doses greater than 4 g is small. The correlation of therapeutic efficacy with serum levels of SP remains controversial,[53,123,171,172] but the impracticality of their routine measurement makes the question moot.

Once symptomatic and proctoscopic remission has been achieved, it is reasonable to attempt a reduction to a dose of 2 g daily that then is continued indefinitely. If the disease reactivates, then a higher dose (2 to 4 g daily) will be required.

SASP may also be beneficial in severe ulcerative colitis. The acute symptoms (nausea, abdominal pain, anorexia) of the disease may mimic intolerance to the drug or be aggravated by the introduction of the medication, however, especially in patients who are unable to eat. Furthermore, with severe diarrhea and rapid transit time,[54,66] or with the co-administration of antibiotics,[67] the bacterial splitting of SASP into the active moiety 5-ASA is impaired and the drug's efficacy reduced. Therefore, it seems appropriate to withhold SASP until the patient is stabilized, is eating, and the diarrhea is controlled prior to the gradual introduction of SASP.

Several drug interactions with SASP have been recognized.[43] The impaired splitting of the azo bond with co-administration of antibiotics already was mentioned. The inhibition of absorption of folates from the diet leads us to routinely prescribe folic acid 1 to 2 mg daily. The simultaneous administration of SASP and ferrous sulfate results in decreased blood levels of SASP attributed to a physical interaction (chelation) between SASP and the iron.[173] Although the bioavailability of iron was not shown to be influenced by simultaneous administration of SASP, nor was there an effect on the overall metabolism of SASP, it is still reasonable to administer iron products separately from SASP.[43] Studies in volunteers have demonstrated interference with the bioavailability of digoxin, with a mean reduction of serum digoxin levels by 25%.[174] SASP also may potentiate the effect of concomitantly administered warfarin (Coumadin*), oral hypoglycemic agents, phenylbutazone, and other highly protein-bound agents, indicating the need for caution in their combined use.[175]

Management of Intolerance and Allergy

As described previously, symptoms of intolerance to SASP, such as nausea, vomiting, and headache, are related to the irritant effects of SASP on the digestive tract or to serum levels of SP that depend on the total dose and acetylator status.[123] Also as indicated earlier, we routinely advise patients to take the drug with meals to avoid dyspeptic symptoms. If this is not sufficient, then the enteric-coated preparation may be better tolerated.[61,124] Das and co-workers also have described successful reintroduction of SASP to patients with intolerance, minor skin rashes, or reticulocytosis after discontinuing the drug for one to two weeks, and then initiating therapy with 125 to 250 mg daily for a week with gradual increments of 125 mg daily each week until a maintenance dose of 2 g daily is achieved.[121,123,176]

In three subsequent reports, desensitization protocols have been described for patients with allergic skin rashes or fevers. Holdsworth was able to desensitize 7 out of 8 patients by beginning with 1 mg daily and progressively doubling the dose daily, with one week long plateaus at doses of 10 mg and 100 mg.[177] This schedule required 23 days before the normal tablet strength of 500 mg was achieved, and if a reaction occurred the patients were instructed to continue using the medication until the symptoms resolved. Purdy et al. successfully desensitized 100% of 13 patients by using SASP suspension in a similar dose schedule (Table 21-5), requiring from 32 days to six months to reach a dosage of 2 g.[178] They reported clinical improvement in 11 out of 13 patients during therapy, with 2 out of 13 remaining unchanged. Korelitz et al. used three different dosage schedules depending upon the severity of the allergic reactions:[179]

1. ¼ tablet a day for three days, ¼ tablet twice a day for three days, ¼ tablet three times a day for three days, etc.
2. 1/8 tablet a day for one week, 1/8 tablet twice a day for the second week, etc.
3. 1/4 tablet a day for one week, 1/4 tablet twice a day for one week, etc.

They were able to desensitize 40 out of 47 (85%) patients, including 13 out of 20 who had a recurrence of their sensitivity reaction during the reintroduction program. The authors emphasized the value of an attempt at desensitization as all 17 patients with ulcerative colitis remained well on SASP alone (12 out of 17) or on SASP with intermittent steroids (5 out of 17). *None of the reports advocated attempts at desensitization in patients with severe reactions to SASP such as frank hemolysis, agranulocytosis, hepatotoxicity, and pulmonary reactions, however.* We have found a schedule using SASP suspen-

TABLE 21-5. *Sulfasalazine Desensitization Schedule*

Day	Dose
Solution 1, 1 mg/mL	
1	1 mg = 1 mL
2	2 mg = 2 mL
3	4 mg = 4 mL
4	8 mg = 8 mL
5-11	10 mg = 10 mL
Solution 2, 20 mg/mL	
12	20 mg = 1 mL
13	40 mg = 2 mL
14	80 mg = 4 mL
15-21	100 mg = 5 mL
22	200 mg = 10 mL
23	400 mg = 20 mL
24	800 mg = 40 mL
500 mg sulfasalazine tablets	
25-31	1000 mg = 2 tablets
32+	2000 mg = 4 tablets

*DuPont Pharmaceuticals, Wilmington, DE.

sion beginning with 1 to 50mg daily (depending upon the severity of the reaction) with doubling of the dose every three days to be simple and effective. If reactions recur, the dose can be maintained until resolution in the case of mild episodes, or discontinued and gradually reintroduced, beginning with lower doses (e.g., 1mg) with longer time intervals (five days to a week) between doubling. *Again, such desensitization is not warranted for patients with severe reactions.**

Pregnancy, Lactation, and Children†

Concern over the possibility of kernicterus or congenital malformations has been raised by the appearance of SASP and its metabolites (especially SP) in cord serum, amniotic fluid, and breast milk.[53] Several large clinical series, however, have failed to identify evidence of harmful effects upon the fetus in utero or nursing infants.[180-184] Furthermore, a report from the American College of Gastroenterology supports the continued use of SASP during pregnancy and breast feeding.[185]

Sulfasalazine can be used safely in children, although modifying the dose to 1.5 to 2.0g/m²/day (40 to 70mg/kg/day) minimizes dose related toxicity associated with total SP metabolite concentration of greater than 50µg/ml.[186]

5-ASA Drugs

Despite the documented benefit of SASP for ulcerative colitis, the frequency of adverse effects and intolerance, and its less than total efficacy have led to the development of more effective and less toxic derivatives. Because the identification of 5-ASA as an active moiety and SP as the toxic derivative, a new generation of SASP-like drugs without the sulfa component has emerged, with 5-ASA as the prototype. A variety of preparations currently are being investigated in trials in Europe and the United States. Although at this time none are approved for general use in the United States, several of these products are available in Canada as well as in Europe. Hence, a discussion of the preparations described in the literature follows.

5-ASA ENEMAS. Azad Khan and co-workers were the first to describe the beneficial effects of rectally administered 5-ASA for patients with mild to moderate ulcerative proctosigmoiditis.[79] 700mg of 5-ASA in 100 ml of a neutral (pH 7.0) isotonic solution administered once daily for two weeks produced symptomatic improvement in 75% of patients, sigmoidoscopic responses in 64%, and histologic improvement in 30%; these results were similar to those in patients treated with SASP suspensions, but significantly better than those with SP enemas. Campieri et al. were the first to use high-dose 5-ASA enemas in a double-blind controlled trial of 4g 5-ASA compared to 100mg hydrocortisone (as the succinate salt) enemas in 86 patients over 2 weeks.[187] They found 5-ASA to be superior by producing clinical remission in 93%, sigmoidoscopic remission in 93%, and histologic improvement in 77% of patients, compared to 57%, 54%, and 53% with hydrocortisone. The same group subsequently reported a four year experience in which 144 patients were treated for 327 therapeutic cycles with 2 to 4g of 5-ASA in 100ml for two to four weeks, with clinical improvement after 88% of the therapeutic cycles.[188,189] Forty-four of their patients were either allergic to or intolerant of SASP. Only five of these were unable to tolerate 5-ASA enemas because of skin rash or diarrhea.[190] The pioneering work with high dose 5-ASA enemas from the Bologna group also has documented retrograde flow of the enemas to the splenic flexure,[191] as well as the absence of significant plasma accumulation of 5-ASA after a month of continuous treatment.[192]

Excellent confirmatory results have been reported from uncontrolled studies using high dose 5-ASA enemas in patients with refractory distal colitis.[193-198] We noted symptomatic and proctoscopic improvement in 12 out of 22 patients.* Of the nonresponders, 7 out of 10 had disease proximal to the splenic flexure, 2 were unable to retain the enemas, and 1 patient had a rectal stricture.[193]† We also found the enemas to be useful when tapering or discontinuing steroid therapy in patients who were previously considered to be steroid dependent.[194] d'Albasio and colleagues found intermittent 4g 5-ASA enemas to be effective in maintaining remissions in patients by administering the drug for the first week of the month over one year.[199] Further

---

*Editors' note: see Meyers, S., et al.: Gastroenterology 93:1255, 1987.
†See Chapters 12, 17, and 23.

*Editors' note: See also Hanauer, S. B., et al.: Gastroenterology, *92*:1424, 1987. The authors concluded that a requirement for persistent 5-ASA therapy for maintenance in such patients probably exists, but further trials are needed.
†Editors' note: See also Sutherland, L. R., et al.: Gastroenterology, *92*:1894, 1987, this discusses 5-ASA enemas that are well-tolerated and effective.

work is needed to clarify the optimum dose, tapering, and maintenance schedules for these new products.

The question of optimal dosages for all patients remains unanswered as a number of studies have examined lower dose regimens. While several authors report approximately 50% effectiveness with 700mg to 1g enemas,[200,201] Powell-Tuck et al. found no short-term differences between 1 and 2g doses,[202] and a Danish group reported 77% clinical remissions in a group of 53 patients treated with 1g daily doses;[203] results approaching the effectiveness of high dose enemas. The nature of the study populations (that is, age, proximal extent of disease, chronicity of symptoms, and response to prior therapy) needs to be better defined prior to recommending guidelines of treatment. Nevertheless, the use of the enemas has been well tolerated in all of the previously mentioned series with only local irritation, rare instances of inability to retain the enemas, and occasional diarrhea, skin rashes, or hair loss being reported as side effects.[204] Furthermore, the pH of the buffered suspension can influence the kinetic pattern of metabolism, greater absorption being documented with neutral compared with acidic suspensions.[200] Although high doses have caused nephrotoxicity in rats,[200,205] such effects have not been recognized in numerous human trials.[74]

5-ASA SUPPOSITORIES. In a small, open study, Klotz et al. administered 500mg 5-ASA suppositories three times daily with clinical improvement comparable to oral SASP, 1g t.i.d.,[80] while van Hees and colleagues used an even lower dose (200mg suppository) twice daily over four weeks with superior efficacy to SP.[206] Follow-up German studies of the Dr. Falk GmbH and Co. (Freiburg, West Germany) product have confirmed the effectiveness of the 1.5g daily dose of suppositories in inducing both clinical and sigmoidoscopic improvement with active disease,[207] and of lower doses (250mg t.i.d.) for maintaining remission.[208] In an Italian study, 5-ASA suppositories administered twice daily compared favorably to a 2g nightly enema,[209] and controlled trials are currently being done in the United States, using a 250mg preparation produced by Reid-Rowell, with preliminary results of excellent efficacy during acute disease, as well as in open maintenance studies (Dr. Lowell Borgen, personal communication). Again, final recommendations on the use of these locally acting products cannot be made at this time although we expect that these new agents will add to the therapeutic armamentarium, especially for distal inflammatory bowel disease.

4-ASA ENEMAS. Because of the instability of 5-ASA solutions, a similar salicylate, 4-(para)-aminosalicylic acid (4-ASA; PAS), a drug that has been widely available and used for many years for the treatment of tuberculosis, has been tested in enema form for distal ulcerative colitis. The agent is more stable in suspension than 5-ASA, was as effective as 5-ASA enemas in 2g doses,[210] and was superior to placebo in 1g and 2g doses.[211,212] Continued comparative trials are underway.*

ORAL 5-ASA PREPARATIONS. The effectiveness of 5-ASA as a therapeutic agent in IBD has led to the development of a variety of products, devoid of the sulfa moiety, which deliver 5-ASA to the site of intestinal inflammation. Delivery systems rely either on the azo bond (Fig. 21-7), which requires bacterial action for reduction, or slow-release preparations, which will bypass the rapid absorption of 5-ASA from the proximal bowel.[53,74]

---

*Editors' note: See also Ginsberg, A. L., et al.: Gastroenterology, 92:1406, 1987; the enema treatment in this case was successful in 10 of 12 patients.

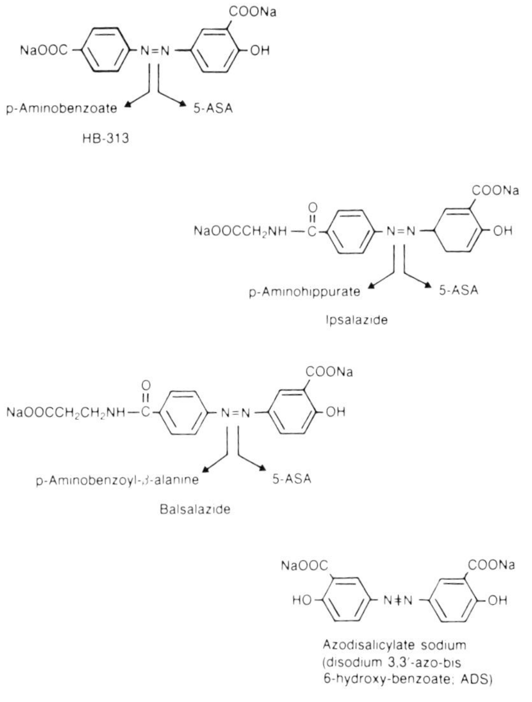

FIG. 21-7. Azo-bond preparations.

Azo-Bond Preparations

AZODISALICYLATE (OLSALAZINE, DIPENTUM*). A logical alternative to SASP is the dimer of two 5-ASA molecules attached by the same azo bond. Studies in normal volunteers have demonstrated only minimal absorption of the intact molecule with serum levels of less than 2.7µg/ml following a 250mg dose, and less than 12µg/ml after 2g/day; low serum levels of 5-ASA (0.8µg/ml) and Ac-5-ASA (1.1µg/ml); the majority (median 34%) of the drug being recovered as 5-ASA or Ac-5-ASA in the feces.[213] Subsequent evaluations of orally administered azodisalicylate have documented the need for an intact gastrointestinal tract with a normal bacterial flora for effective splitting of the azo bond,[100,214] its long serum half-life of 6 to 10 days,[215] and detectable serum levels for up to three weeks after withdrawal.[213] Fecal recovery of total 5-ASA was virtually identical to an equimolar dose of SASP.[215] After rectal administration, urinary recovery of the parent drug and its metabolites was less than 4% of the administered dose.[216]

To date, clinical studies with azodisalicylate have been limited, but encouraging. The Oxford group has begun to investigate both oral and rectal administration in randomized placebo trials. Preliminary findings in patients with mild, distal UC demonstrated improvement in 19 out of 29 patients, compared with 12 out of 28 on placebo. For the oral trial, 13 out of 20 patients improved with the drug compared to 8 out of 20 with placebo.[217] Three quarters of their patients who had been intolerant of SASP could tolerate azodisalicylate.[218] In an open, compassionate-use study for those intolerant or unresponsive to SASP, 52 UC patients were treated and remission was noted in 19, improvement in 20, no change in 8, and worsening in 5. Approximately 25% of the group withdrew from therapy because of worsening of diarrhea, lack of effect, tremors (1 patient), or rash and metallic taste (1 patient).[219]

In Sweden, azodisalicylate, 500mg b.i.d., was evaluated against placebo to prevent relapse of UC in 101 patients who were previously SASP intolerant or allergic and had been successfully put into remission with azodisalicylate. Within six months, 12 out of 52 patients (23%) in the active group versus 22 out of 49 (45%) of the placebo group had relapsed,[220] an experience similar to that with SASP.[51,52]† The same group observed 160 patients with active UC who had previously been intolerant or allergic to SASP and were treated in an open trial with azodisalicylate.[221] The only significant side effect was diarrhea that caused 20 patients (12.5%) to discontinue treatment; an additional 13% experienced transient diarrhea or loose stools not severe enough to stop treatment. Another small randomized trial showed benefit of azodisalicylate over placebo in 30 patients with mild to moderate UC. Again, 13% of the azodisalicylate group were withdrawn because of diarrhea.[222] This most distressing effect has been recognized in patients with ileostomies,[214] and is likely a result of net water and ion secretion from the small bowel. To define the ultimate clinical merit of these findings will require more extensive investigations and clinical experience.

OTHER AZO-BOND PRO-DRUGS OF 5-ASA. Four additional species of 5-ASA preparations have been described, all with limited clinical experience. p-Aminobenzoate (HB-313), p-aminohippurate, 4-aminobenzoylglycine (ABG, Ipsalazide), 4-aminobenzoyl-B-alanine (ABA, Balsalazide*), and a sulfanilamidoethylene polymer (BW75Y) have been used as replacement carrier molecules for SP to deliver the pro-drugs to where enzymatic cleavage by bacterial azo reductase releases 5-ASA.[53,74,223,224] It is to be expected that these preparations will be most useful for colonic inflammation, and will depend upon sufficiently slow intestinal and colonic transit and an intact bacterial population for their proper breakdown and availability of 5-ASA. More extensive studies of the specific pharmacologic and toxicologic properties of the parent compounds and carrier molecules are needed.

Ipsalazide and Balsalazide have been tested in experimental animals and healthy volunteers.[225] In the human studies, the pharmacokinetics of 5-ASA were comparable to that with SASP. Serum concentrations of Ipsalazide and Balsalazide were not detectable, and ABA was not identifiable.[225] While treatments with Balsalazide has been recognized to reverse male infertility caused by SASP,[226] results of a completed, controlled, therapeutic trial have been promised.[225] Salicylabenzoic acid (HB-313) has only been described in a single, brief communication and requires further scrutiny.[227] BW73y has been investigated in cats and it has similar deliveries of 5-ASA to the colon, blood, and urine

---

*Pharmacia Laboratories, Piscataway, NJ 08854. See also, Meyers, S., et al.: Gastroenterology, 93:1255, 1987.

†Editors' note: See also Sandberg-Gertzén, H., et al.: Gastroenterology, 90:1024, 1986; the drug azodisal sodium was found to be effective for maintenance therapy in this study.

*Editors' note: See also McIntire, P. B., et al.: Gut, 27:1271, 1986; Balsalazide was to be more effective and had fewer side effects than sulfasalazine according to this comparison study.

as SASP, and it was a more effective therapy than SASP or 5-ASA in the guinea pig model of carageenan-induced cecitis.[228] In an open trial involving 10 patients with active UC who were intolerant or allergic to SASP, the compound was well-tolerated, with clinical improvement described in 7 patients,[229] and comparable plasma concentrations of 5-ASA and metabolites to those achieved with SASP.[230] Potential problems with BW734, including inadequate dispersion of the compound in the stool, orange staining caused by the coloring of the analine compound, and persorption of the compound into mucosal macrophages, have led to discontinuation of further clinical trials (C.S. Winans, personal communication).

ORAL NON-LINKED 5-ASA. Three pharmaceutical preparations formulated to delay or sustain the release of 5-ASA independent of bacterial action are currently being investigated. A slow-release oral preparation of 5-ASA (Salofalk*) recently has been marketed in West Germany. In patients with active inflammatory bowel disease treated with 500mg t.i.d., steady state plasma concentrations of 5-ASA and Ac-5-ASA averaged 0.7 and 1.2μg/ml (comparable to levels with SASP) with fecal recovery of 5-ASA at 35%.[53,73] In a randomized controlled trial with 5-ASA, 0.5g t.i.d., or 1g SASP t.i.d., involving 30 patients with active UC, a morphologic remission was achieved in 60% of the patients with 5-ASA compared to 53% with SASP; symptoms and bowel movements normalized in 86% of both groups.[231]

Another slow release 5-ASA tablet (Pentasa†) has been prepared by coating microgranules of 5-ASA with a semipermeable membrane of ethylcellulose that releases 5-ASA in a pH-dependent manner throughout the length of the gut.[71] Release also is dependent upon the rate of intestinal transit.[232] In ileostomy patients, approximately 50% had been released from the granules in the small bowel. In healthy subjects, about 35% of the drug is absorbed in the small intestine, 25% in the colon, and 40% of the 24 hour dose is recovered in the feces.[71] Pentasa has been evaluated in an open trial in 18 patients with Crohn's disease (10 with colonic disease) at a dose of 500mg t.i.d. for 6 weeks. Improvement was noted in 13 patients (77%), without side effects.[233] Clinical trials for ulcerative colitis are now in progress in the United States, Canada, Denmark, and Italy.

In another preparation recently marketed in Great Britain and Canada (Asacol[R]*), 400mg of 5-ASA is coated with an acrylic based resin (Eudragit-S) that delays the release until the luminal pH is above 7 (usually within the terminal ileum or colon).[234] In patients with ulcerative colitis, nearly complete breakdown of the tablets occurred with peak serum concentrations by 6 hours of 2.3μg/ml after a 3.2g dose.[235] In UC patients in remission, urinary recovery of the drug was approximately 20 to 25%, mainly as Ac-5-ASA, as was the case with SASP.[236] In therapeutic trials, Asacol[R], at a mean dose of 2.7g daily, was equally as beneficial as SASP (mean dose 2.3g daily) in preventing relapse (in 78% and 80% respectively) in 57 patients with UC in remission followed over 6 months.[237,238] The drug was well-tolerated without side effects in most patients, including those who were previously intolerant or allergic to SASP, although a few patients complained of nausea, abdominal discomfort, and feelings of unreality.[239] Asacol[R] has been of benefit in open studies of patients with active ulcerative colitis and has been well-tolerated,[240–243] although exacerbations of diarrhea have occurred in several patients who reacted similarly to SASP.[243] Despite the potential for nephrotoxicity observed in rats receiving 10 to 30 times the dose prescribed in human studies, long-term toxicity has not been reported.[74,244] Furthermore, SASP-induced infertility has been reversed after changing treatment to 5-ASA.[159,160]

Clearly, we are entering an era of therapeutic alternatives to the conventional first-line therapy for ulcerative colitis. The ultimate agent(s) of choice and mode of administration (rectal and/or oral) will depend upon the extent, severity, and response to prior therapy. The advantages of one preparation over another have not yet been clarified. Schedules for tapering and their role and doses of these preparations for maintaining remissions have not been elucidated. It is likely that combined therapy (an oral plus rectal agent, or steroids plus 5-ASA derivatives will be useful in certain situations. We await reports on the ever-expanding experience with these promising new products.

Steroids and ACTH

Mechanism of action

Thirty-five years have passed since the initial report by Truelove and Witts stating that corti-

---

* Dr. Falk GmbH & Company; Freiburg, West Germany.
† Ferring A/S; Vanlose, Denmark

* Tillotts Laboratory

sone was effective in a controlled trial in ulcerative colitis,[245] yet the mechanism of action of steroids in inflammatory bowel disease remains uncertain. The anti-inflammatory activity of glucocorticoid steroids has been studied intensively in animal and human models. The hormones act in a large number of sites with many different actions.[246] At a cellular level, glucocorticoid steroids interact with specific receptors located within the cytosol of a variety (if not all) of nucleated cells. After an allosteric change, the steroid-receptor complex moves into the nucleus, binds to segments of DNA, and, in an undetermined manner, causes synthesis of an RNA that reaches the cytoplasm and results in protein synthesis. One such protein inhibits phospholipases and prevents the liberation of arachidonic acid and the prostaglandin and lipoxygenase products (see Fig. 21-6).[247] Suppression of the release of growth factors such as interleukin-1 and interleukin-2 inhibits the proliferation of lymphoid cells. Steroids also inhibit the release of other lymphokines and inflammatory proteases (collagenase, elastase, plasminogen activators) by a host of cells, but especially from monocytes, macrophages, and basophils. Corticosteroids also induce changes in inflammatory cell traffic that can prevent their accumulation at local sites of inflammation. Again, the effect is not simple and may result from the impaired release of chemotactic mediators in the tissues, changes in vascular endothelial cells that reduce their "stickiness," and/or the inhibition of adherence and migration of inflammatory cells to and through the vascular endothelium. In addition, steroids are potent vasoconstrictors that increase microvascular tone and decrease permeability, stabilize lysosomal membranes, and facilitate adrenergic responses to sympathetic stimuli and circulating catecholamines.[246,247] The lack of an experimental animal model for inflammatory bowel disease has hindered the study of steroid actions in inflammatory bowel disease, although, in ulcerative colitis, corticosteroids have been shown to inhibit prostaglandin synthesis in vitro in tissue cultures of rectal biopsies from patients, and in vivo by using equilibrium dialysis techniques.[248,249]

Several other aspects of steroid therapy must be considered before an adequate understanding of their action can be achieved. The biologic activities of cortisone, hydrocortisone, and the synthetic glucocorticoids probably are different, as are the biologic effects of the drugs on endogenous cortisol secretion.[250] Furthermore, ACTH treatment is even more complex because of the release of a variety of glucocorticoid, mineralocorticoid, and androgen products.[251] The biologic effects probably differ between single synthetic preparations and endogenously produced and metabolized products. Likewise, the available information on drug levels usually pertains to body fluids rather than tissues where the anti-inflammatory activity appears to correlate best with steroid concentrations.[252] Determinations of plasma levels may not adequately reflect the therapeutic activity (and potential for side effects). These correlate best with free drug levels rather than the protein-bound proportion that may relate to levels of transcortin and albumin, as well as the particular dose schedule and route of administration. Few of these factors have been adequately investigated as they pertain to ulcerative colitis.[250,253]

Clinical Trials

As applies to many conditions, "anecdotal" clinical experience with steroid therapy (including ACTH) for ulcerative colitis far exceeds the documentation of its effect in controlled therapeutic trials. Nevertheless, a variety of clinical studies have led to several empiric approaches that are applicable to the majority of clinical situations the treating physician may confront. We shall first review the few controlled trials before detailing the role of steroid therapy in specific clinical settings. Both systemic and local steroid therapy will be described.

SYSTEMIC THERAPY. Truelove and Witts were the first to examine steroid therapy in a controlled fashion in ulcerative colitis.[245] They compared 109 patients treated with cortisone (100mg/day) to 101 subjects treated with placebo over a six week period. They included a spectrum of patients with mild to severe disease and found cortisone to be superior in all groups, although the effect was less favorable in more severely ill patients. Lennard-Jones et al. later confirmed the benefit of oral prednisone over placebo in patients with mild to moderate colitis.[254]

Subsequently, Truelove and Witts compared intramuscular ACTH-gel (80 units daily) to oral cortisone (200mg daily) and found similar benefits with each.[255] A somewhat greater benefit for patients treated with ACTH for relapsing colitis (compared with equal efficacy for first attacks), was offset by a higher relapse rate during the subsequent year. Kaplan et al. treated 22 hospitalized patients who had Crohn's disease or ulcerative colitis in a double-blind manner by administering either intravenous ACTH (40 units daily) or hydrocortisone (300mg daily), and found the drugs to be equally effective in inducing clinical remissions in those not receiving prior steroids, although the patients who had received prior steroids seemed to benefit more from the hydrocortisone.[256] Powell-Tuck et al. confirmed the superiority of the effect of intravenous hydrocortisone (400mg daily) over intramuscular ACTH-gel (80 units daily) in patients previously treated with steroids.[257] Neither of the aforementioned studies could correlate plasma cortisol levels with the clinical responses.[256,257] Finally, in the largest comparative, controlled trial of ACTH to date, the Mount Sinai group randomized 66 patients with strictly defined, severe ulcerative colitis to receive either intravenous ACTH (120 units daily) or intravenous hydrocortisone (300mg daily).[258] Patients were prospectively stratified according to previous oral corticosteroid therapy, and the medication was administered continuously over 24 hours to avoid questions regarding intermittent dosing. In this study, clear benefits were apparent for those receiving ACTH who had not previously received oral steroids (63% versus 27% response), whereas hydrocortisone therapy benefited a greater proportion of patients who had been exposed to prior steroid therapy (53% versus 25%). Hence, while both steroids and ACTH are beneficial in acute, severe ulcerative colitis, the clinical outcome appears to differ depending upon the prior treatment. Once again, the improvement observed in this study could not be correlated with serum cortisol or dehydroepiandrosterone levels in either treatment group, suggesting that alternative factors, such as other adrenal hormones or the rate of adrenal response, may influence the therapeutic outcome.[251,258]

Additional evidence for the effectiveness of ACTH in acute ulcerative colitis came from studies at the Beth Israel Hospital in Boston and at the University of Chicago.[259,260]

Further evidence for a therapeutic role for systemic steroids comes from retrospective studies by Truelove and Witts and Hartong et al.[261,262] The former documented reduced colectomy and mortality rates in steroid treated patients; the latter noted an improved outcome in such individuals. Despite these results, controversy over the length of medical therapy for acutely ill patients treated with steroid therapy was sustained by results from a Scandinavian study that showed that prolonging therapy beyond two weeks yielded no higher proportion of patients entering remission and avoiding surgical treatment, and the operative death rate increased.[263] These findings led the Oxford and Swedish groups to treat patients intensively with intravenous steroids (equivalent to 40mg prednisone), fluids, and nutritional support over a 5 day period, after which time patients were recommended to undergo colectomy if they had not improved.[264-266] Sixty percent of the patients in the Oxford series and 56% in the Swedish study group improved enough to avoid surgical intervention, with a median time to remission of 8 to 10 days in the latter study.

Although intensive intravenous therapy was found to be effective in over 90% of patients with mild to moderate ulcerative colitis,[265] in most of such cases parenteral steroids are not necessary. Oral steroid therapy is effective in the majority of those less severely ill with ulcerative colitis, as initially demonstrated by Truelove and Witts.[245] Seventy percent of the steroid treated patients either entered remission or improved during a six week course of 100mg of cortisone daily. Compared to SASP, prednisone (with or without hydrocortisone enemas) works faster and has an equal overall response rate for patients with mild or moderate colitis.[47,254]

Two reports of intra-arterial prednisolone administered directly into the mesenteric system in adults and children with severe ulcerative colitis warrant further investigation in patients unresponsive to standard intensive therapy.[267,268]

The optimum dose of steroids has not been extensively evaluated by "dose-ranging" studies.[250] Two-thirds of outpatients treated with 40 or 60mg of prednisone daily in divided doses improved over three weeks, compared to one-third of those treated with 20mg daily.[269] The benefit was rapid, with most responders improving within two weeks. The maximum response with minimum side effects at 40mg daily led to the recommendation of the intermediate dose. The St. Mark's group subsequently compared 40mg in a single dose to 10mg given four times a day. No difference was observed either in response rates or side effects, leading the authors to recommend 40mg as a single morning dose because it is convenient and adrenal suppression is less.[270] Although this approach is reasonable for the majority of patients, the use of divided doses of steroids for those who fail to respond to a single dose daily or for patients with persistent nocturnal symptoms should not be abandoned.

Maintenance Therapy

Unlike the situation with sulfasalazine in ulcerative colitis, which has been shown to be effective both for the induction of remissions and maintenance therapy, it is difficult to find evidence in favor of chronic maintenance therapy to prevent relapses using steroid therapy alone. Kirsner and colleagues described a large clinical experience with corticosteroids and ACTH, in which many patients required chronic continuous therapy to maintain a sustained response.[260] Nevertheless, controlled trials of cortisone, 50mg daily,[261] and prednisone, 15mg daily,[271] showed no evidence of a decreased relapse rate. In the former study, the relapse rate at 10 months was 50% in both drug-treated and placebo groups; in the latter trial, 60% of the steroid and placebo-treated groups had relapsed by six months.

In one series of nine patients at Johns Hopkins, an alternate day regimen of prednisone, 25 to 120mg, prescribed over 11 to 20 months, was comparable in effect to the daily administration of prednisone, 15 to 60mg in divided doses, and was associated with less adrenal suppression.[272] Supplemental sulfasalazine obscured the potential benefit of the intermittent regimen, however. The St. Mark's group has since reported a double-blind crossover study of 24 patients with frequently relapsing colitis who also were continued on sulfasalazine in addition to 40mg of prednisone on alternate days, or placebo.[273] The cumulative likelihood of no relapse after three months was significantly better with prednisone (80%) than during the placebo period (40%). Hence, only in a small, select group of patients who frequently relapsed despite SASP treatment, has relatively short-term, alternate day, maintenance therapy with prednisone been shown to be efficacious. For the majority of patients with active colitis who respond to steroid therapy with complete remission, the steroids should be expeditiously tapered (see the following) and sulfasalazine, or an alternative 5-ASA derivative, should be maintained. A minority of patients with chronic persistent or frequently relapsing colitis may require continuous steroid treatment, in which case an alternate day regimen should be tried at the minimal dose that prevents recurrent activity. Although many patients may not tolerate such a schedule and will require chronic, low-dose daily therapy, the alternate day schedule has been shown to reduce adrenal suppression and the likelihood of side effects.[273]

Local Steroids

Shortly after systemic steroid therapy became recognized as an effective therapy for ulcerative colitis, the local administration of hydrocortisone was found to be useful in open and placebo-controlled trials.[274-277] Even in these early clinical studies, the careful observational techniques documented the lag between clinical, sigmoidoscopic, and histologic improvement that has been found in subsequent reports.[278] In the controlled trial of hydrocortisone hemisuccinate enemas (100mg in 120ml saline) by Truelove, clinical and sigmoidoscopic improvement was noted in 60% of patients by one week, with up to 72% of patients achieving "remission" by the end of three weeks. No differences were encountered between patients treated with maintenance therapy of a rectal drip on two consecutive nights each week ("weekend maintenance therapy"), as 5 out of 13 patients in both the hydrocortisone and control groups relapsed during the six month trial period.[276] Subsequent studies also performed by Truelove at Oxford found that local corticosteroid therapy induced a more rapid clinical remission than a comparable oral dose,[279] and that a rectal drip of hydrocortisone hemisuccinate could be a useful adjunct to systemic corticosteroid therapy for patients with more extensive and severe ulcerative colitis.[280]

Once the efficacy of hydrocortisone retention enemas was described, additional preparations were tested and questions arose as to the extent of the proximal spread of the enemas, to what degree did systemic absorption occur, and whether the benefit was derived from a topical effect of the enema solution or from the systemic absorption. After Matts found prednisolone-21-phosphate to be an effective treatment for ulcerative colitis when administered via a dispensable plastic bag, he investigated the retrograde spread of 100ml of barium suspension in normal controls and patients with ulcerative colitis when instilled via a plastic bag or through a slow-drip infusion.[281] No obvious difference existed between the two techniques, with proximal penetration to the mid-descending colon occurring in most of the patients, and in many cases the splenic or hepatic flexures were reached.[282] Swarbrick and colleagues found the proximal spread of steroid enemas to be greater in patients with active disease, with a rough correlation between enema volume and the distance reached.[283] On the contrary, low volumes of hydrocortisone foam are less likely to migrate as far as the descending colon.[284,285] Most recently, 60ml hydrocortisone enemas radiolabelled with technetium were shown to penetrate for a distance equal to or greater than the extent of disease involvement in 7 out of 8 patients with mainly left-sided colitis.[286]

The degree to which systemic absorption and adrenal suppression occur depends upon the preparation and dose, as well as the degree of colonic inflammation and length of time for which the enema is retained. Separate studies have been made of the absorption into the plasma, the urinary levels of the drug, or the adrenal suppression after administration of hydrocortisone,[287-289] prednisone,[290] prednisolone,[290-295] betamethasone,[294,295] or methylprednisolone enemas.[296] Studies using these drugs have been insufficient to document consistent advantages of one preparation over another when absorption (adrenal suppression) versus efficacy are compared. In general, the absorption is less than that of an equivalent dose administered by mouth,[292,297] but as much as three-fourths of a rectal dose may be absorbed.[290]

The beneficial topical effects as compared to effectiveness resulting from systemic absorption recently has been clarified by employing preparations of prednisolone enemas that have different absorptive capacities but equal therapeutic efficacy.[298,299] Prednisolone metasulfobenzoate is poorly absorbed, yet has therapeutic effects equal to prednisolone phosphate enemas, and a greater effect than the oral dose of prednisolone that provides equal plasma levels.[300] Likewise, beclomethasone enemas produce topical effects without interference with the hypothalamic pituitary axis.[301,302] Most recently, tixocortol pivalate, a nonglucocorticoid, non-mineralocorticoid steroid with local and topical anti-inflammatory activity,[303] has been found in a large, multicenter trial to have an efficacy equal to hydrocortisone enemas for left-sided colitis,[304] and may be useful in high doses for patients with refractory proctosigmoiditis.[305] Tixocortol is rapidly metabolized after absorption and has essentially no systemic effects, as measured by routine laboratory studies of blood counts, serum chemistries, determinations of cortisol, or influence upon the hypothalamic-pituitary-adrenal axis.[303]

Topical steroids also can be administered in a foam suspension that may be useful for patients with distal proctitis in whom proximal penetration is not necessary.[284] Such a formulation is well-tolerated, may be prescribed to ambulatory patients more often than the single nocturnal enema application, and provides an efficacy equal to hydrocortisone or prednisolone 21-phosphate enemas and greater patient preference and a less disturbing impact on the quality of life.[306,307] A suppository form of prednisolone-21 phosphate, at a dose of 10mg nightly, also has been effective in 75% of patients with proctitis treated over three weeks, compared to 40% receiving placebo.[308]

Adverse Effects

The complications of steroid therapy are well-known and have been reviewed previously as pertains to general use and to inflammatory bowel disease.[309-311] The long-term complications seen in patients with inflammatory bowel disease range from psychologic dependence,[312] to growth retardation.[260,310] The prevalence of side effects is dose- and chronicity-related, and complications are seen more frequently in debilitated and malnourished (especially hypoalbuminemic) patients. Abnormalities of fat distribution ("moon face") can be anticipated with moderate to high dose therapy, and the absence of such features is likely to correlate with an inadequate therapeutic response. The glucocorticosteroids are catabolic hormones and loss of muscle mass is to be expected with long-term treatment, although muscle weakness and fatigue are usually only seen either with high dose therapy or when treatment is complicated by hypokalemia aggravated by the mineralocorticoid effects of some products (cortisone and hydrocortisone more so than prednisone, prednisolone, or methylprednisolone) (Table 21-6). Bone loss and osteoporosis are long-term complications that may be hastened by milk-free or low calcium diets. Osteonecrosis (aseptic necrosis) can complicate high dose steroid therapy and is, to date, an irreversible and most troublesome, debilitating disorder that may only be recognized after dose reduction or discontinuation of treatment (personal observation).

Gastrointestinal side effects must be closely monitored in patients with ulcerative colitis. Whether peptic ulceration is caused by steroid therapy remains controversial,[313] but such ulceration must be considered in patients with unexpected gastrointestinal hemorrhage on steroid therapy.[314] In seriously ill patients, steroid therapy can mask colonic (or proximal gastrointestinal) perforations, so careful clinical and noncontrast radiographic observations are essential.[315] Despite early concerns over the effect

TABLE 21-6. *Steroids Commonly Used in Ulcerative Colitis.*

	Relative Anti-inflammatory Potency	Relative Sodium Retaining Potency	Appropriate Equivalent Dose (mg)
Hydrocortisone	1	1	20
Prednisone	4	0.8	5
Prenislolone	4	0.8	5
Methylprednisolone	5	0.5	4
Triamcinolone	5	0	4
Betamethasone	2.5	0	0.75
Topically Active			
Beclomethasone Diproprionate	500	0	*
Prednisolone Metasulphobenzoate	4	0.8	20*
Tixocortol Pivalate	300	0	250-1000*

*Doses utilized in clinical trials

of steroid therapy on patients who require surgical intervention, most surgical complications in patients treated with steroids appear to relate to the underlying illness or severe debilitation, rather than to the steroid therapy.[316,317]

Finally, withdrawal of steroid therapy must be carefully monitored for evidence of hypothalamic-pituitary-adrenal suppression, disease recrudescence, emotional or physical dependence (including myalgias, arthralgias, or increasing diarrhea in the absence of active inflammation), or subclinical adrenal suppression that may persist for months after withdrawal and only manifest under stressful situations.[318] A protocol for steroid withdrawal has been proposed,[319] although each patient requires an individualized approach (see specific approaches that follow).

Immunomodulation

The positive effects of corticosteroids and the concept of an immunologic cause or contribution to the inflammatory response in ulcerative colitis led to an early trial of immunosuppressants in inflammatory bowel disease.[320,321] Unfortunately, just as the etiology and pathogenesis of ulcerative colitis remain obscure, the currently available techniques of immune monitoring have not permitted a suitable, comprehensive assessment of pathogenetically important immune cell activities (including patterns of circulation, proportions of cells in tissues and their function), no correlation between treatment-induced immune modification and therapeutic benefit.[322] Many of the available agents and therapies either do not have the same quantitative and/or qualitative effects on specific immune cells, or function in such a way that the dichotomy between immune suppression and stimulation is obscured, and the clinical experience has been based on empirical trials. No study, as yet, has adequately monitored the immune profiles of patients with ulcerative colitis treated with immunomanipulative therapies. Furthermore, the concern over long-term consequences of immunosuppressive therapy, most significantly the potential for intercurrent malignancies, has deterred widespread trials (especially long-term) for a disorder potentially "cured" by colectomy.

Immunosuppressive Drugs

Azathioprine is metabolized in the liver to its active form 6-mercaptopurine (6-MP), a purine analog that interferes with DNA synthesis. These agents have been used most often in inflammatory bowel disease because they have relatively few short-term effects and have been used clinically in many patients with organ transplantation and other autoimmune disorders. Bean was the first to describe the use of 6-MP in a patient with ulcerative colitis who seemed to respond.[320] Korelitz and colleagues subsequently treated 25 patients, who had not responded to steroid and sulfasalazine, with 50 to 200mg of 6-MP a day for 10 to 52 months.[323] They reported that 15 of them had complete responses, 8 improved and only 2 required colectomy. Radiologic improvement occurred in 13 out of 18 patients, and toxicity was minimal. No *controlled* trials of 6-MP have been described.

Azathioprine has been used in several controlled studies. Jewell and Truelove administered either azathioprine (2.5mg/kg) or placebo to 80 patients with acute attacks of ulcerative colitis, along with corticosteroids over a one year period. They found no added benefit from combining azathioprine with the standard course of steroids, although it was suggested (with no statistical significance) that the patients treated with azathioprine relapsed less often during the subsequent year.[324] Neither Rosenberg et al. nor Caprilli and colleagues were able to identify dramatic influences of azathioprine in controlled trials of patients with ulcerative colitis,[325,326] although the University of Chicago group was able to document a potential steroid-sparing role.[325] Kirk and Lennard-Jones found a similar steroid-sparing effect, as well as a reduction in disease activity, in a group of 44 patients with active chronic ulcerative colitis who were randomized to receive azathioprine with prednisolone or prednisolone and placebo.[327] These studies and the retrospective series of Theodur et al. suggest that these drugs may have a role in patients with troublesome active disease for whom standard therapy has been unsuccessful, or chronic steroid therapy is needed to control symptoms, or when surgical treatment is deemed inappropriate.[328]

The short-term toxicity of the drugs in the dose range of 2 to 2.5mg/kg has been minimal. Mild reactions include nausea, hair loss, and transient peripheral neuropathy. More pronounced abdominal pain and vomiting may herald pancreatitis that seems to be mild and an idiosyncratic reaction, as is fever, skin rash, and hepatitis that have occurred in the same individuals.[329,330] Bone marrow suppression is uncommon at these low doses, but blood counts should be monitored at monthly intervals.

The concern over the potential for malignant complications of the use of such drugs has been reviewed in a mixed series of patients where the risk of lymphoma, especially, seems to be enhanced in Crohn's disease compared to the general population.[331,332] These reports ignore the general predisposition towards hematologic malignancies in ulcerative colitis, however.[333] Present and associates have presented their 15 year experience with 277 patients with inflammatory bowel disease treated over 554 patient years with 6-MP therapy and with 1939 years of follow-up.[334] Toxic reactions were rare and neoplasms were identified no more frequently than would be anticipated in the general population.

Apparently, cyclosporine was used successfully in a single patient with ulcerative colitis and controlled trials of this immunosuppressive agent are anticipated.[335] Antilymphocyte globulin was noted to be useful in a few case reports,[336,337] but was not more effective than standard intensive therapy in a randomized series.[338,339]

Immunostimulation

Levamisole, a known stimulant of polymorphonuclear cell function, was evaluated by Hermanowicz and colleagues in comparative studies with sulfasalazine alone or in combination, or corticosteroids alone, for patients with acute ulcerative colitis.[340,341] Despite a paradoxic depression of polymorphonuclear cell chemotaxis and a fall in the disease activity index, fewer patients went into remission on levamisole therapy and the relapse rate was greater. Ascorbic acid was evaluated as an additional treatment in their second report and was associated with worsening disease activity.[341] Neither transfer factor, BCG, nor interferon have been tested in a controlled fashion in ulcerative colitis.

Other Therapies
Mast Cell Stabilizers

The observation that the intense local inflammation in the colonic mucosa is partially composed of increased numbers of eosinophils and mast cells encouraged speculation that an immediate hypersensitivity reaction may degranulate mast cells and release toxic substances with additional inflammatory recruitment.[342] Supporting evidence for this concept included the finding of elevated histamine levels in the mucosa during clinical relapse and led to a series of trials involving sodium cromoglycate,[22,343-349] PRD-92,[350] and N-(3, 4-dimethoxycinnamoyl) anthranilic acid;[351] drugs known to stabilize mast cell membranes and inhibit the release of histamine and other toxic intracellular compounds. Despite an early report of benefit,[22] subsequent studies have not shown a positive role for these drugs in either active disease or as a maintenance therapy, although a very limited role may be conceived in a small subset of patients who cannot tolerate sulfasalazine despite attempts at desensitization.[352]

Miscellaneous Agents

Because the mechanism of mucosal hemorrhage in ulcerative colitis is poorly understood, attempts to reduce the enhanced local fibrinolytic activity have used both ϵ-aminocaproic acid and tranexamic acid. The former drug appeared to be beneficial only in uncontrolled trials, and its use was hampered by its severe side effects of nausea, vomiting, and diarrhea.[353,354] In the small trials of tranexemic acid, either by mouth,[355] or in enema form,[356] although a diminution of bleeding occurred, sigmoidoscopic changes did not differ from placebo.

Lechin et al. have reported success in a double-blind study of clonidine in 45 patients randomly treated during five successive six-week periods with clonidine, prednisone, sulfasalazine, or placebo.[357] Both clonidine (0.3mg t.i.d.) and prednisone (20mg t.i.d.) were superior to sulfasalazine (1.5g t.i.d.). Clonidine was chosen because it reduces intestinal motility and inhibits noradrenaline release as well as decreasing plasma ACTH levels through a central nervous system effect. Successfully treated patients were found to have improved symptoms and sigmoidoscopic examinations, raised cortisol plasma levels in relapse with return to normal during remission, and improved sigmoid tone after therapy.[357] This work followed the successful treatment with thioproperazine of 19 patients with ulcerative colitis. Adverse side effects precluded further studies, however.[358] Epidemiologic evidence suggesting that cigarette smoking may have a protective role in patients with ulcerative colitis raises the unusual possibility that nicotine may have a beneficial effect in colitis either because of its central or peripheral vascular effects.[359] Whether any of these pharmacologic agents will have a continuing role in the therapeutic armamentarium requires much further investigation.

Sucralfate, a surface active polysulphated disaccharide effective in healing gastroduodenal ulcers, has been tried in 10% enema solution in 15 patients with distal colitis.[360] Good or excellent results were described in 11 patients, sufficient to warrant a double-blind, controlled trial that has not been completed at this time.

Antimicrobial Therapy

It has long been recognized that antibiotics had no significant impact on the remission rate in ulcerative colitis.[361] The recognition that sulfasalazine was effective in ulcerative colitis led to renewed speculation regarding the potential for antibacterial therapy. Indeed, many patients who were intolerant of sulfasalazine tolerated phthalylsulfathiazole with favorable clinical results (J. Kirsner, unpublished data), and in rheumatoid arthritis the controversy over the effective moiety continues.[81] Furthermore, although an infective agent in ulcerative colitis has not been demonstrated directly, the inflammatory reaction in one animal model using guinea pigs fed carageenan can be aborted by pretreatment with metronidazole.[362] Unfortunately, in the only reported trial of antibiotics alone for chronic ulcerative proctitis, metronidazole was not an effective therapy.[363]*

One dramatic study used whole-gut irrigation as antiendotoxemic therapy in 4 patients who had been unresponsive to conservative treatment, with apparently good short-term results.[364] This rationale originated from the positive experience using whole-gut irrigation to prepare for surgical procedure of the large bowel, because of lowered bacterial contamination. For the most part, however, experienced clinicians have moved away from antibiotic therapy in ulcerative colitis,[171,253,365] either because of its lack of efficacy, the relationship of flare-ups to antibiotic exposure,[31] or the fear of inducing antibiotic-associated diarrhea. In this regard, it is our general policy to give vancomycin or metronidazole in the treatment of sulfasalazine- or antibiotic-associated pseudomembranous colitis complicating ulcerative colitis.

Even in the intensive therapeutic studies of ulcerative colitis, antibiotic therapy was of no sustained benefit.[266,366] Hence, broad spectrum antibiotic therapy would appear to be more appropriate for patients with severe, acute ulcerative colitis, for patients with toxic megacolon (see the following), or surgical treatment.

Total Parenteral Nutrition†

The clinical experience with total parenteral nutrition (TPN) is continually expanding and the role for TPN and bowel rest has gradually evolved to that of adjunctive therapy.[367-372] In a controlled trial of TPN and bowel rest, Dickinson et al. found no primary therapeutic effect in the 27 ulcerative colitis patients who were randomly chosen to receive standard therapy with

---

* Editors' note: See also Chapman, R. W., et al.: Gut, 27:1210, 1986; this study showed no advantage if intravenous metronidazole is used as an adjunct to corticosteroid therapy.
† See also Chapter 24.

or without TPN and bowel rest, with a regular schedule of steroid tapering.[373] To concentrate on the primary effect alone, however, would ignore a valuable therapeutic adjunct in seriously ill individuals who may benefit from the improved nutrition, stabilization of symptoms, diminished rate of infections, decreased requirement for blood and albumin, reversal of growth retardation in children, and, at worst, as preparation for colectomy if medical management should fail.[370,374,375] *

Intensive parenteral nutrition has been an important aspect of the management of patients with severe ulcerative colitis.[265,266,370,375] A trial of TPN and bowel rest is recommended for patients with ulcerative colitis who are unresponsive to steroids and sulfasalazine, for stabilizing severely ill patients with impending toxic megacolon, for malnourished individuals who may require colectomy (with TPN continued through the immediate postoperative period), and for children with growth retardation who do not meet other criteria for colectomy. Jarnerot and colleagues also found the intensive intravenous regimen to be helpful in patients with mild to moderate colitis.[266] The failure rate for patients correlates poorly with the length of treatment and depends upon the willingness of the patient and physician to forego further medical therapy.[266,370,376] The only predictor of failure for TPN in our series of 38 ulcerative colitis patients receiving TPN was the transfusion requirement.[376] The recurrence rate for severely ill patients who do respond is no worse than for patients with mild to moderate disease,[266] and many patients enjoy long or permanent remissions on sulfasalazine maintenance.

Approaches to Clinical Situations

This section describes the overall approach at the University of Chicago for the management of patients with ulcerative colitis, based upon the extent and severity of the illness. As emphasized earlier, important information includes an assessment of an individual's symptoms; nutritional state; laboratory studies including blood counts, serum chemistries, iron stores; and endoscopic examination with biopsies when indicated. The categorization is not rigid, because the course and the response of the individual patient vary.

Ulcerative Proctitis

Patients with ulcerative proctitis are troubled mainly by rectal bleeding; diarrhea is less of a problem. Constipation with the daily passage of blood or blood-tinged mucopus devoid of stool is not uncommon. At proctoscopy, the rectum is diffusely inflamed.

Most patients respond to rectal steroids over a course of several weeks. For distal disease (e.g., limited to 15cm or so), hydrocortisone acetate 10% foam (Cortifoam*), 80mg, can be administered via a special rectal applicator once or twice daily for several weeks, followed by bedtime applications every other day for an additional week or two. Hydrocortisone suspension enemas (Cortenema†) of 60ml provide 100mg of hydrocortisone and are best tolerated when administered nightly at bedtime for several weeks, and then every other night until tapered. Over the short-term course of three to six weeks (with tapering), adrenal suppression is rarely a problem.[377] Patients with mild disease who respond rapidly may wish to defer further treatment pending the outcome of their course.

For patients who rapidly relapse or have more severe symptoms of proctitis, the addition of sulfasalazine is helpful for the active disease, and as maintenance therapy in divided doses of 2 to 4g daily. Sulfasalazine is best tolerated when taken with meals to avoid gastric irritation and nausea, and may be prescribed in an enteric-coated form (Azulfidine-EN) for patients with symptoms of intolerance. If the side effects remain intolerable, the suspension form (Azulfidine suspension) allows a more gradual schedule of dose increments beginning at low initial doses (e.g., 50 to 100mg q.i.d.). Daily doses of 1mg of folic acid also should be prescribed.

With improvement, the enemas are gradually decreased and the sulfasalazine continued indefinitely, although the dose usually can be reduced to 2g daily. Some patients may require up to 3 to 4g daily to maintain the remission. Approximately 15% of patients may be refractory to the combination of local hydrocortisone and sulfasalazine. For these individuals, the therapeutic options are now expanding. Methyl-

---

*Editors' note: See also Matuchansky, C.: Gut, 27:81, 1986; this author emphasizes that the precise place of TPN as a sole or adjunct-treatment for IBD has yet to be defined. McIntyre, P. B., et al.: Gut, 27:481, 1986; "bowel rest" did not influence the outcome in severe ulcerative colitis treated with intravenous prednisolone in this study.

*Reed & Carnick; Piscataway, NJ 08854
†Reid-Rowell Inc; Atlanta, GA 30318

prednisolone enemas (Medrol EnPak*) can be administered in variable amounts of water (generally 50 to 100ml) and provide 40mg of the drug. Alternatively, the addition of oral steroids at the equivalent dose of 20 to 40mg of prednisone daily may initiate a remission. High dose (4g) 5-ASA enemas are most efficacious for patients with distal colitis and are of benefit even in refractory cases. These may be used alone and the dose and/or frequency of administration gradually reduced after symptomatic and proctoscopic improvement. It has been our experience that the disease will flare up after tapering the treatment (sometimes into more extensive colitis) to an extent that maintenance therapy may be necessary, similar to the results of sulfasalazine therapy. Suppositories of 500mg 5-ASA inserted t.i.d. also may be therapeutic for patients with colitis limited to the rectum. Tixocortol pivalate enemas can be useful for patients with active disease, using high doses (up to 1g) for "refractory" patients.

Dietary advice for patients with proctitis depends on the individual's symptoms. Bland, low residue diets, supplemented by antidiarrheal drugs, will benefit those with a tendency towards diarrhea. Constipated patients may find high fiber diets, psyllium supplements, or stool softeners useful, together with antispasmodics to alleviate lower abdominal cramping. For patients with more severe rectal pain or tenesmus, warm sitz baths often are helpful.

Left-sided Colitis

Patients with disease limited to the left colon typically present with an intermediate and variable course. Mild to moderate symptoms without systemic manifestations of colitis are treated with sulfasalazine 2 to 4g daily, supplemented with folic acid. Steroid enemas may be useful for symptoms of tenesmus or rectal bleeding, and these can be tapered as soon as symptoms (and proctoscopic changes) resolve. Sulfasalazine is continued on a maintenance schedule.

Patients with limited anatomic involvement may be quite ill, and hospitalization may be indicated for those who do not respond rapidly to outpatient management, or for patients who present with severe anorexia, nausea, vomiting, fever, bleeding, or anemia. In this situation, they should be stabilized in the same manner as for those with acute pan-colitis, *prior* to any invasive endoscopic procedures. Often a limited

*Upjohn Co; Kalamazoo, MI 49001

proctoscopy will confirm the presence of severe mucosal disease, and a post-procedure "flat-plate" abdominal radiograph will provide an approximation of the extent of colonic involvement by outlining the ulcerated, ahaustral bowel with a small amount of insufflated air.

In the presence of chronic, persistent symptoms, therapeutic doses of 3 to 6g of sulfasalazine daily are prescribed, together with either hydrocortisone enemas (Cortenema) or methylprednisolone enemas (Medrol EnPak) administered nightly or twice daily. If these fail or are poorly tolerated (e.g., cannot be retained), then oral steroids in doses equivalent to 20 to 40mg of prednisone are prescribed. Patients often respond maximally to their first exposure to steroids, and tapering too rapidly may be followed by a flare-up that will respond submaximally to a similar starting dose. Hence, both the symptoms and the mucosal changes should be resolved prior to tapering. The reduction schedule then is proportional to the duration of the symptoms preceding the introduction of the drug. Patients with acute disease of less than a month's duration usually respond rapidly and may be "tapered" over one to two months. Those with longstanding disease require a more gradual reduction schedule. Decreasing doses of prednisone above 20mg by 5mg monthly and by 2.5mg monthly at levels below 20mg may be necessary for those with chronic symptoms. A combination of oral and local steroids often is helpful for patients with refractory distal colitis. Many of these patients will be able to "taper" easily to a threshold dose of prednisone (usually below 20mg) and then may require a more gradual tapering along with adjunctive steroid enemas.

Many patients who are resistant to the standard approach described previously will improve with the administration of high-dose 5-ASA or high-dose tixocortol pivalate enemas. Those whose symptoms persist despite these adjuncts require more individualized, often combined approaches. Some will respond to the intensive intravenous regimen used by Jarnerot in which patients are hospitalized with a "nothing by mouth" regimen of parenteral nutrition, combined systemic and local steroids, and sulfasalazine.[266] Patients whose response is hampered by a threshold level of steroids below which they experience flare-up may benefit by the introduction of an immunosuppressive drug and subsequent attempts at steroid "tapering." Alternative day steroids should be tried for patients with long-standing steroid dependence, although the results usually are not satisfactory. Progressive or continuous disease, or the inability to "taper" steroids may be indications for surgical procedure (approximately 10% of these patients).[4]

Individualized dietary advice depends upon the patient's symptoms. Lactose intolerance should be considered in those with gaseousness, distention, or diarrhea. Likewise, a reduction in "hard roughage" will be useful for patients with frequent loose stools. Avoidance of spices and concentrated or acidic juices may provide symptomatic relief. Iron deficiency is not uncommon and oral doses of iron then are indicated. As mentioned earlier, calcium supplements should be considered for patients on milk-free diets or on steroids. Symptomatic therapy with antispasmodics, antidiarrheals, and/or bulk forming agents may be useful and allow further reduction of steroids. Some patients who are unable to retain steroid enemas will be helped by a preceding dose of loperamide or deodorized tincture of opium (5 to 10 drops per dose).

Extensive Disease

Ulcerative colitis proximal to the splenic flexure can be expected in approximately one-quarter of all patients at presentation and in 30% of patients after ten years.[378] These patients account for the majority of hospitalizations and operations. Again, management of the individual patient will be guided by the severity of disease during the current flare-up, as well as the response to prior medical therapy.

Acute Colitis

Patients with extensive ulcerative colitis who present with *mild* symptoms usually can be managed as outpatients. Those who present with a first attack will be evaluated with stool cultures to examine for ova, parasites, and C. difficile toxin, as the nature of the colitis is being established. Most will tolerate a colonoscopy or air contrast barium enema to document the proximal extent of the disease. Laboratory studies will substantiate the nutritional status, degree of anemia, and iron stores.

Once the diagnosis has been confirmed, these patients should be started on a program of sulfasalazine with eventual doses of 2 to 4g daily. For those who are intolerant, a schedule of desensitization is warranted and it is hoped that alternative, sulfa-free derivatives of 5-ASA soon will be generally available. Folic acid is supplemented and dietary advice to minimize diarrhea is helpful. Antispasmodics or carefully monitored antidiarrheal agents may be added for symptomatic relief.

Most of the mildly ill patients will respond to sulfasalazine alone. If the patient does not rapidly improve over several days to weeks, however, or if clinical deterioration is evident, steroid therapy should be added, using prednisone at a dose of 20 to 40mg daily. If hematochezia, tenesmus, or significant rectal urgency continue to be troublesome, steroid enemas can be added. Once clinical and sigmoidoscopic improvement is attained, the steroids can be gradually "tapered." For mild, acute cases such "weaning" usually can be achieved rapidly over several weeks (or as long as it takes to achieve remission). Once the steroids are "tapered," the patient is continued on a maintenance dose of sulfasalazine.

Moderate to Severe Colitis

These attacks require more careful clinical judgement to determine the optimal setting for treatment. Significant weight loss, fever, arthritis, greater than six bloody bowel movements daily accompanied by severe mucosal changes and/or evidence of dehydration, significant anemia, electrolyte imbalances, or a rapidly deteriorating course necessitate prompt hospitalization. If the patient is less severely ill, reliable, able to remain in close contact with the physician, and has a suitable supportive at-home environment, outpatient therapy can be pursued. Oral steroids, topical steroids, and sulfasalazine are combined with symptomatic treatment of diarrhea and abdominal pain with close attention to nutrition and emotional support.

Prednisone (or its equivalent), at a dose of 40mg, should be instituted promptly as sulfasalazine is gradually introduced to achieve an eventual dose of 3 to 4g daily. Steroid enemas can be useful to reduce rectal urgency and hemorrhage, even in the presence of more proximal disease. These individuals require a reduction in their physical activities until the disease is brought under control. Bedrest, initially, will help to reduce the frequency of the passage of stool. Dietary adjustments to reduce the residue reaching the colon are useful, and a lactose-free diet should be considered until the ability to digest milk products has been established. Low residue, liquid supplements can provide additional calories during the initial period of therapy.*

---

*Editors' note: See also Gassull, M. A., et al.: Gut, *27*:76, 1986; and Rhodes, J., and Rose, J.: Gut, *27*:471, 1986.

The judicious use of antispasmodics or antidiarrheals requires careful day to day evaluations until the course is stabilized. A poor response or progression of symptoms will necessitate hospitalization, with the same treatment as for severe disease. Otherwise, as the patient improves the steroid dose can be gradually reduced. Prednisone is maintained at 40mg for two to four weeks, and then gradually tapered by 2.5 to 5mg daily every week. We do not usually reduce below 20mg for six to eight weeks, and then gradually as tolerated thereafter; generally by 5mg every two to four weeks. Once the steroids are completely tapered, the sulfasalazine can be reduced, assuming no clinical worsening, to a maintenance dose of 2g daily.

Until alternate preparations generally are available and more is known of their effects, desensitization to sulfasalazine is definitely warranted for intolerant or allergic patients (see earlier). If patients remain intolerant or if allergic manifestations recur, then a trial of gradually tapering or alternate day steroids will be necessary. The addition of an immunosuppressant occasionally can be useful. Until then, either intermittent courses of steroids or an empiric trial of maintenance antibiotics (e.g., metronidazole or a sulfonamide) may be necessary despite the negative results in controlled trials.

Severe Colitis

The severely ill patient with ulcerative colitis requires immediate hospitalization. Severe illness exists if the patient is hypotensive, dehydrated, febrile in excess of 40°C, if the diarrhea exceeds more than 10 to 12 stools daily, if rectal bleeding is continuous or occurs between bowel movements, if severe protein depletion and wasting or edema are present, or if colonic dilatation or evidence of serosal inflammation (signs of peritoneal irritation) exists. Evidence of perforation (free abdominal air) requires immediate surgical treatment (see also Chaps. 14, 25, and 26).

Such an individual requires the prompt institution of general resuscitative measures to correct fluid and electrolyte imbalances (especially hypokalemia) and transfusions to maintain the hematocrit above 30%. Nasogastric suction is indicated in the presence of small intestinal ileus or colonic dilatation. *As stressed earlier, anticholinergics, antidiarrheals, and narcotic analgesics should be withheld if the course is deteriorating, as they may induce colonic dilatation and/or mask peritoneal signs in a debilitated patient (especially those on chronic steroids).*

We recommend an intensive medical regimen similar to that described by the Oxford group,[265] and further applied by Jarnerot et al.[266] The patient is placed on a total intravenous regimen with no oral feedings except for sips of water and no oral medications except for those essential for other conditions that cannot be given parenterally. Sulfasalazine is usually withheld because of the relatively frequent side effects when taken without food; however, if previously the drug has been well tolerated, an attempt at continuing the therapy is warranted. Parenteral nutritional support is instituted either by a peripheral vein or by a central vein, if the patient is significantly malnourished and will require more prolonged nutritional repletion. In addition to the standard regimen of electrolytes, dextrose, amino acid, and lipid solutions, albumin is administered to those with severe hypoalbuminemia (e.g., below 2.5g/dl) as an empiric means of hastening the clinical response to medical management, or, at least, to improve the plasma protein concentration in preparation for surgical intervention.

Intravenous steroids should be administered to patients who have been receiving continuous steroid therapy. Either 40 to 60mg of prednisolone-21-phosphate daily, 32 to 48mg of methylprednisolone daily, or 200 to 300mg of hydrocortisone daily is prescribed, according to the size of the patient and severity of the illness. The patient who is not responding to similar doses in an oral program is given a different steroid parenterally, administered either as a constant infusion over 24 hours or in four doses by way of slow intravenous drip. Patients who have never received previous steroid therapy may benefit from intravenous ACTH therapy, 80 to 120 units daily.[253,258] A rectal steroid preparation (e.g., 60ml of Cortenema or 60ml of Medrol Enpak, nightly or b.i.d.) also is prescribed.

As we have indicated, the use of antibiotics in IBD remains a matter of controversy. Broad spectrum antibiotics should be given to patients with progressively severe colitis and an impending toxic megacolon, or to those requiring surgical treatment. We consider that antibiotics probably are useful in patients with acute ulcerative colitis that is severe enough to warrant intensive bowel rest and parenteral nutritional support. We suggest either a combination of metronidazole and an aminoglycoside, or a second generation cephalosporin alone; but tetracycline, chloramphenicol, ampicillin and doxycycline also have been used.[265,266] In such situations, vitamin K needs to be replaced as part of the intravenous nutritional support. Continuing symptoms require reinvestigation of stool for the presence of C. difficile toxin. The antibiotics are discontinued when the patient improves and oral intake and sulfasalazine therapy are resumed.

Patients treated in this manner are constantly observed for signs of deterioration that would indicate the need for surgical intervention (see Chaps. 14, 25, and 26). In addition to frequent auscultation of the abdomen for evidence of the presence and quality of peristaltic activity, daily plain film radiographs of the abdomen are advisable to detect evidence of an impending toxic dilatation until the patient stabilizes. Daily electrolyte and hemograms are essential in the severely ill.

Intensive therapy is continued for approximately five days. If the patient responds by rapid clinical improvement, a gradually increasing oral regimen is instituted, beginning with small quantities (30 to 60ml/hr) of an isosmotic, low residue supplement such as diluted Ensure* or Sustacal,† gradually advancing to full strength solutions, and, eventually, to a low residue diet.

If a favorable response is apparent but the patient has not yet "turned the corner," intravenous therapy is continued for an additional two to seven days. If no improvement occurs, surgical intervention is indicated. Occasionally, patients will improve gradually such that continued central hyperalimentation is maintained for up to four to six weeks. In our series of patients with complicated, tertiary ulcerative colitis, approximately 50% of them have been able to avoid surgical therapy during the immediate hospitalization. Such an approach should not be considered routine, however, and it requires the support of a nutrition service capable of monitoring severe inflammatory bowel disease, and comprehensive medical and surgical resources. After the acute phase of the intensive intravenous program, oral feeding is instituted commencing with elemental feedings (as discussed earlier), followed by a more liberal liquid diet for several days, and eventually a full, low residue maintenance diet. The rate of progression is proportional to the length of time the patient has been NPO and the severity of the colitis. A carefully prescribed oral hyperalimentation regimen will be important for the undernourished patient.

*Ross Laboratories; Columbus, OH 43216
†Mead Johnson Nutritional; Evansville, IN, 47721

Oral steroids are initiated as the intravenous therapy is completed, using the same daily dose. The steroids are then gradually decreased over weeks and months. After discharge, the patient usually can reduce the prednisone by 5mg every week or two until 20mg is reached, and then by 2.5mg every two weeks or so. Rectal steroids are decreased as soon as the patient has improved and the proctoscopic findings have begun to resolve. An alternate night schedule of steroid enemas for one to two weeks, followed by twice weekly and then weekly treatments, usually is successful. If clinical symptoms or proctoscopic findings of active disease persist, the weaning process must be more gradual.

As the oral program is reinstituted, sulfasalazine is prescribed in incremental doses according to the patient's tolerance, usually beginning with 500mg once or twice daily. The dose is gradually advanced to 3 or 4g daily and continued until the steroids are "tapered," at which point the medication can be reduced to the maintenance range of 2 to 3g daily in 2 to 4 divided doses. Residual symptoms of bowel irritability, spasm, or minor diarrhea can be treated with nonspecific measures as for mild to moderate disease.

Toxic Megacolon*

The development of colonic dilatation in the midst of acute ulcerative colitis is a medical emergency with an overall mortality of up to 30%.[379,380] The sudden extension of mucosal inflammation through all layers of the bowel wall to the serosa is associated with the clinical signs of direct visceral tenderness, which can be indistinguishable from a localized and walled off, or free perforation. Often the condition is heralded by a diminution in diarrhea, or the passage of a bloody discharge or clots devoid of stool associated with progressive abdominal distention and hollow, hypoactive bowel sounds. Despite longstanding awareness of the problem, only a few predisposing factors have been identified. Provocative medications include anticholinergics, diphenoxylate with atropine loperamide and opiates.[381] Electrolyte abnormalities, particularly hypokalemia, occur commonly in severe ulcerative colitis and have been implicated in the occurrence of toxic megacolon.[381,382] The role of corticosteroids has been controversial[381,383] and, in our experience, is unlikely to be a factor. Additional putative factors are manipulations of the colon such as barium studies

*See Chapter 14.

or colonoscopy. It is important to recognize that toxic dilatation can occur with severe left-sided ulcerative colitis, although it has most commonly been associated with pan-colonic disease.[380]

The diagnosis is suspected clinically in any severely ill colitic patient who presents or manifests abdominal tenderness (with or without guarding) associated with distension, often with fevers, diaphoresis, and evidence for dehydration; unfortunately, many or all of these may be masked by high-dose steroid therapy. The crucial examination is a plain abdominal roentgenogram demonstrating a distended, gas-filled colon with absent haustrations and outlined "islands" of residual mucosa surrounded by extensive ulcerations. We emphasize that *no* minimal diameter should be regarded as a requirement for the diagnosis of toxic megacolon. Rather, serial measurements demonstrating dilated (usually greater than 6cm) colon with features of severe ulceration that do not improve, or worsen, in association with clinical symptoms and signs of the "toxic state," as outlined already, are sufficient to cause alarm. Furthermore, colonic dilatation is not an invariable antecedent of perforation,[384] the latter being the major determinant of the outcome of any severe attack.[379,380]

The medical treatment of toxic megacolon is the same as described for severe extensive colitis with the addition of the following: the patient is best managed in an intensive care setting with medical-surgical consultations; support with fluids, electrolytes, albumin, fresh frozen plasma (if clotting studies are abnormal), and transfusions; broad spectrum antibiotics; and intravenous corticosteroids administered at doses equivalent to 40 to 80mg daily of prednisolone (32 to 60 mg methylprednisolone). A nasogastric tube is inserted and, twice daily, abdominal flat plate and upright radiographs are performed.

Signs of perforation are an immediate indication for surgical intervention (see Chaps. 14, 25, and 26). Likewise, any deterioration should lead to an emergency colectomy with the understanding that the complication of a perforation greatly increases the morbidity and mortality. Furthermore, the failure to improve over 24 to 72 hours is an indication for colectomy. Meyers and Janowitz point out that early colectomy for patients who do not improve within 72 hours minimizes the risk of perforation and reduces the mortality to less than 6%.[385] With good, early instituted management a successful medically induced outcome can be achieved in up to 52% of patients, with low mortality.[386] Unfortunately, many of the medically treated patients are destined for further medical or surgical complications, including the potential for recurrent episodes of toxic megacolon.[380,387]

Refractory Disease

While most patients with ulcerative colitis will respond to medical therapy, several patterns of refractory disease may emerge. Some patients will respond initially to the introduction of steroids and sulfasalazine, but tend to develop recurrent flare-ups as steroids are reduced. These individuals may benefit from a more gradual reduction of steroids over many months, with the implementation of an alternate day dosing schedule to reduce the long-term side effects. Some may require a higher dose of maintenance sulfasalazine, such as 4 to 6g daily, to prevent relapse. In a few situations, the addition of immunosuppressive medication may facilitate the steroid withdrawal.

Other patients may fall into a pattern of *chronic persistent* colitis in which symptoms improve with higher doses of steroids, but the mucosa never heals completely. These individuals may do just as well without steroid therapy. Others may respond to a change to a different steroid preparation (e.g., from prednisone to hydrocortisone). Infrequently, the colitis worsens with sulfasalazine (sometimes with the aggravation being masked by simultaneous steroid treatment), and stopping the drug is useful. Again, an immunosuppressant can be added, or rectal steroids or 5-ASA enemas can be combined with oral steroids and sulfasalazine. If sulfa sensitivity is diagnosed, then a change to an oral 5-ASA product may be feasible. Occasionally, even patients with milder disease will improve with hospitalization and a course of intensive, intravenous therapy sufficient to induce a remission.[266] In many such circumstances, the initial response to high-dose steroids will be the most complete, so tapering too rapidly may subsequently necessitate even higher doses to attain the same clinical response.

Because ulcerative colitis is potentially curable by way of colectomy, the point at which surgical intervention becomes mandatory is a matter of clinical judgement (see Chaps. 25 and 26). Often patients hitherto considered to be refractory to medical management respond favorably to this comprehensive approach outlined earlier. In others, an operation is unavoidable. Despite the advances in surgical techniques, however, neither a permanent ileostomy nor an ileoanal pull-through assure optimal medical, social, or psychological outcomes. In some instances, a final attempt at maximal medical therapy, limited in time, with a failure to respond provides the patient and the family with evidence of the absolute need for surgical therapy.

Maintenance Medical Therapy

For most patients who respond to medical therapy, the induction of a remission is only the beginning of a long-term medical program. Once the steroid therapy has been tapered, all attempts should be made to maintain the response because, short of a proctocolectomy, therapy does not eliminate the possibility of a recurrence and medical supervision is required indefinitely.

As already indicated, whenever possible patients with quiescent disease are maintained on sulfasalazine, 2g daily (or the minimal dose required to prevent relapse), in two to four divided doses. Folic acid supplements should be maintained, with dietary advice for symptoms of colonic irritability (e.g., low residue diet for diarrhea). Asymptomatic patients without proctoscopic evidence of inflammation should consult their physician every six months and proctoscopic exams should be performed yearly with screening blood counts and blood chemistries. Follow-up of the quiescent patient is directed to controlling the disease and also to general measures of health maintenance. The patient should be instructed to contact the physician as soon as a flare-up is suspected and to recognize associated conditions such as inflammatory eye disorders, arthritis, or skin changes of erythema nodosum or pyoderma gangrenosum, which may herald an attack of colitis.

In patients with long-standing ulcerative colitis, the physician must always be alert for the complication of carcinoma of the colon. Current practice recommends screening colonoscopic examinations after ten years of disease with multiple mucosal biopsies for dysplasia (see Chap. 15).

Intestinal Complications*

Bowel complications such as perforation, persistent hemorrhage, and carcinoma require surgical treatment. *Post-inflammatory polyps* present as filiform projections, mucosal bridges and occasionally form a "forest" or mass-like lesion and indicate prior disease. Such lesions pose difficulties in distinguishing between flat mucosa, dysplastic masses, adenomatous polyps, and cancers if they occur in mass-like configurations. Occasionally these lesions tend to be the site of hemorrhage in the midst of otherwise quiescent disease. Rarely these lesions can be so large as to cause bowel obstruction. Strictures in ulcerative colitis, once considered benign and reversible because of muscular hypertrophy,[388] recently have been demonstrated sometimes to be associated with dysplasia and cancer.[389] Any area of narrowing should be evaluated with colonoscopic biopsies and/or brushings for pathologic/cytologic analysis. The presence of high-grade dysplasia within a stricture is an indication for a colectomy.

Extraintestinal Complications*

The presence of certain extraintestinal manifestations of ulcerative colitis, such as iritis, episcleritis, peripheral arthritis, erythema nodosum, or pyoderma gangrenosum, often are indications for more vigorous medical treatment of the diseased bowel and most respond to therapy for the colitis. Specifically, local and systemic steroids will control the ocular lesions, but these should be monitored by an ophthalmologist to assure complete recovery. The peripheral arthropathy will almost always respond to satisfactory treatment of the colitis with either sulfasalazine or steroids. Occasionally, a nonsteroidal anti-inflammatory drug may be necessary, requiring the patient to be monitored closely for signs of increased bleeding or peptic ulceration. Likewise, the less severe skin lesions of erythema nodosum almost always respond to therapy aimed at control of the colitis. Interim treatment with analgesics and occasional nonsteroidal anti-inflammatory drugs, and elevation of the legs, may provide symptomatic relief. Pyoderma gangrenosum is a much more difficult lesion to treat.[390,391] Local and systemic steroid treatment may be necessary and unremitting skin ulceration may occasionally require colectomy. Fortunately, these disorders now appear to be less common, possibly because of earlier detection and treatment of the inflammatory bowel disease.

Other extracolonic manifestations, such as uveitis, sacroiliitis, ankylosing spondylitis, and hepatobiliary disease (pericholangitis, sclerosing cholangitis), pursue a course independent of

*See also Chapters 14, 15.

*See also Chapter 16.

the colitis. Therapy, including proctocolectomy, has little impact upon the natural history of these disorders.

The Approach to the Inflammatory Bowel Disease Patient and Family

A physician who accepts the role as the primary doctor for patients with IBD must, from the outset, understand their perspectives and concerns. Most patients are afflicted while young and inexperienced with serious or chronic ailments. Often, the first symptoms are bleeding or diarrhea that may be accompanied by a loss of control of bowel function. These symptoms initiate fear of cancer and cause the emotional upheaval associated with decreased control of excretory function. Often, the patient, at least subconsciously, generates fears of death and isolation, prior to seeking medical attention. It is not unusual for these symptoms to be so worrisome that, paradoxically, they are hidden from parents or other family members until their revelation becomes unavoidable. Seeking answers and consolation from the physician, the patient almost immediately undergoes experiences that further expose his vulnerability. For example, the patient may be concerned that the disorder's cause is not known; that no medical cure is available; that successful treatment may be associated with disfiguring (steroid) side effects; or that, if treatment fails, it might be required of the patient to "wear a bag;" or that the condition is associated with a long-term risk of cancer. Thus confronted, the patient then turns to family and friends who usually have never heard of the condition, or are under the impression that "colitis" is an emotional disorder.

From this perspective, it is easy to understand how colitis induces a sense of isolation and why Lennard-Jones points out that "the care of patients with colitis demands from the doctor, knowledge, availability, ingenuity, understanding and emotional resource."[365] To this we would add *optimism*, the converse of all of the concerns, fantasies, and information the patient has experienced. These qualities also must be transmitted to the family who need to be transformed from awestruck, fearful observers (Is it contagious? Will we catch it? How could we have prevented this? Is it transmitted to the children?) into active participants in the care and support of their loved one.

Many patients suffer from a lack of understanding about ulcerative colitis. The provision of a diagnosis and a handful of prescriptions is insufficient. Rather, an educational conference with the patient with family members present is essential to avoid suboptimal therapy because of misunderstanding or inadequate explanations regarding diet, medication, or lifestyle. Also, it is critical to allow the family to ask questions and allay their fears. Hopefully, this can be accomplished with adequate uninterrupted time allotted by the physician. This single conference setting can be an important focal point to which the entire group can refer, where all information is both transmitted and received so misinterpretation and failed communication can be minimized.

The doctor also needs to be available for the patient and family on a 24-hour basis. The uncertainty imposed by an unpredictable illness and the added emotional swings accompanying high-dose steroids leave the patient continually "exposed," with few other resources. Certainly, this is an even greater reason to involve the family from the onset and makes either local support groups or those initiated by the National Foundation for Ileitis and Colitis (New York) helpful for patients, families, and the often overburdened doctor. Yet, the patient, who continues to regard the physician as the major source of truthful information, medical care, and often solace, should be able to feel that this source is available when any problems arise.

The doctor also must be the focusing agent for the patient (and family) as the patient is directed through the many aspects of the medical system that now involves dieticians, nutritionists, physical therapists, social workers, psychiatric, and surgical consultants. With no single responsible guide, the patient will easily become lost in this "morass," and the medical care will likely become unfocused, confused, and distorted.

Despite the potential downfalls, an optimistic, resourceful physician will find tremendous reward in successfully directing the most challenging patient through these troublesome periods. Even if medical treatment fails and the patient is actually confronted with surgical therapy, the availability and support of the doctor will become a critical factor in the patient's acceptance and adaptation to surgical treatment. If the support is absent, this can lead to further feelings of abandonment and isolation.

The ingenuity and resourcefulness of the physician as pertaining to all aspects of the patient's care, are necessary to create an individual program of management. Clearly, the appropriate diet, changes in lifestyles, ability to take medications, and support from the family are different for each patient and will demand an approach requiring the physician to be aware of concerns over life events at school, on the job, relating to recreational capabilities, and the timing of pregnancies. The treatment of patients with IBD is often most challenging to the physician, but the success of such an effort is extremely personally rewarding.

References

1. Kirsner, J. B.: Problems in the differentiation of ulcerative colitis and Crohn's disease of the colon: The need for repeated diagnostic evaluation. Gastroenterology, 68:187, 1975.
2. Kirsner, J. B., Deutsch, S., and Hanauer, S. B.: Selected individual therapeutic problems in inflammatory bowel disease. Am. J. Gastroenterol., 79:368, 1984.
3. Kirsner, J. B., and Shorter, R. G.: Recent developments in "nonspecific" inflammatory bowel disease—part I. N. Engl. J. Med., 306:775, 1982.
4. Farmer, R. G.: Long-term prognosis for patients with ulcerative proctosigmoiditis (ulcerative colitis confined to the rectum and sigmoid colon). J. Clin. Gastroenterol., 1:47, 1979.
5. Edwards, F. C., and Truelove, S. C.: The course and programs of ulcerative colitis. Part II. Long-term prognosis. Gut, 4:309, 1963.
6. Truelove, S. C., and Witts, I. J.: Cortisone in ulcerative colitis. Report on therapeutic trial. Br. Med. J., 2:1041, 1955.
7. Lennard-Jones, J. E., Ritchie, J. K., Hilder, W., and Spicer, C. C.: Assessment of severity in colitis: A preliminary study. Gut, 16:579, 1975.
8. Powell-Tuck, J., et al.: Correlations between defined sigmoidoscopic appearances and other measures of disease activity in ulcerative colitis. Dig. Dis. Sci., 27:533, 1982.
9. Hodgson, H. J. F.: Assessment of drug therapy in inflammatory bowel disease. Br. J. Clin. Pharmacol., 14:159, 1982.
10. Fagan, E. A., et al.: Serum levels of C-reactive protein in Crohn's disease and ulcerative colitis. Eur. J. Clin. Invest., 12:351, 1982.
11. Descos, L., et al.: Assessment of appropriate laboratory measurements to reflect the degree of activity of ulcerative colitis. Digestion, 28:148, 1983.
12. Dearing, W. H., McGuckin, W. F., and Elveback, L. R.: Serum alpha$_1$-acid glycoprotein in chronic ulcerative colitis. Gastroenterology, 56:295, 1969.
13. Buckell, N. A., et al.: Measurements of serum proteins during attacks of ulcerative colitis as a guide to patient management. Gut, 20:22, 1979.
14. Jensen, K. B., et al.: Serum orosomucoid in ulcerative colitis. Its relation to clinical activity, protein loss and turnover of albumin and IgG. Scand. J. Gastroenterol., 11:177, 1976.
15. Weeke, B., and Jarnum, S.: Serum concentrations of 19 serum proteins in Crohn's disease and ulcerative colitis. Gut, 12:297, 1971.
16. Andre, C., et al.: Biological measurements of Crohn's disease activity: A reassessment. Hepatogastroenterology, 32:135, 1985.
17. Saverymuttu, S. H., Hodgson, H. J. F., and Chadwick, V. S.: Comparison of fecal granulocyte excretion in ulcerative colitis and Crohn's colitis. Dig. Dis. Sci., 29:1000, 1984.
18. Saverymuttu, S. H., et al.: Indium 111-granulocyte scanning in the assessment of disease extent and disease activity in inflammatory bowel disease. A comparison with colonoscopy, histology, and fecal indium 111-granulocyte excretion. Gastroenterology, 90:1121, 1986.
19. Roediger, W. E. W., et al.: Colonic bicarbonate output as a test of disease activity in ulcerative colitis. J. Clin. Pathol., 37:704, 1984.
20. Meyers, S., et al.: Fecal alpha$_1$-antitrypsin measurement: An indicator of Crohn's disease activity. Gastroenterology, 89:13, 1985.
21. Baron, J. H., Connell, A. M., and Lennard-Jones, J. E.: Variation between observers in describing mucosal appearances in proctocolitis. Br. Med. J., 1:89, 1964.
22. Heatley, R. V., et al.: Disodium cromoglycate in the treatment of chronic proctitis. Gut, 16:559, 1975.
23. Morson, B. C., and Dawson, I. M. P.: Gastrointestinal Pathology. Oxford, England, Blackwell Scientific Publications, 1979.
24. Spiro, H. M.: Patient and physician in the management of inflammatory bowel disease. J. Clin. Gastroenterol., 7:117, 1985.
25. Colcher, S. D.: Family structure, stress and individual adjustment to ulcerative colitis. Ph.D. Dissertation, Evanston, Illinois, Northwestern University.
26. Isgar, B., Harman, M., Kaye, M. D., and Whorwell, P. J.: Symptoms of irritable bowel syndrome in ulcerative colitis in remission. Gut, 24:190, 1983.
27. Awouters, F., Niemegeers, C. J. E., and Janssen, P. A. J.: Pharmacology of antidiarrheal drugs. Annu. Rev. Pharmacol. Toxocol., 23:279, 1983.
28. Shea, C. D., and Pounder, R. E.: Loperamide, diphenoxylate, and codeine phosphate in chronic diarrhea. Br. Med. J., 1:524, 1980.
29. Pelemans, W., and Vantrappen, G.: A double blind crossover comparison of loperamide with diphenoxylate in symptomatic treatment of chronic diarrhea. Gastroenterology, 70:1030, 1976.
30. Tytgat, G. N., et al.: Effect of loperamide on fecal output and composition in well established ileostomy and ileorectal anastomosis. Dig. Dis. Sci., 22:669, 1977.
31. Engbaek, J., et al.: The constipating effect of diphenoxylate (Retardin^R) in ulcerative colitis. Scand. J. Gastroenterol., 10:695, 1975.
32. Read, M., and Read, N. W.: Anal sphincter function in diarrhea: influence of loperamide. Clin. Res. Rev. 1:219, 1981.
33. Durbin, T., et al.: Clonidine and lidamidine (WHR-1142) stimulates sodium and chloride absorption in the rabbit intestine. Gastroenterology, 82:1352, 1982.
34. Lechin, F., et al.: Treatment of ulcerative colitis with clonidine. J. Clin. Pharmacol., 25:219, 1985.
35. Guillemin, R., et al.: Neural Modulation of Immunity. New York, Raven Press, 1985.
36. Rampton, D. S., McNeil, N. I., and Sarner, M.: Analgesic ingestion and other factors preceding relapse in ulcerative colitis. Gut, 24:187, 1983.
37. Rampton, D. S., and Sladen, G. E.: Relapse of ulcerative proctocolitis during treatment with non-steroidal anti-inflammatory drugs. Postgrad. Med. J., 57:297, 1981.
38. Campieri, M., et al.: Prostaglandins, indomethacin, and ulcerative colitis. Gastroenterology, 78:193, 1980.
39. Kaplan, M. A., Fochios, S. E., and Korelitz, B. I.: Dependence on narcotics and other supplemental drugs in pa-

tients with inflammatory bowel disease. Gastroenterology, *90*: 1483, 1986.
40. Svartz, N.: Salazopyrin, a new sulfanilamide preparation. A. Therapeutic results in rheumatic polyarthritis. B. Therapeutic results in ulcerative colitis. C. Toxic manifestations in treatment with sulfanilamide preparations. Acta Med. Scand., *110*: 577, 1942.
41. Svartz, N.: The treatment of 124 cases of ulcerative colitis with salazoprine and attempts at desensitization in cases of hypersensitiveness to sulpha. Acta Med. Scand. (Suppl.), *206*: 465, 1948.
42. Svartz, N.: The treatment of ulcerative colitis. Gastroenterologia, *86*: 683, 1956.
43. Peppercorn, M. A.: Sulfasalazine: Pharmacology, clinical use, toxicity, and related new drug development. Ann. Intern. Med., *3*: 377, 1984.
44. Moertel, C. G., and Bargen, J. A.: A critical analysis of the use of salicylazosulfapyridine in chronic ulcerative colitis. Ann. Intern. Med., *51*: 879, 1959.
45. Baron, J. H., Connell, A. M., and Lennard-Jones, J. E.: Sulphasalazine and salicylazo-sulphadimidine in ulcerative colitis. Lancet, *1*: 1094, 1962.
46. Dick, A. P., Grayson, M. J., Carpenter, R. G., and Petrie, A.: Controlled trial of sulphasalazine in the treatment of ulcerative colitis. Gut, *5*: 437, 1964.
47. Truelove, S. C., Watkinson, G., and Draper, G.: Comparison of corticosteroid and sulphasalazine therapy in ulcerative colitis. Br. Med. J., *2*: 1708, 1962.
48. Truelove, S. C., Lee, E. G., Willoughby, C. P., and Kettlewell, M. G. W.: Further experience in the treatment of severe attacks of ulcerative colitis. Lancet, *1*: 1086, 1978.
49. Misiewicz, J. J., et al.: Controlled trial of sulphasalazine in maintenance therapy for ulcerative colitis. Lancet, *2*: 185, 1965.
50. Riis, P., et al.: The prophylactic effect of salazosulphapyridine in ulcerative colitis during long-term treatment: a double-blind trial on patients asymptomatic for one year. Scand. J. Gastroenterol., *8*: 71, 1973.
51. Dissanayake, A. S., and Truelove, S. C.: A controlled therapeutic trial of long-term maintenance treatment of ulcerative colitis with sulphasalazine (salazopyrin). Gut, *14*: 923, 1973.
52. Azad Khan, A. K., et al.: Optimum dose of sulphasalazine for maintenance treatment of ulcerative colitis. Gut, *21*: 232, 1980.
53. Klotz, U.: Clinical pharmacokinetics of sulphasalazine, its metabolites, and other prodrugs of 5-aminosalicylic acid. Clin. Pharmacokinet., *10*: 285, 1985.
54. Peppercorn, M. A., and Goldman, P.: Distribution studies of salicylazosulfapyridine and its metabolites. Gastroenterology, *64*: 240, 1973.
55. Schroder, H., Lewkonia, R. M., and Price-Evans, D. A.: Metabolism of salicylazosulfapyridine in healthy subjects and in patients with ulcerative colitis: Effects of colectomy and of phenobarbital. Clin. Pharmacol. Ther., *14*: 802, 1973.
56. Das, K. M., et al.: Small bowel absorption of sulfasalazine and its hepatic metabolism in human beings, cats, and rats. Gastroenterology, *77*: 280, 1979.
57. Khan, A. K. A., Truelove, S. C., and Aronson, J. K.: The disposition and metabolism of sulphasalazine (salicylazosulphapyridine) in man. Br. J. Clin. Pharm., *13*: 523, 1982.
58. Das, K. M., et al.: The metabolism of salicylazosulphapyridine in ulcerative colitis. Gut, *14*: 631, 1973.
59. Ashworth, M., et al.: A comparison of serum concentrations of sulphasalazine and some of its metabolites after therapy by the oral or rectal route. Pharmatherapeutica, *3*: 551, 1984.
60. Ryde, E. M., and Lima, J. J.: Bioavailability study on oral sulfasalazine suspension compared to tablets in healthy volunteers. Curr. Ther. Res., *29*: 728, 1981.
61. Pieniaszek, H. J., et al.: Relative systemic availability of sulfapyridine from commercial enteric-coated and uncoated sulfasalazine tablets. J. Clin. Pharmacol., *19*: 39, 1979.
62. Khan, A. K. A., Nurrazzaman, M., and Truelove, S. C.: The effect of the acetylator phenotype on the metabolism of sulphasalazine in man. J. Med. Genet., *20*: 30, 1983.
63. Peppercorn, M. A., and Goldman, P.: The role of intestinal bacteria in the metabolism of salicylazosulfapyridine. J. Pharmacol. Exp. Ther., *181*: 555, 1972.
64. Khan, A. K. A., et al.: Tissue and bacterial splitting of sulphasalazine. Clin. Sci., *64*: 349, 1983.
65. Das, K. M., Eastwood, M. A., McManus, J. P. A., and Sircus, W.: The role of the colon in the metabolism of salicylazosulphapyridine. Scand. J. Gastroenterol., *9*: 137, 1974.
66. Van Hees, P. A. M., et al.: Influence of intestinal transit time on azo-reduction of salicylazosulphapyridine (Salazopyrin). Gut, *20*: 300, 1979.
67. Houston, J. B., Day, J., and Walker, J.: Azo reduction of sulphasalazine in healthy volunteers. Br. J. Clin. Pharmacol., *14*: 395, 1982.
68. Schroder, H., and Campbell, D. E. S.: Absorption, metabolism, and excretion of salicylazosulfapyridine in man. Clin. Pharmacol. Ther., *13*: 539, 1972.
69. Ireland, A., Priddle, J. D., and Jewell, D. P.: Acetylation of 5-aminosalicylic acid by human colonic epithelial cells. Gastroenterology, *90*: 1471, 1986.
70. Pieniaszek, H. J., and Bates, T. R.: Capacity-limited gut wall metabolism of 5-aminosalicylic acid, a therapeutically active metabolite of sulfasalazine, in rats. J. Pharm. Sci., *68*: 1323, 1979.
71. Rasmussen, S. N., et al.: 5-aminosalicylic acid in a slow-release preparation: Bioavailability, plasma level, and excretion in humans. Gastroenterology, *83*: 1062, 1982.
72. Meese, C. O., Fischer, C., and Klotz, U.: Is N-acetylation of 5-aminosalicylic acid reversible in man? Br. J. Clin. Pharmacol., *18*: 612, 1984.
73. Klotz, U., Maier, K. E., Fischer, C., and Bauer, K. H.: A new slow-release form of 5-aminosalicylic acid for the oral treatment of inflammatory bowel disease: biopharmaceutic and clinical pharmacokinetic characteristics. Arzneimittelforschung, *35*: 636, 1985.
74. Bondesen, S.: Personal communication, 1987.
75. Nielson, O. H., and Bondesen, S.: Kinetics of 5-aminosalicylic acid after jejunal instillation in man. Br. J. Clin. Pharmacol., *16*: 738, 1983.
76. Svartz, N.: The pathogenesis and treatment of ulcerative colitis. Acta Med. Scand., *141*: 172, 1951.
77. Cooke, E. M.: Fecal flora of patients with ulcerative colitis during treatment with salicylazosulfapyridine. Gut, *10*: 565, 1969.
78. West, B., et al.: Effects of sulphasalazine on faecal flora in patients with inflammatory bowel disease. Gut, *15*: 950, 1974.
79. Azad Khan, A. K., Piris, J., and Truelove, S. C.: An experiment to determine the active therapeutic moiety of sulphasalazine. Lancet, *2*: 892, 1977.
80. Klotz, U., Maier, K., Fischer, C., and Heinkel, K.: Therapeutic efficacy of sulfasalazine and its metabolites in patients with ulcerative colitis and Crohn's disease. N. Engl. J. Med., *303*: 1499, 1980.
81. Pullar, T., Hunter, J. A., and Capell, H. A.: Which compo-

nent of sulphasalazine is active in rheumatoid arthritis? Br. Med. J., 290:1535, 1985.
82. Donowitz, M.: Arachidonic acid metabolites and their role in inflammatory bowel disease. An update requiring addition of a pathway. Gastroenterology, 88:580, 1985.
83. Hawkey, C. J., and Rampton, D. S.: Prostaglandins and the gastrointestinal mucosa: are they important in its function, disease, or treatment. Gastroenterology, 89:1162, 1985.
84. Sharon, P., Ligumsky, M., Rachmilewitz, D., and Zor, U.: Role of prostaglandins in ulcerative colitis: enhanced production during active disease and inhibition by sulfasalazine. Gastroenterology, 75:638, 1978.
85. Ligumsky, M., et al.: Enhanced thromboxane A_2 and prostacyclin production by cultured rectal mucosa in ulcerative colitis and its inhibition by steroids and sulfasalazine. Gastroenterology, 81:444, 1981.
86. Racusen, L. C., and Binder, H. J.: Effect of prostaglandin on ion transport across isolated colonic mucosa. Dig. Dis. Sci., 25:900, 1980.
87. Rachmilewitz, D.: Prostaglandins and diarrhea. Dig. Dis. Sci., 25:897, 1980.
88. Zifroni, A., Treves, A. J., Sachar, D. B., and Rachmilewitz, D.: Prostanoid synthesis by cultured intestinal epithelial and mononuclear cells in inflammatory bowel disease. Gut, 24:659, 1983.
89. Rachmilewitz, D., Ligumsky, M., Haimovitz, A., and Treves, A. J.: Prostanoid synthesis by cultured peripheral blood mononuclear cells in inflammatory diseases of the bowel. Gastroenterology, 82:673, 1982.
90. Rampton, D. S., Sladen, G. E., and Youlten, L. J. F.: Rectal mucosal prostaglandin E_2 release and its relation to disease activity, electrical potential difference, and treatment in ulcerative colitis. Gut, 21:591, 1980.
91. Lauritsen, K., et al.: Effects of sulphasalazine and disodium azodisalicylate on colonic PGE_2 concentrations determined by equilibrium in vivo dialysis of faeces in patients with ulcerative colitis and healthy controls. Gut, 25:1271, 1984.
92. Smith, P. R., Dawson, D. J., and Swan, C. H.: Prostaglandin synthetase activity in acute ulcerative colitis: effects of treatment with sulphasalazine, codeine phosphate, and prednisolone. Gut, 20:802, 1979.
93. Hawkey, C. J., and Truelove, S. C.: Inhibition of prostaglandin synthetase in human rectal mucosa. Gut, 24:213, 1983.
94. Gilat, T., et al.: Prostaglandins and ulcerative colitis. Gastroenterology, 76:1083, 1979.
95. Campieri, M., et al.: Prostaglandins, indomethacin and ulcerative colitis. Gastroenterology, 78:193, 1980.
96. Rampton, D. S., and Sladen, G. E.: Prostaglandin synthesis inhibitors in ulcerative colitis: flubiprofen compared with conventional treatment. Prostaglandins, 21:417, 1981.
97. Hoult, J. R. S., and Moore, P. K.: Sulphasalazine is a potent inhibitor of prostaglandin 15 hydroxy dehydrogenase: a possible basis for therapeutic action in ulcerative colitis. Br. J. Pharmacol., 64:6, 1978.
98. Hoult, J. R. S., and Page, H.: 5-aminosalicylic acid, a cofactor for prostacyclin synthesis. Lancet, 2:255, 1981.
99. Gould, S. R., et al.: Studies of prostaglandins and sulphasalazine in ulcerative colitis. Prostaglandins Med., 6:165, 1981.
100. Lauritsen, K., et al.: Colonic azodisalicylate metabolism determined by in vivo dialysis in healthy volunteers and patients with ulcerative colitis. Gastroenterology, 86:1496, 1984.
101. Goldin, E., and Rachmilewitz, D.: Prostanoids cytoprotection for maintaining remission in ulcerative colitis: failure of 15 (R), 15-methylprostaglandin E_2. Dig. Dis. Sci., 28:807, 1983.
102. Stenson, W. F.: Pharmacology of sulfasalazine. Viewpoints Dig. Dis., 16:13, 1984.
103. Sharon, P., and Stenson, W. F.: Enhanced synthesis of leukotriene B_4 by colonic mucosa in inflammatory bowel disease. Gastroenterology, 86:453, 1984.
104. Hammarstrom, S.: Leukotrienes. Annu. Rev. Biochem., 52:355, 1983.
105. Stenson, W. F., and Lobos, E.: Sulfasalazine inhibits the synthesis of chemotactic lipids by neutrophils. J. Clin. Invest., 69:494, 1982.
106. Sircar, J. C., Schwender, C. F., and Carethers, M. E.: Inhibition of soybean lipoxygenase by sulfasalazine and 5-aminosalicylic acid: A possible mode of action in ulcerative colitis. Biochem. Pharmacol., 32:170, 1983.
107. Allgayer, H., Eisenberg, J., and Paumgartner, G.: Soybean lipoxygenase inhibition: studies with sulphasalazine metabolites N-acetylaminosalicylic acid, 5-aminosalicylic acid and sulphapyridine. Eur. J. Clin. Pharmacol., 26:449, 1984.
108. Hawkey, C. J., and Rampton, D. S.: Benoxaprofen in the treatment of active ulcerative colitis. Prostaglandins Leukotrienes Med., 10:405, 1983.
109. Siegel, M. I., et al.: Arachidonate metabolism via lipoxygenase and 12L-hydroperoxy-5, 8, 10, 14-icosatetraenoic acid peroxidase sensitive to anti-inflammatory drugs. Proc. Natl. Acad. Sci. USA, 72:308, 1980.
110. Kelly, J. P., Johnson, M. C., and Parker, C. W.: Effect of inhibitors of arachidonic acid metabolism on mutogenesis in human lymphocytes: possible role of thromboxanes and products of the lipoxygenase pathway. J. Immunol., 122:1563, 1979.
111. Bland, P. W., et al.: Isolation and purification of human large bowel mucosal lymphoid cells: effect of separation technique on functional characteristics. Gut, 20:1037, 1979.
112. Holm, G., and Perlmann, P.: Cytotoxicity of lymphocytes and its suppression. Antibiot. Chemother., 15:295, 1969.
113. Thayer, W. R. Jr., Charland, C., and Field, C. E.: Effects of sulfasalazine on selected lymphocyte subpopulations in vivo and in vitro. Dig. Dis. Sci., 24:672, 1979.
114. Rubinstein, A., Das, K. M., Melamed, J., and Murphy, R. A.: Comparative analysis of systemic immunologic parameters in ulcerative colitis and idiopathic proctitis: effects of sulfasalazine in vivo and in vitro. Clin. Exp. Immunol., 33:217, 1978.
115. Holdstock, G., Ershler, W. B., and Krawitt, E. L.: Defective lymphocyte IgA production in inflammatory bowel disease. Clin. Immunol. Immunopathol., 24:47, 1982.
116. Molin, L., and Stendahl, O.: The effect of sulfasalazine and its active components on human polymorphonuclear leukocyte function in relation to ulcerative colitis. Acta Med. Scand., 206:451, 1979.
117. Rhodes, J. M., Bartholomew, T. C., and Jewell, D. P.: Inhibition of leucocyte motility by drugs used in ulcerative colitis. Gut, 22:642, 1981.
118. Stenson, W. F., Mehta, J., and Spilberg, I.: Sulfasalazine inhibition of binding of N-formyl-methionyl-leucyl-phenylalanine (FMLP) to its receptor on human neutrophils. Biochem. Pharmacol., 33:407, 1984.
119. Del Soldato, P., et al.: A possible mechanism of action of sulfasalazine and 5-aminosalicylic acid in inflammatory bowel diseases: interaction with oxygen free radicals. Gastroenterology, 89:1215, 1985.
120. Lauterburg, B. H.: 5-aminosalicylic acid (5-ASA) sca-

venges superoxide anion radicals: an additional mode of action in ulcerative colitis (CUC). Gastroenterology, 90:1514, 1986.
121. Taffet, S. L., and Das, K. M.: Sulfasalazine: adverse effects and desensitization. Dig. Dis. Sci., 28:833, 1983.
122. Schroder, H., and Price-Evans, D. A.: Acetylator phenotype and adverse effects of sulphasalazine in healthy subjects. Gut, 13:278, 1972.
123. Das, K. M., Eastwood, M. A., McManus, J. P. A., and Sircus, W.: Adverse reactions during salicylazosulfapyridine therapy and the relation with drug metabolism and acetylator phenotype. N. Engl. J. Med., 289:491, 1973.
124. Nielsen, O. H.: Sulfasalazine intolerance: A retrospective survey of the reasons for discontinuing treatment with sulfasalazine in patients with chronic inflammatory bowel disease. Scand. J. Gastroenterol., 17:389, 1982.
125. Misiewicz, J. J., et al.: Controlled trial of sulphasalazine (Azulfidine [salicylazosulfapyridine]) in maintenance therapy for ulcerative colitis. Lancet, 1:185, 1965.
126. Mihas, A. A., Goldenberg, D. J., and Slaughter, R. L.: Sulfasalazine toxic reactions: hepatitis, fever, and skin rash with hypocomplementemia and immune complexes. J. Am. Med. Assoc., 239:2590, 1978.
127. Griffiths, I. D., and Kane, S. P.: Sulphasalazine induced lupus syndrome in ulcerative colitis. Br. Med. J., 2:1188, 1977.
128. Rafoth, R. J.: Systemic granulomatous reaction to salicylazosulfapyridine (Azulfidine) in a patient with Crohn's disease. Am. J. Dig. Dis., 19:465, 1974.
129. Gulley, R. M., Mirza, A., and Kelly, C. E.: Hepatotoxicity of salicylazosulfapyridine. Am. J. Gastroenterol., 72:561, 1979.
130. Caravatti, C. M., and Hooker, T. H.: Acute massive hepatic necrosis with fatal liver failure. Am. J. Dig. Dis., 16:803, 1971.
131. Sotolongo, R. P., et al.: Hypersensitivity reactions to sulfasalazine with severe hepatotoxicity. Gastroenterology, 75:95, 1978.
132. Jacobs, E., Paulet, P., and Rahier, J.: Hypersensitivity reaction to sulfasalazine—another case [letter]. Gastroenterology, 75:1193, 1978.
133. Namias, A., Bhalotra, R., and Donowitz, M.: Reversible sulfasalazine-induced granulomatous hepatitis. J. Clin. Gastroenterol., 3:193, 1981.
134. Chester, A. C., Diamond, L. H., and Schreiner, G. E.: Hypersensitivity to salicylazosulfapyridine: renal and hepatic toxic reactions. Arch. Intern. Med., 138:1138, 1978.
135. Block, M. B., Genant, H. K., and Kirsner, J. B.: Pancreatitis as an adverse reaction to salicylazosulfapyridine. N. Engl. J. Med., 282:380, 1970.
136. Sulfasalazine-induced lung disease (editorial). Lancet, 2:504, 1974.
137. Mosely, R. H., et al.: Sulfasalazine-induced pulmonary disease. Dig. Dis. Sci., 9:901, 1985.
138. Williams, T., Eidus, L., and Thomas, P.: Fibrosing alveolitis, bronchiolitis obliterans, and sulfasalazine therapy. Chest, 81:766, 1982.
139. Tydd, T. F., and Dyer, N. H.: Sulphasalazine lung. Med. J. Aust., 1:570, 1976.
140. Eade, O. E., et al.: Pulmonary function in patients with inflammatory bowel disease. Am. J. Gastroenterol., 73:154, 1980.
141. Hamshidi, K., et al.: Azulfidine agranulocytosis with bone marrow megakaryocytosis, histiocytosis, and plasmocytosis. Minn. Med., 55:545, 1972.
142. Wheelan, K. R., Cooper, B., and Stone, M. J.: Multiple hematologic abnormalities associated with sulfasalazine. Ann. Intern. Med., 97:726, 1982.
143. Davies, G. E., and Palek, J.: Selective erythroid and megakaryocytic aplasia after sulfasalazine administration (letter). Arch. Intern. Med., 140:1122, 1980.
144. Pounder, R. E., Craven, E. R., Henthorn, J. S., and Bannatyne, J. M.: Red cell abnormalities associated with sulphasalazine maintenance therapy for ulcerative colitis. Gut, 16:181, 1975.
145. Goodacre, R. L., et al.: Hemolytic anemia in patients receiving sulfasalazine. Digestion, 17:503, 1978.
146. Van Hees, P. A., Van Elferen, L. W., Van Rossum, J. M., and Van Tongeren, J. H.: Hemolysis during salicylazosulfapyridine therapy. Am. J. Gastroenterol., 70:501, 1979.
147. Franklin, J. L., and Rosenberg, I. H.: Impaired folic acid absorption in inflammatory bowel disease: effects of salicylazosulfapyrine (Azulfidine). Gastroenterology, 64:517, 1973.
148. Halsted, C. H., Gandhi, G., and Tamura, T.: Sulfasalazine inhibits the absorption of folates in ulcerative colitis. N. Engl. J. Med., 305:1513, 1981.
149. Longstreth, G. F., and Green, R.: Folate status in patients receiving maintenance doses of sulfasalazine. Arch. Intern. Med., 143:902, 1983.
150. Swinson, C., et al.: Role of sulphasalazine in the aetiology of folate deficiency in ulcerative colitis. Gut, 22:456, 1981.
151. Selhub, J., Dhar, G. J., and Rosenberg, I. H.: Inhibition of folate enzymes by sulfasalazine. J. Clin. Invest., 61:221, 1978.
152. Reisenauer, A. M., and Halsted, C. H.: Human jejunal brush border folate conjugase: characteristics and inhibition by salicylazosulfapyridine. Biochem. Biophys. Acta, 659:62, 1981.
153. Baum, C. L., Selhub, J., and Rosenberg, I. H.: Antifolate actions of sulfasalazine on intact lymphocytes. J. Lab. Clin. Med., 97:779, 1981.
154. Toth, A.: Reversible toxic effect of salicylazosulfapyridine on semen quality. Fertil. Steril., 31:538, 1979.
155. Birnie, G. G., McLeod, T. I. F., and Watkinson, G.: Incidence of sulphasalazine-induced male infertility. Gut, 22:452, 1981.
156. Hudson, E., et al.: Sperm size in patients with inflammatory bowel disease on sulfasalazine therapy. Fertil. Steril., 38:77, 1982.
157. Toovey, S., et al.: Sulphasalazine and male infertility: reversibility and possible mechanism. Gut, 22:445, 1981.
158. O'Morain, C., Smethurst, P., Dore, C. J., and Levi, A. J.: Reversible male infertility due to sulphasalazine: studies in man and rat. Gut, 25:1078, 1984.
159. Cann, P. A., and Holdsworth, C. D.: Reversal of male infertility on changing treatment from sulphasalazine to 5-aminosalicylic acid. Lancet, 1:1119, 1984.
160. Shaffer, J. L., Kershaw, A., and Berrisford, M. H.: Sulphasalazine-induced infertility reversed on changing treatment to 5-aminosalicylic acid. Lancet, 1:1240, 1984.
161. Neeman, A., et al.: Salazopyrine-induced tachycardia. Biomed., 33:1, 1980.
162. Attar, A., and Anuras, S.: Sulfasalazine and hair loss. Gastroenterology, 80:1102, 1981.
163. Wallace, I. W.: Neurotoxicity associated with a reaction to sulfasalazine. Practitioner, 204:850, 1970.
164. Smith, M. D., Gibson, G. E., and Rowland, R.: Combined hepatotoxicity and neurotoxicity following sulphasalazine administration. Aust. N. Z. J. Med., 12:76, 1982.
165. Werlin, S. L., and Grand, R. J.: Bloody diarrhea—a new complication of sulfasalazine. J. Pediatr., 92:450, 1978.

166. Schwartz, A. G., Targan, S. R., Saxon, A., and Weinstein, W. M.: Sulfasalazine-induced exacerbation of ulcerative colitis. N. Engl. J. Med., *306*: 409, 1982.
167. Adler, R. D.: Sulfasalazine-induced exacerbation of ulcerative colitis (letter). N. Engl. J. Med., *307*: 315, 1982.
168. Ring, F. A., Hershfield, N. B., Machin, G. A., and Scott, R. B.: Sulfasalazine-induced colitis complicating idiopathic ulcerative colitis. Can. Med. Assoc. J., *131*: 43, 1984.
169. Ruppin, J., and Domschke, S.: Acute ulcerative colitis—a rare complication of sulfasalazine therapy. Hepatogastroenterology, *31*: 192, 1984.
170. Pokorney, B. H., and Nichols, T. W.: Pseudomembranous colitis: A complication of sulfasalazine therapy in a patient with Crohn's colitis. Am. J. Gastroenterol., 76: 374, 1981.
171. Sack, D. M., and Peppercorn, M. A.: Drug therapy of inflammatory bowel disease. Pharmacotherapy, *3*: 158, 1983.
172. Azad Khan, A. K., and Truelove, S. C.: Circulating levels of sulphasalazine and its metabolites and their relation to the clinical efficacy of the drug in ulcerative colitis. Gut, *21*: 706, 1980.
173. Das, K. M., and Eastwood, M. A.: Effect of iron and calcium on salicylazosulfapyridine metabolism. Scott. Med. J., *18*: 45, 1973.
174. Juhl, R. P., et al.: Effect of sulfasalazine on digoxin bioavailability. Clin. Pharmacol. Ther., *20*: 387, 1976.
175. Das, K. M.: Pharmacotherapy of inflammatory bowel disease: Part 1—sulfasalazine. Postgrad. Med., *74*: 141, 1983.
176. Taffet, S. L., and Das, K. M.: Desensitization of patients with inflammatory bowel disease to sulfasalazine. Am. J. Med., *73*: 520, 1982.
177. Holdworth, C. D.: Sulphasalazine desensitization. Br. Med. J. (Clin. Research), *282*: 110, 1981.
178. Purdy, B. H., Philips, D. M., and Summers, R. W.: Desensitization for sulfasalazine skin rash. Ann. Intern. Med., *100*: 512, 1984.
179. Korelitz, B. I., Present, D. H., Rubin, P. H., and Fochios, S. E.: Desensitization to sulfasalazine after hypersensitivity reactions in patients with inflammatory bowel disease. J. Clin. Gastroenterol., *6*: 27, 1984.
180. Willoughby, C. P., and Truelove, S. C.: Ulcerative colitis and pregnancy. Gut, *21*: 469, 1980.
181. Mogadam, M., et al.: Pregnancy in inflammatory bowel disease: Effect of sulfasalazine and corticosteroids on fetal outcome. Gastroenterology, *80*: 72, 1981.
182. Nielsen, O. H., Andreasson, B., Bondesen, S., and Jarnum, S.: Pregnancy in ulcerative colitis. Scand. J. Gastroenterol., *18*: 735, 1983.
183. Baiocco, P. J., and Korelitz, B. I.: The influence of inflammatory bowel disease and its treatment on pregnancy and fetal outcome. J. Clin. Gastroenterol., *6*: 221, 1984.
184. Jarnerot, G., and Into-Malmberg, M. B.: Sulphasalazine treatment during breast feeding. Scand. J. Gastroenterol., 14: 869, 1979.
185. Lewis, J. H., and Weingold, A. B.: The use of gastrointestinal drugs during pregnancy and lactation. Am. J. Gastroenterol., *80*: 912, 1985.
186. Goldstein, P. D., Alpers, D. H., and Keating, J. P.: Sulfapyridine metabolites in children with inflammatory bowel disease receiving sulfasalazine. J. Pediatr., *95*: 638, 1979.
187. Campieri, M., et al.: Treatment of ulcerative colitis with high-dose 5-aminosalicylic acid enemas. Lancet, *2*: 270, 1981.
188. Campieri, M., et al.: High-dose 5-aminosalicylic acid enemas in the treatment of ulcerative colitis. Intern. Med., 5: 164, 1984.
189. Lanfranchi, G. A., et al.: Treatment of ulcerative colitis patients with high-dose 5-ASA enemas. Report of 2 years in an out-patient clinic. Gastroenterology (Abstract), *86*: 1151, 1984.
190. Campieri, M., et al.: 5-aminosalicylic acid as rectal enemas in ulcerative colitis in patients unable to take sulphasalazine. Lancet, *1*: 403, 1982.
191. Campieri, M., et al.: 5-aminosalicylic acid for the treatment of inflammatory bowel disease. Gastroenterology, *89*: 701, 1985.
192. Campieri, M., et al.: Topical administration of 5-aminosalicylic acid enemas in patients with ulcerative colitis. Studies on rectal absorption and excretion. Gut, *26*: 400, 1985.
193. Hanauer, S. B., Schultz, P. A., and Kirsner, J. B.: Treatment of refractory proctitis with 5-ASA enemas. Gastroenterology, *88*: 1412, 1985.
194. Hanauer, S. B., and Schultz, P. A.: Efficacy of 5-ASA enemas for steroid dependent ulcerative colitis. Gastroenterology, *90*: 1449, 1986.
195. Barber, G. B., et al.: Refractory distal ulcerative colitis responsive to 5-aminosalicylate enemas. Am. J. Gastroenterol., *80*: 612, 1985.
196. Sandgren, J. E., McPhee, M. S., and Greenberger, N. J.: Refractory distal ulcerative colitis: response to therapy with 5-aminosalicylic acid (5-ASA enemas). Gastroenterology, *86*: 1230, 1984.
197. Jansens, J., et al.: 5-aminosalicylic acid enemas are effective in patients with resistant ulcerative rectosigmoiditis. Gastroenterology, *84*: 1198, 1983.
198. Friedman, L. S., et al.: 5-aminosalicylic acid enemas in refractory distal ulcerative colitis: A randomized controlled trial. Gastroenterology, *88*: 1388, 1985.
199. d'Albaso, G., et al.: Long-term maintenance therapy in ulcerative colitis. A controlled trial with intermittent 5-aminosalicylic acid (5-ASA) enemas. Second International Symposium on Inflammatory Bowel Diseases. Jerusalem, 1985.
200. Bondesen, S., et al.: 5-aminosalicylic acid enemas in patients with active ulcerative colitis. Scand. J. Gastroenterol., *19*: 677, 1984.
201. Wyman, J. B., et al.: 5-aminosalicylic acid retention enemata for long term therapy of inflammatory bowel disease. Gastroenterology, *88*: 1636, 1985.
202. Powell-Tuck, J., and Parkins, R. A.: Controlled comparison of enemas containing 1 gm and 2 gm 5-aminosalicylic acid in patients with ulcerative proctosigmoiditis. Gut, *25*: A1143, 1984.
203a. Austin, C. A., et al.: Exacerbation of diarrhoea and pain in patients treated with 5-aminosalicylic acid for ulcerative colitis [letter]. Lancet, *1*: 917, 1984.
203. Bondesson, S., and a Danish 5-ASA Study Group: Topical 5-aminosalicylic acid versus prednisolone in ulcerative proctosigmoiditis. Gastroenterology, *90*: 1350, 1986.
204. Kutty, P. K., et al.: Hair loss and 5-ASA enemas. Ann. Intern. Med., *97*: 785, 1982.
205. Calder, I. C., et al.: Nephrotoxic lesions from 5-aminosalicylic acid. Br. Med. J., *1*: 152, 1972.
206. Van Hees, P. A., Bakker, J. H., and Van Tongeren, J. H. M.: Effect of sulphapyridine, 5-aminosalicylic acid, and placebo in patients with idiopathic proctitis: A study to determine the active therapeutic moiety of sulphasalazine. Gut, *21*: 632, 1980.
207. Maier, K., et al.: 5-aminosalicylsaure bei colitis ulcerosa und morbus Crohn. Dtsch. Med. Wochenschr., *107*: 1131, 1982.

208. Maier, K., et al.: 5-aminosalicysaure—ein neues behandlungsprinzip bei colitis ulcerosa und morbus Crohn. Verdauungskrankheiten, *1*:62, 1983.
209. Campieri, M., et al.: A controlled trial on the efficacy and compliance of 5-ASA suppositories in distal ulcerative sigmoiditis. Gastroenterology, *90*:1364, 1986.
210. Campieri, M., et al.: A double-blind clinical trial to compare the effects of 4-aminosalicylic acid to 5-aminosalicylic acid in topical treatment of ulcerative colitis. Digestion, *29*:204, 1984.
211. Gandolfo, J., et al.: Treatment of distal colitis with 4-ASA enemas. Gastroenterology, *88*:1391, 1985.
212. Selby, W. S., Bennett, M. K., and Jewell, D. P.: Topical treatment of distal ulcerative colitis with 4-aminosalicylic acid enemas. Digestion, *29*:231, 1984.
213. Willoughby, C. P., et al.: Distribution and metabolism in healthy volunteers of disodium azodisalicylate, a potential therapeutic agent for ulcerative colitis. Gut, *23*:1081, 1982.
214. Sandberg-Gertzen, H., Ryde, M., and Janerot, G.: Absorption, metabolism and excretion of a single 1 gm dose of azodisal sodium in subjects with ileostomy. Scand. J. Gastroenterol., *18*:107, 1983.
215. Van Hogezand, R. A., et al.: Disposition of disodium azodisalicylate in healthy subjects. Gastroenterology, *88*:717, 1985.
216. Sandberg-Gertzen, H., Ryde, M., and Jarnerot, G.: Absorption and excretion of azodisal sodium and its metabolites in man after rectal administration of a single 2-g dose. Scand. J. Gastroenterol., *18*:571, 1983.
217. Ireland, A., et al.: Azodisalicylate for the treatment of active ulcerative colitis. Gut, *26*:45, 1985.
218. Ireland, A., and Jewell, D. P.: Olsalazine in patients intolerant of sulphasalazine. Gastroenterology (Abstract), *90*:1471, 1986.
219. Gabel, L. P., Turlein, D., and Moore, M.: Compassionate use of Dipentum (azodisal sodium) in medically-refractory IBD patients. Second International Symposium on Inflammatory Bowel Diseases. Jerusalem, 1985.
220. Jarnerot, G., and Sandberg-Gertzen, H.: Azodisal sodium (ADS), Dipentum,[R] as relapse prevention in ulcerative colitis. A double-blind placebo controlled study. Gastroenterology, *88*:1432, 1985.
221. Sandberg-Gertzen, H., and Jarnerot, G.: A tolerance study of azodisal sodium Dipentum,[R] in sulphasalazine intolerant patients with ulcerative colitis. Gastroenterology, *88*:1568, 1985.
222. Hetzel, D. J., et al.: Azodisalicylate (ADS) in the treatment of ulcerative colitis: A controlled trial and assessment of drug disposition. Gastroenterology, *88*:1418, 1985.
223. Goerg, K. J., et al.: Effect of azodisalicylate and HB313 on water and ion transfer in the rat ileum in vivo and in vitro. Gastroenterology, *88*:1397, 1985.
224. Friedman, G.: Sulfasalazine and new analogues. Am. J. Gastroenterol., *81*:141, 1986.
225. Chan, R. P., et al.: Studies of two novel sulfasalazine analogs, ipsalazide and balsalazide. Dig. Dis. Sci., *28*:609, 1983.
226. McIntyre, P. B., and Lennard-Jones, J. E.: Reversal with balsalazide of infertility caused by sulphasalazine. Br. Med. J., *288*:1652, 1984.
227. Bartalsky, A.: Salicylazobenzoic acid in ulcerative colitis. Lancet, *1*:960, 1982.
228. Brown, J. P., et al.: A polymeric drug for treatment of inflammatory bowel disease. J. Med. Chem., *26*:1300, 1983.
229. Garretto, M., Riddell, R. H., and Winans, C. S.: Treatment of chronic ulcerative colitis with poly-ASA: A new nonabsorbable carrier for release of 5-aminosalicylic in the colon. Gastroenterology, *84*:1162, 1983.
230. Lashner, B. A., et al.: Release of 5-aminosalicylic acid (5-ASA) from BW73Y: in vitro and in vivo studies in humans. Gastroenterology, *86*:1154, 1984.
231. Maier, K., et al.: Successful management of chronic inflammatory gut disease with oral 5-aminosalicylic acid. Dtsch. Med. Wochenschr., *110*:363, 1985.
232. Sanchez, G., et al.: The influence of intestinal transit time on 5-ASA from Pentasa[R]. Gastroenterology, *90*:1373, 1986.
233. Rasmussen, S. N., et al.: Treatment of Crohn's disease with peroral 5-aminosalicylic acid. Gastroenterology, *85*:1350, 1983.
234. Dew, M. J., et al.: An oral preparation to release drugs in the human colon. Br. J. Clin. Pharmacol., *14*:405, 1982.
235. Dew, M. J., et al.: Colonic release of 5-aminosalicylic acid from an oral preparation in active ulcerative colitis. Br. J. Clin. Pharmacol., *16*:185, 1983.
236. Dew, M. J., et al.: Comparison of the absorption and metabolism of sulphasalazine and acrylic-coated 5-aminosalicylic acid in normal subjects and patients with colitis. Br. J. Clin. Pharmacol., *17*:474, 1984.
237. Dew, M. J., et al.: Maintenance of remission in ulcerative colitis with oral preparation of 5-aminosalicylic acid. Br. Med. J., *285*:1012, 1982.
238. Dew, M. J., et al.: Maintenance of remission in ulcerative colitis with 5-aminosalicylic acid in high doses by mouth. Br. Med. J., *287*:23, 1983.
239. Dew, M. J., et al.: Treatment of ulcerative colitis with oral 5-aminosalicylic acid in patients unable to take sulphasalazine (letter). Lancet, *2*:801, 1983.
240. Habal, F. M., and Greenberg, G. R.: Oral 5-aminosalicylic acid in the treatment of ulcerative colitis. Gastroenterology, *88*:1409, 1985.
241. Schroeder, K. W., and Tremaine, W. J.: Oral 5-aminosalicylic acid (Asacol) for treatment of symptomatic ulcerative colitis (CUC). Gastroenterology, *90*:1620, 1986.
242. Tremaine, W. J., and Schroeder, K. W.: Oral 5-aminosalicylic acid (Asacol) tolerance versus oral sulfasalazine tolerance in patients with chronic ulcerative colitis. Gastroenterology, *90*:1670, 1986.
243. Austin, C. A., et al.: Exacerbation of diarrhoea and pain in patients treated with 5-aminosalicylic acid for ulcerative colitis. Lancet, *1*:917, 1984.
244. Diener, U., et al.: Renal function was not impaired by treatment with 5-aminosalicylic acid in rats and man. Naunyn Schmiedebergs Arch. Pharmacol., *326*:278, 1984.
245. Truelove, S. C., and Witts, L. J.: Cortisone in ulcerative colitis: Final report on a therapeutic trial. Br. Med. J., *2*:1041, 1955.
246. Claman, H. N.: Anti-inflammatory effects of corticosteroids. Clin. Immunol. Allergy, *4*:317, 1984.
247. Schleimer, R. P.: The mechanism of anti-inflammatory steroid action in allergic diseases. Ann. Rev. Pharmacol. Toxicol., *25*:381, 1985.
248. Hawkey, C. J., and Truelove, S. C.: Effect of prednisolone on prostaglandin synthesis by rectal mucosa in ulcerative colitis: investigation by laminar flow bioassay and radioimmunoassay. Gut, *22*:190, 1981.
249. Lauritsen, K., et al.: Effects of systemic prednisolone on arachidonic acid metabolism determined by equilibrium in vivo dialysis of rectum in severe relapsing ulcerative colitis. Gastroenterology, *88*:1466, 1985.
250. Lennard-Jones, J. E.: Toward optimal use of corticosteroids in ulcerative colitis and Crohn's disease. Gut, *24*:177, 1983.

251. Peppercorn, M. A.: Role of corticotropin therapy in ulcerative colitis: the controversy continues. Gastroenterology, 85:472, 1983.
252. Swartz, S. L., and Dluhy, R. G.: Corticosteroids: clinical pharmacology and therapeutic use. Drugs, 16:238, 1978.
253. Meyers, S., and Janowitz, H. D.: Systemic corticosteroid therapy of ulcerative colitis. Gastroenterology, 89:1189, 1985.
254. Lennard-Jones, J. E., et al.: An assessment of prednisone, salazopyrine, and topical hydrocortisone hemisuccinate used as outpatient treatment for ulcerative colitis. Gut, 1:217, 1960.
255. Truelove, S. C., and Witts, L. J.: Cortisone and corticotropin in ulcerative colitis. Br. Med. J., 1:387, 1959.
256. Kaplan, H. P., et al.: A controlled evaluation of intravenous adrenocorticotropic hormone and hydrocortisone in the treatment of acute colitis. Gastroenterology, 69:913, 1975.
257. Powell-Tuck, J., Buckell, N. A., and Lennard-Jones, J. E.: A controlled comparison of corticotropin and hydrocortisone in the treatment of severe proctocolitis. Scand. J. Gastroenterol., 12:971, 1977.
258. Meyers, S., et al.: Corticotropin versus hydrocortisone in the intravenous treatment of ulcerative colitis. A prospective, randomized, double-blind clinical trial. Gastroenterology, 85:351, 1983.
259. Zetzel, L., and Atin, H. L.: ACTH and adrenalcorticosteroids in the treatment of ulcerative colitis. Am. J. Dig. Dis., 3:916, 1958.
260. Spencer, J. A., et al.: Immediate and prolonged therapeutic effects of corticotrophin and adrenal steroids in ulcerative colitis. Gastroenterology, 42:113, 1982.
261. Truelove, S. C., and Witts, L. J.: Cortisone and corticotropin in acute ulcerative colitis. Br. Med. J., 2:387, 1959.
262. Hartong, W. A., et al.: Treatment of toxic megacolon. Dig. Dis. Sci., 23:195, 1977.
263. Schjonsby, H., et al.: Intensive treatment in severe attacks of ulcerative colitis. Acta Med. Scand. (Suppl.), 603:43, 1977.
264. Truelove, S. C., and Jewell, D. P.: Intensive intravenous regimen for severe attacks of ulcerative colitis. Lancet, 1:1067, 1974.
265. Truelove, S. C., et al.: Further experience in the treatment of severe attacks of ulcerative colitis. Lancet, 2:1086, 1978.
266. Jarnerot, G., Rolny, P., and Sandberg-Gertzen, H.: Intensive intravenous treatment of ulcerative colitis. Gastroenterology, 89:1005, 1985.
267. Hirai, Y., Takamatsu, H., Nakagawa, T., and Koide, T.: The selective administration of corticosteroid into the mesenteric arteries in children with ulcerative colitis: A preliminary report. J. Pediatr. Gastroenterol. Nutr., 3:478, 1984.
268. Momoshima, S., et al.: Intra-arterial prednisolone infusion therapy in ulcerative colitis. A. J. R., 145:1057, 1985.
269. Baron, J. H., et al.: Out-patient treatment of ulcerative colitis. Br. Med. J., 2:441, 1962.
270. Powell-Tuck, J., Brown, R. L., and Lennard-Jones, J. E.: A comparison of oral prednisolone given as single or multiple daily doses for active proctocolitis. Scand J. Gastroenterol., 13:833, 1978.
271. Lennard-Jones, J. E., et al.: Prednisone as maintenance treatment for ulcerative colitis in remission. Lancet, 1:188, 1965.
272. Cocco, A. E., and Mendeloff, A. I.: An evaluation of intermittent corticosteroid therapy in the management of ulcerative colitis. Johns Hopkins Med. J., 120:162, 1967.
273. Powell-Tuck, J., Brown, R. L., Chambers, T. J., and Lennard-Jones, J. E.: A controlled trial of alternate day prednisolone as a maintenance treatment for ulcerative colitis in remission. Digestion, 22:263, 1981.
274. Truelove, S. C.: Treatment of ulcerative colitis with local hydrocortisone. Br. Med. J., 2:1267, 1956.
275. Truelove, S. C.: Treatment of ulcerative colitis with local hydrocortisone hemisuccinate sodium. Br. Med. J., 1:1437, 1957.
276. Truelove, S. C.: Treatment of ulcerative colitis with local hydrocortisone hemisuccinate sodium: A report on a controlled therapeutic trial. Br. Med. J., 2:1072, 1958.
277. Watkinson, G.: Treatment of ulcerative colitis with topical hydrocortisone hemisuccinate sodium. Br. Med. J., 2:1077, 1958.
278. Spencer, J. A., and Kirsner, J. B.: Experience with short and long-term courses of local adrenal steroid therapy for ulcerative colitis. Gastroenterology, 42:669, 1962.
279. Truelove, S. C.: Systemic and local corticosteroid therapy in ulcerative colitis. Br. Med. J., 1:464, 1960.
280. Truelove, S. C.: Local corticosteroid treatment in severe attacks of ulcerative colitis. Br. Med. J., 2:102, 1960.
281. Matts, S. G. F.: Local treatment of ulcerative colitis with prednisolone-21-phosphate enemata. Lancet, 1:517, 1960.
282. Matts, S. G. F., and Gaskell, K. H.: Retrograde colonic spread of enemata in ulcerative colitis. Br. Med. J., 2:614, 1961.
283. Swarbrick, E. T., Loose, H., and Lennard-Jones, J. E.: Enema volume as an important factor in successful topical corticosteroid treatment of colitis. Proc. R. Soc. Med., 67:753, 1974.
284. Farthing, M. J. G., Rutland, M. D., and Clark, M. L.: Retrograde spread of hydrocortisone containing foam given intrarectally in ulcerative colitis. Br. Med. J., 2:822, 1979.
285. Hay, D. J., Sharma, H., and Irving, M. H.: Spread of steroid-containing foam after intrarectal administration. Br. Med. J., 1:1751, 1979.
286. Jay, M., et al.: Retrograde spreading of hydrocortisone enema in inflammatory bowel disease. Dig. Dis. Sci., 31:139, 1986.
287. Liddle, G. W.: Fluorohydrocortisone, new investigative tool in adrenal physiology. J. Clin. Endocrinol., 16:557, 1956.
288. Nabarro, J. D. N., et al.: Rectal hydrocortisone. Br. Med. J., 2:272, 1957.
289. Scherman, L. F., Tenner, R. J., and Schoettler, J. L.: Treatment of ulcerative colitis with hydrocortisone alcohol retention enemas. A topical and systemic anti-inflammatory agent. Dis. Colon Rectum, 10:43, 1967.
290. Halvorsen, S., Myren, J., and Aakvaag, A.: On the absorption of prednisone and prednisolone disodium phosphate after rectal administration. Scand. J. Gastroenterol., 4:581, 1969.
291. Powell-Tuck, J., et al.: Plasma prednisolone levels after administration of prednisolone-21-phosphate as a retention enema in colitis. Br. Med. J., 1:193, 1976.
292. Lee, A. H., et al.: Plasma prednisolone levels and adrenocortical responsiveness after administration of prednisolone-21 phosphate as a retention enema. Gut, 20:349, 1979.
293. Elliott, P. R., et al.: Prednisolone absorption in acute colitis. Gut, 21:49, 1980.
294. Matts, S. G. F., et al.: Adrenal cortical and pituitary function after intrarectal steroid therapy. Br. Med. J., 2:24, 1963.
295. Anonymous: Betamethasone 17-valerate and prednisolone 21-phosphate retention enemas in proctocolitis. A multicentre trial. Br. Med. J., 3:84, 1971.

296. Spencer, J. A., Kirsner, J. B., and Palmer, W. L.: Rectal absorption of 6-alpha-^{14}C-H$_3$ prednisolone. Proc. Soc. Exp. Biol. Med., *103*:74, 1960.
297. Misiewicz, J. J., et al.: Comparison of oral and rectal steroids in the treatment of proctocolitis. Proc. R. Soc. Med., *57*:561, 1964.
298. Lee, A. H., et al.: Rectally administered prednisolone—evidence for a predominantly local action. Gut, *21*:215, 1980.
299. McIntyre, P. B., et al.: Therapeutic benefits from a poorly absorbed prednisolone enema in distal colitis. Gut, *26*:822, 1985.
300. Hamilton, I., et al.: A comparison of prednisolone enemas with low-dose oral prednisolone in the treatment of acute distal ulcerative colitis. Dis. Colon Rectum, *27*:701, 1984.
301. Kumana, C. R., et al.: Beclomethasone dipropionate enemas for treating inflammatory bowel disease without producing Cushing's syndrome or hypothalamic pituitary adrenal suppression. Lancet, *1*:579, 1982.
302. Levine, D. S., and Rubin, C. E.: Topical beclomethasone dipropionate enemas improve distal ulcerative colitis and idiopathic proctitis without systemic toxicity. Gastroenterology, *88*:1473, 1985.
303. Larochelle, P., et al.: Tixocortol pivalate, a corticosteroid with no systemic glucocortoid effect after oral, intrarectal, and intranasal application. Clin. Pharmacol. Ther., *33*:343, 1983.
304. Hanauer, S. B., Kirsner, J. B., and Barrett, W. E.: The treatment of left sided ulcerative colitis with tixocortol pivalate (TP). Gastroenterology, *90*:1449, 1986.
305. Friedman, G.: Treatment of refractory proctosigmoiditis and left-sided colitis with a rectally-instilled nonglucocorticoid, nonmineralocorticoid steroid. Gastroenterology, *88*:1388, 1985.
306. Ruddell, W. S., et al.: Treatment of distal ulcerative colitis (proctosigmoiditis) in relapse: comparison of hydrocortisone enemas and rectal hydrocortisone foam. Gut, *21*:885, 1980.
307. Sommerville, K. W., et al.: Effect of treatment on symptoms and quality of life in patients with ulcerative colitis: comparative trial of hydrocortisone acetate foam and prednisolone-21 phosphate enemas. Br. Med. J., *291*:866, 1985.
308. Lennard-Jones, J. E., et al.: A double blind controlled trial of prednisolone-21-phosphate suppositories in the treatment of idiopathic proctitis. Gut, *3*:207, 1962.
309. Streeten, D. H. P., and Phil, D.: Corticosteroid therapy: II. Complications and therapeutic indications. J. Am. Med. Assoc., *232*:1046, 1975.
310. Goldstein, M. J., Gelzayd, E. A., and Kirsner, J. B.: Some observations on the hazards of corticosteroid therapy in patients with inflammatory bowel disease. Trans. Am. Acad. Ophthalmol. Otolaryngol., *71*:254, 1967.
311. Singleton, J. W.: Medical therapy of inflammatory bowel disease. Med. Clin. North Am., *64*:1117, 1980.
312. Kimball, C. P.: Psychological dependency on steroids? Ann. Intern. Med., *75*:111, 1971.
313. Conn, H. O., and Blitzer, B. L.: Non-association of adrenocorticosteroid therapy and peptic ulcer. N. Engl. J. Med., *294*:473, 1976.
314. Diethelm, A. G.: Surgical management of complications of steroid therapy. Ann. Surg., *185*:251, 1977.
315. ReMine, S. G., and McIlrath, D. C.: Bowel perforation in steroid treated patients. Ann. Surg., *192*:581, 1980.
316. Ewart, W. B., and Lennard-Jones, J. E.: Corticosteroids in preoperative medical management of ulcerative colitis: Do they affect surgical success? Lancet, *2*:60, 1960.
317. Prohaska, J. V., Dragstedt, L. R. II, and Thompson, R. G.: Ulcerative colitis: Surgical problems in corticosteroid treated patients. Ann. Surg., *154*:408, 1961.
318. Dixon, R. B., and Christy, N. P.: On the various forms of corticosteroid withdrawal syndrome. Am. J. Med., 68:224, 1980.
319. Byyny, R. L.: Withdrawal from glucocorticoid therapy. N. Engl. J. Med., *295*:30, 1976.
320. Bean, R. H. D.: The treatment of chronic ulcerative colitis with 6-MP. Med. J. Aust., *2*:592, 1962.
321. Sachar, D. B., and Present, D. H.: Immunotherapy in inflammatory bowel disease. Med. Clin. North Am., *62*:173, 1980.
322. Spreafico, F.: Problems and challenges in the use of immunomodulating agents: A general introduction. Int. Arch. Allergy Appl. Immunol., *76*:108, 1985.
323. Korelitz, G. I., Glass, J. L., and Wisch, N.: Long-term immunosuppressive therapy of ulcerative colitis. Am. J. Dig. Dis., *18*:317, 1973.
324. Jewell, D. P., and Truelove, S. C.: Azathioprine in ulcerative colitis: final report on controlled therapeutic trial. Br. Med. J., *4*:627, 1974.
325. Rosenberg, J. L., et al.: A controlled trial of azathioprine in the management of chronic ulcerative colitis. Gastroenterology, *69*:96, 1975.
326. Caprilli, R., Carratu, R., and Babbini, M.: A double-blind comparison of the effectiveness of azathioprine and sulfasalazine in idiopathic proctocolitis. Am. J. Dig. Dis., *20*:115, 1975.
327. Kirk, A. P., and Lennard-Jones, J. E.: Controlled trial of azathioprine in chronic ulcerative colitis. Br. Med. J., *284*:1291, 1982.
328. Theodur, E., Niv, Y., and Bat, C.: Imuran in the treatment of ulcerative colitis. Am. J. Gastroenterol., *76*:262, 1981.
329. Singleton, J. W., et al.: National Cooperative Crohn's Disease Study: Adverse reactions to study drugs. Gastroenterology, *77*:870, 1979.
330. Present, D. H., et al.: Treatment of Crohn's disease with 6-mercaptopurine: A long term randomized double blind study. N. Engl. J. Med., *302*:981, 1980.
331. Kinlen, L. J., et al.: Collaborative United Kingdom-Australian study of cancer in patients treated with immunosuppressive drugs. Br. Med. J., *2*:1461, 1979.
332. Kinlen, L. J.: Incidence of cancer in rheumatoid arthritis and other disorders after immunosuppressive treatment. Am. J. Med., *78*:44, 1985.
333. Hanauer, S. B., et al.: Acute leukemia following inflammatory bowel disease. Dig. Dis. Sci., *27*:545, 1982.
334. Present, D. H., et al.: Short and long-term toxicity to 6-mercaptopurine in the management of inflammatory bowel disease. Gastroenterology, *88*:1545, 1985.
335. Gupta, S., Keshavarzian, A., and Hodgson, H. J.: Cyclosporin in ulcerative colitis. Lancet, *2*:1277, 1984.
336. Oberling, F., and Hiebel, G.: Intravenous ALS in the treatment of severe rectocolitis. N. Engl. J. Med., *285*:409, 1971.
337. Marmont, A., et al.: The treatment of autoimmune blood diseases with antilymphocyte globulin. Postgrad. Med. J., *52*:139, 1976.
338. Heyworth, M. F., and Truelove, S. C.: A therapeutic trial of anti-lymphocytic globulin in acute ulcerative colitis. Digestion, *20*:121, 1980.
339. Heyworth, M. F., and Truelove, S. C.: Failure of antilymphocytic globulin in acute ulcerative colitis. Lancet, *1*:1060, 1981.
340. Hermanowicz, A., Nowak, A., and Gajos, L.: Controlled therapeutic trial of levamisole and sulphasalazine in acute ulcerative colitis. Gut, *25*:534, 1984.

341. Hermanowicz, A., Sliwinski, Z., and Kaczor, R.: Effect of long-term therapy with sulphasalazine, levamisole, corticosteroids and ascorbic acid and of disease activity on polymorphonuclear leukocyte function in patients with ulcerative colitis. Hepatogastroenterology, *32*:81, 1985.
342. Babb, R. R.: Cromolyn sodium in the treatment of ulcerative colitis. J. Clin. Gastroenterol., *2*:229, 1980.
343. Mani, V., et al.: Treatment of ulcerative colitis with oral disodium cromoglycate. Lancet, *2*:439, 1976.
344. Binder, V., et al.: Disodium cromoglycate in the treatment of ulcerative colitis and Crohn's disease. Gut, *22*:55, 1981.
345. Dronfield, M. W., and Langman, M. J. S.: Comparative trial of sulphasalazine and oral sodium cromoglycate in the maintenance of remission in ulcerative colitis. Gut, *19*:1136, 1978.
346. Willoughby, C. P., et al.: Comparison of disodium cromoglycate and sulphasalazine as maintenance therapy for ulcerative colitis. Lancet, *1*:119, 1979.
347. Whorwell, P. J., et al.: A double-blind controlled trial of the effect of sodium cromoglycate in preventing relapse in ulcerative colitis. Postgrad. Med. J., *57*:436, 1981.
348. Bucknell, N. A., et al.: Controlled trial of sodium cromoglycate in chronic persistent ulcerative colitis. Gut, *19*:1140, 1978.
349. Hovdenak, N., et al.: Local sodium cromoglycate is ineffective in ulcerative proctosigmoiditis. Scand. J. Gastroenterol, *20*:75, 1985.
350. Davies, P. S., Rhodes, J., Counsell, B., and Evans, B. K.: Maintenance of remission in ulcerative colitis. Am. J. Gastroenterol., *74*:150, 1980.
351. Hara, M., et al.: Treatment of ulcerative colitis with oral N-(3,4-dimethoxycinnamoyl) anthranilic acid. Second International Symposium on Inflammatory Bowel Diseases. Jerusalem, 1985.
352. Allan, R. N.: Sodium cromoglycate in proctitis and ulcerative colitis (editorial). Br. Med. J., *284*:70, 1982.
353. Salter, R. H., and Read, A. E.: Epsilon-aminocaproic acid therapy in ulcerative colitis. Gut, *11*:585, 1970.
354. Mowat, N. A. G., et al.: Epsilon-aminocaproic acid therapy in ulcerative colitis. Am. J. Dig. Dis., *18*:959, 1973.
355. Hollanders, D., Thomson, J. M., and Schofield, P. F.: Tranexamic acid therapy in ulcerative colitis. Postgrad. Med. J., *58*:87, 1982.
356. Kondo, M., et al.: Treatment of ulcerative colitis by the direct administration of an antifibrinolytic agent as an enema. Hepatogastroenterology, *28*:270, 1981.
357. Lechin, F., et al.: Treatment of ulcerative colitis with clonidine. J. Clin. Pharmacol., *25*:219, 1985.
358. Lechin, F., et al.: Treatment of ulcerative colitis with thioproperazine. J. Clin. Gastroenterol., *4*:445, 1982.
359. Jick, H., and Walker, A. M.: Cigarette smoking and ulcerative colitis. N. Engl. J. Med., *308*:261, 1983.
360. Carling, L., and Kagevi, I.: Sucralfate enema—a new therapy for inflammatory bowel disease. Scand. J. Gastroenterol., *20*:37, 1985.
361. Rice-Oxley, J. M., and Truelove, S. C.: Ulcerative colitis. Course and prognosis. Lancet, *1*:663, 1950.
362. Onderdonk, J. A., et al.: Protective effect of metronidazole in experimental ulcerative colitis. Gastroenterology, *74*:521, 1978.
363. Davies, P. S., et al.: Metronidazole in the treatment of chronic proctitis: a controlled trial. Gut, *18*:680, 1977.
364. Wellmann, W., Fink, P. C., and Schmidt, F. W.: Whole-gut irrigation as antiendotoxinaemic therapy in inflammatory bowel disease. Hepatogastroenterology, *31*:91, 1984.
365. Lennard-Jones, J. E.: Medical treatment of ulcerative colitis. Postgrad. Med. J., *60*:797, 1984.
366. Lerer, P., et al.: Predicting therapeutic outcomes of severe ulcerative colitis. Gastroenterology, *88*:1471, 1985.
367. Babb, R. R.: The role of total parenteral nutrition in the treatment of inflammatory bowel disease. Am. J. Gastroenterol., *70*:506, 1978.
368. Driscoll, R. H., and Rosenberg, I. H.: Total parenteral nutrition in inflammatory bowel disease. Med. Clin. North. Am., *62*:185, 1978.
369. Weser, E.: Total parenteral nutrition and bowel rest in inflammatory bowel disease. Gastroenterology, *79*:1337, 1980.
370. Elson, C. O., et al.: An evaluation of total parenteral nutrition in the management of inflammatory bowel disease. Dig. Dis. Sci., *25*:42, 1980.
371. Holm, I.: Benefits of total parenteral nutrition (TPN) in the treatment of Crohn's disease and ulcerative colitis. Acta Chir. Scand., *147*:271, 1981.
372. Sales, D. J., and Rosenberg, I. H.: Total parenteral nutrition in inflammatory bowel disease. Prog. Gastroenterol., *3*:299, 1981.
373. Dickinson, R. J., et al.: Controlled trial of intravenous hyperalimentation and total bowel rest as an adjunct to the routine therapy of acute colitis. Gastroenterology, *79*:1199, 1980.
374. Harford, F. J. Jr., and Fazio, V. W.: Total parenteral nutrition as primary therapy for inflammatory bowel disease of the bowel. Dis. Colon Rectum, *21*:555, 1978.
375. Diehl, J. T., Steiger, E., and Hoolei, R. D.: The role of intravenous hyperalimentation in intestinal disease. Surg. Clin. North Am., *63*:11, 1983.
376. Hanauer, S. B., et al.: Can response of ulcerative colitis to total parenteral nutrition be predicted? Gastroenterology (Abstract), *86*:1106, 1984.
377. Farmer, R. G., and Schumacher, O. P.: Treatment of ulcerative colitis with hydrocortisone enemas. Dis. Colon Rectum, *13*:355, 1970.
378. Ritchie, J. K., Powell-Tuck, J., and Lennard-Jones, J. E.: Clinical outcome of the first ten years of ulcerative colitis and proctitis. Lancet, *1*:1140, 1978.
379. Binder, S. C., Patterson, M. D., and Glotzer, D. J.: Toxic megacolon in ulcerative colitis. Gastroenterology, *66*:909, 1974.
380. Greenstein, A. J., et al.: Outcome of toxic dilatation in ulcerative colitis and Crohn's colitis. J. Clin. Gastroenterol., *7*:137, 1985.
381. Truelove, S. C., and Marks, C. G.: Toxic megacolon. Clin. Gastroenterol., *10*(1):107, 1981.
382. Caprilli, R., et al.: Risk factors in toxic megacolon. Dig. Dis. Sci., *25*:817, 1980.
383. Meyers, S., and Janowitz, H. D.: The place of steroids in the therapy of toxic megacolon. Gastroenterology, *75*:729, 1978.
384. Goligher, J. C., Hoffman, D. C., and de Dombal, F. T.: Surgical treatment of severe attacks of ulcerative colitis, with special reference to the advantages of early operation. Br. Med. J., *4*:703, 1970.
385. Meyers, S., and Janowitz, H. D.: The management of toxic megacolon. J. Clin. Gastroenterol., *1*:345, 1979.
386. Katzka, I., Katz, S., and Morris, E.: Management of toxic megacolon: the significance of early recognition in medical management. J. Clin. Gastroenterol., *1*:307, 1979.
387. Grant, C. S., and Dozois, R. R.: Toxic megacolon: ultimate fate of patients after successful medical management. Am. J. Surg., *147*:106, 1984.

388. Goulston, S. J. M., and McGovern, V. J.: The nature of benign strictures in ulcerative colitis. N. Engl. J. Med., *281*:290, 1969.
389. Hanauer, S. B., Turner, B. C., and Frank, P. H.: Do truly benign strictures occur in ulcerative colitis? Gastroenterology, *88*:1412, 1985.
390. Powell, F. C., Schroeter, A. L., Su, W. P. D., and Perry, H. O.: Pyoderma gangrenosum: A review of 86 patients. Q. J. Med., *55*(217):173, 1985.
391. Read, A. E.: Pyoderma gangrenosum. Q. J. Med., *55*(217):99, 1985.

22 · Medical Therapy of Crohn's Disease

SAMUEL MEYERS, M.D. AND DAVID B. SACHAR, M.D.

At present, no cure for Crohn's disease exists. This goal must await better understanding of the etiology or pathogenesis of this complex, mysterious disorder. Medical therapy, however, may offer comfort to patients and improve their lives. The aims of medical programs are, at least, to maintain nutritional status and provide symptomatic relief, and, at best, to reduce or reverse the bowel inflammation itself. Several dietary, psychologic, and pharmacologic approaches are available to achieve these goals.

Diet and Nutrition

A "Crohn's disease diet" does not exist. When offering dietary advice to patients with this condition, however, one should bear in mind two rules. The first is, "eat well and maintain adequate caloric intake." The second is, "avoid only those foods that clearly provoke symptoms or complications." The rules may sound simple, but it is extraordinary how often they are ignored.

For example, a high proportion of Crohn's disease patients have been advised to adhere to unnecessarily bland and restrictive diets, such as "no fried foods" or "no dairy products." These admonitions leave few appetizing choices on the approved list for patients who already have trouble enjoying food and maintaining adequate nutrition. An equally common mistake is committed by patients who blame every flare-up of their symptoms on whatever they have eaten most recently, and consequently they add more and more foods to their proscribed list. Crohn's disease, of course, frequently undergoes spontaneous exacerbations and remissions. If patients eliminated from their diets everything they happened to eat the day preceding an episode of abdominal pain or diarrhea, they would soon starve. Excessive dietary roughage may precipitate obstruction in a stenotic segment of ileum, or aggravate bleeding from a friable colonic mucosa. Some patients may be consistently lactose intolerant; others may find that alcohol provokes diarrhea or that chili peppers irritate their perianal lesions. Most people with Crohn's disease, however, should be encouraged to eat whatever they can tolerate and enjoy.

On the other hand, because Crohn's disease patients often find their overall food intake limited by abdominal discomfort, diarrhea, or anorexia, and because they are sometimes prone to the malabsorption of certain nutrients, they may suffer a variety of curable nutritional defects.* When systematically evaluated, patients may turn out to have reversible anemias, electrolyte deficiencies, jejunal bacterial outgrowth, or impairments of carbohydrate, fat, nitrogen, and vitamin B_{12} absorption.[1] Malnutrition is surprisingly common in patients with Crohn's disease,[2] and it can be corrected or prevented if its patho-

---

*Editors' note: see also Clark, M. I.: Gut, *27 (Suppl.1)*:72, 1986; and Koretz, R. L.: Gut, *27*:85, 1986.

physiologic basis is appreciated.[3] Specific physiologic derangements predispose to electrolyte loss,[4] vitamin D malabsorption,[5] zinc depletion,[6-13] ascorbic acid deficiency,[14] disturbances of bile acid and vitamin B_{12} metabolism,[15] impaired folic acid absorption,[16-18] nicotinic acid deficiency,[19] hypocalcemia,[20] depletion of magnesium,[21,22] and many other metabolic complications.[23] These various physiologic vulnerabilities present many special challenges to the medical, surgical, and nursing teams caring for patients critically ill with inflammatory bowel disease.[24] Although the disease itself is often responsible for these nutritional disturbances, some metabolic problems, particularly trace metal deficiencies, can be accentuated during parenteral hyperalimentation.[25,26] In general, nutritional problems are particularly intense and prevalent following surgical resections.[22,27,28] The most aggressive efforts to reverse nutritional disturbances have focused on various regimens of parenteral hyperalimentation.[29-36] The published experience with this therapeutic modality ranges from isolated anecdotal case reports,[37,38] to detailed studies of the clinical and laboratory responses in series of patients.[39,40] Some series emphasize the effects of total parenteral nutrition (TPN) as primary therapy,[41,42] others concentrate specifically on the use of TPN to forestall surgical intervention,[43] and still others focus exclusively on the radiographic and endoscopic reversal of colonic lesions.[44] Many reports are interested in the results of TPN for special populations of Crohn's disease patients, such as pregnant women,[45-48] or children and adolescents with growth failure (see also Chaps. 23 and 24).[49-52] A particularly important advance has been the development of techniques for performing TPN at home.[53,54]

Because the use of TPN is the principal topic of Chapter 24, it will not be considered in any detail here, although one general point is worth making. A review of the proliferating literature on the subject is distressing because few studies evaluate TPN in controlled trials;[55] few distinguish between its short-term and long-term outcomes or between its roles as primary versus supportive therapy;[56,57] and few pay attention to the impact of concomitant medical or surgical treatments,[58,59] or to "sober assessment" of the costs, benefits, risks, and practical feasibilities of different avenues of nutritional support.[60]*

Like TPN, dietary supplements have also been studied extensively in the treatment of Crohn's disease. Regimens have been devised to correct caloric deprivation,[61] intestinal protein loss,[62,63] growth retardation,[64,65] and impaired immune function.[66] Other dietary prescriptions have been based on avoiding specific food intolerances.[67,68] The most effort, however, has been expended on the search for diets that may benefit the course of the underlying inflammatory bowel disease itself. Based on the hypothesis that high sugar and/or low fiber intake might be involved in the etiology of Crohn's disease,[69,70] even independent of secondary alterations in taste acuity,[71] a wealth of literature has developed (primarily in Great Britain and West Germany) concerning the management of Crohn's disease with sugar-free and/or fiber-enriched diets.[72-76] All these studies are somewhat consistent, emphasizing high sugar intake among Crohn's disease patients and suggesting a therapeutic benefit to sugar-free diets. The triviality of the statistically "significant" differences between patients and controls, however, and the inadequacies of controlled designs in the clinical trials all leave us with considerable uncertainty regarding the clinical and biologic importance of these findings.†

An even more popular and widespread approach to dietary management of Crohn's disease has been the use of the elemental diet. Some series have concentrated on continuous enteral tube feedings either as treatment for children and adolescents with growth failure,[77-79] as long-term management for short bowel or intestinal failure,[80] or even as primary therapy for the acute phase of the disease.[81] More attention, however, has been given to the use of standard elemental diets without tube feedings. Elemental diets have been employed to reduce gastrointestinal protein loss,[63] to control perianal or enterocutaneous fistulas,[82,83] or to control other specific complications of Crohn's disease.[84] It has been suggested that elemental diets might be a first-line treatment of choice, perhaps preferable to steroids for inducing remissions in acute exacerbations of disease.[85-91] What seems to be happening in most of these cases, though, is not any specific therapeutic action of the elemental diet. Rather, the diet appears to tide the patient over acute bouts of illness, by maintaining hydration and nutritional intake, while the disease undergoes spontane-

---

*Editors' note: see also Matuchansky, C.: Gut, *27 (Suppl. 1)*: 81, 1986; Greenberg, G. R.: Gastroenterology, *88*:1405, 1985; these studies found TPN to be a useful adjunct but not to be superior to defined formula diets or partial parenteral nutrition and oral food.

†Editors' note: see also Ritchie, J. K., et al.: Gut, *27*:A1278, 1986; this study shows no clear therapeutic merit of an unrefined carbohydrate, fiber rich diet in Crohn's disease.

ous remission. The role of the elemental diet, therefore, is probably more supportive than directly therapeutic. Its primary benefit is to restrain the physician from unnecessarily prescribing toxic drug therapies while the disease settles down on its own. The elemental diet is useful among other therapies, but the management of each patient will still require a diverse approach.[92]

Psychotherapy

The psychiatric and psychologic aspects of inflammatory bowel disease are so important that they merit a separate discussion (see Chap. 11), although they are important enough to be mentioned also as a component of the general medical treatment of Crohn's disease.* General emotional and psychologic support are, of course, essential in the management of any chronic incurable illness. It is important to develop sensitivity and sophistication in recognizing and treating the depression that often accompanies Crohn's disease.[93] Although the use of formal individual psychotherapy, group and family therapy, and especially modern antidepressive medication can be tremendously beneficial in this condition, the physician must be alert to the psychiatric diagnosis.

Sulfasalazine

Clinical Studies

Sulfasalazine has become the most widely prescribed agent for the treatment of Crohn's disease. Its use is supported by several small clinical studies, as well as by more recent controlled trials (Table 22-1). A Scandinavian, multicenter trial compared sulfasalazine (0.5 g three times daily for the first three days, then 1 g three times daily) to placebo.[94] The study was performed in a double-blind fashion, with a double crossover, in four periods of one month each. The initial selection of therapy was randomized; the following periods then alternated. Among 12 patients with disease relapse after prior surgical resection, sulfasalazine therapy was not superior to the placebo. Perhaps the treatment periods of only one month were too short to demonstrate adequately the full benefit of sulfasalazine in this group. In a second group without prior surgical therapy, however, symptomatic improvement was demonstrated.

In the United States, the National Cooperative Crohn's Disease Study (NCCDS) was a placebo-controlled, randomized, multicenter cooperative trial.[95] Seventy-four patients received sulfasalazine (1g/15kg body weight, with a maximum daily dose of 5 g) for a 17 week study period. Sulfasalazine resulted in a superior symptomatic improvement for those patients with colonic involvement, whether or not the small bowel was involved, but was not effective against disease confined to the small bowel. If the patients were on prednisone at the beginning of the study and then randomized to sulfasalazine, they were unlikely to improve. The NCCDS used the Crohn's Disease Activity Index (CDAI) (see also Chap. 9) to determine drug response rates. This index has been of proven value in determining clinical disease activity; however, it is largely determined by subjective feelings of the patients or variables not necessarily related to gut inflammatory disease activity.†

Van Hees et al. conducted a randomized, placebo-controlled trial for 26 weeks using an activity index thought better to reflect inflammatory activity.[96] Thirteen patients who received sulfasalazine (6 g/day) responded better to therapy than the 13 receiving placebo. Disease located in the small or large bowel responded equally well; however, the small number of patients studied makes it difficult to derive definitive conclusions from the data.

A European cooperative study (ECCDS),[97] provides data on a group of patients that may be compared to the United States trial (NCCDS),[96] although the methodologic details were not identical. The Europeans divided 452 patients into 160 who were previously treated and 292 who were previously untreated. Sulfasalazine was given to 42 patients in the former group and 75 in the latter; thus, 117 patients constituted the sulfasalazine group. Fifty-four patients had active disease (defined by a CDAI ≥ 150) and were treated with sulfasalazine (3g/day) for six weeks. Therapy was repeated one or two times if the CDAI did not fall below 150. If the CDAI did not fall after the third therapy cycle, the patient was withdrawn as a drug failure. Remission rates were calculated by several types of statistical methods. Improvement with sulfasalazine was modest and was only revealed by a life-table analysis based on "failure and relapse," a sensitive type of analysis that is similar to the method used in the NCCDS.[96] After 100 days of therapy 58% of patients were well, compared to 42% who received placebo. After 70 days, 22% of those remaining on therapy were well, compared to

---

*Editor's note: see also Drossman, D. A., et al.: Gastroenterology, *92*:1375, 1987.

†See also Chapter 33.

TABLE 22-1. *Summary of Clinical Studies of Sulfasalazine in Crohn's Disease.*

Clinical Trial	Number of Patients	Dosage (g/day)	Patients with Prior Surgical Treatment	Disease Activity	Total Trial Duration	Small Bowel Disease	Colon Disease	Small and Large Bowel Disease
Anthonisen et al.[94]	31	3	12	Active	4 months	yes	—	yes
NCCDS[95] Part I								
Phase 1	74	1g/15kg	27	Active	17 weeks	no	yes	no
Phase 2	19	1g/15kg	—	Inactive	2 years	no	no	no
Part II	58	1g/15kg	32	Inactive	2 years	no	no	no
Van Hees et al.[96]	26	6	1	Active	26 weeks	yes	yes	yes
ECCDS	117	3	16	Active	2 years	no	yes	yes
				Inactive	—	no	no	no
Multicentre Trial[98]	43	3	32	Inactive	1 year	no	no	no
Wenchert et al.[99]	66	3	66	Inactive	18 months	no	no	no

ECCDS = European Cooperative Crohn's Disease Study; NCCDS = National Cooperative Crohn's Disease Study, U.S.A.

10% of the placebo group. Although the differences between sulfasalazine and placebo achieved statistical significance ($p < 0.05$) by this life-table method of analysis, other methods gave conflicting results. Sulfasalazine was not effective when only the small bowel was involved, but it did result in significant improvement in patients with colonic disease. Although therapy was effective in the patient group as a whole, in the smaller, previously untreated group, no effect was demonstrated. Previous surgical treatment in this and several prior studies did not affect the efficacy of sulfasalazine.[95,96]

A British multicenter trial demonstrated no benefit of sulfasalazine as treatment for reducing the relapse rate after resection or in asymptomatic patients with established disease.[98] Sulfasalazine (3g/day) was compared to placebo during a one year study period. A Scandinavian trial compared sulfasalazine (3g/day) with placebo for an 18 month period among 66 patients within one month of disease resection.[99] The treated group had a cumulative relapse rate of 13%, compared to a 45% relapse rate in the placebo group. Despite this difference, the study groups were too small to demonstrate statistical significance. The NCCDS examined the effect of sulfasalazine for quiescent Crohn's disease.[95] Nineteen patients who achieved remission during the initial study period continued therapy for up to two years. The majority of patients entering this study (Part I, Phase II) remained in remission with no significant differences between the sulfasalazine and placebo treated groups. Fifty-eight patients (Part II) received sulfasalazine to maintain preexistent remission or to prevent recurrence after surgical extirpation. Therapy in this group also produced no difference from those receiving placebo. The ECCDS similarly showed no benefit of drug treatment for patients with quiescent disease at entry to the study.[97] Thus, no benefit of sulfasalazine is apparent in preventing relapse either in postoperative patients or among those with quiescent disease.

The effect of the combination of sulfasalazine and prednisone has been evaluated by the NCCDS.[100] This combination was compared to that of prednisone and placebo among patients with active disease for eight weeks. The combination was less effective than prednisone alone. Patients who were in remission at the end of eight weeks were rerandomized to receive either the two drugs together or prednisone plus placebo, and repeated attempts to withdraw prednisone were made over the next six months. Sulfasalazine showed no prednisone-sparing effect. The addition of sulfasalazine to 6-methylprednisolone in the ECCDS also offered no advantage in the therapy of active or quiescent disease.[97] The combination of sulfasalazine (3g/day for 16 weeks, then 1.5g/day for 17 weeks) and prednisone (15mg/day) for 2 weeks, then 10mg/day for 14 weeks, and for the last 17 weeks 5mg/day) also conferred no advantage over placebo on the prevention of postoperative Crohn's disease recurrence.[101]

Recommendations for Therapy

Despite the lack of support from controlled trials, we use sulfasalazine in the therapy of both small and large bowel Crohn's disease, as well as for disease recurrence after prior surgical resection. We feel that this drug is especially useful for those patients with mild to moderate disease activity. It is used either alone as the first-line agent, or in combination with corticosteroids or other drugs. It is hoped that the addition of sulfasalazine will allow the use of corticosteroids in a lower dose for a shorter period of time. Sulfasalazine therapy should be initiated slowly and given with meals to minimize dyspepsia, which is a common adverse effect. Starting with 500 mg the first day, one 500 mg tablet should be added each day until the therapeutic dose of up to 6 g/day is achieved, given in three or four divided doses. Those patients who complain of persistent dyspepsia may better tolerate an enteric coated tablet, although children may prefer the suspension. Therapy is continued for as long as the disease remains active. Once clinical remission is achieved, observation of the patient free of drug therapy is attempted. Corticosteroids, if used in combination, are gradually reduced and once this therapy is discontinued, if the patient remains well over several months, the sulfasalazine is also stopped.

Pharmacology*

Sulfasalazine is a conjugate of 5-aminosalicylic acid (5-ASA), a salicylate analogue, and sulfapyridine, a sulfonamide, linked by an azo-bond. After oral ingestion, up to one-third of the drug is absorbed from the upper gastrointestinal tract. An extensive enterohepatic circulation exists, with much of the absorbed sulfasalazine being taken up by the liver and excreted unmetabolized in the bile. The remainder enters the

*See also Chapter 21.

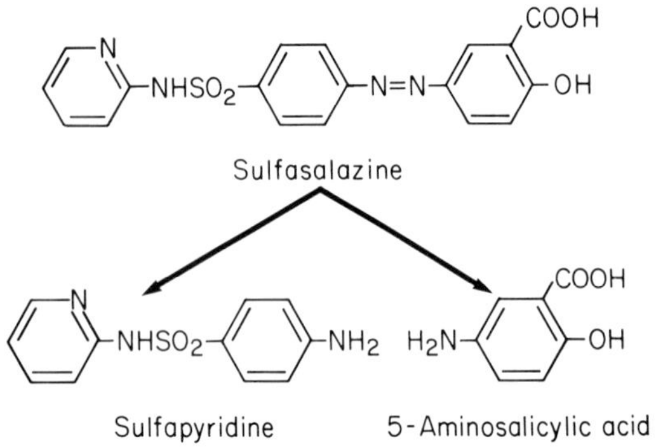

FIG. 22-1. Metabolism of Sulfasalazine.

colon where the azo-bond is cleaved by colonic bacteria to yield 5-ASA and sulfapyridine (Fig. 22-1).[102-107] The 5-ASA is poorly absorbed from the colon and is excreted primarily in the feces.[108] The sulfapyridine is efficiently absorbed from the colon and, when transported to the liver, is acetylated, hydroxylated, conjugated with glucuronic acid, and excreted in the urine.[108,109] When 5-ASA and sulfapyridine are administered as single agents orally, both are absorbed in the small bowel and excreted in the urine.[102] It is suggested that the parent drug may act as a vehicle for delivery of one or more of its metabolites to the distal disease sites. Recovery of the drug primarily as 5-ASA in the feces has raised the possibility that this metabolite is the therapeutically active moiety of sulfasalazine, whereas the demonstration that sulfapyridine is the principal portion of the drug found in the serum has suggested that this component may be responsible for most of the drug's toxicity. The rate of acetylation of the sulfapyridine varies considerably among individual patients and is a major determinant of serum sulfapyridine levels. Thus, persons who are genetically slow acetylators tend to have higher serum levels and experience more toxic side effects.[109] Crohn's disease patients may have an increase in their small bowel microbial population, allowing the release of 5-ASA in this location as well as in the colon. These patients theoretically may derive some therapeutic benefit from sulfasalazine for their small bowel Crohn's disease.

The exact mechanisms of action of sulfasalazine, its components, or its metabolites remain unclear. Theories have included drug-induced changes in the bowel connective tissue,[110,111] an antibacterial action,[112] effects on systemic and local immunity,[113] or on the phagocytic process and polymorphonuclear cell function.[114,115] Inhibition of prostaglandin synthesis by blocking the cyclooxygenase pathway has been demonstrated with sulfasalazine, 5-ASA, and the 5-ASA metabolite N-acetyl-5-aminosalicylate.[116-120] Prostaglandins are important mediators of inflammation and their levels are increased in acute colitis. Other more potent and specific prostaglandin inhibitors have not been successful in the therapy of inflammatory bowel disease, however, despite their ability to reduce colonic prostaglandin levels.[121] An alternate hypothesis has used data showing that sulfasalazine inhibits prostaglandin F_2 breakdown and that low doses of 5-ASA enhance prostacyclin formation.[122] Increased local levels of prostaglandins may act in a cytoprotective manner. Although most cells contain cyclooxygenase, some cells, especially inflammatory neutrophils, contain an alternate pathway for arachidonic acid metabolism, the lipoxygenase pathway. Sulfasalazine and its active metabolite 5-ASA block this pathway and thereby reduce synthesis of potent inflammatory mediators, including leukotrienes and certain hydroxyfatty acids. This inhibition may account for some of the anti-inflammatory effects of sulfasalazine.[124,125]

Adverse Effects and Desensitization*

The incidence of side effects among patients treated with sulfasalazine is approximately 20%.[126] In the NCCDS,[127] the adverse effects were evaluated prospectively. They were severe enough to withdraw the drug or reduce its dosage in 4% of the patients. Surprisingly, none of the side effects occurred significantly more frequently with sulfasalazine than placebo. Only 1% of the patients in the ECCDS withdrew from the study because of side effects, and the incidence of these effects again was similar in the placebo-treated group.[97]

The most common but least severe adverse reactions include nausea, vomiting, anorexia, heartburn, epigastric distress, and diarrhea. Serious adverse reactions are uncommon. These include various skin eruptions,[128-130] iridocyclitis,[131] pancreatitis,[132] hepatotoxicity,[133-137] pulmonary complications,[138-142] sinus tachycardia,[143] hematopoietic effects,[144-148] generalized allergic reactions,[149-150] drug-induced connective tissue disease,[151] neurotoxicity,[152] and reversible male infertility.[153-161] Bloody diarrhea

*See also Chapter 21.

with fever and rash resembling an acute flare-up of colitis also has been described.[131]

The common side effects, including nausea, vomiting, and headache, have been directly related to the level of sulfapyridine in the serum.[126] Thus, these effects occur most often among patients receiving larger sulfasalazine doses (over 4g/day) or who are slow acetylators. The occurrence of hemolysis in many patients also seems related to serum sulfapyridine levels.[162] Most of the uncommon, severe side effects are hypersensitivity reactions, not related to the dose or sulfasalazine, acetylator status, or serum sulfapyridine levels.

Patients intolerant to sulfasalazine because of vomiting, headache, or hemolysis can generally be treated by lowering their daily dose by about 50%.[126] An alternative is to discontinue therapy for 1 to 2 weeks and then to resume at a dose of 0.25 to 0.5 g/day for a period of 7 to 10 days, then gradually increasing by 0.25 g at weekly intervals to a maintenance dosage of 2g/day.[163] The dyspeptic side effects may occasionally be overcome more easily by the use of enteric-coated tablets.[164] In more difficult cases, such as those who experience fever and rash caused by the drug, desensitization may still be successful. Treatment should be begun with a daily dose of 1/8 of a tablet or 1/2 teaspoon of suspension (62.5mg) and slowly increased to a therapeutic dose over 4 weeks or more.[165,166] The oral suspension is usually used to facilitate the administration of the small doses required for desensitization. Those who have suffered severe hypersensitivity reactions, such as anaphylaxis or agranulocytosis, should *not* be rechallenged.

Exacerbation of disease activity associated with sulfasalazine or antibiotic therapy should provoke stool examinations for clostridium difficile toxin. In general, the treatment of significant pseudomembranous colitis complicating such therapy warrants the use of vancomycin or metronidazole.

Drug Interactions

Sulfasalazine inhibits the absorption of folic acid and is a competitive inhibitor of the jejunal brush border enzyme folate conjugase.[167,168] These effects result in folate malabsorption with reduced serum levels. Sulfasalazine also interferes with the bioavailability of digoxin, causing a mean decrease of approximately 25% of serum digoxin levels.[169] The mechanism of this effect is unknown. Concurrent administration of cholestyramine or ferrous sulfate may reduce the metabolism of sulfasalazine,[170-171] as a result of physical interaction between the drugs. Although the exact effect of these interactions on the clinical efficacy of sulfasalazine is unclear, administering the drugs separately would be prudent. Antibiotics may also diminish sulfasalazine metabolism.[108] This is caused by diminution of the gut flora responsible for sulfasalazine azo-bond reduction. Again, the effect of this phenomenon on the clinical effectiveness of sulfasalazine is unknown.

Pregnancy and Nursing*

Sulfasalazine does cross the placenta, and mean concentrations in cord serum are approximately half of those in maternal serum. The concentration of sulfapyridine is identical in maternal and cord blood, whereas both maternal and cord serum levels of 5-ASA are negligible.[172] Despite the exposure of the fetus to sulfasalazine and its metabolites, no evidence of fetal harm is apparent.[173,174]

The concentration of sulfasalazine in milk in the breast has been reported to vary from negligible amounts to approximately 30% of that found in the maternal serum.[172,175] The concentration of free sulfapyridine is up to 50% of that in maternal serum, while 5-ASA concentration is negligible.[175] Because exposure of the neonate is small and both sulfapyridine and sulfasalazine have only weak bilirubin-displacing capacities, minimal effects on the child would be expected.[175] Indeed, no reports of kernicterus related to sulfasalazine have ever been published.

The evidence suggests that sulfasalazine can be used to treat Crohn's disease during pregnancy, and that treated patients whose disease has been made less active have fewer fetal complications.[173] No evidence exists to suggest that therapy must be stopped near the time of delivery or that use by a nursing mother will harm the infant.

Sulfasalazine-related Drugs

The preponderance of evidence suggests that 5-ASA is the active therapeutic agent in sulfasalazine.[176] A word of caution regarding this hypothesis, however, must be given. Evidence exists that sulfasalazine has pharmacologic properties distinct from 5-ASA and may itself

*See also Chapter 17.

have a therapeutic action.[177-179] Nonetheless, the suggested therapeutic benefit of 5-ASA has led to the development of agents designed to deliver 5-ASA alone to active disease sites.

An enema form of 5-ASA may be prepared but has an unstable shelf life, is inconvenient for some patients, and probably would benefit most patients with right-sided Crohn's colitis or small bowel disease. Suppositories containing 5-ASA have been used, but they are only applicable to localized rectal Crohn's disease.[180] These limitations have led to development of oral forms of 5-ASA. Because 5-ASA is absorbed in the proximal small bowel and either excreted in the urine or metabolized in the liver with biliary excretion, it was necessary to develop a preparation that could deliver 5-ASA intact to the colon.[181] A water soluble polymer has been produced that links 5-ASA by an azo-bond to an inert polysulfanilamide "backbone." In rat studies, this preparation delivered similar amounts of 5-ASA to the colon, blood, and urine, as did sulfasalazine, and it requires bacterial azo-bond reduction similar to sulfasalazine.[182] Three other analogues of sulfasalazine linking 5-ASA by an azo-bond to structures other than sulfapyridine have also been synthesized.[183,184] The most promising may be osalazine sodium, in which two molecules of 5-ASA are linked to each other through an azo-bond (Fig. 22-2). After being split by bacterial azoreductases, this drug delivers twice the molar amount of 5-ASA to the colonic lumen than does sulfasalazine, with negligible serum concentrations.[185] Small intestinal metabolism of osalazine sodium is minimal.[186] Thus, its role in the therapy of Crohn's disease may be limited to those with colonic involvement, as has been suggested for sulfasalazine.[95,97]

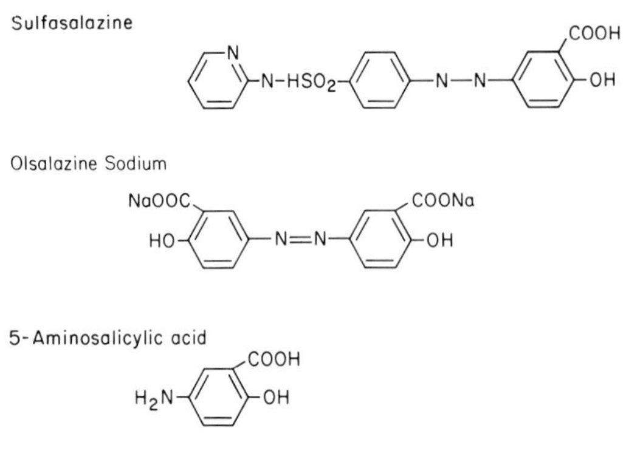

Fig. 22-2. Formula of Sulfasalazine, osalazine sodium, and 5-Aminosalicylic Acid (5-ASA).

Sustained-release preparations of 5-ASA have been developed that obviate the need for the bacterial cleavage of azo-bonds. In one form, 5-ASA microgranules are coated with a semipermeable membrane of ethyl cellulose. Another preparation coats 5-ASA with an acrylic resin. The 5-ASA is then released in the ileum and cecum at a pH of 7 or above. These slow-release forms allow drug appearance in the small and large bowel and may have promise in Crohn's disease therapy.[187-188]

Clinical Studies

5-ASA suppositories (1.5g/day) were given to 4 patients (2 with rectal involvement) with active Crohn's disease, as part of a 6-week randomized trial.[180] Fifty percent of this small group had a remission. The slow-release microgranule form of 5-ASA was studied in 12 patients with active Crohn's disease.[186] Six patients received 1.5g 5-ASA daily, and six received placebo. Despite a slight reduction in disease activity, as measured by the fecal excretion of[111] Indium-labelled autologous granulocytes, no statistically significant difference from the placebo group occurred. This preparation was further studied in an open trial among 18 patients with small bowel Crohn's disease, two of whom also had colonic involvement.[190] The 5-ASA (1.5g/day) was given for 6 weeks, and 13 patients improved (72%), 3 worsened (17%), and two were unchanged (11%). No side effects were observed. At this time, no major reports have been published of the effectiveness of any of the new forms of 5-ASA in Crohn's disease.

Corticosteroids

Clinical Studies

These agents are widely used for the treatment of active symptomatic Crohn's disease. Early uncontrolled clinical studies supported their use and were later confirmed by more rigorous controlled trials (Table 22-2). Good initial symptomatic response was obtained in 75 to 90% of patients treated with 30 mg/day of prednisone or its equivalent.[191-193] Fever, pain, and diarrhea subsided, appetite and well-being improved, and in the majority the hematocrit, sedimentation rate, and serum seromucoid levels returned toward normal. These favorable clinical responses were not necessarily associated with radiologic improvement. Although it appeared that steroid therapy produced satisfactory short-term bene-

TABLE 22-2. *Summary of Clinical Studies of Corticosteroids in Crohn's Disease.*

Clinical trial	Number of Patients	Dosage mg/day	Patients with Prior Surgical Treatment	Disease Activity	Total Trial Duration	Small Bowel Disease	Colon Disease	Small and Large Bowel Disease
NCCDS[95]								
Part I								
Phase 1	85	¼ mg/kg–¾ mg/kg	32	Active	17 weeks	yes	no	yes
Phase 2	28	¼ mg/kg	—	Inactive	2 years	yes	no	yes
Part II	61	¼ mg/kg	27	Inactive	2 years	no	no	no
ECCDS[97]	113	48 mg with predetermined reduction over 6 wk to 12 mg	30	Active	2 years	yes	yes	yes
Smith et al.[193]	33	7.5 mg	22	Inactive	3 years	no	no	no
Bergman and Krause[101]	187	15 mg decreasing to 5 mg-combined with sulfasalazine	187	Inactive	33 weeks, with 3 year follow-up	no	no	no

ECCDS = European Cooperative Crohn's Disease Study; NCCDS = National Cooperative Crohn's Disease Study, U.S.A.

fit, it was suspected that such therapy would not alter the long-term course of the disease.

The NCCDS was the first controlled, prospective double-blind study of corticosteroid therapy.[95] Eighty-five patients received prednisone in doses determined by their disease activity (¼ mg/kg to ¾ mg/kg). At the completion of the 17 week study period, prednisone was found to be significantly more effective than placebo for disease involving the small bowel. The cumulative percentage of patients achieving remission was 60% with prednisone therapy but less than 30% with placebo. Although such results were *not* demonstrated when the disease was confined to the colon, the total number of such patients was small, which may have allowed a beneficial effect to be overlooked. The extraintestinal complications and perianal disease of patients in the NCCDS were not responsive to prednisone therapy. Beginning the study with sulfasalazine therapy seemed to blunt the response to prednisone.

The ECCDS confirmed these American results.[97] One hundred-thirteen patients received 6-methylprednisolone for the therapy of active Crohn's disease. Therapy was initiated with 48 mg/day and reduced over 6 weeks to 12 mg/day. Although the initial dosage was higher than that used by the NCCDS,[95] the dosage reduction schedule was faster and automatic. This therapy cycle continued for 6 weeks but could be repeated 2 times if the disease was active (CDAI was ≥150) and if none of the criteria of treatment failure were present. 6-methylprednisolone was significantly more effective than placebo in the treatment group as a whole, both in patients previously treated and in those previously untreated. The drug was also superior to placebo in patients with all localizations of disease. Patients who achieved remission (CDAI of >150) after therapy could be continued on 6-methylprednisone (8 mg/day) for a period up to 2 years. Such continued therapy helped to maintain the remission of patients.[97] The NCCDS had also found some long-term benefit from continued prednisone therapy for periods up to two years.[95] According to the ECCDS lifetable analysis method,[90] almost 80% of patients were in remission after 100 days and about 35% at 700 days compared to 15% and 8%, respectively, for the placebo group.

The role of corticosteroid therapy both in quiescent disease and after surgical resection has been examined in several trials. The long-term effect of prednisone, 7.5 mg/day for up to 3 years after bowel resection, with or without residual disease, has been examined.[193] In each study, subjects treated with prednisone fared no better than those taking placebo. Both the United States and European controlled trials showed no benefit of corticosteroid therapy for those with inactive disease.[95,97] Clearly, prophylactic steroid therapy is *not* indicated in Crohn's disease.

Although all studies show that the combination of steroids with sulfasalazine appears to offer no benefit, many clinicians continue to combine these agents. Perhaps they are right, or perhaps they are only frustrated by the lack of proven therapeutic alternatives for their patients. The inability to withdraw corticosteroids after 1 to 2 years of continuous therapy is a relative indication for surgical intervention. Prolonged use of alternate day corticosteroid doses may be an option in selected cases, but we find this often fails to adequately control active disease.

In ill patients who are not responding to therapy or not tolerating oral therapy, parenteral corticoids can be used. The most common agents include prednisolone, betamethasone, hydrocortisone, and adrenocorticotropic hormone (ACTH). No adequate studies have been done to prove which of these agents is superior. Studies performed in severe ulcerative colitis may offer some guidance. Hydrocortisone has been found to be superior for patients who have been continuously on corticosteroids immediately prior to intravenous therapy (30 days or more), and ACTH has been found to be superior for those *not* on such therapy (see Chap. 21).[195] We administer intravenous therapy as a continuous infusion, mixing either hydrocortisone or ACTH with 5% dextrose and water. The mixture is then infused over each 24 hours (daily dose of 300 mg hydrocortisone or 120 units ACTH) for 7 to 14 days. Once the optimal benefit is achieved, the intravenous therapy is discontinued and oral prednisone instituted, as previously outlined.

Recommendations for Therapy

Corticosteroids are used for treatment of either small or large bowel Crohn's disease; however, such therapy should not be initiated in the presence of major suppurative complications such as an intra-abdominal or perianal abscess. In the case of such abscesses, initial therapy with antibiotics is safer and more useful. Corticosteroids may be introduced later if needed, once the infection is controlled. Therapy is initiated with 45 to 60 mg/day of prednisone, given in divided doses. This high dose is continued for approximately 10 to 14 days and then tapered 5 mg every 7 to 10 days. The reduction should be made from the last dose of the day. Thus, as lower doses are achieved more will be administered in the morning, which helps to minimize the side effects. If a relapse of disease activity occurs, the prednisone dose will need to be raised again. Once the disease is controlled, the tapering process is resumed. Clinical experience suggests that as the dose of corticosteroids is reduced, recrudescence of symptoms within one year occurs in at least one-third of patients.[191,192] In the NCCDS, the withdrawal of steroids in quiescent disease was *not* associated with more relapses than their continuation.[95] In acute symptomatic disease, however, withdrawal of steroids caused the condition to deteriorate more often than occurred with continued therapy. Thus, withdrawal is attempted from patients with quiescent Crohn's disease and is usually successful.

Pharmacology

Synthetic glucocorticoids, such as prednisone or prednisolone, are the most commonly used for the treatment of Crohn's disease. These drugs are absorbed in the upper small intestine after oral ingestion. Even though drug levels of these and natural corticosteroids can be measured, the results are difficult to interpret in clinical terms because the biologic effects of the drug on endogenous cortisol secretion, or on experimentally induced inflammation, persist longer than would be predicted from plasma levels. The plasma half-life of prednisolone after intravenous administration is 3 or 4 hours, but the biologic half-life is 18 to 36 hours.[196-198] Furthermore, although anti-inflammatory activity appears to be quantitatively related to the concentration of active steroid in the tissue,[196] no clear relation has been observed between the plasma level and the therapeutic response in inflammatory bowel disease.[199,200] The situation is further complicated by the fact that both therapeutic activity and liability to side effects are related *not* to *total* drug levels, but rather to drug levels unbound to protein. The main binding proteins are corticosteroid-binding globulin and albumin.

Absorption of oral prednisolone has been found to be reduced in patients with Crohn's disease.[201] These observations differ from an earlier report of normal mean peak levels and areas under the curve after oral prednisolone.[202] The later study, however, had greater variation in the patients in this latter study than among the controls, and included more patients with predominantly colonic disease than the earlier report.

Mechanism of Action

The mechanism by which corticosteroids exert their clinical usefulness is unknown. In experimentally induced inflammation, corticosteroids decrease capillary permeability, reduce migration of macrophages and polymorphonuclear cells into the inflamed area, interfere with phagocytosis of antigens by macrophages, stabilize lysosomal membranes, and inhibit cell-mediated immunity. Some data suggest that corticosteroids inhibit prostaglandin synthesis by decreasing the availability of the prostaglandin precursor; arachidonic acid.[203]

Adverse Effects

The toxicity of corticosteroid therapy at the doses used to suppress active Crohn's disease is appreciable. In addition, this therapy has been suggested to increase the overall mortality rate and the need for surgical treatment.[191,192] The NCCDS provided important information regarding the incidence and severity of corticosteroid side effects during the course of therapy for Crohn's disease.[127] Contrary to earlier clinical reports, the incidence of Crohn's disease complications, such as perianal disease, intraabdominal abscess, peritonitis, and bowel perforation or fistulae, did not increase. A large number of adverse effects, however, were noted among those patients being treated for active disease, including facial mooning (47%), acne (30%), ecchymoses (17%), petechial bleeding (6%), and striae (6%). When the lower maintenance doses were evaluated, moon face was seen among 25%, hirsutism in 8%, and striae in 7%. Other minor side effects reported by the patients occurred with similar frequency among those receiving corticosteroids or placebo. More serious side effects, which were noted more commonly among those receiving prednisone for active disease, included infection (27%) and hypertension (13%). Peptic ulcer and severe emotional disturbances were also frequently seen. These complications generally responded to the withdrawal or reduction of the prednisone dose and specific therapy for the complication. Despite this fact, perforated ulcers and hypertension associated with cerebrovascular accidents pose potential life-threatening situations. In this study no patient suffered more than one major adverse effect, in contrast to other clinical data.[191] Steroid toxicity sufficient to result in withdrawal from the NCCDS occurred in 18% of the patients receiving therapeutic doses for active disease over 17 weeks,[127] compared to a 6% withdrawal rate among the corresponding placebo group. The ECCDS also provided valuable information regarding the side effects that can be expected during steroid therapy of Crohn's disease.[97] The effects were similar to those found in the United States study,[127] but only facial mooning occurred with significantly more frequency than the side effects noted in the placebo group. Five patients were withdrawn from the study because of side effects related to 6-methylprednisolone. Three patients who received 6-methylprednisolone died of septic complications, two during the course of the study and one a few months after withdrawal from the study. All three of these patients had a palpable abdominal mass. Thus, the presence of such a mass with its usually associated suppuration may increase the potential risk associated with corticosteroid therapy. Steroids may also mask the clinical signs of an abscess, resulting in delay of specific therapy.

Pregnancy*

Corticosteroids are known to cause fetal abnormalities in animals. Treated mice have delivered offspring with an increased incidence of cleft palate, and have a high abortion rate and small litter size.[204] Studies in humans, however, have failed to demonstrate significant harmful effects.[205] The use of steroids does not appear to adversely affect the course and outcome of pregnancy.[206-208] In a national survey that included patients with ulcerative colitis and Crohn's disease, the incidence of fetal complications in those receiving drugs during pregnancy was even less than in the general population.[173] Medications, including corticosteroids, seem to participate as "innocent bystanders," with disease activity playing the predominant role in determining fetal outcome.[209,210] Fetal complications appear more commonly when the mother's disease is active rather than quiescent during pregnancy.

Antibiotics

Broad-Spectrum†

Bacterial overgrowth commonly occurs in the small intestine of Crohn's disease patients. This may be secondary to a stricture, internal fistula, or prior surgical therapy, especially if the ileocecal valve has been removed. An antibiotic such as tetracycline is often useful in reducing the malabsorption, gaseous distension, and flatulence that may result from bacterial overgrowth. Most physicians would also use broad spectrum antibiotics to treat clear-cut suppurative complications of Crohn's disease, such as an intra-abdominal abscess. The use of antibiotics for the *primary* therapy of active Crohn's disease may, however, raise some eyebrows. Many physicians now favor the use of a variety of antibiotics including ampicillin, sulfonamides, cephalosporins, tetracycline, and paromomycin. In the absence of extensive clinical trials, this practice is used in desperation. On the other hand, a rationale for using antibiotics as primary therapy of Crohn's disease is suggested by the abnormal intestinal flora found among many of these patients,[212,213] as well as by the bacteria demonstrated in the bowel wall and mesenteric lymph nodes.[214,215] In one clinical report that supports the use of antibiotics,[211] ampicillin, tetracycline, clindamycin, cephalothin, or erythromycin were used continuously among 44 patients. Symptomatic improvement occurred in 41 (93%) who were treated for six months or longer. Radiologic follow-up demonstrated improvement in 57% of those for whom post-therapy roentgenograms were available. These changes occurred within weeks in some patients, over a period of years in others. Patients with perianal fistulae or recurrence after surgical treatment usually made up the therapeutic failures. A six week prospective, randomized study, however, found that using metronidazole, co-trimoxazole (a sulfonamide derivative), or both was no better than placebo.[216] The clinical or hematologic parameters did not improve and the fecal flora compared to the placebo was not affected.

It has been postulated that a cell wall-deficient organism, perhaps a mycobacterium or corynebacterium, might be involved in the pathogenesis of Crohn's disease.[217-219] This hypothesis led to a controlled double-blind trial of sulfadoxine and pyrimethamine combination therapy.[217] Sulfadoxine is a long-acting sulfona-

---

*See also Chapter 17.

†See also Chapter 21.

mide that has been used in various infections, including M leprae. Pyrimethamine is similar to trimethoprim but longer lasting, and acts sequentially with sulfonamides to block folic acid metabolism. A total of 51 patients received either active drugs or placebo over a 12 month period. No benefit from the use of these antibiotics was demonstrated.

Anti-tuberculous Therapy

As indicated earlier, some have implicated a cell wall deficient mycobacterium in the etiology of Crohn's disease.[218,219]* A strain of mycobacterium kansasii has been cultured from lymph nodes. This organism was sensitive in vitro to rifampicin, ethambutol, and ethionomide.[219] These results prompted a controlled trial of rifampicin and ethambutol among 27 patients over a 2 year period. The patients received either active drugs or placebo for one year, with a subsequent one year cross-over period. The response to the active drugs compared to placebo was not significantly different.[220] Two European uncontrolled trials have, however, suggested benefit from therapy with isoniazid, rifampicin, and streptomycin,[221] or with rifampicin alone.[222] Further trials with these and other medications might seem warranted, but this is dubious, based on available data.†

Metronidazole

This antibiotic has received a great deal of attention since Ursing and Kamme reported its uncontrolled use in 5 patients with Crohn's disease.[223] After 4 weeks of treatment, 4 of the 5 improved, and corticosteroids and sulfasalazine could be withdrawn in 3 of the patients. One patient required four months of therapy before improvement was noted. Other uncontrolled trials have appeared and support the beneficial action of metronidazole.[224-226] Despite preliminary data from uncontrolled trials suggesting benefit,[227] published completed studies comparing metronidazole to placebo fail to confirm the earlier clinical experience.[228,229] Both controlled trials did note that metronidazole seemed most effective in the subgroup of patients with colonic Crohn's disease.

In Sweden a randomized, double-blind trial compared metronidazole (800 mg/day) to sulfasalazine (3 g/day).[230] No difference in efficacy was noted between these two drugs when clinical disease activity was evaluated. The reduction of the plasma orosomucoid, however, was more pronounced in the metronidazole group. Those patients with active disease despite sulfasalazine therapy clinically improved when switched to metronidazole. Such improvement was not seen in patients treated with metronidazole who were switched to sulfasalazine. In fact, the plasma concentration of orosomucoid increased in this group. This study suggested that metronidazole is slightly more effective than sulfasalazine, each being more beneficial for colonic than small bowel Crohn's disease. Adverse reactions were seen in 36 of the 78 patients studied, 18 in each treatment group. Nausea, anorexia, and fatigue were the most common complaints. The frequency or type of adverse reactions were not different between the two drugs. In our experience, the dosage of metronidazole used in this report was well tolerated and may represent a valuable therapeutic option. This drug would be especially useful for those patients who are allergic, intolerant, or unresponsive to sulfasalazine.

The possible benefit of metronidazole, especially for colonic Crohn's disease, led to the study of this therapy in perineal Crohn's disease. Bernstein et al. used this drug (20 mg/kg) in 21 consecutive patients with chronic, unremitting perineal disease.[232] Improvement occurred in 20 patients and complete healing occurred in 10 of 18 patients maintained on therapy. A subsequent report from this group included 26 patients, 17 of whom were also in their initial study.[233] All patients initially showed a good clinical response to the drug, with 10 experiencing complete healing. Dose reduction or drug discontinuation, whether in response to healing or the occurrence of side effects, was not successful in the majority of cases, however. Metronidazole therapy was successfully discontinued in only 28% of those in whom cessation of therapy was attempted. Those patients in whom the drug was gradually discontinued seemed to have a better chance of healing than those in whom therapy was stopped abruptly. When dosage reduction was associated with disease exacerbation, a prompt response was achieved with the reinstitution of full dose therapy. The effect of therapy

---

*Editors' note: See also Chapter 3. These, and other mycobacteria, are probably opportunistic organisms in Crohn's disease.

†Editors' note: A controlled trial of rifampicin and ethambutol in Crohn's disease showed no benefit, however (Shaffer, J. L., et al.: Gut, 25:203, 1984). See also Afdhal, N. H., et al.: Gastroenterology, 92:1284, 1987; this trial found the drug clofazimine to be ineffective in disease and in maintaining remission.

persisted for long periods, up to 36 months. Among the 15 patients observed for at least 12 months, only one suffered a disease exacerbation while on full dosage. Another patient treated for 8 months had an increase in disease activity while on full dosage.

Even in the high doses used for perineal disease, the drug was generally well tolerated.[232,233] One or more minor reactions, however, did occur in over 90% of patients, including gastrointestinal disturbances, metallic taste, glossitis, furry tongue, urticaria, vaginal and urethral burning, dark urine, and a reversible neutropenia. A disulfiram-like reaction may occur in response to alcohol ingestion. Nervous system side effects such as headache, ataxia, vertigo, encephalopathy, and seizures were uncommon or rare. Peripheral neuropathy with paresthesias occurred in 50% of patients, however, and it developed approximately six months after the initiation of drug therapy. This complication was dose-related and generally disappeared after dose reduction. Rarely, however, paresthesias may continue over prolonged periods even after discontinuation of the drug, which can be distressing. A similar incidence of peripheral neuropathy has been reported in a pediatric population treated for Crohn's disease.[234] A potential problem with continued metronidazole therapy is its carcinogenicity in rodents and its mutagenicity in bacteria.[235,236] In humans no cases of cancer attributable to metronidazole have been reported,[237] nor have chromosomal aberrations been observed.[238] Another potential problem is illustrated by a case report of a liver abscess that was caused by metronidazole-resistant streptococcus milleri. This organism spread from a perianal abscess during metronidazole therapy.[239]

The mechanism of action of metronidazole in the therapy of Crohn's disease is unknown. To the extent that infectious complications contribute to a particular case, reduction in the bacterial number would be useful. This action would also decrease any component of small bowel bacterial overgrowth and its attendant symptoms. Lowering bacterial counts could also reduce direct bacterial invasion of the gut wall and regional lymph nodes, endotoxin levels, antigen-antibody reactions, or other potential factors that may be of significance in disease pathogenesis or persistence. Among Crohn's disease patients, sulfasalazine and, particularly, metronidazole have been reported to significantly reduce concentrations of gut bacteroides species.[240,241] Metronidazole also suppresses cell-mediated immunity, especially granuloma formation.[242] Whether other antibiotics have beneficial actions by similar or other mechanisms remains to be determined.

Immunosuppressive Therapy*

No medical treatment of Crohn's disease has aroused more controversy than immunosuppressive therapy[243] with three possible reasons for this dispute. One has been the failure of a large multicenter study to prove the superiority of azathioprine over placebo with statistical certainty.[95] A second reason is the passionate enthusiasm with which immunosuppressive therapy has been advocated.[244,245] The third reason is an understandably pervasive fear of the short- and long-term toxicity of antimetabolites and cytotoxic drugs.[246-249]

The truth is, however, that a review of the literature on immunotherapy of inflammatory bowel disease reveals more consensus than controversy.[250,251] It is now virtually indisputable that immunosuppressives are effective adjuncts in the management of Crohn's disease. Seven separate randomized, controlled trials of azathioprine or 6-mercaptopurine have all shown some benefits in treating certain patients with active Crohn's disease,[252-257] or in maintaining their remissions.[258] The effects of 6-mercaptopurine in reducing steroid dependency and healing fistulas are particularly striking.[257,259] The failure of the National Cooperative Crohn's Disease Study (NCCDS) to demonstrate a benefit of azathioprine over placebo seems to have been attributable to certain features of the study design, such as its short duration, its use as a single agent, and the insensitivities of the method of clinical assessment.[95,250,260]

The most critical issue concerning the use of immunosuppressives is not their effectiveness but their potential toxicity. The problem can be clarified only by thorough quantitation of adverse reactions in large series of patients during long-term treatment.[261]† Leukopenia can be controlled by careful monitoring. Opportunistic infections are surprisingly infrequent. Development of neoplasia is the most worrisome question, but the risk is still not clearly established.[262] Of all the reported side-effects, the

---

*See also Chapter 21.

†Editors' note: See also Nyman, M., Hansson, I. and Eriksson, S.: Scand. J. Gastroenterol., *20*:1197, 1985; This study showed effective steroid-sparing with no serious side effects in 42 patients.

most troublesome is acute pancreatitis.[247] The increased risk of this complication undoubtedly is a direct consequence of both azathioprine and 6-mercaptopurine.[95,257,261] Fortunately, it is always rapidly reversible and never fatal.

In summary, immunosuppressive drugs must be counted among the useful adjunctive therapies for patients with Crohn's disease. Their major role is in the patient who is steroid-dependent, or the patient who is afflicted by perianal or enteric fistulae and is not a candidate for surgical therapy. Although most experience has been with azathioprine and 6-mercaptopurine, the potential role of cyclosporine has yet to be established.[263-266]*

Miscellaneous Therapeutic Approaches

Immunostimulants

Cell-mediated immunity is impaired in some patients with Crohn's disease.[267] This observation has suggested the therapeutic use of immunostimulants. Oral administration of Bacille Calmette-Guérin (BCG) vaccine has been used to stimulate the immune response. Controlled trials, however, have shown no benefit from this agent in the therapy of Crohn's disease.[268,269] Levamisole and transfer factor are other agents capable of stimulating immunity.[270,272] Controlled trials also have shown no evidence of therapeutic efficacy for Crohn's disease. It has been claimed that levamisole has a role in maintaining a remission attained by other conventional medical therapies,[272] but this has not been confirmed in controlled trials.[273,274] Interferon has an immune stimulatory activity, and a preliminary clinical trial in five patients led to speculation on a role in the therapy of Crohn's disease.[275] Recently, the 7S-immunoglobulin preparation vennimun (Behring, FRG) has been used in the treatment of a small number of patients with Crohn's disease or CUC with claimed but unproven benefits.†

Disodium Cromoglycate

It was suggested, but not proven, that this mast-cell stabilizer might have a beneficial effect in the therapy of ulcerative colitis. In Crohn's disease, however, controlled trials showed no benefit over placebo.[276-278]

Plasmaphoresis

This technique has been used in a clinical study of six patients with Crohn's disease.[279] The symptoms in one patient were controlled by this therapy alone, and in the five others, steroid requirements were reduced. Clinical relapses were also managed in these patients by plasmaphoresis without increasing their steroid dose. A reduction in circulating soluble immune complexes may be a possible basis for the benefit of this therapy. Although this approach is not likely to become a first-line therapy, further study is clearly indicated.

Vitamin A

This vitamin was reported to ameliorate clinical symptoms, as well as to improve impaired intestinal permeability in one patient with Crohn's disease.[280] The known effect of vitamin A in supporting normal intestinal epithelium and mucus production may explain its beneficial action.[281] A long-term, double-blind study found no significant effect of vitamin A in preventing relapse of Crohn's disease.[282] More studies may better define any possible therapeutic role for vitamin A in this disease.

Gut Irrigation

To cause a simultaneous reduction in the bacterial microflora of the bowel and removal of bacterial antigens, whole gut irrigation has been used to treat Crohn's disease.[283,284] Through a tube positioned in the jejunum, 18 L of normal saline were infused over two hours. Improvement in symptoms and laboratory data were reported from these small, uncontrolled reports. This therapy is unconventional and may theoretically be associated with significant fluid and electrolyte changes or with exacerbation of obstruction. Therefore, we do not support its use in the absence of controlled trials that confirm its proposed benefit.

Superoxide Dismutase

Superoxide dismutase (SOD) packaged in liposomes was given subcutaneously to three patients with Crohn's disease and applied locally to skin lesions on two others.[285] Beneficial results were briefly reported. Superoxide dismu-

---

*Editors' note: see also Parrott, H. R., et al.: Gut, 27:A1277, 1986; This study found only low efficacy in the 11 cases studied. Peltekian, K. M. et al.: Gastroenterology, 92:1571, 1987. Authors of this report concluded, from a study of 10 patients, that the drug is safe and effective for Crohn's disease.

†Editors' note: Rohr G., et al.: Gastroenterology 92:1599, 1987.

tase acts as an O_2 scavenger and may protect against the spontaneous chromosomal instability present in Crohn's disease, as well as in other autoimmune diseases. These results are clearly preliminary and have yet to be confirmed.

Therapeutic Measures for Upper Gastrointestinal Tract Disease

Local steroid preparations are useful for Crohn's disease involving the mouth. Disease of the gastroduodenal area may require systemic steroid therapy. Sulfasalazine can be effective but it may have an irritant action upon the already diseased upper bowel. A low residue or liquid diet may be required if the disease has resulted in pyloric or duodenal stenosis. If obstruction does not respond promptly to medical therapy, surgical bypass of the diseased area will provide palliation. The upper gastrointestinal tract disease is generally accompanied by disease in more distal areas. The therapy is generally guided by the principles previously discussed, usually with similar responses from all diseased areas.[286]

"The Placebo Lesson"

For a disease with such a variable and protracted course as Crohn's disease, we need to know a great deal about its natural history if we are to properly evaluate any standard or proposed therapy. Unfortunately, we do not have the needed information. Patients do not remain untreated, either by our current drugs or surgical procedures, to allow evaluation of their course. The only exceptions, we believe, are the placebo groups of some clinical trials of medical therapy in this disease. Despite the many limitations and biases inherent in the study of these patients, valuable information can be learned,[287] and pertinent data from clinical trials in Crohn's disease regarding patients treated with placebo are shown in Table 22-3.

Patients sick enough to require treatment for Crohn's disease can get better with no specific "active" drug therapy. Indeed, when patients are observed for approximately 4 months, somewhere between 25 and 40% have gone into remission. Even after longer periods of observation, about 20% remain well after 1 year and 10% after 2 years.[95-97] Maintenance studies of patients already in remission, regardless of how they came into remission, show that up to 75% of them will continue to be in remission at the end of 1 year and up to 63% after 2 years.[95,97,98,268,277,288] Thus, sick patients with Crohn's disease may get better not only with a variety of medical or surgical approaches, but also with no active drug treatment. Having gotten better, they may continue well for at least a year or even longer. This information should temper our enthusiasm for the medicines we are currently using with their limited efficacy and their known toxicities.

Approach to the Patient

The careful therapeutic studies performed in patients with Crohn's disease provide a framework on which to base therapy. Further work is necessary, however, to better define our therapeutic options and answer many additional questions. Pending these studies, much of our current therapy program is more art than science, acquired through experience. The first step in choosing therapy is to make an assessment of the disease activity in an individual patient. No uniform measurement of disease activity is available. The NCCDS used the Crohn's Disease Activity Index, which has been of proven value.[95]* Others, however, have derived indices thought to better reflect bowel inflammatory activity.[96] We prefer a simple index based on clinical criteria and done in a single office visit.[289] A variety of laboratory measurements may be used in conjunction with this clinical index. We find serum C-reactive protein or orosomucoid valves and, especially, random fecal alpha-1-antitrypsin levels most useful (see also Chap. 9).[290]

Mild to Moderate Disease Activity†

Ambulatory patients with mild to moderate Crohn's disease activity should be given sulfasalazine as initial therapy. The dose is slowly increased to a level of up to 6g/day, if tolerated. Because approximately 60% of patients will achieve a good response within 6 weeks,[95] this seems to be a reasonable time period before drawing conclusions about the final results of this therapy. If successful, treatment is continued until a full clinical remission is secured. Metronidazole is an alternative (up to 20mg/kg if tolerated), especially in those patients who are allergic or intolerant to sulfasalazine or who have failed on this therapy. Metronidazole would be especially attractive for the patient with predominantly colonic disease and/or perineal complications.

* Editors' Note: However, see the caveat raised in Chapter 33.
† See also Chapter 9.

TABLE 22-3. Summary of Placebo Groups in Crohn's Disease Therapeutic Trials.

Clinical Trial	Number of Patients	Disease Location — Small Bowel	Colon	Small & Large Bowel	Number with Prior Surgical Treatment	Disease Activity	Total Trial Duration	Achieved Remission — Study Period	Percentage	Maintained Remission — Study Period	Percentage
NCCDS[95] Part I	77	25	9	43	25	Active	2 years	17 weeks	26	1 year	75
								1 year	18		
								2 years	12	2 years	63
Part II	101	43	9	48	18		2 years	—	—	1 year	64
										2 years	40
ECCDS[97]	101	33	24	53	18	Active[58]	2 years	100 days	42	100 days	71
								300 days	18	300 days	52
								700 days	9	700 days	35
						Inactive[52]	—	—	—	—	—
Van Hees et al.[96]	13	5	5	3	2	Active	0.5 year	26 weeks	8	—	—
Multicenter Trial[98]*	22	2	0	20	20	Inactive	1 year	—	—	1 year	36
Burnham et al.[268]	26	4	4	18	10	Inactive	0.5 year	—	—	0.5 year	65
Binder et al.[277]	14	3	2	9	—	Inactive	1 year	—	—	1 year	21
Müller et al.[288]	30	9	6	15	21	Inactive	4 years	—	—	1 year	66
										2 years	40
										3 years	19
										4 years	15

ECCDS = European Cooperative Crohn's Disease Study; NCCDS = National Cooperative Crohn's Disease Study. *Eleven patients with all known disease resected were omitted from the final analysis. (Adopted from Meyers, S., and Janowitz, H. D.: "Natural history" of Crohn's disease. An analytic review of the placebo lesson. Gastroenterology, 87:1189, 1984.)

Antibiotics are considered as initial therapy in those symptoms caused by bacterial small bowel overgrowth, or with evidence of suppuration such as fever or abdominal tenderness. We ususaly do not combine antibiotics with sulfasalazine. The former agents theoretically interfere with sulfasalazine metabolism and efficacy.

Those who fail therapy with sulfasalazine or antibiotics, will generally require steroids. Prednisone (45 to 60mg/day) should be given. This dose is continued for 7 to 14 days and then tapered over approximately 2 months as the symptoms improve. Continuing high doses of prednisone for prolonged periods is not advisable. We often use sulfasalazine combined with prednisone, especially while the latter is being tapered, despite the lack of supportive evidence from controlled trials.

A variety of preparations, including antidiarrheals, anticholinergics, tranquilizers, and analgesics, may be of symptomatic benefit. During periods of active disease, avoiding fresh fruits and vegetables is advised to reduce diarrhea and episodes of intestinal obstruction. A trial of avoidance of lactose-containing milk products may be worthwhile. Proper nutritional balance and adequate rest are important but strict bed rest is not necessary.

Severe Disease Activity*

Patients with severe disease will generally require corticosteroids and hospitalization. Oral feedings are allowed if they are tolerated, but sicker patients will require bowel rest or even nasogastric suction. Intravenous fluids and electrolytes will be required to insure adequate hydration. If a full diet cannot be reinstituted within 10 to 14 days, total parenteral nutrition should be considered. If any suspicion of a suppurative complication is present, antibiotics are given after all appropriate cultures are collected. Sulfasalazine is generally not helpful. Its onset of action is slow and it may be poorly tolerated because of the side effects of gastric intolerance. Although corticosteroids will usually be necessary, extreme caution should be used if any suspicion exists of an abscess complicating this severe disease. Hydrocortisone (300mg/day) or ACTH (120 units/day), given as a continuous intravenous infusion, may be used, especially for those patients not able to tolerate oral therapy. Preferably those not already on steroid therapy should be given ACTH. After 7 to 14 days of intravenous infusions, therapy is continued with 45 to 60mg of oral prednisone, as described for those with less severe disease. Antibiotics, sulfasalazine, or corticosteroids may be used either alone or in combination, as described earlier. Those patients who do not improve promptly with vigorous medical therapy should be considered for surgical treatment. This is especially true for those with complications such as profuse bleeding, abdominal infection, or toxic megacolon.

Crohn's Disease in Remission

Once clinical activity has subsided with medical therapy, attempts to withdraw steroids must be made. When this aim is accomplished, sulfasalazine and other drugs are also discontinued. In contrast to the situation in ulcerative colitis, the Crohn's disease patient in remission requires no therapy. No drug has been conclusively proven to be useful in the prevention of subsequent disease exacerbation.†

Unfortunately, many patients treated with steroids cannot have these withdrawn without a flare-up of their disease activity. Continued therapy may be required to suppress chronic symptoms. Antibiotics or sulfasalazine are often used in the hope of sparing steroids, despite the lack of supporting evidence for their efficacy in this role. Immunosuppressive agents may be useful adjuncts in selected cases to allow steroid withdrawal. However, in general we consider surgical intervention preferable to immunosuppressive therapy or long-term steroids.

References

1. Beeken, W. L.: Remediable defects in Crohn's disease: a prospective study of 63 patients. Arch. Intern. Med., 135:686, 1975.
2. Gerson, C. D.: Small bowel malfunction and malnutrition. Mt. Sinai J. Med., 50:119, 1983.
3. Rutgeerts, P., Ghoos, Y., Vantrappen, G., and Eyssen, H.: Ileal dysfunction and bacterial overgrowth in patients with Crohn's disease. Eur. J. Clin. Invest., 11:199, 1981.
4. Hawker, P. C., McKay, J. S., and Turnberg, L. A.: Electrolyte transport across colonic mucosa from patients with inflammatory bowel disease. Gastroenterology, 79:508, 1980.
5. Compston, J. E., and Creamer, B.: Plasma levels and intestinal absorption of 25-hydroxyvitamin D in patients with small bowel resection. Gut, 18:171, 1977.

---

*See also Chapter 9.

†Editors' note: However, see also Brignola, C., et al.: Gastroenterology; 92:1327, 1987; the authors of this study claim that the drug methylprednisolone is effective in preventing relapse.

6. Solomons, N. W., Rosenberg, I. H., Sandstead, H. H., and Vo-Khactu, K. P.: Zinc deficiency in Crohn's disease. Digestion, 16:87, 1977.
7. Sturniolo, G. C., Molokhia, M. M., Shields, R., and Turnberg, L. A.: Zinc absorption in Crohn's disease. Gut, 21:387, 1980.
8. McClain, C., Souter, C., and Zieve, L.: Zinc deficiency: A complication of Crohn's disease. Gastroenterology, 78:272, 1980.
9. Fleming, C. R., Huizenga, K. A., and McCall, J. T.: Zinc nutrition in Crohn's disease. Dig. Dis. Sci., 26:865, 1981.
10. Sandiford, J. A., and Alexander, R.: Zinc deficiency in Crohn's disease. J. R. Coll. Surg. Edinb., 26:357, 1981.
11. Anonymous: Zinc deficiency in Crohn's disease. Nutr. Rev., 40:109, 1982.
12. Tiomny, E., et al.: Serum zinc and taste acuity in Tel-Aviv patients with inflammatory bowel disease. Am. J. Gastroenterol., 77:101, 1982.
13. McClain, C., Su, L. C., Gilbert, H., and Cameron, D.: Zinc-deficiency-induced retinal dysfunction in Crohn's disease. Dig. Dis. Sci., 28:85, 1983.
14. Gerson, C. D., and Fabry, E. M.: Ascorbic acid deficiency and fistula formation in regional enteritis. Gastroenterology, 67: 428, 1974.
15. Farivar, S., et al.: Tests of bile-acid and vitamin B_{12} metabolism in ileal Crohn's disease. Am. J. Clin. Pathol., 73:69, 1980.
16. Hoffbrand, A. V., Stewart, J. S., and Mollin, D. L.: Folate deficiency in Crohn's disease: Incidence, pathogenesis, and treatment. Br. Med. J., 2:71, 1968.
17. Franklin, J. L., and Rosenberg, I. H.: Impaired folic acid absorption in inflammatory bowel disease: Effects of salicylazosulfapyridine (Azulfidine). Gastroenterology, 64:517, 1973.
18. Elsborg, L., and Larsen, L.: Folic deficiency in chronic inflammatory bowel diseases. Scand. J. Gastroenterol., 14:1019, 1979.
19. Pollack, S., et al.: Pellagra as the presenting manifestation of Crohn's disease. Gastroenterology, 82:948, 1982.
20. Howdle, P. D., Bone, I., and Losowsky, M. S.: Hypocalcaemic chorea secondary to malabsorption. Postgrad. Med. J., 55:560, 1979.
21. Main, A. N. H., et al.: Mg deficiency in chronic inflammatory bowel disease and requirements during intravenous nutrition. J. P. E. N., 5:15, 1981.
22. Hessov, I., Hasselblad, C., Fasth, S., and Hulten, L.: Magnesium deficiency after ileal resection for Crohn's disease. Scand. J. Gastroenterol., 18:643, 1983.
23. Turnberg, L.: Pathophysiology and management of some medical complications of Crohn's disease. Ann. R. Coll. Surg. Engl., 64:105, 1982.
24. Stotts, N. A., Fitzgerald, K. A., and Williams, K. R.: Care of the patient critically ill with inflammatory bowel disease. Nurs. Clin. North Am., 19:61, 1984.
25. de Leeuw, I., Peeters, R., and Croket, A.: Acquired trace element deficiency during total parenteral nutrition in a man with Crohn's disease. Acta Clin. Belg., 33:227, 1978.
26. Main, A. N. H., et al.: Clinical experience of zinc supplementation during intravenous nutrition in Crohn's disease: value of serum and urine zinc measurements. Gut, 23:984, 1982.
27. Brotman, M.: Inflammatory disease of the bowel: treatable physiologic disorders following surgery. Dis. Colon Rectum, 19:588, 1976.
28. Gerson, C. D., Cohen, N., and Janowitz, H.: Small intestinal absorptive function in regional enteritis. Gastroenterology, 64:907, 1973.
29. Allardyce, D. B.: Preoperative parenteral feeding in Crohn's disease: preoperatively, to induce remission, and at home. Am. Surg., 44:510, 1977.
30. Babb, R.: The role of total parenteral nutrition in the treatment of inflammatory bowel disease. Am. J. Gastroenterol., 70:506, 1978.
31. Driscoll, J. H., Jr., and Rosenberg, I. H.: Total parenteral nutrition in inflammatory bowel disease. Med. Clin. North Am., 62:185, 1978.
32. Elson, C. O., et al.: An evaluation of total parenteral nutrition in the management of inflammatory bowel disease. Dig. Dis. Sci., 25:42, 1980.
33. Descos, L., and Vignal, J.: Total parenteral nutrition in the management of Crohn's disease. World J. Surg., 4:161, 1980.
34. Bos, L. P., and Weterman, I. T.: Total parenteral nutrition in Crohn's disease. World. J. Surg., 4:163, 1980.
35. Holm, I.: Benefit of total parenteral nutrition (TPN) in the treatment of Crohn's disease and ulcerative colitis. Acta Chir. Scand., 147:271, 1981.
36. Kushner, R. F., and Craig, R. M.: Intense nutritional support in inflammatory bowel disease: A review. J. Clin. Gastroenterol., 4:511, 1982.
37. Jacobson, S. J., Gabrielsson, N., and Granqvist, S.: Crohn's disease of the appendix: remission obtained by total parenteral nutrition. J. P. E. N., 5:145, 1981.
38. Sanedler, M., et al.: Home parenteral nutrition in a patient with Crohn's disease. S. Afr. Med. J., 61:972, 1982.
39. Houcke, J., et al.: Nutrition parenterale exclusive: Resultats dans 45 poussees aigues de la maladie de Crohn. Nouv. Presse Med., 9:1361, 1980.
40. Meryn, S., et al.: Influences of parenteral nutrition on serum levels of proteins in patients with Crohn's disease. J. P. E. N., 7:553, 1983.
41. Harford, F. J., and Fazio, V. W.: Total parenteral nutrition as primary therapy for inflammatory disease of the bowel. Dis. Colon Rectum, 21:555, 1978.
42. Muller, J. M., Keller, H. W., Erasmi, H., and Pichlmaier, H.: Total parenteral nutrition as the sole therapy in Crohn's disease—a prospective study. Br. J. Surg., 70:40, 1983.
43. Terrizzi, G., Arnulfo, G., Bertoglio, E., and Berti Riboli, E.: La nutrizione parenterale totale nel trattamento del morbo di Crohn e della colite ulcerosa in fase acuta od iperacuta. Minerva Dietol. Gastroenterol., 28:237, 1982.
44. Fuchigami, T., et al.: Effects of total parenteral nutrition on colonic lesions in Crohn's disease: Radiographic and endoscopic study. Gastroenterol. Jpn., 17:521, 1982.
45. Anonymous: Intravenous feeding to sustain pregnancy in patient with Crohn's disease. Br. Med. J., 283:1221, 1981.
46. Benny, P. S., et al.: The biochemical effects of maternal hyperalimentation during pregnancy. NZ Med. J., 88:283, 1978.
47. Hew, L. R., and Deital, M.: Total parenteral nutrition in gynecology and obstetrics. Obstet. Gynecol., 55:4, 1980.
48. Tresadern, J. C., Falconer, G. F., Turnberg, L. A., and Irving, M. H.: Maintenance of pregnancy in a home parenteral nutrition patient. J. P. E. N., 8:199, 1984.
49. Layden, T., et al.: Reversal of growth arrest in adolescents with Crohn's disease after parenteral alimentation. Gastroenterology, 70:1017, 1976.
50. Kelts, D. G., et al.: Nutritional basis of growth failure in children and adolescents with Crohn's disease. Gastroenterology, 70:1017, 1976.
51. Anonymous: Parenteral nutrition in the correction of growth failure in chronic inflammatory bowel disease. Nutr. Rev., 38:118, 1980.
52. Motil, K. J., et al.: Whole body leucine metabolism in adolescents with Crohn's disease and growth failure during

nutritional supplementation. Gastroenterology, *82*:1359, 1982.
53. Khursheed, N., et al.: Total parenteral nutrition at home: Studies in patients surviving 4 months to 5 years. Gastroenterology, *71*:943, 1976.
54. Strobel, C. T., Byrne, W. J., and Ament, M. E.: Home parenteral nutrition in children with Crohn's disease: An effective management alternative. Gastroenterology, *77*:272, 1979.
55. Dickinson, R. J., et al.: Controlled trial of intravenous hyperalimentation and total bowel rest as an adjunct to the routine therapy of acute colitis. Gastroenterology, *79*:1199, 1980.
56. Seashore, J. H., Hillemeier, A. C., and Gryboski, J. D.: Total parenteral nutrition in the management of inflammatory bowel disease in children: A limited role. Am. J. Surg., *143*:504, 1982.
57. Shiloni, E., and Freund, H. R.: Total parenteral nutrition in Crohn's disease: Is it a primary or supportive mode of therapy? Dis. Colon Rectum, *26*:275, 1983.
58. Lerebours, E., et al.: Etude de l'utilite d'une corticotherapie au cours des poussees aigues de maladie de Crohn traitees par alimentation parenterale totale prolongee. Gastroenterol. Clin. Biol., *6*:19, 1982.
59. Homer, D. R., Grand, R. J., and Colodny, A. H.: Growth, course and prognosis after surgery for Crohn's disease in children and adolescents. Pediatrics, *59*:717, 1977.
60. Rosenberg, I. H.: Nutritional support in inflammatory bowel disease. (Letter). Gastroenterology, *77*:393, 1979.
61. Harries, A. D., et al.: Controlled trial of supplemented oral nutrition in Crohn's disease. Lancet, *1*:887, 1983.
62. Beeken, W. L., Busch, H. J., and Sylvester, D. L.: Intestinal protein loss in Crohn's disease. Gastroenterology, *62*:207, 1972.
63. Logan, R. F. A., Gillon, J., Ferrington, C., and Ferguson, A.: Reduction of gastrointestinal protein loss by elemental diet in Crohn's disease of the small bowel. Gut, *22*:383, 1981.
64. Kirschner, B. S., et al.: Reversal of growth retardation in Crohn's disease with treatment emphasizing oral nutritional restitution. Gastroenterology, *80*:10, 1981.
65. Anonymous: Nutritional supplementation and growth retardation in juvenile Crohn's disease: A new approach. Nutr. Rev., *40*:199, 1982.
66. Harries, A. D., Danis, V. A., and Heatley, R. V.: Influence of nutritional status on immune functions in patients with Crohn's disease. Gut, *25*:465, 1984.
67. Workman, E. M., Alun-Jones, V., Wilson, A. J., and Hunter, J. O.: Diet in the management of Crohn's disease. Hum. Nutr. Appl. Nutr., *38*:469, 1984.
68. Kirschner, B. S., DeFavaro, M. V., and Jensen, W.: Lactose malabsorption in children and adolescents with inflammatory bowel disease. Gastroenterology, *81*:829, 1981.
69. Kasper, H., and Sommer, H.: Dietary fiber and nutrient intake in Crohn's disease. Am. J. Clin. Nutr., *32*:1898, 1979.
70. Mayberry, J. F., et al.: Diet in Crohn's disease: Two studies of current and previous habits in newly diagnosed patients. Dig. Dis. Sci., *26*:444, 1981.
71. Penny, W. J., et al.: Relationship between trace elements, sugar consumption, and taste in Crohn's disease. Gut, *24*:288, 1983.
72. Heaton, K. W., Thornton, J. R., and Emmett, P. M.: Treatment of Crohn's disease with an unrefined-carbohydrate, fibre-rich diet. Br. Med. J., *2*:764, 1979.
73. Brandes, J. W., and Lorenz-Meyer, H.: Zuckerfreie diat: Eine neue perspektive zur behandlung des morbus Crohn? Z. Gastroenterol., *19*:1, 1981.

74. Brandes, J. W., Korst, H. A., and Littmann, K. P.: Zuckerfreie diat als langzeit-bzw. Intervallbehandlung in der remissionsphase des Morbus Crohn—eine prospektive studie. Leber Magen Darm, *12*:225, 1982.
75. Lorenz-Meyer, H., and Brandes, J. W.: Gibt es eine diatetische behandlung des Morbus Crohn in der remision? Dtsch. Med. Wochenschr., *108*:595, 1983.
76. von Riemann, J. F., and Kolb, S.: Zuckerarme und faserreiche kost bei Morbus Crohn. Fortschr. Med., *102*:67/37, 1984.
77. Navarro, J., et al.: Prolonged constant rate elemental enteral nutrition in Crohn's disease. J. Pediatr. Gastroenterol. Nutr., *1*:542, 1982.
78. Morin, C. L., Roulet, M., Roy, C. C., and Weber, A: Continuous elemental enteral alimentation in children with Crohn's disease and growth failure. Gastroenterology, *79*:1205, 1980.
79. Morin, C. L., et al.: Continuous elemental enteral alimentation in the treatment of children and adolescents with Crohn's disease. J. P. E. N., *6*:194, 1982.
80. Main, A. N. H., et al.: Home enteral tube feeding with a liquid diet in the longterm management of inflammatory bowel disease and intestinal failure. Scott. Med. J., *25*:312, 1980.
81. Lochs, H., et al.: Is tube feeding with elemental diets a primary therapy of Crohn's disease? Klin. Wochenschr., *62*:821, 1984.
82. Calam, J., Crooks, P. E., and Walker, R. J.: Elemental diets in the management of Crohn's perianal fistulae. J. P. E. N., *4*:4, 1980.
83. Steffee, W. P., and Shipps, T. B.: Improvement of Crohn fistulas with a peptide diet. Clin. Ther., *3*:280, 1980.
84. Russell, R. I., and Hall, M. J.: Elemental diet therapy in the management of complicated Crohn's disease. Scott. Med. J., *24*:291, 1979.
85. Stober, B., Nutzenadel, W., and Ullrich, F.: Elementardiat bei Morbus Crohn. Monatsschr. Kinderheilkd., *131*:721, 1983.
86. Axelsson, C., and Jarnum, S.: Assessment of the therapeutic value of an elemental diet in chronic inflammatory bowel disease. Scand. J. Gastroenterol., *12*:89, 1977.
87. O'Morain, C.: Elemental diets in the treatment of Crohn's disease. Proc. Nutr. Soc., *38*:403, 1979.
88. O'Morain, C., Segal, A. W., and Levi, A. J.: Elemental diets in treatment of acute Crohn's disease. Br. Med. J., *281*:1173, 1980.
89. O'Morain, C.: Crohn's disease treated by elemental diet. J. R. Soc. Med., *75*:135, 1982.
90. O'Morain, C., Segal, A. M., Levi, A. J., and Valman, H. B.: Elemental diet in acute Crohn's disease. Arch. Dis. Child., *53*:44, 1983.
91. O'Morain, C., Segal, A. W., and Levi, A. J.: Elemental diet as primary treatment of acute Crohn's disease: A controlled trial. Br. Med. J., *288*:1859, 1984.
92. Werlin, S. L.: Growth failure in Crohn's disease: An approach to treatment. J. P. E. N., *5*:250, 1981.
93. Helzer, J. E.: Psychiatric aspects of inflammatory bowel disease. IBD News, *6*:1, 1985.
94. Anthonisen, P., et al.: The clinical effect of salazosulphapyridine (Salazopyrin^R) in Crohn's disease. Scand. J. Gastroenterol., *9*:549, 1974.
95. Summers, R. W., et al.: National Cooperative Crohn's Disease C D Study: Results of drug treatment. Gastroenterology, *77*:847, 1979.
96. Van Hees, P. A. M., et al.: Effect of sulphasalazine in patients with active Crohn's disease: A controlled double-blind study. Gut, *22*:404, 1981.
97. Malchow, H., et al.: European Cooperative Crohn's Dis-

ease Study (ECCDS): Results of drug treatment. Gastroenterology, 86:249, 1984.
98. Multicenter trial. Sulfasalazine in asymptomatic Crohn's disease. Gut, 18:69, 1977.
99. Wenckert, A., et al.: The long-term prophylactic effect of salazosulphapyridine (Salazopyrine[R]) in primarily resected patients with Crohn's disease. A controlled double-blind trial. Scand. J. Gastroenterol., 13:161, 1978.
100. Singleton, J. W., et al.: A trial of sulfasalazine as adjunctive therapy in Crohn's disease. Gastroenterology, 77:887, 1979.
101. Bergman, L., and Krause, N.: Postoperative treatment with corticosteroids and salazosulphapyridine (Salazopyrin[R]) after radical resection for Crohn's disease. Scand. J. Gastroenterol., 11:651, 1976.
102. Schroder, H., and Campbell, D. E. S.: Absorption, metabolism and excretion of salicylazosulfapyridine in man. Clin. and Pharmacol. Ther., 13:539, 1972.
103. Das, K. M., Chowdhury, J. R., Zapp, B., and Fara, J. W.: Small bowel absorption of sulfasalazine and its hepatic metabolism, in human beings, cats and rats. Gastroenterology, 77:280, 1979.
104. Peppercorn, M. A., and Goldman, P.: The role of intestinal bacteria in the metabolism of salicylazosulfapyridine. J. Pharmacol. Exp. Ther., 181:555, 1972.
105. Azad Khan, A. K., et al.: Tissue and bacterial splitting of sulfasalazine. Clin. Sci., 64:349, 1983.
106. Schroder, H., Lewkonia, R. M., and Price Evans, D. A.: Metabolism of salicylazosulfapyridine in healthy subjects and in patients with ulcerative colitis: Effects of colectomy and of phenobarbitol. Clin. Pharmacol. Ther., 14:802, 1973.
107. Das, K. M., Eastwood, M. A., McManus, J. P., and Sircus, W.: The role of the colon in the metabolism of salicylazosulfapyridine. Scand. J. Gastroenterol., 9:137, 1974.
108. Peppercorn, M. A., and Goldman, P.: Distribution studies of salicylazosulfapyridine and its metabolites. Gastroenterology, 64:240, 1973.
109. Das, K. M., and Eastwood, M. D.: Acetylation polymorphosis of sulfapyridine in patients with ulcerative colitis and Crohn's disease. Clin. Pharmacol. Ther., 18:514, 1975.
110. Levine, M. D., Kirsner, J. B., and Klotz, A. P.: A new concept of the pathogenesis of ulcerative colitis. Science, 114:552, 1951.
111. Hanngren, A., et al.: Distribution and metabolism of salicyl-azo-sulfapyridine: II. A study with S[35]-salicyl-azo-sulfapyridine and S[35]-sulfapyridine. Acta Med. Scand., 173:391, 1963.
112. West, B., et al.: Effects of sulfaphasalazine on fecal flora in patients with inflammatory bowel disease. Gut, 15:960, 1974.
113. Holm, G., and Perlmann, P.: Cytotoxicity of lymphocytes and its suppression. Antibiot. Chemother., 15:295, 1969.
114. Molin, L., and Stendahl, O.: The effect of sulfasalazine and its active components on human polymorphonuclear leukocyte function in relation to ulcerative colitis. Acta Med. Scand., 206:451, 1979.
115. Stenson, W. F., Mehta, J., and Spilberg, J.: Sulfasalazine inhibits the binding of formylmethionylleucylphenylalanine (FMLP) to its receptor on human neutrophils. Biochem. Pharmacol., 33:407, 1984.
116. Gould, S. R.: Prostaglandins, ulcerative colitis and sulfasalazine. Lancet, 2:988, 1975.
117. Gould, S. R.: Assay of prostaglandin-like substances in feces and their measurement in ulcerative colitis. Prostaglandins, 11:489, 1976.
118. Sharon, P., Ligumoky, M., Rachmilewitz, D., and Zor, U.: Role of prostaglandins in ulcerative colitis; enhanced production during active disease and inhibition of sulfasalazine. Gastroenterology, 75:638, 1978.
119. Harris, D. W., Smith, P. R., and Swan, C. H. J.: Determination of prostaglandin synthetase activity in rectal biopsy material and its signficance in colonic disease. Gut, 19:875, 1978.
120. Smith, P. R., Dawson, D. J., and Swan, C. H. J.: Prostaglandin synthetase activity in acute ulcerative colitis: Effects of treatment with sulfasalazine, codeine phosphate and prednisolone. Gut, 20:802, 1978.
121. Campieri, M., Lanfranchi, G. A., and Bozzocchi, G.: Salicylate other than 5-aminosalicylic acid ineffective in ulcerative colitis. Lancet, 2:993, 1978.
122. Hoult, J. R. S., and Moore, P. K.: Effects of sulfasalazine and its metabolites on prostaglandin synthesis, inactivation and actions on smooth muscle. Br. J. Pharmacol., 68:19, 1980.
123. Hoult, J. R. S., and Page, H.: 5-aminosalicylic acid, as cofactor for colonic prostacyclin synthesis (Letter). Lancet, 2:255, 1981.
124. Stenson, W. F., and Lobos, E.: Sulfasalazine inhibits the synthesis of chemotactic lipids by neutrophils. J. Clin. Invest., 69:494, 1982.
125. Sircar, J. C., Schwender, C. F., and Carethers, M. E.: Inhibition of soybean lipoxygenase by sulfasalazine and 5-aminosalicylic acid: A possible mode of action in ulcerative colitis. Biochem. Pharmacol., 32:170, 1983.
126. Das, D. M., Eastwood, M. A., McManus, J. P., and Sircus, W.: Adverse reactions during salicylazosulfapyridine therapy and the relation with drug metabolism and acetylator phenotype. N. Engl. J. Med., 289:491, 1973.
127. Singleton, J. W., et al.: National Cooperative Crohn's Disease Study: Adverse reactions to study drugs. Gastroenterology, 77:870, 1979.
128. Strom, J.: Toxic epidermal necrolysis (Lyell's syndrome). Scand. J. Infect. Dis., 1:209, 1969.
129. Das, K. M., and Sternlieb, I.: Salicylazosulfapyridine in inflammatory bowel disease. Am. J. Dig. Dis., 20:971, 1975.
130. Hensen, E. J., Class, E. H., and Vermer, B. J.: Drug-dependent binding of circulating antibodies in drug-induced toxic epidermal necrolysis (letter). Lancet, 2:151, 1981.
131. Schwartz, A. G., Targan, S. R., Saxon, A., and Weinstein, W. M.: Sulfasalazine-induced exacerbation of ulcerative colitis. N. Engl. J. Med., 306:409, 1982.
132. Block, M. B., Genant, H. K., and Kirsner, J. B.: Pancreatitis as an adverse reaction to salicylazosulfapyridine. N. Engl. J. Med., 282:380, 1970.
133. Kanner, R. S., Tedesco, F. J., and Kalser, M. H.: Azulfidine (sulfasalazine)-induced hepatic injury. Am. J. Dig. Dis., 23:956, 1978.
134. Jacobs, E., Paulet, P., and Rahier, J.: Hypersensitivity reaction to sulfasalazine—another case (letter). Gastroenterology, 75:1193, 1978.
135. Callen, J., and Soderstrom, R. M.: Granulomatous hepatitis associated with salicylazosulfapyridine therapy. South. Med. J., 71:1159, 1978.
136. Namias, A., Bhalotra, R., and Donowitz, M.: Reversible sulfasalazine-induced granulomatous hepatitis. J. Clin. Gastroenterol., 3:193, 1981.
137. Gulley, R. M., Mirza, A., and Kelly, C. E.: Hepatotoxicity of salicylazosulfapyridine: A case report and review of the literature. Am. J. Gastroenterol., 72:561, 1979.
138. Jones, G. R., and Malone, D. N. S.: Sulfasalazine-induced lung disease. Thorax, 27:713, 1972.

139. Davies, D., and MacFarlane, A.: Fibrosing alveolitis and treatment with sulfasalazine. Gut, 15:185, 1974.
140. Tydd, T. E.: Sulfasalazine lung. Med. J. Aust., 1:570, 1976.
141. Beliner, S., et al.: Salazopyrin-induced eosinophilic pneumonia. Respiration, 39:119, 1980.
142. Wang, K. K., Bowyer, B. A., Fleming, C. R., and Schroeder, K. W.: Pulmonary infiltrates and eosinophilia associated with sulfasalazine. Mayo Clin. Proc., 59:343, 1984.
143. Neeman, A., et al.: Salazopyrine-induced tachycardia (letter). Biomedicine, 33:1, 1980.
144. Jamohidi, K., et al.: Azulfidine agranulocytosis with bone marrow, megakaryocytosis, histiocytosis and plasmacytosis. Minn. Med., 55:545, 1972.
145. Davies, G. E., and Palek, J.: Selective erythroid and megakaryocytic aplasia after sulfasalazine administration (letter). Arch. Intern. Med., 140:1122, 1980.
146. Schneider, R. E., and Beeley, L.: Megaloblastic anemia associated with sulfasalazine treatment. Br. Med. J., 1:1638, 1977.
147. Cohen, S. M., Rosenthal, D. S., and Karp, P. J.: Ulcerative colitis and erythrocytic G6PD deficiency: Salicylazosulfapyridine provoked hemolysis. J. Am. Med. Assoc., 205:528, 1968.
148. Gabov, E. P.: Hemolytic anemia as adverse reaction to salicylazosulfapyridine (letter). N. Engl. J. Med., 289:1372, 1973.
149. Griffiths, I. D., and Kane, S. P.: Sulfasalazine-induced lupus syndrome in ulcerative colitis. Br. Med. J., 2:1188, 1977.
150. Mihas, A. A., Goldberg, D. J., and Slaughter, R. L.: Sulfasalazine toxic reactions: Hepatitis, fever, and skin rash with hypocomplementemia and immune complexes. J. Am. Med. Assoc., 239:2590, 1978.
151. Reid, J., Holt, S., Housley, E., and Snedden, D. J.: Raynaud's phenomenon induced by sulfasalazine. Postgrad. Med. J., 56:106, 1980.
152. Wallace, I. W.: Neurotoxicity associated with a reaction to sulfasalazine. Practitioner, 204:850, 1970.
153. Levi, A. J., Fisher, A. M., Hughes, K., and Hendry, W. F.: Male infertility due to sulfasalazine. Lancet, 2:276, 1979.
154. Toth, R.: Male infertility due to sulfasalazine (letter). Lancet, 2:904, 1979.
155. Toth, A.: Reversible toxic effect of salicylazosulfapyridine on semen quality. Fertil. Steril., 31:538, 1979.
156. Griene, J.: Male infertility due to sulfasalazine (letter). Lancet, 2:464, 1979.
157. Traub, A. J., Thompson, W., and Carville, J.: Male infertility due to sulfasalazine (letter). Lancet, 2:639, 1979.
158. Collen, M. J.: Azulfidine-induced oligospermia. Am. J. Gastroenterol., 74:441, 1980.
159. Levi, A. J., Toovey, S., and Hudson, E.: Male infertility due to sulfasalazine. Gastroenterology, 80:1208, 1981.
160. Cosentini, M. J., Chey, W. Y., Takihara, H., and Cockett, A. T. K.: The effects of sulfasalazine on human male fertility potential and seminal prostaglandins. J. Urol., 132:682, 1984.
161. Morain, C. O., Smethurst, P., Dore, C. J., and Levi, A. J.: Reversible male infertility due to sulfasalazine: Studies in man and rat. Gut, 25:1078, 1984.
162. Van Hess, P. D., Van Elferen, L. W., Van Rossum, J. M., Van Tongeen, J. H.: Hemolysis during salicylazosulfapyridine therapy. Am. J. Gastroenterol., 70:501, 1978.
163. Taffet, S. L., and Das, K. M.: Sulfasalazine adverse effects and desensitization. Dig. Dis. Sci., 28:833, 1983.
164. Nielsen, O. H.: Sulfasalazine intolerance: A retrospective survey of the reasons for discontinuing treatment with sulfasalazine in patients with chronic inflammatory bowel disease. J. Clin. Gastroenterol., 6:27, 1984.
165. Korelitz, O. J., Present, D. H., Rubin, P. H., and Fochios, S. E.: Desensitization to sulfasalazine after hypersensitivity reactions in patients with inflammatory bowel disease. J. Clin. Gastroenterol., 6:27, 1984.
166. Purdy, B. H., Philips, D. M., and Summers, R. W.: Desensitization for sulfasalazine skin rash. Ann. Intern. Med., 100:512, 1984.
167. Franklin, J. L., and Rosenberg, J. H.: Impaired folic acid absorption in inflammatory bowel disease: Effects of salicylazopyridine (Azulfidine). Gastroenterology, 64:517, 1973.
168. Reisenauer, A. M., and Halsted, C. H.: Human jejunal brush border folate conjugase: Characteristics and inhibition by salicylazopyridine. Biochim. Biophys. Acta, 659:62, 1981.
169. Juhl, R. P., et al.: Effect of sulfasalazine on digoxin bioavailability. Clin. Pharmacol. Ther., 20:387, 1976.
170. Pieniaszek, H. J., and Bates, T. R.: Cholestyramine-induced inhibition of salicylazopyridine (sulfasalazine) metabolism by rat intestinal microflora. J. Pharmacol. Exp. Ther., 198:240, 1976.
171. Das, K. M., and Eastwood, M. A.: Effect of iron and calcium on salicylazosulfapyridine metabolism. Scott. Med. J., 18:45, 1976.
172. Azad Khan, A. K., and Truelove, S. C.: Placental and mammary transfer of sulfasalazine. Br. Med. J., 11:1553, 1979.
173. Mogadam, M., Dobbins, W. C., Korelitz, B. I., and Ahmed, S. W.: Pregnancy in inflammatory bowel disease: Effect of sulfasalazine and corticosteroids on fetal outcome. Gastroenterology, 80:72, 1981.
174. Willoughby, C. P., and Truelove, S. C.: Ulcerative colitis and pregnancy. Gut, 21:469, 1980.
175. Jarnerst, G., and Into-Malmberg, M. B.: Sulfasalazine treatment during breast feeding. Scand. J. Gastroenterol., 14:869, 1979.
176. Van Hees, P. A. M., Bakker, J. H., and Van Tongeren, J. H. M.: Effect of sulfapyridine, 5-aminosalicylic acid and placebo in patients with idiopathic proctitis. A study to determine the active therapeutic moiety of sulfasalazine. Gut, 21:632, 1980.
177. Stenson, W. F.: Pharmacology of sulfasalazine. Viewpoints Dig. Dis., 16:13, 1984.
178. Stenson, W. F., and Lobos, E. A.: Inhibition of platelet thromboxane synthetase by sulfasalazine. Biochem. Pharmacol., 33:2205, 1983.
179. Riis, P., et al.: The therapeutic effect of methyl-salazosulfapyridine verus salazosulfapyridine in active ulcerative colitis. Scand. J. Gastroenterol., 14:647, 1979.
180. Klotz, U., Maier, K., Fischer, G., and Heinkel, K.: Therapeutic efficacy of sulfasalazine and its metabolites in patients with ulcerative colitis and Crohn's disease. N. Engl. J. Med., 303:1449, 1980.
181. Shafh, A., Chowdhury, J. R., and Das, K. M.: Absorption, enterohepatic circulation and excretion of 5-aminosalicylic acid in rats. Am. J. Gastroenterol., 77:297, 1982.
182. Brown, T. P., McGarraugh, G. V., and Parkinson, J. M.: A polymeric drug for the treatment of inflammatory bowel disease. J. Med. Chem., 26:1300, 1983.
183. Bartalsky, A.: Salicylazobenzoic acid in ulcerative colitis (letter). Lancet, 1:960, 1982.
184. Chan, R. P., et al.: Studies of two novel sulfasalazine analogs, ipsalazide and balsalazine. Dig. Dis. Sci., 28:609, 1983.
185. Lauritsen, K., Hansen, J., Ryde, M., and Rask-Madsen, J.: Colonic azodisalicylate metabolism determined by in vivo dialysis in healthy volunteers and patients with ulcerative colitis. Gastroenterology, 86:1496, 1984.

186. Sandberg-Gertzén, H., Ryde, M., and Järnerot, G.: Absorption and excretion of a single 1 g dose of azodisalsodium in subjects with ileostomy. Scand. J. Gastroenterol., *18*:107, 1983.
187. Rasmussen, S. N., et al.: 5-aminosalicylic acid in a slow-release preparation: Bioavailability, plasma level, and excretion in humans. Gastroenterology, *83*:1062, 1982.
188. Dew, M. J., et al.: Maintenance of remission in ulcerative colitis with 5-aminosalicylic acid in high doses by mouth. Br. Med. J. (Clin. Res.), *287*:23, 1983.
189. Saverymuttu, S., et al.: Evaluation of short-term treatment of Crohn's disease with slow release 5-aminosalicylic acid. Gut, *25*:A552, 1984.
190. Rasmussen, S. N., et al.: Treatment of Crohn's disease with peroral 5-aminosalicylic acid. Gastroenterology, *85*:1350, 1983.
191. Sparberg, M., and Kirsner, J. B.: Long-term corticosteroid therapy for regional enteritis: An analysis of 58 courses in 54 patients. Am. J. Dig. Dis., *11*:865, 1966.
192. Cooke, W. T., and Fielding, J. F.: Corticosteroid or corticotrophin therapy in Crohn's disease. Gut, *11*:921, 1970.
193. Jones, J. H., and Lennard-Jones, J. F.: Corticosteroids and corticotrophin in the treatment of Crohn's disease. Gut, *7*:181, 1966.
194. Smith, R. C., et al.: Low dose steroids and clinical relapse in Crohn's disease: A controlled trial. Gut, *19*:606, 1978.
195. Meyers, S., Sachar, D. B., Goldberg, J. D., and Janowitz, H. D.: Corticotrophin versus hydrocortisone in the intravenous treatment of ulcerative colitis. A prospective, randomized, double-blind clinical trial. Gastroenterology, *85*:351, 1983.
196. Swartz, S. L., and Dluhy, R. G.: Corticosteroids: Clinical pharmacology and therapeutic use. Drugs, *16*:238, 1978.
197. Pickup, M. E.: Clinical pharmacokinetics of prednisone and prednisolone. Clin. Pharmacokinet., *4*:111, 1979.
198. Al-Habet, S., and Rogers, H. J.: Pharmacokinetics of intravenous and oral prednisolone. Br. J. Clin. Pharmacol., *10*:503, 1980.
199. Kaplan, et al.: A controlled evaluation of intravenous adrenocorticotropic and hydrocortisone in the treatment of acute colitis. Gastroenterology, *69*:91, 1975.
200. Powell-Tuck, J., Buckell, N. A., and Lennard-Jones, J. E.: A controlled comparison of corticotrophin and hydrocortisone in the treatment of severe proctocolitis. Scand. J. Gastroenterol., *12*:971, 1977.
201. Shaffer, J. A.: Absorption of prednisolone in patients with Crohn's disease. Gut, *24*:182, 1983.
202. Tanner, A. R., Halliday, J. W., and Powel, L. W.: Serum prednisolone levels in Crohn's disease or celiac disease following oral prednisolone administration. Digestion, *21*:310, 1981.
203. Hawkeye, C. J., and Truelove, S. C.: Effect of prednisolone on prostaglandin synthesis by rectal mucosa in ulcerative colitis: Investigation by laminar flow bioassay and radioimmunoassay. Gut, *22*:190, 1981.
204. Fraser, F. C., and Fainstat, T. D.: Production of congenital defects in offspring of pregnant mice treated with cortisone: progress notes. Pediatrics, *8*:527, 1951.
205. Bongiovanni, A. M., and McPadden, A. J.: Steroids during pregnancy and possible fetal consequences. Fertil. Steril., *11*:186, 1959.
206. Vender, R. J., and Spiro, H. M.: Inflammatory bowel disease and pregnancy. J. Clin. Gastroenterol., *4*:231, 1982.
207. Fielding, J. F.: Pregnancy and inflammatory bowel disease. Ir. J. Med. Sci., *151*:194, 1982.
208. Willoughby, C. P., and Truelove, S. C.: Ulcerative colitis and pregnancy. Gut, *21*:469, 1980.
209. Barocco, P. J., and Korelitz, B. I.: The influence of inflammatory bowel disease and its treatment on pregnancy and fetal outcome. J. Clin. Gastroenterol., *6*:211, 1984.
210. Khosla, R., Willoughby, C. P., and Jewell, D. P.: Crohn's disease and pregnancy. Gut, *25*:52, 1984.
211. Moss, A. A., Carbone, J. V., and Kressel, H. Y.: Radiologic and clinical assessment of broad-spectrum antibiotic therapy in Crohn's disease. Am. J. Roentgenol., *131*:787, 1978.
212. Keighley, M. R., Arabi, Y., and Dimock, F.: Influence of inflammatory bowel disease on intestinal flora. Gut, *17*:1099, 1978.
213. Ambrose, N. S., Youngs, D., Burdon, D. W., and Keighley, M. R.: Changes in intestinal microflora in Crohn's disease. Br. J. Surg., *69*:681, 1982.
214. Aluwihare, A. P.: Electron microscopy in Crohn's disease. Gut, *12*:509, 1971.
215. Ambrose, N. S., Johnson, M., Burdon, D. W., and Keighley, M. R.: Incidence of pathogenic bacteria from mesenteric lymph nodes and ileal serosa during Crohn's disease surgery. Br. J. Surg., *71*:623, 1984.
216. Ambrose, N. S., et al.: Antibiotic therapy for the treatment in relapse of intestinal Crohn's disease. A prospective randomized study. Dis. Colon Rectum, *28*:81, 1985.
217. Elliott, P. R., et al.: Sulphadoxine-pyrimethamine therapy in Crohn's disease. Gut, *25*:132, 1982.
218. Burnham, W. R., Lennard-Jones, J. E., Stanford, T. L., and Bird, R. G.: Mycobacteria as a possible cause of inflammatory bowel disease. Lancet, *2*:693, 1978.
219. Donnelly, B. J., Delaney, P. V., and Healy, T. M.: Evidence for a transmissible factor in Crohn's disease. Gut, *18*:360, 1977.
220. Shaffer, J. L., et al.: Controlled trial of rifampicin and ethambutol in Crohn's disease. Gut, *25*:203, 1984.
221. Paris, J., et al.: Resultats a distance du traitement de la maladie de Crohn par la medication antituberculeuse. Lille Medical, *23*:494, 1978.
222. Toulet, J., Rousselet, J., and Viteau, J. M.: La rifampicine dans le traitement de la maladie de Crohn (letter). Gastroenterol. Clin. Biol., *3*:209, 1979.
223. Ursing, B., and Kamme, C.: Metronidazole for Crohn's disease. Lancet, *1*:775, 1975.
224. Kasper, H., Sommer, H., and Kuhn, H. A.: Therapy of Crohn's disease with metronidazole. An uncontrolled trial. Acta Hepatogastroenterol., *26*:217, 1979.
225. Hildebrand, H., Berg, N. O., Hoevals, J., and Ursing, B.: Treatment of Crohn's disease with metronidazole in childhood and adolescence. Gastroenterol. Clin. Biol., *4*:19, 1980.
226. Jakobovits, J., and Schuster, M. M.: Metronidazole therapy for Crohn's disease and associated fistulae. Am. J. Gastroenterol., *79*:533, 1984.
227. Keighley, M. R. B.: Infection and the use of antibiotics in Crohn's disease. Can. J. Surg., *27*:438, 1984.
228. Allan, R., and Cooke, W. T.: Evaluation of metronidazole in the management of Crohn's disease (abstract). Gut, *18*:A422, 1977.
229. Blichfeldt, P., Blomhoff, J. P., Gjone, M., and Gjone, E.: Metronidazole in Crohn's disease. A double blind crossover clinical trial. Scand. J. Gastroenterol., *13*:123, 1978.
230. Ursing, B., et al.: A comparative study of metronidazole and sulfasalazine for active Crohn's disease: The cooperative Crohn's disease study in Sweden. II. Result. Gastroenterology, *83*:550, 1982.
231. Schneider, M. U., Strobel, S., Rieman, J. F., and Dembling, L.: Metronidazol in der behandlung des morbus Crohn. Dtsch. Med. Wochenschr., *106*:1126, 1981.

232. Bernstein, L. H., Frank, M. S., Brandt, L. J., and Boley, S. J.: Healing of perineal Crohn's disease with metronidazole. Gastroenterology, 79:357, 1980.
233. Brandt, L. J., Bernstein, I. H., Boley, S. J., and Frank, M. S.: Metronidazole therapy for perineal Crohn's disease: a follow-up study. Gastroenterology, 83:383, 1982.
234. Duffy, L. F., et al.: Peripheral neuropathy in Crohn's disease patients treated with metronidazole. Gastroenterology, 88:681, 1985.
235. Rustia, M., and Shubik, P.: Induction of lung tumors and malignant lymphomas in mice by metronidazole. J. Natl. Cancer Inst., 48:721, 1972.
236. Speck, W. I., Stein, A. B., and Rosenkranz, H. S.: Mutagenicity of metronidazole: presence of several active metabolites in human urine. J. Natl. Cancer Inst., 56:283, 1976.
237. Beard, C. M., et al.: Lack of evidence for cancer due to metronidazole. N. Engl. J. Med., 301:519, 1979.
238. Mitelman, F., Stombeck, B., and Ursing, B.: No cytogenic effect of metronidazole (letter). Lancet, 1:1249, 1980.
239. Hatoff, D. E.: Perineal Crohn's disease complicated by pyogenic liver abscess during metronidazole therapy. Gastroenterology, 85:194, 1983.
240. Krook, et al.: Relation between concentrations of metronidazole and bacteroides spp in faeces of patients with Crohn's disease and healthy individuals. J. Clin. Path., 34:645, 1981.
241. Krook, A., Jarnerot, G., and Danielsson, D.: Clinical effect of metronidazole and sulfasalazine on Crohn's disease in relation to changes in fecal flora. Scand. J. Gastroenterol., 16:569, 1981.
242. Grove, D. I., Mahmond, A. A. F., and Warren, K. S.: Suppression of cell mediated community by metronidazole (abstract). Clin. Res., 24:285, 1976.
243. Lennard-Jones, J. E., and Singleton, J. W.: The azathioprine controversy. Dig. Dis. Sci., 26:364, 1981.
244. Korelitz, B. I.: The role of immunosuppressives. Mt. Sinai J. Med., 50:144, 1983.
245. Korelitz, B. I.: Pharmacotherapy of inflammatory bowel disease. Postgrad. Med., 74:165, 1983.
246. Lee, F. L., Murray, S. M., Prior, J., and Shreeve, D. R.: Primary liver cell cancer occurring in association with Crohn's disease treated with prednisolone and azathioprine. Hepatogastroenterology, 30:188, 1983.
247. Sturdevant, R. A. L., et al.: Azathioprine-related pancreatitis in patients with Crohn's disease. Gastroenterology, 77:883, 1979.
248. Steckman, M. L.: Treatment of Crohn's disease with mercaptopurine: What effects on fertility. (letter). N. Engl. J. Med., 303:817, 1980.
249. Anonymous: Azathioprine and 6-mercaptopurine for Crohn's disease. Lancet, 2:298, 1980.
250. Sachar, D. B., and Present, D. H.: Immunotherapy in inflammatory bowel disease. Med. Clin. N. Am., 62:173, 1978.
251. Blaker, F., and Schafer, K. H.: Immunosuppressive therapie unspezifischer enterocolitiden. Klin. Pediatr., 195:13, 1983.
252. Willoughby, J. M. T., et al.: Controlled trial of azathioprine in Crohn's disease. Lancet, 2:944, 1971.
253. Rhodes, J., et al.: Controlled trial of azathioprine in Crohn's disease. Lancet, 2:1273, 1971.
254. Watson, W. C., and Butovsky, M.: Azathioprine in management of Crohn's disease: a randomized cross-over study (abstract). Gastroenterology, 66:796, 1974.
255. Klein, M., et al.: Treatment of Crohn's disease with azathioprine: a controlled evaluation. Gastroenterology, 66:916, 1974.
256. Rosenberg, J. L., et al.: A controlled trial of azathioprine in Crohn's disease. Am. J. Dig. Dis., 20:721, 1975.
257. Present, D. H., et al.: Treatment of Crohn's disease with 6-mercaptopurine: A long-term, randomized, double-blind study. N. Engl. J. Med., 302:981, 1980.
258. O'Donoghue, D. P., et al.: Double-blind withdrawal trial of azathioprine as maintenance treatment for Crohn's disease. Lancet, 2:955, 1978.
259. Korelitz, B. I., and Present, D. H.: Favorable effect of 6-mercaptopurine on fistulae of Crohn's disease. Dig. Dis. Sci., 30:58, 1985.
260. Korelitz, B. I., and Present, D. H.: Shortcomings of the National Crohn's Disease Study: The exclusion of azathioprine without adequate trial (letter). Gastroenterology, 80:193, 1981.
261. Present, D., Meltzer, S. J., Wolke, A., and Korelitz, B. I.: Short and long term toxicity to 6-mercaptopurine in the management of inflammatory bowel disease. Gastroenterology, 88:1545, 1985.
262. Kinlen, L. J., Sheil, A. G. R., Peto, J., and Doll, R.: Collaborative United Kingdom-Australasian sudy of cancer in patients treated with immunosuppressive drugs. Br. Med. J., 2:1461, 1979.
263. Allison, M. C., and Pounder, R. E.: Cyclosporin for Crohn's disease (letter). Lancet, 1:902, 1984.
264. Bianchi, P. A., Mondelli, M., Quarto di Palo, F., and Ranzi, T.: Cyclosporin for Crohn's disease (letter). Lancet, 1:1241, 1984.
265. Cohen, D. J., et al.: Cyclosporine: A new immunosuppressive agent for organ transplantation. Ann. Intern. Med., 101:667, 1984.
266. Dannecker, G., Malchow, H., Niessen, K. H., and Ranke, M. B.: Morbus Crohn: erste erfahrungen mit Cyclosporin a bei einer Adoleszenten. Dtsch. Med. Wochenschr., 110:339, 1985.
267. Meyers, S., Sachar, D. B., Taub, R. N., and Janowitz, H. D.: Dinitrochlorobenzene (DNCB) in inflammatory bowel disease: family and postoperative studies. Gut, 19:249, 1978.
268. Burnham, W. R., et al.: Oral BCG vaccine in Crohn's disease. Gut, 20:299, 1979.
269. Rahban, S., et al.: BCG treatment of Crohn's disease. Am. J. Gastroenterol., 71:196, 1979.
270. Wesdorp, E., et al.: Levamisole in Crohn's disease. A double-blind controlled trial. Digestion, 18:186, 1978.
271. Vicary, F. R., Chambers, J. D., and Dhillon, P.: Double-blind trial of the use of transfer factor in the treatment of Crohn's disease. Gut, 20:408, 1979.
272. Seagal, A. W., Levi, A. J., and Loewi, G.: Levamisole in the treatment of Crohn's disease. Lancet, 2:382, 1977.
273. Swarbrick, E. T., and O'Donoghue, D. P.: Levamisole in Crohn's disease (letter). Lancet, 1:392, 1979.
274. Modigliani, R., et al.: Effect du levamisole sur la prevention des poussees evolutines de la maladie de Crohn quiescent: un essai prospectif multicentrique controle sur 155 malades. Gastroenterol. Clin. Biol., 7:683, 1983.
275. Vanhappen, G., Coremans, G., Billiau, A., and DeSomer, P.: Treatment of Crohn's disease with interferon. A preliminary clinical trial. Acta Clin. Belg., 35:238, 1980.
276. Williams, S. E., Grundman, M. J., Baker, R. D., and Turnberg, L. A.: A controlled trial of disodium cromoglycate in the treatment of Crohn's disease. Digestion, 20:395, 1980.
277. Binder, V., et al.: Disodium cromoglycate in the treatment of ulcerative colitis and Crohn's disease. Gut, 22:55, 1981.
278. Franchi, F., et al.: Insuccesso del disodiocromoglicato della terapia de 17 pazienti affetti da malattie infiam-

matorie croniche dell'intestino. Minerva Dietol. Gastroenterol., *28*:285, 1982.
279. Holdstock, G. E., Fisher, J. A., Hamblin, T. J., and Loehry, C.: Plasmapheresis in Crohn's disease. Digestion, *19*:197, 1979.
280. Skogh, M., Sundquist, T., and Tagesson, C.: Vitamin A in Crohn's disease (letter). Lancet, *1*:766, 1980.
281. Dvorak, A. M.: Vitamin A in Crohn's disease. Lancet, *1*:1303, 1980.
282. Wright, J. P., et al.: Vitamin A therapy in patients with Crohn's disease. Gastroenterology, *88*:512, 1985.
283. Wellman, W., and Schmidt, F. W.: Intestinal lavage in the treatment of Crohn's disease: a pilot study. Klin. Wochenschr., *60*:371, 1982.
284. Wellman, W., Fink, P. C., and Schmidt, F. W.: Whole-gut irrigation as antiendotoxinaemic therapy in inflammatory bowel disease. Hepatogastroenterology, *31*:91, 1984.
285. Emerit, J., Loeper, J., and Chomette, G.: Superoxide dismutase in the treatment of post-radiotherapeutic necrosis and of Crohn's disease. Bull. Eur. Physiopath. Resp., *17*:287, 1981.
286. Fitzgibbons, T. J., et al.: Management of Crohn's disease involving the duodenum including duodenal cutaneous fistula. Arch. Surg., *115*:1022, 1980.
287. Meyers, S., and Janowitz, H. D.: "Natural history" of Crohn's disease. An analytic review of the placebo lesson. Gastroenterology, *87*:1189, 1984.
288. Müller, J. M., Keller, H. W., Erasmi, H., and Pichlmaier, H.: Total parenteral nutrition as the sole therapy in Crohn's disease—a prospective study. Br. J. Surg., *70*:40, 1983.
289. Harvey, R. F., and Bradshaw, J. M.: A simple index of Crohn's disease activity. Lancet, *1*:514, 1980.
290. Meyers, S., et al.: Fecal alpha-1-antitrypsin measurement: an indicator of Crohn's disease activity. Gastroenterology, *89*:13, 1985.

23 · Medical Management of Inflammatory Bowel Disease in Children

BARBARA S. KIRSCHNER, M. D.

Children and adolescents constitute an important group of patients with chronic inflammatory bowel disease. Retrospective analysis of 844 patients with ulcerative colitis and 489 patients with Crohn's disease demonstrated that approximately 20% of each group had the onset of symptoms before 15 years of age.[1] Most children are diagnosed between the ages of 5- and 16-years-old; rarely, children under 2-years-old are affected.[2] Successful therapeutic intervention requires the physician to recognize the special needs of pediatric patients.

Approach to the Pediatric Patient

Other chapters in this text have described the multisystemic nature of both ulcerative colitis and Crohn's disease. Children, have to adapt not only to the unpredictability of recurrent gastrointestinal symptoms, but also to the complicating features of malaise, joint pain, disturbances in growth and sexual maturation, and absenteeism from school, all of which cause them to feel different from their peers.

Because only 20 to 25% of pediatric patients have a family history of inflammatory bowel disease, many children and their parents have no prior knowledge of these disorders. If the family history of inflammatory bowel disease is positive, parents often feel guilty for having passed it to their child. One must be available to discuss these concerns, often over a period of several visits. The disease process, tests, and procedures must be explained truthfully to the child or teenager, taking care to minimize discomfort. This can establish trust in the pediatric patient that may enhance cooperation with medical management.

The physician may need to be an advocate for the child or teenager if the parents are overly protective or restrictive in activities. Role models such as sports heroes or public figures (former President Eisenhower) can help encourage young patients to participate in outside activities as fully as tolerated. Physicians must recognize the importance of teachers in the life of pediatric patients with inflammatory bowel disease. Gym activities may need to be modified and bathroom privileges granted without attracting attention to the child during class.

Although general therapeutic approaches to childhood inflammatory bowel disease exist, periodic visits are necessary not only to assess disease activity and the response to medical management, but also to evaluate the effect of these illnesses on school attendance and peer and family relationships. The goals of therapy are the control of gastrointestinal symptoms and the restitution, as far as possible, of a feeling of well-being.

Large multicenter cooperative studies, such as the National Cooperative Crohn's Disease

Study, European Cooperative Crohn's Disease Study, and Swedish Cooperative study, have not been performed in children.[3-5] At the present time, however, no evidence exists to suggest that the response to medications differs between children and adults.

Ulcerative Colitis

Medical Management

MILD DISEASE. If ulcerative colitis is mildly active, children generally respond to sulfasalazine, which initially may be combined with a topical corticosteroid enema or foam. In order to minimize side effects, sulfasalazine is begun at approximately 25 to 40 mg/kg/day, and is increased to 75 mg/kg/day (maximum 4 g/day) if symptoms are not improved. Topical rectal preparations may be given at bedtime for 2 to 4 weeks as needed. At the onset of therapy, spicy foods and roughage (seeds, nuts, and popcorn) are avoided. Folic acid supplementation (1 mg/day) is recommended because of impaired folate absorption with sulfasalazine.

MODERATE DISEASE. When the frequency of abdominal cramping and diarrhea is greater than with mild disease, corticosteroid medications are indicated.[6] Depending upon the severity of the illness, these preparations are given either orally (as prednisone) or intravenously as methylprednisone or hydrocortisone. The usual pediatric dose is 1.0 to 2.0 mg/kg/day (prednisone equivalent). Sulfasalazine is initially withheld if oral intake is restricted because of potential gastrointestinal irritation. It should be noted that a few children have experienced worsening of bloody diarrhea after sulfasalazine.[7] Intravenous fluids may be necessary to decrease intestinal motility. Hematologic status (hemoglobin, hematocrit, white blood cell count with determination of the percent band forms) and serum albumin must be closely monitored.

Prednisone is initially administered on a daily basis (usually for 4 to 8 weeks) until cramping and hematochezia subside and proctoscopic or sigmoidoscopic evidence of improvement occurs. Prednisone is then gradually tapered every 1 to 2 weeks by 2.5 to 5.0 mg/day on the alternate day, until every other day prednisone therapy is achieved.[8] Doses of prednisone as high as 40 to 50 mg as a single morning dose every other day allow normal growth in children with ulcerative colitis.[8]

Although roughage (raw fruits and vegetables, seeds, nuts, and popcorn) is restricted during the early phase of treatment, it can be added to the diet as signs of disease activity improve. Clinically significant lactose intolerance should be specifically evaluated by inquiring about the presence of borborygmi, bloating, flatulence, or change in stools after the ingestion of milk or large amounts of dairy products. The likelihood of lactose malabsorption in IBD is greater in children whose ethnic group has a high prevalence of lactase deficiency.[9] Performance of the lactose breath hydrogen test or lactose tolerance test will help to determine whether it is necessary to limit dietary lactose. Because calories, protein, calcium, and phosphorus are important nutrients in growing children, dairy products should not be eliminated from the diet of pediatric patients without documenting intolerance. Commercially available lactase-hydrolyzed milk and hard cheeses (swiss, muenster, cheddar) are usually tolerated by these children.

Some pediatric gastroenterologists judiciously use antispasmodic agents, such as loperamide or diphenoxylate with atropine, to help control symptoms in patients with mild or moderate disease.[10] Other physicians rarely, if ever, prescribe these medications because of concern for inducing toxic megacolon. During school hours, small doses of these preparations (2 mg before school and at lunch time) may be useful in some patients to provide symptomatic relief.

Although newer drugs are currently undergoing clinical trials in adults with ulcerative colitis, no results have been published in children. These include 6-mercaptopurine,[11] tixocortal and oral and rectal 5-aminosalicylic acid.[14-15]

SEVERE DISEASE. Children with severe ulcerative colitis usually have pronounced abdominal tenderness, frequent bloody stools, anemia, fever, and hypoalbuminemia. Aggressive medical support is necessary and usually consists of nothing by mouth, intravenous fluids and corticosteroids (see previous section), often broad spectrum antibiotics, albumin infusions (1 g/kg/day), and packed red blood cells, if necessary. The abdomen must be observed frequently for distention, increased tenderness, or hypoactive bowel sounds. Abdominal roentgenograms are taken as indicated to exclude the development of toxic megacolon (see Chap. 14). The response to this comprehensive medical approach was reviewed in 14 children with severe ulcerative colitis and 5 children with severe Crohn's colitis.[16] Only 8 children improved; the response was evident within 12 days of the onset of medical therapy in most cases. Successful therapy occurred more often in those having their first attack of colitis (83% response) than in children who were previously treated (31% response). Unfortunately, relapse was common; only one of the eight who responded initially was doing well 24 months after hospitalization. Complications were greater in children who received medical therapy for more than 12 days, despite a lack of clinical response.

More favorable results were reported by Seashore et al.[17] These authors used total parenteral nutrition and intravenous steroids in eight children with severe ulcerative colitis. Four became asymptomatic in 7 to 20 days and four required surgical intervention. During the follow-up period, two of the four responders remained well and two required additional therapy. The authors emphasized that they were unable to discern any specific clinical or laboratory features that helped to predict who would respond to this form of therapy.

Surgical Intervention.*

Although the emphasis of this chapter concerns the medical treatment of inflammatory bowel disease in children, surgical treatment is indicated at times. Some of the indications are similar to those for adults, and they include hemorrhage, suspected perforation or abscess, and toxic megacolon unresponsive to medical therapy. In addition, intractable disease, necessitating high doses of corticosteroids daily and resultant growth failure, is another reason to recommend surgical intervention.[18]

Interestingly, the frequency of colectomy in children with ulcerative colitis has decreased significantly during the last two decades. Michener et al. reported that 48.9% of children with ulcerative colitis underwent colectomy during the period of 1955 to 1965, but only 26.2% had this procedure performed from 1965 to 1974.[19] This change is undoubtedly a reflection of the availability of improved medical therapy and the use of colonoscopy rather than "prophylactic colectomy" for cancer surveillance. In a review of 336 patients with ulcerative colitis diagnosed prior to 21 years of age, 9 developed adenocarcinoma of the colon at least 11 years after the diagnosis of ulcerative colitis. Similarly, in the review by Greenstein of 279 patients with ulcerative colitis, no colon cancer was observed prior to 10 years after the initial diagnosis (see also Chap. 15).[20]

When surgical treatment is indicated, the standard procedure has been total colectomy with ileostomy. Alternative procedures that are now available are often requested by teenagers. Techniques continue to be modified as improvements in results are sought. The continent ileostomy (Kock pouch) and other reservoir procedures are discussed elsewhere in this text (see Chap. 29). Some reviews describe the results of total colectomy with rectal mucosectomy and ileoanal anastomosis in children.[21-23] The frequency of patient satisfaction and risk of complications continue to be evaluated,† but rectal continence and gradual decrease in stool frequency appear to occur in most patients.

Crohn's Disease

The treatment of Crohn's disease must be individualized, based upon the relative severity of symptoms and any accompanying extraintestinal manifestations. In children, the approach to intervention must include not only control of gastrointestinal complaints but also an ongoing assessment of linear growth and weight gain, dietary intake, intensity of arthralgias and arthritis, malaise, and frequency of school absences.

Medical Treatment

No evidence has been found to suggest that children or adolescents with Crohn's disease will respond differently to available medications than adult patients. The National Cooperative Crohn's Disease Study (NCCDS) excluded patients under 15 years and the European Cooperative Crohn's Disease Study limited enrollees to those over 18 years, however.[3-4] These studies demonstrated that prednisone induced remissions more rapidly and consistently than sulfasalazine. Although sulfasalazine was effective in Crohn's colitis, it was often ineffective when Crohn's disease was limited to the small bowel. Some patients with small bowel involvement do improve with sulfasalazine, however, including those with growth failure.[5,24] This drug usually is used in combination with prednisone or methylprednisolone.

*See Chapters 25 to 27.

†Editor's note: See also, Berry R., et al. Postoperative development of Crohn's disease (CD) in young patients undergoing the rectal pull-through procedure for ulcerative colitis (UC). Gastroenterology 92; 1315, 1987.

CORTICOSTEROIDS. Corticosteroid medications are frequently effective in Crohn's disease, with 76% of adult patients achieving improvement or remission within 8 weeks.[3] Because of the well known growth suppression that often follows daily administration of corticosteroids in children, alternate-day regimens are used whenever possible in pediatric patients.[8,25] In general, prednisone or its equivalent is given in a dose of 1.0 to 1.5 mg/kg/day until disease activity diminishes. Initially, the drug may be given in divided doses, but later as a single morning dose. In approximately 4 to 8 weeks, the dosage is lowered on the alternate morning by 2.5 to 5.0 mg/week.

It should be understood by physicians and explained to parents that linear growth is usually normal on the alternate-day regimen, if the disease is relatively quiescent.[7,25] Studies of growth hormone secretion in 14 children who were treated with a single dose of prednisone on alternate days were similar to normal children.[26] Cortisol secretion was suppressed on the day of glucocorticoid therapy, but normal on the following day. The undesirable cosmetic side effects of glucocorticoid therapy (round facies, acne) also regress after 1 to 2 months of alternate day treatment.

Once clinical remission has been achieved, it is unclear whether the alternate-day therapy should be continued or gradually tapered. Patients often have a recurrence of clinical symptoms and an elevation of the sedimentation rate when the dose is lowered below a certain level. Thus, although several studies, including the cooperative studies, indicate that corticosteroids are not useful in quiescent disease,[3,4,27] they may be helpful in preventing increases in disease activity in low-grade, chronically active disease. Therefore, in practice, some pediatric gastroenterologists continue alternate-day prednisone therapy in an attempt to suppress chronically active symptoms, at least while the potential for continuing linear growth is present.[24,25,28] For patients with anal disease, topical therapy with corticosteroid foam or enemas may be useful in alleviating the need for daily systemic therapy.

SULFASALAZINE AND NEWER DERIVATIVE MEDICATIONS. Sulfasalazine is particularly useful in children with Crohn's disease because of its potential for decreasing the corticosteroid dose. Although the drug is most effective in colonic or ileocolonic disease, it can diminish symptoms in some patients with small bowel disease.[5,24] The usual dose is 50 to 75 mg/kg in 2 to 4 doses per day, although smaller dosages are often effective and should be tried if side effects, such as headaches occur. In one study of 67 pediatric patients with Crohn's disease using sulfasalazine, 2.5% developed hemolytic anemia, and 15% demonstrated pruritic dermatitis. Headaches are not uncommon and can be improved by starting at a lower dose and gradually increasing to the recommended level.

Newer preparations, such as 5-aminosalicylic acid taken orally, appear to be as effective as sulfasalazine in active Crohn's disease and are accompanied by fewer side effects.[14,29] The dimer azodisalicylate has been used in a small number of patients with medically refractory disease with some success. The future role of these medications will need to await the results of on-going investigations.

METRONIDAZOLE. Perianal complications may respond to therapy with metronidazole.[30] The frequency of peripheral neuropathy in 13 pediatric patients who received this medication for 4 to 11 months was assessed by neurologic examination and nerve conduction studies.[31] Sensory peripheral neuropathy was detected by these methods in 11 of the 13 children (85%), although only 6 of them were symptomatic. When the drug was discontinued, complete resolution or improvement occurred in 8 of 9 patients evaluated 5 to 13 months later.

6-MERCAPTOPURINE AND AZATHIOPRINE. The effectiveness of 6-mercaptopurine (6-MP) in adult patients with Crohn's disease has prompted its use in pediatric patients with complicated disease.[32] Although toxicity appears to be infrequent, the long-term malignant potential for malignancy is not certain.[11] Therefore, the indications for the use of these drugs should include steroid dependency and medical intractability (particularly with no focally resectable disease). We tend to restrict its use to patients with extensive disease, particularly those with previous intestinal resection. The recommended dose of 6-MP is 1.5 mg/kg/day. Patients must be monitored for leukopenia.

Limited "anecdotal" experience suggests that additional immunosuppressive medications, such as cyclosporine, may be useful in severe cases of Crohn's disease.[33-34] Further studies are needed, however, to determine the indications (if any) for using this drug in children with inflammatory bowel disease.*

---

*Editor's note: See, Parrott, H. R., et al. Treatment of Crohn's disease with cyclosporin-A: A report of 11 cases. Gut 27; A1277, 1986. The drug appeared to be of low efficacy in this group of adults with active disease. However, Peltekian K.M. et al., Gastroenterology 92: 1571, 1987, favor its use.

ENTERIC INFECTIONS. The potential role of enteric infectious agents to precipitate relapses in patients with IBD must be considered when a patient suffers a sudden increase in gastrointestinal symptoms. Salmonella, shigella, and campylobacter may produce signs and symptoms suggestive of increased disease activity.

Clostridium difficile cytopathic toxin was reported to occur in the stool in up to 19% of patients with chronic IBD, including a few patients with no history of antibiotic exposure.[35] The toxin was not found in any of 25 patients classified as having mild disease but was present in 2 of 19 with moderate disease and 9 of 15 with severe disease. Prompt improvement in clinical signs and symptoms occurred within 72 hours in 5 of 8 patients treated with vancomycin, 250 mg orally 4 times daily for 10 days. Other groups have not observed any relationship between the presence of C. difficile toxin and the severity of the IBD.[36] The diarrheal symptoms of children with C. difficile toxin who do not have inflammatory bowel disease often resolve spontaneously without specific therapy.[37] It is my opinion, however, that the child with moderate or severe IBD and toxin-positive stools should receive vancomycin therapy, 0.5 to 2.0 g/day for 10 to 14 days,[38] or metronidazole 20 mg/kg/day (maximum of 1.5 g/day).[39]*

Parents frequently inquire whether viral infections will cause a recurrence of active disease. The study by Gebhard et al. demonstrated that most relapses of IBD were not accompanied by a rise in serologic titer or stool antigen for rotavirus, Norwalk agent, or adenovirus.[40] In the few cases where these viruses were found (8 of 77 patients), however, symptoms of relapse occurred and lasted much longer than would have been expected from viral enteritis alone. Grill observed that rotavirus infection in a child with an ileostomy was associated with large fluid losses and hyponatremia.[41]

DISEASE ACTIVITY INDICES. As mentioned elsewhere (see Chaps. 9, 22, and 33), a number of clinical scoring systems have been proposed to quantitate disease activity to evaluate changes in an individual's course as well as for use in cooperative clinical trials. The indices derived from adult populations are not entirely applicable to pediatric patients, however, because they require weekly diaries, do not include growth failure, include measurement of the usage of antidiarrheal agents that are used less frequently in children, and are based in part on higher hematocrit levels than are normal for young children.[42] The rating systems suggested by pediatric investigators include a subjective Disease Activity Rating (from I to VI) that is based predominantly upon severity of symptoms,[25] a Disease Activity Score (from 0 to 11) determined by physical signs and selected laboratory tests,[43] and the Lloyd-Still-Green Clinical Scoring System, which is the most comprehensive and includes an assessment of general activity, physical findings, height and weight changes, and laboratory tests.[44] Each study found good correlation between the more cumbersome clinical scores and simpler subjective ratings. Thus, the role of activity indices in the routine management of children with inflammatory bowel disease remains to be determined.

Nutritional Intervention

The importance of nutritional assessment† and support has been highlighted by studies of the etiology of growth failure. Although the general tenets of nutritional support pertain both to ulcerative colitis and Crohn's disease, the availability of curative surgical therapy for intractable disease in the ulcerative colitis group has resulted in most clinical studies having a preponderance of patients with Crohn's disease. Growth failure is frequently reversed by augmenting caloric intake, whether by enteral or parenteral means, which has prompted much investigation into the role of nutritional support in Crohn's disease (see also Chap. 24).[24,45-52]

GROWTH FAILURE AND DELAYED PUBERTY. Impaired linear growth is more common in Crohn's disease than in ulcerative colitis. It occurs in approximately 35% of all pediatric patients and perhaps as many as 85% of all prepubertal patients with Crohn's disease.[25,46,53,54] By comparison, most studies indicate that only 6 to 12% of children with ulcerative colitis have growth failure prior to corticosteroid therapy.[46]

Because children (prior to sexual maturation) usually grow at least 5 cm/year,[55] rates under this level should be investigated for factors that may be suppressing growth. These include chronic undernutrition or prolonged daily corticosteroid therapy. Sequential records of height and weight are necessary for pediatric patients with inflammatory bowel disease. Standardized growth charts have been prepared by the National Center for Health Statistics

---

* Editor's note: See also, Bartlett, J. G. Treatment of clostridium difficile colitis. Gastroenterology 89; 1192, 1985. Major problems with vancomycin therapy are relapses and cost.

† Editor's note: See also, Dionigi, R., et al. Diagnosing malnutrition. Gut, 27(S1): 5, 1986.

(NCHS).[56] Plotting the current height and weight percentile against previous levels will clarify if the child is showing growth failure (by crossing height percentile lines) or is genetically short (persistently below the fifth percentile, but growing at a normal rate).

Estimating skeletal age by using a wrist film will document the delay in skeletal maturation that is often seen in these children.[57] The same film can be used to estimate growth potential (predicted adult stature).[58] Delayed or arrested pubertal development usually accompanies impaired linear growth; therefore, pubertal maturation should be assessed to determine whether delay is present. Pubertal staging is based upon the character, amount, and distribution of pubertal hair, as well as breast contour in girls and testicular size in boys. The most frequently used criteria are those of Tanner.[59,60] Guidelines for assessing anthropometric and nutritional status with disease activity are listed in Table 23-1.

METHODS OF NUTRITIONAL SUPPORT. The indications for nutritional intervention are described elsewhere in this text (see Chap. 24). Therefore, this discussion will review therapeutic approaches that have been useful in controlling disease activity and reversing the growth failure in pediatric patients.

TABLE 23-1. *Assessment of Disease Activity, Anthropometry and Nutritional Status in Children with Chronic Inflammatory Bowel Disease.*

Disease Activity
  Gastrointestinal symptoms: frequency and severity
  Physical signs of gastrointestinal disease: abdominal tenderness, mass, fistula
  Extraintestinal disease: fever, arthritis/arthralgia, anemia
  Laboratory tests: erythrocyte sedimentation rate or
      C-reactive protein
      CBC with differential count
      stool hemoccult
      fecal α_1-antitrypsin, if available[43,68]
Anthropometry
  Weight and height percentiles: (NCHS)[56]
  Arm anthropometry: skinfold, muscle area[67]
  Pubertal stage[59,60]
  Bone age (if growth impairment)[57]
Nutritional status
  Dietary intake evaluation[64]
  Total protein, albumin
  RBC indices: iron/iron binding capacity,
      folate and vitamin B_{12} as indicated
  Plasma zinc in growth-impaired patients

Following the pioneer work in total parenteral nutrition (TPN) by Dudrick,[61-62] its application to decreasing the symptoms of active Crohn's disease in children was described.[63] In 1976, Layden et al. reported that parenteral nutritional support reversed growth impairment in four adolescents with Crohn's disease.[45] Keits later substantiated this observation in hospitalized children,[47] as did Strobel, who extended the hospital care to home total parenteral nutrition (TPN).[48]

Although intravenous nutritional support is clearly effective in decreasing disease activity and promoting growth, similar results have been demonstrated using enteral nutrition.† We reported that medical management and supplementation with liquid formulas that raised the daily caloric intake from 54 to 91% of the Recommended Daily Allowance (RDA) were sufficient to improve growth velocity and achieve pre-illness height percentile in 7 adolescents with Crohn's disease.[24,64] These supplements provided an additional 600 to 1200 kcal above the dietary intake and were usually employed for approximately the first 3 months of treatment. For patients who are unable to tolerate this regimen, continuous nasogastric infusion of elemental formulas can be effective.[49-52] Older children can be taught to pass soft 5 to 8 Fr feeding tubes for this purpose. To date, no studies have used gastrostomy or jejunostomy feedings specifically to improve growth in children with IBD.

RECOMMENDATIONS. Recommendations regarding caloric and protein intake used in the studies discussed in the previous section are summarized in Table 23-2. It should be noted that caloric recommendations on a per kilogram basis at the onset of therapy are much higher than for healthy children, because these children have usually lost weight. It has not been documented that the daily caloric requirements (based on height and age) are higher than for normal children, however. In the few instances where basal metabolic rates were measured, they were not greater than those observed in normal children.[47]

Recommendations for protein intake follow the guidelines for calories (Table 23-2); protein intake in most studies has been similar to that of healthy children and protein catabolism has not been found to be greater than for healthy controls.[50,65] Because enhanced enteric protein loss

Heatley, R. V. Assessing nutritional state in inflammatory bowel disease. Gut *27(S1)*: 61, 1986.

TABLE 23-2. *Daily Calorie and Protein Intakes That Successfully Reverse Growth Failure in Crohn's Disease.*

Reference	Calorie Intake	Protein Intake	Route of Administration
Layden[45]	75 kcal/kg	1.66 g/kg	IV
Kelts[47]	95 kcal/kg	not specified	IV
Strobel[48]	60 to 80 kcal/kg	not specified	IV
Kirschner[24]	2200 to 3000 kcal*	50 to 60 g	PO
Motil[51]	93 kcal/kg	3.5 g/kg	PO + NG
O'Morain[50]	50 to 75 kcal/kg	50 to 75 g	NG
Navarro[52]	130 to 150% R. D. A.	2.5 to 3.0 g/kg	NG

*Adapted from National Research Council: Recommended Daily Allowance. Washington, D. C., National Academy of Sciences, 1980.

frequently occurs in these children, however,[24,43,45,48,66] it is important to monitor protein status with regard to visceral proteins (albumin, prealbumin) and somatic protein (arm muscle circumference or the area calculated by anthropometry).[67] Some studies have shown that enteric protein loss can be estimated by measuring fecal α_1-antitrypsin (A-1AT) concentrations.[43,68] Either random specimens or 72-hour stool collections can be used to determine A-1AT levels and intestinal clearance. Concentrations correlate well with serum albumin levels and the extent of small bowel disease, but not with disease activity. Some authors have suggested that an increase in enteric protein loss may precede and predict clinical relapse.[48]

Iron deficiency anemia is common in children with IBD and is usually accompanied by microcytosis. Therapeutic doses (5 mg/kg/day) of oral iron are indicated when this complication is observed. Patients who do not respond to oral supplementation may require parenteral administration. Intravenous administration of iron dextran complex has been employed in selected patients.[69] Test doses are mandatory to decrease the risk of anaphylactic reactions.

An area of controversy is the role of zinc deficiency in contributing to the growth failure and delayed sexual maturation of children with inflammatory bowel disease. Solomons et al. reported that the average plasma zinc level was lower in growth-impaired than in normally-growing teenagers with Crohn's disease.[70] The two groups overlapped, however, possibly because of the strong correlation of the zinc concentration with the level of serum albumin. McClain found low serum zinc concentrations in 40% of patients with Crohn's disease, including five adolescents with growth failure.[71] Subsequently, Nishi et al. observed that 7 of 14 children with growth failure had low plasma zinc levels (less than 0.7 μg/ml), but so did 3 of 7 with normal height.[72] Therefore, the possibility of zinc deficiency must be considered, and supplementation with oral zinc sulfate or chloride (200 mg/day) undertaken if blood levels are low.

Mineral imbalance involving calcium, magnesium, and phosphorus may be present in older children with IBD. Large intravenous magnesium requirements were noted in a 14-year-old boy with Crohn's disease who developed seizures associated with a serum magnesium of 0.9 mg/dl.[73] Motil et al. studied 6 growth-retarded adolescents with Crohn's disease before and after oral nutritional therapy.[74] The patients were in negative magnesium balance prior to nutritional support. Calcium, phosphorus, and nitrogen balance were positive at the onset, but retention improved with treatment. Urinary phosphorus fell, however, suggesting enhanced renal conservation of phosphorus, perhaps because of increased use of intermediates in energy metabolism or tissue repletion. Thus, these mineral levels should be monitored in children with active inflammatory bowel disease.

NUTRITION AND GROWTH-PROMOTING HORMONES. The mechanism(s) by which nutritional support contributes to the reversal of growth suppression is uncertain. Growth hormone levels are normal in most growth-impaired children with IBD, whether fasting or after measurements following provocative tests.[75,76] The growth promoting activity of growth hormone is mediated through peptides called somatomedins. Circulating somatomedin levels are modulated by nutrient intake, falling with fasting or undernutrition, and rising with refeeding.[77] We have shown that somatomedin-C levels are low in poorly-growing children with IBD, and rise with nutritional support in those who show improved growth.[78] Further study is necessary before recommending routine measurements of this hormone in children with IBD. The pubertal growth spurt occurs in response to sex hormones. Gonadotrophins are also modulated by nutrient status. This is reflected by the delay in sexual maturation that frequently accompanies impaired linear growth, and by the secondary amenorrhea that follows significant weight loss. Whether growth impairment is caused by alterations in the levels of these hormones resulting from chronic undernutrition is under investigation.

In order for normal growth to occur, disease activity and nutritional intake must be adequate for a prolonged period of time, until skeletal maturation is complete. At different times, an individual child may require a change in therapy such as hospital or home TPN, a trial of 6-mercaptopurine, or metronidazole, or intestinal resection to achieve these goals.

Surgical Intervention

Surgical treatment may be indicated for Crohn's disease with growth failure if a localized area of resectable disease is present, but its success in reversing growth failure has been variable. Wesson et al. reported that 10 of 15 children demonstrated improved growth following surgical intervention.[79] Despite gains in height, Homer et al. observed that only 2 of 11 prepubertal children with Crohn's disease demonstrated an increase in height percentile following bowel resection.[80] These two patients were not only prepubertal (and thus had sufficient time to allow for growth) but also free of disease recurrence for more than two years. Limited information exists to suggest that patients who receive preoperative TPN may have a greater growth response following intestinal resection than those who do not receive it.[81] An assessment of skeletal age combined with an estimation of growth potential may provide a more accurate prediction of the expected growth response to therapy than has been previously reported.[58]

The care of children and adolescents with chronic inflammatory bowel disease must not only take into account medical control of gastrointestinal and extraintestinal symptoms, but also be aware of the normal growth and progression of puberty. The importance of nutritional support in impairment in these areas has been established. The impact of the disease on family and peer relationships and school attendance form an integral part of the overall treatment of this age group.

References

1. Rogers, B. H. G., Clark, L. M., and Kirsner, J. B.: The epidemiologic and demographic characteristics of inflammatory bowel disease: An analysis of a computerized file of 1400 patients. J. Chronic Dis., 24:743, 1971.
2. Gryboski, J. D., and Spiro, H. M.: Prognosis in children with Crohn's disease. Gastroenterology, 74:807, 1978.
3. Summers, R. W., et al.: National Cooperative Crohn's Disease Study: Results of drug treatment. Gastroenterology, 77:847, 1979.
4. Malchow, H., et al.: European Cooperative Crohn's Disease Study (ECCDS): Results of drug treatment. Gastroenterology, 86:249, 1984.
5. Ursing, B., et al.: A comparative study of metronidazole and sulfasalazine for active Crohn's disease: The cooperative Crohn's disease study in Sweden. II Result. Gastroenterology, 83:550, 1982.
6. Truelove, S. C., Watkinson, G., and Draper, G.: Comparison of corticosteroid and sulfasalazine therapy in ulcerative colitis. Br. Med. J., 2:1708, 1962.
7. Werlin, S. L., and Grand, R. J.: Bloody diarrhea—a new complication of sulfasalazine. J. Pediatr., 92:450, 1978.
8. Sadeghi-Nejad, A., and Senior, B.: The treatment of ulcerative colitis in children with alternate-day corticosteroids. Pediatrics, 43:840, 1968.
9. Kirschner, B. S., DeFavaro, M. V., and Jensen, W.: Lactose malabsorption in children and adolescents with inflammatory bowel disease. Gastroenterology, 81:829, 1981.
10. Galambos, J. T., Hersh, T., Schroder, S., and Wenger, J.: Loperamide: A new antidiarrheal agent in the treatment of chronic diarrhea. Gastroenterology, 70:1026, 1976.
11. Present, D. H., Meltzer, S. J., Wolke, A., and Korelitz, B. I.: Short and long-term toxicity to 6-mercaptopurine in the management of inflammatory bowel disease. Program of the Second International Symposium on Inflammatory Bowel Disease, Jerusalem, Israel, 1985.
12. Larochele, P., et al.: Tixocortal pivalate, a corticosteroid with no systemic glucocorticoid effect after oral, intrarectal and intranasal application. Clin. Pharmacol. Ther., 33:343, 1983.
13. Willoughby, C. P., et al.: Distribution and metabolism in healthy volunteers of disodium azodisalicylate, a potential therapeutic agent for ulcerative colitis. Gut, 23:1081, 1982.
14. Klotz, U., et al.: Oral treatment of inflammatory bowel disease with 5-aminosalicylic acid (5-ASA): Its clinical pharmacokinetics and therapeutic efficacy. Program of the Second International Symposium on Inflammatory Bowel Disease, Jerusalem, Israel, 1985.
15. Campieri, M., et al.: Treatment of ulcerative colitis with high-dose 5-aminosalicylic acid enemas. Lancet, 2:270, 1981.
16. Werlin, S. L., and Grand, R. J.: Severe colitis in children and adolescents: diagnosis, course, and treatment. Gastroenterology, 73:828, 1977.
17. Seashore, J. H., Hillemeier, A. C., and Gryboski, J. D.: Total parenteral nutrition in the management of inflammatory bowel disease in children: A limited role. Am. J. Surg., 143:504, 1982.
18. Berger, M., Gribetz, K., and Kopel, F. B.: Growth retardation in children with ulcerative colitis: the effect of medical and surgical therapy. Pediatrics, 55:459, 1975.
19. Michener, W. M., Farmer, R. G., and Mortimer, E. A.: Long-term prognosis of ulcerative colitis with onset in childhood or adolescence. Clin. Gastroenterol., 1:301, 1979.

20. Greenstein, A. J., et al.: Cancer in universal and left-sided ulcerative colitis: Factors determining risk. Gastroenterology, 77:290, 1979.
21. Fonkalsrud, E. W., Ament, M. E., and Byrne, W. J.: Clinical experience with total colectomy and endorectal mucosal resection for inflammatory bowel disease. Gastroenterology, 77:16, 1979.
22. Telander, R. L., and Perrault, J.: Total colectomy with rectal mucosectomy and ileoanal anastomosis for chronic ulcerative colitis in children and young adults. Mayo Clin. Proc., 55:420, 1980.
23. Perrault, J., and Telander, R.: Rectal mucosectomy and ileo-anal anastomosis (RMIAA) in young patients. Pediatr. Res., 18:208A, 1984.
24. Kirschner, B. S., et al.: Reversal of growth retardation in Crohn's disease with therapy emphasizing oral nutritional restitution. Gastroenterology, 80:10, 1981.
25. Whittington, P. F., Barns, H. V., and Bayless, T. M.: Medical management of Crohn's disease in adolescence. Gastroenterology, 72:1338, 1977.
26. Sadeghi-Nejad, A., and Senior, B.: Adrenal function, growth, and insulin in patients treated with corticoids on alternate days. Pediatrics, 43:277, 1969.
27. Smith, R. C., et al.: Low dose steroids and clinical relapse in Crohn's disease: A controlled trial. Gut, 19:606, 1978.
28. Silverman, A., and Roy, C. C.: Pediatric Clinical Gastroenterology. 3rd Ed. St. Louis, C. V. Mosby, 1983.
29. Rasmussen, S. N., et al.: Treatment of Crohn's disease with peroral 5-aminosalicylic acid. Gastroenterology, 85:1350, 1983.
30. Bernstein, L. H., Frank, M. S., Brandt, L. J., and Boley, S. J.: Healing of perineal Crohn's disease with metronidazole. Gastroenterology, 79:357, 1980.
31. Duffy, L. F., et al.: Peripheral neuropathy in Crohn's disease patients treated with metronidazole. Gastroenterology, 88:681, 1985.
32. Present, D. H., et al.: Treatment of Crohn's disease with 6-mercaptopurine. N. Engl. J. Med., 302:981, 1980.
33. Allison, M. C., and Pounder, R. E.: Cyclosporin for Crohn's disease. Lancet, 1:902, 1984.
34. Bianchi, P. A., Mondelli, M., Quarto di Palo, F., and Ranzi, T.: Cyclosporin for Crohn's disease. Lancet, 1:1242, 1984.
35. Trnka, Y. M., and LaMont, J. T.: Association of Clostridium difficile toxin with symptomatic relapse of chronic inflammatory bowel disease. Gastroenterology, 80:693, 1981.
36. Meyers, S., et al.: Occurrence of Clostridium difficile toxin during the course of inflammatory bowel disease. Gastroenterology, 80:697, 1981.
37. Thompson, C. M., Gilligan, P. H., Fisher, M. C., and Long, S. S.: Clostridium difficile cytotoxin in a pediatric population. Am. J. Dis. Child., 137:271, 1983.
38. Viscidi, R. P., and Bartlett, J. G.: Antibiotic-associated pseudomembranous colitis in children. Pediatrics, 67:381, 1981.
39. Cherry, R. D., et al.: Metronidazole: An alternate therapy for antibiotic-associated colitis. Gastroenterology, 82:849, 1982.
40. Gebhard, R. L., et al.: Acute viral enteritis and exacerbations of inflammatory bowel disease. Gastroenterology, 83:1207, 1982.
41. Grill, B. B., Andiman, W. A., and Gryboski, J. D.: Rotavirus-induced electrolyte losses in a patient with ileostomy. Am. J. Dis. Child., 137:1127, 1983.
42. Best, W. R., Becktel, J. M., Singleton, J. W., and Kern, F.: Development of a Crohn's disease activity index. National cooperative Crohn's Disease Study. Gastroenterology, 70:439, 1976.
43. Thomas, D. W., Sinatra, F. R., and Merritt, R. J.: Fecal α_1-antitrypsin excretion in young people with Crohn's disease. J. Pediatr. Gastroenterol. Nutr., 2:491, 1983.
44. Lloyd-Still, J. D., and Green, O. C.: A clinical scoring system for chronic inflammatory bowel disease in children. Dig. Dis. Sci., 24:620, 1979.
45. Layden, T., et al.: Reversal of growth arrest in adolescents with Crohn's disease after parenteral alimentation. Gastroenterology, 70:1017, 1976.
46. Kirschner, B. S., Voinchet, O., and Rosenberg, I. H.: Growth retardation in children with inflammatory bowel disease. Gastroenterology, 75:504, 1978.
47. Kelts, D. G., et al.: Nutritional basis of growth failure in children and adolescents with Crohn's disease. Gastroenterology, 76:720, 1979.
48. Strobel, C. T., Byrne, W. J., and Ament, M. E.: Home parenteral nutrition in children with Crohn's disease: An effective management alternative. Gastroenterology, 77:272, 1979.
49. Morin, C. L., Roulet, M., Roy, C. C., and Weber, A.: Continuous elemental enteral alimentation in children with Crohn's disease and growth failure. Gastroenterology, 79:1205, 1980.
50. O'Morain, C., Segal, A. W., and Levi, A. J.: Elemental diets in the treatment of acute Crohn's disease. Br. Med. J., 281:1173, 1980.
51. Motil, K. J., Grand, R. J., Maletskos, C. J., and Young, V. R.: The effect of disease, drug and diet on whole body protein metabolism in adolescents with Crohn's disease. J. Pediatr., 101:343, 1982.
52. Navarro, J., et al.: Prolonged constant rate elemental enteral nutrition in Crohn's disease. J. Pediatr. Gastroenterol. Nutr., 1:541, 1982.
53. Burbige, E. J., Huang, S. H., and Bayless, T. M.: Clinical manifestations of Crohn's disease in children and adolescents. Pediatrics, 55:866, 1975.
54. Kanof, M. D., and Bayless, T. M.: Decreased height velocity in Crohn's disease. Gastroenterology, 88:1437, 1985.
55. Tanner, J. M., and Davies, P. S. W.: Clinical longitudinal standards for height and height velocity for North American children. J. Pediatr., 107:317, 1985.
56. National Center for Health Statistics Percentiles. National Center for Health Statistics (NCHS), Hyattsville, Maryland, 1980.
57. Greulich, W. W., and Pyle, S. I.: Radiologic Atlas of Skeletal Development of the Hand and Wrist. 2nd Ed. Palo Alto, Stanford University Press, 1959.
58. Kirschner, B. S., et al.: Prediction of growth potential of children and adolescents with chronic inflammatory bowel disease. Gastroenterology, 86:1135, 1984.
59. Tanner, J. M.: Growth at Adolescence. 2nd Ed. Oxford, Blackwell Scientific Publications, 1962.
60. Behrman, R. E., and Vaughn, V. C. III: Nelson Textbook of Pediatrics. 12th Ed. Philadelphia, W. B. Saunders, 1983.
61. Dudrick, S. J., Wilmore, D. W., Vars, H. M., and Rhoads, J. E.: Long-term parenteral nutrition with growth development, and positive nitrogen balance. Surgery, 64:134, 1968.
62. Dudrick, S. J., Wilmore, D. W., Vars, H. M., and Rhoads, J. E.: Can intravenous feeding as the sole means of nutrition support growth in the child and restore weight loss in an adult? An affirmative answer. Ann. Surg., 169:974, 1969.
63. Cohen, M. I., et al.: The role and effect of parenteral nutri-

tion on the liver and its use in chronic inflammatory bowel disease in childhood. Adv. Exp. Med. Biol., 46:214, 1974.
64. National Research Council: Recommended Dietary Allowance. Washington, D. C., National Academy of Sciences, 1980.
65. Motil, K. J., et al.: Whole body leucine metabolism in adolescents with Crohn's disease and growth failure during nutritional supplementation. Gastroenterology, 82:1359, 1982.
66. Beeken, W. L.: Absorptive defects in young people with regional enteritis. Pediatrics, 52:69, 1973.
67. Frisancho, A. R.: New norms of upper limb fat and muscle areas for assessment of nutritional status. Am. J. Clin. Nutr., 34:2540, 1981.
68. Grill, B., Hillemeier, A. C., and Gryboski, J. D.: Fecal α_1-antitrypsin clearance in patients with inflammatory bowel disease. J. Pediatr. Gastroenterol. Nutr., 3:56, 1984.
69. Reed, M. D., Bertino, J. S., and Halpin, T. C.: Use of intravenous iron dextran injection in children receiving total parenteral nutrition. Am. J. Dis. Child., 135:829, 1981.
70. Solomons, N. W., Rosenberg, I. H., Sanstead, H. H., and Vo-Khactu, K. P.: Zinc deficiency in Crohn's disease. Digestion, 16:87, 1977.
71. McClain, C., Soutor, C., and Sieve, L.: Zinc deficiency: A complication of Crohn's disease. Gastroenterology, 78:272, 1980.
72. Nishi, Y., et al.: Zinc status and its relation to growth retardation in children with chronic inflammatory bowel disease. Am. J. Clin. Nutr., 33:2613, 1980.
73. Grand, R. J., and Colodny, A. H.: Increased requirement for magnesium during parenteral therapy for granulomatous colitis. J. Pediatr., 81:788, 1972.
74. Motil, K. J., Altchuler, S. I., and Grand, R. J.: Mineral balance during nutritional supplementation in adolescents with Crohn's disease and growth failure. J. Pediatr., 107:473, 1985.
75. Gotlin, R. W., and Dubois, R. S.: Nyctohemeral growth hormone levels in children with growth retardation and inflammatory bowel disease. Gut, 14:191, 1973.
76. Tenore, A., et al.: Basal and stimulated serum growth hormone concentrations in inflammatory bowel disease. J. Clin. Endocrinol. Metab., 44:622, 1977.
77. Phillips, L. S., and Young, H. S.: Nutrition and somatomedin. I. Effect of fasting and refeeding on serum somatomedin activity and cartilage growth activity in rats. Endocrinology, 99:304, 1976.
78. Kirschner, B. S., and Sutton, M. M.: Longitudinal studies of somatomedin-C (SM-C) in growth-retarded children with Crohn's disease (CD). Pediatr. Res., 18:202A, 1984.
79. Wesson, D. E., and Shandling, B.: Results of bowel resection for Crohn's disease in the young. J. Pediatr. Surg., 16:449, 1981.
80. Homer, D. R., Grand, R. J., and Colodny, A. H.: Growth, course, and prognosis after surgery for Crohn's disease in children and adolescents. Pediatrics, 59:717, 1977.
81. Lake, A. M., Kim, S., Mathis, R. K., and Walker, W. A.: Influence of preoperative parenteral alimentation on postoperative growth in adolescent Crohn's disease. J. Pediatr. Gastroenterol., 4:182, 1985.

24 · Nutritional Consequences and Therapy in Inflammatory Bowel Disease

KURSHEED N. JEEJEEBHOY, M.D.
MICHAEL J. OSTRO, M.D.

Malnutrition frequently occurs in patients with inflammatory bowel disease (IBD). It is important to be aware of this and its accompanying complications, because the potential problems associated with malnutrition may be even more debilitating than the underlying disease process. Unfortunately, until parenteral nutrition became available, it was difficult to treat malnutrition in these patients because of exacerbating intestinal symptoms and/or a limitation of the ability to eat an oral diet. The use of parenteral nutrition suggested clinically that refeeding with nutrients that bypassed the bowel seemed to reduce the activity of Crohn's disease, and certainly improved the nutritional well-being of the patient. The improvement in the activity of disease was attributed to bowel rest. Bowel rest is achieved by keeping the patient nil per os (NPO), in the belief that not feeding orally will reduce motility and secretion. Based on this concept, it was assumed that keeping patients with Crohn's disease NPO was important in improving disease activity. Recent evidence suggests that renourishment may be more important than bowel rest, however. This controversy will be discussed in the "Primary Therapy" section.

In this chapter, two main issues will be discussed. First, the genesis and treatment of malnutrition in inflammatory bowel disease (IBD), and second, the potential role of nutrition in improving disease activity (primary therapy).

Etiology of Malnutrition in Inflammatory Bowel Disease*

The malnutrition may be caused by a combination of factors listed in Table 24-1. First, patients with IBD often have decreased oral intake of food. This is frequently because of anorexia secondary to the presence of chronic inflammation, debility, depression, or side effects of medications. Nausea and vomiting may also contribute to decreased oral intake. In addition, a conditioned response to avoid eating may exist because eating precipitates unpleasant symptoms such as vomiting, abdominal pain, and diarrhea. Inadequate caloric intake is the most common cause of weight loss in patients with IBD.

Secondly, patients with IBD may have increased nutritional requirements. Fever, when present, can increase the basal metabolic rate by 12% for every degree centigrade that body temperature elevates. Ongoing active inflammation and stress, both physical and emotional, may also increase the basal metabolic rate via mechanisms that are not well known. In addition, increased nutrition may be required not only to correct the deficiencies, but also to promote growth in children and adolescents. Nutrition must always be considered when treating children and adolescents with IBD, because significant growth retardation can occur not only from the effects of the disease process and the use of

*See also Chapters 21, 22, and 23.

TABLE 24-1. *Causes of Malnutrition in Inflammatory Bowel Disease.*

Inadequate Intake of Nutriment
   Anorexia, nausea, vomiting
   Avoidance of unpleasant symptoms (nausea, vomiting, diarrhea, abdominal pain)
Increased Requirements
   Fever
   Physical and emotional stress
   Promotion of growth
   Active inflammation
   Repletion of stores
Decreased Absorption
   Decreased absorptive capacity
     previous bowel resections
     bypassed bowel
     inflammation of bowel
   Stagnant-loop syndrome
     stricture
     fistulae
     surgical blind loop
Excessive Gastrointestinal Losses
   Water and electrolytes
   Blood
   Trace elements
   Protein
   Bile salts
Miscellaneous
   Protein catabolism secondary to steroids
   Rapid intestinal transit time
   Toxic depression of metabolism caused by presence of active inflammation
   Effects of parenteral nutrition without adequate supplementation of trace elements, minerals, or vitamins

steroids, but also as a result of nutritional deficiencies.

Thirdly, absorption of nutrients may decrease because of the decreased absorptive capacity of the bowel (as a result of previous resections, bypassed bowel, and/or inflammation), bacterial overgrowth (caused by stricture, fistulae, or surgical intervention), or rapid intestinal transit time (the result of fistulae or short bowel syndrome).

Fourthly, excessive gastrointestinal losses of nutrients may occur. Fluid and electrolytes can be lost through vomiting, diarrhea, ostomy output, or exudation from intestinal mucosa. Protein, blood, bile salts, and trace elements can also be lost via these routes.

A negative nitrogen balance also may be caused by catabolic effects of drugs such as antibiotics and steroids, which are commonly used in patients with IBD. The presence of active inflammation may lead to toxic depression of the biosynthetic process. Finally, patients given parenteral nutrition without adequate supplementation can develop deficiency of trace elements, minerals, and vitamins.

Specific Deficiencies*

Aside from the deficits in both protein and calories resulting from the causes listed above, special mention of mineral losses and vitamin deficiencies is required, because failure to recognize and correct these losses and deficiencies can lead to serious consequences.

Electrolytes

SODIUM, POTASSIUM, AND CHLORIDE

Severe losses of fluid and electrolytes can occur as a result of diarrhea and/or vomiting. In addition, absorption of water and sodium may be impaired in patients with Crohn's disease.[1]

Significant potassium deficiency may develop even in the presence of a normal plasma level.[2] It usually occurs in those patients with chronic diarrhea. Potassium deficiency may account for nonspecific symptoms such as weakness, lassitude, and depression. Preoperative correction of body potassium has been shown to reduce the complication rate and mortality.[2]

Metals and Trace Elements

CALCIUM

Hypocalcemia commonly occurs in Crohn's disease,[3] usually in association with hypoalbuminemia, but when corrections are made for hypoalbuminemia, true hypocalcemia is rare.

Calcium deficiency may result from decreased intake and/or absorption of calcium or from secondary effects of vitamin D deficiency. Hypocalcemia with clinical tetany can occur secondary to hypomagnesemia,[4] which in turn reduces the ability of parathormone to mobilize bone calcium.

MAGNESIUM

Magnesium deficiency was not widely accepted as a complication of Crohn's disease until 1970, perhaps because the signs and symptoms of hypomagnesemia may have been mistaken for those of hypocalcemia. In 1970, Gerlach, Morowitz, and Kirsner described four patients

---
*See also Chapters 21, 22, and 23.

with symptomatic hypomagnesemia.[4] Relying on serum magnesium levels will lead to underdiagnosis of the condition. Beeken found hypomagnesemia in only 9 of 63 patients,[3] but Main et al. found that 15 of 17 patients admitted to the hospital with severe disease were magnesium deficient when serum and urine levels were used together as indicators of magnesium status.[5]

PHOSPHATE

Hypophosphatemia may occur as a result of insufficient intake and/or absorption. The deficiency syndrome can include muscular weakness, tremors, paraesthesiae, convulsions, and coma. In addition, phosphate,[6] magnesium,[7] and potassium[6] are essential for a positive nitrogen balance to occur. These elements are all driven intracellularly when anabolism occurs. If they are not supplied exogenously, deficiency develops despite intracellular stores.

Deficiencies of various trace elements can occur as a result of either decreased intake or excessive losses in diarrhea or ostomy fluid. In Crohn's disease specifically, zinc deficiency and malabsorption have been described.[8,9] In general, however, these deficiencies usually occur when total parenteral nutrition is given without supplementation of these elements. Zinc,[10] selenium,[11-14] chromium,[15] copper,[16] and molybdenum deficiency syndromes have been found in humans[17] and are described later in this chapter. Iron deficiency may occur in those with chronic occult blood loss, as well as those with overt bleeding.

Vitamins

Deficiency of fat-soluble vitamins (A, D, E, and K) may exist in any situation where steatorrhea is present. There are several causes for steatorrhea in association with IBD, but the two most common are inadequate absorption because of resection or severe inflammation, and reduced intestinal bile salt concentration which causes impaired micelle formation. Reduced intestinal bile salts can occur as a result of bacterial overgrowth or interruption of the enterohepatic circulation of bile salts caused by terminal ileal disease or resection.

Deficiency of water-soluble vitamins, especially C, B_{12}, and folate, may also complicate IBD. Vitamin C deficiency is most commonly a result of decreased intake. Vitamin B_{12} deficiency can occur as a result of extensive terminal ileal disease, resection, or bacterial overgrowth (secondary to intestinal stasis as with fistulae, strictures, or blind loops). Folate deficiency may be related to diffuse inflammation of the small bowel mucosa, extensive small bowel resection, or the use of sulfasalazine, which impairs folate absorption.

The clinical effects and daily requirements of these and other vitamins are discussed later in this chapter.

Physiologic Effects of Malnutrition

Malnutrition can lead to an increased incidence of infection and impaired healing of wounds. In addition, patients with Crohn's disease who are malnourished have been found to have higher activity indices.[18] Nutritional support may not only prevent or reverse the metabolic consequences of malnutrition,[19] but also result in an improved sense of well-being, improved wound healing,[20] and increased resistance to infection.[21] Hence, it is obvious that preventing or reversing malnutrition is the key to successful management of any patient with IBD.

Nutritional Assessment

To determine the need for nutritional support, some assessment of the patient's nutritional status must be made. One of the most widely accepted methods to do this is that of Blackburn et al.,[22] which combines anthropometric measurements with biochemical and hematologic measurements, as well as assessments of anergy and daily caloric intake, to generate a nutritional/metabolic profile.*

INTAKE IN RELATION TO NEEDS. Reduced intake and/or malabsorption are the primary abnormalities that instigate the development of malnutrition. Because prolonged malnutrition and wasting are difficult to correct, it is desirable to detect an imbalance between intake and needs before body composition is significantly altered. Based on this premise, patients should be assessed in regard to their ability to eat and absorb sufficient nutrients to meet their needs. A simple way of making such a judgment is to determine whether the caloric intake is adequate for their needs. In theory, a person should eat 20 to 30% more calories than their calculated resting metabolic rate. As will be shown later, this approach

---

*Editors' note: See also, Dionigi R., et al.: Gut. 27:5, 1986. Heatley R.V.: Gut. 27:61, 1986. Chan A.T.H., et al.: Gastroenterology 91:1986.

also applies to the critically ill patient. The resting metabolic rate can be calculated for the patient by the Harris-Benedict equation.[23] This equation can be easily worked out using a hand calculator at the bedside.

Metabolic Rate (kcal/24 hr):
Males = 66.5 + 13.75 weight (kg) + 5 height (cm) − 6.75 age (yrs)
Females = 655 + 9.56 weight (kg) + 1.8 height (cm) − 4.67 age (yrs)

To this figure, add 20 to 30% to compute a safe intake for the average patient. Add 12% for every degree of temperature above 37°C. If the patient is eating less than this figure, weight will ultimately be lost. The formula will not hold if the patient is malabsorbing. In addition, even if caloric intake is normal, selective losses or malabsorption can cause specific deficiencies. For example, hypomagnesemia, hypocalcemia, metabolic bone disease, and megaloblastic anemia can occur even if caloric absorption is sufficient to meet needs. In this context, we have shown that in patients with a short bowel, the caloric absorption can be assumed to be between 50 to 70% of intake, irrespective of the diet eaten (high fat or high carbohydrate). This statement applies to patients with between 40 and 80 cm of bowel remaining. This estimation will only be for the requirements of calories and protein, however, but not necessarily for electrolytes, divalent ions, trace elements, and water. Depending upon the severity of any existing diarrhea, those nutrients may need to be supplemented separately.*

Anthropometric Measurements

Weight loss below the 5th percentile of the normal range for height suggests malnutrition. Weight has to be taken in the context of the usual body habitus of the patient, however.

Skinfold thickness of the triceps and circumference of the arm muscle that are below the fifth percentile of the normal population suggests significant loss of fat and muscle, respectively. It should be recognized that up to 20% of the normal population may have one of the aforementioned parameters in the malnourished range without being malnourished. Thus, to consider a person as having lost a significant amount of body tissue, he should have a reduction in at least 2 out of the 3 parameters to below the fifth percentile (Table 24-2).

*Editors' note: See also, Ameen, V.Z., et al.: Gastroenterology 92:493, 1987.

TABLE 24-2. *Fifth Percentile of Weight, Triceps Skin-fold, and Arm Muscle Circumference for Adults of Medium Habitus.*

Sex	Age (years)	Height (cm)	Weight (kg)	AMC (cm)	TSF (mm)
Male	25-54	157	51	24.5	5.0
		160	52		
		165	59		
		170	62		
		175	63		
		180	64		
		185	70		
	55-74	157	50	22.5	50
		160	51		
		165	56		
		170	59		
		175	62		
		180	68		
		185	68		
Females	25-54	147	41	18.5	13.0
		150	47		
		155	47		
		160	49		
		165	52		
		170	54		
		175	58		
	55-74	147	39	18.6	11.5
		150	41		
		155	43		
		160	43		
		165	43		
		170	45		
		175	46		

Published with permission from Jeejeebhoy, K. N.: Nutrition in gastrointestinal diseases. Medicine International, 1985. Data adapted from Frisancho, R. A.: Am. J. Clin. Nutr., 40:808, 1984; and Bishop, C. W., et al.: Am. J. Clin. Nutr., 34:2530, 1981.

Plasma/Blood Chemistry†

HEMOGLOBIN AND BLOOD FILM. Abnormalities of these will indicate the presence of iron and/or folate and B_{12} deficiency. These deficiencies can be confirmed by the measurements of serum ferritin, folate, and B_{12}.

ELECTROLYTES, MG, CA, AND P. The plasma electrolyte levels can indicate a specific deficiency. Hypokalemia and a reduced bicarbonate level indicate potassium deficiency and base loss respectively. In patients with loss of fluids and electrolytes from a jejunostomy, however, the

†Editors' note: Ingensveek and Carpenter: Int. J. Vitam. Nutr. Res. 55:91, 1985; This study suggested that determinations of orosomucoid and C-reactive protein in sick patients provide a nutritional index and are prognostic indicators.

plasma electrolyte levels may be normal, as the fluid lost has an electrolyte composition close to that of plasma. Hypomagnesemia is a good index of magnesium deficiency and in patients with gastrointestinal disease hypomagnesemia (and, by inference, magnesium deficiency) is often associated with hypocalcemia. Hypocalcemia in these patients results from a functional hypoparathyroidism caused by magnesium deficiency. Thus hypocalcemia in such patients should not be treated simply by giving calcium, but by injecting 12.5 mmols of magnesium per day until the serum magnesium becomes normal.

PLASMA ALBUMIN. Although low plasma albumin is often taken to be a sign of protein deficiency, this is not true, because pure starvation in adults often does not result in hypoalbuminemia. By contrast, gastrointestinal protein loss because of inflammatory and other bowel diseases often causes hypoalbuminemia even when the patient is receiving enough protein. Hence, hypoalbuminemia is more likely to be caused by disease activity or overhydration than to malnutrition.

DELAYED CUTANEOUS HYPERSENSITIVITY. This is not a suitable way of judging the degree of malnutrition because it is altered by a variety of diseases, trauma, drugs, and infections.

SKELETAL MUSCLE FUNCTION. While still an investigational tool, it has been shown that muscle function is a sensitive and specific index of malnutrition. Furthermore, muscle power and contraction-relaxation characteristics return to normal with nutritional support before body composition is restored.[24]

Prevention and Treatment of Malnutrition*

The simplest way to combat malnutrition is to increase the oral intake of nutrients but this may not always be feasible, as severe anorexia, nausea, or vomiting may preclude the provision of nutrients orally. In these situations, other methods of delivering nutrients must be considered. If the gastrointestinal tract is able to absorb nutrients without aggravating symptoms such as abdominal pain and diarrhea, then enteral feeding can be used. When this is not possible, however, intravenous alimentation, delivered peripherally or centrally, must be considered.

*See also Chapters 21, 22, and 23.

Increased Oral Intake

Obviously increasing the oral intake of nutrients would be the simplest and safest way of providing nutritional support. The ideal product should have a high nutrient density, empty easily from the stomach, and not obstruct the bowel. These objectives are met by feeding dietary supplements that are low in fat, high in calorie density, and low in residue. If a modified oral diet, based on these principles and composed of foods that are usually consumed, cannot be tolerated, commercial formulas are available for nutritional supplementation. Each of these preparations contains approximately 100 to 120 cal/per 100 ml. Some contain lactose and should therefore be avoided in patients with lactose intolerance.

A major problem with these supplements is that the more the patient drinks, the less food he can eat, because they commonly result in early satiety. In patients who develop early satiety and cannot increase their total caloric intake adequately, it is necessary to provide caloric supplementation via a route that does not depend on voluntary ingestion. These are listed in Table 24-3.

Enteral Feeding of Defined Formula Diets

As pointed out earlier, several situations do not permit an increase in the voluntary oral intake of nutrients. These include severe anorexia, nausea or vomiting, painful intraoral or pharyngeal lesions, or debility so severe that the patient is too weak to eat. The latter will occur only with severe malnutrition or when another complicating illness is present. In all of these situations, other means of providing nutrition must be considered. The choice is between enteral nutrition using defined formula diets (DFD)'s, and parenteral nutrition.

To be able to use enteral nutrition, the gastrointestinal tract must be able to propel, absorb, and use the provided solutions without the precipitation of severe abdominal cramps or diar-

TABLE 24-3. *Routes Available for Administering Nutrition.*

Oral intake of food
Oral intake of supplemental formulas
Nasogastric or nasojejunal tube feedings
Gastrostomy or jejunostomy tube feedings
Parenteral nutrition—peripheral
     —central

rhea. Many preparations are currently available for enteral delivery and some of those in common use are listed in Table 24-4. These may be delivered via nasogastric or nasojejunal tubes, or via gastrostomy or jejunostomy tubes.* They contain specified amounts of amino acids, hexose sugars, essential fatty acids, vitamins, and minerals, and are absorbed in the upper gastrointestinal tract. Infusion of these solutions has been shown to reduce pancreatic and gastric secretions. Because they are composed of substances that are readily absorbed in the proximal small bowel, they may be used in patients with the short bowel syndrome.

Selection of Patients for Nutritional Support

Once it has been determined that nutritional support is required, one of the following options must be chosen:

1. Maintain the same oral diet or encourage the patient to eat more.
2. Supplement specific nutrients, such as iron, folic acid, vitamin B_{12}, potassium, or magnesium.
3. Feed the patient with artificial nutrient mixtures enterally (naso-gastrically or nasojejunally) or parenterally. These support regimens are chosen for patients unable to eat, absorb, or benefit from a normal diet.

The first of these is chosen when the patient is recognized as anorexic and can be encouraged to eat a normal diet. The second is required when specific micronutrient deficiencies occur that may require individual supplementation. In such patients, protein and calorie absorption is sufficient to meet needs. In the following situations, however, a normal diet is clearly not appropriate:

1. When massive bowel resection or extensive disease results in less than 40 cm of functional small bowel.
2. When chronic bowel obstruction is not amenable to surgical correction. This occurs in patients with extensive Crohn's disease, radiation enteritis, previous extensive peritonitis, or pseudo-obstruction syndrome. The latter may be primary or secondary to diseases such as systemic sclerosis.

3. In patients with associated total or subtotal gastric resection.
4. When severe associated pancreatic insufficiency exists.
5. In fistulous bowel disease, especially with associated malnutrition. In this case, loss of intestinal contents through a fistula or the inability to reduce fistula output on an oral diet makes it necessary to use parenteral nutrition.
6. Following total resection of the ileum and colon with an end-jejunostomy. These patients have lost the segment of bowel necessary to concentrate intestinal contents and eating results in losses of copious amounts of isotonic bowel contents. Parenteral nutrition or supplementation of fluid and electrolytes without protein or calories is necessary to avoid dehydration and malnutrition.

In addition, in the following situations, artificial nutrition is often required:

1. For extreme previous malnutrition and an inability to eat a normal diet.
2. In an unconscious or intubated patient unable to swallow.
3. When there is obstruction to the oropharynx, esophagus, or cardia.
4. In those with sepsis, when the general condition of the patient requires the use of assisted nutritional intake.

Enteral nutrition is the route of choice in the following situations†:

1. For obstructive lesions of the pharynx, esophagus, and cardia that can be bypassed by a fine bore tube or by a gastrostomy or jejunostomy.
2. For anorexic patients with sepsis and trauma, having a gut patent to liquids.
3. When associated pancreatic disease is present without ileus.
4. For chronic low grade bowel obstruction that settles down on a liquid diet but recurs when solid food is eaten.
5. For inflammatory bowel disease with malnutrition.
6. For semiconscious patients.

---

*Editors' note: See also, Rees, R.G.P., et al.: J.P.E.N. *10*:258, 1986. The authors concluded that the omission of such regimens was advantageous to the nutritional effects.

†Editors' note: See also, Jones, B.J.M.: Gut *27 (Suppl.1)*:47, 1986. In this review, the author lists the local complications of large bore nasogastric or nasoenteric feeding tubes and those encountered with fine bore tubes.

TABLE 24-4. *Approximate Composition of Representative Nutritional Supplements*

Supplement	kcal /100 ml	Carbohydrate Source	g/100 ml	Protein Source	g/100 ml	Fats Source	g/100 ml	mOsm/L
Vivonex (Eaton Norwich)	100	Glucose Oligosaccharides	22.6	L-Amino acids	2.0	Safflower oil	0.14	550
Vivonex HN	100	Glucose Oligosaccharides	21.1	L-Amino acids	4.4	Safflower oil	0.87	810
Flexical (Mead-Johnson)	100	Sucrose Dextrins	15.5	Casein hydrolysate	2.68	Safflower oil	3.4	805
Isocal (Mead-Johnson)	106	Corn syrup solids	13.5	Calcium caseinate Soy isolate	3.45	Soy oil	4.4	350
Vital (Ross)	100	Glucose Oligosaccharides Polysaccharides	18.9	Soy, whey Hydrolyzed casein	4.1	Sunflower oil	1.0	450
Ensure (Ross)	106	Corn syrup solids Sucrose	14.4	Calcium caseinate Soy isolate	3.7	Corn oil	3.7	460
Sustacal (Mead-Johnson)	100	Sucrose Corn syrup solids	13.5	Skim milk Na and Ca caseinates Soy isolates	5.1	Soy oil	2.3	625
Sustagen (Mead-Johnson)	160	Corn syrup solids Dextrose	27.2	Nonfat dry milk Powdered whole milk Ca caseinate	9.6	Milk fat	1.4	1620

Data adapted from Belli D. C., Morin C. L., and Roy C. C.: Medicine North America 20:2626, 1985.

Enteral nutrition is contraindicated in the following situations:

1. Patients with vomiting and serious bowel obstruction.
2. Patients with gastric retention, unless the feeding tube can be passed into the small bowel or a jejunostomy created.
3. Severe diarrhea with enteral feeding. This usually occurs in patients with short bowel.
4. When a very short bowel is present.*
5. For the patients with end-jejunostomy and an inability to concentrate intestinal contents.

Parenteral Nutrition

Throughout the ages, physicians have been plagued by the problem of how to deliver vital nutrients to sick patients who are unable to ingest, digest, or absorb a normal oral diet. Over the past two decades, the use of parenteral nutrition has provided the means of preventing or reversing the metabolic consequences of malnutrition in such patients. With the current availability of total parenteral nutrition (TPN), not only can patients be provided with short-term TPN during a period when they cannot accept, absorb, or use oral nutrition, but they can now be maintained on long-term home TPN and live relatively normal and productive lives.†

Total parenteral nutrition is most useful in providing nutrition to patients who develop unpleasant symptoms with enteral feeds. Providing TPN while keeping patients NPO—so called "bowel rest"—may also have a role as primary therapy in Crohn's disease. The use of TPN has enabled the physician to assess better the benefits of bowel rest without further compromising the patient's nutritional status.

Currently, total parenteral nutrition is widely available and technically easy to administer; it should, however, be reserved for situations where the enteral route cannot be used effectively. The two main reasons for this reservation of use of TPN are that parenteral nutrition is relatively expensive compared with enteral nutrition, and a greater potential for serious complications exists with parenteral nutrition.

Even after determining that a patient requires parenteral nutritional support, it is imperative that an expert team consisting of a physician, nurse, and a pharmacist be available so the TPN can be delivered with optimal patient care, thus reducing the risk of complications.

Indications

Eight main indications for the use of TPN in inflammatory bowel disease currently exist.

MALNUTRITION OR THE POTENTIAL FOR MALNUTRITION. It is obvious that a patient who is malnourished should receive additional nutrition. It is not, however, so obvious that active nutritional intervention is necessary to avoid malnutrition in patients suffering from a disease that precludes their nourishing themselves adequately without assistance. Thus, malnutrition or even the potential for its development should be indications for nutritional support.

PREOPERATIVE ADJUVANT THERAPY TO IMPROVE THE NUTRITIONAL STATUS. Surgical treatment in the malnourished patient may be associated with increased morbidity.[25]‡ Hence, such patients should receive nutritional support preoperatively in order to achieve a nutritional state that can withstand such treatment. Because the infusion of low calorie, protein-free solutions has been shown to result in a negative nitrogen balance, it has been suggested that all patients receive nutritional support both pre- and postoperatively. This practice would obviously increase the complexity of managing the average patient requiring surgical intervention. The universal use of parenteral nutrition preoperatively is not supported at the present time, so it is not recommended.

SHORT BOWEL SYNDROME. Following massive resection of the small bowel, the remaining gut may not be able to absorb sufficient amounts of nutrients to maintain nutritional homeostasis. In some of these patients, an oral diet may be possible if extreme measures are used, such as eating every two hours and so defecating approximately as frequently. Thus, the patient would become a "social cripple." Such a patient would obviously benefit from home parenteral nutrition (HPN) despite being able to "get by," from a nutritional standpoint, with an oral diet. With time, the remaining bowel may adapt, resulting in adequate bowel function so that HPN can be discontinued and oral diet resumed.

END-JEJUNOSTOMY SYNDROME. In this condition the patient has lost those areas of ileum and colon where intestinal contents are concen-

---

*Editors' note: However, see Casnes, J., et al.: Am. J. Clin. Nutr., *41*:1002, 1985.
†Detsky, A.S., et al.: J.P.E.N., *10*:49, 1986.

‡Editors' note: See also, Mughal M.M., et al.: J.P.E.N., *11*:40, 1987.

trated. As a consequence, eating results in the loss of copious amounts of isotonic bowel contents. Although nutrients may be absorbed adequately, severe deficiency of fluid and electrolytes, especially magnesium, will ensue. These patients require parenteral fluid and electrolyte supplementation, which can now be provided via HPN.

CHRONIC SMALL BOWEL OBSTRUCTION. Patients with Crohn's disease may have chronic small bowel obstruction caused by multiple strictures not amenable to surgical alleviation. In these patients, eating results in abdominal pain, nausea, and vomiting, and the patients may condition themselves to avoid eating, leading to malnutrition. HPN should be considered in such patients.

GROWTH RETARDATION. (SEE ALSO CHAPTERS 12, 13) An unfortunate consequence of inflammatory bowel disease in childhood and adolescence is cessation of growth and maturation. Severe impairment of linear growth, lack of weight gain, retarded bone development, and delayed puberty occur in about 15 to 30% of patients under age 21 with Crohn's disease, and a smaller percentage with ulcerative colitis.[26,27] These effects are caused by malnutrition. Several studies have demonstrated that the major cause of malnutrition in these patients is decreased caloric intake.[28] Nutritional support, given enterally or parenterally, has resulted in catch-up growth and the onset of puberty.[28,29]*

LONG-TERM THERAPY TO ALLOW CLOSURE OF FISTULAE. Fistulas occasionally close during a brief course of TPN with complete bowel rest, but usually do not. In the past, such patients routinely underwent surgical procedures. Currently, two viable alternatives exist: home enteral nutrition using defined formula diets,[30] and home parenteral nutrition.[31] Although both forms of therapy have resulted in fistula closure in some patients, adequate controlled studies are lacking.

AS PRIMARY THERAPY FOR IBD

Routes of Administration

CENTRAL VENOUS METHOD. Delivering TPN through the central venous route is most satisfactory for patients requiring prolonged infusion or those with poor peripheral veins. This approach allows the infusion of fluids irrespective of the osmolality, is more comfortable for the patient, and avoids repeated venipuncture. The insertion and maintenance of the catheter used for central TPN should be done by an expert team to avoid complications.

PERIPHERAL VENOUS METHOD. The peripheral route may be considered when TPN is required and the following conditions are present: a) the infusion is required for only a short time (10 to 14 days), b) the patient has a predisposition to septicemia or bleeding, c) the patient has traumatized subclavian veins, d) when a central venous catheterization is considered dangerous and inadvisable, or e) in prospective home TPN patients prior to the insertion of a permanent line.

This system requires that 80% of the calories be infused as lipids, as larger amounts of glucose predispose to the development of thrombophlebitis. Preferably, the solutions should be delivered in a 1 to 1.5 : 1 ratio, that is, 1.5 liters of lipid solution and 1 to 1.5 liters of 6% amino acid, 12% dextrose solution.

Nutritional Requirements

PROTEIN REQUIREMENTS. Despite previous beliefs that a positive nitrogen balance could occur only in conjunction with a positive energy balance, Greenberg and Jeejeebhoy showed that a positive nitrogen balance was possible even with hypocaloric infusions in malnourished patients if the amount of amino acid infused was about 2 g/kg of ideal body weight (IBW) per day.[32] Thus, the most important nutrient for creating a positive nitrogen balance is nitrogen as amino acids.

Having recognized the dominant role of amino acids in promoting nitrogen retention, the question arises as to the quantity of amino acids required. Stable adults require only 0.4 g/kg IBW/day of nitrogen to maintain zero balance. The gain in nitrogen is linear over a range from 0.25 to 2 g/kg/day, with increased requirements for increased metabolic rate and decreased requirements with increased energy intake. Roulet et al. showed that septic patients achieved zero or positive nitrogen balance when about 1.5 g of amino acids/kg IBW/day was provided.[33] Thus, it is advisable to start TPN with about 1 to 1.5 g of protein/kg IBW/day.

*Editors' note: See also, Alges, H., et al.: Gastroenterology 92:1291, 1987.

ENERGY REQUIREMENTS. Energy requirements can be predicted from the Harris-Benedict equation (see previous section),[22] based on age, sex, and size, or by indirect calorimetry. From these formulae it appears that roughly 30 kcal/kg IBW/day are required to meet the daily energy requirements. This amount may have to be increased in cases of sepsis or when a weight gain response is desired. The energy requirements of "septic-injured" patients are only 13 to 14% above the predicted value derived from the Harris-Benedict equation.[33,34] Thus, approximately 40 kcal/kg IBW/day should be sufficient to induce a weight gain in such patients.

The major energy sources used in TPN consist of carbohydrates and lipids. Jeejeebhoy et al. showed that nitrogen balance was the same when patients were given 1 g/kg of amino acid per day and 40 kcal/kg/day of nonprotein calories, either as glucose alone or as 83% fat and 17% glucose.[35] Several studies have shown that fat energy is needed and that total body nitrogen can be gained only when fat is provided as part of the nonprotein calories.[36,37] In addition, when glucose is provided as the sole nonprotein calorie source for a prolonged period, a syndrome of essential fatty acid deficiency (EFAD) will develop (vide infra).

Based on these data, it is presently the authors' practice to provide 35 to 40 kcal/kg IBW/day of an equicaloric mixture of glucose and lipid. This regimen is usually tolerated and used well by most patients.

ESSENTIAL FATTY ACID REQUIREMENTS. Linoleic and linolenic acids cannot be synthesized endogenously in humans and, as such, must be provided from external sources. These two fatty acids are present in many natural foods, but if patients are receiving TPN without lipids, they will develop a syndrome of essential fatty acid deficiency (EFAD). This syndrome consists of a red, scaly, eczematoid dermatitis on the face, palms, soles, extremities, chest, and trunk, intertriginous skin with oozing, alopecia, brittle nails, poor wound healing, reduced resistance to infection, thrombocytopenia, fatty infiltration of the liver, and lipid accumulation in pulmonary macrophages. This syndrome can be reversed by the supplementation of linoleic acid, but not by linolenic acid.

All of the lipid solutions commercially available for parenteral infusion contain linoleic acid in such quantities that about 1 to 2 liters per week is sufficient to prevent the development of EFAD.

TRACE ELEMENT REQUIREMENTS. With the increasing use of TPN, several syndromes caused by trace element deficiency have become apparent. Of the trace elements, zinc, copper, chromium, iron, iodine, selenium, cobalt (as vitamin B_{12}), and molybdenum are clearly essential.

Zinc. Zinc is necessary for cell proliferation and has an important role in the maintenance of cellular immunity and delayed hypersensitivity, insulin secretion, and nitrogen retention. Clinical zinc deficiency during unsupplemented TPN has been observed,[38,39] consisting of a scaly pustular rash starting around the mouth and over the articular prominences, and spreading over the entire body. Alopecia, erythema of the palms and soles with desquamation, loss of taste and smell, eye changes (blepharitis and conjunctivitis), behavioral changes, impaired delayed cutaneous hypersensitivity, and resistant skin infections may also occur.[10]

The zinc requirements during TPN have been shown to be about 2.5 to 3.0 mg/day, but higher requirements are seen in patients with diarrhea and ostomies, where they can lose 10 to 20 mg of zinc per liter of fluid.[40]

Copper. Copper deficiency results in a hypochromic, normocytic anemia, leukopenia, and skeletal abnormalities (osteoporosis and metaphyseal irregularities).[16] Shike et al. found the daily requirement to be about 300 μg in patients without diarrhea and 500 μg in patients with substantial fluid losses from the gastrointestinal tract.[41] The dose must be decreased in patients with cholestatic jaundice, because copper is excreted via the biliary tract.

Chromium. Chromium is required for the peripheral action of glucose. Chromium deficiency can lead to weight loss, peripheral neuropathy, ataxia, and glucose intolerance.[15] The neuropathy and glucose intolerance are resistant to large amounts of insulin unless chromium is supplemented.

It appears that 20 μg of chromium per day is sufficient to prevent deficiency, but further balance studies are needed.

Selenium. Selenium is an essential component of the enzyme glutathione peroxidase, which, together with catalase, superoxide dismutase, and vitamin E, provides a line of defense against oxidative damage by peroxides and free radicals. Deficiency of selenium has resulted in life-threatening or even fatal cardiomyopathy.[11-13,42]

In addition, Van Rij et al. described a patient on long-term TPN who developed incapacitating bilateral muscular pain in her quadriceps and hamstring muscles, associated with a significantly decreased plasma selenium level.[14] Complete recovery was achieved within 3 weeks of starting selenium supplementation.

The daily requirements for selenium are not well established but 120 µg per day is enough to prevent deficiency without any untoward effects.*

Iodine. It appears that 120 µg per day of iodine should be supplemented in TPN, but adequate balance studies are lacking. With this dose, neither goiters nor hypothyroidism has been found during long- or short-term TPN. It should, however, be recognized that patients being treated with povidone-iodine in the dressings will absorb sufficient amounts of iodine for their needs.

Manganese. Manganese is a cofactor for many enzymes such as carboxylase and several kinases. Manganese deficiency has resulted in defective growth, reproductive system dysfunction, and CNS abnormalities in other animals, but no documented disease in humans.

The recommended daily requirements are about 0.2 to 0.8 mg/day, but this dose should be decreased in patients with cholestatic jaundice, because manganese is excreted via the biliary tract and accumulation of this element may occur in the basal ganglia.

Molybdenum. Molybdenum is an essential component of several enzymes including sulfite oxidase,[43] which is required for the conversion of sulfite to sulfate. Molybdenum deficiency has been shown to cause neurologic abnormalities. Abumrad et al. described a patient on TPN who received amino acid solutions containing sulfite and developed a comatose state, which was reversed by supplementing the TPN with 300 µg per day of molybdenum.[17]

The daily requirements for molybdenum have not been well established, but it appears that 48 to 96 µg per day are required to maintain molybdenum balance.

Other Trace Elements. Other trace elements, including fluorine, tin, arsenic, silicon, aluminum, vanadium, cadmium, lead, and mercury, have not been shown to be essential in man, so they are not supplemented in TPN.

VITAMIN REQUIREMENTS. Vitamin requirements during TPN, with the exception of a few, have not been studied in detail. Therefore, most current recommendations are based on extrapolations from oral Recommended Daily Allowances and studies using commercially prepared multivitamin preparations.

Water-soluble Vitamins. Several studies have shown that the regular use of routine multivitamin preparations will maintain adequate blood levels of many water-soluble vitamins, including thiamine (B_1), riboflavin (B_2), pyridoxine (B_3), niacin, pantothenic acid, and ascorbic acid (C).[44,45]

THIAMINE (B_1). Thiamine is an integral part of the carboxylase enzyme complex that is necessary for the metabolism of alpha-keto acids such as pyruvate. Some cells, such as neurons, depend exclusively on carbohydrate for their source of energy and as such are particularly vulnerable to thiamine deficiency. Thiamine, given in doses of 5 mg/day, is sufficient for patients receiving TPN.

RIBOFLAVIN. Deficiency of riboflavin (B_2) can lead to photophobia, cheilosis, glossitis, and pruritus of the skin with inflammation, especially of the anogenital region. The recommended daily dose in patients receiving TPN is 5 mg.

NIACINAMIDE. Niacinamide deficiency can lead to the syndrome of pellagra, which consists of erythema and pigmentation of the skin, glossitis, stomatitis, and diarrhea. Delirium and confusion may also develop. The recommended daily dose in patients receiving TPN is 50 mg.

PANTOTHENIC ACID. Disease states caused by pantothenic acid deficiency have not been described in man. Nevertheless, the recommended daily dose for patients receiving TPN is 15 mg.

PYRIDOXINE. Pyridoxine (B_6) deficiency can lead to dermatitis, seborrhea, intertrigo, neuropathy, and changes in mental status. The recommended daily dose in patients receiving TPN is 15 mg.

B_{12} AND FOLIC ACID. Deficiencies of B_{12} and folate have a combination of hematologic, gastrointes-

---

*Editors' note: Martin, R.F., et al.: J.P.E.N. *10*:213, 1986. Lane, H.W., et al.: J.P.E.N. *11*:177, 1987.

tinal, and neurologic manifestations. These two vitamins are not present in many of the multivitamin preparations. The recommended daily dose in patients receiving TPN is 3 to 5 µg of B_{12} and 5 mg of folate, although 600 µg of folate has been shown to be sufficient.

ASCORBIC ACID. Deficiency of ascorbic acid (vitamin C) leads to the syndrome of scurvy, which is characterized by perifollicular hemorrhages in the skin, gingivitis, and infections. The recommended daily dose for patients receiving TPN is about 300 mg.

BIOTIN. Low plasma biotin levels have been found in patients on long-term home TPN, but no deleterious effects were demonstrable. It is recommended that 300 µg be given per day, however.

Fat-soluble Vitamins. Vitamins A, D, E, and K are all fat-soluble vitamins.

VITAMIN A. Large quantities of vitamin A can be stored in the liver and as such it is not surprising that normal serum levels were found in patients on home TPN for 6 months without vitamin A supplementation.[46] It is our current practice to provide 2500 IU/day to our home TPN patients, and 5000 IU/week to our hospitalized patients receiving TPN.

VITAMIN D. In one study, patients receiving vitamin D with their TPN developed metabolic bone disease, hypercalcemia, hypercalciuria, and loss of skeletal calcium. These symptoms resolved after vitamin D was discontinued.[46] In addition, pancreatitis secondary to hypercalcemia related to vitamin D supplementation in patients receiving TPN has occurred.[47] It is our current practice to give 500 IU of vitamin D weekly to our hospitalized TPN patients and none to our home TPN patients.

VITAMIN E. Vitamin E is supplied to patients on TPN in part by vitamin preparations and in part by that present in the lipid solutions. Jeejeebhoy et al. showed that the serum vitamin E levels were almost normal in long-term TPN patients receiving daily lipid infusions.[45] Thurlow et al. described ten patients on TPN who developed increased peroxidase-induced red blood cell hemolysis in vivo and increased platelet aggregation in vitro in conjunction with low serum vitamin E levels.[48] These abnormalities were corrected in seven patients with 50 mg of d,1 alpha-tocopherol daily but not by 25 mg/day. In addition, children and adults with vitamin E deficiency have developed progressive neuromuscular disease characterized by ataxia, dysmetria, areflexia, loss of vibration and proprioception sensations, and a variable ophthalmoplegia, all of which improved dramatically with vitamin E replacement.[49-51] We recommend the provision of 10 IU per day in addition to that in the lipid solutions.

VITAMIN K. Vitamin K is required for the synthesis of several coagulation factors (II, VII, IX, and X). Under normal circumstances it is derived from the diet, mainly plants, and from the gut bacteria. In patients receiving TPN, the production by the gut bacteria may be sufficient as the source of vitamin K, but changes in the bacterial flora of the nonactive gut may occur (especially if the patient is receiving antibiotics), and then supplementation with vitamin K is advisable. Sodium menadiol diphosphate (Synkavite*) given in doses of 10 mg weekly is sufficient.

Current Vitamin Recommendations. It is our current practice to supply for hospital patients a multivitamin preparation containing all of the vitamins except A, D, E, and biotin, 6 days out of every week. On the seventh day, vitamin A (5000 IU), D (500 IU), E (5 IU), and K (10 mg) are added. Patients on home TPN receive daily vitamin A (2500 IU), weekly vitamin K (10 mg), and a multivitamin preparation containing the water-soluble vitamins 6 days out of every week, with biotin (100 µg) 3 days a week.

FLUID AND ELECTROLYTE REQUIREMENTS

Water. As most solutions used for TPN have a caloric density of approximately 1 kcal/ml, about 2 to 3 liters of fluid are required to provide the daily energy requirements. When fluid restriction is necessary, 20% lipid emulsions can be used. Also, 70% dextrose can be added to the solution in a pharmacy to increase the caloric density. These solutions are viscous, and as a result may be difficult to infuse. When abnormal fluid losses result from diarrhea or stomal losses, more fluid must be provided.

Sodium. Approximately 120 mmol/day of sodium are usually provided during TPN, but this can be reduced to 20 to 40 mmol/day if salt restriction is necessary. Severely malnourished

---

*Roche Laboratories, Nutley, N.J.

patients may quickly develop peripheral edema or severe pulmonary edema when refed with a system rich in carbohydrates. It has been shown that feeding carbohydrate induces salt retention,[52] which is exaggerated in malnourished patients who already have an excess of total body water. Thus, refeeding should be performed cautiously in such patients, initially restricting the intake both of sodium and fluid.

Potassium. During TPN, potassium is retained with nitrogen as lean body mass is reformed.[6] Thus at least 90 to 120 mmol of potassium should be provided daily in TPN solutions to avoid hypokalemia and assist positive nitrogen balance. Additional potassium should be provided to those patients receiving vigorous nasogastric suctioning, through which they can lose large amounts of potassium. Lower doses of potassium should be given to patients with renal failure.

Magnesium. Like potassium, magnesium is retained during TPN, especially during the phase of positive nitrogen balance. In fact, a positive nitrogen balance cannot be achieved unless adequate magnesium is provided.[7] Approximately 12 to 15 mmol of magnesium must be provided daily to maintain magnesium balance.

Calcium. As mentioned above, metabolic bone disease and pancreatitis have been observed in patients with hypercalcemia developing during TPN. The hypercalcemia is probably caused by the vitamin D supplementation and not the calcium per se. Currently, we recommend that about 10 to 12 mmol of calcium be provided daily during TPN.

Phosphorus. Positive nitrogen balance cannot be achieved in the absence of phosphate.[6] In addition, hypophosphatemia may lead to serious neurologic symptoms.[53] We recommend that about 10 to 20 mmol of elemental phosphate be provided daily during TPN.

Complications of TPN

The use of TPN is not without risks. The complications can be broadly classified as mechanical or metabolic, and they are listed in Table 24-5.

MECHANICAL COMPLICATIONS. The mechanical complications are mainly related to the insertion and care of the catheter. Damage to the involved or adjacent vessels, to pleural and mediastinal

TABLE 24-5. *Complications of Total Parenteral Nutrition.*

Mechanical
  Sepsis
  Pneumothorax
  Venous thrombosis
  Arterial puncture and laceration
  Air embolism
  Hemothorax
  Hydrothorax
  Catheter embolism
Metabolic
  Hyperglycemia
  Rebound hypoglycemia
  Electrolyte imbalance
  Vitamin deficiencies
  Trace element deficiencies

Tables 1, 3 and 5 are taken from Ostro, M. J., and Jeejeebhoy, K. N.: Nutritional support of patients with inflammatory bowel disease. In: Inflammatory Bowel Disease, edited by I. A. D. Bouchier, G. Watkinson, J. Myren and F. T. de Dombal. Oxford, Oxford University Press, 1985. Published with permission.

spaces, and to distant organs, can be caused by misdirected catheters. Vessel occlusion by thrombus formation can also occur. The most frequent complication related to TPN is sepsis. If strict attention is paid to asepsis, the incidence of catheter-related sepsis may be decreased to 7% or less.[54] The infectious complications can be drastically decreased by observing the following precautions: (1) careful preparation of the TPN solutions by the pharmacy, maintaining strict sterile conditions; (2) aseptic technique employed during insertion of the catheter; (3) aseptic care of the catheter and dressing while they are in place;* and (4) the regulation of TPN by a trained team.

Metabolic Complications. The metabolic complications are mainly related to the composition of the infused solutions.†These complications can be prevented or minimized by careful monitoring of the patient, both clinically and by laboratory testing. Such complications are usually caused by deficits or excesses of various elements or incompatibilities, and they are listed in Table 24-5.

Hyperglycemia results from the infusion of glucose at a rate greater than the rate at which the body can metabolize it. Rebound hypoglycemia occurs if the infusion of glucose (especially at rapid rates) is stopped suddenly, either

---
*Editors' note: See also, Murphy, L.M., Lipman, T.O.: J.P.E.N. *11*:190, 1987.
†Lerebours, E., et al.: J.P.E.N. *11*:45, 1987.

intentionally when discontinuing the infusion, or unintentionally because of mechanical obstruction of the delivery system as a result of blockage or kinking of the tubing.

TPN AS PRIMARY THERAPY FOR CROHN'S DISEASE (BOWEL REST)* Patients with idiopathic inflammatory bowel disease, particularly Crohn's disease, not responding to conventional medical therapy, will improve if kept NPO and given parenteral nutrition. This mode of therapy is conceptually equivalent to diverting the luminal stream away from the inflamed bowel. Obviously if the patient is kept NPO, malnutrition will eventually occur unless parenteral nutrition is provided. The combination of keeping the patient NPO and providing parenteral nutrition is referred to as "bowel rest."

Although the efficacy of bowel rest has not been substantiated by controlled studies,† there is evidence from prospective studies in patients with Crohn's disease that the effect of such therapy is favorable in reducing both the disease activity and the size of inflammatory masses.‡ There may also be a favorable effect on the closure of bowel fistulas in patients with Crohn's disease, but these results are less striking. Various small series indicate a remission rate of between 40 to 80%.[55-58] In 100 patients so treated, we have observed a remission rate of 77% and the improvement was maintained in 54% for over a year.[59] Total parenteral nutrition with bowel rest therapy has *not* been found to be effective as a primary therapeutic modality in the treatment of acute colitis, whether it is caused by ulcerative colitis or Crohn's disease.[60] In a controlled trial, elemental diet was found to be as effective as prednisone in reducing the activity of acute Crohn's disease.[61] It is not known whether bowel rest or nutrition is more important in inducing a remission. Our controlled trial showed that bowel rest per se did not influence the rate of remission.[62] This suggests that nutrition may be important in aiding the resolution of Crohn's disease. Indeed, a study of controlled nutritional supplementation reduced the orosomucoid levels,[63] and another controlled study suggested that nutritional support, rather than bowel rest, is responsible for remission.[64] Further studies are required, however, to confirm this conclusion and to define the best way of delivering nutrition for this purpose, whether enteral or parenteral.*

Patients with inflammatory bowel disease may have a wide range of nutritional disturbances that may be even more detrimental than the underlying disease process itself. Thus, the management of patients with inflammatory bowel disease is not complete without an awareness of their nutritional status. Early assessment and treatment of potential malnutrition are essential, as is the choice of the most appropriate means of providing the required nutrition.†

References

1. Atwell, J. D., and Duthie, H. L.: The absorption of water, sodium and potassium from the ileum of humans showing the effects of regional enteritis. Gastroenterology, 46:16, 1964.
2. Lehr, L., Schober, O., Hundeshagen, H., and Pichlmaier, R.: Body potassium depletion in Crohn's disease requiring specific nutritional preparation for surgery. Scand. J. Gastroenterol., 17(78):497, 1982.
3. Beeken, W. L.: Remediable defects in Crohn's disease. A prospective study of 63 patients. Arch. Intern. Med., 135:686, 1975.
4. Gerlach, K., Morowitz, D. A., and Kirsner, J. B.: Symptomatic hypomagnesemia complicating regional enteritis. Gastroenterology, 59:567, 1970.
5. Main, A., et al.: Vitamin A deficiency in severe Crohn's disease and supplements during nutritional support. Clin. Nutr. (Special suppl.), 1:F34, 1982.
6. Rudman, D., et al.: Elemental balances during intravenous hyperalimentation of underweight adult subjects. J. Clin. Invest., 55:94, 1975.
7. Freeman, J. B.: Magnesium requirements during parenteral nutrition. *In* Parenteral Nutrition/Canada. Present Status and Newer Developments. Edited by G. L. Hill, K. N. Jeejeebhoy, and J. M. Kinney. Princeton, N. J., Communications Media for Education, 1981.
8. Solomons, N. W., Rosenberg, I. H., Sandstead, H. H., and Vo-Khactu, K. P.: Zinc deficiency in Crohn's disease. Digestion, 16:87, 1977.
9. Sturniolo, G. C., Molokhia, M. M., Shields, R., and Turnberg, L. A.: Zinc absorption in Crohn's disease. Gut, 21:387, 1980.
10. Golden, M. H. N., Golden, B. E., Jackson, A. A., and Harland, P. S. E.: Zinc and immunocompetence in protein-energy malnutrition. Lancet, 1:1226, 1978.
11. Keshan Disease Research Group of the Chinese Academy of Medical Sciences, Beijing: Observations on the effect of sodium selenite in prevention of Keshan Disease. Chin. Med. J., 92(7):471, 1979.
12. Keshan Disease Research Group of the Chinese Academy of Medical Sciences, Beijing: Epidemiologic studies of the etiologic relationship of selenium and Keshan Disease. Chin. Med. J., 92(7):477, 1979.
13. Fleming, C. R., et al.: Selenium deficiency and fatal cardi-

---

*See also Chapters 22 and 23.
†Editors' note: See also, McIntyre, B., et al.: Gut 27:481, 1986. The authors found no effect by bowel rest on the patient's outcome.
‡See also: Seidman, E.G., et al.: Gastroenterology 90:1625, 1986.

*See also: Rhodes, J. and Rose, J. (Editorial). Gut 27:471, 1986.
†Editors' note: See also, Howard, L., et al.: J.P.E.N. 10:416, 1986.

omyopathy in a patient on home parenteral nutrition. Gastroenterology, 83:689, 1982.
14. Van Rij, A. M., Thomson, C. D., McKenzie, J. M., and Robinson, M. F.: Selenium deficiency in total parenteral nutrition. Am. J. Clin. Nutr., 32:2076, 1979.
15. Jeejeebhoy, K. N., et al.: Chromium deficiency, glucose intolerance and neuropathy reversed by chromium supplementation in a patient receiving long-term total parenteral nutrition. Am. J. Clin. Nutr., 30:531, 1979.
16. Karpel, J. T., and Peden, V. H.: Copper deficiency in long-term parenteral nutrition. J. Pediatr., 80:32, 1972.
17. Abumrad, N. N., Schneider, A. J., Steel, D., and Rogers, L. S.: Amino acid intolerance during prolonged total parenteral nutrition reversed by molybdate therapy. Am. J. Clin. Nutr., 34:2551, 1981.
18. Dyer, N. H., and Dawson, A. M.: Malnutrition and malabsorption in Crohn's disease with reference to the effect of surgery. Brit. J. Surg., 60:134, 1973.
19. Greig, P. D., Baker, J. P., and Jeejeebhoy, K. N.: Metabolic effects of total parenteral nutrition. Ann. Rev. Nutr., 2:179, 1982.
20. Daly, J. M., Vars, H. C., and Dudrick, S. J.: Effects of protein depletion on strength of colonic anastomoses. Surg. Gynecol. Obstet., 134:15, 1972.
21. Law, D. K., Dudrick, S. J., and Abdou, N. I.: Immunocompetence of patients with protein-calorie malnutrition. Ann. Intern. Med., 79:545, 1973.
22. Harris, J. A., and Benedict, F. G.: Standard basal metabolism constants for physiologists and clinicians. In: A Biometric Study of Basal Metabolism in Man. Carnegie Institution of Washington. Publication no. 279. Philadelphia, J. B. Lippincott, 1919.
23. Blackburn, G. L., et al.: Nutritional and metabolic assessment of the hospitalized patient. J. P. E. N., 1:11, 1977.
24. Russell, D. McR., Atwood, H. L., and Jeejeebhoy, K. N.: Nitrogen versus muscle calcium in the genesis of abnormal muscle function in malnutrition. J. P. E. N., 9:415, 1985.
25. Muller, J. M., Dienst, C., Brenner, V., and Pichlmaier, H.: Preoperative parenteral feeding in patients with gastrointestinal carcinoma. Lancet, 1:68, 1982.
26. Grand, R. J., and Homer, D. R.: Approaches to inflammatory bowel disease in childhood and adolescence. Pediatr. Clin. North Am., 22:835, 1975.
27. McCaffery, T. D., Nasr, K., Lawrence, A. H., and Kirsner, J. B.: Severe growth retardation in children with inflammatory bowel disease. J. Pediatr., 45:386, 1979.
28. Kelts, D. G., et al.: Nutritional basis of growth failure in children and adolescents with Crohn's disease. Gastroenterology, 76:720, 1979.
29. Prader, A., Tanner, J. M., and Wonttarnack, G. A.: Catch-up growth following illness or starvation. J. Pediatr., 62:646, 1963.
30. Main, A. N. H., et al.: Home enteral tube feeding with a liquid diet in the long-term management of inflammatory bowel disease and intestinal failure. Scott. Med. J., 25:312, 1980.
31. Byrne, W. J., Burke, M., Fonkalsrud, E. W., and Ament, M. E.: Home parenteral nutrition: An alternative approach to the management of complicated gastrointestinal fistulas not responding to conventional medical or surgical therapy. J. P. E. N., 3:355, 1979.
32. Greenberg, G. R., and Jeejeebhoy, K. N.: Intravenous protein-sparing therapy in patients with gastrointestinal disease. J. P. E. N., 3:427, 1979.
33. Roulet, M., et al.: A controlled trial of the effect of parenteral nutrition support on patients with respiratory failure and sepsis. Clin. Nutr., 2:97, 1983.
34. Askanazi, J., et al.: Influence of total parenteral nutrition on fuel utilization in injury and sepsis. Ann. Surg., 191:40, 1980.
35. Jeejeebhoy, K. N., et al.: Metabolic studies in total parenteral nutrition with lipid in man: comparison with glucose. J. Clin. Invest., 57:125, 1976.
36. Wolfe, R. R., Durkot, M. J., Allsop, J. R., and Burke, J. F.: Glucose metabolism in the severely burned patient. Metabolism, 20:1031, 1979.
37. McFie, J., Smith, R. C., and Hill, G. L.: Glucose as a nonprotein energy source? A controlled clinical trial in gastroenterological patients requiring intravenous nutrition. Gastroenterology, 80:103, 1981.
38. Kay, R. G., and Tasman-Jones, C.: Acute zinc deficiency in man during intravenous alimentation. Aust. N. Z. J. Surg., 45:325, 1975.
39. Arakawa, T., et al.: Zinc deficiency in two infants during total parenteral alimentation for diarrhea. Am. J. Clin. Nutr., 29:197, 1976.
40. Wolman, S. L., Anderson, G. H., Marliss, E. B., and Jeejeebhoy, K. N.: Zinc in total parenteral nutrition: requirements and metabolic effects. Gastroenterology, 73:458, 1979.
41. Shike, M., et al.: Copper metabolism and requirements in total parenteral nutrition. Gastroenterology, 81:290, 1981.
42. Johnson, R. A., et al.: An occidental case of cardiomyopathy and selenium deficiency. N. Engl. J. Med., 304:1210, 1981.
43. Cohen, H. J., Fridovich, T., and Rajagopalan, K. V.: Hepatic sulfite oxidase. A functional role for molybdenum. J. Biol. Chem., 246:374, 1971.
44. Nichoalds, G. E., Meng, H. C., and Caldwell, M. D.: Vitamin requirements in patients receiving total parenteral nutrition. Arch. Surg., 112:1061, 1977.
45. Jeejeebhoy, K. N., et al.: Total parenteral nutrition at home: studies in patients surviving 4 months to 5 years. Gastroenterology, 71:943, 1976.
46. Shike, M., et al.: A possible role of vitamin D in the genesis of parenteral-nutrition-induced metabolic bone disease. Ann. Intern. Med., 95:560, 1981.
47. Izsak, E. M., Shike, M., Roulet, M., and Jeejeebhoy, K. N.: Pancreatitis associated with hypercalcemia in patients receiving total parenteral nutrition. Gastroenterology, 79:555, 1980.
48. Thurlow, P. M., and Grant, J. P.: Vitamin E, essential fatty acids and platelet function during total parenteral nutrition. J. P. E. N., 4:586, 1980.
49. Guggenheim, M. A., Ringel, S. P., Silverman, A., and Grabert, B. E.: Progressive neuromuscular disease in children with chronic cholestasis and vitamin E deficiency: diagnosis and treatment with alpha tocopherol. J. Pediatr., 100:51, 1982.
50. Rosenblum, J. L., Keating, J. P., Prensky, A. I., and Nelson, J. S.: A progressive neurological syndrome in children with chronic liver disease. N. Engl. J. Med., 304:503, 1981.
51. Howard, L., Ovesen, L., Satya-Murti, S., and Chu, R.: Reversible neurological symptoms caused by vitamin E deficiency in a patient with short bowel syndrome. Am. J. Clin. Nutr., 36:1243, 1982.
52. De Fronzo, R. A.: The effect of insulin in renal sodium metabolism: a review with clinical implications. Diabetologia, 21:165, 1981.
53. Silvas, S. E., and Paragas, P. D.: Paresthesiae, weakness, seizures and hypophosphatemia in patients receiving hyperalimentation. Gastroenterology, 62:513, 1972.
54. Goldmann, D. A., and Maki, D. G.: Infection control in total parenteral nutrition. J. Am. Med. Assoc., 223:1360, 1973.

55. Bos, L. P., Nabe, M., and Weterman, I. T.: Total parenteral nutrition in Crohn's disease; a clinical evaluation. *In* Recent Advances in Crohn's Disease. Edited by A. S. Peña, I. T. Weterman, C. C. Booth, and W. Strober. Boston, Martinus Nijhoff, 1981.
56. Elson, C. O., Layden, T. J., Nemchausky, B. A., and Rosenberg, I. H.: An evaluation of total parenteral nutrition in the management of inflammatory bowel disease. Dig. Dis. Sci., *25*:42, 1980.
57. Fischer, J. E., et al.: Hyperalimentation as primary therapy for inflammatory bowel disease. Am. J. Surg., *125*:165, 1973.
58. Greenberg, G. R., and Jeejeebhoy, K. N.: Total parenteral nutrition in the management of Crohn's disease. *In* Recent Advances in Crohn's Disease. Edited by A. S. Peña, I. T. Weterman, C. C. Booth, and W. Strober. Boston, Martinus Nijhoff, 1981.
59. Ostro, M. J., Greenberg, G. R., and Jeejeebhoy, K. N.: Total parenteral nutrition and bowel rest in the management of Crohn's disease. J. P. E. N., *9*:280, 1985.
60. Dickinson, R. J., et al.: Controlled trial of intravenous hyperalimentation and total bowel rest as an adjunct to the routine therapy of acute colitis. Gastroenterology, *79*:1199, 1980.
61. O'Moran, C., Segal, A. W., and Levi, A. J.: Elemental diet as primary therapy of acute Crohn's disease: a controlled trial. Brit. Med. J., *28*:1859, 1984.
62. Greenberg, G. R., et al.: Controlled trial of bowel rest and nutritional support in the management of Crohn's disease. Gastroenterology, *88*:1405, 1985.
63. Harries, A. D., et al.: Controlled trial of supplemented oral nutrition in Crohn's disease. Lancet, *1*:887, 1983.
64. Lochs, H., et al.: Has total bowel rest a beneficial effect in the treatment of Crohn's disease? Clin. Nutr., *2*:61, 1983.

25 · Indications for Surgery in Inflammatory Bowel Disease: A Gastroenterologist's Opinion

NORTON J. GREENBERGER, M.D.

Several effective drugs are available to treat the inflammatory bowel disorders idiopathic ulcerative colitis and Crohn's disease. These include sulfasalazine, rectal steroid preparations, systemic corticosteroids, metronidazole, azathioprine, and 6-mercaptopurine (see Chaps. 21, 22, and 23). In addition, enteral and total parenteral nutrition are useful therapeutic adjuncts and may help to induce a remission of disease activity (see Chap. 24). Medical therapy of chronic ulcerative colitis (CUC) is frequently successful in effecting a sustained remission or good control of disease activity with minimal limitations of life style. In this regard, approximately 70 to 75% of patients with CUC respond favorably to medical therapy.[1-3] On the other hand, medical therapy of Crohn's disease (CD) is less effective. Although up to 70% of patients with CD respond favorably to short-term (4 months) therapy with drugs such as corticosteroids, a sharp falloff occurs in the response rate over a 2 year period.[4,5] Thus, 50% of CD patients initially responding to corticosteroids failed such medical treatment after 2 years.[4,5] Importantly, the vast majority of CD patients will have a surgical procedure performed within a 10 to 15 year period after the diagnosis of Crohn's disease has been established. Thus, in a detailed review of the literature, Sales and Kirsner found that approximately 60% of 743 CD patients underwent surgical treatment after 10 years.[6]

It is important for physicians to have a clear understanding of the benefits as well as the limitations of medical therapy of ulcerative colitis and Crohn's disease. Similarly, the indications for surgical therapy, its outcome, and special problems associated with the operation for these disorders are important considerations that require a working knowledge of the current literature. It should be emphasized that many patients with idiopathic inflammatory bowel disease pose difficult management problems and the rationale for electing either medical or surgical therapy is often not clear-cut. In this discussion, I have reviewed much of the relevant literature in an attempt to provide reasonable guidelines for considering surgical intervention in these disorders. I have also included several case studies to underscore key points and highlight decision-making processes.

Indications for Surgical Intervention in Chronic Ulcerative Colitis

Failure of Medical Therapy

The most common indication for surgical treatment in chronic ulcerative colitis is failure of medical therapy. In this regard, medical therapy can fail, the response to treatment can be incomplete, or the response to treatment can be satisfactory but with continued requirement for corticosteroids at a dosage that is prohibitive (Tables 25-1 and 25-2). A review of the pertinent literature provides useful guidelines and puts the role of medical and surgical therapy in CUC in proper perspective. In several large series,[1-3,7] the favorable rate of response to corticosteroid therapy has ranged from 42 to 81%. In the study by Kirsner et al., 115 of 240 patients (48%) exhibited a good response and 80 patients (33%) a moderately favorable response to corticosteroids.[1] Similarly, in the series of Edwards and Truelove a remission induced by corticosteroid therapy occurred in 505 of 624 patients (81%).[2] Korelitz and Lindner studied the effect of 274 courses of corticosteroid therapy in 238 patients.[3] In 169 courses (63%) of treatment the response was considered dramatic or favorably impressive. In 63 courses (22%), the patients improved slowly and incompletely. In 42 courses (15%) of therapy, the patients either did not improve or worsened. It is instructive to examine the course of 96 patients who received 105 courses of therapy with either ACTH or corticosteroids and who had an unsatisfactory or an incomplete response. Importantly, 55 of these patients (57%) underwent surgical procedure either during the same admission or at a later date. Only 29 patients (30%) were able to be maintained on medical therapy. These data indicate that a slow or incomplete response to corticosteroid therapy is a poor prognostic sign, and approximately 2/3 of such patients will subsequently undergo colectomy.

A study by Meyers et al. of 66 patients with severe attacks of CUC is of interest.[7] These patients were entered into a randomized controlled trial and given either 300 mg of intravenous hydrocortisone or 120 units of intravenous ACTH per day. The criteria used to assess colitis activity were abdominal tenderness, 9 or more bowel movements per day, pulse rate of 100 or more per minute, and body temperature greater than 37.5°C. Colitis was considered fulminant if the patient had more than 9 bowel movements per day, as well as a temperature >38.0°C, or colonic dilatation (diameter >6.0 cm), or both. Seventeen patients had disease confined to the rectum and sigmoid, 32 to the descending colon, and 17 had universal colitis. Eleven patients were experiencing their first attack and 55 a relapse of their disease. Eighteen patients were judged to have fulminant colitis. Successful response to therapy was rigidly defined as complete amelioration of all symptoms and a reduction in diarrhea to less than or equal to 2 bowel motions per day. The major finding was that 28 of 66 patients (42%) responded to therapy with either corticosteroids or ACTH within 10 days. Several subsets were studied and it was found that: 7 of the 11 patients with first attacks, 21 of 55 patients who were experiencing a relapse in their disease, 7 of 18 patients with fulminant disease, and 21 of 48 with severe disease responded to treatment. The data obtained suggest that intravenous ACTH is more effective for those patients not previously treated with corticosteroids, whereas intravenous hydrocortisone appeared to be more effective for those already receiving corticosteroids. Twenty of the 28 patients who went into remission remained there after one year of therapy. These data underscore the fact that less than half the patients with a *severe* attack of CUC will go into full remission with intensive corticosteroid therapy. As noted above, many such patients with an incomplete response to pharmacologic doses of corticosteroids will subsequently require surgical intervention. An incomplete response to treatment manifested by persistent troublesome diarrhea imposes significant limitations of lifestyle. All too often, a long delay occurs before elective

TABLE 25-1. *Indications for Surgery in Idiopathic Ulcerative Colitis.*

Failure of Medical Therapy
    Frank failure:
        Treacherous nature of first attacks
    Incomplete response:
        Limitations of life style
    Satisfactory response but corticosteroid dosage prohibitive
    Complications of corticosteroid therapy
    Noncompliance with medical regimen
Fulminant Colitis
    With and without toxic megacolon
Perforation
Hemorrhage
    Acute
    Recurrent
Growth Retardation
Carcinoma
    Definite risk factors:
        Long duration disease (>10 years)
        Universal colitis
        Dysplasia
        Dysplasia-associated lesion or mass (DALM)
    Controversial risk factors:
        Onset of disease in childhood
        Continuous active disease
        Clinically severe first attack
    Problem of weighing risk factors if only one or two are present

TABLE 25-2. *Supporting Data Regarding Indications for Surgery in Idiopathic Ulcerative Colitis (CUC).*

Indication/ Complication	Approximate Incidence	Comment
Failure of Medical Therapy		
Frank failure	5–15%	Most CUC patients have intermittent attacks.
Failure after initial response to medical therapy	10%	5–10% have one attack; 75–80% respond well after initial episode; 5–15% have continuous symptoms with remission.
Incomplete response to corticosteroid therapy	Subgroup of groups A and B above	Approximately 65% of patients with an incomplete response to steroids essentially undergo colectomy, often within 1 year.[3]
Severe (Fulminant) Colitis	10–15%	Approximately 75% of patients with fulminant colitis fail to respond to intensive therapy in 2–4 days and undergo colectomy. Mortality rate is ~ 11% without perforation.[8] These are older data and currently survival is increased as a result of earlier surgical intervention.
Toxic megacolon	5–10%	
With perforation (16% of group acute toxic megacolon)	0.9–1.6%[8–10]	
Perforation	3%	Perforation can occur with severe disease but without fulminant colitis or toxic megacolon. Risk of perforation increased with *initial* severe attack.
Hemorrhage		
Massive	3%	
Recurrent		
Growth Retardation		
Carcinoma		
With universal colitis	13%[13]	
Left-sided colitis	5%[13]	

surgery is recommended for such patients. An equally difficult problem concerns the patient who experiences a satisfactory clinical response to corticosteroids but the dosage required to maintain remission is either prohibitive or is associated with troublesome complications. Case Study Number 1 (see the discussion that follows) illustrates this particular problem. It should also be emphasized that long-term corticosteroid therapy can be associated with many complications. These are summarized in Table 25-3. The most important complications of corticosteroid therapy include weight gain, masking of latent diabetes mellitus or aggravation of manifest diabetes, metabolic bone disease with osteopenia and compression fractures, increased irritability and insomnia, and stigmata of hypercorticism. Finally, all patients on long-term corticosteroid therapy need to have periodic ophthalmologic examinations to detect early cataract formation.

CASE STUDY NUMBER 1.: CHRONIC ULCERATIVE COLITIS WITH SATISFACTORY CLINICAL RESPONSE BUT WITH A PROHIBITIVE CORTICOSTEROID DOSAGE AND TROUBLESOME COMPLICATIONS OF THERAPY. In 1975, at the age of 34, this woman developed crampy abdominal pain, diarrhea, rectal bleeding, and tenesmus. Pertinent studies, including sigmoidoscopy, rectal biopsy, and barium enema examination led to a diagnosis of chronic ulcerative colitis. Initial treatment consisted of sulfasalazine in a dosage of 3.0 g per day and folic acid 1.0 mg per day. Because diarrhea, hematochezia, and crampy abdominal pain persisted, however, the patient was started on prednisone in a dosage of 40 mg per day. She responded well to this treatment and corticosteroids were slowly tapered over a 6 month period and discontinued. During the next 2 years, the patient experienced recurrent flare-ups, but such exacerbations responded well to high doses of corticosteroids, that is, 40 to 60 mg of prednisone per day. Importantly, long-term corticosteroid therapy unmasked latent diabetes mellitus and the patient required 30 units of NPH insulin daily to effect reasonable control of hyperglycemia.

TABLE 25-3. *Complications of Corticosteroid Therapy.*

Stigmata of Hypercorticism
  Acne
  Hirsutism
  Moon facies
  Cervicothoracic obesity
  Easy bruisability
  Poor wound healing
Problems Related to Abnormalities in Salt and Water Metabolism
  Sodium retention
  Weight gain (also related to increased appetite and polyphagia)*
  Edema
  Increased blood pressure
  Hypokalemia (can contribute to muscle weakness)
Endocrine—Metabolic Problems
  Unmask latent diabetes*
  Aggravate manifest diabetes*
  Adrenal crisis may occur if medications abruptly discontinued
Musculoskeletal
  Steroid myopathy with muscle weakness
  Osteopenia*
  Compression fractures*
  Aseptic necrosis, femoral head
Gastrointestinal
  Abdominal pain and dyspepsia
  Mask an acute abdomen (especially perforated viscus)
  Exacerbate peptic ulcer disease
Nervous System
  Depression
  Increased irritability*
  Insomnia
  Psychosis
Hematologic
  Leukocytosis
  Neutrophilia
  Lymphocytopenia
Immunologic/Infections
  False-negative skin tests
  Increased susceptibility to infection (opportunistic infections)
  Impaired cell-mediated immunity
  Reactivation of tuberculosis
Miscellaneous
  Premature cataracts

*Most important complications

In June 1980, because of a particularly severe flare-up and increased disease activity accompanied by fever, tachycardia, leukocytosis, severe diarrhea, and hematochezia, the patient was hospitalized at the Kansas University Medical Center. Following the institution of high dose corticosteroid therapy, i.e., 60 mg of prednisone per day, the patient's symptoms gradually improved; however, whenever the corticosteroid dosage was decreased below 35 mg of prednisone per day, she developed diarrhea and hematochezia. In addition, with the higher dosage she experienced recurrent staphylococcal infections of the skin and herpetic keratitis. Because of inability to effect control of the patient's disease with a more modest corticosteroid dosage, and in view of the presence of a serious side effect (i.e., corticosteroid-induced diabetes mellitus), it was decided to carry out elective pancolectomy. Two months after this procedure was performed, all medications had been discontinued and the patient no longer had evidence of carbohydrate intolerance. She had no further difficulties from 1980 to 1986.

Comment. This patient had rather severe chronic ulcerative colitis that initially responded well to conventional therapy; however, corticosteroids unmasked latent diabetes that required the patient to remain on insulin therapy. Later, the dosage of corticosteroids required to maintain the patient in reasonable control, greater than 40 mg of prednisone per day, was prohibitive. Finally, additional troublesome complications, such as staphylococcal skin infections and herpetic keratitis, were felt to be related, at least in part, to corticosteroid therapy. These factors were important considerations in recommending pancolectomy.

Fulminant colitis with or without toxic megacolon

Severe (fulminant) colitis occurs in approximately 10 to 15% of patients with CUC. Toxic megacolon is a potentially lethal complication and develops in about 10 to 20% of patients with severe attacks of CUC (see Chapter 14). Thus, approximately 1 to 6% of all cases of CUC are complicated by the development of toxic megacolon. Current guidelines for management of toxic megacolon are as follows (see also Chapter 14)—(1) patients with toxic megacolon should receive 48 to 72 hours of intensive medical treatment, and (2) patients who have not shown clear-cut objective evidence of progressive improvement within this time should undergo operation. Thus, patients with toxic megacolon and fulminant colitis should rapidly demonstrate a marked decrease in the number of bowel motions per day, obvious improvement in hematochezia, amelioration of fever, tachycardia, signs of toxicity, and abdominal pain, and disappearance of radiographic signs of toxic dilatation. If such objective signs of improvement are lacking, prompt operation is indicated. This policy of aggressive early (within 72 hours) operative intervention in toxic magacolon has resulted in a decrease in the mortality rate from 23% to approximately 5 to 10%.[8-10] The key variable affecting the mortality rate in toxic megacolon is perforation. The mortality rate with medical treatment alone is as high as 80% if perforation has occurred.[8-10] Similarly, the mortality rate with surgical treatment is 42 to 50% if perforation has occurred, compared with 8.7 to 11% without perforation.[8-10]

It should be emphasized that toxic megacolon is not an absolute indication for colectomy. Approximately 25% of such patients will respond to an intensive medical regimen, including pharmacologic doses of corticosteroids, repair of red blood cell, serum protein, intravascular volume, and serum electrolyte abnormalities, antibiotics, and colonic decompression. For further details on the medical treatment of fulminant colitis and toxic megacolon, see Chapters 14 and 21.

The treacherous nature of first attacks and their propensity to progress to fulminant colitis is illustrated by the second case study.

CASE STUDY NUMBER 2: ULCERATIVE COLITIS WITH RAPID PROGRESSION OF DISEASE, ILLUSTRATING THE TREACHEROUS NATURE OF FIRST ATTACKS. In September 1979, this 24-year-old steelworker experienced the onset of diarrhea, hematochezia, and crampy abdominal pain. He consulted his family physician who initiated therapy with an anticholinergic drug. The patient's symptoms persisted and two weeks later he underwent a sigmoidoscopic examination that revealed changes felt to be entirely consistent with the diagnosis of chronic ulcerative colitis. A barium enema examination done shortly thereafter revealed changes involving the left colon; these changes were also felt to be characteristic of ulcerative colitis. The presence of deep collar-button ulcers was also noted, however. The patient was started on sulfasalazine in a dosage of 4.0 g per day. During the next two weeks, he continued to have diarrhea, hematochezia, and abdominal discomfort. He was transferred to another hospital but, unfortunately, the patient's roentgenograms and records were not sent with him. Inadvertently, a repeat barium enema examination was carried out. Surprisingly, this showed the presence of universal colitis with deep ulcerations throughout the colon. After these findings became evident, the patient was transferred to the Kansas University Medical Center. Upon admission, he was noted to have fever, tachycardia, leukocytosis, hypoalbuminemia, and hypokalemia. Accordingly, he was placed on an intensive regimen including intravenous corticosteroids; vigorous rehydration, and repair of serum albumin and serum potassium abnormalities was carried out and, in addition, the patient was made nil per os (NPO). In the next 24 hours, he improved substantially, with regression of fever, tachycardia, and a decrease in the number of bloody bowel motions. During the third day in the hospital, however, it was noted that the patient's pulse rate increased from 78 to 100 beats per minute, and this was accompanied by complaints of abdominal and shoulder pain. A flat film of the abdomen revealed the presence of free air under the diaphragm and a diagnosis of intestinal perforation, masked by corticosteroid therapy, was made. The patient underwent laparotomy and total proctocolectomy was performed. Examination of the surgical specimen revealed the presence of severe pancolitis with a perforation at the hepatic flexure.

Comment. This case exemplifies the treacherous nature of first attacks of ulcerative colitis. This patient had experienced only rare gastrointestinal complaints until September 1979. In a relatively brief period of six weeks, the patient's inflammatory bowel disease progressed from a seemingly localized colitis to a severe life threatening universal colitis. This occurred despite treatment with sulfasalazine and corticosteroids. It is recognized that two serious errors were made in this patient's management. First, in the presence of diarrhea and hematochezia, he was placed on anticholinergic drugs without a firm diagnosis. Subsequently, the clinical features indicated the presence of unstable inflammatory bowel disease. In this setting, it was unfortunate that a repeat barium enema examination was performed. This may have contributed significantly to the rapid progression of disease and the development of fulminant colitis with perforation (see Chap. 14). This case underscores the need for first attacks of ulcerative colitis to be brought under control quickly. This is especially so if certain clinical features such as fever, tachycardia, leukocytosis, more than six grossly bloody bowel motions per day, anemia, and hypokalemia are present.

Perforation*

Perforation is an infrequent complication of idiopathic ulcerative colitis, occurring in approximately 3% of patients. It is most likely to occur with the first attack and is the only major local complication of ulcerative colitis that appears to behave in this manner. The most common site of perforation is the sigmoid colon. The majority of cases occur in patients with a severe attack of ulcerative colitis. In the series of Edwards and Truelove, 20 of 624 patients (3.2%) experienced a perforation.[10] Sixteen such cases occurred with a severe attack, four with an attack that was classified as moderately severe, and none with an attack deemed mild. The evidence that corticosteroids increase the risk of perforation is not convincing. As stressed earlier, perforation remains a serious problem that is underscored by the fact that the operative mortality rate in patients with toxic megacolon and perforation is 42%.[8] By contrast, the mortality rate for patients with toxic megacolon without perforation is 5 to 10%.[8]

Hemorrhage*

Massive hemorrhage occurs infrequently in idiopathic ulcerative colitis. In the classic study by Edwards and Truelove, 21 of 624 patients (3.4%) experienced a massive hemorrhage as defined by sudden bleeding that required urgent blood transfusion, or continued heavy bleeding demanding massive transfusion.[10] Such bleeding can usually be treated by conservative measures and only rarely is an indication for emergency colectomy.

Growth Retardation

See the discussion on growth retardation in the "Crohn's Disease" section of this chapter (see also Chapters 23, 24).

Carcinoma*

DEFINITE RISK FACTORS. Several studies have firmly established that ulcerative colitis predisposes to colonic carcinoma.[11-13] At least five factors are associated with a high risk of subsequent development of cancer in patients with idiopathic ulcerative colitis. These include the following: (1) long duration of disease, (i.e., greater than 10 years); (2) universal colitis or total involvement of the colon; (3) left sided colitis; (4) dysplasia, especially if it is high grade;[14,15] and (5) dysplasia-associated lesion or mass (DALM).[16] In one series of 396 patients with ulcerative colitis followed for as long as 43 years, 3% developed cancer within 10 years after the onset of colitis.[12] Thereafter, cancer developed in 20% of exposed children in each decade, however. The risk was 43%, 35 years after onset of colitis. Greenstein et al. reviewed the records of 276 patients with ulcerative colitis seen between 1960 and 76 at the Mount Sinai Hospital.[13] Adenocarcinoma of the large bowel was present in 26 patients (9.7%). Cancer developed in 13% of the patients with universal colitis but it also occurred in 5% of those with left sided colitis. Nugent et al. provided firm evidence supporting the concept that dysplasia is a significant risk factor in the development of colonic carcinoma.[14] These investigators reviewed the records of 23 patients known to have chronic ulcerative colitis and colonic carcinoma and 57 consecutive patients with ulcerative colitis without malignancy. Dysplasia was identified in all but one of 23 resected colons harboring colonic carcinoma. By contrast, moderate to marked dysplasia was found in specimens from only 10.5% of control cases.

Blackstone et al. performed colonoscopy over a 4 year period on 112 patients with long-standing ulcerative colitis, and found a dysplasia-associated lesion or mass (DALM) in 12.[16] This appeared as either a single polypoid mass (5 cases), a plaque-like lesion (2 cases), or multiple polyps (5 cases). In 7 of these 12 cases, carcinoma was subsequently found. This was particularly true in the 5 cases of single polypoid masses where all 5 contained invasive carcinoma. In none of the cases associated with malignancy did multiple biopsies of the DALM reveal invasive carcinoma. In only 2 of the 7 patients with carcinoma was the dysplasia "severe," being "mild" or "moderate" in the remaining 5. In the 27 patients with dysplasia found incidentally in random biopsies of flat mucosa only one carcinoma was found, in contrast to the 7 cancers in 12 patients with DALM. This difference led Blackstone et al. to regard the finding of DALM, especially a single polypoid mass, as highly significant in patients with long-standing ulcerative colitis. It carries a sufficiently high risk of cancer, thereby constituting a strong indication for colectomy.

---

*See Chapter 14.

†See Chapter 15.

CONTROVERSIAL RISK FACTORS. Other risk factors exist, currently considered controversial, that may be associated with an increased risk of colonic cancer in patients with ulcerative colitis. These include the onset of the disease in childhood,[12] continuous active disease,[11,17] and a clinically severe first attack. Whereas Devroede et al. provided data indicating that onset of disease in childhood is a risk factor,[12] this was not confirmed in the studies by Greenstein et al.[13]

VEXING PROBLEM OF WEIGHING RISK FACTORS FOR DEVELOPING CARCINOMA IF ONLY ONE OR TWO ARE PRESENT. The decision to recommend elective proctocolectomy in patients with idiopathic ulcerative colitis is clear-cut if several of the aforementioned risk factors are present. Thus, in a patient with long-standing disease, (i.e., greater than 10 years), universal colitis, dysplastic lesions demonstrated upon examination of colonic biopsy specimens, and continuous active symptomatic disease, proctocolectomy is clearly indicated. On the other hand, in the majority of cases, the decision is not so obvious. For example, consider the relatively asymptomatic patient with long duration of disease and universal colitis and in whom colonic biopsy specimens reveal *indefinite* evidence for dysplasia. An equally troublesome situation is the patient with disease of less than 10 years duration, segmental disease, such as left sided colitis, but with *definite* dysplasia.

Accumulating evidence supports the concept that the demonstration of unequivocal high-grade dysplasia constitutes a definite indication for colectomy. In the paper by Riddell et al.,[15] colonic biopsy specimens are classified as "negative," "indefinite for dysplasia," and "positive for dysplasia," the latter category including both low-grade dysplasia and high-grade dysplasia. In patients with high-grade dysplasia, colectomy should be considered, especially if dysplasia is confirmed upon examination of repeat biopsy specimens. In patients with low-grade dysplasia, it is important to insure interval follow-up at 6 month intervals. As already indicated, however, if a dysplasia-associated mass lesion is identified, colectomy is also indicated. Although the risk factors outlined in Table 25-1 are helpful in identifying the patient with high risk for developing colonic carcinoma, it should be re-emphasized that many patients will not fit neatly into this scheme. In such cases, serial detailed observations will frequently allow a decision regarding elective proctocolectomy* (see also chapter 15).

Finally, it should be recalled that colorectal cancers in patients with ulcerative colitis are frequently unusual from both a clinical and pathologic point of view. The cancers in such patients are often multiple (10%) and more proximal in distribution (50% in the ascending or transverse colon) than colon cancers in the noncolitis population. Further, the presence of an abdominal mass and intestinal obstruction are significantly more frequent in patients with cancer complicating ulcerative colitis.

Indications for Surgical Intervention in Crohn's Disease

The indications for surgical intervention in Crohn's disease are summarized in Table 25-4

TABLE 25-4. *Indications for Surgery in Crohn's Disease.*

Gastroduodenal Crohn's Disease
  Obstruction
  Hemorrhage
Small Bowel Crohn's Disease
  Failure of medical therapy
    Frank failure
    Incomplete response
      limitations of life-style
    Satisfactory response but corticosteroid dosage prohibitive
    Complications of corticosteroid therapy
    Noncompliance with medical regimen
  Obstruction
    Acute
    Chronic
      with intermittent moderate-to-high-grade obstruction
      with multiple strictures
      with stagnant loop syndrome
  Perforation
  Fistula
    With or without obstruction
    Types
      enteroenteric
      enterocutaneous
      enterovesical
  Abscess
  Hemorrhage
  Carcinoma
    Long-standing disease (>15 years)
    Bypassed gut
  Growth retardation

*Editors' note: See also: Lennard-Jones, J. E.: Gut 27:1403, 1986.

TABLE 25-4. (continued).

Colonic Crohn's Disease
  Failure of medical therapy
  Fulminant colitis
    With and without toxic megacolon
  Hemorrhage
    Acute
    Recurrent
  Growth retardation
  Fistulas
    Enteroenteric
    Enterocutaneous
    Enterovesical
    Enterovaginal
  Obstruction
    Chronic
  Perforation
  Abscess
    Perirectal
    Other
  Florid anal/perianal disease
  Carcinoma

and pertinent supporting data are found in Tables 25-5 and 25-6.

Failure of Medical Therapy

The National Cooperative Crohn's Disease Study (NCCDS) provided important information on the natural history of Crohn's disease and the effectiveness of medical therapy.[4,5] In that study, 569 patients with Crohn's disease were randomized to receive either placebo, prednisone, sulfasalazine, or azathioprine treatment for 4 months. Patients entering remission within a 17 week period, as defined by a Crohn's disease activity index (CDAI) of <150, were randomized to receive either placebo, prednisone, or sulfasalazine during a more prolonged trial lasting 2 years. During the first phase, approximately 32% of the patients receiving placebo achieved a spontaneous remission and approximately half of this group remained in remission

TABLE 25-5. *Supporting Data Regarding Indications for Surgical Treatment in Crohn's Disease.*

Indication/Complication	Approximate Incidence	Comment
Failure of medical therapy[4,20]	• Ileocolic—15/225 (7%) patients • Small intestine—11/130 (8%) patients • Colon—33/127 (26%) patients Totals = 59/482 (12.2%)	Approximately 33% of Crohn's disease patients achieve remission with placebo, and half of these are still in remission after 2 or more years. Remission occurs in 60–75% of patients treated acutely (17 weeks) with corticosteroids. Approximately 70% of this group (42–50% of the total group) remain in remission after 2 years of continuous corticosteroid therapy.
Obstruction[20]	• Ileocolic—79/225 (35%) patients • Small bowel—72/130 (55%) patients • Colon—15/127 (12%) patients Totals = 166/482 (34%)	While patients with obstructive lesions may respond to high-dose intravenous steroids, such responses are often short-lived. High-grade obstructive lesions should be treated surgically, especially in persons with increasing symptoms.
Fistula/Abscess[20]	• Ileocolic—98/225 (44%) patients	Fistulas infrequently heal with corticosteroids. Closure

TABLE 25-5. *(continued).*

	• Small bowel—41/130 (32%) patients • Colon—30/127 (23%) patients Totals = 169/482 (35%)	rate has been as high as 30–40% with 6-mercaptopurine; however, obstruction and active disease are often associated with failure of medical therapy.
Hemorrhage[37,38]	Massive hemorrhage is rare, occurring in about 1% of patients with CD	Massive bleeding not related to: (1) age at onset, duration of, or activity of disease; (2) medical therapy; or (3) clinical pattern. Patients having one such bleed are more likely to experience additional bleeds. Surgical treatment is indicated if life threatening hemorrhage persists despite medical therapy, including selective embolization.
Growth Retardation	15–30% children with CD[39]	22/130 youngsters with inflammatory bowel disease (19-CUC, 3-CD) were growth retarded (< 3rd percentile in height). Significant growth temporally related to intestinal resection occurred in 7 of 11 patients.[39–41]
Perforation[22,23]	Free perforation is a rare complication; 7 cases found in one series of 360 patients.[22] Mt. Sinai Series; 10/627 (1.6%) patients with Crohn's colitis or ileocolitis, and 6/849 (0.7%) patients with small bowel regional enteritis or ileocolitis, experienced a free perforation.[23]	Perforation most likely to occur during an acute exacerbation of chronic disease, particularly in the presence of distal obstruction.
Florid Anorectal and Perineal Disease	Anorectal disease occurred in 21 of 615 (3.4%) patients with Crohn's disease.[20]	Therapy with high dosages of metronidazole (20 mg/kg/day) for up to 20 months results in healing in approximately 60% of patients. However, when metronidazole is discontinued, relapse occurs in about 75% of patients. Reinstitution of metronidazole often results in healing, which is maintained as long as the drug is continued.[42,43]
Carcinoma	12 cases of carcinoma in 449 CD patients (7 colon, 1 rectum, 4 small bowel).[44] Risk of colorectal cancer	CD patients develop colorectal cancer a decade earlier than patients with colorectal carcinoma of the usual type.

TABLE 25-5. *(continued).*

	increased 6- to 24-fold in patients with Crohn's colitis or bypassed gut.[45–48]	Average duration of Crohn's colitis is 24 years. Dysplasia usually present. Mucinous type carcinoma is common.
Gastroduodenal Crohn's disease[49]	2–4% of CD patients have their primary disease confined to the duodenum.	Unrelenting obstruction is the primary indication for operation.

TABLE 25-6. *Fistulas in Crohn's Disease.*

I. Enteroenteric

Series	Number of Patients with CD	Number of Patients with Enteroenteric Fistulas	Number with Ileosigmoidal Fistulas	Mean Age at Diagnosis (years)	Time Before Diagnosis (years)
Broe[24]	348	64 (18.4%)	17 (4.9%)	25	4.4
Greenstein[25]	160	51 (31.8%)	9 (5.6%)		
Fazio[26]	1600		27 (1.7%)		
Block[27]	376		48 (12.7%)		
Givel[28]		99	30	30	7.5

II. Enterovesical

Series	Number of Patients with CD	Number of Patients with Enterovesical Fistulas	Mean age at diagnosis (years)	Time before diagnosis (years)
Talamini[29]	348	16 (4.6%)	31	10
Kyle[30]	440	10 (2.3%)		
Schraut[31]	376	29 (7.7%)		

III. Enterovaginal

Series	Number of Patients with CD	Number of Patients with Fistula	Number of Patients with Enterovaginal Fistula	Comment
Givel[32]	99	16	Rectum—13 Sigmoid—1 Small bowel—1 Ileorectal anastomosis—1	1. Fistulas infrequently demonstrated by x-ray or endoscopy 2. 11/16 did not heal with medical therapy 3. Outcome of surgery "radical"— 8/8 healed "conservative" 0/4 healed
Bandy[34]		15		9/10 undergoing primary repair *without* fecal diversion, healed

TABLE 25-6. (continued)

Korelitz[35]	34	6				2/6 patients with rectal-vaginal fistulas closed with 6-MP, and 1/6 improved

Enterocutaneous

Series	Number of Patients with Enterocutaneous Fistula	Groups	Healed With Medical Therapy	Healed After Surgical Treatment	
				Conservative	Radical
Hawker[36]	39	1. No active disease; (post-operative fistulas)	6/7		
		2. Active disease	1/20	1/8	28/29
Korelitz[35]	8		6/8 healed with 6-MP in dosage of 1.5 mg/kg/day		

after 24 months. By contrast, 78% of the group receiving prednisone attained a Crohn's disease activity index of <150 units, and 52% of the patients receiving sulfasalazine also attained a CDAI of <150 units. In the second part, approximately 68% of the patients receiving prednisone remained in remission, as compared to approximately 53 to 58% of the patients receiving placebo and sulfasalazine. These data indicate that the *initial* treatment with sulfasalazine and prednisone is more effective than placebo in inducing remission in patients with Crohn's disease. The patients most likely to respond to sulfasalazine are patients with: (1) colon-only disease; (2) active disease for less than 6 months; and (3) no prior history of medical or surgical therapy. It is disappointing to note, however, that over the course of 2 years, prednisone therapy did not prove to be superior to placebo or sulfasalazine in maintaining patients in remission. The long-term medical therapy of patients with symptomatic and extensive Crohn's disease is discussed in detail in Chapter 22. It should be emphasized that the majority of patients with the disease either fail medical therapy or require continued treatment with medications such as corticosteroids, metronidazole, azathioprine, and 6-mercaptopurine (Table 25-5). As the data cited previously indicate that corticosteroids are variably effective in maintaining Crohn's disease in remission, the question can be raised as to how long patients should remain on such therapy. Most authorities would argue that failure to respond to medical therapy within

6 months constitutes a treatment failure. Many such patients with an incomplete response are maintained on corticosteroids indefinitely merely for control of symptoms, however. It should be emphasized that if the response is *incomplete* or if the *dosage of corticosteroids required to maintain a patient in remission is prohibitive*, and other indications for surgical therapy exist, then a decision should be made to carry out elective surgery (see also Chapter 26). This recommendation is more clear cut if localized disease is present. The third case study illustrates the problem posed by an incomplete response to medical therapy.

CASE STUDY NUMBER 3: ELECTIVE ILEOCOLECTOMY FOR LOCALIZED CROHN'S DISEASE RESPONDING WELL TO MEDICAL THERAPY. In 1975, at age 24, this young woman presented to the Kansas University Medical Center with complaints of cramping abdominal pain, diarrhea, weight loss, fever, and back pain. Physical examination confirmed the presence of low-grade fever (38.0°C), borderline tachycardia (pulse = 100 beats/min), and weight loss (body weight 45.0 kg). In addition, a tender palpable mass was easily appreciated in the right lower quadrant. Sigmoidoscopic examination was normal to 25 cm. Barium enema studies revealed changes consistent with Crohn's disease involving the cecum and terminal ileum. Upper GI and small bowel series confirmed the presence of distal ileal disease. In addition, a fistulous communication was noted between the ileum and cecum. The hematocrit and hemoglobin levels were 35% and 11.2 g/dl respectively. The white blood cell count was 14,000/mm^3 and the erythrocyte sedimentation rate 45 mm/hour (Wintrobe). The serum albumin was 3.8 g/dl and the serum potassium 4.0 mEq/l. Treatment was initiated with sulfasalazine at a dosage of 3.0 g/day and prednisone at a dosage of 30 mg/day. A dramatic response occurred with amelioration of constitutional symptoms, weight gain of 10 kg, and a decrease in size and tenderness of the right lower quadrant abdominal mass. The prednisone dosage was slowly tapered from 30 mg/day to 10 mg/day over a 6 month period of time. An attempt was then made to change the prednisone regimen from 10 mg/day to 20 mg every other day. Within 2 months of this change, the patient experienced an exacerbation of symptoms that required increasing the prednisone dosage to 20 mg/day. Again, corticosteroids were cautiously tapered over a 12 month period of time from 20 mg/day to 10 mg/day. The regimen was then changed to 20 mg prednisone every other day. Within 3 months after switching the patient to this regimen, she again experienced an exacerbation of disease with recrudescence of abdominal pain, weight loss, and low grade fever. When the prednisone dosage was increased to 20 mg/day, the symptoms resolved. This cycle was repeated once more with the same results. Small bowel enema examination done in 1980 revealed persistence of a fistulous tract between the distal ileum and the cecum. No evidence of dilatation of the ileum was found above the diseased area of distal small bowel. Yearly ophthalmic examinations had revealed no evidence of cataracts until early 1980 when evidence of early cataract formation was noted. Because of the incomplete response to treatment and because of the early development of cataracts, it was recognized that the patient could not remain on corticosteroids indefinitely. Accordingly, she underwent resection of the distal ileum and cecum and an ileotransverse colostomy was fashioned. Her postoperative course was uneventful and the patient has remained asymptomatic.

Comment. This patient had a good albeit incomplete response to therapy with corticosteroids and sulfasalazine. Whenever attempts were made to taper corticosteroids below a dosage of 10 mg/day, however, she experienced an exacerbation of her disease. The development of early cataracts forced her physicians to assess treatment alternatives. The possibility of using azathioprine, 6-mercaptopurine, and metronidazole were discussed with the patient and she chose surgical treatment. This case illustrates a dilemma frequently faced by gastroenterologists treating patients with Crohn's disease. The patient's disease is reasonably controlled with modest doses of corticosteroids; however, whenever an attempt is made to reduce corticosteroids below a critical level, the disease flares. The minimum dosage of corticosteroids calculated to maintain such patients in remission is approximately 0.15 mg prednisone equivalent per kg/day.[18] The question arises as to the likelihood that fistulas will close either spontaneously or in response to corticosteroid therapy (see also Chap. 14). Review of the literature suggests that fistulas, in the presence of an obstructive lesion, rarely heal. The healing rate for fistulas in the absence of an obstructive lesion ranges from 6 to 30%.[19] Thus, in this patient with low-grade obstruction and a fistulous tract, it appeared unlikely that the disease would remit with medical therapy and this influenced the decision to recommend surgical intervention.

Obstruction

Obstruction is one of the most common indications for surgical treatment in Crohn's disease, ranking just behind fistula and abscess formation. In an analysis of 500 patients with Crohn's disease undergoing surgical therapy, 166 (33.2%) had obstruction as their primary indication for surgical therapy.[20,21] If one examines the relationship between the clinical pattern of Crohn's disease and the likelihood of surgical intervention for an obstructive lesion, some interesting data emerge (Table 25-5). In this regard, 72 of 130 patients (55%) with small bowel Crohn's disease developed intestinal obstruction. Similarly, 79 of 225 patients (35%) with ileocolic Crohn's disease underwent surgical procedure because of intestinal obstruction. By contrast, only 15 of 127 patients (12%) with Crohn's disease of the colon only underwent surgical treatment because of obstruction. While patients with obstructive lesions may respond to high-dose intravenous corticosteroid therapy, such responses are often short-lived. High-grade obstructive lesions should be treated surgically, especially in the presence of increasing symptoms. Furthermore, patients with high-grade obstructive lesions and worsening symptoms are at an increased risk of developing perforation. These features are illustrated in the fourth case study.

CASE STUDY NUMBER 4: CROHN'S ILEOCOLITIS, HIGH-GRADE INTESTINAL OBSTRUCTION, AND INTESTINAL PERFORATION MASKED BY CORTICOSTEROIDS. In December 1969, at age 26, this woman developed diarrhea, crampy abdominal pain, and fever. She was hospitalized, a diagnosis of ulcerative colitis was made, and treatment with sulfasalazine was initiated. She was first seen at the Kansas University Medical Center in October 1975, at which time a detailed workup suggested that she had Crohn's ileocolitis. In this regard, sigmoidoscopic examination was normal, barium enema studies showed inflammatory disease involving the right colon and distal ileum, and an upper GI and small bowel follow-through roentgenogram study revealed a normal small bowel except for changes in the distal ileum thought to be characteristic of Crohn's disease. A Schilling test part II revealed only 6% excretion of labeled vitamin B_{12}. Complete blood count (CBC), erythrocyte sedimentation rate, and serum proteins were normal. Therapy with sulfasalazine was continued at a dosage of 1.0 g t.i.d.

In 1976, the patient complained of increased abdominal pain and for the first time a mass was palpable in the right lower quadrant. The erythrocyte sedimentation rate was minimally raised to a value of 44 mm/hr (Wintrobe). Treatment with prednisone at a dosage of 20 mg/day was started.

In January 1977, she developed the abrupt onset of severe right lower quadrant pain. It was thought that she had an incomplete small bowel obstruction, and she was given high-dose parenteral steroids that led to prompt relief of symptoms, decrease in the size of the mass in the right lower quadrant, and amelioration of abdominal pain and tenderness. A small bowel series done at that time showed a stenotic distal ileum with changes comparable to those seen previously. Treatment with prednisone at a dosage of 40 mg/day and sulfasalazine at a dosage of 3.0 g/day was continued. In April 1977, she had a similar presentation, also with prompt resolution of symptoms with intravenous corticosteroids. In June 1977, she once again developed severe right lower quadrant pain. Examination revealed hypoactive bowel sounds and equivocal rebound tenderness in the right lower quadrant. The white blood cell count was 21,000/mm^3. Abdominal plain films revealed no small bowel gas, no air fluid levels, and no evidence of free air under the diaphragm. Blood cultures were drawn, the patient was started on nasogastric suction, and the dose of corticosteroids was again increased. The next day she was clearly better and the white blood cell count had decreased to 9,300/mm^3. On the patient's third day in the hospital, she had the onset of right upper quadrant pain that radiated to the shoulder. The pulse increased from 78 to 96 beats per minute. A chest film revealed free air under the diaphragm. Laparotomy disclosed a ruptured terminal ileum with peritonitis and a subhepatic abscess. She underwent subtotal colectomy and ileostomy.

Comment. This patient experienced a free perforation of the terminal ileum, which is an unusual complication of Crohn's disease (see Chap. 14). In a representative study, only 7 cases of perforation were found in a total series of 360 patients with Crohn's disease.[22] Typically, perforation occurs during an acute exacerbation of the disease and is always associated with distal obstruction caused by a chronic stenosing lesion. The duration of Crohn's disease has ranged from 3 months to over 6 years prior to the occurrence of perforation.[22,23] The perforations occur in a diseased segment of bowel and all are proximal to diseased and narrowed bowel. Little evidence exists that corticosteroids increase the risk of perforation. In the case study above, however, it does appear that corticosteroids masked the perforation, because the only signs pointing to perforation were an increase in the pulse rate and the development of right shoulder pain. The patient's two prior episodes of high-grade obstruction that responded to corticosteroids should have alerted her attending physicians to the increased likelihood that she would sustain a perforation of the distal small bowel. Elective rather than emergency surgical treatment should have taken place.

Fistula/Abscess in Crohn's Disease

Fistula with or without abscess formation is a major indication for surgical treatment in Crohn's disease. That this is a considerable problem is underscored by the data obtained by Farmer et al. in their review of indications for surgical therapy in 500 patients with Crohn's disease (see Chap. 26).[21] In 225 patients with ileocolic Crohn's disease, fistula and abscess were the primary indication for surgical intervention in 98 (44%). Similarly, in 130 patients with small intestinal Crohn's disease, fistula and abscess formation were the major indication for surgical intervention in 41 patients (32%). Finally, in 127 patients with colonic Crohn's disease, fistula and abscess formation were the major indication for surgical intervention in 30 patients (23%).

Patients with Crohn's disease develop 4 different kinds of fistulas (see Chap. 14): enteroenteric, enterovesical, enterovaginal, and enterocutaneous (Table 25-6). The most common of the four is the enteroenteric fistula, which has been noted in 18 to 32% of patients with regional enteritis.[24–28] The most common enteroenteric fistula is the ileosigmoidal fistula. Such fistulas are often present for years before the correct diagnosis is established. Enterovesical fistulas occur less frequently and the incidence has ranged from 2.3 to 7.7% in 3 representative large series of patients with regional enteritis.[29–31] Enterovaginal fistulas are less common; the most frequent subtype of this variety of fistula is rectovaginal.[32–35] Enterovaginal fistulas are infrequently demonstrated by using roentgenograms or endoscopy but can be demonstrated by fistulagrams. The majority of enterovaginal fistulas do not heal with medical therapy. Further, such fistulas rarely heal if "conservative" surgical treatment is carried out that, by definition, does not include resection of diseased bowel. More "radical" surgical procedures, with resection of diseased bowel, often result in healing. It is debatable whether diversion needs to be carried out if primary repair is undertaken. Data on the efficacy of 6-mercaptopurine and azathioprine in effecting closure of rectovaginal fistulas are sparse; no large series of such patients have been studied. Some patients, however, have had such fistulas close while on medical treatment. Enterocutaneous fistulas may heal if no active underlying disease is present. All too often, however, active disease either with or without an abscess is present, and under these circumstances such fistulas infrequently heal with medical treatment. However, Korelitz et al. reported that 6 out of 8 patients with enterocutaneous fistulas healed when administered 1.5 mg/kg/day of 6-mercaptopurine.[35] If such fistulas heal, they do so within 3 to 6 months. Importantly, fistulas often reappear when immunosuppressive therapy is discontinued. All of the aforementioned fistulas constitute valid indications for surgical intervention. The likelihood of success is enhanced if the diseased bowel is resected at the time of the treatment. From a practical point of view, it is often difficult to persuade a patient who is not particularly troubled by an enterocutaneous fistula, and whose disease is otherwise quiescent, to undergo surgical repair. This is especially true if the drainage from the fistula is minimal and the patient already has undergone prior episodes of surgical resection for Crohn's disease. It is in this setting that serious consideration should be given to treatment with agents such as metronidazole, azathioprine, and 6-mercaptopurine.

Little evidence exists indicating that corticosteroids are effective in healing fistulas. For example, in the study by Present et al., fistulas healed in only 6% of the patients receiving corticosteroids compared with 31% of those receiving 6-mercaptopurine.[19] In a subsequent study by the same investigators involving 34 patients with Crohn's disease and fistulas treated with 6-MP, fistulas closed in 13 patients (39%) and another 9 (26%) showed obvious improvement.[35] It should be reemphasized that the long-term response to treatment was good if 6-mercaptopurine was continued, whereas exacerbation frequently followed discontinuation of treatment.

CASE STUDY NUMBER 5: CROHN'S DISEASE COMPLICATED BY RECTOVAGINAL FISTULA. This 41-year-old woman presented to the Kansas University Medical Center in March 1985 for evaluation of Crohn's disease and severe malnutrition. In 1975, the patient had been diagnosed as having Crohn's disease with involvement of the rectum as well as the distal small bowel. Treatment was initiated with sulfasalazine at a dosage of 3.0 g/day and prednisone at a dosage of 30 mg/day, and these medications were subsequently discontinued. She did well and remained in remission until 1981 when she developed diarrhea, fever, crampy abdominal pain, and weight loss. Treatment with corticosteroids was reinstituted. Since 1981, she had been maintained on varying doses of prednisone and had also been on metronidazole at a dosage of 250 mg t.i.d. During this time, she felt improved but never experienced a sustained remission. In February 1984 she required hospitalization elsewhere and received intravenous fluids and hyperalimentation. At that time she was noted to have a rectovaginal fistula with persistent drainage. In addition, she had a perianal abscess drained in November 1984.

When evaluated in March 1985, the patient was having 2 to 5 loose mucoid bowel motions per day, associated with crampy abdominal pain, bloating, and urgency. Rarely, she experienced hematochezia. Her weight had decreased from 125 to 110 to 85 pounds. She had arthralgias involving both the knees and the shoulders. In addition, she had mucocutaneous lesions of the mouth.

Physical examination revealed a cachectic white female with moon facies; her weight was 85 pounds. Vital signs were normal. Pertinent findings included the presence of a 6 × 7 cm, fairly tender, firm mass extending from the umbilicus to just above the bladder. Rectal examination revealed large hemorrhoids and a perirectal fistula. Colonoscopic examination revealed normal mucosa to 13 to 15 cm. However, from 15 cm to 33 cm there was patchy inflammation, erythema, linear ulcerations, and some polypoid lesions. From 33 cm to the cecum no evidence of additional disease existed. Small bowel roentgenograms revealed evidence of ileal disease, with narrowing of the distal 5 to 10 cm; the remainder of the small bowel appeared normal. Tests of intestinal absorptive function revealed a fecal fat excretion of 4.8 g/day. D-xylose test, Schilling test for vitamin B_{12} absorption, and routine chemistries were normal except for a borderline serum albumin of 3.5 g/dl, and a serum zinc of 54 μg/dl. The important finding was the demonstration of a fistulous opening, with a diameter approximately the size of a small pencil, 1 to 2 cm above the anus that communicated directly with the vagina.

The patient was placed on a total parenteral nutrition and during the next 2 weeks gained weight from 36.9 to 45 kg. It was recognized that the patient was significantly anorectic and that this was, at least in part, because of treatment with metronidazole. The patient's corticosteroid dosage was reduced to 17.5 mg/day, and metronidazole dosage was decreased to 250 mg/day. Subsequently, the patient was able to ingest 2,000 calories per day and maintain her weight at approximately 100 pounds. She was also treated with zinc sulfate at a dosage of 220 mg p.o. daily.

Comment. Considerable discussion took place as to whether this patient's rectovaginal fistula should be repaired. The 4 choices with regard to managing a rectovaginal fistula in this case were as follows: (1) to change the diet and add either enteral or parenteral nutrition to effect a weight gain up to the patient's normal weight of 110 pounds; (2) to consider direct closure of the fistula; (3) to consider a diverting colostomy and wait for the fistulas to heal prior to reanastomosis of gut; and (4) to elect for a combination of #2 and #3, (i.e. carry out a diverting colostomy and do a primary repair as well). From a review of the literature, it appears that no particular surgical procedure has a clear superiority. We chose to delay making a recommendation until the patient gained weight to approximately 120 pounds, then recommended direct closure or a combination of diverting colostomy and primary closure.

Hemorrhage*

Occult gastrointestinal bleeding is common in patients with Crohn's disease, especially with ileocolic or colonic involvement. By contrast, acute massive intestinal bleeding is unusual. Crohn and Yarnis found such bleeding in 5 of 540 (0.9%) patients.[36] Farmer et al. describe hemorrhage in 2 of 352 (0.6%) patients with either ileocolic or colonic Crohn's disease.[20] Homan et al. recorded massive intestinal bleeding in 7 of 503 (1.4%) patients.[38] In the latter study, bleeding was not influenced by the age of the patient, the duration of Crohn's disease, the use of corticosteroids, or the activity of disease. Interestingly, patients having one massive bleeding episode are more likely to have at least one additional massive bleed. In general, therapy for such bleeding is unsatisfactory and no uniform agreement has been reached on the efficacy of surgical resection. Surgical treatment should be recommended in patients with Crohn's disease and massive bleeding if the following conditions exist: (1) no other causes or source of bleeding have been demonstrated; (2) bleeding has not slowed following initial stabilization and transfusion of 4 to 6 additional units of blood; (3) bleeding is life-threatening; (4) recurrent massive hemorrhage has occurred; and (5) another concurrent indication for resection of involved intestine obtains. Obviously, not all these conditions need to be present.

The following case study illustrates the problem of recurrent bleeding coupled with another concurrent indication for colectomy.

Case Study Number 6: Long-standing Crohn's colitis with intermittent activity and recurrent rectal bleeding. In 1961, at age 27, this patient, a male physician, was hospitalized at the University of Washington Hospital because of diarrhea, fever, erythema nodosum, and arthritis. Proctosigmoidoscopic examination and barium enema studies revealed the presence of inflammatory disease involving the rectum and cecum. The distal ileum appeared to be normal. These findings led to a diagnosis of Crohn's disease. Treatment with sulfasalazine, oral corticosteroids, and corticosteroid enemas was initiated.

*See Chapter 14.

The patient's symptoms were resolved, and the medications were tapered and discontinued.

In 1964, he was seen at the Kansas University Medical Center with complaints of recurrent fever, arthritis involving the knees and ankles, diarrhea, and hematochezia. Barium enema studies at this time confirmed the presence of disease involving the cecum, ascending colon, splenic flexure, and rectosigmoid. An upper GI and small bowel series were normal. He was started on treatment with prednisone at a dosage of 30 mg/day, which ameliorated his symptoms. In 1965, he developed painless hematochezia without other symptoms. The hematocrit and hemoglobin levels fell from 40% and 13 g/dl to 30% and 10 g/dl, respectively. He was treated with 3 units of packed red blood cells and the prednisone dosage was increased to 80 mg/day; this was subsequently tapered to 40 mg/day.

From 1965 to 1969, he altered his corticosteroid dosage from 60 to 10 mg/day according to the symptoms he experienced; this was done without the supervision of his regular physicians. In 1969 he had the onset of more severe diarrhea and underwent repeat evaluation. Barium enema revealed no changes from the studies obtained in 1965. From 1971 to 1975, he had periodic flare-ups when the dosage of corticosteroids was tapered. If prednisone was tapered from a dosage of 20 mg/day to 20 mg/every other day, he developed recurrent diarrhea, crampy abdominal pain, rectal bleeding, and arthritis.

In 1976, he was admitted to the hospital again complaining of rectal bleeding but without other symptoms. He was found to have a pulse of 120 beats/minute. The hematocrit and hemoglobin levels fell from 40% and 13 g/dl to 35% and 11 g/dl, despite a transfusion of two units of blood. Serum albumin was 3.0 g/dl. Colonoscopy revealed severe involvement of the splenic and hepatic flexures with cobblestoning, ulcerations, and pseudopolyp formation. The cecum and rectosigmoid areas were also involved, but to a lesser degree.

The patient underwent total colectomy and the pathologic study revealed the characteristic changes of Crohn's colitis. A small villous adenoma was also found. Importantly, areas of severe dysplasia were also identified.

Comment. The indications for recommending colectomy to this patient can be summarized as follows: (1) he had long-standing active disease despite treatment with pharmacologic doses of corticosteroids; (2) he had experienced recurrent rectal bleeding that required blood transfusions and hospitalization; and (3) a strong family history of colon carcinoma was present, with his father and a paternal uncle having succumbed to that disease. Any one of these factors should raise the question of elective colectomy. The fact that all 3 were present made the decision more clear-cut. In addition, histopathologic findings upon detailed examination of the colon revealed severe dysplastic changes. If this patient were being evaluated today rather than in 1976, several colonic biopsies would have been obtained and the information gained from such biopsy specimens would have influenced the decision to recommend elective colectomy.

Growth Retardation*

Significant growth retardation has been well documented in children with inflammatory bowel disease (IBD).[39-41] In a representative study, 22 of 130 (17%) youngsters had severe growth retardation, defined by height below the 3rd percentile.[39] Growth failure can occur in the absence of intestinal symptoms, and such unexplained growth failure in children and adolescents should raise the question of IBD. Retarded growth appears to be more prevalent among males with CD when gastrointestinal symptoms begin before age 14, and frequently precedes corticosteroid therapy although steroids are often a contributory factor. In the study by McCaffery et al., only 2 of 20 patients maintained on corticosteroids manifested a percentile growth increment.[39] By contrast, resection of diseased bowel resulted in a temporally related significant growth spurt in 7 of 11 patients. Such growth spurts may be related to additional factors, such as discontinuation of corticosteroids or delayed onset of pubertal growth. Growth retardation in children is related to several factors including nutritional deficiencies, acquired secondary hypopituitarism, corticosteroid therapy, and delayed pubertal growth spurt.[40] When conservative therapy, including parenteral and enteral nutrition, fails, serious consideration should be given to surgical intervention.[41]

Perforation†

Spontaneous or free perforation of the bowel is a rare complication of Crohn's disease. In a rep-

---

*See Chapters 12 and 23.
†See Chapter 14.

resentative study by Steinberg et al.,[22] 7 cases of perforation were recorded in a group of 360 patients (1.9%). In the Mt. Sinai series, 10 out of 627 (1.6) patients with Crohn's colitis or ileocolitis and 6 out of 849 (0.7%) patients with small bowel Crohn's disease or ileocolitis experienced a free perforation.[23] A review of 99 cases of free perforation revealed that the site of perforation was the ileum in 65, the colon in 22, and the jejunum in 12 patients.[23] Two perforations occurred in 3 patients and 4 perforations in one patient. Characteristically, perforation occurs during an acute exacerbation of the disease and is always associated with distal obstruction. The duration of Crohn's disease has ranged from 3 months to over 6 years prior to the occurrence of perforation. It should be emphasized, however, that perforation was the presenting manifestation of the disease in 25 of 84 reported cases.[23] Ninety-six of 99 patients were operated on; the 3 patients treated without surgical intervention died. The mortality rate was high (39%) following simple suture, and considerably lower (3.7%) after resection and anastomosis.

Anorectal and Florid Perineal Disease in Crohn's Disease*

In the study by Farmer et al., anorectal disease occurred in 21 of 615 (3.4%) patients with Crohn's disease.[20] Bernstein et al. also provided important data from 21 patients with chronic unremitting perineal Crohn's disease characterized by persistent drainage, erythema, and induration.[42] These investigators studied the efficacy of high-dose metronidazole therapy (i.e., 20 mg/kg/day) given for up to 20 months. Complete healing occurred in 10 of 18 patients receiving continuous therapy, advanced healing in 5 of 18 patients, and minimal healing in 2 of 18 patients. Side effects of metronidazole therapy were frequent and included anorexia and nausea in 33% of the patients, metallic taste in the mouth in 66% of the patients, and peripheral neuropathy in approximately 30%.

In follow-up studies on the efficacy of metronidazole, Brandt et al. attempted to discontinue the drug in 26 patients with severe perineal Crohn's disease.[43] The cessation of metronidazole therapy resulted in exacerbation of perineal disease in approximately 75% of the patients, however. When such flare-ups occurred, reinstitution of metronidazole therapy in full doses usually resulted in remission of disease. Although the data are incomplete, preliminary studies suggest that metronidazole therapy may remain effective for as long as 36 months. It must be emphasized that the majority of patients need to be maintained on such therapy continuously or perineal disease will relapse. The question arises as to whether long-term metronidazole therapy is associated with mutagenic and carcinogenic effects. To date, however, no cases have been reported in which cancer has been clearly attributable to metronidazole therapy. It is often possible to reduce the dose of metronidazole and maintain improvement in perineal Crohn's disease.

In patients with florid perineal Crohn's disease not responding to metronidazole alone, a 4 to 6 week trial of total parenteral nutrition (TPN) should be considered. The combination of metronidazole and TPN may prove effective where therapy with either alone has failed. Finally, patients with severe perineal disease who have failed the intensive medical therapy previously outlined are candidates for surgical procedures such as diverting the fecal stream or proctocolectomy.

Carcinoma†

For inexplicable reasons, many physicians do not believe that patients with Crohn's colitis are predisposed to develop colorectal carcinoma. Several epidemiologic studies, however, have shown a 6-fold to 24-fold increased risk of colorectal carcinoma in patients with Crohn's disease as compared with the general population.[44–48] More than 80% of the reported cases have occurred in those with grossly evident colorectal involvement by Crohn's disease. A study by Hamilton provided important insights into the problem of carcinoma in patients with Crohn's colitis.[47] The following points warrant emphasis: (1) patients with Crohn's disease develop colorectal cancer a decade earlier than patients with colorectal carcinoma of the usual type (55 years vs. 65 years), and 30% of the cases develop in individuals younger than 40-years-old; (2) the incidence of mucinous carcinoma appears to be increased; (3) the mean duration of Crohn's colitis prior to the development of carcinoma is approximately 24 years; (4) dysplasia was identified in all 10 patients with carcinoma and all of the 10 resected carcinomas were found to be contiguous with areas of high-grade dysplasia; and (5) 20% of the cases occurred in

*See Chapter 14. †See Chapter 15.

patients with a bypassed rectum. Thus, it appears that patients with bypassed segments of colon or rectum are at a particularly increased risk of developing colorectal carcinoma, as are those with long-standing small bowel Crohn's disease who have bypassed areas of diseased small bowel.

Another representative study was that by Weedon et al. who obtained data from 449 patients with Crohn's enteritis, enterocolitis, or colitis.[44] Life-table methods were used to compute survival rates and risk of cancer. Males constituted 63.3% of the series. All subjects were white and 26.5% were Jewish. Cancer was found in 12 patients with Crohn's disease; the primary site was in the colon in 7, in the rectum in 1, and in the small bowel in 4 patients. The interval from onset of Crohn's disease to diagnosis of cancer was 7 to 45 years. The number of cases of colorectal cancer was 20-fold greater than expected (8 colorectal cancers per 356 cases).

These and other data raise the question whether surveillance should be considered for patients with clinically evident colorectal involvement with Crohn's disease or a bypassed segment of colon or rectum, especially if the disease has been present for longer than 10 years.[47,48] Currently, this point is moot.

Gastroduodenal Crohn's Disease*

Involvement of the duodenum in Crohn's disease occurs infrequently. Crohn's disease may be confined to the duodenum or duodenal Crohn's disease may occur in association with Crohn's disease involving the stomach or colon. The latter often takes the form of a duodenal colic fistula. Primary duodenal disease has been reported to occur in approximately 2 to 4% of patients with Crohn's disease. A typical study is that of Murray et al. who reported the presence of Crohn's disease in the duodenum in 70 patients (4.2% of 1670 patients with regional enteritis) followed at the Lahey Clinic over a 30 year period.[49] Of the 70 patients with duodenal Crohn's disease, 22, or approximately 1/3, required surgical treatment. The primary symptoms of duodenal Crohn's disease relate to ulceration and obstruction; thus, pain is present in approximately 3/4 of the patients and symptoms such as nausea, vomiting, and early satiety are also present in the same number of patients. The mean time from the onset of symptoms to the time of diagnosis is approximately 2-1/2 years.

About half the patients have evidence of Crohn's disease in other areas of the gastrointestinal tract. In the study by Murray et al., several patterns of duodenal involvement were noted. Of 22 patients, 9 had involvement of the pylorus and duodenal bulb, 7 had disease limited to the descending duodenum, 3 had disease involving the distal duodenum and proximal jejunum, and 3 had diffuse involvement of the duodenum. Radiographic studies revealed a stricture of the descending duodenum in 12, a deformed bulb in 10, and ulceration or cobblestoning of the duodenum in 6 patients. Approximately 50% of 17 patients treated with antacids and a histamine H_2 receptor blocker (Tagamet†) improved for periods lasting 2 to 9 months.

The primary indication for surgical intervention in Crohn's disease involving the duodenum is unrelenting obstruction. In the series of Murray et al.,[49] 18 of 22 patients underwent a duodenal bypass procedure. A third of the patients who underwent a surgical procedure required a second operation. Hemorrhage is a rare indication for surgical intervention in duodenal Crohn's disease, having occurred in only one patient in this series.[49] Preliminary data suggested that patients with Crohn's disease involving the duodenum are at greater risk for developing pancreatitis as compared to patients with Crohn's disease without duodenal involvement.[49] Patients with duodenal-colic or gastrocolic fistulas in Crohn's disease almost always have significant disease in the colon, and such fistulas often arise from the latter diseased areas.

References

1. Kirsner, J. B., et al: Corticotropin (ACTH) and adrenal steroids in the management of ulcerative colitis: observations in 240 patients. Ann. Intern. Med., *50*:891, 1959.
2. Edwards, F. C., and Truelove, S. C.: The course and prognosis of ulcerative colitis. Gut, *4*:299, 1963.
3. Korelitz, B., and Lindner, A. E.: The influence of corticotrophin and adrenal steroids in the course of ulcerative colitis: a comparison with the presteroid era. Gastroenterology, *46*:671, 1964.
4. Summers, R. W., et al.: National Cooperative Crohn's Disease Study: Results of drug treatment. Gastroenterology, *77*:847, 1979.
5. Mekhjian, H. S., et al.: Clinical features and natural history of Crohn's disease. Gastroenterology, *77*:898, 1979.
6. Sales, D. J., and Kirsner, J. B.: Prognosis of inflammatory bowel disease. Arch. Intern. Med., *143*:294, 1983.
7. Meyers, S., et al.: Corticotropin versus hydrocortisone in the intravenous treatment of ulcerative colitis: prospec-

---

*See Chapters 9 and 22.

†Smith, Kline, and French, Philadelphia, PA 19101

tive, randomized, double-blind clinical trial. Gastroenterology, 85:351, 1984.
8. Binder, S. C., Patterson, J. F., and Glotzer, D. J.: Toxic megacolon in ulcerative colitis. Gastroenterology, 66:909, 1974.
9. Norland, C., and Kirsner, J. B.: Toxic dilatation of colon (toxic megacolon): etiology, treatment and prognosis in 42 patients. Medicine, 48:229, 1969.
10. Edwards, F. C., and Truelove, S. C.: The course and prognosis of ulcerative colitis. III. Complications. Gut, 5:1, 1964.
11. Edwards, F. C., and Truelove, S. C.: The course and prognosis of ulcerative colitis. IV. Carcinoma of the colon. Gut, 5:15, 1964.
12. DeVroede, G. J., et al.: Cancer risk and life expectancy of children with ulcerative colitis. New Engl. J. Med., 285:17, 1971.
13. Greenstein, A. J., et al.: Cancer in universal and left-sided ulcerative colitis: factors determining risk. Gastroenterology, 77:290, 1979.
14. Nugent, F. W., et al.: Malignant potential of chronic ulcerative colitis. Preliminary report. Gastroenterology, 76:1, 1979.
15. Riddell, R. H., et al.: Dysplasia in inflammatory bowel disease: Standardized classification with provisional clinical applications. Hum. Pathol., 14:931, 1983.
16. Blackstone, M. O., Riddell, R. H., Rogers, B. H. G., and Levin, B.: Dysplasia-associated lesion or mass (DALM) detected by colonoscopy in long-standing ulcerative colitis: an indication for colectomy. Gastroenterology, 80:366, 1981.
17. Truelove, S. C.: Ulcerative colitis beginning in childhood. New Engl. J. Med., 285:50, 1971.
18. Whittington, P. F., Barnes, H. V., and Bayless, T. M.: Medical management of Crohn's disease in adolescence. Gastroenterology, 72:1338, 1977.
19. Present, D. H., et al.: Treatment of Crohn's disease with 6-mercaptopurine. A long-term, randomized, double-blind study. New Engl. J. Med., 302:981, 1980.
20. Farmer, R. G., Hawk, W. A., and Turnbull, R. G., Jr.: Clinical patterns in Crohn's disease: Statistical study of 615 cases. Gastroenterology, 68:627, 1975.
21. Farmer, R. G., Hawk, W. A., and Turnbull, R. B., Jr.: Indications for surgery in Crohn's disease: analysis of 500 cases. Gastroenterology, 71:245, 1976.
22. Steinberg, D. W., Cooke, W. T., and Alexander-Williams, J. T.: Free perforation in Crohn's disease. Gut, 14:187, 1973.
23. Greenstein, A. J., Mann, D., and Sacher, D. B.: Free perforation in Crohn's disease. I. A survey of 99 cases. Am. J. Gastroenterol., 80:682, 1985.
24. Broe, P. J., Bayless, T. M., and Cameron, J. L.: Crohn's disease: are enteroenteral fistulas an indication for surgery? Surgery, 91:249, 1982.
25. Greenstein, A. J., Kark, A. E., and Dreiling, D. A.: Crohn's disease of the colon. I. Fistula in Crohn's disease of the colon: classification, presenting features, and management in 63 patients. Am. J. Gastroenterol., 62:419, 1974.
26. Fazio, V. W., Wick, P., and Turnbull, R. J.: The dilemma of Crohn's disease: Ileosigmoidal fistula complicating Crohn's disease. Dis. Colon Rectum, 20:381, 1977.
27. Block, G. E., and Schraut, W. H.: The operative treatment of Crohn's enteritis complicated by ileosigmoid fistula. Ann. Surg., 196:356, 1982.
28. Givel, J. C., et al.: Entero-enteric fistula complicating Crohn's disease. J. Clin. Gastroenterol., 5:321, 1983.
29. Talamini, M. A., Broe, P. J., and Cameron, J. L.: Urinary fistulas in Crohn's disease. Surg. Gynecol. Obstet., 154:553, 1982.
30. Kyle, J., and Murray, C. M.: Ileovesical fistula in Crohn's disease. Surgery, 66:497, 1966.
31. Schraut, W. E., and Block, G. E.: Enterovesical fistula complicating Crohn's ileocolitis. Am. J. Gastroenterol., 79:186, 1984.
32. Givel, J. C., et al.: Enterovaginal fistulas associated with Crohn's disease. Surg. Gynecol. Obstet., 155:494, 1982.
33. Saegesser, F.: Complications uro-genitales de la maladie de Crohn. Helv. Chir. Acta, 46:727–730, 1980.
34. Bandy, L., Addison, A., and Parker, R. J.: Surgical management of rectovaginal fistulas in Crohn's disease. Am. J. Obstet. Gynecol., 147:359, 1983.
35. Korelitz, B. I., and Present, D. H.: Favorable effect of 6-mercaptopurine in fistulae of Crohn's disease. Dig. Dis. Sci., 30:58, 1984.
36. Hawker, P. C., et al.: Management of enterocutaneous fistulae in Crohn's disease. Gut, 24:284, 1983.
37. Crohn, B. B., and Yarnis, H.: Regional Ileitis. 2nd Ed. New York, Grune and Stratton, 1958.
38. Homan, W. P., Tang, C. K., and Thorbjarnason, B.: Acute massive hemorrhage from intestinal Crohn's disease. Arch. Surg., 111:901, 1976.
39. McCaffery, T. D., Nasr, K., Lawrence, A. M., and Kirsner, J. B.: Severe growth retardation in children with inflammatory bowel disease. Pediatrics, 45:386, 1970.
40. Kelts, D. G., Grand, R. J., and Shen, G.: Nutritional basis of growth failure in children and adolescents with Crohn's disease. Gastroenterology, 76:720, 1979.
41. Steinberg, D. M., Allan, R. N., and Thompson, H.: Excisional surgery with ileostomy for Crohn's colitis with particular reference to factors affecting recurrence. Gut, 15:845, 1974.
42. Bernstein, L. H., Frank, M. S., Brandt, L. J., and Boley, S. J.: Healing of perineal Crohn's disease with Metronidazole. Gastroenterology, 79:357, 1980.
43. Brandt, L. J., Bernstein, L. H., Boley, S. J., and Frank, M. S.: Metronidazole therapy for perineal Crohn's disease: a follow-up study. Gastroenterology, 83:383, 1982.
44. Weedon, D. D., et al.: Crohn's disease and cancer. New Engl. J. Med., 289:1099, 1973.
45. Gyde, S. N., et al.: Malignancy in Crohn's disease. Gut, 21:1024, 1980.
46. Greenstein, A. J., et al.: A comparison of cancer risk in Crohn's disease and ulcerative colitis. Cancer, 48:2742, 1981.
47. Hamilton, S. R.: Colorectal carcinoma in patients with Crohn's disease. Gastroenterology, 89:398, 1985.
48. Glotzer, D. J.: The risk of cancer in Crohn's disease. Gastroenterology, 89:438, 1985.
49. Murray, J. J., Schoetz, D. J., Jr., and Nugent, F. W.: Surgical management of Crohn's disease involving the duodenum. Am. J. Surg., 147:58, 1984.

26 · Indications for Operation in Inflammatory Bowel Disease—A Surgeon's Opinion

DONALD J. GLOTZER, M.D.

Operation for inflammatory bowel disease is efficacious and safe, and it is presently the only potentially definitive therapy available. Because "cure" in ulcerative or Crohn's colitis is essentially at the expense of a permanent ileostomy, however and restorative operation for Crohn's disease is frequently followed by recurrent disease, operation should be undertaken only after failure of optimal nonoperative management or in the presence of otherwise unmanageable complications. Thus, a proper consideration of whether or not operation is indicated at a given point in a patient's course requires a comparison of the disabilities imposed by the disease and its nonoperative treatment, on the one hand, with those of the contemplated operation on the other. An understanding of the benefits and limitations of various aspects of medical and surgical treatment is essential, and is the appropriate perspective from which the role of operation must be assessed, not unlike the decisions that must be made about patients who have valvular heart disease. In inflammatory bowel disease, a sympathetic understanding of and insight into the unique physical and emotional consequences of the disease and its treatment are even more pertinent. An unswerving advocacy of either operative or nonoperative treatment is inappropriate and detrimental to the patient.

Crohn's Disease Involving the Foregut and Midgut

In this section the indications for operation, in "classical" regional enteritis,[1] Crohn's disease of the stomach and duodenum, jejunoileitis, and ileocolitis of limited extent are discussed. Acute ileitis is also considered because it may be confused with chronic Crohn's disease. Predominantly colonic Crohn's disease, which is now universally accepted as a true entity,[2-5] is discussed in a subsequent section together with ulcerative colitis because the two diseases often share the same therapeutic problems and, at times, may be difficult to distinguish from one another (see chapter 10).

Acute Ileitis, Considerations Regarding Appendectomy, and Appendicitis

Acute ileitis or ileocolitis (so-called acute Crohn's disease) is usually discovered at laparotomy for suspected appendicitis. Although in this case it is not necessary to consider whether or not an operation is indicated, important therapeutic decisions must be made based on the nature of the process and a clear understanding of its course.

Acute enteritis seldom if ever progresses to chronic Crohn's disease and, in fact, most authorities currently question any pathologic or etiologic relationship between the two.[6-8] A number of reports have clearly documented that acute enteritis will subside in most instances (100% in some series) without specific surgical or medical therapy.[6,8-12] Moreover, a specific etiologic agent, the Yersinia organism, has been implicated in cases of acute ileitis and mesenteric lymphadenitis, particularly in reports from Europe,[8,9,13-15] but also in those from North America.[16] Supporting evidence for causality includes rising hemagglutination titers for Yersinia and the finding of the organism in cultures of the appendiceal stump and feces. It has been estimated that about 50 to 80% of cases of acute enteritis are caused by Yersinia species.[19] Campylobacter species,[17,18] and other intestinal pathogens such as tuberculosis, tularemia, amebiasis, actinomycosis, and infestation with schistosomiasis or the fish nematode anisakis may also be etiologic in some cases of acute ileitis.[19] Now that special culture methods for Yersinia and Campylobacter are available in most hospital laboratories, these organisms should be sought for in cases of acute enteritis.

Despite the clear implication of Yersinia species in the pathogenesis of many cases of acute ileitis, no evidence has been found that it has any causal relationship to chronic Crohn's disease.[8,14,15] Some workers, particularly those in Sweden, contend that progression of non-Yersinia acute enteritis to chronic Crohn's disease can occur, however.[9]

The lack of antecedent symptoms is extremely important in the differential diagnosis of acute enteritis and chronic Crohn's disease. The gross appearance of the two lesions also helps in this differentiation. In both conditions the intestine and adjacent mesentery are inflamed and prominent lymphadenopathy may be found. In acute enteritis, however, the serosal surfaces appear fiery red, edematous, and acutely inflamed rather than fibrotic and opaque with neovascularity. Moreover, the stiff, thickened wall resembling a rubber garden hose, the circumferential encroachment of fat on the intestine, the thickened mesentery, skip areas, and fibrotic, loop-to-loop adhesions suggestive of enteroenteric fistulas are not found in cases of acute enteritis.[19]

Recognition by the surgeon of the true nature of the process (which is based on the previously mentioned considerations), together with his awareness of its self-limited course should obviate an ill-advised bypass procedure or resection for acute enteritis. Whatever the nature of the process, appendectomy usually should be performed if the cecum is normal, despite the concern expressed in the older literature,[20-22] and, more recently, about postoperative fecal fistula after appendectomy for chronic Crohn's disease.[23,24] A number of reports attest to the safety of appendectomy and the infrequent occurrence of postoperative enterocutaneous fistula in the presence of either acute enteritis or chronic Crohn's disease, provided that the cecum at the base of the appendix is not involved by the inflammatory process.[6,11,12,25-27] Violation of this proscription appears to account for the high incidence of complications following appendectomy in one of the recent studies advising against appendectomy when Crohn's disease is found at laparotomy.[23] The diseased ileum rather than the appendiceal stump usually is at fault in the rare fecal fistula that follows appendectomy in chronic Crohn's disease.[24,26] This hazard exists after laparotomy in patients with Crohn's disease whether or not appendectomy is performed, a fact that is not always recognized by those who advise against appendectomy.[24] Indeed, Van Patter et al. found a higher incidence of postoperative fistula when exploration was performed *without* appendectomy.[28] If the appendix is not removed from a patient with either acute ileitis or chronic Crohn's disease, the presence of a right lower quadrant incisional scar might lead to inappropriate treatment if acute appendicitis subsequently develops. If the primary process is chronic Crohn's disease, appendectomy will make the diagnosis much easier and will also simplify the management of the recurrent episodes of right lower quadrant pain which are almost certain to occur.

Increasing numbers of cases of primary Crohn's disease of the appendix are being reported.[29-35] In most of these there has been gross and microscopic evidence of acute inflammation, as well as chronic changes indicative of Crohn's disease. Synchronous Crohn's disease has been present elsewhere in the gastrointestinal tract in only about 25% of patients, and only 10 to 14% subsequently developed such lesions.[34,35] Interestingly, none of the reported patients has developed a postoperative fecal fistula after appendectomy. Gangrenous, ordinary appendicitis can also occur in patients with Crohn's disease,[36] but is seldom diagnosed preoperatively. Occasionally, however, a previously perforated appendix is found at the time of elective or urgent operation for worsening Crohn's disease, an additional argument for appendectomy at the time of discovery of Crohn's disease at laparotomy. Appendectomy is indicated and it is safe for either Crohn's disease of the appendix or the rare instance of gangrenous appendicitis in patients with Crohn's disease, provided that the base of the appendix in the cecum is normal.

Recurrence after Restorative Operation

At the time of Crohn and coworkers' original report, 1 of the 14 patients in the series had already suffered a postoperative recurrence of disease.[5] Although this was attributed to a resection that was too conservative, it is now generally accepted that recurrent disease will eventually develop in the majority of operated patients. The site of recurrence is typically the neoterminal ileum and, curiously, the process usually ends abruptly at the site of anastomosis with the colon, an enigma that is more fully discussed in Chapter 27 on surgical treatment. In a milestone paper, Lennard-Jones and Stalder pointed out that the true incidence of recurrence depends upon whether this is defined by the rate of reoperation, by symptoms, by X-ray documentation, or by a combination of these.[37] Even more important was the introduction by Lennard-Jones and Stalder of actuarial methodology into the analysis of the results of operation in Crohn's disease. Previously, rates of recurrence had been reported as gross rates that did not take into account the length and completeness of the follow-up. In contrast to older literature, in which recurrence rates varied from very low to very high, the currently reported rates of recurrence from one institution to another are rather uniform. Based on X-ray and/or pathologic examination, the rate of recurrence is about 30% at 5 years, 50% at 10 years, and 70% at 15 years.[37-46] If routine X-ray surveillance for postoperative recurrence were carried out, an even steeper climb in the cumulative rate of recurrence would be noted. In fact, Rutgeerts et al.,[47] who routinely endoscoped patients within 1 year of ileocolonic resection for Crohn's disease, found that 72% had already developed recurrent disease. Interestingly the incidence of recurrent disease at 1 year was not significantly different from the 79% rate observed for patients endoscoped 1 to 3 years after operation, or the 77% rate 3 to 10 years post-operatively.

It is this high incidence of recurrent disease after operation that dictates that nonoperative therapy be the primary approach to the treatment of Crohn's disease. Most authorities would agree with the general tenor expressed throughout this chapter that operation should be undertaken only when intensive and optimal nonoperative management has failed or in the face of otherwise unmanageable complications. It is true that some clinicians advocate early "radical" operation to forestall future complications;[7] however, the evidence for an overall improvement in results by the adoption of this policy is by no means convincing. Moreover, despite the attractiveness of the concept, no drug or combination of drugs has been shown to be beneficial as a prophylactic measure after all recognizable disease has been removed (see Chap. 22).[48-50]*

These comments should not be misconstrued to suggest that operation in regional enteritis be avoided or delayed "at all costs" or, for that matter, that a recurrence in a given patient constitutes a failure of the treatment. Quite the contrary—operation offers immediate relief of severe disability or life threatening complications, occasional "cure," and, most often, significant palliation, many times with a prolonged asymptomatic interval. These benefits will be achieved and maximized *only* if proper indications for operation are employed.

Gastric and Duodenal Crohn's Disease

Involvement of the stomach and/or duodenum occurs in 1 to 4% of all cases of Crohn's disease.[51-64] Most often it is seen as "skip" disease in conjunction with the more common sites of involvement such as the terminal ileum and/or the colon, or as part of diffuse involvement of the small intestine.[51-64] Indeed, in the absence of simultaneous or metachronous involvement of other areas of the intestinal tract (although a number of such cases have been reported) the diagnosis of isolated gastric or duodenal Crohn's disease may be difficult because of the frequent lack of specific histologic features. Duodenal Crohn's disease is much more common than gastric involvement. Gastroduodenitis is common, however, and in some series it is more common than isolated involvement of either the duodenum or stomach.

The symptoms of gastroduodenal Crohn's disease are produced primarily by obstruction

---

* Editors' note: See also Gebdes K., et al.: Prospective follow-up of early lesions after ileal resection for Crohn's Disease. Gut, 27:A610, 1986.

secondary to progressive cicatricial stenosis of the lumen.[51-64] Thus, the initial symptoms are usually nausea, vomiting, and early satiety.[64] Epigastric pain is also prominent among the complaints and, over time, is at least as common as nausea and vomiting. It seems likely that acid-peptic digestion plays a part in the generation of some of the symptoms, especially pain, because relief can often be achieved, at least for a time, with antacids and/or H_2 blockers.[64] Because food aggravates the symptoms, the patient tends to restrict the intake of food, resulting in loss of weight. Chronic anemia resulting from occult loss of blood from the ulcerated mucosa or from B_{12} deficiency in gastric disease can also be part of the clinical picture.[65] Sometimes, however, bleeding can be acute and massive (vide infra).[66,67]

Increasing numbers of cases of duodenal Crohn's disease have been reported in which the symptoms, the radiologic findings, and the gross appearance mimic those of bulbar or postbulbar duodenal ulcer.[51,54,64] To add further confusion to the differential diagnosis of these two conditions, the incidence of duodenal ulcer appears to be increased in patients with ileal Crohn's disease, although acid hypersecretion has not been documented consistently nor has it been clearly related to the extent of ileal disease or resection.[68] It is also possible that corticosteroid treatment might be an additional ulcerogenic factor, although the significance of this association has been questioned and is controversial.[69,70] Failure to recognize or to consider the possibility of duodenal Crohn's disease when operation for presumed peptic ulcer is undertaken in patients with Crohn's disease has often led to duodenal fistula after gastric resection or pyloroplasty. Because a fairly characteristic endoscopic picture has been described,[71] gastroduodenoscopy may be helpful in making the differential diagnosis. The microscopic findings after endoscopic biopsy in duodenal Crohn's disease usually prove to be nonspecific, however.[71] Even direct inspection at the time of operation may be of limited usefulness in this distinction. Because of the indeterminate nature of the pathology and because the complication of duodenal fistula is so grave, it is probably best to avoid any operative manipulation of the duodenum should surgical treatment of duodenal disease become mandatory in a patient with Crohn's disease (see Chap. 27). The advantage of establishing a definitive diagnosis of duodenal Crohn's disease by resection or biopsy (often impossible, as already suggested) is not as important as avoiding a duodenal fistula.

The most common indication for operation for gastroduodenal Crohn's disease is failure of nonoperative management. Because the experience with the long-term results of operation in gastroduodenal Crohn's disease is not so great as that for more common sites of involvement, the proper timing of operation is even more difficult to determine. Reports with long-term follow-up clearly indicate, however, that operation for gastroduodenal Crohn's disease, as might be expected, is not definitive in the majority of patients.[63,64] Thus, a recommendation for operation should be predicated on the failure of intensive and careful medical management, including dietary manipulations, antacids, and H_2 blockers, as well as specific pharmacologic agents to bring relief of intractable symptoms of pain and vomiting, inability to eat, and progressive weight loss.

Complications of gastroduodenal Crohn's disease also may mandate operation. Acute pancreatitis as a complication of duodenal disease has been reported.[72] The putative mechanism for the generation of this complication is the reflux of duodenal contents into the pancreatic duct, a phenomenon that has been documented by X-ray study.[72,73] In this setting, drug-induced acute pancreatitis must be considered in the differentia diagnosis. Azathioprine has been documented as a cause of acute pancreatitis in patients with Crohn's disease,[50,74] in patients treated with this drug for renal transplantation[75] or for conditions other than Crohn's disease.[76] The case for sulfasalazine-induced pancreatitis also has been made.[77] Because gastrojejunostomy has been effective in preventing further bouts of pancreatitis,[72] recurrent attacks in patients with duodenal Crohn's disease in the absence of other causes such as gallstones, drugs, or alcoholism represent an indication for operation.

Acute upper gastrointestinal bleeding, sometimes massive, is another complication of gastroduodenal Crohn's disease that may require operative intervention.[66,67] It has not always been clear whether the erosion into the responsible vessel has been the result of the Crohn's process or whether such erosion was peptic in origin. In any event, operation, which has included vagotomy, drainage, and suture of the bleeding vessel, has been effective in preventing exsanguination and death from this rare complication.[66]

The duodenum in patients with Crohn's disease can also be affected by a coloduodenal fistula because of the close proximity of the hepatic flexure region of the colon to the duodenum.[64,78-80] The duodenum in such cases is usually normal and is involved only passively by colonic Crohn's disease or by recurrent disease at the site of an ileocolic anastomosis. The diarrhea, malabsorption, profound weight loss, feculent vomiting, and foul eructations that result from coloduodenal fistula are largely attributed to fecal contamination of the upper gastrointestinal tract, rather than to short-circuiting of the intestinal stream. Resection of the primary site of involvement and secure closure of the duodenum is indicated and is usually effective in eliminating this complication.[64,78]

Small Intestinal Crohn's Disease

The various indications for operation in small intestinal Crohn's disease are listed in Table 26-1.

FAILURE OF MEDICAL MANAGEMENT—THE GENERIC INDICATION FOR OPERATION

In the final analysis, unless there are complications that are life-threatening, the presence of intractable symptoms is the usual reason for the abandonment of nonoperative management, whatever the anatomic distribution of the Crohn's disease. This is somewhat contrary to the position expressed by Farmer and his colleagues, who concluded that the indications for operation in ileal and ileocolonic Crohn's disease tend to be specific (e.g., obstruction, fistula).[81] Specific pathologic processes exist, such as luminal stenosis or penetration of the intestinal wall resulting in sinuses, fistulas, and/or abscesses that may eventually make the patient unresponsive to treatment or limit the rational use of drug therapy. The mere presence of one or more complications, however, does not constitute an indication for operation. Thus, the process of determining the need for operation is in essence the same for patients with ulcerative colitis or with Crohn's disease affecting the small intestine, colon, or both.

Let us consider the fairly typical patient with regional enteritis who has abdominal pain (which may or may not be exacerbated by eating), diarrhea, fever, fatigue, progressive weight loss, and inability to function productively. The roentgenogram may show some narrowing of

TABLE 26-1. *Indications for Definitive Operation in Small Intestinal Crohn's Disease**.

Intractability—failure of non-operative management
    Increasing or persistent symptoms, debility, weight loss and inability to function despite optimal management which might include sulfasalazine, metronidazole, corticosteroids, and possibly azathioprine or 6-mercaptopurine.
    Complications of chronic corticosteroid treatment.
Small intestinal obstruction or unremitting obstructive symptoms.
Internal (enteroenteric, enterovesical) or enterocutaneous fistula.
Inflammatory mass, perforation with localized peritonitis, and abdominal abscess.
Generalized peritonitis from secondary perforation of abdominal abscess or free perforation**.
Obstructive uropathy.
Multiple strictures and stagnant loop syndrome.
Persistent retardation of growth and delayed maturation in children unresponsive to nutritional and drug treatment.
(Carcinoma)**.
(Perirectal sepsis).

* Most indications are relative as explained in the text. The mere presence of a given complication is not necessarily an indication for operation.
** Absolute indication

the lumen of the terminal ileum, an inflammatory mass, or an ileocecal fistula. These demonstrated complications may exist for some time before it is determined that the patient can no longer be adequately or safely managed without operation. If we examine a still more specific indication for operation, obstruction, the same process for determining the need for operation usually takes place: a single bout of acute small bowel obstruction secondary to Crohn's disease rarely mandates emergency operation. Rather, repeated episodes of obstruction or obstructive symptoms not responding to treatment will eventually constitute the indications for an elective operation. Intractable obstructive symptoms can occur when there is neither pronounced dilatation of the proximal intestine nor what appears to be sufficient narrowing radiologically to produce the symptoms. Conversely, a surprising degree of narrowing may be found radiologically (the classic string sign) in patients with minimal symptoms.

Failure of medical management is considered to have occurred when, despite vigorous nonoperative treatment, a "downhill" course and chronic invalidism persist to an extent intolerable to the patient. Such nonoperative treatment may include dietary manipulation, nutritional supplements, systemic antibiotics, and the informed and judicious use of sulfasalazine,[50,82] metronidazole,[83] corticosteroids,[50] or possibly azathioprine or 6-mercaptopurine.[84] In addition to uncontrollable symptoms, complications of corticosteroid therapy such as osteoporosis, hip pain suggesting impending aseptic necrosis, gross Cushingoid features, diabetes, hypertension, mental aberration or frank psychosis, alopecia, atrophy of skin, or myopathy may make continued nonoperative treatment impossible.

In determining that the patient's disease is unresponsive to therapy, it should be remembered that weight loss and diarrhea may be caused by treatable secondary physiologic disturbances. These include bile salt diarrhea and steatorrhea, which latter can be secondary to bacterial overgrowth with bile salt deconjunction and/or a diminished bile salt pool as a result of deficient absorption.[85-90] Proper documentation and treatment of these abnormalities could obviate or postpone operative therapy. Anemia from chronic disease, blood loss, or deficiency of vitamin B_{12} or folic acid is common and contributes to chronic disability. Anemia alone rarely leads to operation, however. Massive hemorrhage is rare in small intestinal Crohn's disease,[91] and it is an even rarer indication for operation.

Persistent fever, toxicity unresponsive to therapy, or bacteremia should always raise the question of a suppurative complication. Although conclusive proof of the presence of undrained pus is often impossible to obtain preoperatively, the radiologic finding of penetration outside the intestinal wall with fistulas or sinus tracts is evidence in favor of this possibility.

The endpoint for the determination of failure of medical management can be somewhat imprecise and subjective, and therefore, variation is to be expected. Extreme variations in practice, however, do not seem to take into account what is known about Crohn's disease and the results of its surgical treatment. Under the same guise of "failure of medical management" I have observed operations performed before scarcely any medical treatment has been administered, or, conversely, operations being postponed for unreasonable and dangerous periods of time. Two extreme examples of the latter will illustrate this point:

Case 1: a 16-year-old female with a right lower quadrant mass varying from the size of a "plum" to "a small orange" was treated with corticosteroids for 2 years, during which time she was never well enough to attend school regularly. The treatment for an exacerbation of symptoms associated with fever and an enlarging right lower quadrant mass consisted of an increase in the dose of corticosteroids. A roentgenogram of the small intestine at this time showed an obvious communication of the ileum with a large abscess cavity.

Case 2: A 31-year-old male who had severe obstructive symptoms and demonstrated ileosigmoid and ileovesical fistulas was treated for an entire year with high doses of corticosteroids and an "elemental" diet. The "elemental" diet was necessary because this was the only nourishment he could tolerate without disabling symptoms.

Although nonoperative treatment is the foundation upon which the therapeutic approach to Crohn's disease must be based, it is also evident that avoiding an operation should never be to the detriment of the patient. A fine line of judgment often is required in an individual case.

OBSTRUCTION

An episode of acute intestinal obstruction complicating ileal Crohn's disease usually does not require emergency or urgent operative management. It is important, especially in patients with previous abdominal operations, to differentiate between obstructions caused by adhesions and those secondary to narrowing of the lumen as a result of enteritis or superimposed obturation from indigestible food residue. The differential diagnosis in this setting is usually not difficult because obstruction from regional enteritis, although it may be high-grade, is most frequently partial, essentially eliminating the possibility of strangulation. In addition, obstruction from Crohn's disease is frequently heralded by augmented symptoms of the disease including accentuated colicky pain and increased diarrhea.

Episodes of obstruction caused by Crohn's disease usually will respond to decompression with a nasogastric or intestinal tube and the intravenous replacement of fluid and electrolyte deficits and ongoing losses. Institution of or increases in dosage of corticosteroids may be of additional benefit in resolution of the obstruction. The use of an "elemental" or other liquid diet in the interval between the acute attack and the resumption of a full diet may be of value in maintaining nutrition. A prolonged period of such nonoperative therapy is not justified and is seldom necessary in patients whose obstructions will speedily resolve. An episode of obstruction sometimes indicates that the degree of cicatricial stenosis is worsening, however, and may indicate the need for operation in the near future. It has been suggested that severe obstruction may predispose to free perforation of the ileum.[92]

It is not unusual for patients with ileal or ileocolonic Crohn's disease to suffer from repeated episodes of acute small intestinal obstruction with shorter and shorter intervals between attacks. This sequence, which is often accompanied by progressive deterioration of the state of health of the patient despite optimal therapy, constitutes a strong indication for surgical treatment.

INTERNAL AND ENTEROCUTANEOUS FISTULAS

Crohn stated that "fistula formation" is the most constant clinical and pathologic phenomenon in ileitis.[93] Fistulas have been reported to occur in from 17 to 48% of patients in various series of operated cases.[94]

Before consideration of specific types of fistulas, a few general observations may be of value. Internal fistulas are the result of luminal penetration, usually with the intermediary complication of an abscess that then ruptures into an adjacent viscus. Similarly, enterocutaneous fistulas usually result from the surgical drainage of an abscess or the spontaneous rupture of an abscess through the abdominal wall. Because the accompanying abscess is usually incompletely drained by the fistula, these tracts must be viewed neither as bland communications nor as mechanisms for bypassing an obstruction. In view of the pathogenesis of fistulas, corticosteroids should be used with great caution, if at all, in their presence (vide infra). A prevalent misconception is that fistulization into an adjacent viscus spreads the disease into that viscus. If such spread occurs at all, it must be rare.

There have been frequent claims or observations of healing of fistulas in response to various therapeutic modalities including intravenous alimentation,[95-97] elemental diets,[98,99] and azathioprine or 6-mercaptopurine.[84,100-103] Claims that a given therapeutic modality can result in healing of a fistulous tract, especially one arising from a diseased segment of intestine, must be examined carefully before being accepted as valid. Many of the reports are anecdotal in nature,[100-103] and/or the definition of healing is often unclear.[84,103] Moreover, the distinction has not always been made between a fistula originating in diseased intestine and one which is a complication of anastomotic failure. It is true that the latter type of fistula frequently will heal in patients with Crohn's disease, just as it does in patients with other conditions, provided that adequate surgical drainage is effected, distal obstruction is not present, and the intestine used for anastomosis is normal.[104-106] Most importantly, as suggested, a difference exists between long-term, solid healing, or permanent cure of an external enteric fistula and "healing-over" of an external opening accompanying reduction of inflammation and temporary cessation of drainage. Especially if the external opening of the fistula is small, spontaneous healing-over is common. Such healing-over concomitant with a given therapeutic manipulation may give rise to false attribution of "cure."

ENTEROENTERIC FISTULA. Ileocecal, ileo right colic, and ileosigmoidal fistulas are the most frequent of the internal fistulas.[28,93] Fistulization can involve any organ to which the inflamed intestine can adhere, however, such as proximal loops of small intestine, duodenum, transverse colon, bladder, vagina, uterus, or fallopian tube. Fistulas may be multiple and extremely complex with involvement of numerous loops of small and large intestine, urinary bladder, and duodenum, especially when Crohn's disease of the colon is also present.

Although a dearth of solid quantitative data exists on the natural history of fistulas in Crohn's disease, it seems clear that some ileoileal, ileocecal, or even small ileosigmoidal fistulas may be tolerated for long periods of time without change or exacerbation of symptoms.[107] In fact, such fistulas are frequently discovered only at a time of operation performed for indications other than the fistula.[107,108] Therefore, the presence of an enteroenteric fistula is a relative but not an absolute indication for operation. In the patient with one or more enteroenteric fistulas who is otherwise reasonably well, nonoperative treatment may be appropriate. Nonoperative treatment of enteroenteric fistulas does entail the risk that the fistulas might become more complex during such management.[107,108] In addition, internal fistulas do, or should, limit choices in nonoperative therapy, particularly the use of corticosteroids.

ENTEROCUTANEOUS FISTULA. These most frequently drain through the scar of a previous laparotomy, although spontaneous drainage through an intact abdominal wall can also occur.[94,108] The umbilicus is an especially likely site for spontaneous fistulization, apparently because the abdominal wall is thinnest at that point and also because the pus may track to the surface by way of the urachal remnant.[109-111] Enterocutaneous fistulas also may result from the external surgical drainage of an abscess when a definitive resection or bypass of the perforated intestine is not performed at the same time.

As is the case with internal fistulas, an enterocutaneous fistula does not constitute an absolute indication for operation. For most patients, however, the choice is not a difficult one to make. It lies between having symptomatic Crohn's disease together with a persistently draining opening on the abdominal wall, and having an operation that will relieve the condition and that, in any event, will probably be necessary in the long run. Our experience with the long-term results of operation in Crohn's disease indicates that patients who had fistulas at the time of operation were no more likely to develop recurrent fistulas as a manifestation of any recurrent disease than those without fistula.[46] Therefore, operative treatment in such patients may permanently cure the annoying and troublesome external fistula, especially if the tract through the abdominal wall is properly managed (See Chap. 27).

ENTEROVESICAL FISTULA. This complication is usually considered an absolute indication for operative treatment because of the consequences of repeated or persistent urinary infection in addition to the symptoms of the intestinal disease itself.[112-114] The resultant urinary tract infections may not be severe and in some patients can be controlled over long periods by antibiotics or urinary antiseptics.[113,114] Moreover, anecdotal reports have told of spontaneous healing or of healing that occurred following various kinds of drug treatment. The majority of patients, however, are not successfully managed over time without operation, and resection, rather than bypass, almost always is necessary to correct this condition.[108,112-114] In our experience, staged procedures seldom add to the ease with which operation can be performed.

EXTENSIVE OR END-STAGE DISEASE COMPLICATED BY FISTULA. At times one encounters patients whose disease is so extensive or whose residual intestine is so limited that the presence of fistulas, including troublesome enterocutaneous communications, would appear to be less disabling than the results of an extensive and crippling resection necessary to deal with the problem. In such patients, attempts at simple interruption of the fistula and closure of the opening in the diseased intestine by one or the other method are seldom, if ever, successful.[94] Provision of adequate surgical drainage and parenteral antibiotics can be helpful in palliative management. Metronidazole also might be tried.[73] Although reservations as to the efficacy of immunosuppressive therapy in closing fistulas were expressed earlier, it is in this type of patient in whom the risk-benefit scale would be tipped in favor of trial of such therapy. Intravenous alimentation or elemental diets may be helpful in these difficult cases, but again, clear-cut documentation of the efficacy of these treatments has not been obtained.[95-99] In a few of these seemingly "inoperable" patients, when all the aforementioned measures have failed, I have undertaken operations that entailed freeing the intestine from one end to the other from adhesions, careful repair of serosal injuries, and one or more conservative resections, with gratifying success in eliminating fistulas and the accompanying sepsis and disability. Obviously, such salvage surgical treatment should be undertaken only as a last resort in the type of patient described, because the result will not always be good.

INFLAMMATORY MASS, ABDOMINAL ABSCESS, AND PERFORATION

Palpable abdominal masses were almost a constant feature of the cases originally described by Crohn et al.[5] In a report 22 years later, Van Patter et al. still reported masses in about one-third of over a thousand operated patients.[28] At the present time, such masses appear to be less prevalent, but when encountered they continue to present a clinical dilemma. These masses may simply be one or more palpable loop of stiff, hose-like intestine together with the thickened mesentery containing large hyperplastic lymph nodes. Abdominal masses in patients with Crohn's disease are often phlegmons or frank abscesses resulting from extraluminal penetrations or perforations, however. A tubular configuration of the mass on physical examination suggests that the mass is the diseased intestine itself, rather than the result of an extraluminal complication. Roentgen studies may be helpful in this differentiation (vide infra).

The development of acute right lower quadrant peritonitis constitutes a fairly common emergency in patients with Crohn's disease. A mass may or may not be present but because of tenderness may not be detectable. Still other patients have a long-standing mass that may have been noted by themselves or their physicians. Patients with localized peritoneal signs and Crohn's disease with or without a mass are usually safely treated with nasogastric suction, intravenous fluids, and intravenous antibiotics, provided that the patient is closely and continuously observed. A progressive decrease in the degree and extent of the local signs, together with improvement of constitutional signs including falling temperature, pulse rate, and leukocytosis, would encourage continued nonoperative treatment. On the other hand, spreading peritonitis or failure to improve constitutes an indication for immediate operation. Assuming that initial treatment is successful in containing and ultimately eliminating the peritoneal signs, subsequent treatment should depend upon whether the underlying inflammatory process is intramural or extramural. Even though this distinction cannot always be made with absolute certainty, an informed assessment of the probable pathology must be made so further treatment can proceed rationally.

The presence on prior roentgenograms of deep sinus tracts or fistulas is indicative of penetration outside the lumen and thus suggests that the exacerbation may be secondary to the development of an abscess. Imaging with ultrasound or computerized tomography may also be helpful, and can be carried out safely at an early stage of treatment. It is preferable, however, to postpone contrast roentgenograms to avoid the possibility of disrupting a sealed-off perforation and extravasating intestinal content and barium into the peritoneal cavity. Furthermore, the main clinical question, whether or not the peritonitis will remain localized and come under control, will not be answered by emergency roentgen studies. Subsequent to the subsidence of all or most of the local signs, contrast studies may be safely obtained. Based on the radiographic findings and clinical course up to that time, a judgment can be made about long-range definitive therapy just as in any patient with Crohn's disease and an abdominal mass. The management strategy just described is analogous to typical protocol in the treatment of suspected diverticulitis.

A diagnosis of a frank abscess represents a clear indication for operation. This diagnosis may sometimes be made on the basis of physical findings that include progressive enlargement of a mass, increasing tenderness and/or erythema, or even the development of fluctuance. The presence of an abscess is usually documented, however, by conventional roentgenograms that show a contrast-filled cavity or an extraluminal mass. Ultrasound or computed tomography can also be helpful in some cases.

I feel that the presence of masses with fistulas and sinus tracts contraindicates treatment with corticosteroids, recognizing that this may be a controversial position. The European drug trial provides strong evidence supporting this position because patients with palpable abdominal masses treated with 6-methylprednisolone were found to suffer from an excess of unfavorable outcomes, including death.[115] Although some abscesses may drain into the lumen and resolve, frequently intra-abdominal abscesses develop into a huge size, the premonitory symptoms of which may be masked by corticosteroid therapy. In other cases, the onset of generalized peritonitis secondary to perforation of the abscess has represented the first clue that such patients were not as well as they seemed. Under corticosteroid treatment, ileovesical or enteroenteric fistulas may develop, also unheralded by increased symptoms.

Thus, in patients with fistulas or deep sinus tracts, particularly those associated with a mass, surgical treatment seems to be a safer alternative for an acute exacerbation of symptoms than treatment with corticosteroids or immunosuppressive agents. On the other hand, resolution of the clinical episode during treatment with systemic antibiotics, perhaps with the addition of a relatively safe drug such as sulfasalazine or metronidazole, suggests an intramural or a relatively minor extraluminal process that may be safely treated by nonoperative means.

PERITONITIS AND FREE PERFORATION

The development of generalized peritonitis in regional enteritis is relatively infrequent, presumably because of the indolent course of the inflammatory process. As in diverticulitis, "perforation," and generalized peritonitis most commonly result from secondary rupture of an abscess into the peritoneal cavity. Free perforation of the intestine, spilling intestinal content into the abdomen, has been reported many times, however, disproving the older dictum that this complication never occurred in Crohn's disease.[91,116-120] The infrequency of free perforation in Crohn's disease is in contrast to the case with ulcerative colitis in which free perforation may well be the ultimate complication of a severe exacerbation or toxic megacolon. A number of free perforations in Crohn's disease have developed in loops of intestine excluded from the fecal stream by surgical bypass.[117,119] Many of the reported cases of free perforation have occurred in patients without a previous diagnosis of Crohn's disease and indeed in those without antecedent symptoms. As emphasized by Waye and Lithgow, some of these patients already have established chronic regional enteritis at the time of perforation, and others may have had a true "acute Crohn's disease," if such exists, or acute enteritis.[117]

Emergency operation is obviously required for both free perforation and secondary rupture of an abscess.

OBSTRUCTIVE UROPATHY

Obstruction of the ureter (usually the right) is a well recognized complication of ileal and ileocecal Crohn's disease.[121,122] The true incidence of this complication is difficult to determine. It is probably not as high as that reported by Block et al. who found obstructive uropathy in 27 of 106 operated cases.[122] These investigators themselves acknowledged that the frequency of this complication in their experience may have been a reflection of the referral of difficult cases, rather than a representation of the true incidence.

Patients with obstructive uropathy may or may not have symptoms specifically referrable to this complication. In a high percentage, some or all of the symptoms are attributable to the inflammatory mass causing the obstruction, such as pain in the hip, flank, and anterior thigh.[121,122] Conversely, Crohn's disease must be considered in the differential diagnosis of any extrinsic right sided ureteral obstruction. Because obstructive uropathy is often occult, ultrasound study of the kidneys should be obtained in any patient with Crohn's disease about to undergo operation, to screen for this complication. In those patients in whom the ultrasound study demonstrates a dilated collecting system, an intravenous pyelogram might be of additional diagnostic help.

Patients with Crohn's disease complicated by obstructive uropathy almost invariably require operation because of the symptoms and signs of the causative inflammatory mass, progressive destruction of renal mass, or both.

CARCINOMA*

The association of carcinoma of the small intestine and regional enteritis had been reported in over 78 patients up to 1985.[123] It is generally concluded that this association is not a chance event and that the usual long duration of the inflammatory changes has predisposed the small intestinal mucosa to neoplasia. Such a causal relationship is even more difficult to establish conclusively than is the case for colonic cancer and colonic inflammatory bowel disease in which some controversy as to the magnitude of risk still exists, especially in Crohn's colitis.[124] Meaningful cohort analyses are not possible because both regional enteritis and sporadic carcinoma of the small intestine, especially the latter, have such a low incidence. However, Hoffman et al. estimated that the risk of small intestinal adenocarcinoma in a patient with regional enteritis is, at a minimum, 6 to 320 times greater than that in a person of the same age and sex without Crohn's disease.[125] Darke et al. calculated that the chance association of the two diseases (based on the prevalence figures of both) is 1 in 1,000,000,000, whereas the reported prevalence is about 1 in 350.[126] Additional evidence for a significant association includes the observations that, compared to sporadic cases, Crohn's disease-associated cancers: (1) tend to occur in patients 1 or 2 decades younger; (2) are more likely to be found in the distal (inflamed) intestine rather than in the jejunum, where sporadic cases more commonly occur; (3) have a male/female predominance, whereas usually the ratio is 1 to 1; (4) may be multifocal rather than unifocal; and (5) are more likely to be poorly differentiated, of the signet ring type, and grossly invisible.[123,127,128] The fact that mucosal dysplasia also has been found in a number of cases can be taken as additional evidence that Crohn's disease predisposes to carcinoma.[128,129]

Almost all of the reported cases of carcinoma have been found unexpectedly at operation or at autopsy. These flat tumors are virtually impossible to detect by radiographic examination in the already distorted intestine. Small intestinal adenocarcinomas complicating Crohn's disease are generally incurable, with only 3 patients (with

*See also Chapter 15.

incidentally found cancers) who survived 5 years or more after operation.[123] Nonetheless an awareness of the possible association may lead the astute clinician to suspect carcinoma in the patient with long-standing quiescent disease who develops rapidly increasing obstructive symptoms. Although a few cases have been reported of the simultaneous discovery of the two diseases,[127] the duration of Crohn's disease before the development of carcinoma has usually been long, averaging about 16 to 18 years.[123,128] Nevertheless, the low absolute incidence of carcinoma suggests that no role for prophylactic resection or even routine surveillance exists.[124] On the other hand, because 30 to 40% of the reported cases have occurred in bypassed segments of small intestine,[128,130] prophylaxis of a sort can be practiced by using resection, whenever feasible, rather than bypass in surgical treatment.

PERINEAL COMPLICATIONS

Perineal complications occur frequently during the course of Crohn's disease and may antedate clinically detectable intestinal disease.[131,132] When patients are carefully examined, significant lesions (fissures, abscesses, sinuses, or fistulas) are found in as many as 75% of Crohn's patients as compared to only 6% of control patients.[133] Perineal complications, particularly abscesses and fistulas, are more common in patients with colonic or ileocolonic disease than in those who have small intestinal disease alone.[132-134] These problems are particularly frequent when the rectum is involved.[132-134]

Even though these complications are among the most frequent and troublesome found in Crohn's disease, the presence of perirectal sepsis alone is seldom an indication for definitive surgical therapy of the intestinal disease. The exception is the patient with colonic Crohn's disease who has severe rectal involvement, in which case the fistulas are particularly destructive and difficult to treat. In patients with small intestinal Crohn's disease and right sided ileocolitis, fistulas and abscesses are usually the result of suppurative infection in an anal crypt gland, identical with the pathogenesis in patients without underlying inflammatory disease. They are not, as has been suggested in the past,[135] enterocutaneous lesions secondary to heavy, diseased ileum sinking into the pelvis and perforating through to the perineum. Perirectal abscesses and fistulas associated with rectal Crohn's disease can result from a transmural perforation of an ulcerating lesion and thus the lesions in some of these patients may have a different pathogenesis from the usual.

Although perianal abscesses and fistulas have received much emphasis as a diagnostic trait of Crohn's disease, the local treatment of these complications has usually been given little more attention than the brief and cryptic advice for extreme conservatism. These admonitions have resulted in a widely prevalent policy of "benign neglect." Such an ultraconservative approach (sitz baths, antibiotics, inadequate drainage) often results not only in unnecessary suffering, but also in extension of the suppurative process to produce a "watering pot" perineum and destruction of the sphincter mechanism. Even such treatment as metronidazole may fall into the category of "benign neglect" when the lesion is small and amenable to surgical correction,[136,137] especially because this treatment lacks conclusive proof of efficacy,[138] entails drug side effects and the possibility of severe septic complications in the presence of undrained pus.[139] Many patients with rectal Crohn's disease, extensive or high level fistula, or even a normal rectum and active ileitis undergo the usual treatment for fistula, laying open the entire tract, including the crypt of origin—fistulotomy, fistulectomy, which may result in an indolent unhealed wound. Nevertheless, completely noninterventionist treatment of these complications by physicians and surgeons has been overemphasized.

For abscesses of any magnitude, adequate external drainage under general or regional anesthesia is advisable followed by careful aftercare to prevent premature closure of the wound. This conventional method of dealing with suppuration often has been followed by control of sepsis and normal healing. An attempt to identify and lay open the crypt of origin in the presence of a large abscess is not recommended; however, established fistulas in patients without rectal Crohn's disease, even if these are extensive and complex, can often be treated definitively by marsupialization of all the fistulous tracts and laying open the crypt of origin. Even extensive wounds of this type may heal without incident. In a number of cases it has been gratifying to find that even though the external tracts were extensive and involved the groin, labia, or scrotum, the tract through the sphincter was superficial and that simply laying-open the tracts resulted in total healing. Little or no evidence exists to legitimize the fear expressed in older literature that attempts at surgical treatment of perirectal complications would cause a flare-up of intestinal disease.[140] On the other hand, some evidence supports the oft claimed adverse effect of intestinal disease on the perirectal complications and their surgical treatment.[141,142] It is prudent practice to have the intestinal disease under good medical or surgical control before attempting any local treatment.[140] Obviously, such operations are at increased risk, and the possible benefits and drawbacks must be understood by patient and physician.

Support for the views expressed in this section can be found in the publications of Lockhart-Mummery,[135,143] Sohn,[140] Bergstrand,[143,144] and their associates. On the other hand, Alexander-Williams and his colleagues argue for "conservative" treatment of fistulas, although even they agree that adequate surgical drainage of abscesses is necessary and, moreover, many of their patients with low level fistulas were managed successfully by operation.[134,145,146]

The question of fecal diversion by colostomy for control of extensive perianal fistulas and sepsis in Crohn's disease is frequently raised. If perianal sepsis complicates rectal Crohn's disease, diversion with colostomy or subtotal colectomy and ileostomy has been of little or no benefit in spontaneous healing of the fistula tracts and, in fact, extension rather than healing may occur.[132,135,147,148] The same is true in patients with proximal disease (terminal ileum) and perirectal sepsis. In both cases, temporary fecal diversion has not been followed by spontaneous permanent healing that would allow subsequent restoration of intestinal continuity, nor has diversion allowed lasting local healing after fistulectomy.[132,135,147,148] I have used *permanent* end-sigmoid colostomy, in conjunction with adequate local drainage, in a few such patients with otherwise unmanageable, advanced local disease, and I have seen good patient satisfaction with use of this technique.

In the long-term treatment of patients with extensive perianal lesions of Crohn's disease, it should be kept in mind that both adenocarcinoma and squamous cell (or cloacogenic) carcinoma have been reported as presumed complications.[149,150]

DIFFUSE JEJUNOILEITIS, PROXIMAL ENTERITIS, MULTIPLE STRICTURES, AND STAGNANT LOOP SYNDROME

Extensive involvement of the proximal small intestine has been reported to occur in 3 to 10% of all patients with regional enteritis.[151] In the analysis of their experience with jejunoileitis, Cooke and Swan made the distinction between patients with diffuse, almost universal involvement of the small intestine at the time they were first seen, and those with segmental or single strictures of the proximal intestine.[151] Although this classification may be important insofar as the prognosis and course are concerned, if surgical therapy is considered the importance of this distinction often vanishes. Malabsorption, protein-losing enteropathy, and edema are common manifestations of jejunoileitis. Symptoms in patients with this form of Crohn's disease do not necessarily include diarrhea, presumably because the terminal ileum may not be affected.[151,152]

The dilemma of the proper operative treatment of patients with such widespread involvement of the small intestine serves to epitomize the view that surgical therapy in Crohn's disease is essentially palliative. Not only is the surgeon confronted with the problem of dealing with a disease with a high rate of postoperative recurrence, but he must recognize at the outset that the manifest areas of disease cannot, in practical terms, be fully eradicated. Fortunately, many of these patients may go on for years in fairly reasonable health, often with little or no "specific" treatment. Others may require mainly nutritional and dietary manipulation. I participated in the care of a patient with diffuse Crohn's disease whose course spanned 50 years. He never required (or would accept) pharmacologic treatment in any form, and his experience with surgical treatment was confined to an incision and drainage of a small perirectal abscess (healed without chronic fistula) and a ureterolithotomy for uric acid stones.

Because extirpation of all known areas of disease in jejunoileitis frequently is not possible or reasonable, surgical therapy has to be directed toward the relief of specific problems that are otherwise unmanageable. Nevertheless, operation becomes necessary in more than half of these patients, and, in the experience of Cooke and Swan, the average number of operations per patient was 2.2.[151] This figure is comparable to that for all patients with Crohn's disease.

Despite recognized diffuse or localized proximal or distal (colonic) involvement, severe disease in the terminal ileum may require resection, either during an exacerbation unresponsive to medical management or because of local complications such as obstruction, abscess, or fistula. Such operations may be followed by years of reasonably good health even though residual diffuse proximal disease is present and despite the slight involvement of the intestine at the site of anastomosis.

Stagnant loop syndrome, secondary to single or multiple strictures, that is poorly responsive to courses of broad-spectrum antibiotics is sometimes an indication for operation in jejunoileitis. The results of resection or strictureplasty of one or more strictures can be extremely gratifying in the management of these patients.

Successful correction of severe protein-losing enteropathy by resection of a limited segment of proximal ileum involved by severe enteritis has been reported.[153]

GROWTH RETARDATION AND INFANTILISM

Severe growth retardation (<3rd percentile in height) has been found in as many as 30% of children with inflammatory bowel disease, especially those with Crohn's disease.[154-157] The majority of these children have small intestinal (Crohn's) disease but this complication can also be seen in ulcerative colitis as well.[154-156] Although a complete eludication of all the factors responsible for retarded growth and development in inflammatory bowel disease has not been found, a good deal has been learned in recent years about the important role of nutrition in the pathogenesis of the disease.[158-162] Deficits of thyroid hormone, growth hormone, or somatomedin have not been documented,[154,159] and, furthermore, the administration of human growth hormone was ineffective in reversing growth arrest.[163] These children have been shown to have sizable nitrogen and caloric deficits as a result of their often subnormal intake in the face of possible malabsorption, increased losses caused by disease, and the normal or increased daily requirements for maintenance and growth.[154,159,162] It is known that such deficits in children without inflammatory bowel disease can result in delayed growth and maturation.[164-167] High dose corticosteroid therapy is another detrimental factor because growth retardation is a well-known complication of this therapy in children treated with steroids for other conditions.[168,169]

A number of investigators have demonstrated striking spurts in growth in stunted children with inflammatory bowel disease who have been given adequate calories and nitrogen through "therapeutic nutrition." The latter can be given by the intravenous or oral route, either as the sole source of nutrition or as supplements.[158-162] Growth spurts have also been achieved in some affected children concomitant with substantial improvement of symptoms as a result of corticosteroid therapy even though these agents are well-known growth retardants.[170,171] For similar reasons operation can produce clinically significant growth spurts,[172-177] but this is by no means a uniform result even if carried out before puberty.

Because of its striking effectiveness in reversing this complication, nutritional therapy rather than operation or drugs has become the mainstay of therapy. In conjunction with the provision of adequate nutrition, sulfasalazine, corticosteroids, or operation are used to deal with otherwise intractable symptoms or complications and to maintain the improvement in the rate of growth. Every-other-day steroids appear to be useful in treating some growth retarded children with Crohn's disease because this regimen has the potential for minimizing the growth retardant properties of corticosteroids.[171] Whittington et al. reported growth spurts or maintenance of height percentile in 69% of their patients under this regimen.[171]

It is important to emphasize that whatever the therapy, it should be administered promptly and intensively before puberty, or longitudinal growth may be eliminated by closure of epiphyses.[177] All too often growth retardation is not recognized early or the underlying inflammatory bowel disease is not diagnosed in a timely manner. It would be even more tragic to persist with high-dose corticosteroid treatment in the face of recognized and unabated growth arrest in the mistaken belief that the ultimate goal is to avoid operation. Surgical treatment should be strongly considered for growth retardation if it persists despite maximal medical-nutritional treatment, or when high-dose daily corticosteroids are required to control symptoms.[154]

SYSTEMIC COMPLICATIONS

The extraintestinal complications of inflammatory bowel disease occur in small intestinal Crohn's disease as well as in ulcerative colitis and Crohn's disease of the colon; however, because they are associated with small intestinal disease less frequently, they will be discussed below in conjunction with colonic disease. In any event, since the advent of corticosteroid treatment, these complications seldom are the sole indication for operation.

Colonic Inflammatory Disease

Panproctocolectomy and ileostomy "cures" ulcerative colitis and restores normal life expectancy.[178,179] Despite its salutary effect, operation is indicated only after failure of nonoperative therapy or in cases with life-threatening complications, because of the handicaps imposed by either a permanent ileostomy or an alternative procedure (see the following). Thus, when surgical treatment is being considered as a therapeutic option, the trade-offs between disability of disease and its treatment must be carefully weighed against those of the operation. The emergence of Crohn's disease of the colon as a specific entity during the past 25 years has further increased the complexity of the determination of the proper indications for operation for colonic inflammatory bowel disease, because colonic Crohn's disease has a somewhat different course from ulcerative colitis, has unique complications, and sometimes recurs postoperatively.[2-5]

Operative intervention would be used more liberally for colonic inflammatory bowel disease, especially in ulcerative colitis, if an effective procedure that spared the anal sphincter was available. The Aylett operation (colectomy and ileoproctocolectomy) does not meet this criterion, although occasionally the result can be superb.[180-185] Similarly, at least in the author's opinion, the result of the ileoanal pull-through procedures on the average are not good enough to change the indications for and timing of operation in ulcerative colitis (See Chapters 27 and 29),[186-188] and such procedures are contraindicated in Crohn's disease because of the potential for postoperative recurrence.

In view of these considerations, this discussion of the indications for operation in colonic inflammatory bowel disease is undertaken with the assumption that panproctocolectomy will be the "Gold standard" for ulcerative colitis and for Crohn's disease affecting the rectum and substantial portions of the colon. These indications are summarized in Table 26-2.

*Ileostomy and Its Alternatives**

The reluctance of patients to accept operation for inflammatory bowel disease is often based on lack of knowledge and unreasonable fears that, regrettably, are sometimes unconsciously intensified by their physicians. An unwillingness on the part of the physician even to mention operation, especially ileostomy, presumably to avoid upsetting the patient and exacerbating the symptoms, may actually enhance the patient's concern. Rather than provoking anxiety, a frank but tactful discussion of the various modalities of treatment is reassuring to most patients. Patients often do not realize that full health can be restored by operation, and are unaware of the exact nature of an ileostomy and that few physical and social limitations are imposed thereby.

When operation is under consideration, the patient must be made aware of the advantages and disadvantages of several alternative operations that must be compared with continued nonoperative management. Available surgical alternatives include panproctocolectomy and conventional ileostomy, the Kock reservoir ileostomy,[189] various other pouch procedures, the Aylett operation, and the ileoanal pull-through procedures. Especially in the acutely ill patient,

---

TABLE 26-2. *Indications for Definitive Operation in Colonic Inflammatory Bowel Disease.*

Intractability—failure of non-operative management.
    Persistent or increasing symptoms, debility and inability to function socially and economically despite optimal management (failure of corticosteroids, sulfasalazine, and ? immunosuppressives).
    Complications of chronic corticosteroid treatment.
    Retardation of growth and maturation in children unresponsive to nutritional and drug treatment.
Fulminating colitis or toxic megacolon which fails to respond promptly to optimal therapy.
Perforation.
Pericolonic abscess, internal (enteroenteric, enterovesical) or enterocutaneous fistula in Crohn's disease.
Unremitting hemorrhage (uncommon).
Carcinoma, high grade dysplasia on biopsy (?), or high statistical probability of carcinoma.
Stricture.
    Obstructive symptoms in Crohn's disease and in ulcerative colitis (rare).
    Unresolved differential diagnosis with carcinoma.
Anal and perianal complications.
    Severe and destructive abscesses and fistulas failing to respond to local surgical therapy and systemic management.
    Stricture (rare).
Unremitting cutaneous and systemic complications (arthritis, uveitis, liver disease, pyoderma, erythema nodosum, etc.) (rare).

---

*See Chapters 27, 28, and 29.

a subtotal colectomy and ileostomy must also be mentioned because it will generally solve the immediate problem and allow a less pressured consideration of the alternatives at a later time when the patient's health and clarity of thought are restored. Moreover, leaving the rectum in situ has the additional advantage of allowing the patient to experience living with an ileostomy before being irretrievably committed to it. Further discussion of these various alternatives can be found in Chapters 27, 28, and 29.

Especially in adults, there have been relatively few severe or insurmountable problems in adjustment to conventional ileostomy when both the patient and the physician recognize that all nonoperative methods of treatment have failed, and the advantages and disadvantages of various alternative operations have been discussed in great detail. Under these circumstances, operation, which typically includes permanent ileostomy, is usually accepted by the patient as a reasonable trade-off for devastating symptoms and chronic debility. Personal contact with an attractive, well-adjusted "ileostomy patient" of the same sex and similar age often has a salubrious effect on the emotional state of the potential candidate for operation. Similar discussions with patients who have had one of the alternative procedures can be important in choosing the right operation for a particular individual.

Ulcerative Colitis

The course of ulcerative colitis varies from indolent and benign, chronic and debilitating, to acute and fulminating, and its character is subject to abrupt changes. In its severe and extensive form ulcerative colitis is potentially fatal, especially if therapy is inappropriate. The excellent study of Edwards and Truelove showed systematically what experienced clinicians had long before suspected: once a patient has had an attack of verified ulcerative colitis, further attacks can be expected almost without exception.[190] Moreover, patients having a severe or moderately severe first attack frequently already have involvement of the entire colon, and it is in these cases that the cumulative fatality rate is almost 30% in 15 years, with a continuing subsequent increment.

URGENT OPERATION FOR SEVERE DISEASE

Based on mortality statistics alone,[191,192] an argument could be made for operation during a severe first attack in the patient with universal colitis. Randomized trial of such therapy was considered worthwhile by such authorities as Edwards and Truelove,[190] but such a study has not been done. Rigid use of early operation in severe first attacks would fail to take into account those patients who might ultimately avoid operation, and such a plan presumes that the patient who fails to respond to medical treatment cannot be identified in time to prevent fatality. Even if the premise were proved that the largest number of lives could be saved by a policy of early intervention during a severe first attack, the quality of postoperative life must also be considered. Such a program might be equated to one of routine, prophylactic, bilateral simple mastectomy to prevent breast cancer in highly susceptible females.

Goligher and associates, noting the high rate of mortality of severe attacks in the previous decade, observed a reduction in the overall fatality rate from 11.3 to 1.3% after introduction of a policy of selective early operation.[192] In this study, the proportion of patients going into remission with nonoperative management was only slightly smaller than in the previous 10 years. Therefore, the improvement in the mortality rate did not appear to be at the expense of subjecting large numbers of patients to unnecessary operation. Although admittedly not randomized, Goligher's study strongly supports a policy of early surgical intervention after failure of medical treatment in the seriously ill patient.

INTRACTABILITY

Intractability is the most frequent indication for operation in ulcerative colitis. Conceptually, it is clear that when medical management has failed, operation is required. In Crohn's disease of the small intestine, however, the practical application of this indication is not so simple. Similar to the treatment of other chronic illnesses, such as heart disease or duodenal ulcer, reasonable differences of opinion can exist in an individual case, even among the most experienced clinicians. Surgeons and physicians should not be advocates of their particular disciplines. It is as inexcusable for the surgeon treating ulcerative colitis to be unaware of the effectiveness of nonoperative treatment, even in fulminating disease, as it is for the physician to take untoward risks by going to extraordinary lengths to save an already destroyed colon.

Too frequently, physicians are not sufficiently aware of the limitation of life's activities imposed by chronic debility and the necessity for living in close proximity to a bathroom. In addition, the severe physical and psychologic side effects of corticosteroid therapy are sometimes not given sufficient weight. Patients who are unable to function productively because of frequent exacerbations, intractable diarrhea, or multiple hospitalizations despite optimal treatment are candidates for elective operation.

Even in these days of cost-conscious medical care, it is necessary to hospitalize patients with exacerbations that do not respond to out-patient therapeutic manipulations. Such patients typically are treated in the hospital by the parenteral administration of optimal doses of corticosteroids, nothing by mouth (or clear liquids only), and intravenous fluids. At times, parenteral antibiotics are added to the regimen on an empiric basis. The use of azathioprine can also be considered because dramatic remissions have occasionally followed institution of this therapy. A frequent error in the management of such patients, especially in the past, has been the failure to provide for and to monitor nutrition and body weight. During prolonged attempts to bring about a remission, the provision of adequate calories and nitrogen, usually by central parenteral nutrition, will prevent the patient from lapsing imperceptibly into a situation that makes him a formidable operative risk. A lack of response of such patients to an optimal regimen over a reasonable period of time, e.g., two to three weeks, constitutes indication for semi-elective operation.

Patients with ulcerative colitis are frequently treated with corticosteroids for many years, a practice that may lead to all of the well-known and sometimes devastating complications of the hyperadrenal state. The studies by Truelove and Witts and Lennard-Jones and associates have shown that in patients in remission, a dose of corticosteroids low enough to avoid serious side effects was not better than placebo in preventing exacerbations.[193,194] This is in contrast to chronic sulfasalazine therapy that has clearly been shown to reduce the frequency of attacks in such patients,[195] even over long periods,[196] although some disagreement exists about the latter.[197] These data suggest that the optimal method of use of corticosteroids in ulcerative colitis should be to bring about a remission and then to "wean" the patient as quickly as possible, perhaps with the addition of maintenance sulfasalazine. Unfortunately, not all patients can be weaned from steroids without the development of intolerable symptoms. In some of these patients the concomitant use of sulfasalazine, which has already been mentioned, or perhaps even azathioprine[198,199] may allow the gradual reduction and ultimate omission of the steroids.[198,199] The alternative, which is probably practiced too frequently, is to accept the potentially serious side effects of relatively high-dose chronic steroid therapy. Especially in these days of informed consent, if "maintenance" corticosteroid therapy is practiced, it behooves the physician periodically to spell out the potential side effects of this treatment. Failure to achieve a remission together with an unwillingness on the part of the patient to accept chronic debility and/or the side effects of chronic steroids are strong indications for elective operation.

Growth retardation in children with ulcerative colitis represents a subgroup of patients with intractable symptoms. This complication is seen most often with small intestinal or ileocolonic Crohn's disease, but it also occurs in children with ulcerative colitis.[154,156] By extrapolation from data derived primarily from growth retarded children with Crohn's disease, growth spurts should be achievable by providing adequate nutrition. Control of symptoms by careful management with corticosteroids may also be followed by growth.[156,170] Although colectomy in such children has not always been followed by catch-up growth, at least as reported in the past,[154,156,170,172-175] a clear-cut failure to grow, as assessed by carefully kept growth charts while on adequate nonoperative treatment, suggests the need for colectomy before the epiphyses are closed.

FULMINATING COLITIS, TOXIC MEGACOLON, AND PERFORATION

The severe attack of ulcerative colitis, fulminating ulcerative colitis, and toxic megacolon represent closely related segments in the spectrum of disease severity. In general, attempts to decide whether or not a roentgenogram of the abdomen demonstrates a "true" toxic megacolon is an unrewarding exercise. Fulminating colitis can be as devastating and can be followed by the identical complications as in toxic megacolon, including perforation.

It is hoped that acute perforation, which is a medical disaster, can be prevented by appropriate management. Should perforation occur it constitutes an absolute indication for operation. Table 26-3 shows that the operative mortality rate for toxic megacolon essentially quadruples in the event of a perforation, 40% compared with

TABLE 26-3. *Collected Data on Toxic Megacolon Compiled from Major Series in the Literature.*

Author	Year	Total Cases	Total Survived	Successful Medical Management	Medical Deaths due to Perforation	Medical Deaths	Medical Failure due to Perforation	Surgical Survival without Perforation	Surgical Survival with Perforation
Lumb (200)	1955	7	3	1	0	0	3	1/3	1/3
McConnell (201)	1958	26	20	13	2	7	4+?	12/13	2/4
Roth (202)	1959	12	9	5 (1 c̄ perf)	0	1	3	3/3	1/3
Korelitz (203)	1960	16	13	5	0	2	5	6/6	4/5
Peskin (204)	1960	9	7	0	0	0	7	2/2	5/7
Sampson (205)	1961	14	10	0			4	8/10	2/4
McInerney (206)	1962	36	26	23	4	5	9	2/3	1/5
Smith (207)	1962	11	9	1	1	2	4	6/6	3/3
Rowe (208)	1963	10	9	1	0	0	5	4/5	4/4
Silverberg (209)	1964	4	3	0	1	1	1	3/3	0
Prohaska (210)	1964	16	11	—		—	9	7/7	4/9
Edwards (211)	1964	10	7	6	0	3	?	0/1	1/1
Ferrante (212)	1965	6	6	2	0	0	1	5/5	1/1
McElwain (213)	1965	9	9	4	0	0	1	4/4	1/1
Odyniec (214)	1967	37	33	13	0	1	9	?	?
Neschis (215)	1968	12	10	4	0	0	?	?	?
Jalan (216)	1969	55	30	7	4	24	16	18/22	4/12
Foley (217)	1970	28	19	0	0	0	12	14/16	7/12
Adams (218)	1973	16	13	3	0	0	5	8/8	2/5
Binder (219)	1974	18	17	1	0	0	3	13/14	3/3
Scott (220)	1975	17	16	0	0	0	7	10/10	6/7
Koudahl (221)	1975	21	15	1	0	0	6	9/14	5/6
Hartong (222)	1977	29	26	10	0	1	0	16/18?	—
Sirinek (223)	1977	42	35	10	1	1	10	?	?
Roys (224)	1977	10	7	1	0	1	3	6/6	1/3
Greenstein (225)	1985	61	51	11	1	2?	9	26/26?	13/22?
Total		532	414	122	14	51	139	183/205	71/120
			(78% of total)	(23% of total)		(10% of total)	(26% of total)	(89%)	(60%)

11%. Furthermore, careful study of the collected statistics reveals that for every patient with toxic megacolon who goes into remission with nonoperative management, more than one will perforate (23% remitted; 29% perforated). Nevertheless, the presence of toxic megacolon per se is not an absolute indication for operation because it has been demonstrated that some patients recover without operation.[219,226] Corticosteroids clearly have been demonstrated to be effective in ameliorating acute attacks of ulcerative colitis,[193,227,228] regardless of the severity,[227] although a randomized trial has never been done to assess treatment of toxic megacolon.[229] It should be remembered that only a relatively small proportion (which varies from series to series) of those who have a remission remain well for 1 or more years.[193,226,230] Therefore, the risk of prolonged nonoperative treatment must be weighed carefully against the benefits of a remission that may be short-lived (see also Chapters 14, 21, and 22).

The patient with toxic megacolon should be placed on optimal medical treatment immediately.[219] This includes nasogastric suction, replacement of fluid, serum protein, erythrocyte and electrolyte deficits, and, perhaps most importantly, optimal doses of corticosteroids. Although no serious objections to their use have been found, at our institution we do not employ nasointestinal tubes, such as the Miller-Abbott or Cantor types, in the treatment of toxic megacolon because no evidence of their superiority over a nasogastric tube exists and the usual time frame of treatment does not allow for their placement well into the small intestine. Corticosteroids are given parenterally in a dose level of 60 to 80 mg of prednisolone per 24 hours or an equivalent amount of another suitable preparation. Adrenocorticotrophic hormone may be used in patients whose adrenals are not suppressed by recent treatments with corticosteroids.[231] We prefer intramuscular corticosteroids or a constant intravenous infusion with an infusion pump over bolus intravenous doses, which have a short half-life, recognizing clearly that no study demonstrates the superiority of more constant blood levels over periodic "peaks and valleys"; constant vigilance must be exercised to make certain the patient is actually receiving the medication as ordered. A rectal tube also may be helpful in some cases. In addition, it may be worthwhile to change the position of the patient frequently from supine to prone to eliminate "gas trapping" in the colon, as described by Present et al.[232] We usually administer parenteral broad-spectrum antibiotics (typically ampicillin and chloramphenicol, or gentamicin and metronidazole), although their efficacy in this situation has not been proved. The possibility that overgrowth of Clostridium difficile may be responsible for an exacerbation leading to toxic megacolon must be kept in mind, because when this organism has been found and treated appropriately, abatement of the megacolon has resulted.[233]

Substantial and progressive improvement should ensue promptly if nonoperative management of toxic megacolon is to be continued. Although it is advisable to obtain daily abdominal films, it should be kept in mind that the roentgenogram is only one of many features that require close monitoring. Lack of significant objective improvement within a period of 24 to 72 hours or any deterioration in vital signs, physical examination, or radiologic findings during this time constitutes an indication for immediate operation. The management of fulminating colitis and severe attacks is similar, although the time table may be altered by the severity of the original manifestations of the disease.

A frequent error in the management of these patients is the failure to institute the full therapy (including maximum doses of corticosteroids) as soon as a severe or fulminating attack is recognized. Unless this is done, the doubt will continue late into the course of treatment that further medical therapy might result in remission, a position that sometimes encourages additional dangerous delay.

The medical treatment of toxic megacolon also is considered in Chapter 14 on the treatment of local complications in idiopathic colitis.

The proper surgical therapy for fulminant ulcerative colitis or toxic megacolon has been the subject of considerable debate and is considered in detail in the next chapter. In brief, I have favored subtotal colectomy and ileostomy with exteriorization of the rectosigmoid as a mucous fistula. Generally speaking, it is not necessary to resort either to tube cecostomy, as advocated by Klein and associates,[234] or to the multiple "ostomy" procedure of Turnbull.[235] If the timing of the operation is planned according to the principles just outlined, the pathologic state of the colon usually allows safe excision. Furthermore, the more severely the colon is diseased, the greater the concern about the possibility of perforation *despite* the presence of multiple stomas, a complication that I have observed. Even in Turnbull's report,[235] 4 of 42 patients so treated (almost 10%) required reoperation in the immediate postoperative period, and an additional patient died of "necrotizing vasculitis" of the intestine.

HEMORRHAGE

Massive bleeding from the colon is an infrequent complication of ulcerative colitis, occurring in only 21 of the 654 cases in the experience of Edwards and Truelove.[236] Operation to arrest unrelenting hemorrhage is required even less infrequently. In my experience, massive bleeding usually occurs in the patient with fulminating colitis or toxic megacolon. Colonic hemorrhage in general is more likely to cease spontaneously than that from the stomach or duodenum where the blood supply is richer and where ulceration tends to penetrate deeper into the wall of the viscus. However, after replacement of the blood volume deficit (as judged by the vital signs, central venous pressure, urine output, and rising hematocrit), the requirement of more than 1,000 ml of blood per 24 hours over a 2 to 3 day period should be adequate warning that the bleeding will in all likelihood not cease. As mentioned, many such patients have fever, abdominal tenderness and other signs of severe inflammation in addition to hemorrhage, which weigh additionally in favor of operation.

If emergency operation is required for patients with bleeding, the question arises as to whether resection of the rectum as well as the abdominal colon will be necessary to control the hemorrhage. In the past I have attempted to make this decision on the basis of whether or not active bleeding from the rectum could be seen by sigmoidoscopy just prior to operation. Because the rectal mucosa in such patients is friable and oozy, thereby making it difficult to distinguish between blood coming from the proximal bowel and that extravasating locally, sometimes I have wrongly concluded that the rectum was not bleeding actively at the time of subtotal colectomy only to find that reoperation was required to remove the rectum because of massive postoperative bleeding. Sigmoidoscopy is nevertheless worthwhile in this setting because if massive diffuse hemorrhage from the rectum is seen, proctectomy is mandatory, whereas if no local bleeding is encountered the rectum may be retained if intraoperative considerations suggest that the procedure be terminated. Rarely, a discrete bleeding point may be found by sigmoidoscopy and controlled by suture or judicious fulguration, techniques appropriate for the extraperitoneal rectum.

CANCER AND PRECANCER

Carcinoma is a generally recognized and feared complication of long-standing ulcerative colitis and, when found, obviously constitutes an absolute indication for colectomy. Too frequently these tumors are at an advanced stage with no hope for cure when the diagnosis is made, a circumstance resulting in large part from the fact that the early symptoms of the carcinoma are identical to those of ulcerative colitis. Compared to sporadically developing colon cancers, carcinomas complicating ulcerative colitis tend to occur more frequently and at an earlier age (vide infra), to be multifocal and submucosal, harder to see endoscopically, and are not so likely to develop in the distal colon and rectum.[237-240] Although in the past they were believed to be inherently more malignant, several reports now suggest that, Dukes' stage for stage, their prognosis is similar to that of sporadic carcinoma,[241-243] indicating that the overall poor prognosis of such tumors complicating CUC results from their usual discovery at a late stage. In considering treatment of the patient with colitis and carcinoma of the colon, it should be noted that obstructing carcinoma of the colon can be the cause of a type of colitis that occurs proximal to the lesion and can be fairly extensive.[244] This association between obstruction carcinoma and colitis must be sharply distinguished from carcinoma complicating idiopathic ulcerative colitis or Crohn's disease, because failure to do so will lead to unnecessarily radical operation.

Although it has been accepted for a number of years that carcinoma is, in fact, a complication of ulcerative colitis much controversy still exists about the magnitude of the risk,[245-248] and the optimal strategy for dealing with the problem.[211,212,249] The epidemiologic assessment of the likelihood of patients with ulcerative colitis developing carcinoma carries with it a number of pitfalls and methodologic problems that were enumerated by Sackett and Whelan.[250] Despite the numerous reports on the subject that have appeared through the years, few, if any, are free of the various types of hidden statistical bias.[246]

Despite the difficulties of producing a scientifically perfect study on the risk of cancer, it is necessary to have some sense of the level of the risk. The incidence of cancer appears to be a function of the duration of the disease. It is generally accepted that up until about 8 years of disease, the risk of a patient with ulcerative colitis developing carcinoma is no greater than that of the general population. Subsequently, depending on the study, the risk is variously estimated to rise cumulatively (in patients with universal colitis) by 0.3 to 2% each year.[237-239,245-248] The risk of cancer is roughly correlated with the extent of disease, and thus those with universal colitis are subject to the greatest hazard.[237] Those with disease confined to the left colon appear to be at a lesser, but nevertheless substantial, risk.[251] Onset in childhood has also been cited as an independent risk factor,[180,237] but this is somewhat controversial and may reflect at least in part an increased prevalence of universal colitis in this age group.[251,252] Edwards and Truelove also cited fulminating onset and continuous symptoms as additional risk factors but, again, it is difficult to ascertain whether or not these are independent variables.[237]

Obviously, then, cancers should be found at an early, curable stage or, better yet, the patient destined to develop invasive cancer should be identified and subjected to a prophylactic colectomy. The value of the rigid sigmoidoscope as a surveillance instrument is limited by the extent of its reach, especially because these cancers tend to be located in the proximal colon. The sensitivity of the radiologic detection of carcinoma in patients with ulcerative colitis is poor because of the already distorted colon and the frequent submucosal position of the tumors. Therefore, barium studies have been given up for cancer surveillance in ulcerative colitis. Carcinoembryonic antigen (CEA) has also been abandoned as a cancer detection technique because of lack of sensitivity and specificity.[253-255]

In a seminal study Morson and Pang found extensive premalignant changes ("precancer") in 100% of 23 colons with cancers complicating ulcerative colitis (see Chap. 15).[256] Because these changes frequently were found in flat mucosa remote from the tumor, especially in the left colon and rectum, these investigators proposed that the presence of the precancer lesion (dysplasia) in random rectal biopsies could pinpoint patients who actually harbored, or were likely to develop, carcinoma. After their initial report a large number of studies appeared that variably confirmed or denied the usefulness of this test as a method of detecting cancer.[240,257-264] Morson and Pang even in their first publication on the subject stressed that the absence of dysplasia in rectal biopsies could not be relied upon to *exclude* carcinoma. With regard to false-positives, the presence of precancer in the rectal mucosa has been associated with as few as 20% to as many as 71% associated carcinomas.[260,261] These studies were all retrospective and, therefore, cannot be used to ascertain the value of the test for prospective surveillance.

It is now generally accepted that dysplasia is focal in location and can occur in the proximal colon remote from the rectum, frequently only in the immediate vicinity of a tumor. As our understanding of the dysplastic lesion increased, the colonoscope came into general use and could be used not only to find invasive tumors but also to perform multiple biopsies searching for precancer. This instrument now occupies for many a position of central importance for diagnosing invasive cancer, for "excluding" it and for predicting its future development.

Pathologists have had difficulty in agreeing upon the proper criteria for the diagnosis of dysplasia and its degree of severity. This alone has accounted for much of the variability in the prevalence of false-positive and false-negative associations between dysplasia and invasive cancer. The presence of active inflammation in the area of biopsy is an important confounding factor because, especially to the unwary, reactive regenerative mucosal changes can easily be confused with neoplastic ones. An important cooperative study by knowledgeable gastrointestinal pathologists has gone a long way toward standardizing both the criteria and the nomenclature (Table 26-4).[265] It is revealing that in the process of developing the criteria for the presence of dysplasia there was at first tremendous interobserver variability in the blinded assessment of given microscopic slides. Even subsequent to the publication of this study, I have observed disagreement among pathologists. Therefore, it seems prudent to have key slides reviewed by two pathologists especially knowl-

TABLE 26-4. *Standardized Nomenclature for Colonic Biopsies in Inflammatory Bowel Disease (Inflammatory Bowel Disease-Dysplasia Morphology Study Group)*

Negative
  Normal mucosa
  Inactive (quiescent) colitis
  Active colitis
Indefinite
  Probably negative (probably inflammatory)
  Unknown
  Probably positive (probably dysplastic)
Positive
  Low-grade dysplasia
  High-grade dysplasia

edgeable in this area before far-reaching decisions are made based on the diagnosis of dysplasia.

Colonoscopy as a method of discovering already invasive carcinomas has some real limitations.[266,267] Cook and Goligher, as well as many others, have emphasized that only the minority of carcinomas complicating ulcerative colitis resemble ordinary carcinomas on gross examination.[240] Most such cancers resemble fibrous strictures or flat plaques, or may be macroscopically unrecognizable. Because of this and other considerations to be discussed, when colonoscopy is performed, multiple random biopsies should be taken every 10 cm along the colon in search of the dysplastic lesion. In addition, biopsies should be taken of any area of raised polypoid mucosa because such lesions "draw attention to the possibility of dysplastic changes or carcinoma."[268] In most instances "dysplasia associated mucosal masses" (DALM) even in the presence of low grade dysplasia were found to be associated with cancer in 7 out of 12 cases.[269] In 27 patients with similar degrees of dysplasia that occurred in flat mucosa only 1 carcinoma was found.[269] In my experience with DALMs that are discovered in the process of doing *surveillance* colonoscopy the yield in finding invasive carcinoma at the time of colectomy has not been impressive. On the other hand, until the lesion is removed in its entirety (which in this instance usually would mean a colectomy) the burden of proof would be on the physician choosing not to recommend that the colon be removed.

As a test for the current presence of cancer the precancer lesion has a relatively low predictive value, because invasive cancer will be found in only ⅓ to, at most, ½ of colons removed solely for the finding of dysplasia.[247,264,269-272] It is generally assumed that even if the colon does not contain a cancer the patient almost inevitably would have developed one, but this has not always been the case over reasonably long periods of followup.[260,269,272]

There have now been several publications on the results of prospective colonoscopic surveillance for cancer of high risk patients with ulcerative colitis.[247,269-273] It is clear that such surveillance programs do not produce the ideal result, the total prevention of cancer. In a number of instances, cancer and precancer appeared simultaneously, precluding a prophylactic colectomy before the development of invasive cancer.[269,272,273] Moreover, the tumors detected in these surveillance studies were by no means always at a curable stage and were not even accompanied invariably by high-grade dysplasia. On the other hand, those patients in the studies who did not develop dysplasia or cancer could have been spared a prophylactic colectomy because they were all in the high risk group on the basis of extent of colitis and duration of disease.

Because the early diagnosis of carcinoma can be difficult even with invasive surveillance techniques, consideration must still be given to the merits of prophylactic operation. Even in the more conservative and well conceived epidemiologic studies, the risk of carcinoma after 10 years of disease is rather substantial and exceeds the operative risk. Individual patients place different values on the amount of cancer risk they are willing to take to avoid the obvious drawbacks of operation, including the psychological disability of an ileostomy. Although in the 10 to 20 year interval prophylactic operation may be justifiable on the basis of saving the greatest number of lives, the increment in saving lives when operative mortality is subtracted is relatively small. Such an eminent authority as J.C. Goligher, who had strongly recommended prophylactic colectomy for patients with universal colitis of 10 or more years duration,[274] now recommends colonoscopic surveillance as a better alternative.[275] Whether or not surveillance can be proved to be cost effective in the societal sense, it certainly is a good alternative for the individual patient with disease of 10 to 20 years' duration. In patients under surveillance, most authorities at the present time would recommend colectomy on the basis of one or more biopsies showing definite high-grade dysplasia. The case for colectomy solely on the basis of a biopsy showing low-grade dysplasia is less compelling unless it is part of a DALM, but at the least follow-up would be indicated. After 20 years or more of disease a stronger rationale for prophylactic colectomy rather than surveillance exists because of the exponential shape of the cumulative incidence curve. Moreover, some patients elect to have colectomy rather than surveillance at the outset because the fear of cancer is overriding, they do not want to tolerate periodic colonoscopy or the locale of their home or their lifestyle make surveillance difficult.

A strong case can be made for prophylactic colectomy after 10 years of disease in childhood-onset ulcerative colitis. Devroede et al. found that children, after 10 years of disease, developed carcinoma at a rate of 20% per decade, reaching 43% at 35 years.[180] Among those with universal colitis the risk was even higher, facts that suggested to the authors at least consideration of prophylactic colectomy. More recently, Prior et al. confirmed that early age of onset was associated with an increased risk of developing cancer, eliminating from consideration cancer found on the patient's initial encounter,[276] which was not the case with the Devroede study.

In my experience, a decision for or against operation based solely on the question of prophylaxis against cancer does not arise as often as this discussion would seem to indicate. By the time the patient has had ulcerative colitis long enough for cancer to be a statistically important risk, often additional factors such as the suboptimal response to nonoperative therapy, with limitation of lifestyle and work, may make the decision in favor of operation an easier one to make.

When operation is carried out for carcinoma, or even for prophylaxis against carcinoma, I feel that there is no place for a procedure other than one that removes all susceptible mucosa whether this be a panproctocolectomy with conventional or Kock ileostomy, or an ileoanal pull-through procedure. In 1 series of 9 patients with limited resection for carcinoma, exactly one-third developed metachronous carcinoma.[277] Given this degree of risk, it would not be wise to leave in a defunctionalized rectal stump.

STRICTURE

Benign colonic or rectal strictures in ulcerative colitis, in contrast to those in Crohn's disease of the colon, occur infrequently and develop late in the course of the disease.[278] Although strictures may occasionally require treatment because of obstructive symptoms, this is exceedingly rare. It is surprising how narrow a stricture may appear without producing significant symptoms, perhaps because such strictures frequently represent hypertrophy and thickening of the muscularis mucosae rather than being the result of fixed fibrosis.[279]

The major clinical dilemma is that of differentiating a benign stricture from carcinoma. A stricture of long duration as ascertained by prior barium radiographs is less likely to be a carcinoma. A symmetric appearance also suggests an inflammatory narrowing, but the presence of asymmetry strongly suggests carcinoma.[278] Because benign strictures usually occur in the left colon, a right-sided stricture suggests malignancy.[279] Colonoscopy together with brushings for cytology and biopsy of the lesion and its immediate vicinity can be useful in ascertaining the nature of such strictures. Obviously, however, a positive result is more definitive than a negative one and, thus, it is not surprising that failure of colonoscopy in ascertaining the true nature of colonic strictures has been reported on a number of occasions.[265,280,281] In one study the instrument could not traverse the stricture in almost half the cases and, in addition, a perforation occurred that was attributed to extreme bowing of the colonoscopy during too vigorous attempts to pass the narrowed area.[281] Although brushings for cytology and biopsy for dysplasia will add to the diagnostic accuracy in both traversable and nontraversable strictures,[281] the burden of proof is on the individual who contends that a stricture, whatever its appearance by roentgenogram and colonoscopy, is not malignant (see also Chap. 15).

Anal stricture is not uncommon in long-standing ulcerative colitis, but it is seldom a solitary indication for operation.

PERIANAL FISTULAS AND ABSCESSES

With the emergence of Crohn's disease of the colon as an entity, it has become obvious that a large proportion of the perianal fistulas and abscesses complicating colonic inflammatory bowel disease occur (almost by definition) in patients with Crohn's disease rather than ulcerative colitis. Small and uncomplicated anal fistulas occur in patients with ulcerative colitis, however, as do small, low-level rectovaginal fistulas. Adequate drainage of anorectal abscesses that rarely may complicate ulcerative colitis is not only permissible, but mandatory. A definitive surgical attack on the fistula of origin in the presence of active colitis is seldom advisable or necessary, however. When the disease is quiescent and the symptoms of the fistula are sufficiently distressing, such operative therapy may be undertaken even though the risk of failure to heal is considerably higher. Attempts to cure rectovaginal fistulas associated with ulcerative colitis are seldom if ever successful and, therefore, these lesions are best managed nonoperatively.

Anal fistulas and abscesses are seldom factors leading to definitive colonic operation in ulcerative colitis, in contrast to the case with Crohn's disease of the colon in which they can be important indications for operation by themselves because of their extensive and destructive nature.

SYSTEMIC (EXTRAINTESTINAL) COMPLICATIONS OF INFLAMMATORY BOWEL DISEASE

Greenstein et al. reported that one or more remote ("colitis-related," e.g., joint, skin, eye) complications occurred in 36% of 700 patients with inflammatory bowel disease.[282] These were more common in ulcerative colitis and Crohn's disease involving the colon (42%) than in small intestinal Crohn's disease (23%), and the musculoskeletal complications were the most frequent, followed by those in the skin, eye, and mouth.[282] These complications are discussed in detail in Chapter 16, but a few points pertaining to operation will be emphasized here.

The cutaneous manifestations (such as pyoderma gangrenosum and erythema nodosum) usually regress and do not recur after a totally extirpative operation, such as total colectomy and ileostomy,[235,282,283] but exceptions do exist. The specific "colitic" arthritis or arthropathy of ulcerative colitis usually parallels the activity and extent of disease, and has almost invariably been cured by operation.[284-287] Because about half these reported patients with putative ulcerative colitis undoubtedly had Crohn's disease of the colon (because the reports antedated the recognition of the latter), "curative" operation in Crohn's disease would be expected to have the same salutary effect. Attacks of iritis and uveitis may occur during periods of quiescence of Crohn's disease or ulcerative colitis, but are unlikely to recur after operation,[288,289] (despite an association with HLA-B-27 antigen[290]), an important consideration because repeated attacks of uveitis may result in blindness. The association of ankylosing spondylitis (usually with HLA-B-27 histocompatibility antigen) with ulcerative colitis or Crohn's disease is currently thought to reflect a common genetic predisposition to colitis and spondylitis rather than representing a complication of the bowel disease. Its course is independent of the bowel disease (indeed, the onset may antedate it by years) and so it is not surprising that colectomy is of no benefit in improving or arresting the course of the spondylitis.[283-286,290] Similarly, the course of true, "fixed" rheumatoid arthritis is not affected favorably by colectomy.[283-287]

Fortunately, with the exceptions mentioned, these various systemic complications usually subside when the bowel disease is controlled by nonoperative treatment and, therefore, presently operation is required less frequently for their treatment than it was before the advent of corticosteroid therapy.

The liver disease of colonic inflammatory bowel disease (typically and most specifically pericholangitis) unfortunately is not so clearly responsive to any modality of treatment, whether corticosteroids, broad-spectrum antibiotics, or operation.[291-293] Eade and associates, however, have provided uncontrolled evidence that the liver disease in some instances may improve, or at least does not become worse, after colectomy in both ulcerative and Crohn's colitis.[292,293] Because it seems clear from the data of Mistilis that liver disease is frequently progressive without operation, leading to cirrhosis,[295] colectomy must be seriously considered in a patient with pericholangitis.[296] It is generally thought that the course of sclerosing cholangitis is not favorably affected by colectomy.[297,298] In one report a combination of colectomy, duct dilatation, and long-term transhepatic stenting appeared to be beneficial, although it is by no means clear that colectomy was a key element in the success of the treatment regimen.[299] Ultimately, a hepatic allograft offers the best hope for patients with primary sclerosing cholangitis.*

If operation becomes necessary, in whole or in part, because of any of these systemic complications, the entire colon and rectum should be removed, preferably by a one-stage procedure.

Crohn's Disease of the Colon

Crohn's disease of the colon is now an accepted entity and accounts for 50% or more of all cases of idiopathic colitis.[299-303] In previous years most of these cases of Crohn's colitis and ileocolitis were diagnosed and treated as ulcerative colitis. Clinical examination and endoscopic and/or radiologic studies usually suffice to differentiate Crohn's disease from ulcerative colitis, although occasionally the diagnosis is established only after pathologic examination of an operative specimen. The distinguishing features of Crohn's disease of the colon and ulcerative colitis are detailed elsewhere in this book (see Chap. 10).

A diagnosis of Crohn's disease of the colon rather than ulcerative colitis has an important bearing on any discussion of indications for operation for several reasons: (1) the distribution of lesions in Crohn's disease may lend itself to a restorative operation without the need for panproctocolectomy and ileostomy, (2) the

---

*Editors' note: See also, Helzberg, J. H., et al.: Gastroenterology 92:1869, 1987.

course and complications of the two diseases can be different, and (3) the possibility of recurrent Crohn's disease after operation is an additional risk that must be considered, although the rate of postoperative recurrence is lower and the quality of life and prospects for long-term rehabilitation are better than was previously thought.[301,302,304-306]

CHRONIC DISEASE AND INTRACTABILITY IN UNIVERSAL CROHN'S COLITIS AND ILEOCOLITIS

Intractability is the most frequent indication for operation in Crohn's disease of the colon, as it is in ulcerative colitis. This is somewhat contrary to the view that single specific complications leading to operation can usually be identified in the ileocolonic pattern of presentation (see earlier discussion on small intestinal disease).[85] When surgical treatment is being considered for the patient with Crohn's disease of the colon on the basis of intractability, the anticipated result of operation obviously influences the advisability of operation at that particular time. Specifically, if it were true that, despite the handicaps of an ileostomy, the patient then faced a likelihood of early ileal recurrence and progressive proximal extension of disease, an ultraconservative policy regarding operation, which was previously advised, might be warranted.[3,4] Hence, in the following paragraphs the rate of recurrence and the prospects for long-term rehabilitation after operation for Crohn's disease of the colon are considered.

My studies of the comparative courses of patients with Crohn's disease of the colon and ulcerative colitis after operation first raised serious doubts as to the validity of the claim that major differences existed between the two in the long-term outcome after surgical treatment, causing a different threshold for operative intervention to be justified. Prior to my initial report in 1967, no distinction was made between the recurrence rate after resection and anastomosis and that following colectomy and ileostomy. A number of studies document a substantial difference between the two types of operation.[301,302,306,308,309] The recurrence rate in those patients whose disease distribution is such that colectomy and ileostomy is required to extirpate the areas of involvement is rather low. Conversely, patients with limited disease that allows resection and anastomosis with reestablishment of intestinal continuity realize this advantage at the expense of at least a 75% chance of developing recurrent disease, a figure comparable to the recurrence rate of classical Crohn's disease.[302,306]

Subsequent studies by others recognized the flaw in comparing restorative procedures with panproctocolectomy, but still reported rates of recurrent disease after colectomy and ileostomy of as high as 33 to 46%.[310,311] However, these reports did not take into account additional problems. The most important of these had to do with the proportion of those with colonic inflammatory bowel disease diagnosed as Crohn's colitis as opposed to ulcerative colitis. In a given study the number of patients assumed to have one or the other entity depends not only upon the criteria used for diagnosis but, also more importantly, upon whether or not the *entire* population of patients with inflammatory bowel disease has been analyzed.[302] It has been found that more than 50% of patients with colonic inflammatory disease coming to operation have Crohn's disease,[298-301] whereas those reporting high recurrence rates after operation noted only an 11 to 12% relative incidence of Crohn's disease.[310,311] This fact makes it likely that many of the patients in these studies who were thought to have ulcerative colitis (and doing well) in fact had Crohn's disease of the colon. This large difference in the denominator of the fraction, *patients developing recurrence/those at risk*, by itself would seem to account for the high rates of recurrence reported.[304]

Another problem in studies comparing the outcome of operation in Crohn's and ulcerative colitis involves the definition of recurrence after ileostomy, that is, the differentiation between intrinsic inflammatory bowel disease of the ileum and problems associated with the ileostomy itself (e.g., ileostomy dysfunction and postcolectomy ileitis).[312] Needless to say, the problem of differentiating these types of ileal inflammation is considerable. Ileitis may occur after colectomy for such noninflammatory diseases as familial polyposis in which the diagnosis cannot be ambiguous.[313-315] If ileitis is found after colectomy for ulcerative colitis (which generally is assumed to be cured after operation) it tends either to be attributed to ileostomy dysfunction or postcolectomy ileitis, or the original diagnosis is changed to that of Crohn's disease. If these same problems occur after ileostomy for Crohn's disease, there is a tendency to attribute them to recurrent disease, resulting in a falsely elevated rate of recurrence. Thus, in my studies (in which many of the patients were operated upon before the days of primary maturation of the ileostomy), I compared rates and types of ileostomy revisions in side-by-side comparisons of ulcerative colitis and Crohn's ileocolitis. If combined clinical, distributional, and histologic criteria were used for diagnosis, although the prevalence of ileostomy revisions in patients with Crohn's disease was higher than in ulcerative colitis, the difference was not statistically significant.[301,302,304] When ileal inflammation did occur after operation for either disease, it usually responded to one or more resections of the affected intestine and revision of the ileostomy. After the first two postoperative years the probability of ileostomy revision was approximately the same in both diseases.[302] Moreover, the chances of ultimate rehabilitation of the patients in each group were good.

The use of the relative rates of ileostomy revisions to compare the postoperative courses of Crohn's disease and ulcerative colitis (as already explained) has been confusing to other workers who mistakenly conclude that I believe that Crohn's disease never recurs following ileostomy. Therefore, for purposes of comparison with other studies I have estimated that 16% of my patients with ileostomy and colectomy for Crohn's disease had ileostomy revisions for what appeared to be a true prestomal recurrence of granulomatous ileitis.[302,304] Other large studies have reported even lower rates of recurrence, ranging from 3 to 14.8%.[306,308,309,316] Goligher has reviewed his long-term results in 162 patients with colonic Crohn's disease treated by colectomy and ileostomy, and found, somewhat contrary to his previous belief, a much more favorable postoperative course that included a rate of recurrence of 14.8%, a good response to re-resection for prestomal Crohn's disease, and a good to excellent "corrected" (subtracting intercurrent disease) patient satisfaction score in 96.5% of patients.[306]

A great deal of rapprochement has become apparent between the conflicting points of view in this controversy. Clearly some patients with colonic Crohn's disease develop recurrent "regional enteritis" after colectomy and ileostomy, but workers from the various centers, including mine, now appear to agree that the course in most such cases is favorable and that the quality of life after operation is generally good.[304-306,317,318]

Because of these considerations, I continue to employ approximately the same end point for the determination of intractability to nonoperative management in Crohn's disease of the colon as for ulcerative colitis, even when the extent of the Crohn's disease dictates total colectomy and ileostomy. Perhaps the main point should be that when ileostomy is employed as part of the treatment of inflammatory bowel disease of the colon of either type, it is because all available nonoperative treatments have been exhausted and have failed. Therefore, whatever the presumed prognosis, further procrastination is unjustified and hazardous.

ANASTOMOTIC PROCEDURES

Segmental resection with intestinal anastomosis for Crohn's colitis or ileocolitis has a recurrence rate of approximately 75 percent within 15 years.[46,301,302,306] This recurrence rate, high as it is, does not justify the uniform employment of the more radical total colectomy and ileostomy as the primary operation, even though such a procedure may eventually become necessary. The distinct chance of obtaining long-term palliation without the necessity of ileostomy has obvious merit. This is especially true for the adolescent or young adult who has not yet matured socially or psychosexually. Furthermore, long-term "cures" may indeed sometimes result after partial colectomy and anastomosis, but this has been observed only in disease confined to the right side of the colon and terminal ileum.[301,302] The absolute number of patients I have treated in this way is relatively small, so that this statement should not be misconstrued as proscription against ileosigmoidal or ileorectal anastomosis when left-sided colonic involvement is present.

Colocolic anastomoses have been reported to have a distinctly higher rate of recurrence than ileocolonic anastomoses.[308] Nevertheless, if careful study documents only limited colonic involvement, it would seem unjustifiable to recommend an extensive resection based on the high rate of recurrence because the site of recurrence can be variable and the conserved absorbing surface of the colon may prove to be useful in the future.

Although the results of ileoproctostomy for colonic Crohn's disease are somewhat less encouraging than those in ulcerative colitis,[183,306] critical assessment of these results is impossible because a clear separation of the two diseases has not always been made. One can only be somewhat skeptical of the diagnosis of cases of ulcerative colitis without rectal involvement reported in some series of Aylett operations. Thus, the chance of a satisfactory result of ileoproctostomy in Crohn's disease of the colon and ulcerative colitis is probably about the same, that is, 25 to 30%. The risk of the future development of carcinoma in the rectum is possibly less for the patient with Crohn's disease. Although the prognosis after this operation is not optimistic in terms of freedom from recurrent disease, it has great merit in the younger and less mature patient.

In the event of a recurrence after an anastomotic procedure, conversion to an ileostomy and total colectomy provides an excellent chance for ultimate rehabilitation.[306]

COLOSTOMY FOR LEFT-SIDED OR RECTAL DISEASE

Occasionally, the inflammatory process involves only the distal colon, either in Crohn's disease or ulcerative colitis. In these patients, operation with transverse colostomy and excision of the left colon and rectum has been advocated.[319] In our experience, over the long run, the proximal colon has almost invariably become diseased whether in ulcerative or Crohn's colitis, and subsequent operation has been uniformly necessary.[301] Furthermore, an ileostomy is esthetically more pleasing and easier to manage than a transverse colostomy. Thus, any physiologic advantage of leaving in the ileocecal valve and right colon is outweighed by the considerations just enumerated. Therefore, we do not advocate this procedure for any patient with inflammatory disease of the colon, even if anatomically feasible.

In view of the fact that a sigmoid colostomy may be somewhat easier to manage than an ileostomy and conserving intestine in Crohn's disease has merit, sigmoidostomy and rectal excision should be considered when severe disease that is confined to the rectum requires operative treatment. Ritchie and Lockhart-Mummery reported a series of 26 such patients with excellent results and a recurrence rate of only 4.2%.[309]

ILEOSTOMY FOR DIVERSION

Oberhelman and associates and Truelove, Lee, and coworkers have advocated a diversionary ileostomy for Crohn's disease of the colon, either with the intent of subsequent restoration of intestinal continuity when inflammation subsides, or as a first stage procedure for seriously ill and debilitated patients.[320-323] McIlrath also had some limited success with diversion for Crohn's disease.[324] Although a few patients in these various series have undergone subsequent closure of the ileostomy with long-term success, these are but a small proportion of the total. Burman et al. and Jones and associates found that diversion of the fecal stream was ineffective for control of colonic or rectal disease, much less a good method for restoring useful function to a diseased segment of intestine.[148,308] In fact, inflammation frequently progressed in Burman's cases despite proximal diversion,[148] but it is possible that diversion colitis (which was unrecognized at that time) contributed to this outcome, particularly with regard to rectal disease.[325] My experience with diversionary ileostomy is limited but unfavorable. Moreover, I have not found the need for performing staged procedures using diversionary ileostomy as the preliminary procedure. Oberhelman stated that diverting ileostomy should be regarded as experimental, a viewpoint that is difficult to dispute on the basis of the accumulated experience with this procedure.[320]

CONCOMITANT EXTENSIVE JEJUNOILEITIS AND COLITIS

An occasional patient with more or less universal Crohn's disease of the colon will also be found to have extensive disease of the proximal small intestine. This combination is now regarded as an example of granulomatous ileocolitis rather than coexisting regional enteritis and ulcerative colitis, as diagnosed in the past. I have treated two patients with extensive enterocolitis with severe and active disease in the colon and almost universal but inactive involvement of the small intestine. Total colectomy and ileostomy performed in these two patients interrupted what appeared to be almost certain fatal outcomes, presumably by removing the site of the most active inflammatory process. This strategy is analogous in many respects to the surgical management of jejunoileitis.

SPECIFIC COMPLICATIONS NECESSITATING OPERATION

Although in the early publications on Crohn's disease of the colon it was thought that carcinoma and toxic megacolon did not occur,[3,4] accumulated experience has indicated clearly that the potential for all possible complications of ulcerative colitis also exists in Crohn's colitis, including both these dreaded ones. Beyond these, the hallmark feature of the Crohn's lesion to produce burrowing sinuses, abscesses, and fistulas gives rise to further complications that are unique to this entity and often constitute indications for operation. In the following sections differences between the courses of Crohn's disease of the colon and ulcerative colitis are discussed as they influence management and indications for operative intervention.

CARCINOMA. Data from several large cohort studies of patients seem to establish that Crohn's disease of the colon is associated with a risk of developing colonic carcinoma that exceeds that of the general population,[326-328] although not all workers have come to the same conclusion.[324-331] These analyses are subject to all the various types of hidden statistical biases already mentioned in the discussion of neoplasia in ulcerative colitis.[246,250] Moreover, because Crohn's disease of the colon has been generally recognized for only about 25 years, it is difficult to ascertain retrospectively the exact population at risk for developing carcinoma, a problem that exists not only for Crohn's disease but for ulcerative colitis as well.[125] Nevertheless, at this time it is reasonable to conclude that a risk of cancer in Crohn's colitis exists that exceeds that in the general population but it may be lower than in ulcerative colitis.[146] One reason that has been proposed for this difference is that patients with Crohn's disease may require operation more frequently than in ulcerative colitis and somewhat earlier in their course. Thus, the apparent lower incidence of carcinoma in Crohn's disease could result from a shorter exposure to a carcinogenic stimulus;[332] however, even if true, this is of only theoretic interest to the clinician who is primarily interested in the risk to the patient who still retains his colon.

Several reports are now available of the association of dysplasia with colonic cancer complicating Crohn's disease.[333-335] The invasive tumors do not always arise in inflamed mucosa and the time of diagnosis of cancer in a few cases has been simultaneous with that of Crohn's disease rather than after exposure to long-term disease. Because of the occurrence of the dysplastic lesion in patients with Crohn's disease and cancer, surveillance has been suggested,[335,336] but the problems and the logistics of such a strategy are considerable and even more complex than is the case in ulcerative colitis, primarily because the magnitude of the cancer risk may be lower and the identification of a highly susceptible group of patients is difficult. For similar reasons, despite the apparent increased risk of carcinoma, no solid data strongly support the use of prophylactic colectomy for the prevention of cancer in long-standing disease.

Nevertheless, an awareness of the possibility of complicating colon cancer must be part of the management of patients with Crohn's disease of the colon. I have observed invasive carcinoma or severe dysplasia in areas of long-standing stricture or fistulization, both of which have been observed by others.[337,338] In some cases biopsy or brushings of such areas searching for carcinoma or dysplasia may be warranted. The evidence for an increased risk of carcinoma in colonic Crohn's disease would also appear to favor resection over bypass when operation is indicated. This would include the excision of permanently defunctionated segments such as the rectum after subtotal colectomy and ileostomy although this cannot be advised nearly so strongly as in ulcerative colitis. Nevertheless, complicating carcinoma in retained rectal stumps in Crohn's disease has been reported on a number of occasions.[335,337,339] The development of anal carcinoma in patients with perirectal complications must be kept in mind in the management of patients with these lesions.

STRICTURE. In Crohn's disease, stricture formation is not uncommon and often occurs early in the course of the disease.[1-4,278] Whereas the patient with ulcerative colitis who bears a stricture is a prime cancer suspect, the same is not necessarily the case for an individual who has a colonic stricture in Crohn's disease. Nevertheless, stenoses occurring in patients with Crohn's colitis can represent complicating carcinoma that may develop in either inflamed or in normal mucosa. Moreover, as already pointed out, carcinomas can arise in long-standing, benign strictures, presumably as a result of chronic irritation and repair.

Despite all of this, most colonic strictures in Crohn's disease are benign and may be managed nonoperatively if they are not so narrow as to cause obstructive symptoms and reasonable attempts to exclude carcinoma have been made.

TOXIC MEGACOLON, FULMINATING DISEASE, PERFORATION, AND HEMORRHAGE. Toxic megacolon complicating Crohn's disease of the colon is currently being reported to occur in from 2.3 to 6.4% of patients (in one report as high as 11% in the colitis pattern).[226,340-342] The incidence of megacolon in Crohn's disease has been reported as both lower and higher than in ulcerative colitis. Free colonic perforation in the absence of toxic megacolon may also occur in Crohn's disease involving the colon as it may in both regional enteritis and ulcerative colitis.[343-345] Although bleeding is not as common a symptom of Crohn's disease as it is of ulcerative colitis, massive bleeding has been the indication for colectomy in a number of cases in our experience.

Although subtle differences may be found in the incidence and pathogenesis of these complications in Crohn's disease and ulcerative colitis, the same criteria for management that would be appropriate in ulcerative colitis apply to their management in Crohn's disease.

ABSCESSES, INTERNAL AND ENTEROCUTANEOUS FISTULAS, AND INFLAMMATORY MASSES. Fistulas and abscesses represent pathognomonic features of Crohn's disease of the colon that serve to distinguish it from ulcerative colitis. If present, an abdominal abscess represents an obvious indication for operation that should include definitive treatment of the underlying intestinal lesion. The management of inflammatory masses of indeterminate nature and the various types of fistulas involves the same considerations as with small intestinal Crohn's disease (previous section). Again it is emphasized, although these complications are not absolute indications for operation, they do, or should, place some constraints upon the drugs should be used for treatment. Specifically, corticosteroid treatment is clearly contraindicated in the presence of undrained pus such as an abscess and, because of the possibility of a suppurative process, should be used with caution or not at all in the presence of other extraluminal complications. Thus, in the presence of inflammatory masses and internal fistulas, failure to respond to management with systemic antibiotics, sulfasalazine, metronidazole, and possibly immunosuppressive therapy is an indication for operation.

PERIANAL AND PERIRECTAL ABSCESSES, FISTULAS, AND DEEP FISSURES (ANAL LESIONS). These are common in predominantly colonic Crohn's disease. Their primary management has been covered in the preceding discussions of midgut Crohn's disease and ulcerative colitis.* Because of their high incidence, multiplicity, and destructive capacity, they constitute rather frequent indications for definitive operation in colonic Crohn's disease, in contrast to the situation in ulcerative colitis or more proximal Crohn's disease. Fistulas and deep fissures (and, at times, the ill-advised and ill-conceived operative treatment of these lesions) may destroy the anal sphincter mechanism and thus lead to fecal incontinence, an additional clear indication for operation. In contrast to internal fistulas, corticosteroid treatment is not necessarily interdicted in the presence of perianal sepsis because any progression of the inflammatory process can be monitored more easily. Metronidazole and immunosuppressives have been reported to be helpful in the management of perianal fistulas, but my admittedly limited experience has not been favorable with either.[75,137,138,104]

If proctocolectomy is required in a patient who has multiple anorectal fistulas, serious consideration should be given to staging the procedure. Although, in my experience, total diversion of the fecal stream has not always prevented progression of the perianal fistulas (see above), a decrease in the overall inflammatory reaction and improved nutrition may allow a safer operation and more rapid healing of the perineal wound when the rectal segment is removed at a later date.

Systemic complications have been discussed previously under ulcerative colitis.

In conclusion, in chronic idiopathic inflammatory bowel disease, operation is a highly effective modality of treatment. However, operative treatment may impose a physical and psychological burden, such as occurs with an ileostomy, or may incur the threat of postoperative recurrence. Therefore, perhaps more so than in any other type of disease, the degree of disability or threat to life must be weighed carefully against the anticipated results of operation. Those having the responsibility for making such decisions must be aware of the efficacy and the limitations of medical and surgical therapy, and must have an in-depth understanding of the problems imposed by chronic diseases and their treatment.

References

1. Crohn, B. B., Ginzburg, L., and Oppenheimer, G. D.: Regional ileitis: A pathologic and clinical entity. J. Am. Med. Assoc., *191*:825, 1932.
2. Lockhart-Mummery, H. E., and Morson, B. C.: Crohn's disease (regional enteritis) of the large intestine and its distinction from ulcerative colitis. Gut, *1*:87, 1960.
3. Lockhart-Mummery, H. E., and Morson, B. C.: Crohn's disease of the large intestine. Gut, *5*:493, 1964.

---

*Editors' note: See also, van Dongen, L. M., and Lubbers E.-J. C.: Arch. Surg. *121*:1187, 1986.

4. Lindner, A. E., et al: Granulomatous colitis: A clinical study. N. Engl. J. Med., 269:379, 1963.
5. Janowitz, H. D., Lindner, A. E., and Marshak, R. H.: Granulomatous colitis: Crohn's disease of the colon. J. Am. Med. Assoc., 191:825, 1965.
6. Gump, F. E., Lepore, M., and Barker, H. G.: A revised concept of acute regional enteritis. Ann. Surg., 166:942, 1967.
7. Wenckert, A., Brahme, F., and Nilsson, R.: Operationsindikationer vid Crohns sjukdom. Nord. Med., 83:334, 1970.
8. Sjostrom, B.: Acute terminal ileitis and its relationship to Crohn's disease. In Regional Enteritis (Crohn's Disease). Edited by A. Engel and T. Larrson. Stockholm, Nordiska Bokhandelns Forlag, 1971.
9. Jess, P.: Acute terminal ileitis: A review of recent literature on the relationship to Crohn's disease. Scand. J. Gastroenterol., 16:321, 1981.
10. Schofield, P. F.: The natural history and treatment of Crohn's disease. Ann. R. Coll. Surg. Engl., 36:258, 1965.
11. Atwell, J. D., Duthie, H. L., and Goligher, J. C.: The outcome of Crohn's disease. Br. J. Surg., 52:966, 1965.
12. Banks, B. M., Zetzel, L., and Richter, H. S.: Morbidity and mortality in regional enteritis. Report of 168 cases. Am. J. Dig. Dis., 14:369, 1969.
13. Daniels, J. J. H. M.: Enteral infection with Pasteurella pseudotuberculosis. Isolation of the organism from human faeces. Br. Med. J., 2:997, 1961.
14. Winblad, S., Nilehn, B., and Sternby, N. H.: Yersinia enterocolitica (Pasteurella X) in human enteric infections. Br. Med. J., 2:1363, 1966.
15. Vantrappen, G., et al: Yersinia enteritis. Med. Clin. North Am., 66:639, 1982.
16. Weber, J., Finlayson, N. B., and Mark, J. B.: Mesenteric lymphadenitis and terminal ileitis due to Yersinia pseudotuberculosis. N. Engl. J. Med., 283:172, 1970.
17. Blaser, M. J., and Reller, L. B.: Campylobacter enteritis. N. Engl. J. Med., 305:1444, 1981.
18. Ho, H. D., et al: Campylobacter enteritis. Early diagnosis with Gram's stain. Arch. Intern. Med., 142:1858, 1982.
19. Morain, C. O.: Acute ileitis. Br. Med. J., 283:1075, 1981.
20. Colcock, B. P., and Vansant, J. H.: Surgical treatment of regional enteritis. N. Engl. J. Med., 261:435, 1960.
21. Maingot, R.: Abdominal Operations. 4th Ed. New York, Appleton-Century-Crofts, 1961.
22. Cattell, R. B.: Regional enteritis. Gastroenterology. 36:398, 1959.
23. Fonkalsrud, E. W., Ament, M. E., and Fleisher, D.: Management of the appendix in young patients with Crohn's disease. Arch. Surg., 117:11, 1982.
24. Simonowitz, D. A., Rusch, V. W., and Stevenson, J. K.: Natural history of incidental appendectomy in patients with Crohn's disease who required subsequent bowel resection. Am. J. Surg., 143:171, 1982.
25. Jackson, B. B.: Chronic regional enteritis. A survey of one hundred twenty-six cases treated at the Massachusetts General Hospital from 1937 to 1954. Ann. Surg., 148:81, 1954.
26. Marx, F. W.: Incidental appendectomy with regional enteritis. Advisability. Arch. Surg., 88:546, 1964.
27. Kovalcik, P., et al: The dilemma of Crohn's disease: Crohn's disease and appendectomy. Dis. Colon Rectum, 20:377, 1977.
28. Van Patter, W. N., et al: Regional enteritis. Gastroenterology, 26:345, 1954.
29. Hall, J. H., and Hellier, M. D.: Crohn's disease of the appendix presenting as acute appendicitis. Br. J. Surg., 56:390, 1969.
30. Ewen, S. W. B., et al: Crohn's disease initially confined to the appendix. Gastroenterology, 60:853, 1971.
31. Weiss, Y., and Durst, A. L.: Crohn's disease of the appendix: Presentation of a case with review of the literature. Am. J. Gastroenterol., 63:333, 1975.
32. Brown, W. K., and Peters, R. W.: Crohn's disease of the appendix presenting as lower intestinal hemorrhage and cecal mass. Am. J. Gastroenterol., 65:349, 1976.
33. Green, G. I., Broadrick, G. L., and Collins, J. L.: Crohn's disease of the appendix presenting as acute appendicitis. Am. J. Gastroenterol., 65:74, 1976.
34. Yang, S. S., et al: Primary Crohn's disease of the appendix: Report of 14 cases and review of the literature. Ann. Surg., 189:334, 1979.
35. Lindhagen, T., et al: Crohn's disease confined to the appendix. Dis. Colon Rectum, 25:805, 1982.
36. Korelitz, B. I., and Sommers, S. C.: Perforated nongranulomatous appendicitis in the course of regional enteritis. Gastroenterology, 64:1020, 1973.
37. Lennard-Jones, J. E., and Stalder, G. A.: Prognosis after resection of chronic regional ileitis. Gut, 8:332, 1967.
38. de Dombal, F. T., Burton, I., and Goligher, J. C.: The early and late results of surgical treatment for Crohn's disease. Br. J. Surg., 58:805, 1971.
39. de Dombal, F. T., Burton, I., and Goligher, J. C.: Recurrence of Crohn's disease after primary excisional surgery. Gut, 12:519, 1971.
40. de Dombal, F. T.: The results of surgical treatment for Crohn's disease. Br. J. Surg., 59:826, 1972.
41. Williams, J. A., Fielding, J. F., and Cooke, W. T.: A comparison of results of excision and bypass for ileal Crohn's disease. Gut, 13:973, 1972.
42. Homan, W. P., and Dineen, P.: Comparison of the results of resection, bypass, and bypass with exclusion for ileocecal Crohn's disease. Ann. Surg., 187:530, 1978.
43. Mekhjian, H. S., et al: National Cooperative Crohn's Disease Study: Factors determining recurrence of Crohn's disease after surgery. Gastroenterology, 77:907, 1979.
44. Higgens, C. S., and Allan, R. N.: Crohn's disease of the distal ileum. Gut, 21:933, 1980.
45. Karesen, R., et al: Crohn's disease: Long-term results of surgical treatment. Scand. J. Gastroenterol., 16:57, 1981.
46. Trnka, Y. M., et al: The long-term outcome of restorative operation in Crohn's disease: Influence of location, prognostic factors and surgical guidelines. Ann. Surg., 196:345, 1982.
47. Rutgeerts, P., et al: Natural history of recurrent Crohn's disease at the ileocolic anastomosis after curative surgery. Gut, 25:665, 1984.
48. Bergman, L., and Krause, U.: Postoperative treatment with corticosteroids and salazosulphapyridine (Salazopyrin) after radical resection for Crohn's disease. Scand. J. Gastroenterol., 11:651, 1976.
49. Wenckert, A., et al: The long-term prophylactic effect of salazosulphapyridine (Salazopyrin) in primarily resected patients with Crohn's disease: A controlled double blind trial. Scand. J. Gastroenterol., 13:161, 1978.
50. Summers, R. W., et al: National Cooperative Crohn's Disease Study: Results of drug treatment. Gastroenterology, 77:847, 1979.
51. Jones, G. W., Jr., Dooley, M. R., and Shoenfield, L. J.: Regional enteritis with involvement of the duodenum. Gastroenterology, 51:1018, 1966.
52. Fielding, J. F., et al.: Crohn's disease of the stomach and duodenum. Gut, 11:1001, 1970.
53. Wise, L., et al.: Crohn's disease of the duodenum. Am. J. Surg., 121:184, 1971.
54. Farmer, R. G., Hawk, W. A., and Turnbull, R. B., Jr.:

Crohn's disease of the duodenum (Transmural duodenitis): Clinical manifestations. Report of 11 cases. Am. J. Dig. Dis., *17*:191, 1972.
55. Silva, J. R., and Thomas, J. M.: Isolated regional enteritis of the duodenum. Am. J. Gastroenterol., *57*:349, 1972.
56. Johnson, F. W., and Delaney, J. P.: Regional enteritis involving the stomach. Arch. Surg., *105*:434, 1972.
57. Beaudin, D., et al.: Crohn's disease of the stomach: A case report and review of the literature. Dig. Dis., *18*:623, 1973.
58. Haggitt, R. C., and Meissner, W. A.: Crohn's disease of the upper gastrointestinal tract. Am. J. Clin. Pathol., *59*:613, 1973.
59. Tootla, F., et al.: Gastroduodenal Crohn disease. Arch. Surg., *111*:855, 1976.
60. Nugent, F. W., Richmond, M., and Park, S. K.: Crohn's disease of the duodenum. Gut, *18*:115, 1977.
61. AbuRahma, A. F.: Gastroduodenal Crohn's disease. South Med. J., *72*:551, 1979.
62. Frandsen, P. J., Jarnum, S., and Malmstrom, J.: Crohn's disease of the duodenum. Scand. J. Gastroenterol, *15*:683, 1980.
63. Ross, T. M., Fazio, V. W., and Farmer, R. G.: Long-term results of surgical treatment for Crohn's disease of the duodenum. Ann. Surg., *197*:399, 1983.
64. Murray, J. J., et al: Surgical management of Crohn's disease involving the duodenum. Am. J. Surg., *147*:58, 1984.
65. Kraus, J., and Schneider, R.: Pernicious anemia caused by Crohn's disease of the stomach. Am. J. Gastroenterol., *71*:202, 1979.
66. Paget, E. T., et al.: Massive upper gastrointestinal tract hemorrhage. A manifestation of regional enteritis of the duodenum. Arch. Surg., *104*:397, 1972.
67. Kim, U. S., Zimmerman, M. J., and Weiss, M.: Massive upper gastrointestinal hemorrhage associated with Crohn's disease of the stomach and duodenum. A case report. Am. J. Gastroenterol., *59*:244, 1973.
68. Sanders, M. G., and Schimmel, E. M.: The relationship between granulomatous bowel disease and duodenal ulcer. Dig. Dis. Sci., *17*:1100, 1972.
69. Conn, H. O., and Blitzer, B. L.: Nonassociation of adrenocorticosteroid therapy and peptic ulcer. N. Engl. J. Med., *294*:473, 1976.
70. Messer, J., et al.: Association of adrenocorticosteroid therapy and peptic-ulcer disease. N. Engl. J. Med., *309*:21, 1983.
71. Danzi, J. T., et al.: Endoscopic features of gastroduodenal Crohn's disease. Gastroenterology, *70*:9, 1976.
72. Legge, D. A., Hoffman, H. N., II, and Carlson, H. C.: Pancreatitis as a complication of regional enteritis of the duodenum. Gastroenterology, *61*:834, 1971.
73. Barthelemy, C. R.: Crohn's disease of the duodenum with spontaneous reflux into the pancreatic duct. Gastrointest. Radio., *8*:319, 1983.
74. Nogueira, J. R., and Freedman, M. A.: Acute pancreatitis as a complication of Imuran therapy in regional enteritis. Gastroenterology, *62*:1040, 1972.
75. Kawanishi, H., Rudolph, E., and Bull, F. E.: Azathioprine-induced acute pancreatitis. N. Engl. J. Med., *289*:357, 1973.
76. Guillaume, P., Grandjian, E., and Male, P. J.: Azathioprine-associated acute pancreatitis in the course of chronic active hepatitis. Dig. Dis. Sci., *29*:78, 1984.
77. Block, M. B., Genant, H. K., and Kirsner, J. B.: Pancreatitis as an adverse reaction to salicylazosulfapyridine. N. Engl. J. Med., *282*:380, 1970.
78. Goldwasser, B., Mazor, A., and Wiznitzer, T.: Enteroduodenal fistula in Crohn's disease. Dis. Colon Rectum. *24*:485, 1981.

79. Wilk, P. J., Fazio, V., and Turnbull, R. B., Jr.: The dilemma of Crohn's disease: Ileoduodenal fistula complicating Crohn's disease. Dis. Colon Rectum, *20*:387, 1977.
80. Smith, T. R., and Goldin, R. R.: Radiographic and clinical sequelae of the duodenocolic anatomic relationship: Two cases of Crohn's disease with fistulization to the duodenum. Dis. Colon Rectum, *20*:257, 1977.
81. Farmer, R. G., Hawk, W. A., and Turnbull, R. B., Jr.: Indications for surgery in Crohn's disease. Analysis of 500 cases. Gastroenterology, *71*:245, 1976.
82. Peppercorn, M.: Sulfasalazine: Pharmacology, clinical use, toxicity, and related new drug development. Ann. Intern. Med., *101*:377, 1984.
83. Ursing, B., et al.: A comparative study of metronidazole and sulfasalazine for active Crohn's disease: The cooperative Crohn's disease study in Sweden: II. Result. Gastroenterology, *83*:558, 1982.
84. Present, D. H., et al.: Treatment of Crohn's disease with 6-mercaptopurine. N. Engl. J. Med., *302*:981, 1980.
85. Meihoff, W. E., and Kern, F., Jr.: Bile salt malabsorption in regional ileitis, ileal resection, and mannitol-induced diarrhea. J. Clin. Invest., *47*:245, 1976.
86. Krone, C. L., et al.: Studies on the pathogenesis of malabsorption. Lipid hydrolysis and micelle formation in the intestinal lumen. Medicine, *47*:89, 1968.
87. Vince, A., et al.: Bacteriological studies in Crohn's disease. J. Med. Microbiol., *5*:219, 1972.
88. Smith, A. N.: Clinical pathophysiology. *In* Regional Enteritis (Crohn's Disease) Edited by A. Engel and T. Larrson. Stockholm, Nordiska Bokhandelns Forlag, 1971.
89. Hess-Thayson, E.: Clinical diagnosis. *In* Regional Enteritis (Crohn's Disease) Edited by A. Engel and T. Larrson. Stockholm, Nordiska Bokhandelns Forlag, 1971.
90. Kristensen, M., et al.: Short bowel syndrome following resection for Crohn's disease. Scand. J. Gastroenterol., *9*:559, 1974.
91. Williams, J. A.: Progress report: The place of surgery in Crohn's disease. Gut, *12*:739, 1971.
92. Nasr, K., et al.: Free perforation in regional enteritis. Gut, *10*:206, 1969.
93. Crohn, B. B.: Regional Ileitis. New York, Grune and Stratton, 1949.
94. Steinberg, D. M., Cooke, W. T., and Williams, J. A.: Abscess and fistulae in Crohn's disease. Gut, *14*:865, 1973.
95. Fischer, J. E., Foster, G. S., and Abel, R. M.: Hyperalimentation as a primary therapy for inflammatory bowel disease. Am. J. Surg., *125*:165, 1973.
96. Vogel, C. M., Corwin, T. R., and Baue, A. E.: Intravenous hyperalimentation in the treatment of inflammatory disease of the bowel. Arch. Surg., *108*:460, 1974.
97. MacFadyen, B. V., Dudrick, S. J., and Ruberg, R. L.: Management of gastrointestinal fistulas with parenteral hyperalimentation. Surgery, *74*:100, 1973.
98. Bury, K. D., Stephens, R. V., and Randall, H. T.: Use of a chemically defined, liquid elemental diet for nutritional management of fistulas of the alimentary tract. Am. J. Surg., *121*:174, 1971.
99. Voitk, A. J., et al.: Elemental diet in the treatment of fistulas of the alimentary tract. Surg. Gynecol. Obstet., *137*:68, 1973.
100. Brooke, B. N., Hoffman, D. C., and Swarbrick, E. T.: Azathioprine for Crohn's disease. Lancet, *1*:612, 1969.
101. Brooke, B. N., Javett, S. L., and Davison, O. W.: Further experience with azathioprine for Crohn's disease. Lancet, *2*:1050, 1970.
102. Drucker, W. R., and Jeejeebhoy, K. N.: Azathioprine: An adjunct to surgical therapy of granulomatous enteritis. Ann. Surg., *172*:618, 1970.
103. Korelitz, B. I., and Present, D. H.: Favorable effect of

103. 6-mercaptopurine on fistulae of Crohn's disease. Dig. Dis. Sci., *30*:58, 1985.
104. Sheldon, G. F., Gardiner, B. N., Way, L. W., and Dunphy, J. E.: Management of gastrointestinal fistulas. Surg. Gynecol. Obstet., *133*:385, 1971.
105. Webster, M. W., Jr., and Carey, L. C.: Fistulae of the intestinal tract. In Current Problems in Surgery. Chicago, Year Book Medical Publishers, 1976.
106. Reber, H. A., Roberts, C., Way, L. W., and Dunphy, J. E.: Management of external gastrointestinal fistulas. Ann. Surg., *188*:460, 1978.
107. Broe, P. J., Bayless, T. M., and Cameron, J. L.: Crohn's disease. Are enteroenteral fistulas an indication for surgery? Surgery, *91*:249, 1982.
108. Greenstein, A. J., Kark, A. E., and Dreiling, D. A.: Crohn's disease of the colon: I. Fistula in Crohn's disease of the colon, classification, presenting features and management in 63 patients. Am. J. Gastroenterol., *63*:419, 1974.
109. Hiley, P. C., Cohen, N., and Present, D. H.: Spontaneous umbilical fistula in granulomatous (Crohn's) disease of the bowel. Gastroenterology, *60*:103, 1971.
110. Rentz, T. W., Jr., et al.: Crohn's disease with spontaneous ileoumbilical and ileovesical fistula. Dig. Dis. Sci., *24*:316, 1979.
111. Davidson, E. D.: Crohn's disease with spontaneous cutaneous-urachovesicoenteric fistula. Dig. Dis. Sci., *25*:460, 1980.
112. Kyle, J., and Murray, C. M.: Ileovesical fistula in Crohn's disease. Surgery, *66*:497, 1969.
113. Talamini, M. A., Broe, P. J., and Cameron, J. L.: Urinary fistulas in Crohn's disease. Surg. Gynecol. Obstet., *154*:553, 1982.
114. Greenstein, A. J., et al.: Course of enterovesical fistulas in Crohn's disease. Am. J. Surg., *147*:788, 1984.
115. Malchow, H., et al.: European Cooperative Crohn's Disease Study (ECCDS): Results of drug treatment. Gastroenterology, *86*:249, 1984.
116. Sewell, J. H.: Acute perforation of the small intestine in regional enteritis. Am. J. Gastroenterol., *47*:148, 1967.
117. Waye, J. D., and Lithgow, C.: Small bowel perforation in regional enteritis. Gastroenterology, *53*:625, 1967.
118. Kyle, J., et al.: Free perforation in regional enteritis. Am. J. Dig. Dis., *13*:275, 1968.
119. Alavi, I. A., Printen, K., and Steigmann, F.: Free perforation in chronic regional enteritis. Am. J. Dig. Dis., *14*:420, 1969.
120. Mogadam, M., and Priest, R. J.: Necrotizing enteritis in Crohn's disease of the small bowel. Gastroenterology, *56*:337, 1969.
121. Present, D. H., et al.: Obstructive hydronephrosis: A frequent but seldom recognized complication of granulomatous disease of the bowel. N. Engl. J. Med., *280*:523, 1969.
122. Block, G. E., Enker, W. E., and Kirsner, J. B.: Significance and treatment of occult obstructive uropathy complicating Crohn's disease. Ann. Surg., *178*:322, 1973.
123. Collier, P. E., Turowski, P., and Diamond, D. L.: Small intestinal adenocarcinoma complicating regional enteritis. Cancer, *55*:516, 1985.
124. Glotzer, D. J.: The risk of cancer in Crohn's disease. Gastroenterology, *89*:438, 1985.
125. Hoffman, J. P., Taft, D. A., Wheelis, R. F., and Walker, J. H.: Adenocarcinoma in regional enteritis of the small intestine. Arch. Surg., *112*:606, 1977.
126. Darke, S. G., Parks, A. G., Grogono, J. L., and Pollack, D. J.: Adenocarcinoma in Crohn's disease: A report of two cases and analysis of the literature. Br. J. Surg., *60*:169, 1973.
127. Fresko, D., Lazarus, S. S., Dotan, J., and Reingold, M.: Early presentation of carcinoma of the small bowel in Crohn's disease (Crohn's carcinoma). Case reports and review of the literature. Gastroenterology, *82*:783, 1982.
128. Perzin, K. H., et al.: Intramucosal carcinoma of the small intestine arising in regional enteritis (Crohn's disease): Report of a case studied for carcinoembryonic antigen and review of the literature. Cancer, *54*:151, 1984.
129. Simpson, S., Traube, J., and Riddell, R. H.: The histologic appearance of dysplasia (precarcinomatous change) in Crohn's disease of the small and large intestine. Gastroenterology, *81*:492, 1981.
130. Greenstein, A. J., et al.: Patterns of neoplasia in Crohn's disease and ulcerative colitis. Cancer, *46*:403, 1980.
131. Gray, B. K., Lockhart-Mummery, H. E., and Morson, B. C.: Crohn's disease of the anal region. Gut, *6*:515, 1965.
132. Homan, W. P., Tang, C. K., and Thorbjarnarson, B.: Anal lesions complicating Crohn's disease. Arch. Surg., *111*:1333, 1976.
133. Fielding, J. F.: Perianal lesions in Crohn's disease. J. R. Coll. Surg. Edinb., *1717*:32, 1972.
134. Alexander-Williams, J., and Buchman, P.: Perianal Crohn's disease. World J. Surg., *4*:203, 1980.
135. Lockhart-Mummery, H. E.: Anal lesions of Crohn's disease. Clin. Gastroenterol., *1*:377, 1972.
136. Bernstein, L. H., Frank, M. S., Brandt, L. J., and Boley, S. J.: Healing of perineal Crohn's disease with metronidazole. Gastroenterology, *79*:357, 1980.
137. Brandt, L. J., Bernstein, L. H., Boley, S. J., and Frank, M. S.: Metronidazole therapy for perineal Crohn's disease: A follow-up study. Gastroenterology, *83*:383, 1982.
138. Sachar, D. B.: Metronidazole for Crohn's disease—breakthrough or ballyhoo? Gastroenterology, *79*:393, 1980.
139. Hatoff, D. E.: Perineal Crohn's disease complicated by pyogenic liver abscess during metronidazole therapy. Gastroenterology, *85*:194, 1983.
140. Sohn, N., Korelitz, B. I., and Weinstein, M. A.: Anorectal Crohn's disease: Definitive surgery for fistulas and recurrent abscesses. Am. J. Surg., *139*:394, 1980.
141. Heuman, R., Bolin, T., Sjodahl, R., and Tagesson, C.: The incidence and course of perianal complications and arthralgia after intestinal resection with restoration of continuity for Crohn's disease. Br. J. Surg., *68*:528, 1981.
142. Hellers, G., Bergstrand, O., Ewerth, S., and Holmstrom, B.: Occurrence and outcome after primary treatment of anal fistulae in Crohn's disease. Gut, *21*:525, 1980.
143. Marks, C. G., Ritchie, J. K., and Lockhart-Mummery, H. F.: Anal fistulas in Crohn's disease. Br. J. Surg., *68*:525, 1981.
144. Bergstrand, O., et al.: Outcome following treatment of anal fistulae in Crohn's disease. Acta Chir. Scand., *500*:43, 1980.
145. Buchman, P., et al.: Natural history of perianal Crohn's disease: Ten year follow-up: A plea for conservatism. Am. J. Surg., *140*:642, 1980.
146. Williams, J. A.: Perianal Crohn's disease. In The Management of Crohn's Disease. Edited by I. T. Weterman, A. S. Peña, and C. C. Booth. Amsterdam, Exerpta Medica, 1976.
147. Burman, J. H., et al.: The effect of diversion of intestinal contents on the progress of Crohn's disease of the large bowel. Gut, *12*:11, 1971.
148. Williams, N. S., MacFie, J., and Celestin, L. R.: Anorectal Crohn's disease. Br. J. Surg., *66*:743, 1979.
149. Chaikhouni, A., Regueyra, F. I., and Stevens, J. R.: Adenocarcinoma in perianal fistulas of Crohn's disease. Dis. Colon Rectum, *24*:639, 1981.
150. Slater, G., Greenstein, A. J., and Aufses, A. H.: Anal carci-

noma in patients with Crohn's disease. Ann. Surg., *199*:348, 1984.
151. Cooke, W. T., and Swan, C. H., Jr.: Diffuse jejuno-ileitis of Crohn's disease. Q. J. Med., *43*:583, 1974.
152. Truelove, S. C.: Course and prognosis. *In* Regional Enteritis (Crohn's Disease) Edited by A. Engel and T. Larrson. Stockholm, Nordiska Bokhandelns Forlag, 1971.
153. Warshaw, A. L., Waldman, T. A., and Laster, L.: Protein-losing enteropathy and malabsorption in regional enteritis: Cure by limited ileal resection. Ann. Surg., *178*:578, 1973.
154. Kirschner, B. S., Voinchet, O., and Rosenberg, I. H.: Growth retardation in inflammatory bowel disease. Gastroenterology, *75*:504, 1978.
155. McCaffrey, T., et al.: Severe growth retardation in children with inflammatory bowel disease. Pediatrics, *45*:386, 1970.
156. Berger, M., Gribetz, D., and Korelitz, B.I.: Growth retardation in children with ulcerative colitis: The effect of medical and surgical therapy. Pediatrics, *55*:459, 1975.
157. Grand, R. J., and Homer, D. R.: Approaches to inflammatory bowel disease in childhood and adolescence. Pediatr. Clin. North Am., *22*:835, 1975.
158. Layden, T., et al.: Reversal of growth arrest in adolescents with Crohn's disease after parenteral alimentation. Gastroenterology, *70*:1017, 1976.
159. Kelts, D. G., et al.: Nutritional basis of growth failure in children and adolescents with Crohn's disease. Gastroenterology, *76*:720, 1979.
160. Strobel, C. T., Byrne, W. J., and Ament, M. E.: Home parenteral nutrition in children with Crohn's disease: An effective management alternative. Gastroenterology, *77*:272, 1979.
161. Morin, C. L., Roulet, M., Roy, C. C., and Weber, A.: Continuous elemental enteral alimentation in children with Crohn's disease and growth failure. Gastroenterology, *79*:1205, 1980.
162. Kirschner, B. S., et al.: Reversal of growth retardation in Crohn's disease with therapy emphasizing oral nutritional restitution. Gastroenterology, *80*:10, 1981.
163. McCaffrey, T. D., Jr., et al.: Effect of administered human growth hormone on growth retardation in inflammatory bowel disease. Am. J. Dig. Dis., *19*:411, 1974.
164. Viteri, F. E., and Arroyave, G.: Protein-calorie malnutrition. *In* Modern Nutrition in Health and Disease. 5th Ed. Edited by R. S. Goodhart and M. E. Shils. Philadelphia, Lea & Febiger, 1973.
165. Frish, R. E.: Weight at menarche. Similarity for well-nourished and undernourished girls at different ages, and evidence for historical constancy. Pediatrics, *50*:445, 1972.
166. Gopalan, C., et al.: Effect of calorie supplementation on growth of undernourished children. Am. J. Clin. Nutr., *26*:563, 1973.
167. Simmons, J., et al.: Relation of caloric deficiency to growth failure in children on hemodialysis and the growth response to caloric supplementation. N. Engl. J. Med., *285*:653, 1971.
168. Blodgett, F. F., et al.: Effects of prolonged cortisone therapy on the statural growth, skeletal maturation and metabolic status of children. N. Engl. J. Med., *254*:636, 1956.
169. Van Mettre, T., Miermann, W., and Rosen, L.: A comparison of the growth suppressive effect of cortisone, prednisone, and other adrenal cortical hormones. J. Allergy, *31*:531, 1960.
170. Voinchet, O., Kirsner, J. B., and Rosenberg, I. H.: Growth retardation in children with inflammatory bowel disease: evaluation of surgical therapy. Gastroenterology, *64*:816, 1973.
171. Whittington, P. E., Barnes, H. V., and Bayless, T. M.: Medical management of Crohn's disease in adolescence. Gastroenterology, *72*:1338, 1977.
172. Davidson, S.: Infantilism in ulcerative colitis. Arch. Intern. Med., *64*:1187, 1939.
173. Benson, R. E., and Bargen, J. A.: Chronic ulcerative colitis as a cause of retarded sexual and gonadic development. Gastroenterology, *1*:147, 1943.
174. Lyons, A. S., and Baronofsky, I. D.: Surgical treatment of ulcerative colitis in pubertal years. Surg. Clin. North Am., *40*:999, 1960.
175. Frey, C. F., and Weaver, D. K.: Colectomy in children with ulcerative and granulomatous colitis: operative indications and results. Arch. Surg., *104*:414, 1972.
176. Block, G. E., Moosa, A. R., and Simonowitz, D.: The operative treatment of Crohn's disease in childhood. Surg. Gynecol. Obstet., *144*:713, 1977.
177. Homer, D. R., Grand, R. J., and Colodny, A. H.: Growth, course and prognosis after surgery for Crohn's disease in children and adolescents. Pediatrics, *59*:717, 1977.
178. Daly, D. W.: Outcome of surgery for ulcerative colitis. Ann. R. Coll. Surg. Engl., *42*:38, 1968.
179. Devroede, G. J., et al.: Cancer risk and life expectancy of children with ulcerative colitis. N. Engl. J. Med., *285*:17, 1971.
180. Aylett, S.: Diffuse ulcerative colitis and its treatment by ileorectal anastomosis. Ann. R. Coll. Surg. Engl., *27*:260, 1960.
181. Baker, W. N. W.: The results of ileorectal anastomosis at St. Mark's Hospital from 1953 to 1968. Gut, *11*:235, 1970.
182. Baker, W. N. W.: Ileo-rectal anastomosis for Crohn's disease of the colon. Gut, *12*:427, 1971.
183. Watts, J. McK., and Hughes, E. S. R.: Proceedings IV World Congress of Gastroenterology. Edited by P. Riis, P. Anthonisen, and H. Baden. Copenhagen, The Danish Gastroenterological Association, 1970.
184. Jagelman, D. G., Lewis, C. B., and Rowe-Jones, D. C.: Ileorectal anastomosis appreciation by patients. Br. Med. J., *1*:756, 1969.
185. Adson, M. A., Cooperman, A. M., and Farrow, G. M.: Ileorectostomy for ulcerative disease of the colon. Arch. Surg., *104*:424, 1972.
186. Taylor, B. M., et al.: The endorectal ileal pouch-anal anastomosis. Current clinical results. Dis. Colon Rectum, *27*:347, 1984.
187. Rothenberger, D. A., Buls, J. G., Nivatvongs, S., and Goldberg, S. M.: The Parks S ileal pouch and anal anastomosis after colectomy and mucosal proctectomy. Am. J. Surg., *149*:390, 1985.
188. Schoetz, D. J., Jr., Coller, J. A., and Veidenheimer, M. C.: Ileoanal reservoir for ulcerative colitis and familial polyposis. Arch. Surg., *121*:404, 1986.
189. Kock, N. G.: Continent ileostomy. Prog. Surg. *12*:180, 1973.
190. Edwards, F. C., and Truelove, S. C.: The course and prognosis of ulcerative colitis. Gut, *4*:299, 1963.
191. Watts, J. McK., de Dombal, F. T., and Goligher, J. C.: Early results of surgery for ulcerative colitis. Br. J. Surg., *53*:1005, 1966.
192. Goligher, J. C., et al.: Early surgery in the management of severe ulcerative colitis. Br. Med. J., *3*:193, 1967.
193. Truelove, S. C., and Witts, L. J.: Cortisone and corticotrophin in ulcerative colitis. Br. Med. J., *1*:387, 1959.
194. Lennard-Jones, J. E., et al.: Prednisone as maintenance treatment for ulcerative colitis in remission. Lancet, *1*:188, 1965.
195. Misiewcz, J. J., et al.: Controlled trial of sulphasalazine in maintenance therapy for ulcerative colitis. Lancet, *1*:185, 1965.

196. Dissanayake, A. S., and Truelove, S. C.: A controlled trial of long-term maintenance treatment of ulcerative colitis with sulfasalazine (Salazopyrine). Gut, *14*:923, 1973.
197. Riis, P., et al.: The prophylactic effect of salazosulphapyridine in ulcerative colitis during long-term treatment. Scand. J. Gastroenterol., *8*:71, 1973.
198. Jewell, D. P., and Truelove, S. C.: Azathioprine in ulcerative colitis: Final report on controlled therapeutic trial. Br. Med. J., *4*:627, 1974.
199. Rosenberg, J. L., et al.: A controlled trial of azathioprine in the management of chronic ulcerative colitis. Gastroenterology, *69*:96, 1975.
200. Lumb, G., Protheroe, R. H. B., and Ramsay, G. S.: Ulcerative colitis with dilatation of the colon. Br. J. Surg., *43*:182, 1955.
201. McConnell, F., Hanelin, J., and Robbins, L. L.: Plain film diagnosis of fulminating ulcerative colitis. Radiology, *71*:674, 1958.
202. Roth, J. L. A., Valdes-Dapena, A., Stein, G. N., and Bockus, H. L.: Toxic megacolon and ulcerative colitis. Gastroenterology, *37*:239, 1959.
203. Korelitz, B. I., and Janowitz, H. D.: Dilatation of the colon. A serious complication of ulcerative colitis. Ann. Intern. Med., *53*:153, 1960.
204. Peskin, G. W., and Davis, A. V. O.: Acute fulminating ulcerative colitis with colonic distention. Surg. Gynecol. Obstet., *110*:269, 1960.
205. Sampson, P. A., and Walker, F. C.: Dilatation of the colon in ulcerative colitis. Br. Med. J., *2*:1119, 1961.
206. McInerney, G. T., Sauer, W. G., Baggenstoss, A. H., and Hodgson, J. R.: Fulminating ulcerative colitis with marked colonic dilatation: A clinicopathologic study. Gastroenterology, *42*:244, 1962.
207. Smith, F. W., Law, D. H., Nickel, W. F., Jr., and Sleisenger, M. H.: Fulminant ulcerative colitis with toxic dilation of the colon: Medical and surgical management of eleven cases with observations regarding etiology. Gastroenterology, *42*:233, 1962.
208. Rowe, R. J.: Dilatation of the colon (toxic megacolon) in acute fulminating ulcerative colitis. Dis. Colon Rectum, *6*:23, 1963.
209. Silverberg, D., and Rogers, A. G.: Toxic megacolon in ulcerative colitis. Can. Med. Assoc. J., *90*:357, 1964.
210. Prohaska, J. V., Greer, D., Jr., and Ryan, J. F.: Acute dilatation of the colon in ulcerative colitis. Arch. Surg., *89*:24, 1964.
211. Edwards, F. C., and Truelove, S. C.: The course and prognosis of ulcerative colitis. III. Complications. Gut, *5*:1, 1964.
212. Ferrante, W. H., and Egger, J.: Toxic megacolon complicating chronic ulcerative colitis. South. Med. J., *58*:969, 1965.
213. McElwain, J. W., Alexander, R. M., and MacLean, M. D.: Toxic dilatation of the colon in ulcerative colitis. Arch. Surg., *90*:133, 1965.
214. Odyniec, N. A., Judd, E. S., and Sauer, W. G.: Toxic megacolon. Significant improvement in surgical management. Arch. Surg., *94*:638, 1967.
215. Neschis, M., Siegelman, S. S., and Parker, J. G.: Diagnosis and management of the megacolon of ulcerative colitis. Gastroenterology, *55*:251, 1968.
216. Jalan, K. N., et al.: An experience of ulcerative colitis. I. Toxic dilation in 55 cases. Gastroenterology, *57*:68, 1969.
217. Foley, W. J., Coon, W. W., and Bonfield, R. E.: Toxic megacolon in acute fulminant ulcerative colitis. Am. J. Surg., *120*:769, 1970.
218. Adams, J. T.: Toxic dilatation of the colon. A surgical disease. Arch. Surg., *106*:678, 1973.
219. Binder, S. C., Patterson, J. F., and Glotzer, D. J.: Toxic megacolon in ulcerative colitis. Gastroenterology, *66*:909, 1974.
220. Scott, H. W., et al.: Surgical management of toxic dilatation of the colon in ulcerative colitis. Ann. Surg., *129*:647, 1975.
221. Koudahl, G., and Kristensen, M.: Toxic megacolon in ulcerative colitis. Scand. J. Gastroenterol., *10*:417, 1975.
222. Hartong, W. A., Arvanitakis, C., Skibba, R. M., and Klotz, A. P.: Treatment of toxic megacolon. A comparative review of 29 patients. Am. J. Surg., *22*:195, 1977.
223. Sirinek, K. R., Tetirick, C. E., Thomford, N. R., and Pace, W. G.: Total proctocolectomy and ileostomy. Procedure of choice for acute toxic megacolon. Arch. Surg., *112*:518, 1977.
224. Roys, G., Kaplan, M. S., and Juler, G. L.: Surgical management of toxic megacolon. Am. J. Gastroenterol., *68*:161, 1977.
225. Greenstein, A. J., et al.: Outcome of toxic dilatation in ulcerative colitis and Crohn's disease. J. Clin. Gastroenterol., *7*:137, 1985.
226. Grant, C. S., and Dozois, R. R.: Toxic megacolon: Ultimate fate of patients after successful medical management. Am. J. Surg., *147*:106, 1984.
227. Truelove, S. C., and Witts, L. J.: Cortisone in ulcerative colitis: Final report on a therapeutic trial. Br. Med. J., *2*:1041, 1955.
228. Lennard-Jones, J. E., et al.: An assessment of prednisone, salazopyrin and topical hydrocortisone hemisuccinate used as an outpatient treatment for ulcerative colitis. Gut, *1*:217, 1960.
229. Meyers, S., and Janowitz, H. D.: The place of steroids in the therapy of toxic megacolon. Gastroenterology, *75*:729, 1978.
230. Almy, T. P., and Lewis, L. M.: Ulcerative colitis: A report of progress based on the recent literature. Gastroenterology, *45*:515, 1963.
231. Meyers, S., Sachar, D. B., Goldberg, J. D., and Janowitz, H. D.: Corticotropin versus hydrocortisone in the intravenous treatment of ulcerative colitis. A prospective, randomized, double-blind clinical trial. Gastroenterology, *85*:351, 1983.
232. Present, D. H., et al.: The medical management of toxic megacolon: Technique of decompression with favorable longterm follow-up. Gastroenterology, *80*:1255, 1981.
233. Bolton, R. P., and Read, A. E.: Clostridium difficile in toxic megacolon complicating acute inflammatory bowel disease. Br. Med. J., *285*:475, 1982.
234. Klein, S. H., et al.: Emergency cecostomy in ulcerative colitis with acute toxic dilation. Surgery, *47*:399, 1960.
235. Turnbull, R. B., Jr., Hawk, W. A., and Weakley, F. L.: Surgical treatment of toxic megacolon: Ileostomy and colostomy to prepare patients for colectomy. Am. J. Surg., *122*:325, 1971.
236. Edwards, F. C., and Truelove, S. C.: The course and prognosis of ulcerative colitis. III. Complications. Gut, *5*:1, 1964.
237. Edwards, F. C., and Truelove, S. C.: The course and prognosis of ulcerative colitis. IV. Carcinoma of the colon. Gut, *5*:15, 1964.
238. Goldgraber, M. B., and Kirsner, J. B.: Carcinoma in ulcerative colitis. Cancer, *17*:657, 1964.
239. Welch, C. E., and Hedberg, S. E.: Colonic cancer in ulcerative colitis and idopathic colonic cancer. J. Am. Med. Assoc., *191*:111, 1965.
240. Cook, M. G., and Goligher, J. C.: Carcinoma and epithelial dysplasia complicating ulcerative colitis. Gastroenterology, *68*:1127, 1975.
241. Hughes, R. G., et al.: The prognosis of carcinoma of the

colon and rectum complicating ulcerative colitis. Surg. Gynecol. Obstet., 146:46, 1978.
242. Lavery, I. C., et al.: Survival with carcinoma arising in mucosal ulcerative colitis. Ann. Surg., 195:508, 1982.
243. van Heerden, J. A., and Beart, R. W., Jr.: Carcinoma of the colon and rectum complicating chronic ulcerative colitis. Dis. Colon Rectum, 23:155, 1980.
244. Glotzer, D. J., Roth, S. I., and Welch, C. E.: Colonic ulceration proximal to obstructing carcinoma. Surgery, 56:950, 1964.
245. Katzka, I., Brody, R. S., Morris, E., and Katz, S.: Assessment of colorectal cancer risk in patients with ulcerative colitis: Experience from a private practice. Gastroenterology, 85:22, 1983.
246. Whelan, G.: Cancer risk in ulcerative colitis: Why are results in the literature so varied? Clin. Gastroenterol., 9:469, 1980.
247. Brostrom, O.: The role of cancer surveillance in long-term prognosis of ulcerative colitis. Scand. J. Gastroenterol., 88:40, 1983.
248. Butt, J. H., Lennard-Jones, J. E., and Ritchie, J. K.: A practical approach to the risk of cancer in inflammatory bowel disease. Reassure, watch or act? Med. Clin. North Am., 64:1203, 1980.
249. Yardley, J. H., Ransohoff, D. F., Riddell, R. H., and Goldman, H.: Cancer in inflammatory bowel disease: How serious is the problem and what should be done about it? Gastroenterology, 85:197, 1983.
250. Sackett, D. L., and Whelan, G.: Cancer risk in ulcerative colitis. Scientific requirements for the study of prognosis. Gastroenterology, 78:1632, 1980.
251. Greenstein, A. J., et al.: Cancer in universal and left-sided ulcerative colitis: Clinical and pathologic features. Gastroenterology, 77:290, 1979.
252. Truelove, S. C.: Ulcerative colitis beginning in childhood. N. Engl. J. Med., 285:50, 1971.
253. Rule, A. H., et al.: Tumor associated (CEA-reacting) antigen in patients with inflammatory bowel disease. N. Engl. J. Med., 287:24, 1972.
254. Dhar, P., et al.: Carcinoembryonic antigen (CEA) in colon cancer: Use in preoperative and postoperative diagnosis and prognosis. J. Am. Med. Assoc., 221:31, 1972.
255. Moore, T. L., Kantrowitz, P. A., and Zamcheck, N.: Carcinoembryonic antigen (CEA) in inflammatory bowel disease. J. Am. Med. Assoc., 222:944, 1972.
256. Morson, B. C., and Pang, L. S. C.: Rectal biopsy as aid to cancer control in ulcerative colitis. Gut, 8:423, 1967.
257. Goulston, S. J. M., and McGovern, V. J.: The value of rectal biopsies. Med. J. Aust., 1:1234, 1972.
258. Evans, D. J., and Pollock, D. J.: In-situ and invasive carcinoma of the colon in patients with ulcerative colitis. Gut, 13:566, 1972.
259. Hulten, L., Kewenter, J., and Ahren, C.: Precancer and carcinoma in chronic ulcerative colitis. A histological and clinical investigation. Scand. J. Gastroenterol., 7:663, 1972.
260. Yardley, J. H., and Keren, D. F.: "Precancer" lesions in ulcerative colitis. Cancer, 34:835, 1974.
261. Myrvold, H. E., Kock, N. G., and Ahren, C.: Rectal biopsy and precancer in ulcerative colitis. Gut, 15:301, 1974.
262. Teague, R. H., and Read, A. E.: Polyposis in ulcerative colitis. Gut, 16:792, 1975.
263. Gewertz, B. L., Dent, T. L., and Appelman, H. D.: Implications of precancerous rectal biopsy in patients with inflammatory bowel disease. Arch. Surg., 3:326, 1976.
264. Dobbins, W. O., III: Current status of the precancer lesion in ulcerative colitis. Gastroenterology, 73:1431, 1977.
265. Riddell, R. H., et al.: Dysplasia in inflammatory bowel disease: Standardized classification with provisional clinical applications. Hum. Pathol., 14:931, 1983.
266. Crowson, T. D., Ferrante, W. F., and Gathright, J. B., Jr.: Colonoscopy: Inefficacy for early carcinoma detection in patients with ulcerative colitis. J. Am. Med. Assoc., 236:2651, 1976.
267. Katz, S., et al.: Cancer in chronic ulcerative colitis. Diagnostic role of segmental colonic lavage. Am. J. Dig. Dis., 22:355, 1977.
268. Butt, J. H., et al.: Macroscopic lesions in dysplasia and carcinoma complicating ulcerative colitis. Dig. Dis. Sci., 28:18, 1983.
269. Blackstone, M. O., Riddell, R. H., Rogers, B. H. G., and Levin, B.: Dysplasia-associated lesion or mass (DALM) detected by colonoscopy in long-standing ulcerative colitis: An indication for colectomy. Gastroenterology, 80:366, 1981.
270. Nugent, F. W., and Haggett, R. C.: Results of a long-term surveillance program for dysplasia in ulcerative colitis. Gastroenterology, 86:1197, 1984.
271. Morson, B. C.: Dysplasia in ulcerative colitis. Scand. J. Gastroenterol. 88:36, 1983.
272. Lennard-Jones, J. E., Morson, B. C., Ritchie, J. K., and Williams, C. B.: Cancer surveillance in ulcerative colitis. Experience over 15 years. Lancet, 2:149, 1983.
273. Lennard-Jones, J. E., et al.: Cancer in colitis: Assessment of the individual risk by clinical and histological criteria. Gastroenterology, 73:1280, 1977.
274. Goligher, J. C.: Surgery of the Anus, Rectum and Colon. 3rd Ed. London, Baillière Tindall, 1975, p. 880.
275. Goligher, J. C.: Surgery of the Anus, Rectum and Colon. 5th Ed. London, Baillière Tindall, 1984, p. 856.
276. Prior, P., et al.: Cancer morbidity in ulcerative colitis. Gut, 23:490, 1982.
277. Hulten, L., Kewenter, J., and Kock, N. G.: The long-term results of partial resection of the large bowel for intestinal carcinomas complicating ulcerative colitis. Scand. J. Gastroenterol., 6:601, 1971.
278. Marshak, R. H., Block, L., and Wolf, B. S.: The roentgen findings in strictures of the colon associated with ulcerative and granulomatous colitis. Am. J. Roentgenol., 90:709, 1963.
279. Goulston, S. J. M., and McGovern, V. J.: The nature of benign strictures in ulcerative colitis. N. Engl. J. Med., 281:290, 1969.
280. Max, M. H., and Knutson, C. O.: Colonoscopy in patients with inflammatory colonic strictures. Surgery, 84:551, 1978.
281. Forde, K. A., and Treat, M. R.: Colonoscopy in the evaluation of strictures. Dis. Colon Rectum, 28:699, 1985.
282. Greenstein, A. J., Janowitz, H. D., and Sachar, D. B.: The extra-intestinal complications of Crohn's disease and ulcerative colitis: A study of 700 patients. Medicine, 55:401, 1976.
283. Johnson, M. C., and Wilson, H. T. H.: Skin lesions in ulcerative colitis. Gut, 10:255, 1969.
284. Fernandez-Herlihy, L.: The articular manifestations of chronic ulcerative colitis. Gut, 10:255, 1969.
285. Bywaters, E. G. L., and Ansell, B. M.: Arthritis associated with ulcerative colitis, a clinical and pathological study. Ann. Rheum. Dis., 17:169, 1958.
286. McEwen, L., et al.: Arthritis accompanying ulcerative colitis. Am. J. Surg., 33:923, 1962.
287. Wright, V., and Watkinson, G.: The arthritis of ulcerative colitis. Br. Med. J., 2:670, 1965.

288. Korelitz, B. I., and Coles, R. S.: Uveitis (iritis) associated with ulcerative and granulomatous colitis. Gastroenterology, 52:78, 1967.
289. Hopkins, D. J., et al.: Ocular disorders in a series of 332 patients with Crohn's disease. Br. J. Ophthalmol., 58:732, 1974.
290. Morris, R. I., et al.: HL-A-W27: A useful discriminator in the arthropathies of inflammatory bowel disease. N. Engl. J. Med., 290:1117, 1974.
291. Wright, V., and Watkinson, G.: Sacroiliitis and ulcerative colitis. Br. Med. J., 2:675, 1965.
292. Mistilis, S. P., Skyring, A. P., and Goulston, S. J. M.: Effect of long-term tetracycline therapy, steroid therapy and colectomy in pericholangitis associated with ulcerative colitis. Aust. Ann. Med., 14:489, 1970.
293. Eade, M. N., Cooke, W. T., and Brooke, B. N.: Liver disease in ulcerative colitis: II. The long-term effect of colectomy. Ann. Intern. Med., 72:489, 1970.
294. Eade, M. N., Cooke, W. T., Brooke, B. N., and Thompson, H.: Liver disease in Crohn's colitis. A study of 21 consecutive patients having colectomy. Ann. Intern. Med., 74:518, 1971.
295. Mistilis, S. P.: Pericholangitis and ulcerative colitis: I. Pathology, etiology and pathogenesis. Ann. Intern. Med., 63:1, 1965.
296. Cooperman, A. M., and Judd, E. S.: The role of colectomy in hepatic disease accompanying ulcerative and granulomatous colitis. Current status of a continuous problem. Mayo Clin. Proc., 47:36, 1972.
297. Chapman, R. W., et al.: Primary sclerosing cholangitis: A review of its clinical features, cholangiography and hepatic histology. Gut, 21:870, 1980.
298. Schrumpf, E., et al.: Sclerosing cholangitis in ulcerative colitis. A follow-up study. Scand. J. Gastroenterol., 17:33, 1982.
299. Wood, R. A., and Cuschieri, A.: Is sclerosing cholangitis complicating ulcerative colitis a reversible condition? Lancet, 2:716, 1980.
300. Hawk, W. A., Turnbull, R. B., Jr., and Farmer, R. G.: Regional enteritis of the colon: Distinctive features of the entity. J. Am. Med. Assoc., 201:738, 1967.
301. Glotzer, D. J., et al.: Comparative features and course of ulcerative and granulomatous colitis. N. Engl. J. Med., 282:582, 1960.
302. Fawaz, K. A., et al.: Ulcerative colitis and Crohn's disease of the colon—a comparison of the long-term postoperative courses. Gastroenterology, 71:372, 1976.
303. Janowitz, H. D., and Sachar, D. B.: New observations in Crohn's disease. In Annual Review of Medicine. Selected Topics in the Clinical Sciences, Vol. 27. Edited by W. P. Creger. Palo Alto, Annual Reviews, 1976.
304. Glotzer, D. J.: Recurrence in Crohn's colitis: The numbers game. World J. Surg., 4:173, 1980.
305. Meyers, S., et al.: Quality of life after surgery for Crohn's disease: A psychosocial survey. Gastroenterology, 78:1, 1980.
306. Goligher, J. C.: The long-term results of excisional surgery for primary and recurrent Crohn's disease of the large intestine. Dis. Colon Rectum, 28:51, 1985.
307. Glotzer, D. J., Stone, P. A., and Patterson, J. F.: Prognosis after surgical treatment of granulomatous colitis. N. Engl. J. Med., 277:273, 1967.
308. Jones, J. H., Lennard-Jones, J. E., and Lockhart-Mummery, H. E.: Experience in the treatment of Crohn's disease of the large intestine. Gut, 7:448, 1966.
309. Ritchie, J. K., and Lockhart-Mummery, H. E.: Non-restorative surgery in the treatment of Crohn's disease of the large bowel. Gut, 14:263, 1973.
310. Korelitz, B. I., et al.: Recurrent regional ileitis after ileostomy for granulomatous colitis. N. Engl. J. Med., 287:110, 1972.
311. Steinberg, D. M., et al.: Sequelae of colectomy and ileostomy: Comparison between Crohn's colitis and ulcerative colitis. Gastroenterology, 68:33, 1975.
312. Knill-Jones, R. P., Morson, B., and Williams, R.: Prestomal ileitis: clinical and pathological findings in five cases. Q. J. Med., 39:287, 1970.
313. Dennis, C., and Karlson, K. E.: Surgical measures as supplements to the management of the idiopathic ulcerative colitis: Cancer, cirrhosis and arthritis as frequent complications. Surgery, 32:892, 1952.
314. Counsell, B.: Lesions of the ileum associated with ulcerative colitis. Br. J. Surg., 44:276, 1956.
315. Loygue, J., Florent, R., and Got, R.: Lesions de intestine grele et rectocolite ulcerohemorrhagique. Arch. Med. Appar. Dig., 48:308, 1959.
316. Nugent, F. W., et al.: Prognosis following colonic resection for Crohn's disease of the colon. Gastroenterology, 65:398, 1973.
317. Greenstein, A. J., and Sachar, D. B.: Invited commentary. World J. Surg., 4:180, 1980.
318. Allan, R., Steinberg, D. M., Alexander-Williams, J., and Cooke, W. T.: Crohn's disease involving the colon: An audit of clinical management. Gastroenterology, 73:723, 1977.
319. Topuzlu, C., Andrews, W. E., Gladstone, A. A., and MacKay, A. G.: Preservation of the ascending colon in the surgical treatment of ulcerative colitis. Surg. Gynecol. Obstet., 127:831, 1968.
320. Oberhelman, H. A., Jr., Kahatsu, S., Taylor, K. B., and Kivel, R. M.: Diverting ileostomy in the surgical management of Crohn's disease of the colon. Am. J. Surg., 115:231, 1968.
321. Truelove, S. C., Ellis, H., and Webster, C. U.: Place of a double-barreled ileostomy in ulcerative colitis and Crohn's disease of the colon: A preliminary report. Br. Med. J., 1:150, 1965.
322. Lee, E.: Split ileostomy in the treatment of Crohn's disease of the colon. Ann. R. Coll. Surg. Engl., 56:94, 1975.
323. Harper, P. H., et al.: Split ileostomy and ileocolostomy for Crohn's disease of the colon and ulcerative colitis. A 20 year survey. Gut, 24:106, 1983.
324. McIlrath, D. C.: Diverting ileostomy or colostomy in the management of Crohn's disease of the colon. Arch. Surg., 103:308, 1971.
325. Glotzer, D. J., Glick, M. E., and Goldman, H.: Proctitis and colitis following diversion of the fecal stream. Gastroenterology, 80:438, 1981.
326. Weedon, D. D., et al.: Crohn's disease and cancer. N. Engl. J. Med., 289:1099, 1973.
327. Gyde, S. N., et al.: Malignancy in Crohn's disease. Gut, 21:1024, 1980.
328. Greenstein, A. J., et al.: A comparison of cancer risk in Crohn's disease and ulcerative colitis. Cancer, 48:2742, 1981.
329. Prior, P.: Malignancy in Crohn's disease. Br. J. Prev. Soc. Med., 26:59, 1972.
330. Fielding, J., Prior, P., Waterhouse, J. A., and Cooke, W. D.: Malignancy in Crohn's disease. Scand. J. Gastroenterol., 7:3, 1972.
331. Hellers, G. K. G., Bergstrand, O. L., and Ewerth, S. J.: Malignancy in Crohn's disease in Stockholm County. Ital. J. Gastroenterol., 11:131, 1979.
332. Thayer, W. R., Jr.: Summary: Carcinoma and granulomatous disease. Gastroenterology, 55:554, 1968.
333. Craft, C. F., Mendelsohn, G., Cooper, H. S., and Yardley,

J. H.: Colonic "precancer" in Crohn's disease. Gastroenterology, *80*:578, 1981.
334. Simpson, S., Traube, J., and Riddell, R. H.: The histologic appearance of dysplasia (precarcinomatous change) in Crohn's disease of the small and large intestine. Gastroenterology, *81*:492, 1981.
335. Hamilton, S. R.: Colorectal carcinomas in patients with Crohn's disease. Gastroenterology, *89*:398, 1985.
336. Cooper, D. J., Weinstein, M. A., and Korelitz, B. I.: Complications of Crohn's disease predisposing to dysplasia and cancer of the intestinal tract. Considerations of a surveillance program. J. Clin. Gastroenterol., *6*:217, 1984.
337. Traube, J., et al.: Crohn's disease and adenocarcinoma of the bowel. Dig. Dis. Sci., *25*:939, 1980.
338. Korelitz, B. I.: Carcinoma of the intestinal tract in Crohn's disease: Results of a survey conducted by the National Foundation for Ileitis and Colitis. Am. J. Gastroenterol., *78*:44, 1983.
339. Lavery, I. C., and Jagelman, D. G.: Cancer in the excluded rectum following surgery for inflammatory bowel disease. Dis. Colon Rectum, *25*:522, 1982.
340. Buzzard, A. J., Baker, W. N. W., Needham, P. R. G., and Warren, R. E.: Acute toxic dilatation of the colon in Crohn's colitis. Gut, *15*:416, 1974.
341. Farmer, R. G., Hawk, W. A., and Turnbull, R. B.: Clinical patterns in Crohn's disease: A statistical study of 615 cases. Gastroenterology, *68*:627, 1975.
342. Grieco, M. D., Bordan, D. L., Geiss, A. C., and Beil, A. R., Jr.: Toxic megacolon complicating Crohn's colitis. Ann. Surg., *191*:75, 1980.
343. Fisher, J., Mantz, F., and Calkins, W. G.: Colonic perforation in Crohn's disease. Gastroenterology, *71*:835, 1976.
344. Orda, R., Goldwaser, B., and Witznitzer, T.: Free perforation of the colon in Crohn's disease: Report of a case and review of the literature. Dis. Colon Rectum, *25*:145, 1982.
345. Greenstein, A. J., and Aufses, A. H., Jr.: Differences in pathogenesis, incidence and outcome of perforation in inflammatory bowel disease. Surg. Gynecol. Obstet., *160*:63, 1985.

27 · The Surgical Management of Idiopathic Inflammatory Bowel Disease

DONALD J. GLOTZER, M.D.

Historic Perspective

The interesting history of the surgical treatment of inflammatory bowel disease will not be recounted in great detail because a number of excellent accounts have been published.[1-7] A brief review, however, will serve not only to provide insight and perspective but also to emphasize the continuing need to reassess operative strategy in light of evolving knowledge and new techniques.

The basic surgical maneuvers available to the surgeon for dealing with diseased or damaged organs are rather limited and have included decompression, provision of access, bypass, extirpation, repair, nervous system ablation, and, in recent years, replacement. With the exception of the last, most of these approaches have been used at various times in inflammatory bowel disease, only to be modified, abandoned, or used again in revised form. Undoubtedly, this evolution will continue in the future.

Sporadic attempts to relieve ulcerative colitis by venting with colostomy took place in the late nineteenth century,[8] but colostomy did not gain wide acceptance as a method of treatment. The principle of venting was revived some years ago in the form of tube cecostomy for the treatment of toxic megacolon syndrome,[9] and more recently by the Turnbull multiple "ostomy" procedure.[10] Appendicostomy was first carried out by Weir in 1902 for the purpose of providing access to the colon so that it could be irrigated with various medicaments.[11] For many years thereafter appendicostomy apparently was the operation of choice and was still performed as late as the 1940's.[12] The surgical principle of access to the intestine conceivably could be revived in the future to provide a route for topical treatment with the newer steroid preparations that have little or no systemic absorption or effect, or with the active moiety of sulfasalazine, 5-aminosalicylate.[13-15]

Ileostomy was first used for the treatment of ulcerative colitis by Brown of St. Louis in 1913 with the concept of putting the diseased intestine to rest.[16] This goal was similar to that of the earlier advocates of colostomy. The initial hope that the ileostomy could subsequently be closed was met with disappointment in most cases and in time it became recognized that ileostomy, once established, would be permanent. Therefore, during the 1940's and 1950's, as surgeons and physicians realized that full health would not be restored to most patients until the entire diseased colon including the rectum was removed, ileostomy was used increasingly as the initial step of a staged colectomy. The principle of ileostomy for diversion and bowel rest was resurrected somewhat in the 1960's by Oberhelman et al. and Truelove et al. for Crohn's disease of the colon, with the hope of allowing subsequent closure of the stoma in some patients or as an initial therapeutic maneuver for seriously ill patients.[17,18]

In the 1950's, with the advent of antibiotics, improved anesthetic techniques, and increased understanding of fluid and electrolyte therapy, surgeons gradually abandoned piecemeal removal of the diseased colon in favor of a single stage abdominal colectomy and ileostomy. This approach was popularized and shown to be safe and superior by Miller, Ripstein, Goligher, Crile, Ravitch, and others.[19-23] Some of these pioneers were able to perform panproctocolectomy safely at a single stage in a few patients.[20,21] Subsequently this procedure became the "gold standard" in the surgical treatment of ulcerative colitis, and so it remains today. Unfortunately, however, one-stage panproctocolectomy occasionally has been applied indiscriminately, and a definite place remains for subtotal (abdominal) colectomy and ileostomy in the very ill patient. Concomitant with the development of extirpative surgical treatment for ulcerative colitis, improvements in methods of constructing the ileostomy and in stomal care allowed the full realization of the goal of total restoration of health and longevity in ulcerative colitis.[24-28]

Now that it has been demonstrated by Daly and others that total extirpation of the colon essentially "cures" ulcerative colitis, recent emphasis has been placed on trying to improve on the quality of life provided by a conventional ileostomy.[29,30] These efforts include the continent ileostomy pioneered by Kock,[31] and various ileoanal pull through procedures for maintaining anal sphincteric continence that are currently enjoying a great deal of attention and popularity.[32-34] Sphincter saving procedures are not new, however. Through the years this worthy goal has been championed by Corbett and especially by Aylett, both of whom had a degree of success in treating ulcerative colitis with ileorectal anastomosis despite the fact that the rectal mucosa is and remains diseased.[35,36]

Based on the unproved hypothesis that ulcerative colitis is of psychosomatic origin, vagotomy,[37] pelvic autonomic nerve interruption,[38] and even psychosurgical procedures have all been used with perhaps predictable lack of success.[39-40]

The first operations for regional enteritis were resections.[41] Because of the problem of recurrence after operation and because of lesser operative mortality and morbidity, the bypass principle as developed and advocated by Garlock et al. became the preferred procedure in many centers.[42] Resection has again regained ascendancy, not only because modern metabolic and anesthetic management has obviated the advantage in mortality and morbidity gained by the lesser procedures, but also because of late complications involving the bypassed segment. Increasingly, however, the goal of achieving total ablation of all gross disease (and, therefore, "cure") by sufficiently wide resection has been abandoned in favor of the concept of removing just enough intestine to deal with the problem at hand. Repair of obstructing lesions by strictureplasty is a more recent extension of an emerging concept of palliative surgical therapy that is gaining favor.[43,44]*

Beginning in the late 1950's, the entity of Crohn's disease of the colon began to be clearly separated from that of ulcerative colitis and eventually was accepted as a distinct disease by most physicians.[45-47] The recognition of Crohn's disease of the colon has ended much taxonomic confusion in many patients who did not fit into the mold of either ulcerative colitis or classic regional enteritis. Problems have arisen, however, about the indications for and timing of operation in the two types of colitis, and the nature and management of postcolectomy ileitis in ulcerative colitis and Crohn's disease of the colon (see also Chapter 26).

The artificial gut concept with home intravenous alimentation has gained a modest amount of success and clinical applicability for the patient with Crohn's disease with severely limited residual small intestine.[48,49] Although work is actively in progress in this area,[50] transplantation of intestine for replacement of the irretrievably damaged small intestine has not yet proved to be clinically feasible, however.

Choice of Operation

The choice of the operative procedure best suited for a particular patient depends upon the type of disease, the presence of any complications, the metabolic state of the patient, and lifestyle considerations. In addition, the operative findings and the patient's intraoperative condition may modify the choice during the procedure. Table 27-1 outlines some of the points to be discussed in the following sections.

---

*(Editors' note: see also Fazio, V. W., and Galandivk, S.: Dis. Colon Rectum, *28*:512, 1985., and Pace, B. W., Bank, S., and Wise, L., Arch. Surg., *119*:861, 1984.

TABLE 27-1. *Choice of Operation in Inflammatory Bowel Disease.*

Type of Disease	Special Circumstance	Type of Operation
Gastroduodenal Crohn's Disease	None	Posterior gastrojejunostomy (? with vagotomy)
	Acute hemorrhage	Posterior gastrojejunostomy with vagotomy and suture of bleeding point
	Recurrent pancreatitis	Posterior gastrojejunostomy (? with vagotomy)
Jejunoileitis	None	Resection(s) and end-to-end anastomosis
	Stricture(s)	One or more resections (? or strictureplasties)
Acute ileitis	None	Appendectomy only (if cecum normal)
Classical regional enteritis	None	Resection and ileoascending colostomy
	Free perforation or generalized peritonitis	
	Minimal contamination	Resection and ileoascending colostomy
	Marked contamination	Resection with temporary ileo-ostomy and mucous fistula
	Large abscess or difficult resection	Exclusion ileotransverse colostomy or ileoascending colostomy
	Obstructive uropathy	Resection and ileoascending colostomy (? ureterolysis)
Ulcerative colitis	None	Proctocolectomy and ileostomy (? Ileoanal pull-through procedure or Aylett operation)
	Carcinoma or high carcinoma risk	Proctocolectomy and ileostomy (? Ileoanal pull-through procedure)
	Extreme nutritional depletion or toxicity; toxic megacolon; perforation	Subtotal colectomy and ileo-ostomy with subsequent second-stage proctectomy or ? ileoanal pull-through procedure or Aylett operation
	Extreme aversion to ileo-ostomy	Ileoanal pull-through procedure, Aylett operation, Kock's pouch
Crohn's disease of colon	Segmental disease and/or spared rectum	Resection and anastomosis (ileocolostomy, colocolostomy or ileoproctostomy)
	Universal colitis or destroyed sphincter apparatus	Proctocolectomy and ileostomy (staged or unstaged)

Classical Regional Enteritis and Ileocolitis of Limited Extent

Most surgeons currently favor resection of the affected segment over exclusion bypass. This is because the two procedures can now be carried out with about equal safety and late problems can occur with the excluded segment after bypass including carcinoma, reactivation of disease, and free perforation. The hope once held that the excluded segment would heal while defunctioned and then become available for subsequent use has been realized only on rare occasions.[51] At one time it was claimed that exclusion bypass had a lower rate of recurrence than resection,[42,52] but now the opposite view is generally held.[53,54] The fact is that it is impossible to prove the point one way or the other because all the available studies are retrospective. Our own data[55] and those of other workers[56] indicate similar rates of recurrence, and suggest on that basis that exclusion bypass remains an acceptable operation if and when specifically indicated. The same data, however, suggest that resection will have a better result in the long run because of problems indigenous to the bypassed segment.[55]

Specific indications for bypass might include, firstly, the presence of a large abscess, in which case the bypass can be performed through a left-sided incision without entering the abscess, which can then be drained extraperitoneally; and, secondly, the rare instance in which the inflammatory process is so severe that the mass and the right colon cannot be mobilized and removed without endangering adjacent structures such as the ureter. On the other hand, in the presence of obstructive uropathy the risks inherent in resection must be accepted, even though the mass is rather solidly adherent to the retroperitoneum, because the bypass procedure may not relieve the ureteral obstruction.[57]

When gross peritoneal contamination has occurred, the use of exteriorization with temporary end-ileostomy and mucous fistula rather than primary anastomosis should be strongly considered in order to avoid anastomotic leakage. Restoration of intestinal continuity can be more safely accomplished at a subsequent second stage operation.

Nonexclusion bypass, such as side-to-side ileotransverse colostomy, has been condemned as a procedure that leads to a rate of recurrence in the range of 90%.[54,58] No universal agreement has been reached on this point, however, and bypass in continuity and exclusion bypass apparently have been used interchangeably by some clinicians.[53,59,60] Nonexclusion bypass was used with great success for obstructing ileal Crohn's disease in the extraordinary circumstance of President Eisenhower's illness, and the surgeons involved, apparently reacting to the clamor that arose at the time of the operation, published a case report some years later vindicating their choice of operation.[61] The principle of nonexclusion bypass is used with success in gastroduodenal Crohn's disease, but admittedly this is usually to obviate obstructive symptoms rather than acute inflammatory complications. Because the preponderance of opinion favors exclusion bypass and almost nothing can be gained by performing bypass in continuity, the former is preferred in the rare instance in which bypass is indicated.

Jejunoileitis

The operation of choice is usually a limited resection (with close resection margins and end-to-end anastomosis) of one or more segments judged to be the cause of intractable symptoms or complications. If the problem is chronic obstruction, especially if strictures are multiple and the amount of remaining intestine is limited, one or more strictureplasties may be necessary.[43,44] Most strictures can be dealt with just as effectively and perhaps more safely with a short resection and end-to-end anastomosis, however.

Acute Enteritis

The intraoperative considerations when acute enteritis is encountered were discussed in Chapter 26.

Chronic Ulcerative Colitis

Considered only from the standpoint of lasting restoration to health, the procedure of choice for ulcerative colitis is a proctocolectomy and ileostomy. This can be carried out either as a one-stage procedure or as a staged operation leaving in situ the rectum to be removed at a subsequent time. Factors favoring the one-stage procedure: (1) it can be carried out safely in the majority of elective operations so that the mortality and morbidity of a second operation can be avoided, and (2) the threat of complications arising in the rectum, such as inflammation, bleeding, or neoplasia, is obviated immediately. The advantages of a staged operation include the following: (1) safety in cases of fulminating colitis, toxic megacolon, and/or severe nutritional depletion; (2) less hazard to normal sexual function in the male in the face of severe local inflammation or time factors that would preclude the careful dissection along the wall of the rectum necessary to avoid damage to the presacral plexus and the nervi erigentes; and (3) when the patient (or parent) is undecided about the merits of permanent ileostomy versus a restorative procedure, is emotionally unprepared to accept the finality of a proctectomy, or does not wish to accept the risk of damage to sexual function at the particular time.

Despite the fact that the rectum only rarely requires removal in the early postoperative period, clearly it should not be permanently retained as a defunctioned organ in ulcerative colitis. Many studies have shown that the retained rectum often becomes sufficiently symptomatic and annoying to require removal because of ongoing or recurrent inflammation or systemic complications.[62-65] The risk of carcinoma, however, is the most cogent reason for removal because the threat of this complication is not mitigated by the defunctionation. It is the responsibility of the surgeon and the physician caring for the patient to assure that this tragic complication does not occur.

Currently several alternatives to panproctocolectomy and conventional Brooke ileostomy exist that are advocated as putative means of improving the quality of postoperative life. These include: (1) procedures for saving the sphincter, such as subtotal colectomy and ileoproctostomy or various types of ileonal pull-through operations; and (2) the construction of a reservoir (continent) ileostomy.

The oldest of these procedures is subtotal colectomy with ileorectal anastomosis, as enthusiastically advocated by Aylett who used this procedure as his standard operation for ulcerative colitis and by whose name the procedure is generally known.[35,66] Most surgeons using this procedure have not come close to reproducing Aylett's 83% rate of excellent results. His claim (without supporting data) that the rectum usually heals after this procedure has not been confirmed. Further drawbacks of the Aylett operation include a high rate of complications, intolerable diarrhea, and/or continued activity of disease in a significant number, and a cumulative risk of developing carcinoma that is in the range of 6% at 20 years after onset of disease and 15% at 30 years.[67,68] Nevertheless, the results of this procedure obtained by a number of independent observers suggest that as many as 25 to 50% of patients chosen for this operation may have sufficiently good long-term results to justify its use in selected patients who understand the risk to benefit ratio.[69-76] In these different studies, the proportion of patients having ileorectal anastomosis among those requiring operation for inflammatory bowel disease has varied considerably, ranging from 9 to 96% (the latter figure being Aylett's). Moreover, it is not always easy to ascertain from the published reports the relative numbers of patients having ulcerative colitis and Crohn's disease. I have had excellent results with this procedure in a small number of highly selected, carefully informed patients with ulcerative colitis who had minimally inflamed rectums and short duration disease so that complicating cancer has been only a remote risk.

Kock's reservoir ileostomy (when functioning properly) is considered advantageous by its advocates because it enhances self-esteem and body image, making the patient feel or be more attractive as a sexual partner and avoids peri-ileostomy skin problems.[31,78] I have not recommended this procedure because of the published record of success and failure and the added risk of morbidity and mortality over conventional ileostomy.[79-87] The rate of failure to produce total continence for feces and gas with the initial procedure is significant and, therefore, there is a rate of revision that is variable but usually high. The lack of continence may result from fistulas in the valve, but it is usually caused by dislodgement of the nipple valve that also may make it difficult or impossible to catheterize and empty the pouch. The development of mucosal enteritis in and proximal to the pouch is also a common complication. More devastating or repeated complications may require excision of the reservoir and conversion to a much more proximal than normal Brooke ileostomy. The fact that stomal occlusive devices have been developed for the purpose of maintaining an external pouchless state further speaks to the point that this procedure is not always trouble-free.[88] Nevertheless, some patients request it and are happy with the immediate and/or long-term outcome; however, many of the staunchest advocates of Kock's pouch have shifted their allegiance to the newer ileoanal pull-through procedures.

Ravitch and Sabiston described "anal ileostomy" in 1947 as a sphincter-saving procedure for use in patients with ulcerative colitis or familial polyposis, but they subsequently abandoned it.[89] In their procedure the full thickness of the ileum was anastomosed to the dentate line after the diseased mucosa was removed from a short segment of rectum. I devised a modification that employed a longer muscular tube of rectum that I lined with a mucosal tube of ileum in the hope of achieving near normal rectal motility and sensation,[90] thereby improving on Ravitch and Sabiston's poor functional results. I was also disappointed with the results, however, especially with the degree of nocturnal continence. Martin et al. revived interest in this procedure with their publication in 1977 of good results in 17 children with ulcerative colitis.[91] Subsequently Parks combined the concept of rectal mucosal stripping with that of constructing a pouch of ileum to provide a fecal reservoir.[92] Fifty percent of his patients with his "S" configuration pouch were unable to defecate spontaneously.[92] This problem has been essentially eliminated by: (1) the use of a "J" configuration pouch popularized by Utsonomiya,[93] (2) an "S" pouch with a shorter efferent limb than Parks',[33] or (3) a pouch devised by Fonkulsrud featuring parallel isoperistaltic limbs.[94] The functional results in some of these patients have been quite good and, in some instances, superb; however, this procedure in comparison with panproctocolectomy and ileostomy requires considerably more operating in terms of stages, takes longer to perform, carries with it a substantially higher risk of major complications (many of which require operation to correct), and, in contrast, usually requires a long adjustment period before the patient achieves an ultimate result that may or may not be good.[32-34,94] It is difficult from the published literature to get a clear picture of just how good the functional results are in the *average* patient, not in the least because of vaguely defined, or complete lack of, terms for continence. About 33% of patients have some degree of incontinence at night, as do 10 to 15% during the day. About 20% wear a pad and many cannot distinguish gas from feces. The number of bowel movements averages 4 to 6 per 24 hours, which, if not exceeded, is an acceptable number to most patients. Five percent or more of patients have required takedown of the pouch because of complications or unacceptable functional results. Needless to say if the ileoanal reservoir is removed, the resultant ileostomy will lie significantly more proximal than it would if it were done as the primary procedure. Goligher, who expresses high hopes for this procedure in the future, had good to excellent results in exactly half of his patients.[1] How one views the anticipated outcome of this procedure is analogous to determining whether a glass is half full or half empty.

For the majority of patients with ulcerative colitis I continue to recommend unstaged or staged proctocolectomy as the best choice of operation.

Crohn's Colitis and Ileocolitis Involving Substantial Portions of the Colon

The choice of operation in Crohn's disease of the colon depends upon the anatomic extent and distribution of disease (determined by the appropriate studies) and the overall management strategy in a given patient.

If the gross disease spares portions of the colon and spares the rectum, a resection with restoration of intestinal continuity is possible. While the rate of recurrence is high after such procedures (about 75% in our experience),[55,95,96] success or failure cannot be measured by the recurrence rate alone. Freedom from an ileostomy for a number of years, particularly in a child or young person, may buy valuable time for social and psychosexual maturation. Ileoproctostomy for Crohn's disease of the colon possibly carries a lower risk of the subsequent development of carcinoma than in ulcerative colitis, but the incidence of subsequent perianal sepsis is higher.[72]

In patients requiring operation for Crohn's disease of the colon that involves the rectal segment, or if the anal sphincter apparatus has been destroyed by fistulas, perianal sepsis, or ill-advised operation, proctocolectomy with ileostomy (proximal to any ileal involvement) is the operation of choice. Whether panproctocolectomy is done in one or two stages is governed by many of the same considerations as those already described for ulcerative colitis. In addition to these, because of the frequent presence of severe perirectal complications, a two-stage operation may be indicated more often than in ulcerative colitis. Even though diversion of the fecal stream does not usually result in total healing of these fistulas,[97,98] the surrounding sepsis often clears, especially after adequate drainage, so that proctectomy can be carried out at a second stage with lower risk of infection and injury to the autonomic nervous system. The improved nutrition following subtotal colectomy may further add to the safety of the second stage operation that usually is performed 6 to 12 months later.

The Kock pouch and ileoanal pull-through procedures are contraindicated in Crohn's disease because of the problem of postoperative recurrence.*

Colostomy for disease confined to the left colon and rectum or to the rectum alone, and diverting ileostomy for extensive colitis have been discussed in Chapter 26.

Gastroduodenal Crohn's Disease

Many of the considerations in the choice of operation for gastroduodenal Crohn's disease were discussed in Chapter 26. The operation of

---

*Editors' note: However, Blum, R. J., et al. (in Surg. Gynecol. Obstet., *162*:105, 1968) suggest that the Kock's pouch may be considered for a highly selected few who have had no signs of disease activity for at least 5 years.

choice is usually a posterior gastrojejunostomy that is functionally a bypass-in-continuity but, nevertheless, is effective in relieving intractable symptoms (vide supra). A somewhat controversial issue in the choice of operation is whether or not to add a vagotomy of one or the other type in an attempt to avoid marginal ulceration, which has been reported to occur in 25 to 40% of those patients who have been followed over the long-term.[99,100] Certainly a strong theoretic case can be made for adding a vagotomy because gastroenterostomy is potentially an ulcerogenic preparation in the experimental animal.[101] Moreover, marginal ulceration does, in fact, have a substantial incidence in patients undergoing gastroenterostomy for problems other than ulcer disease.[102,103] Certainly, if the patient has proved or suspected peptic ulcer disease vagotomy would be mandatory, because postoperative marginal ulceration would be likely. The debate in the literature is whether or not the incidence of marginal ulcer justifies the additional operating and the risk of increased postoperative diarrhea, and whether or not this complication, in fact, can be prevented by doing the vagotomy.[99,100] Apparently little can be lost by adding the vagotomy, especially using the highly selective technique that has been helpful in avoiding postoperative diarrhea after the surgical treatment of peptic ulcer disease.

If operation in gastroduodenal Crohn's disease is required for hemorrhage, suture of the bleeding site with non-absorbable material is indicated in addition to vagotomy and gastroenterostomy. If the operative indication is recurrent pancreatitis, other possible causes such as gallstones, drugs, and alcoholism should be excluded before any procedure is recommended.

Psychologic Preparation of the Patient and Obtaining Informed Consent

During severe exacerbations of inflammatory bowel disease, ideally the surgeon should be involved in the patient's care at an early stage, even if operation is not necessarily imminent. This affords the patient the opportunity to interact with the surgeon as an individual and to develop confidence and trust well ahead of any operation that may become indicated. It also allows the surgeon to develop an in-depth understanding of the patient's disease, emotional makeup, and social situation. During these encounters the patient should be reassured by verbal and nonverbal means that operation will be undertaken only if all *reasonable* nonoperative measures have been exhausted. Such rapport is invaluable in the management of these patients. A secretive or noncommunicative attitude on the part of the surgeon relative to sensitive issues, such as the possibility of an ileostomy or the possibility in the long run of postoperative recurrence, is completely unjustified, even for the young patient. Such an approach can only foster hostility and resentment, present and future. The prospective surgical candidate must be given sufficient time to pose (often over and over again) the many questions that are raised by an impending operation.

The expected immediate benefits and risks of the contemplated operation, as well as the long-term prognosis, should be explained to the patient in a gentle and unhurried fashion. In cases of universal colitis, factual discussions about the nature of an ileostomy and life after an ileostomy, as outlined in Chapters 28 and 29, should take place. The alternatives to ileostomy must be carefully described and their advantages and disadvantages fully outlined. Frank, open disclosure is usually more reassuring than deleterious in the continued medical management of these patients, as was discussed in Chapter 26. Exposure to a well-adjusted patient with an ileostomy or one of its alternatives is often an enormous emotional boost to a prospective operative candidate.

There are few places in medicine or surgery where truly informed consent is more rewarding both to the patient and the physician.

Management of Corticosteroids

The majority of patients coming to operation are receiving, or have in the past received, treatment with corticosteroids, but, in general, this should not pose a major or insurmountable problem in the surgical treatment of inflammatory bowel disease. Because these agents have now been shown to be effective not only in ulcerative colitis but also in Crohn's disease,[104-107] their well-known side effects must be accepted with equanimity by the operating surgeon, provided they have been used appropriately. Clearly, adverse effects of steroids on wound healing have been documented both in man and in experimental animals.[108-114] Under corticosteroid treatment the formation of granulation tissue and the rate of gain of tensile strength of sutured wounds are reduced, but these effects are dose-related and refer to a given time in the healing process. Even so, the *eventual* strength of healing achieved in experimental animals under corticosteroids is near normal. The relative doses given in many experimental situations often far exceed even the large doses sometimes used in the clinical setting. Hunt and associates have shown that vitamin A and anabolic steroids mitigate the adverse effects on wound healing of corticosteroids given on an acute basis in experimental animals, but no data are available to support their use in the clinical situation.[115,116] From a practical standpoint, anastomotic and wound disruptions as well as sepsis have not been serious problems, and fear of these complications should not interdict the proper use of corticosteroids or contraindicate needed operation. By recognition and understanding of these adverse effects of corticosteroids, the surgeon can prevent problems by careful attention to methods of wound closure and anastomosis (vide infra) and by the appropriate use of local, luminal, and systemic antibiotics.

Because corticosteroid therapy even in small doses (e.g., 7.5 mg prednisone per day or equivalent) if given over long periods has been shown to alter drastically the response of the adrenal glands to stress,[117,118] patients under current or recent treatment with these agents must receive exogenous steroids intraoperatively and postoperatively. The blunting of the pituitary-adrenal response to stress may continue long after the cessation of corticosteroid treatment.[119] Because the rate of recovery is variable from individual to individual,[119,120] if corticosteroid treatment has been used within 1 or 2 years of operation it is safest to assume that relative adrenal insufficiency is present and that steroids must be given during and after operation. If steroid treatment is even more remote, it may nevertheless be preferable to "cover" the patient unless preoperative testing has shown that the adrenal glands can respond normally to corticotropin and that the hypothalamus and pituitary can normally sense and respond to a deprivation of hydroxycorticoid.

The maximum output of the adrenal gland to the greatest stress has been measured to be the equivalent of about 240 mg of hydrocortisone per 24 hours.[117] It is reasonable, therefore, to administer about 300 mg hydrocortisone phosphate or its equivalent on the day of operation (larger amounts are unnecessary) and to taper the dose subsequently, as the requirements are expected to diminish. One such scheme is outlined in Table 27-2.

Generally, patients who have received short-term corticosteroid therapy, or those who have received this therapy remotely, can be totally weaned from these agents while in the hospital or shortly thereafter. On the other hand, the longer the duration of previous therapy, the longer it may take the pituitary-adrenal axis to recover. Great merit exists in the use of alternate-day single-dose corticosteroid coverage to prevent adrenal crisis and steroid withdrawal symptoms during at least a portion of the roughly 6 to 9 months or longer it may take for total recovery in patients who have been on really long-term suppressive therapy.[119] Even after successful weaning, all patients who have received recent or even remote suppressive corticosteroid treatment must be cautioned that major illness or trauma may require renewed

TABLE 27-2. *Scheme for Management of Corticosteroid Therapy.*

Day of Operation	Postoperative Day 1	Postoperative Days 3-7	Subsequent Postoperative Days
Two hours before operation: Hydrocortisone phosphate or hemisuccinate 100 mg IM	Hydrocortisone phosphate or hemisuccinate 50 mg IM q6h*	Taper hydrocortisone gradually to 100 mg/24h in divided doses (usually in 50 mg increments q48h)	Taper hydrocortisone[†] to 75 mg/24h and then wean quickly if short term prior treatment or long interval since last suppressive treatment
During operation: Continuous IV drip of hydrocortisone phosphate or hemisuccinate at rate of 100 mg q6h			Taper more gradually if on long-term suppressive treatment just prior to operation. Consider use of q.o.d. therapy
Postoperatively: Administer hydrocortisone phosphate or hemisuccinate 75 mg IM q6h*			

*See text regarding intravenous use.
[†]As gastrointestinal function returns fully and enteral absorption seems assured, equivalent oral dose of prednisone or similar drug should be substituted.

corticosteroid coverage to prevent adrenal crisis. The steroid withdrawal syndrome,[121] consisting of malaise, low-grade fever, myalgia, anorexia, and nausea, may require reinstitution of therapy or increase in dosage. A peculiar desquamation of the skin of the tips of the fingers may provide an additional diagnostic clue to this entity. Occasionally, high fever may result from rapid decrease in corticosteroid doses, especially in those with prior treatment of long duration. It is important to understand that steroid withdrawal syndrome is distinct from adrenocortical insufficiency and that it may occur in the presence of normal cortisol levels and in the absence of postural signs and hypotension. It follows that pharmacologic rather than physiologic amounts of corticosteroids may be required to reverse the symptoms of steroid withdrawal syndrome.

Preoperative Preparation of the Patient

The nutritional status and needs of acutely and chronically ill patients with inflammatory bowel diseases are immensely important, especially in those who are actual or potential candidates for operation. Operations on the gastrointestinal tract inevitably carry with them a period of nonfunction so that a loss of 5 to 10 pounds of body mass can be anticipated even after an uncomplicated major operation. Therefore, it is useful in evaluating the patient and planning therapy to assess the nutritional status. Measurement of serum albumin and transferrin levels are valuable in this respect as are rather simple to perform anthropomorphic measurements. A surprisingly high incidence of protein and caloric malnutrition is found in hospitalized patients in general,[122] and many patients with inflammatory bowel disease are among the worst in this regard. It appears that this is not the result of excessive energy expenditure caused by the mucosal inflammatory process because the resting energy requirement in non-septic colitis patients is not greater than normal, especially if the predicted needs are estimated on the basis of the actual body composition.[123,124] *

Consideration of all these issues is especially important in those patients hospitalized for a period of intensive medical management of a subacute or acute exacerbation of colonic inflammatory bowel disease because if the trial fails, operation is the only remaining therapeutic option. Because the treatment of these patients often includes "bowel rest," further nutritional depletion will occur unless nutritional needs are met, perhaps making the patient a poorer operative risk. Caloric and protein requirements can be partially met by the administration of fat emulsions and amino acids by way of a peripheral vein.[125] In practical terms, however, not only is this "hypocaloric," even using 20% fat emulsions, but, more importantly, the amino acids tend to sclerose the patient's veins, making future access difficult. Increasingly, therefore, at our institution we tend to administer nutrition through a central line with hypertonic glucose,[126] amino acids, and fat emulsions, the latter to prevent essential fatty acid deficiency. This allows the time-frame for nonoperative management to be expanded somewhat and to be less pressured, including dealing with the operating room schedule, so that this modality can be tried to the optimal extent. Admittedly, the therapeutic benefit of the added nutrition is difficult to document.* For example, in a randomized controlled trial in patients with colitis in exacerbation, the addition of total parenteral nutrition to the regimen did not result in a greater number of remissions.[127] Controlled trials of total parenteral nutrition for preventing postoperative complications also have either failed to show an overall benefit,[128] or the benefit demonstrated in inflammatory bowel disease specifically amounted only to an increased rate of healing of perineal wounds.[129] Therefore, although we are more likely to use this method of treatment today than in the past, the only justification that is based on solid data is that it will prevent further nutritional depletion while other therapy is taking place, the value of which must be taken on faith. There may be some severely depleted patients who from the onset are operative candidates who, therefore, potentially could benefit by a period of preoperative preparation with nutritional therapy. It remains to be demonstrated, however, who these patients are. Therefore, if operation is already clearly indicated in such patients, I generally tend to proceed forthwith, possibly using postoperative nutritional support.

Some form of mechanical preparation of the colon is essential for most patients with Crohn's disease or ulcerative colitis undergoing elective operation. In recent years, I have tended to pre-

---

*Editors' note: See also, Chan, A. T. H., et al.: Gastroenterology 91:75, 1986.

*Editors' note: See also, Shanehogue, L. K. R., et al.: Br. J. Surg., 74:172, 1982.

fer an iso-osmotic electrolyte and PEG lavage solution (Golytely*) for this purpose because it is effective, reduces time in the hospital, obviates starvation as part of the preparation, and is well tolerated and accepted by the patient.[130,131] It can be used even in patients with rather high-grade stenosis, provided they are monitored carefully. Usually 4 liters of solution at room temperature are administered by mouth, or by way of a small nasogastric tube, over 3 to 4 hours on the morning prior to operation. If conventional bowel preparation is preferred, the use of an "elemental diet" rather than a clear liquid diet to reduce fecal bulk may lessen nutritional depletion during the period of preparation.[132] Purgation, if used, should be gentle, and if a rectal anastomosis is contemplated, saline or tap water enemas should be given the night before operation. Mechanical preparation of the colon rarely is necessary in patients with colonic inflammatory bowel disease who are candidates for emergency operation, because of the excessively liquid consistency of their stools.

Reduction of intestinal bacterial flora by oral antibiotics has now been conclusively shown in many studies (carried out primarily in patients with colonic carcinoma) to reduce infectious complications.[133-135] Nutritionally depleted patients on corticosteroids for inflammatory bowel disease stand to benefit even more by this type of preparation than do those with carcinoma. The author uses the regimen described by Nichols et al. that consists of 1 g each of erythromycin base and neomycin, given by mouth at 1, 2, and 11 p.m. the afternoon and evening prior to operation.[136] This treatment produces a dramatic reduction not only in the aerobic, but also in the anaerobic fecal flora.

If possible, the patient is instructed by a respiratory physiotherapist in the necessity for and the methods of postoperative pulmonary toilet. Correction of any abnormalities of body fluid and electrolyte content is mandatory as is correction of major deficits in red cell mass. The patient should be hydrated intravenously overnight before operation with one or more liters of crystalloid solution, depending upon the state of hydration. The night just prior to operation may also be the final opportunity to replete potassium stores that are not infrequently low in this group of patients because of abnormally high losses from the intestine and kidney as a result of diarrhea and corticosteroid treatment. At times, because of large requirements and limited time, a central venous line may be necessary for the administration of potassium salts.

The pre- and postoperative administration of low-dose heparin or heparin-dihydroergotamine combination may be worthwhile for prophylaxis against thromboembolism.[137,138] Initiation of low-dose heparin therapy at the time of admission should be considered, especially in patients who largely will be bedridden, because it has been shown that thrombosis may begin preoperatively.[139] Intermittent pneumatic compression boots may be substituted for low-dose heparin or used in addition to it.[140] We also usually administer preoperative prophylactic antibiotics based on principles enunciated by Burke and first demonstrated to be effective in patients by Polk and Lopez-Mayor.[141,142] In patients without septic complications, cefazolin sodium (1.0 g) is administered intravenously 2 hours before operation or at the time of the call to the operating room. Two additional doses are given at 8-hour intervals and then the antibiotic is discontinued. If actual septic complications exist, such as fistulas and abscesses, or if significant contamination occurs intraoperatively, broader spectrum, more potent intravenous regimens can be employed by adding metronidazole (500 mg) or substituting gentamicin (1.5 mg/kg) and clindamycin (600 mg), or, alternatively, a regimen consisting of ampicillin (1.0 g) and chloramphenicol (500 mg) can be given at the appropriate intervals. If the organisms and their antibiotic sensitivities are known, the regimen is tailored accordingly. If the septic focus is totally removed by the operation, these antibiotics are used only prophylactically, that is they are perioperatively a so-called "antibiotic umbrella." On the other hand, if a septic focus to treat remains, the antibiotics should be continued for a longer period of time, as dictated by clinical response and past experience with such treatment. Intraoperative irrigation of the operative site and wound with a neomycin/bacitracin solution may be of additional benefit.[143] A #14 nasogastric tube should be placed in most patients preoperatively or after anesthetic induction. A larger tube is unnecessary and is more uncomfortable for the patient. Intramuscular corticosteroid (as already discussed) is administered 2 hours prior to operation.

Intraoperative Physiologic and Metabolic Management

The anesthesiologist responsible for intraoperative management must be knowledgeable about the physiologic derangements likely to be en-

*Braintree Laboratories, Inc., Braintree, MA, 02184

countered. Because each patient is unique, it would be presumptuous and misleading to set down rigid guidelines for the intraoperative management of the patients. Moreover, the guidelines for preoperative preparation discussed previously should hardly be regarded as exhaustive or "routine." The fluid and electrolyte losses of patients undergoing, for example, a proctocolectomy and ileostomy are enormous, and must be replaced pari passu with ongoing losses. It is preferable to replace blood loss with packed red blood cells, in keeping with good blood banking principles, and perhaps with a lesser risk of transfusion hepatitis.[144] If operation is carried out unhurriedly and carefully, transfusion of red blood cells is seldom needed during a typical resection for Crohn's disease or an abdominal colectomy. At times, even a proctocolectomy can be completed without sufficient losses to require transfusion.

The anesthesiologist is guided by continuous EKG monitoring, by frequent blood gas measurements, and by hourly measurement of the intraoperative urine output from an indwelling urethral catheter, especially if the latter is necessary for the technical conduct of the operation (e.g., a proctectomy). In selected cases, continuous intra-arterial pressure measurement or the determination of "filling pressures" through a catheter placed in the superior vena cava or the pulmonary artery may be deemed necessary for safe management. Osmotic diuresis caused by hyperglycemia is not an uncommon cause of high urinary outputs in these steroid-treated, stressed patients, and, unless suspected, may lead to the false presumption that adequate replacement of volume has taken place. If an inlying catheter is not needed, either technically or physiologically, postoperative urinary bladder distension can be prevented by extra peritoneal sterile aspiration of the bladder with a long spinal needle attached to a closed sterile system (Fig 27-1). In operations involving intestinal anastomosis, our anesthesiologists are re-

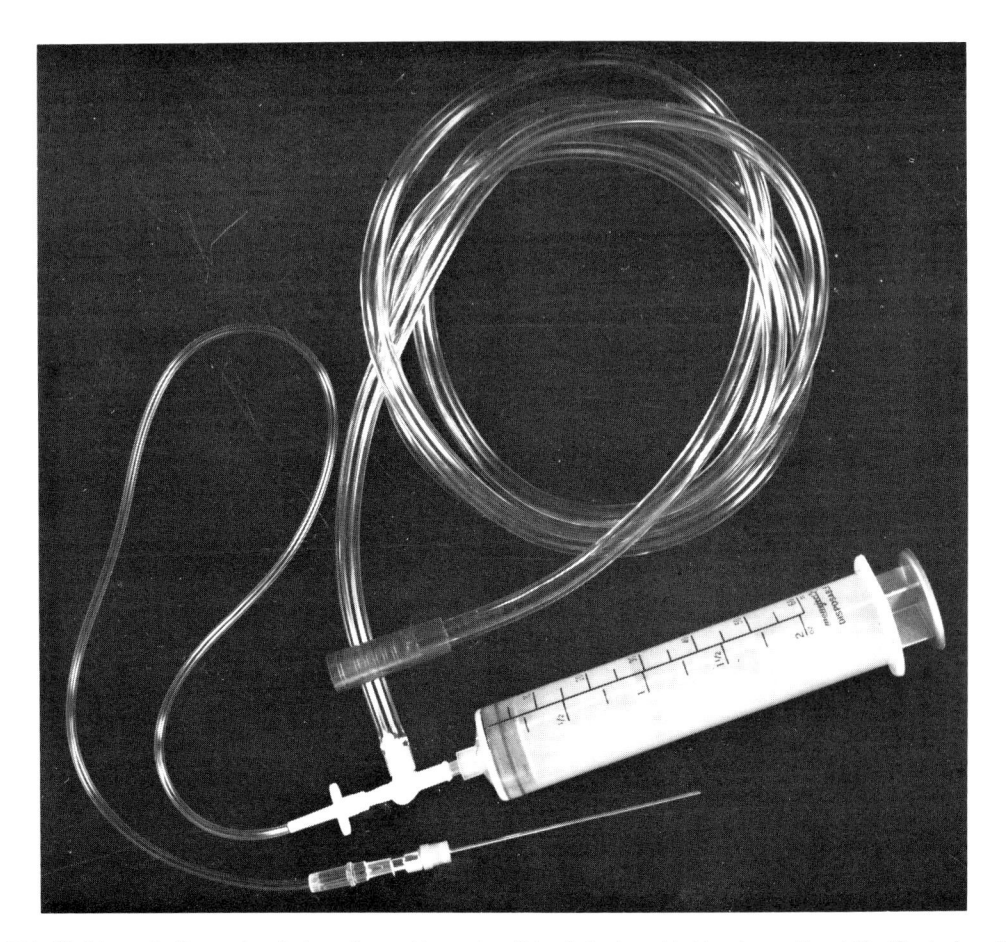

FIG. 27-1. Bladder aspiration system that may be used to empty a distended urinary bladder at operation. A No. 19 spinal needle is introduced into the bladder extraperitoneally, guided by a palpating hand. The bladder is aspirated by a 60-ml syringe connected to a system of tubing via a 3-way stopcock that allows the urine to be measured and discarded off the field.

quested not to reverse relaxants with the use of neostigmine because of evidence suggesting that parasympathomimetic agents produce significant stress on the anastomosis.[145] Thus, because these patients are allowed to recover spontaneous ventilation before extubation, mechanical ventilation is sometimes required for brief periods in the recovery room.

Technique of Intestinal Anastomosis

A consensus about the optimal technique for intestinal anastomosis undoubtedly will never exist. An essential feature, however, is that blood supply must be preserved not only within the mesentery but also by avoiding excessive removal of fat from the intestine during preparation for anastomosis. When a discrepancy exists between the circumference of the cut ends of ileum and colon, I see little place for closure of the end of the colon and anastomosis of the end of the ileum to the side of the colon, even though the blind end of the colon is of the "self-emptying" variety. It is also not necessary to deal with the problem of size discrepancy by making an antimesenteric slit that may only increase contamination and also may interfere with blood supply. I prefer to divide the intestine almost straight across, with the mesenteric side only slightly longer than the antimesenteric side. Any discrepancy in the sizes of the lumens (which can be quite large) can be overcome by serially halving the distance between previously placed sutures after starting at each end of the intestine (the so-called "divide and conquer" technique), as illustrated in Figure 27-2. The clamp on the larger segment of intestine should be removed first to avoid tearing as the sutures are tied.

Closure of Abdominal Incisions in Inflammatory Bowel Disease

As in the case of intestinal anastomosis, rigid rules cannot be set down for subjects as controversial as the optimal suture for or method of wound closure. It should be remembered, however, that patients with inflammatory bowel disease are prime subjects for wound disruption because of nutritional depletion, corticosteroid therapy, and infectious complications. Much can be said for the use of mass closure techniques,[146,147] such as all layer stay sutures (such as #5 Teflon-coated Dacron) in conjunction with a layered closure or, probably better yet, for a Smead-Jones type of closure (using 0 polypropylene or 0 siliconized braided Dacron), both of which techniques have been demonstrated to be superior in a randomized controlled clinical trial to at least one type of layered abdominal closure.[146] In the presence of gross contamination, the skin and subcutaneous tissues should be left open for delayed primary closure, or for healing by second intention. The former can be accomplished in the patient's room 72 to 96 hours later with the use of sterile adhesive strips or stainless steel staples (after local infiltration anesthesia), if the wound appears clean at that time. In the presence of moderate wound contamination, irrigation and scrubbing of the wound with local antibiotics,[143,148] together with systemic antibiotic treatment, may prevent infection as effectively as delayed primary closure.[148] Primary closure is particularly advantageous (if successful) in patients with open stomas on the abdomen that threaten the success of the delayed primary closure technique.[148]

Anastomotic Procedures for Crohn's Disease

Problem of Recurrence

The incidence of recurrence of regional enteritis or ileocolitis is at least 50% within 10 years and 75% within 15 years.[55] Recurrent disease in both ileitis and ileocolitis characteristically develops in the neoterminal ileum and ends abruptly at the anastomosis with the colon. Initial colonic disease makes it more likely that local or distant colonic recurrence will occur as well, but even in ileocolitis, 86% of the recurrences in our experience are in the neoterminal ileum.[55] The cause of this high recurrence rate and the reasons for its typical location are still enigmatic. Especially in the past, it has been suggested that recurrence may be caused by unrecognized retention of skip disease not detected by examination of resection margins. Although some recurrences conceivably might develop on this basis, the hypothesis does not readily explain the characteristic site of recurrent disease in the terminal ileum rather than in a more random distribution. A second possible mechanism that may be at work is that recurrence is caused by some factor related to the juxtaposition of the ileum to the colon, or to an inherent propensity (perhaps subliminal disease) of the ileum juxtaposed to the colon to develop this type of inflammation.

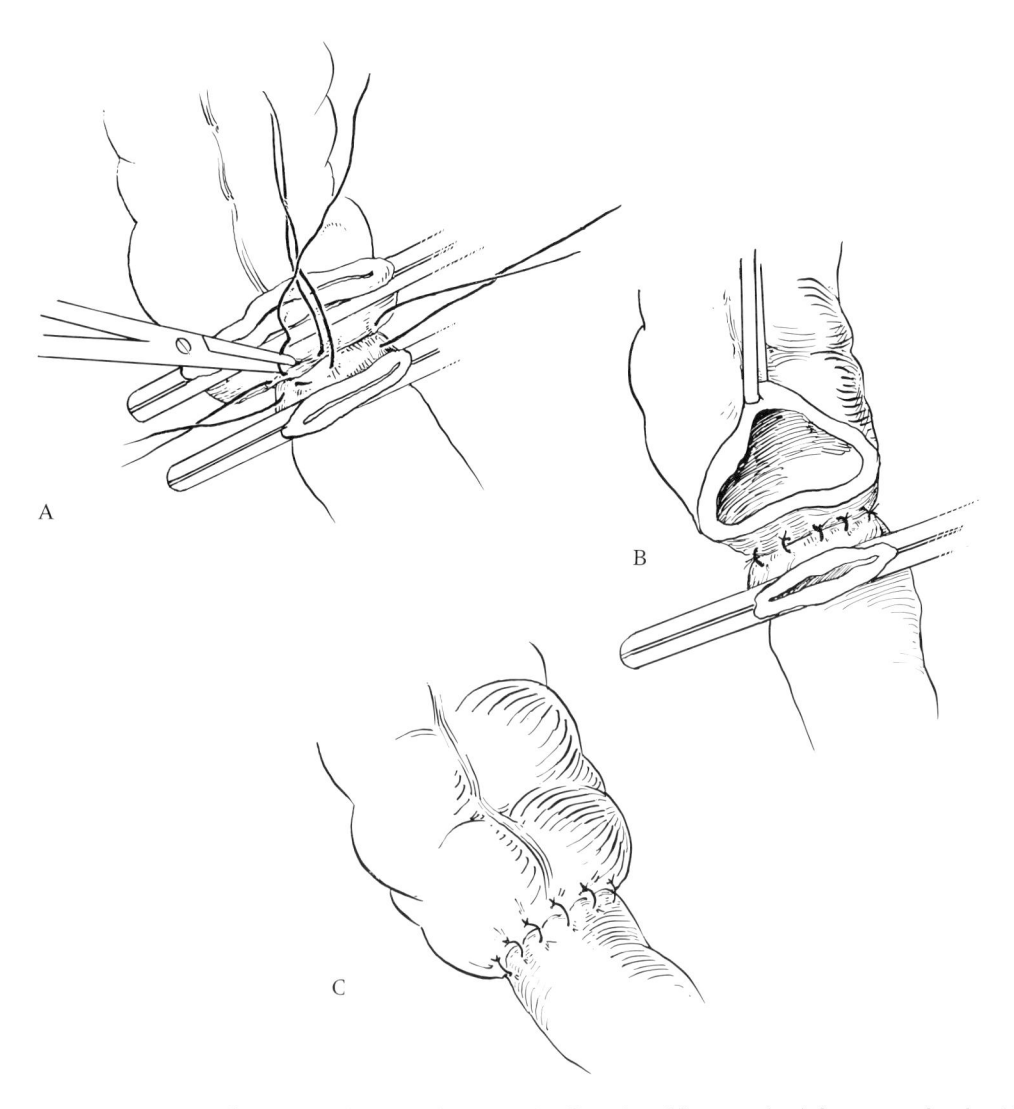

FIG. 27-2 "Divide-and-conquer" technique of end-to-end anastomosis of intestine of disparate size. A. Sutures are placed at either end and then in the middle. Subsequent sutures are placed midway between the previous sutures so that the discrepancy is taken up proportionately throughout. B. As the posterior outer row of sutures is tied, the clamp on the larger end is removed to prevent tearing. C. Completed anastomosis.

Thirdly, although not excluding the aforementioned mechanisms, a growing body of evidence exists that Crohn's lesions are present in grossly and light microscopically normal areas of intestine both at the site of anastomosis and throughout the intestine. This evidence includes the demonstration of abnormalities in ostensibly normal intestine, including aphthous ulcers by careful roentgenogram techniques,[149] cellular abnormalities,[150] and functional changes,[151,152] although some of these abnormalities can occur in the small intestine in ulcerative colitis as well.[150,153] Dvorak and associates have demonstrated widespread electron microscopic abnormalities in "normal" intestine in Crohn's disease both by scanning and transmission techniques.[154-156]

A study by Rutgeerts et al. seems to indicate that recurrent disease becomes manifest much sooner than had been previously supposed on the basis of the usual types of clinical observation.[157] These workers routinely surveyed the site of anastomosis by colonoscopy within 1 year of operation in patients who had had resection for ileitis and ileocolitis. The 72% incidence of recurrence they found was not significantly different from the rates observed 1 to 3 years and 3 to 10 years postoperatively. The longer the interval postoperatively the more the lesions became severe, extensive, and stenotic. This study lends some support to the view long held by many gastroenterologists that operation may "cause" or hasten recurrence and thereby "spread" Crohn's disease. In fact, I have observed clinical evidence of recurrence in the immediate postoperative period in 3 instances, but fortunately this appears to be rare. In fact, some patients apparently never develop recurrent disease, and in many of those who do, the clinical manifestations do not appear until years after operation. The data already cited would not support a policy of early "radical" operation to forestall recurrent disease and complications however,[158] or encourage the application of less than stringent indications for operation for this disease.

Surgical Strategy and Principles

CHOICE OF INCISION

The typical operative incision for classical Crohn's disease of the small intestine is a vertical right paramedian or midline incision, although some surgeons prefer transverse incisions. Special circumstances should modify the position of the wound. A suspected right lower quadrant abscess or the presence of a large inflammatory mass should suggest a left-sided incision: (1) to avoid entry into a pus filled cavity and contaminating the entire abdomen, and (2) to permit free entry into the abdomen and keep wound contamination to a minimum. The presence of colonic involvement is another factor favoring a left-sided incision because it will allow for optimal placement of an ileostomy should this ultimately become necessary. Because of this latter consideration, it has even been suggested that left-sided incisions be used for all cases of Crohn's disease,[1] but my data have indicated that if only ileitis is present, the patient is unlikely to require an ileostomy at any time during the course of his disease.[55]

LYMPH NODES

Some authors have advised removing all "involved" lymph nodes in Crohn's disease and suggest that by doing so postoperative recurrence can be minimized. The experienced and observant surgeon, however, knows that to remove all enlarged lymph nodes in most cases would require sacrifice of the blood supply to practically the entire small intestine. Therefore, removal of lymph nodes is neither technically feasible in most cases, nor is the procedure desirable because the hypothesis upon which it is based is completely unproved.

RESECTION MARGINS

The optimal length of normal intestine that should be resected proximal and distal to diseased areas remains controversial. Because recurrence usually develops in the ileum rather than in the colon,[55,159] the common practice of extending the distal margin of resection to the transverse colon, as is typical in surgical procedure for cancer, is not warranted in Crohn's disease unless preoperative or intraoperative evidence of colonic involvement is present that requires a resection of this extent. Instead, to conserve absorbing surface, the distal anastomosis should be made in the ascending colon in the case of ileitis, and just distal to colonic involvement in ileocolitis.

Although most surgeons experienced in the surgical treatment of inflammatory bowel disease would agree with the aforementioned recommendation about the distal margin of resection, a heated debate is still going on about the optimal proximal resection margin. At one time, Garlock, Crohn, and colleagues advocated the resection of 2 feet of normal intestine proximal to the diseased colon area to forestall or minimize recurrent disease.[42] Van Patter et al. were the first to show that no improvement occurred in recurrence rates by increasing the amounts of grossly normal intestine resected proximal to the disease, however.[160] Several investigators have concluded that even if the resection margin is microscopically diseased, this does not adversely affect the actuarially determined rate of recurrence.[162-164] Moreover, I showed that increasing the length of microscopically normal intestine resected proximal to the disease did not favorably affect the cumulative rate of development of recurrent disease (see Fig. 27-3).[55] Nevertheless, some clinicians still advocate "radical" operation and wide resection margins based on data showing lower rates of recurrence for patients operated upon in this manner.[165-168] It is not possible at this time to reconcile these divergent conclusions. In some cases, the differing results might have to do with the concept of "radical" and "non-radical" operation used by Scandinavian surgeons because it is not always clear from their articles whether "non-radically" operated patients were so

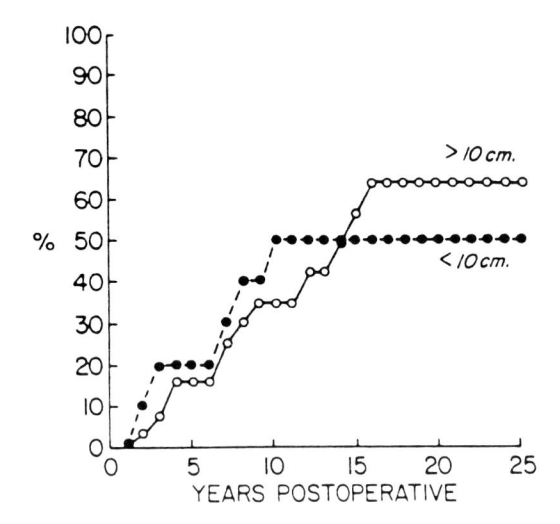

FIG. 27-3 Calculated cumulative recurrence rates for resections in patients with ileitis having proximal resection margins greater or less than 10 cm. The curves are not significantly different. (Reproduced from Trnka et al[55] by permission)

dubbed because they had a purposely less extensive operation or because their disease was so widespread that it was necessary to leave some behind.[165-167] In other studies, which concluded that wide margins of resection were preferable, the authors did not use actuarial methods for the analysis of the relative rates of recurrence so that the data may be criticized as not being "state of the art."[165,166] Neither of these objections apply to the study by Lindhagen et al., however.[168] In this, the authors' policy was to achieve a 10 cm microscopically disease-free margin and "to operate fairly early after diagnosis in an attempt to forestall serious complications." In those patients in whom macroscopically disease-free margins were achieved, about 33% were microscopically normal, 33% proved to have minor inflammation, and 33% had major inflammatory lesions such as "ulcers, crypt abscesses, and/or giant granuloma." Patients with "major inflammatory lesions" in the resection margin had approximately twice the rate of recurrence at 10 years (determined actuarially) than the other two groups (70% vs 35 to 40%). It still may be possible to reconcile this study with many of the others, however, by recognizing that the authors operated earlier in the course of the disease (possible starting time bias), and that their patients with minor inflammatory changes in the margin did about as well as those with normal margins.

At operation the assessment of the proximal extent of disease is often exceedingly difficult, because serosal changes may either overestimate or underestimate the extent of mucosal disease. Although gross "fat wrapping" of the wall of the bowel, in general, is helpful to determine the extent of disease, slight encroachment of fat on the mesenteric border of the small intestine is sometimes found for a considerable distance proximal to light microscopically involved intestine. This slight fatty overgrowth can be a nonspecific finding, and is encountered in other diseases. Therefore, fat wrapping should be used only as a rough guide to the extent of mucosal disease and may be ignored if the intestine in question is soft and pliable and contains no grossly visible disease when the specimen is opened by the pathologist. Edematous intestine with a slightly reddened surface is usually diseased. If an error must be made in the preliminary estimate of mucosal disease, it is better to underestimate because more intestine can be excised if the opened specimen reveals gross extension to the margin of resection. Because of the aforementioned considerations I do not employ rapid microscopic section in an attempt to achieve inflammation-free margins. In fact, one study indicated a high error rate when such attempts were made, and, moreover, it provided additional data indicating that patients having what proved to be involved margins on permanent section did no worse than those with clean margins.[164] The choice of the resection margin based on the pattern of lymphatics seen after the injection of vital dye is based on the unproven hypotheses that Crohn's disease results from lymphatic obstruction and that a lower rate of recurrence can actually be achieved by finding a segment of intestine with normal lymphatics.[169]

FISTULAS

This complication is a hallmark of Crohn's disease. Fistulas may involve any adjacent organ or structure, including loops of small and large intestine, the abdominal wall, and the urogenital system. The process of fistulization does not spread the enteritic process into the organ into which the fistula penetrates, although obviously fistulas between two adjacent diseased segments do occur frequently. The technical management of these various types of fistulas is crucial for optimal results and it is discussed in sections that follow under modifications imposed by complications.

OBSTRUCTIVE UROPATHY

Usually it is wise to perform a preoperative abdominal ultrasound in order to be aware of any obstructive uropathy that, if found, can be further documented by intravenous pyelography.[57,170] Routine preoperative intravenous pyelography is probably not cost-effective because screening for obstruction by ultrasound is cheaper and less invasive and developmental anomalies such as double ureter are infrequent. If this particular anomaly is present, the two ureters will be found in a single sheath and therefore will not be in more than the usual jeopardy. When obstructive uropathy is present, resection rather than bypass is indicated because the latter does not always bring relief of this complication.[57,170] On the other hand, the question of whether or not to perform a ureterolysis, as advocated by Block et al., may be an academic one in most cases because unroofing and exposure of the ureter is required for safe removal of the type of inflammatory mass giving rise to this complication.[57]

Individual Operations

ILEOCOLIC RESECTION FOR ILEAL OR ILEOCOLONIC CROHN'S DISEASE

On occasion, I have seen patients with classic regional enteritis in whom ileal resection alone had been previously performed by other clinicians, and the less-than-optimal results have strengthened my conviction that the ileocecal area should always be resected. Although in some cases the terminal inch or two of ileum may appear normal or less involved than the ileum immediately proximal, I have not observed an anatomic distribution of disease in the terminal ileum that would make it wise or even safe to attempt preservation of this segment. Some patients have diffuse jejunoileitis with a terminal ileum that is normal or less severely involved than elsewhere (vide supra), and this, of course, represents an exception to the recommendation for routine resection of the ileocecal area.

With important exceptions the technique is essentially that used for resection for adenocarcinoma of the right colon. At operation the abdomen should be carefully explored, particularly noting any areas of "skip disease" in the colon, proximal small bowel, and stomach and duodenum. If ileocolectomy is elected, the right colon is mobilized from the retroperitoneum in standard fashion after carefully identifying and preserving the right ureter. Even in the presence of large inflammatory masses or obstructive uropathy it is usually possible, by a combination of sharp and blunt dissection, to mobilize the colon from the retroperitoneum in this manner, and to free any ileal loops adherent to the pelvic peritoneum. Reasonable judgement must be employed, however, and, if any real anxiety exists about entering a large abscess cavity, destroying normal intestine, or injuring vital structures such as the ureter, the exclusion bypass principle should be considered.

Following mobilization, the proposed sites of proximal and distal transection are selected and marked with silk sutures (Fig. 27-4A). In the ileum, an area just proximal to the gross involvement (perhaps 3 or 4 cm) will suffice, based on the considerations discussed earlier, and, if there is no colonic involvement, a point in the proximal ascending colon just above the cecum with a suitable blood supply is marked. Because the operation is not being carried out for cancer, a wide resection of mesentery is neither necessary nor desirable. It is usually possible to preserve blood supply to the ascending colon by dissection around or even through the enlarged lymph nodes. The blood supply to the ileum and cecum is interrupted relatively close to the intestine, as already mentioned (Fig. 27-4A), using nonabsorbable ligatures or sutures. If pus is encountered, absorbable sutures and ligatures should be used to avoid suture sinuses that: (1) can be a source of morbidity, and (2) have mimicked recurrent disease with fistula formation.[171] If the colon is involved, the site of distal transection should be distal to the extent of gross disease in an area where a good blood supply can be preserved. The specimen is moved off the field and examined by the pathologist, who pays particular attention to the areas of involvement, the proximal resection edge, the distal resection edge, and possible areas of involvement of the colon. If the resection margins are grossly free of disease, an anastomosis between the ileum and the colon is fashioned and the mesenteric defect is closed (Fig. 27-4B). A small amount of bacitracin-neomycin solution is placed in the operative area and the excess is aspirated.[143]

Although the procedure just described may not be as neat as a standard right hemicolectomy, preservation of as much colon as possible may be helpful in avoiding postoperative diarrhea.

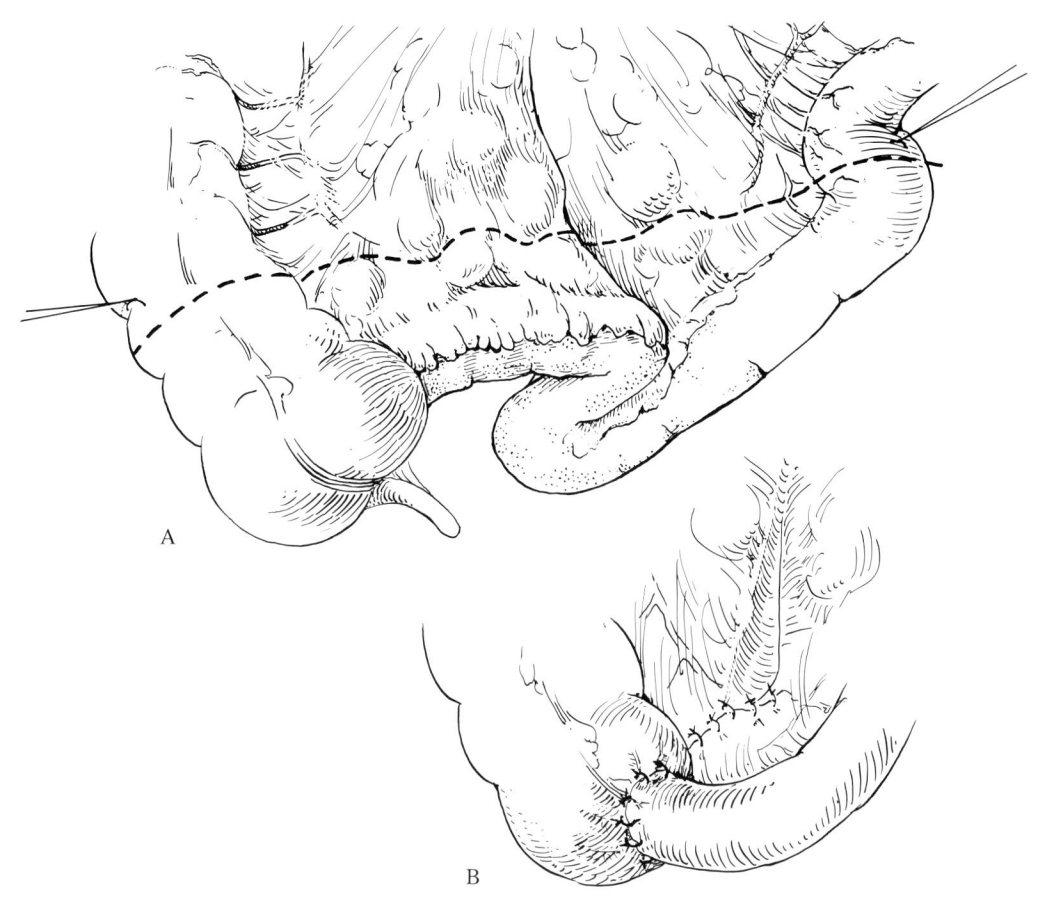

Fig. 27-4. Resection operation for regional enteritis. A. A point 8 to 10 in. proximal to gross disease is chosen for the proximal resection edge; the distal margin can be in the ascending colon if the colon is not involved. The mesenteric vessels are ligated in such a manner that the blood supply to the ascending colon is preserved. As illustrated, it is not necessary, or indeed possible, to remove all enlarged lymph nodes. B. An end-to-end ileoascending colostomy is performed and the mesenteric defect is closed.

MODIFICATIONS OF ILEOCOLECTOMY TECHNIQUE IMPOSED BY COMPLICATIONS

The presence of complications may alter the technique of the operation to a greater or lesser extent.

OBSTRUCTION. Obstruction usually requires minimal change in operative technique. In fact, the dilated ileum more nearly approximates the diameter of the colon, making the anastomosis easier than in the elective operation. Primary anastomosis in the face of obstruction is also *safe* because the dilated small intestine holds sutures well and does not represent a contraindication to primary anastomosis, as would a dilated and obstructed colon. When high-grade obstruction is present, the application of a noncrushing clamp a few centimeters proximal to the anastomotic site after milking intestinal contents proximally, will help to minimize bacterial contamination and the risk of infection. An alternative is the use of the closed anastomosis.

FREE PERFORATION. Resection of the involved intestine is preferred over attempted closure of the perforation in an area of disease involvement. If significant peritonitis is present, exteriorization of the ileum as an ileostomy and of the distal cut end of the colon as a mucous fistula should be strongly considered as a better alternative to primary anastomosis with its increased risk of failure in this circumstance.

FISTULAS. The ileum in regional enteritis or ileocolitis is frequently found to be adherent to the sigmoid colon. If these adherent loops are separated, it is common to encounter a small, often pinpoint fistulous opening into the colon. If the colonic wall is soft and uninvolved (as it frequently is), the defect may simply be closed with sutures and covered with adjacent fat; however, the affected segment of sigmoid should be excised if: (1) intrinsic sigmoid involvement is present, (2) a large defect in the wall of the sigmoid results from the separation of the loops, or (3) the wall is inflamed and rigid.

Fistulization into the right colon or cecum and/or an immediately adjacent ileal loop is best treated by excision of the entire inflammatory mass without any attempt to separate the adherent loops as long as this does not entail sacrifice of long segments of intestine. On the other hand, if there is an adherent loop of uninvolved (or involved) intestine that is more than a few inches proximal, the proximal intestine should be preserved even though contamination of the operative field may occur during transection of fistulas and small abscesses. Nevertheless, sorely needed intestine may be preserved by separating an adherent loop and then doing a local debridement and lateral repair of the adherent area, the excised fistula, or any defect created, or by performing an additional resection with end-to-end anastomosis.

In the presence of ileovesical fistula, the same basic principles used for intestinal fistulas can be applied; fortunately, the fistula is usually at the dome of the bladder so that its excision does not unduly jeopardize the trigonal structures. If the site of bladder adherence is small and soft, the wall adjacent to the opening simply can be debrided and closed by suture inversion. When significant induration of the bladder wall is present, it is prudent to mobilize the bladder wall and to resect a portion rather than to attempt a simple closure of this cartilage-like tissue. After repair the bladder should be drained for 14 to 21 days either with a suprapubic cystotomy or with an indwelling Foley catheter. Rarely the opening into the bladder is so minute that it cannot be identified, in which case it will usually heal without complication if the bladder is decompressed, as just described.

The tract of an enterocutaneous fistula may not heal following resection of the involved intestine if it is simply drained and allowed to remain in place. The wall of the fistulous tract often is so fibrotic and rigid that a persistent draining sinus, a recurrent abscess, or even a recurrent fistula may result from such a practice, even if a drain is left in place for a prolonged period. I prefer to excise the fistulous tract back to normal tissue through all layers of the abdominal wall, insofar as this is anatomically feasible. The peritoneum and posterior fascia then are closed from within using absorbable sutures. The external portion of the tract is loosely packed with gauze to allow secondary healing to occur, a process that usually proceeds at an astoundingly rapid rate.

ABSCESSES. Small, often unsuspected abscesses within the leaves of the colonic or ileal mesentery or between two loops of intestine are frequently resected without having been entered. At other times the diseased intestine is part of the wall of an abscess that may be further bordered by the anterior or lateral abdominal wall, the urinary bladder, or the retroperitoneum. The management will vary depending upon whether or not the abscess is diagnosed preoperatively, its size and its accessibility to extraperitoneal drainage.

Large collections are often diagnosable by physical examination or by imaging with computerized tomography or ultrasound, and can be drained extraperitoneally by a minor operation, or percutaneously if there is a safe "window."[172] After surgical or percutaneous drainage, the fact that a fistula does not ensue immediately does not obviate the need for definitive operation, as has been suggested.[173]

An alternative to a preliminary drainage of a large abscess followed by later definitive operation is the use of the exclusion bypass principle (vide infra). Even if it is not known preoperatively that a large abscess is present, it may be possible to suspect one before the incision is made. The abdomen should always be carefully palpated after induction of anesthesia, and if a large mass is discernible an abscess should be suspected. In the presence of a large mass, the incision should be placed on the left side well away from the mass, a practice that will help avoid uncontrolled entry into pus and, in any event, will permit easier access to the abdomen, even if resection is indicated. With the incision away from the abscess, exclusion bypass can then be performed and the abscess can be drained extraperitoneally through a separate small incision (vide infra).

In many instances, abscesses of intermediate size either are not accessible to extraperitoneal drainage or they cannot be diagnosed preoperatively. In other cases, resection may be essential, whether or not such an abscess is present. In performing resection in the face of an abscess, contamination can be minimized by keeping in mind that the most adherent part of the mass will usually be at the abscess site, and by being prepared to suction up the pus through a small initial entry hole so that it does not flow throughout the operative field during the mobilization of this adherent area. In such cases, as discussed earlier, septic complications can be minimized by careful choice of antibiotic regimens and techniques of wound closure, and by adherence to other sound principles of surgical technique. Because of satisfaction with the results, I increasingly tend to prefer resection over bypass, even in the presence of abscesses.

PROXIMAL SKIP LESIONS. In regional enteritis the lesion often dwindles in a segmental fashion as one proceeds proximally up the ileum from the main site of disease involvement. Such scattered lesions can and should be encompassed with the ileocecal resection, and their removal will usually not add materially to the length of the intestine that is sacrificed. At times, however, gross skip lesions may be at a distance proximal to the terminal ileal disease. Especially in light of emerging knowledge about the extent of the Crohn's lesion and its postoperative behavior, it would be contraindicated to sacrifice a sizable segment of normal intestine in order to encompass such a lesion in a single resection that includes the terminal ileal disease. For that matter, one should not feel compelled to resect such an area provided it is non-stenotic and is causing no other local complications. If it does appear to require resection because of stenosis or other complications, a separate resection is preferred, even though by so doing it will be necessary to perform two anastomoses. This policy is consistent with the strategy of dealing with concomitant gastroduodenal skip disease in a patient requiring operation for distal disease, that is, it would not be wise to attack it surgically merely because of its presence and the fact that the abdomen is open.

EXCLUSION BYPASS

Exclusion bypass is usually performed in the presence of a large, densely adherent inflammatory mass or huge abscess. This procedure is diagrammed in Figure 27-5. The uninvolved intestine is traced into the inflammatory mass and the most distal free portion of intestine is selected for anastomosis, using the aforemen-

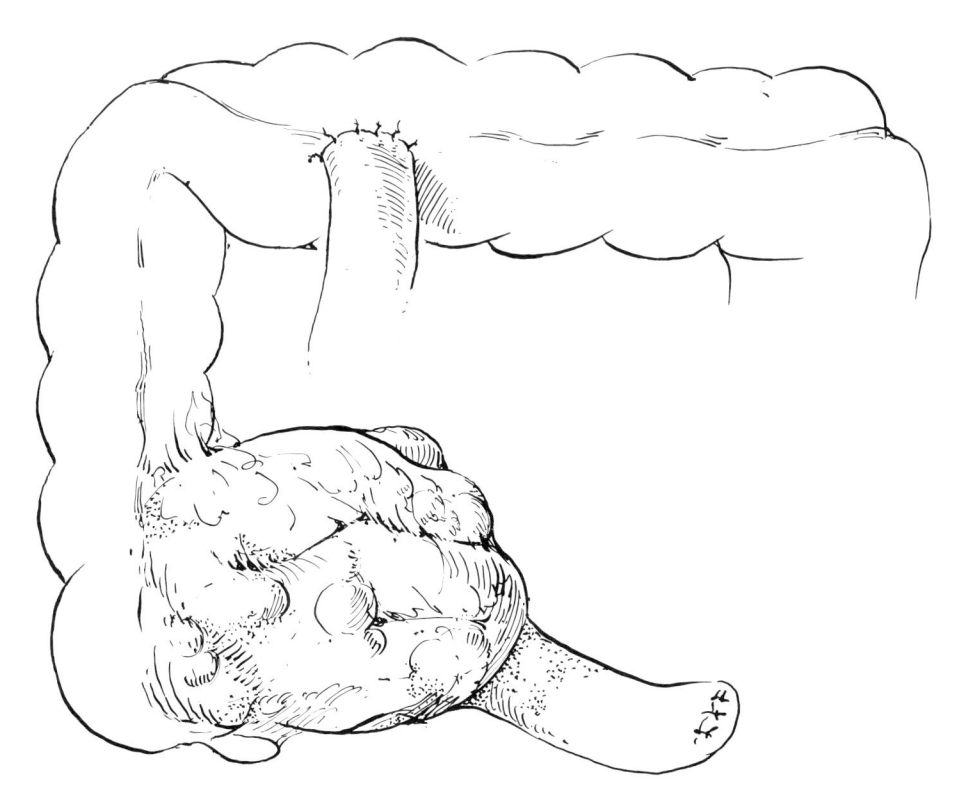

FIG 27-5. Exclusion bypass for regional enteritis. The ileum is transected in an area of normal-appearing intestine just proximal to any inflammatory mass. The distal cut end of ileum is closed (if obstruction is present, this must be vented) and the proximal cut end is anastomosed to the transverse colon, end-to-side (ascending colon would be preferable, local pathology permitting).

tioned criteria. The mesentery of the small intestine is divided only to an extent that allows the ileum to reach the colon comfortably and in such a fashion that the blood supply to neither the proximal nor the excluded distal bowel is endangered. Usually the complication that dictates selection of this procedure will also make necessary an anastomosis between the ileum and the transverse colon. If circumstances allow, however, the ascending colon may be used to take advantage of the additional water-absorbing capacity of this segment. When the tranverse colon is used for the distal side of the anastomosis, the omentum is dissected from the anterior wall of the colon and the anastomosis is made to one of the tenia of the colon. The mesentery of the ileum must be oriented properly to avoid a twist. While it is often impossible to close the "trap" between the ileal mesentery and the transverse colon and its mesentery, this trap usually is easily closed after anastomosis of the ileum to the ascending colon, a further advantage of this procedure over anastomosis to the transverse colon, when all other things are equal.

The distal cut end of ileum is closed if there is no obstruction. In the presence of distal obstruction it is mandatory either to bring the ileum to the abdominal wall as a mucous fistula or to close it and vent the bowel with a tube enterostomy by the Witzel or Stamm technique so that closed loop obstruction and disruption of the suture line do not occur. It is possible that some free perforations reported after exclusion bypass for regional enteritis are caused by development of a closed loop proximal to an area of cicatricial contracture.[174] If a tube enterostomy is used, the intestine around the point of emergence should be sutured to the under surface of the abdominal wall to avoid leakage.

STRICTUREPLASTY

The techniques described are essentially those of Lee and Alexander-Williams and co-workers.[43,44,175] If this operation is deemed suitable for a short stricture, the narrowing is incised along the antimesenteric border entering the non-strictured part proximally and distally (Fig. 27-6A). The closure technique is similar to that of a Heineke-Mickulicz pyloroplasty. Traction sutures are placed at the center of the incision on either side, and the enterotomy is then closed transversely with one layer of synthetic absorb-

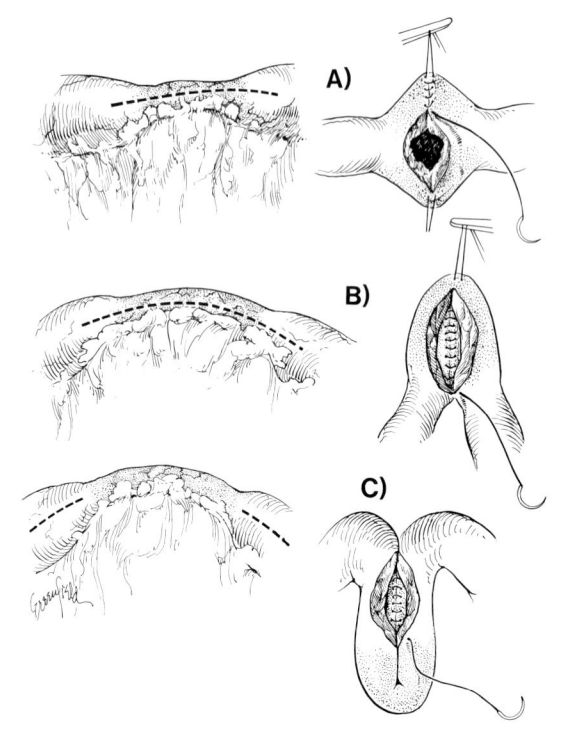

FIG. 27-6. Strictureplasty. A. Short strictures can be relieved by longitudinal incision followed by transverse closure in the manner of a Heineke-Mickulicz pyloroplasty. Longer strictures can be dealt with by: B. A long enterotomy with closure in the manner of a Finney pyloroplasty; or C. Short incisions just proximal and distal to the narrowed segment with anastomosis in the fashion of a Jaboulay pyloroplasty. (After Lee and Papaioannou[44] and Alexander-Williams[175]).

able sutures in an end-on manner, with interrupted or continuous technique (Fig. 27-6A).

For longer strictures, other techniques of strictureplasty are more suitable. In one of these, a long incision through the entire stricture is made closer to the mesenteric border than for a short stricture. The long enterotomy is then closed in the manner of a Finney pyloroplasty (Fig. 27-6B), again with absorbable suture material; for long strictures, however, Lee seems to prefer longitudinal incisions made just proximal and distal to the stricture, which openings are then joined in the fashion of a Jaboulay pyloroplasty (Fig. 27-6C).[44] Alternatively, Lee sometimes performed a short resection of the most thickened part with end-to-end anastomosis using intestine affected by disease, representing a technique consistent with the principle of minimal, palliative surgical therapy but not, in strict terms, a strictureplasty.

Operative Technique for Inflammatory Bowel Disease Involving All or Substantial Portions of the Colon

Total Colectomy and Ileostomy

SITE OF THE ILEOSTOMY

Proper placement of the ileostomy is of immense importance for subsequent ease of management of the stoma and must therefore receive careful attention (see also Chap. 28). If possible, during preoperative teaching a sample appliance should be placed on the patient's abdomen and the optimal site thus determined should be marked with indelible ink or silver nitrate. The advantages of preoperative application of an appliance can largely be attained by careful observation of the transverse crease of the abdominal wall produced by bending the patient's torso, while also considering the position of the umbilicus, the anterior superior spine, the lateral border of the rectus, and previous scars in the area. Ideally the ileostomy is situated just within the rectus sheath (Fig. 27-7) because this may help avoid paraileostomy hernia. Rigid adherence to the placement, however, may bring the ileostomy too far medially in some patients. The optimal site is usually slightly above and medial to the midpoint of a line drawn between the anterior superior spine and the umbilicus. This position has the following advantages: (1) it avoids impingement of the face plate of the ileostomy appliance upon the anterior superior spine or the umbilicus, (2) it is low enough to avoid the bend of the abdomen, (3) it preserves a slim waistline, and (4) it is high enough to avoid the tendency for the face plate to be forced off when the thigh is flexed during sitting. The main disadvantage of this site is that if a belt is worn it tends to ride up over the iliac crest, pulling cranially on the appliance and eventually displacing it. This potential disadvantage can be ameliorated by taping down the face plate and using non-skid attachments to the belt, or by using a rubber belt, especially at night. In any event, with the use of the newer light-weight semi-disposable appliances by most patients a belt is usually not required for secure application.

CONDUCT OF OPERATION

Proctocolectomy is described as a sequential procedure (i.e., with separate abdominal and perineal phases) because I usually perform it in this manner. Although a two-team or single-team, synchronous approach is used successfully by some, I find that the positions for this approach are a little awkward for both the abdominal and perineal phases and, therefore, I seldom use it because it is not particularly suited to my style or temperament. In any event, the basic maneuvers in the sequential and synchronous methods are the same.

The patient is placed in the supine position with an indwelling urethral catheter in place. The mark used to designate the optimal site of the ileostomy, if made with indelible ink or silver nitrate, should survive skin preparation. A long left paramedian incision is made extending from the pubic symphysis to the xyphoid, the incision in the upper abdomen gradually curving almost to the midline (Fig. 27-7). The abdomen is carefully explored with particular attention not only

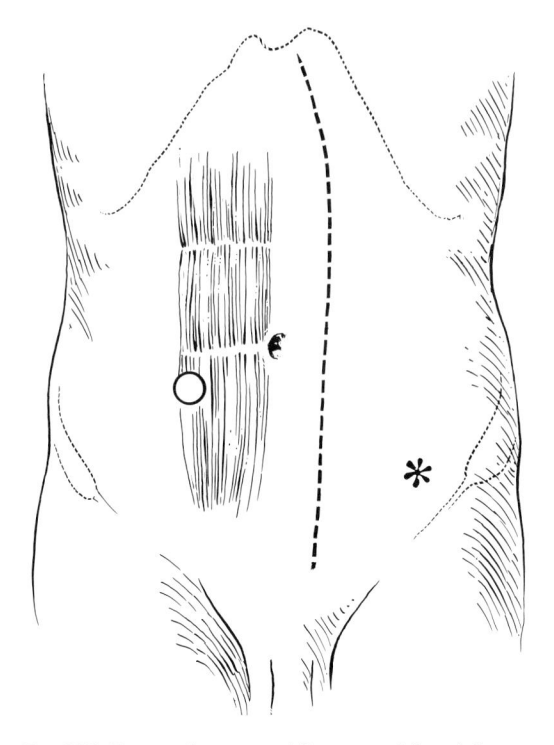

FIG. 27-7. Proctocolectomy and ileostomy. A long left paramedian muscle-retracting incision is made from pubic symphysis to xiphoid. Circle indicates preferred site for ileostomy, the aperture for which should be just within the rectus sheath. The site chosen must allow an appliance to be worn that will avoid the anterior superior spine, umbilicus, and the torso crease. Asterisk indicates site of mucous fistula if operation is completed as abdominal colectomy and ileostomy.

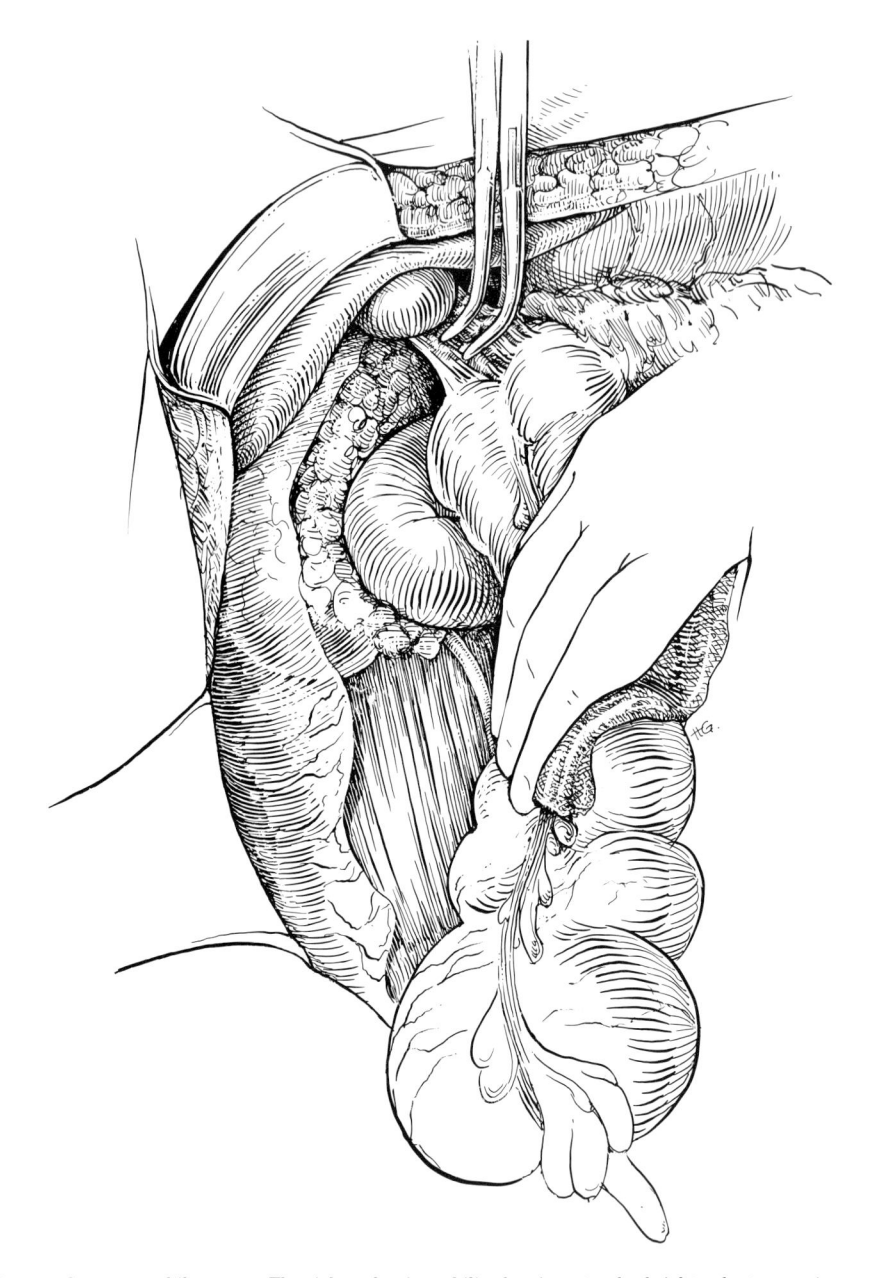

FIG. 27-8. Proctocolectomy and ileostomy. The right colon is mobilized as in a standard right colectomy using gentle traction over gauze. Innumerable small vessels in "avascular" line of Toldt are easily controlled with electrocautery. The attachments of the hepatic flexure are transected between clamps and ligated.

to the extent and degree of colonic involvement, but also to the presence of complications such as perforation, possible liver metastases, and gallstones. The initial inspection should be performed before manipulation of the intestine, because handling makes subtle serosal changes less obvious. It should be emphasized that the appearance of the serosal surface of the colon usually grossly underestimates the extent and severity of the mucosal disease. In cases of Crohn's disease, the extent of any small intestinal involvement is assessed as described earlier, and any "skip" disease in the proximal small bowel, duodenum, and stomach is noted. At this time a tentative site for ileal transection may be marked with a superficially placed silk suture. Having chosen the type and extent of operation, the colon is mobilized from right to left, freeing the colon along the line of peritoneal reflection (Fig. 27-8). Traction on the colon by the surgical

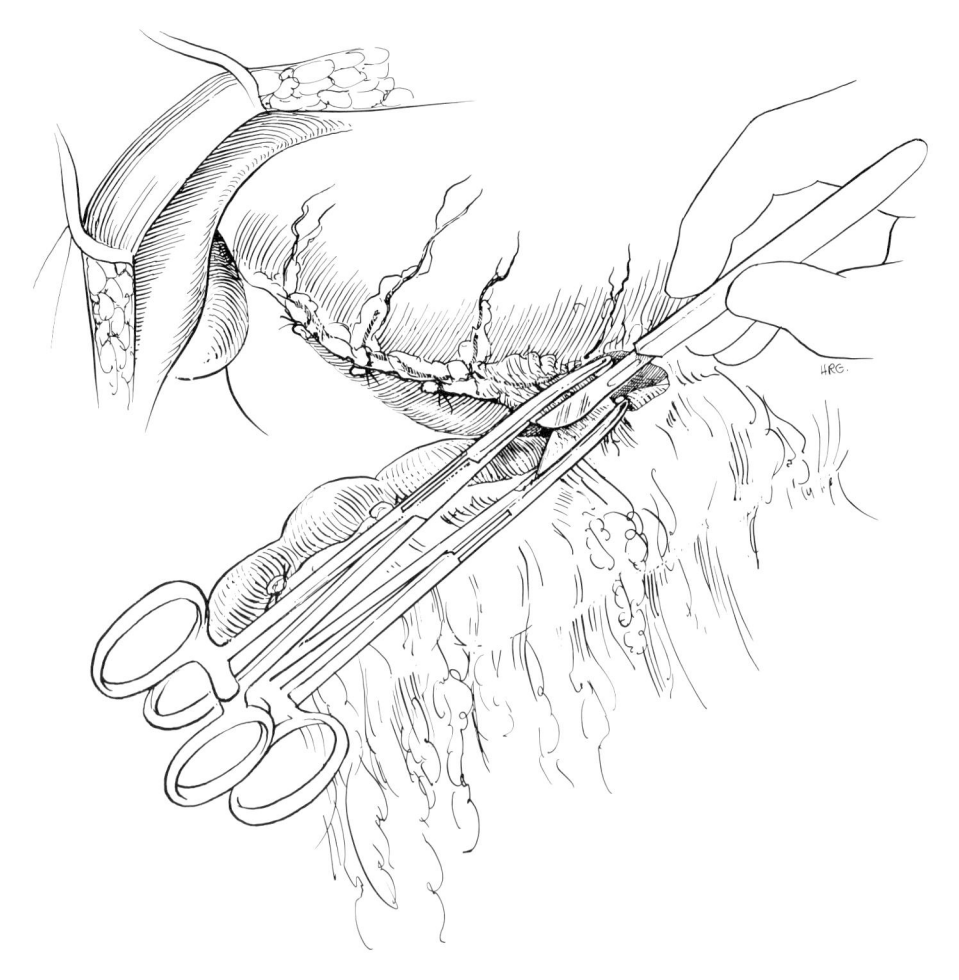

FIG. 27-9. Proctocolectomy and ileostomy. The greater omentum is removed with the colon. The omental branches of the gastroepiploic vessels are severed between clamps and ligated, preserving the gastroepiploic blood supply to the stomach.

assistant must be gentle and over moist gauze to avoid perforating it particularly in toxic megacolon. Multiple small blood vessels in this "avascular" plane of the peritoneal reflection bleed significantly in the face of an inflamed colon, but this is quickly and easily controlled by the electrosurgical unit. The right ureter and duodenum are carefully exposed and preserved. The attachments of the hepatic flexure of the colon to the posterior abdominal wall and duodenum contain sizable blood vessels, and as in any colonic resection, these are divided between clamps and ligated. The greater omentum is excised with the colon, leaving intact the gastroepiploic vessels along the greater curve of the stomach (Fig. 27-9). I see no advantage in preserving the omentum, because it is a potential source of postoperative adhesions in an operation already noteworthy for problems with adhesive obstruction. In addition, dissection of the omentum from an inflamed colon is time-consuming, troublesome, and may unroof sealed-off perforations.

When the omentum has been divided one-half to two-thirds of the way to the splenic flexure, attention is directed to freeing the splenic flexure. This is facilitated by first widely mobilizing the left colon from its attachments to the posterior parietal peritoneum (Fig. 27-10). With progressive mobilization of the left colon medially, traction on the splenic attachments and consequent splenic injury can be avoided, because the attachments to the spleen and omentum are approached from underneath. This maneuver and the use of an adequate abdominal incision makes freeing the splenic flexure relatively easy, even in the presence of toxic megacolon. Moreover, this step of the operation is frequently aided by the usual foreshortening of the colon caused by the inflammatory process.

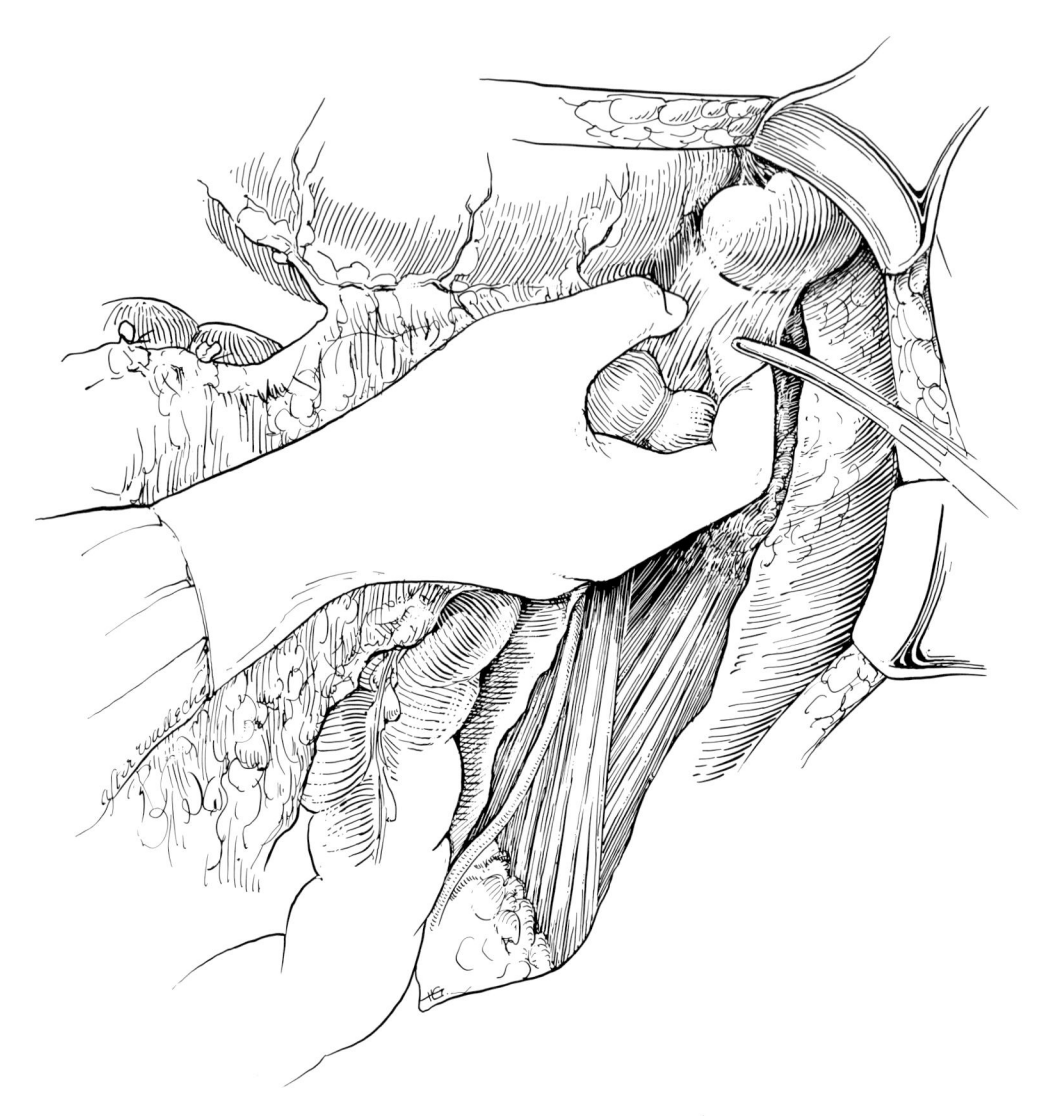

FIG. 27-10. Proctocolectomy and ileostomy. The greater omentum has been detached about two-thirds of the way to the splenic flexure. Mobilization of the splenic flexure is greatly facilitated by first widely mobilizing the left colon and retracting it to the right. The attachments of the splenic flexure can then be identified and approached from inferiorly and posteriorly, staying well away from the spleen and avoiding traction injury. Attachments of the spleen to the colon, which contain small vessels, are beginning to be clamped and ligated in the illustration. The remaining attachments of the greater omentum typically will be ligated from left to right.

As the sigmoid and rectum are approached, the left ureter should be identified and a final decision as to a one- or two-stage procedure must be made (Fig. 27-11).

COMPLETION AS A SUBTOTAL COLECTOMY. If completion as a subtotal colectomy is elected, mobilization of the colon stops at a point that removes the maximal amount of colon but still allows the distal end to be brought out as a mucous fistula without tension. Usually, this point is near the rectosigmoid junction. Some surgeons prefer closure of the distal cut end of rectum to the creation of a mucous fistula.[176] Although this allows somewhat more colon to be removed and obviates the temporary annoyance of a mucous fistula, such a closure may be tenuous and, therefore, hazardous if the colon is severely diseased. In addition, subsequently the second-stage proctectomy may be rendered more difficult if an adequate length of colon is not available on which to apply traction and thus facilitate the pelvic dissection.

The blood supply to the colon is divided and

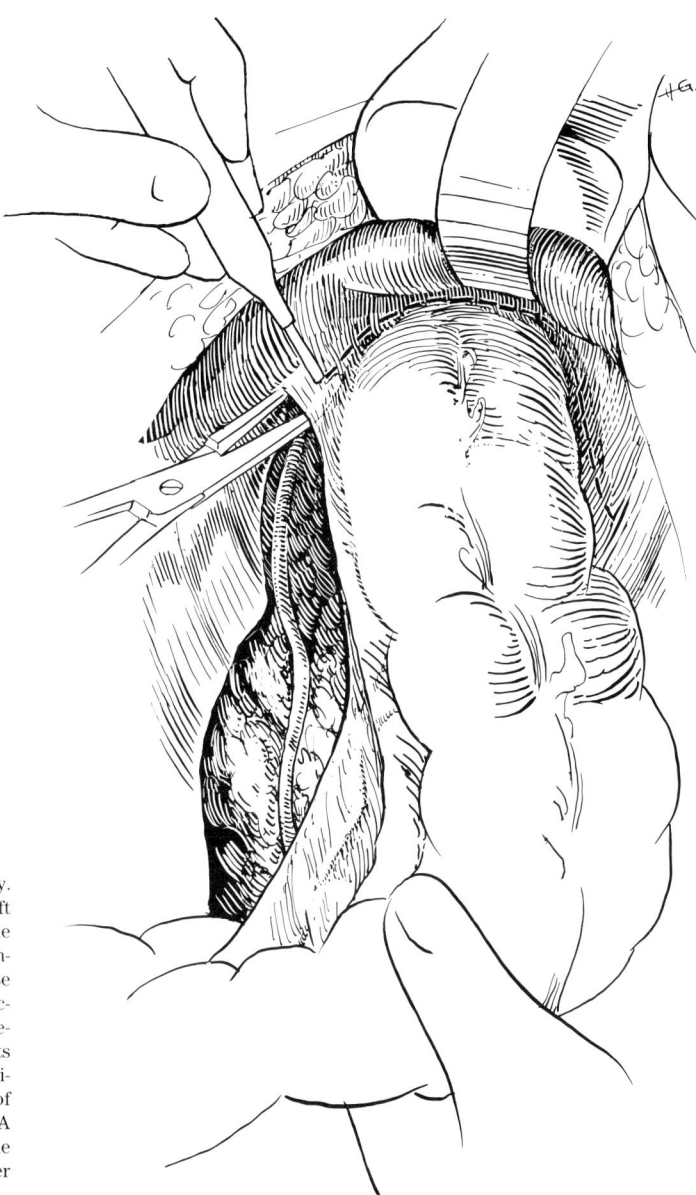

FIG. 27-11. Proctocolectomy and ileostomy. The surgeon is standing on the patient's left and looking downward into the pelvis. The dissection of the rectum is begun by continuing the peritoneal incision caudally, close to the rectum, in the groove between the rectum and the lateral pelvic wall. The left ureter is carefully identified throughout its length and preserved. The peritoneal incision is carried over the anterior surface of the rectum in the cul-de-sac of Douglas. A similar peritoneal incision is made on the right side of the rectum and the right ureter is identified and protected from harm.

ligated from right to left as described in the following, and the initial steps for ileostomy construction are completed with particular attention to preservation of the blood supply to the ileum. Division of the blood supply to the rectosigmoid should be accomplished in a manner to assure the viability of the mucous fistula. The chosen site for division of the sigmoid is transected after the application of a Stone or DeMartel type clamp distally and an Allen intestinal clamp proximally. It is preferable to bring the mucous fistula onto the abdominal wall through a separate stab wound rather than through the lower end of the incisional wound (Fig. 27-7). Although a segment of colon 3 to 6 cm longer is required for delivery of the mucous fistula through a separate stab wound, subsequent wound infection and ventral hernia may be thus avoided. The stab wound is made only large enough to accept the rectosigmoid without strangulation. The clamp on the mucous fistula is left in place postoperatively to keep the intestine from retracting into the abdomen. The potential for intra-abdominal migration of the distal cut end of the rectum can also be lessened by underwrapping the clamp with sponge gauze that seals to the serosa. Premature (less than 10 to 14 days) removal of this gauze, or removal of the clamp before it separates spontaneously by necrosis, has resulted in unnecessary complications. Sole reliance on the clamp and the gauze, however, without adequate mobilization of the colon is condemned.

COMPLETION AS A PROCTOCOLECTOMY. Particularly if a one-stage procedure is chosen, ligation of the blood supply to the colon should be postponed for as long as possible to avoid possible migration of bacteria through the dying intestinal wall during the relatively long dissection. In contrast to good practice in proctectomy for carcinoma, the sigmoid mesentery over the great vessels, sacral promontory, and upper hollow of sacrum *must not be freed* in the plane of Waldeyer's fascia. Rather, it is essential that the dissection for inflammatory bowel disease pro-

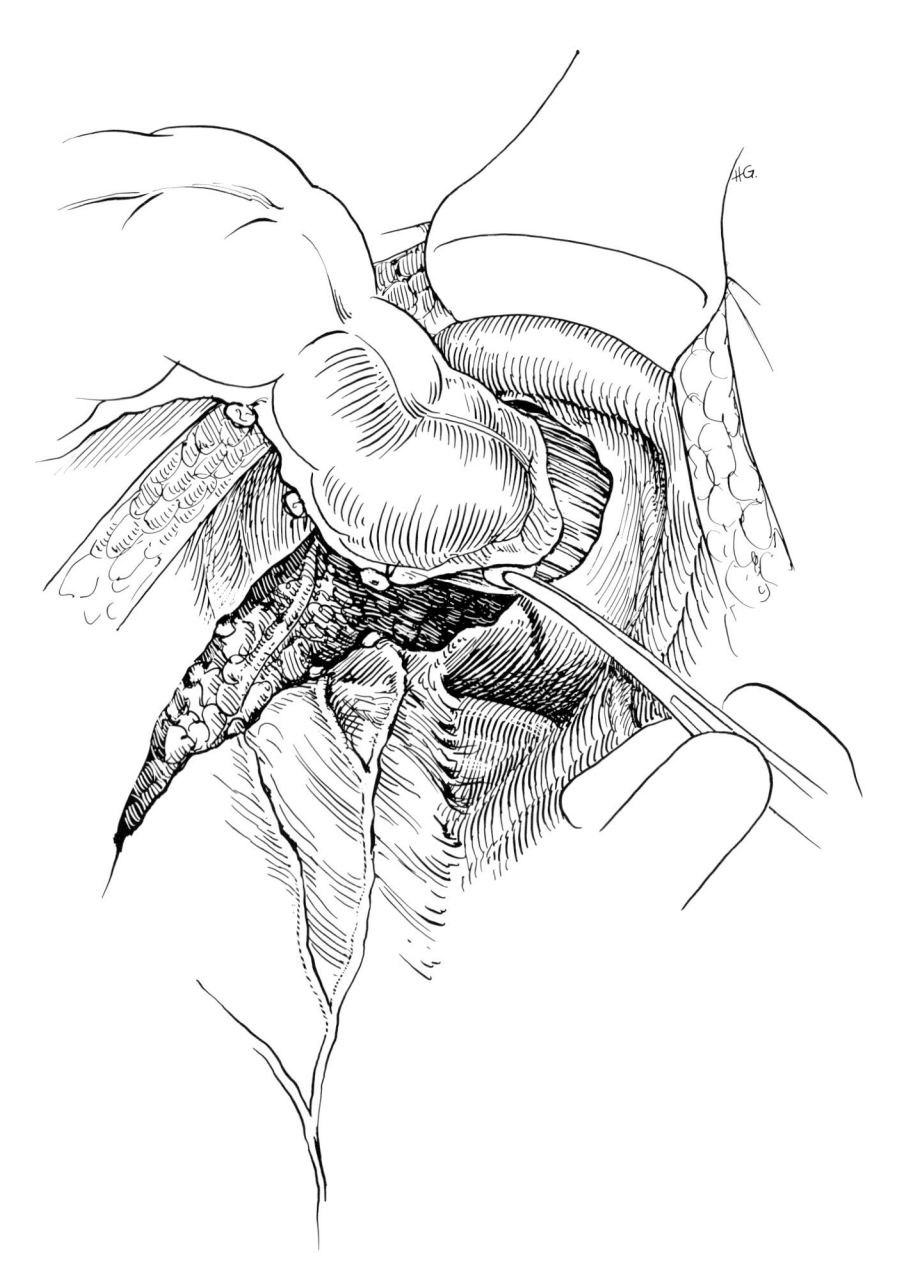

FIG. 27-12. Proctocolectomy and ileostomy. In freeing the rectum posteriorly, the blood supply to the rectum is severed close to the wall of the rectum in order to avoid injury to the hypogastric nerves, leaving a portion of the mesentery of the rectosigmoid over the bifurcation of the great vessels, sacral promontory, and upper sacrum.

ceed close to the wall of the rectum thereby sparing the autonomic nervous system responsible for normal sexual and bladder function, especially the presacral nerves and nervi erigentes (Fig. 27-12).

The peritoneum is incised on both sides of the rectum and the incisions are joined anteriorly in the cul-de-sac of Douglas (Fig. 27-11). The mesentery of the rectum is divided and ligated with absorbable sutures, in contrast to the preferred use of nonabsorbable sutures during the remainder of the procedure. If nonabsorbable sutures are used in the pelvic portion of the dissection, this could lead to development and perpetuation of a perineal sinus if they should become infected. As the operator proceeds distally, the vessels behind the rectum, which divide into two parallel rows, are individually ligated. Farther inferiorly, the dissection enters the presacral plane and ends at the tip of the coccyx (Fig. 27-13A). The rectum is separated anteriorly from the bladder, seminal vesicles, and prostate in the male, and uterine cervix and posterior vagina in the female (Fig. 27-13B). Anterior dissection in the female is aided by a traction suture of heavy catgut placed into the fun-

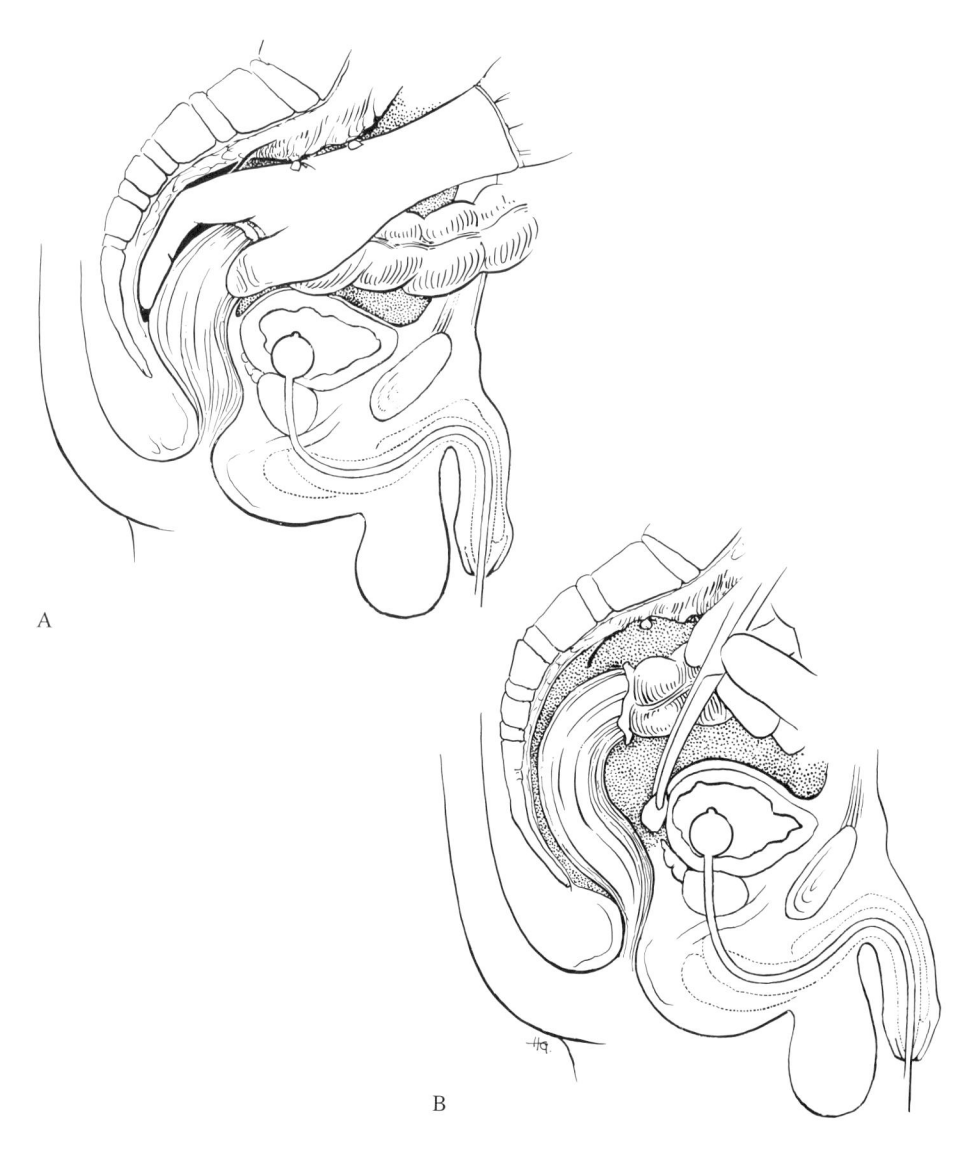

FIG. 27-13. Proctocolectomy and ileostomy. A. The rectum is being mobilized posteriorly by blunt dissection. Note the residual mesentery over the sacral promentory. B. Posterior mobilization has been completed and the anterior surface of the rectum is being separated from the bladder, seminal vesicles, and prostate (cervix and vagina in female). The plane of dissection is established in the midline and "worked" laterally.

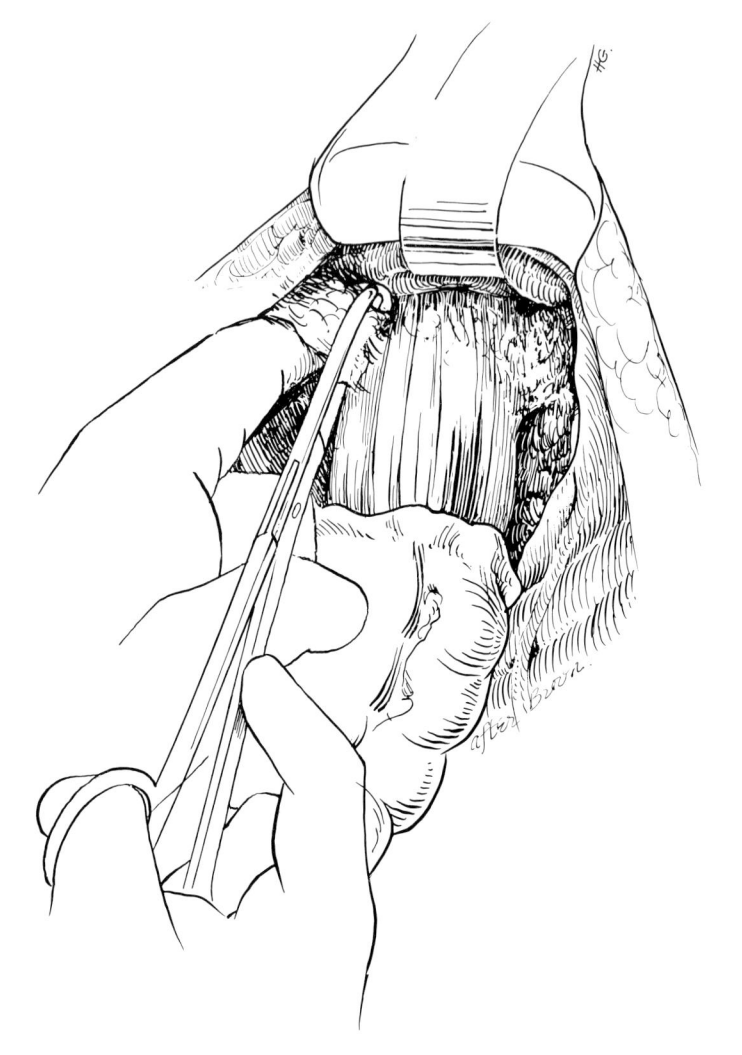

FIG. 27-14. Proctocolectomy and ileostomy. After complete mobilization posteriorly and then anteriorly, the lateral stalks are isolated and divided close to the rectum in order to avoid injury to the nervi erigentes and ligated. The first clamp is being applied. The second will be even closer to the rectum. Absorbable suture material will be used lest an infected, nonabsorbable suture contribute to a persistent perineal sinus.

dus of the uterus. The lateral stalks are ligated as close to the rectum as possible to avoid injury to the nervi erigentes in males, and to prevent interference with bladder innervation (Fig. 27-14). Mobilization of the rectum has been completed when the entire circumference of the rectum down to the level of the levator ani muscles has been freed, at which point the perineum can be felt to be mobile (Fig. 27-15).

LIGATION OF BLOOD SUPPLY OF COLON AND PREPARATION OF ILEUM FOR ILEOSTOMY. When the blood supply to the colon is ready to be serially ligated prior to its removal, the site of contemplated division of the ileum should be reassessed, especially in terms of the blood supply to the portion to be used for the ileostomy. It is helpful to view the blood supply by transilluminating the mesentery with the operating room light. In the usual case of ulcerative colitis, the site of division can be close to the ileocecal valve, so close that it will be necessary to remove the terminal ileal antimesenteric fat pad in order to minimize the bulk of ileum that is to be brought through the abdominal wall to construct the ileostomy. The advantage of ileal division at this level (over and above conservation of maximum length) is that within the mesentery at this point a small vessel usually runs parallel to the ileum (Fig. 27-16A) that makes it possible to produce a straight segment of ileum for construction of the ileostomy with minimal hazard of devascularization (Fig. 27-16B). Although Counsell and others have described regression of backwash ileitis in ulcerative colitis if the ileostomy is constructed in this segment (an observation that I can confirm),[177] in the presence of ileitis, whatever its presumed etiology, it is probably wisest at the present time to sacrifice the segment of inflamed intestine because Crohn's disease of the colon can closely mimic ulcerative colitis. In Crohn's disease, all the involved ileum is excised with close margins (3 or 4 cm), consistent with the practice described earlier in small intestinal disease.

The mesentery, especially of the right colon, is serially divided fairly close to the bowel not only to preserve the blood supply to the ileum, as already discussed, but also to aid in the fixation of the ileostomy and in reperitonealization of the denuded posterior parieties (Fig. 27-17). When the ligation of the blood supply is accom-

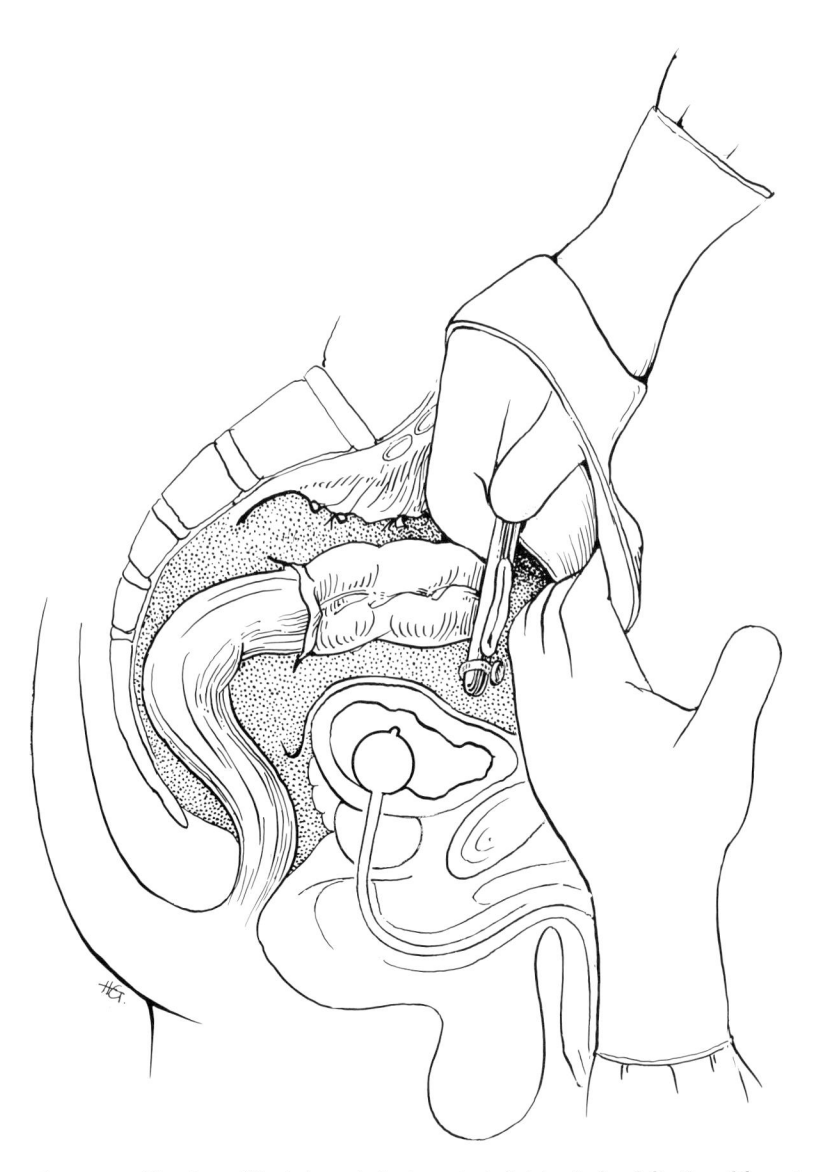

FIG. 27-15. Proctocolectomy and ileostomy. Stippled area indicates extent of abdominal mobilization of the rectum—beyond tip of coccyx posteriorly and beyond prostate in male and to perineal body in female. The perineum feels quite mobile at this point. The rectum has been divided from the rest of the colon, using a Harvey Stone type of clamp as illustrated or a ligature of umbilical tape to prevent fecal spill. A rubber glove is being everted over the rectum and will be securely tied in place over the bowel to prevent contamination from the cut end.

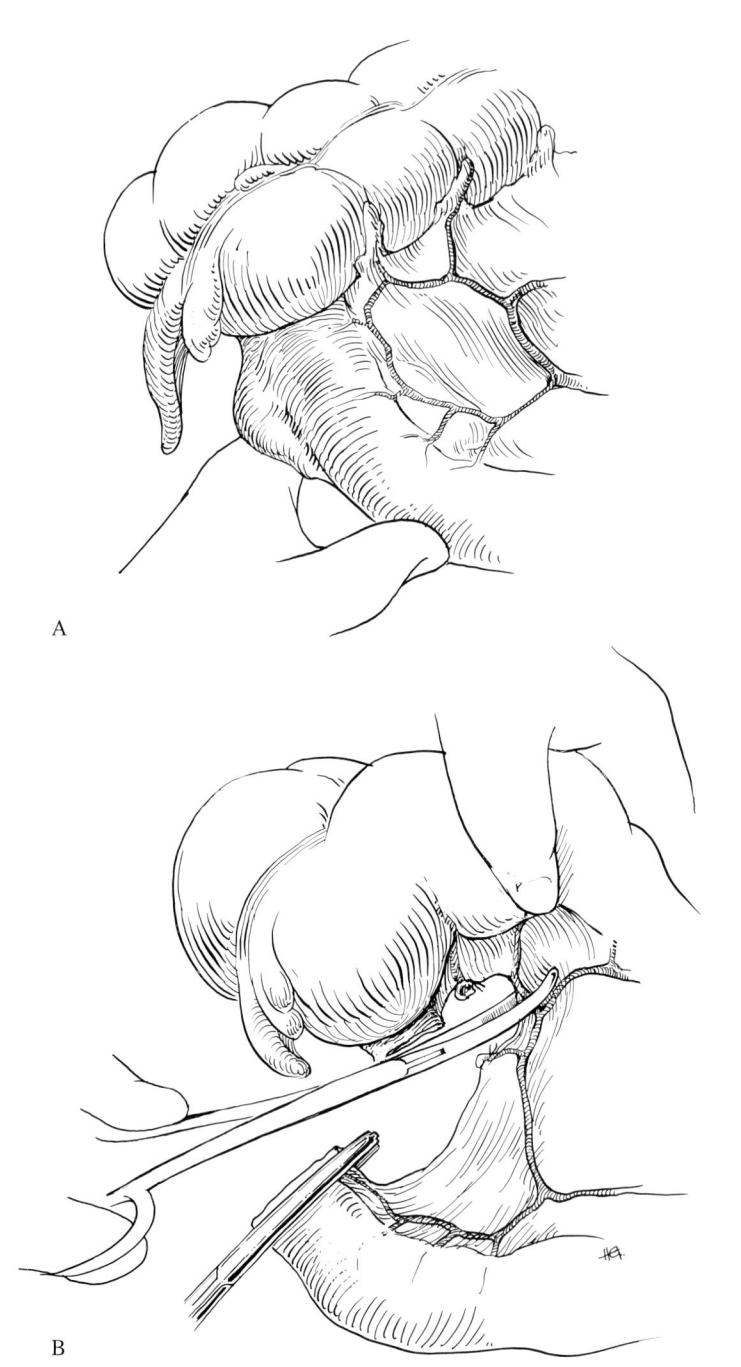

FIG. 27-16. Proctocolectomy and ileostomy. Division of blood supply to colon is begun. A: Note small vessel running parallel to the very terminal ileum opposite the antimesenteric fat pad. B: Antimesenteric fat pad has been excised and the blood supply to the terminal ileum is preserved by dividing blood supply close to the colon.

plished and completion as a subtotal colectomy is elected, the aforementioned steps for creation of the mucous fistula are taken. If proctocolectomy is being carried out, the rectum is divided as low as possible either between tightly tied lengths of umbilical tape or between clamps, the lower one of which should be of the Harvey Stone or DeMartel type. A rubber glove is placed over the cut end of rectum (Figs. 27-15 and 27-18), tied tightly in place, and the rectum placed into the hollow of the sacrum (Fig. 27-18). The specimen is removed from the field and examined by the pathologist. Gross examination is sufficient for determination of the adequacy of

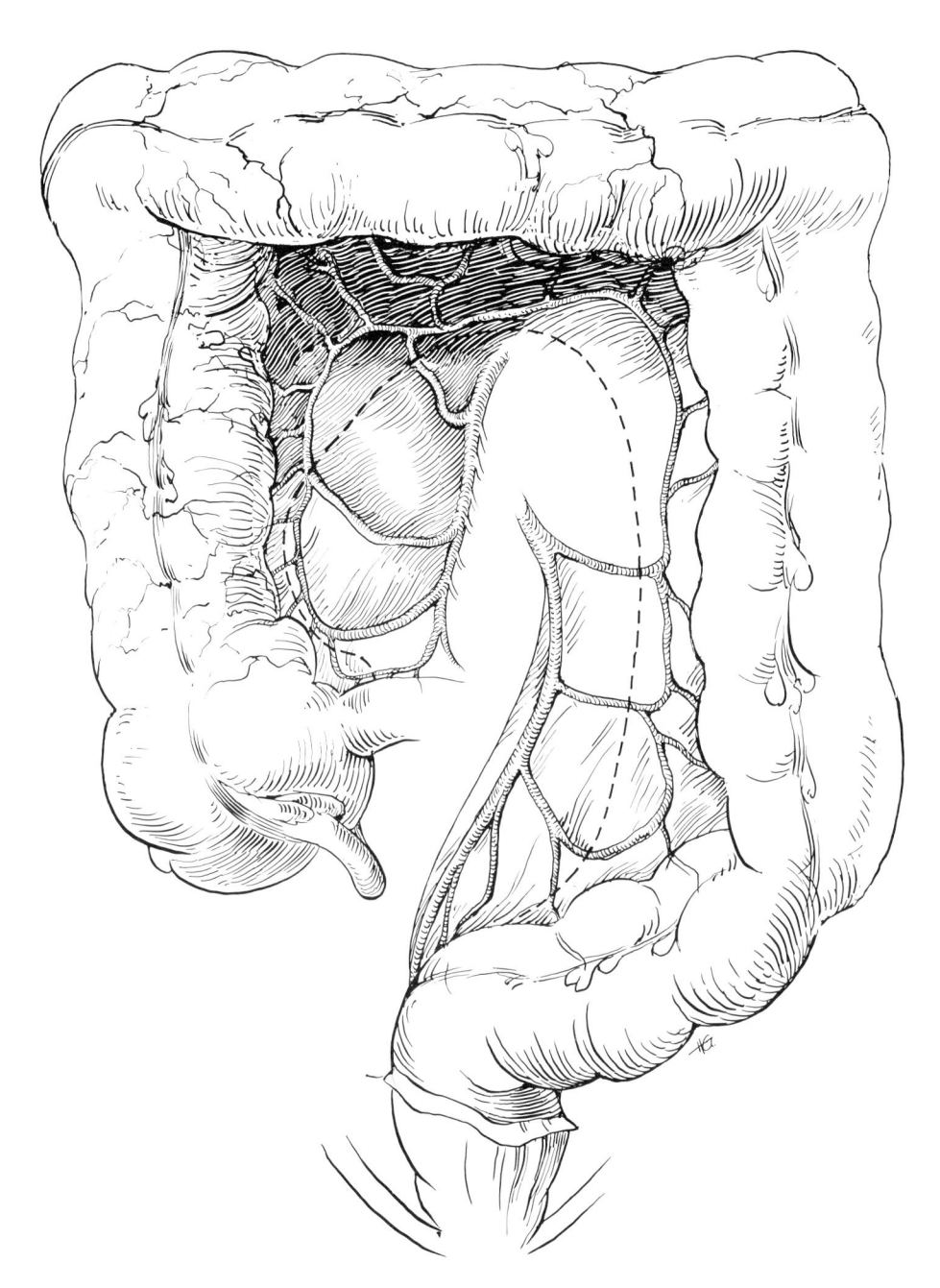

FIG. 27-17. Proctocolectomy and ileostomy. Diagram of approximate sites of division of blood supply to the colon. The division is close to the right colon to prevent devascularization of the ileum. Close division elsewhere will preserve mesentery for reperitonealization (optional).

the resection margin in patients with Crohn's disease and, as noted earlier, rapid section adds nothing to this decision. If unsuspected carcinoma is seen in the colon, further lymph node dissection can be carried out at this point.

In the case of known or strongly suspected carcinoma, the mesenteric dissection is widened so that ligation of the major vessels at the root of the mesocolon is accomplished. The pelvic dissection should be the same as that employed in radical cancer excision, accepting the hazard of injury to the presacral nerve and nervi erigentes.

CONSTRUCTION OF THE ILEOSTOMY. The ileostomy can be fashioned either by bringing the ileum straight through the abdominal wall (the Brooke method),[25] or by bringing it under a tunnel of the lateral parietal peritoneum as described by Goligher.[178] For most cases, I have come to prefer Goligher's extraperitoneal ileostomy for the following reasons: (1) the opening in the abdominal muscles and fascias may be made somewhat larger with the hope that ileostomy dysfunction might be less frequent; (2) the mesentery of the ileum can be brought through more "comfortably" without being compromised by the ring of peritoneum; (3) with a conventional Brooke ileostomy, the sutures between the mesentery and the lateral abdominal wall used to prevent herniation may tear loose; and (4) internal herniation, paraileostomy herniation, and prolapse are probably less likely to occur.

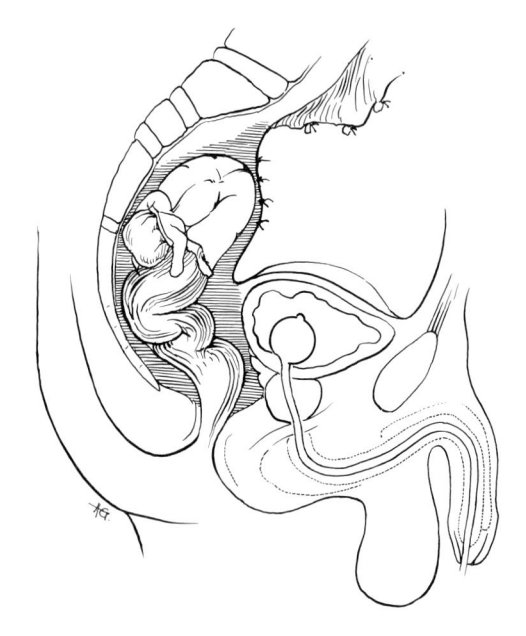

FIG. 27-18. Proctocolectomy and ileostomy. The divided rectum, with everted rubber glove tied over it, has been placed below the peritoneal floor which has been closed with continuous or interrupted absorbable sutures.

Extraperitoneal Ileostomy. The cut edge of the lateral peritoneal reflection within the abdomen

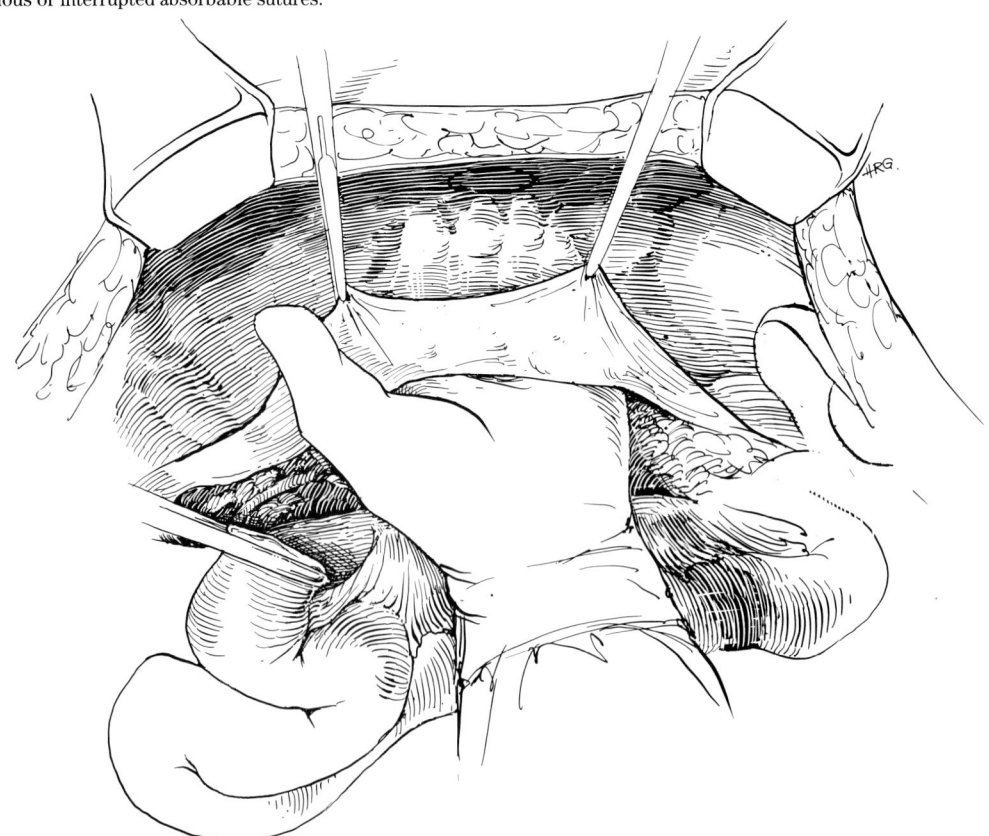

FIG. 27-19. Proctocolectomy and ileostomy. Construction of retroperitoneal ileostomy is begun by widely freeing up the right posterior, lateral and anterior parietal peritoneum in caudad and cephalad directions beyond the site of the proposed ileostomy (circle). (After Goligher[178].)

is grasped, and, with sharp and blunt dissection, the peritoneum is widely and carefully freed from the posterior, lateral, and anterior abdominal wall to a point where the contemplated site of ileostomy is undermined (Fig. 27-19). Anteriorly, as the lateral rectus sheath is approached, the peritoneum is often densely adherent to the posterior rectus sheath so that dissection must proceed carefully in this region to avoid making an opening in the peritoneum. The entire right peritoneal reflection usually requires mobilization to make room for the ileum and its mesentery.

The skin at the previously chosen site for ileostomy is grasped and held up with a Kocher clamp (Fig. 27-20). A button of skin roughly the size of a nickel (2 cm diameter) is excised with a scalpel held parallel to the skin, a maneuver that makes a perfect circle (Figs. 27-20 and 27-21A). Because the skin retracts, the nickel-sized defect enlarges to the size of a quarter (2.5 cm diameter). A larger hole may be necessary if the ileum is dilated, but care must be taken not to render the final opening larger than necessary, which will, because of tension, lead to separation of the ileum from the skin postoperatively. The subcutaneous fat is excised to the same circumference as the skin (Fig. 27-21B). So that the path created through the skin and fascia will be in a straight line, leftward traction is exerted on the skin and on two Kocher clamps previously placed on the fascia at the right edge of the abdominal incision (Fig. 27-20). A button of fascia slightly smaller than the skin defect is then excised or, alternatively, cruciate incisions are made (Fig. 27-21C) and a clamp is used to split the muscle (Fig. 27-21D) so that the clamp emerges into the extraperitoneal space of the

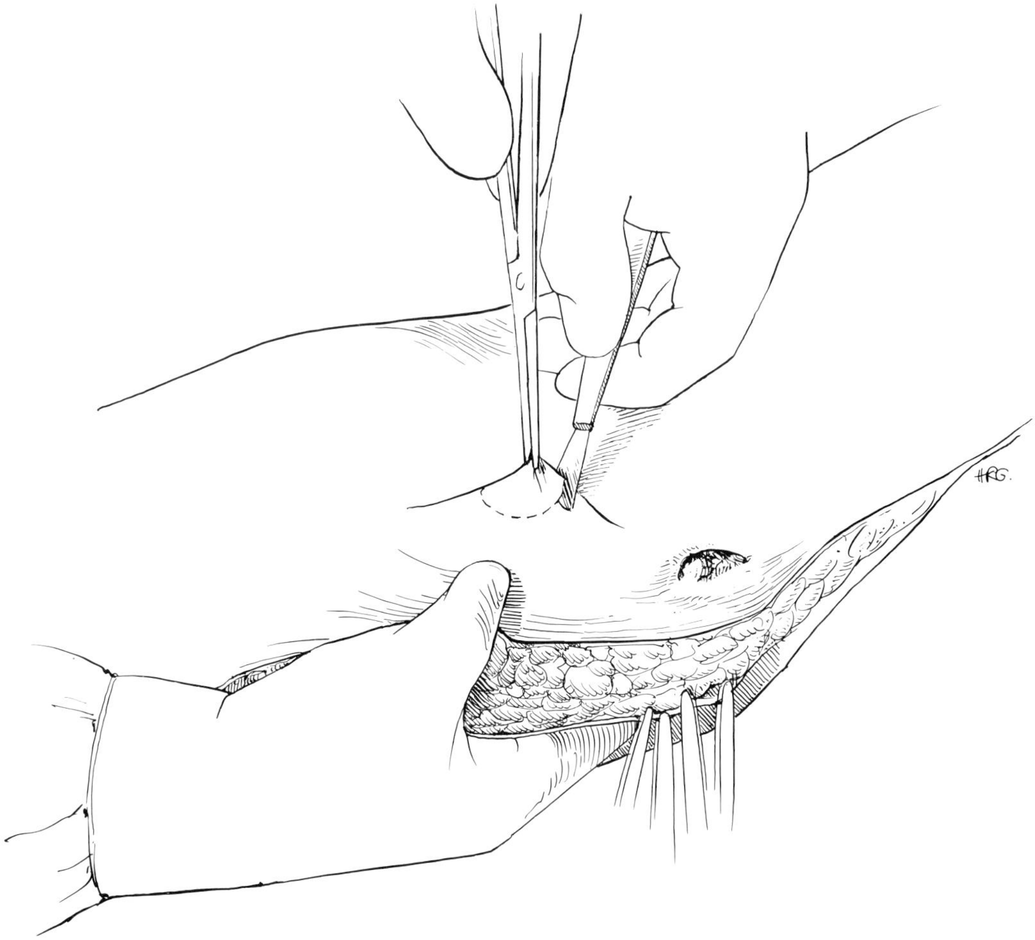

FIG. 27-20. Proctocolectomy and ileostomy. A button of skin is excised at the preselected site in right lower quadrant. Traction on fascia (clamps), skin and subcutaneous tissue (surgeon's thumb) assures straight path through abdominal wall.

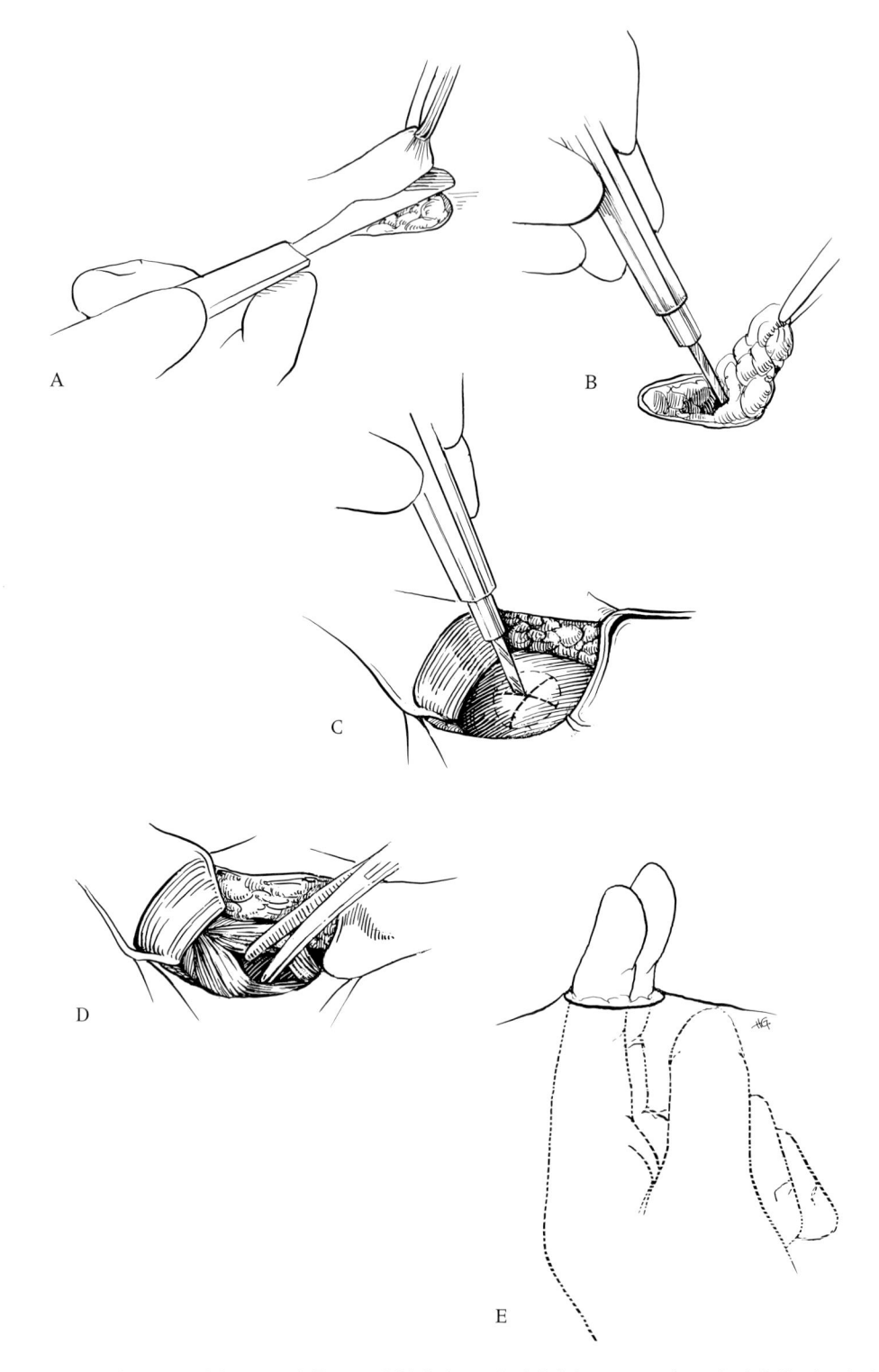

FIG. 27-21. Proctocolectomy and ileostomy. A: Button of skin being excised. B: Subcutaneous fat excised. C: Cruciate incision in fascia (with traction on fascia being maintained). "Dog ears" may be excised. D: Fibers of rectus abdominis muscle split. E: Opening to accommodate two fingers.

right flank. The opening is enlarged to approximately 1 1/2 to 2 fingers depending on the size of the fingers and the diameter of the ileum and its mesentery (Fig. 27-21E). Using an intestinal clamp placed from the outside in, the ileum is brought under the freed peritoneum through the opening for the ileostomy, care being taken not to twist the mesentery, which should lie in its normal orientation (Fig. 27-22A). The peritoneum must have been freed sufficiently to accommodate the mesentery comfortably. At this point, at least 3.5 to 4 cm of ileum must comfortably protrude above the level of the skin because the ileum must be turned back upon itself to "mature" the ileostomy (Fig. 27-22B). A completed ileostomy that projects about 2 cm above skin level is ideal. To maintain this degree of protrusion the mesentery should be fixed to the anterior fascia within the ileostomy wound by several sutures of chromic catgut (Fig. 21-22B). If the mesentery is oriented correctly, these sutures will be in the cephalad quadrant of the wound. The clamp on the intestine is underwrapped temporarily with moist gauze further to maintain the protrusion, and is fixed to the drape with a towel clamp to prevent torsion during reperitonealization and closure (Fig. 27-23). Reperitonealization is begun by sewing the cut edge of the lateral peritoneum to the ileal mesentery with interrupted fine silk sutures (Fig. 27-23). This line of sutures is continued onto the serosa of the intestine, with care being taken to place them superficially and not into the lumen lest a fistula result. The sutures continue caudally and then posteriorly beneath the ileum to close the medial peritoneum beneath the intes-

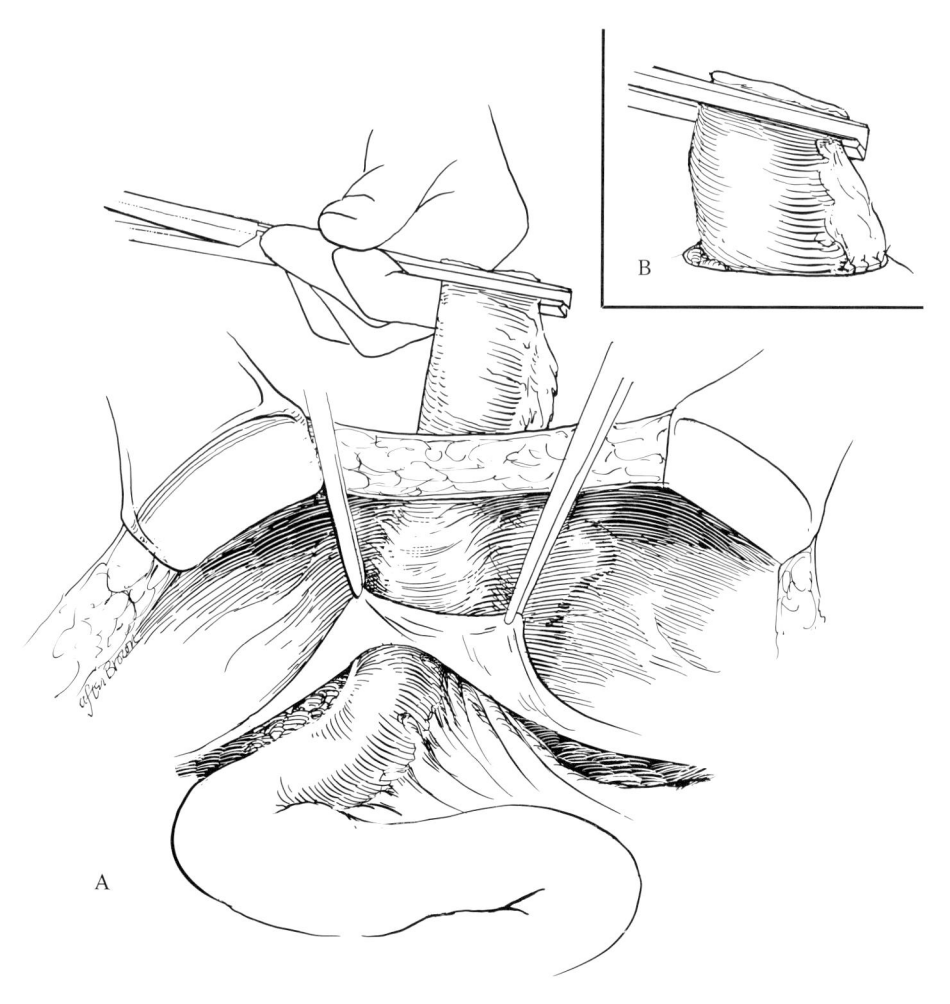

FIG. 27-22. Proctocolectomy and ileostomy. A: Ileum and mesentery drawn through retroperitoneal tunnel and abdominal wall. Note that mesentery lies comfortably within the freed peritoneum. B: Approximately 4 cm of ileum comfortably protrudes above the skin and the ileal mesentery has been sutured to the fascia within the aperture for the ileostomy. (After Goligher[178].)

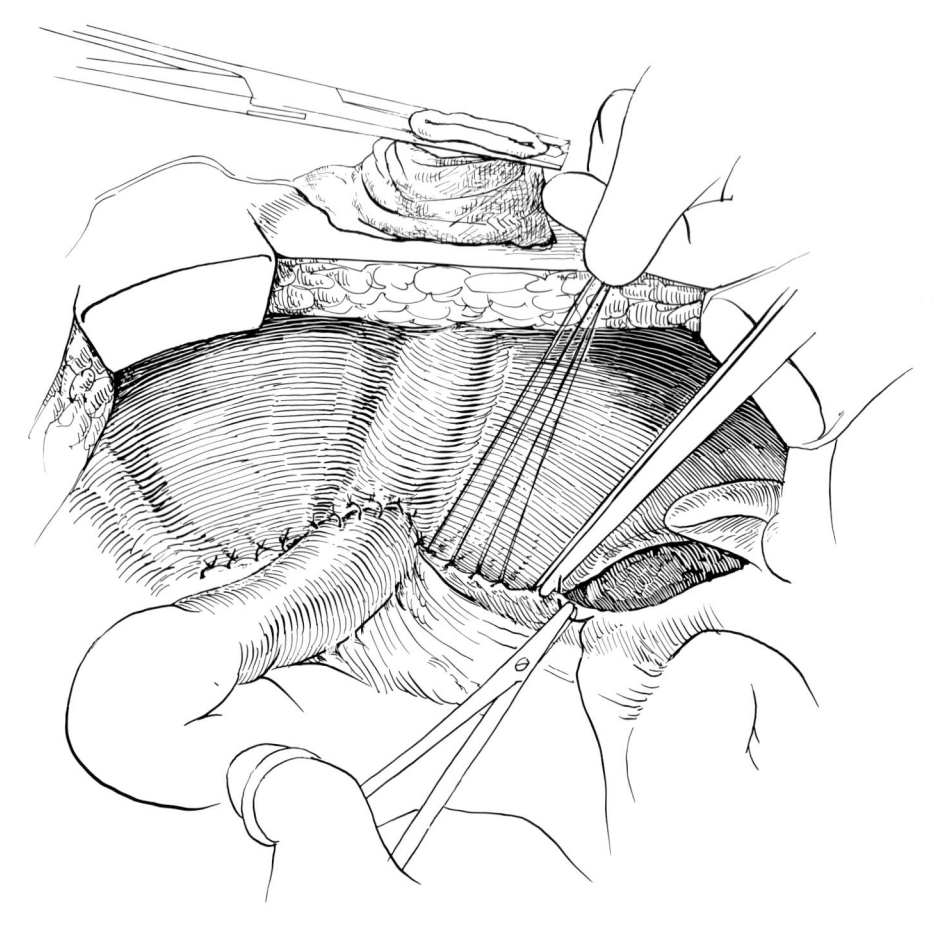

FIG. 27-23. Proctocolectomy and ileostomy. The clamp on the ileum has been temporarily underwrapped with gauze to maintain protrusion. The parietal peritoneum is sutured to the underlying ileal mesentery and ileum. Suture line is continuous with pelvic peritoneal closure. Not shown is continuation of sutures beneath (caudad and dorsad to) the ileum utilizing the pelvic peritoneum and transected right colon mesentery. Sutures must not enter lumen of ileum. (After Goligher[178].)

tine and its mesentery. If panproctocolectomy is being performed, the suture line is continuous with the closure of the peritoneal floor.

Brooke ileostomy. The siting and method of making the abdominal wound for the ileostomy are similar to those for an extraperitoneal ileostomy, except that the tract directly traverses the peritoneum that has been left intact. One has a little less latitude for error in establishing the diameter of the tract. In this technique, the large defect between the ileum and the lateral abdominal wall must be closed to prevent possible herniation of intestine into the trap and consequent small intestinal obstruction and strangulation. The cut edge of the ileal mesentery is sutured with interrupted silk to the lateral and anterior peritoneum. This suture line continues cephalad and is continuous with one that unites the cut edge of the right mesocolon to the lateral peritoneum to cover the denuded posterior parietes. Further sutures between the mesentery and the lateral peritoneum can often be placed caudad to the ileostomy to more securely and completely close the lateral defect. I place no sutures in the ileum itself as it emerges through the peritoneum, although this is practiced by others. If the latter is done care must be taken not to pierce the entire wall and enter the lumen. Secure fixation of the ileal mesentery and the reperitonealization of the right gutter (or the use of the retroperitoneal technique) probably are an important factor in the prevention of ileostomy prolapse that was seen commonly in the past.

"Maturation" of the Ileostomy. Although the abdomen is usually closed before this step is carried out, maturation of the ileostomy will be described at this point for the sake of clarity.

Currently, the Brooke technique, in which the entire wall is turned back on itself, is used by almost all surgeons, including me.[25] The mucosal grafting procedure of Crile and Turnbull, which is subject to the potential complications of devascularization and sloughing of the mucosa, is not particularly advantageous.[24] After the clamp is removed from the intestine by excising the crushed end (Fig. 27-24A), everting sutures are placed in each of four quadrants in the following manner. Using 3-0 chromic catgut on a small intestinal needle, a suture is taken either through the full thickness of skin or into the dermis, through the serosa and superficial muscle of the ileum at the level of the skin (the mesentery cranially), and finally through the full thickness of the cut end of the ileum (Fig. 27-24B). As the four sutures are tied, the ileum will become and remain everted (Fig. 27-24C and D). The remaining portion of the circumference of the cut end of ileum is joined to the skin or dermis with multiple interrupted sutures, thus completing the construction of the ileostomy. Because this step actually takes place after abdominal closure and with a sterile dressing or other form of wound protection already in place, it is permissible and desirable at this point to perform a digital examination of the ileostomy as a check on the adequacy of the lumen. An appliance is placed on the ileostomy as the final step in abdominal colectomy or the abdominal phase of a proctocolectomy (see Chapter 28).

It should be noted that the mesentery from the ileum to be used as the stoma is not ligated and removed for fear of devascularizing the intestine. This restriction in some cases tends to make the stoma somewhat bulbous cranially, with a tendency to flex in a cephalad direction. Both of these problems can be minimized by preserving the straight vessel paralleling the terminal ileum, as described earlier, and/or by division of a few arcades selected to interfere least with blood supply after carefully observing the pattern of blood vessels with the operating light shining through the mesentery. Every effort must be made to avoid a compromised blood supply to the ileum, and if this is recognized or suspected, the abdomen should be reopened and the ileostomy completely reconstructed if necessary. *A cyanotic ileostomy is a potential catastrophe.* Figure 27-25 shows a healed ileostomy ideally situated and with the proper amount of protrusion.

REPERITONEALIZATION AND CLOSURE OF THE ABDOMEN. Reperitonealization is begun after the ileum is brought through the abdominal wall for the ileostomy. First the pelvic floor is closed, usually with running synthetic absorbable sutures, interrupted in several places. The use of absorbable sutures for this purpose is advised because I treated a patient for a chronic perineal sinus that had persisted until silk sutures that were used for pelvic peritoneal closure and had become infected were removed. It is my custom to free the peritoneum over the pelvic floor to facilitate its descent in the presacral space. I believe that this descent is the mechanism by which normal obliteration of the presacral space takes place,[179,180] and, therefore, this maneuver may aid in the prevention of a persistent perineal sinus.[179] For the same theoretic reasons, others who employ primary closure of the perineal wound have, in some cases, left the pelvic peritoneal floor completely open and, interestingly, have not observed the late complication of perineal hernia.[181,182]

Frequently I reperitonealize the remainder of the raw surfaces in the abdomen using the mesocolon if this is sufficiently wide, although conceivably this practice might promote rather than prevent postoperative adhesions if one believes that the results of an experimental study of adhesion formation are applicable to this problem.[183] In doing completion proctectomies after abdominal colectomy and ileostomy, however, I have been pleased with the appearance of the serosal surfaces in my patients. I am particularly careful to suture the cut edge of omentum to the cut edge of the transverse mesocolon to leave no raw edges that may tether the distal stomach to the anterior abdominal wall and impair gastric emptying by producing an exaggerated "J" shape in a full stomach.

The abdomen is then closed (see earlier), a dressing is applied, and the ileostomy is matured as already described.

PERINEAL PHASE OF PROCTOCOLECTOMY. The patient is then ready for the perineal phase of the operation. This may be carried out with the patient in the Sim's, the lithotomy, or the jacknife (Buie) position, depending upon the preference of the surgeon and on any special local pathologic circumstances. After preparation, the anus is closed tightly with a heavy silk suture placed in a purse-string fashion. An incision around the anus is made that is rounded anteriorly and elliptical posteriorly (Fig. 27-26A). Although the excision of skin need not be excessive, it should be wide enough to completely excise the anal sphincters. A special attempt to minimize the

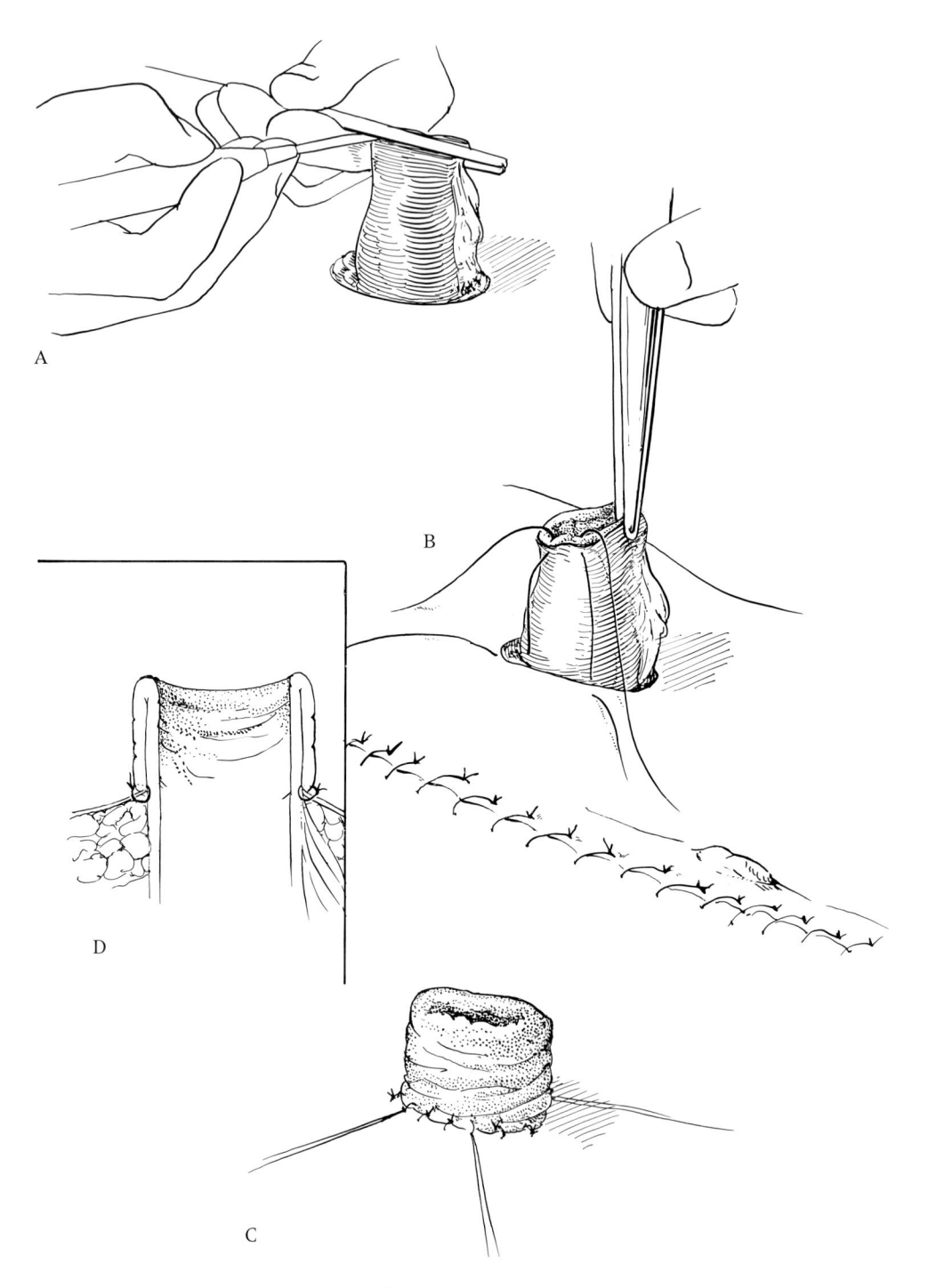

FIG. 27-24. Proctocolectomy and ileostomy. A: "Crush" produced by clamp is excised. B: Everting sutures of chromic catgut are placed in each of four quadrants, uniting skin (or dermis) with serosa and muscularis of ileum at skin level and the full thickness of cut end of ileum. C: After four quadrant everting sutures are tied, the rest of circumference is united to skin or dermis by interrupted sutures. D: Longitudinal section of completed ileostomy. Proper placement of sutures avoids entering the lumen and thus prevents a fistula.

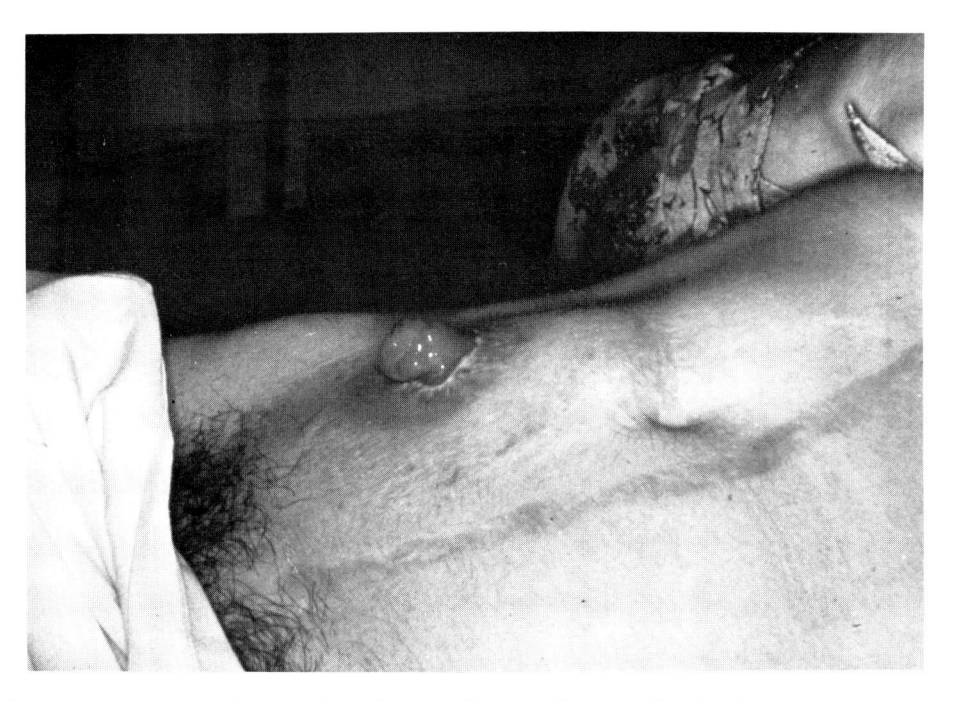

FIG. 27-25. Proctocolectomy and ileostomy. Example of a well situated ileostomy. The site takes into account the umbilicus, torso crease, and bony prominences. The approximately 2 cm protrusion is about ideal. Note the absence of excoriation of skin around the ileostomy.

perineal incision to somehow avoid persistent sinus is not advised and is not based on sound surgical principles. The incision is deepened and the inferior hemorrhoidal vessels are ligated on each side. The presacral space is entered in the midline over the coccyx (Fig. 27-26B) or, alternatively, the coccyx may be excised. The levators are divided relatively close to the rectum on each side in the absence of complicating cancer of the rectum (Fig. 27-26C). The rectum, with its attached rubber glove, is brought out posteriorly and then the anus and lower rectum are dissected from the urogenital diaphragm and the vagina or urethra (Fig. 27-26D). This is the most difficult step of the perineal phase of the operation, and special care must be taken to dissect in the proper plane and in the axis of the rectum to avoid entering either the rectum or the structures anterior to it.* Complete hemostasis is effected by the use of the electrosurgical unit and by vessel ligation and suture with absorbable material. Nonabsorbable sutures are avoided because if sepsis supervenes they may become an important factor in the development and persistence of a perineal sinus. The wound is irrigated with an antibiotic solution. A completed proctectomy is shown diagrammatically in Figure 27-27A.

MANAGEMENT OF THE PERINEAL WOUND. In the absence of perianal and perirectal sepsis and when contamination (as from entering the bowel) has not occurred, it is possible in most instances, after careful hemostasis, to close the perineal wound primarily.[179] I use two suction catheters (#28 plastic chest tubes) placed into the presacral space through anteriorly placed (so that the patient does not lie on the tubes) stab wounds in each buttock (Fig. 27-27B). Other methods of suction have been successfully employed,[181,182] and some surgeons have successfully closed the perineal wound without drainage.[184] No attempt is made to close the levator muscles, because a complete closure of the pelvic diaphragm is usually impossible. The skin edges are closed accurately by a subcuticular suture or synthetic absorbable material or nylon placed in a "pull-out" fashion. Stainless steel staples or sutures may be used in addition to achieve final perfect approximation of the skin (Fig. 27-26B), and then a sterile dressing is applied. The catheters are placed on constant suction at about minus 30 mm Hg pressure by way of a sterile closed system. A

*Editors' note: See also, Berry, A. R., et al.: Br. J. Surg. 73:675, 1985.

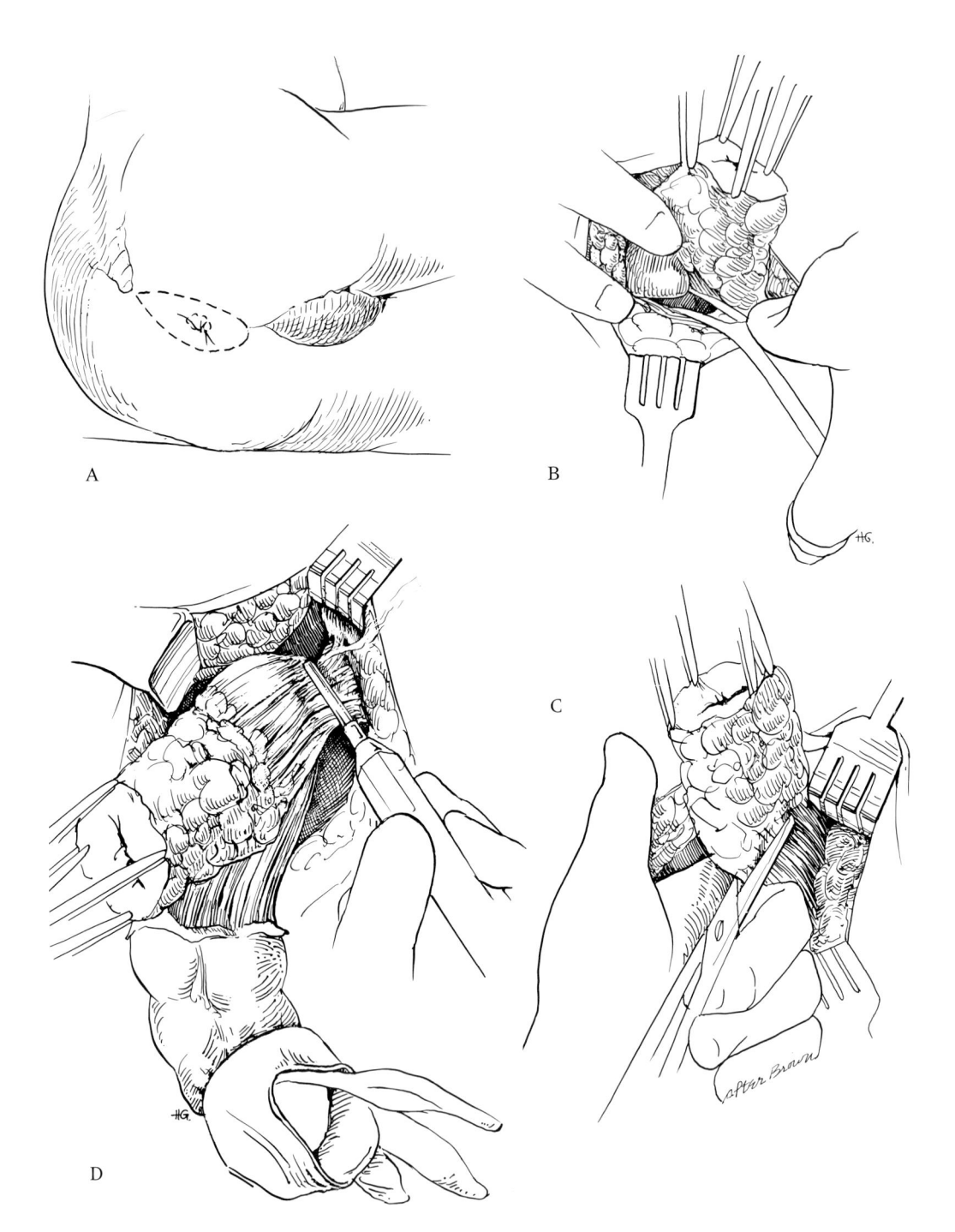

FIG. 27-26. Proctocolectomy and ileostomy. Perineal phase of operation is shown being carried out in Sim's position. A: An ellipse of skin and subcutaneous tissue is excised around the anus, which has been closed by a heavy purse-string suture. B: The dissection is deepened and encompasses the sphincters. Posterior plane which was established in abdominal dissection is entered over the tip of the coccyx (optionally coccyx may be excised). C: Levator ani muscles are divided on each side, close to the rectum. D: The rectal stump with attached rubber glove has been delivered posteriorly and the anterior attachments of the urogenital diaphragm to the rectum are divided, taking care not to enter the rectum.

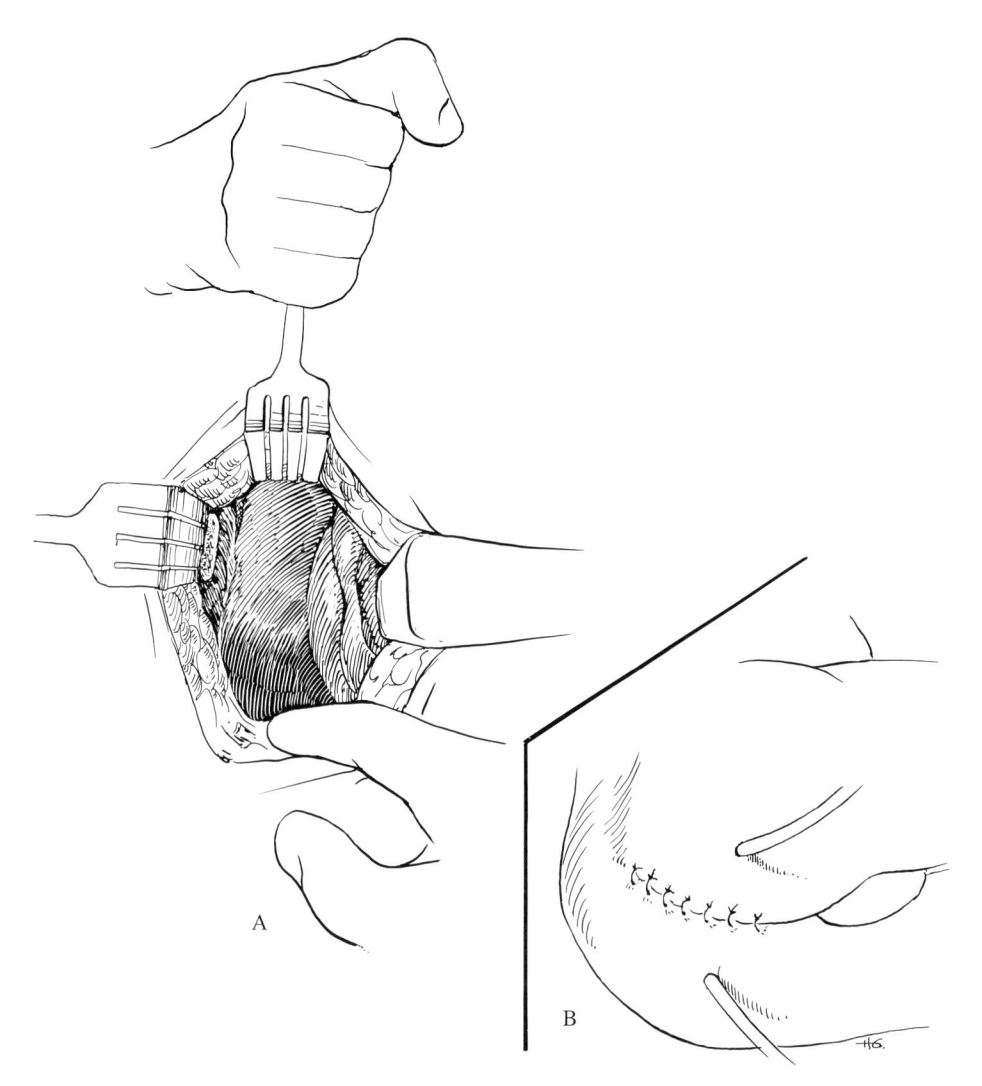

FIG. 27-27. Proctocolectomy and ileostomy. A: Completed perineal phase of dissection is shown. The tip of the sacrum is seen posteriorly (coccyx was removed in this case for ease of exposure); also seen are the prostate, seminal vesicles and bladder. B: Completed closure with suction catheters in place (see text).

closed system for irrigation with sterile saline can also be incorporated. This can be helpful in irrigating out blood and blood clots that appear no matter how "dry" the field appears at the conclusion of the operation.

In the presence of perirectal sepsis and fistulas, each of the tracts is located and either laid open or preferably excised completely, including the fibrotic wall. Two 1-inch, soft rubber drains are placed in the sacral hollow and sutured to the skin. The perineal wound is never closed under these circumstances. Although these wounds are enormous and gaping, they often heal with astounding rapidity, given proper aftercare. Premature closure of the skin before obliteration of the typical presacral space may lead to persistent perineal sinus so that the wide resultant opening after laying open the tracts is an advantage rather than a detriment when extensive perineal sepsis is present.

Even in the absence of perineal sepsis, if primary closure is not elected (e.g., because of contamination) I have given up the practice of partially closing the skin around the rubber drains placed in the sacral hollow. Because these drains are placed to promote drainage, it would seem logical to facilitate free drainage by leaving the skin wide open. Partial skin closure serves only to prevent ready access to the deep portion of the wound for dressings and irrigations, and to potentiate the development of a persistent perineal sinus, one of the features of which is a small external opening in the presence of a long, deep wound.

Secondary (Completion) Proctectomy

The removal of the rectum after a staged panproctocolectomy requires an abdominoperineal operation. Attempts to perform a proctectomy from a solely perineal approach are hazardous, even if the initial phase has left only a small rectal remnant.

The ileostomy is draped out of the field. The skin about the mucous fistula is incised as an ellipse and closed over the mucosa. Instruments and gloves are discarded and a partial repreparation of the skin is carried out. The old incision is opened in its lower portion, excising a wide skin scar if present and deemed advisable. The abdomen is entered and the mucous fistula is freed by dissection from the outside and inside. Once the lower rectosigmoid is mobilized, the dissection and conduct of the remaining portion of the operation are identical to those described previously for the one-stage operation.

Segmental Operations in Crohn's Disease Involving the Colon

In patients with a distribution of disease amenable to restoration of intestinal continuity, consider the following facts and principles: (1) given discontinuous disease (i.e., two isolated segments requiring extirpation), a single resection encompassing the two areas of involvement is preferred to a double resection (if the two segments are relatively close together) to avoid the added risk of two intestinal anastomoses; (2) segmental colonic resection compared with ileocolonic resection appears to have a higher rate of recurrence;[185] (3) the extent of resection is dictated by the extent of disease and not by principles appropriate for cancer therapy; and (4) the results of bypass for the treatment of colonic Crohn's disease have not been favorable.[185] A possible exception to the last principle is the apparent good response of some cases of colonic Crohn's disease to diversionary ileostomy, although clearly this procedure is not generally embraced as an effective operation.[17,18,186-188]

Some of these principles may have to be violated because of the extent, severity, and distribution of the disease. For example, it is not uncommon to find severely diseased ileum together with a skip segment of involvement in the sigmoid colon. For this pattern of involvement, it is preferable to perform an ileocolic resection (as for classic Crohn's disease), together with a separate sigmoid resection.

The best long-term results of segmental resection for Crohn's disease in our experience have been in the right ileocolic distribution of disease. The technique of ileocolic resection has been described earlier, and, as indicated, the distal margin of resection is determined by the distal extent of disease and not by arbitrary levels dictated by patterns of vascular supply or lymphatic drainage, as might pertain in resections for cancer.

Despite the reportedly high rate of recurrence after segmental colon resection with colocolostomy, it would be difficult to justify on this basis a more extensive operation than the appropriate local resection of the disease. After resection of the diseased area and a small margin of normal colon proximal and distal, an end-to-end colocolostomy is performed. Major blood vessels do not need to be ligated in the mesentery as for resection for cancer, so that the excision can be limited to that necessary to remove the disease. The small mesenteric defect is closed with interrupted or running sutures.

Resection and Ileoproctostomy

This procedure has been used in both ulcerative colitis and in Crohn's disease of the colon. In my view, the Aylett procedure is indicated in Crohn's disease only if the rectum appears to be entirely uninvolved. In ulcerative colitis, however, this procedure should be used only for the patient with relatively quiescent disease in the rectal segment, whether such subsidence has occurred spontaneously or after a previous subtotal colectomy and ileostomy. It is not wise to perform this procedure for a patient with proximal colonic carcinoma or for one at high risk for the development of carcinoma.

One further point merits discussion in conjunction with the selection of patients for the Aylett operation. Proctitis can develop in patients with proximal diversion from colostomy or ileostomy, an entity that I have termed "diversion colitis."[189] I have observed a number of patients, including some with Crohn's disease, whose treatment suffered from the false attribution of these changes to idiopathic inflammatory bowel disease. Korelitz and associates have documented the dramatic reversal of severe inflammatory changes in the diverted rectum of some patients with Crohn's disease following reconstitution of intestinal continuity.[190] The differentiation of diversion colitis from idiopathic inflammatory bowel disease can be difficult. The changes of diversion colitis are focal, superficial, and nonspecific; for example, the presence of noncaseating granulomas and sinus tracts is not compatible with this diagnosis. Although the inflammatory reaction is usually not prominent, aphthous ulceration, erosions, and a certain degree of nodularity have been documented as manifestations of diversion colitis.[190,191]

In performing an Aylett operation, the mobilization and resection of the colon are almost identical to that of a subtotal colectomy but the dissection proceeds more distally. Although Aylett makes a point of ligating the superior hemorrhoidal artery for a supposed beneficial effect on the rectal disease, this step is omitted by many other surgeons, including me, because it would not seem to be based on sound principles.[36,66] The anastomosis is performed in the intraperitoneal rectum, just above the peritoneal reflection. The rectum is not mobilized from the sacral hollow, especially in male patients to avoid interfering with ejaculatory function. I use a two layer open anastomosis as in any restorative operation. I use neither drains nor sumps to "protect" the anastomosis in the performance of the Aylett operation, but hasten to add that I consider them superfluous and deleterious after intestinal anastomoses in general. Although many surgeons who perform this procedure use a temporary diversionary loop ileostomy to protect the anastomosis,[36,66] I do not routinely use diversion, in part because of the type of case selected for the operation.

Diversionary Ileostomy in Crohn's Disease

I consider the merits of diversionary ileostomy to be sub judice. The reader is referred to accounts by Oberhelman et al., Lee, and McIlrath for the technical details of their procedure and their results.[17,186,187]

Kock's Ileostomy

Kelly and Dozois discuss this procedure and their technique in Chapter 29.

Ileoanal Pull-through Procedures

The techniques used in the performance of various types of ileoanal pull-through procedures are discussed by Kelly and Dozois in Chapter 29.

Toxic Megacolon and Fulminating Colitis

The management and timing of operation in toxic megacolon and fulminating colitis are discussed in Chapters 14, 21, and 22. Perhaps because of a policy of prompt operative intervention, if a limited course of intensive nonoperative treatment fails I have had to deal with relatively few preoperative or intraoperative perforations.[192] Possibly for the same reason, it has not been necessary to modify operative strategy for the patient with toxic megacolon or fulminating colitis, that is, colectomy and ileostomy have been used in preference to venting of the colon by the multiple "ostomy" procedure or other techniques (Fig. 27-28).[10,193]

In the presence of a preoperative or an intraoperative perforation of the colon, the ileostomy probably should be fashioned by the conventional rather than the retroperitoneal technique to avoid retroperitoneal contamination. Because patients with toxic megacolon are usually

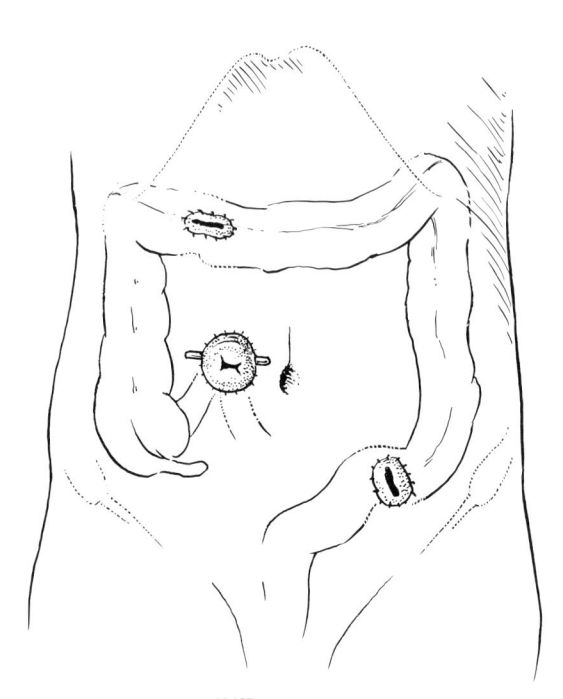

FIG. 27-28. Turnbull's[10,193] multiple-ostomy procedure proposed as alternative to colectomy and ileostomy in severe toxic megacolon. The grossly distended colon has been vented with sigmoidostomy and transversostomy. A loop ileostomy has been established and matured by suture to the skin over a rod in such a manner that the proximal end is "dominant."

extremely ill, I generally prefer a two-stage colectomy. The presence of preoperative or intraoperative perforation would be an additional factor in favor of the two-stage approach because of the fear that the pelvic retroperitoneum could be unnecessarily exposed to contamination. On the other hand, if colonic hemorrhage is one of the manifestations leading to emergency operation, strong consideration should be given to panproctocolectomy because I have seen a number of such patients who required an emergency proctectomy for severe rectal bleeding in the immediate postoperative period. Gentle handling of the colon during operation, especially in dissection about the splenic flexure, is even more mandatory in the presence of toxic megacolon than in the usual elective colectomy. Rough, cavalier technique incurs serious risk of a devastating intraoperative perforation.

Although colectomy is safe in the majority of patients, Turnbull's multiple "ostomy" procedure may be applicable to some patients with a grossly distended colon. For this reason, a diagram depicting the technical goal of the procedure is found in Figure 27-28 and the reader is referred to papers by Turnbull and colleagues on the rationale, technique, and method of management.[10,193]

Postoperative Care

The postoperative care of patients with inflammatory bowel disease differs only in detail from that appropriate for other patients undergoing major abdominal procedures. Most patients will have received corticosteroid treatment, and therefore, these agents must be administered postoperatively and gradually tapered in accordance with a flexible schedule to avoid Addisonian crisis, such as that in Table 27-2. In most cases I prefer to use the intramuscular route of administration to maintain adequate blood levels at all times and because of pragmatic considerations including ease of administration, less chance for missed doses, and inadvertent subcutaneous infiltrations of intravenous infusions. Because the effect of an intravenous bolus of hydrocortisone lasts only about 1 1/2 hours, I do not employ bolus administration and consider it relatively contraindicated. On the other hand, intravenous administration of corticosteroids in a continuous infusion is at least as effective as intramuscular use and, provided an infusion pump is used, this is a perfectly acceptable practice. The dose of corticosteroids should be tapered with all reasonable speed, but it is generally wise to avoid total cessation of steroids until it is clear that no major complications have occurred, gastrointestinal function has returned to the point that a full diet can be tolerated, and the patient is fully ambulatory. Until then the patient should be maintained on the equivalent of 75 to 100 mg hydrocortisone/24 hours.

The period of postoperative ileus in some of these patients may be prolonged, and therefore oral feedings should not be begun according to any predetermined routine, but rather on the basis of the degree of return of gastrointestinal function. The discomfort and the adverse effects on pulmonary toilet of prolonged nasogastric suction may be better tolerated by the patient than are grossly distended loops of intestine. In the clinical assessment of postoperative ileus in patients after a total colectomy, it must be emphasized that abdominal distension may be minimal in the face of considerable small intestine dilatation.

Fluid and electrolyte replacement requirements are best monitored and estimated on the basis of a flow sheet on which is recorded the daily intake and output as well as the body weight measured each morning. In Figure 27-29 an example of a completed flow sheet is reproduced from the chart of a patient who underwent a subtotal colectomy and ileostomy. The weights and the fluid balance data serve as checks on each other, especially in view of the errors inherent in such measurements on a clinical surgical floor. Extrarenal losses of sodium and potassium must be estimated and replaced. Because of the mineralocorticoid effect of high-dose corticosteroid treatment, urinary potassium losses requiring replacement are greater than the usual 30 to 40 mEq/24 hours.

In purely abdominal operations, if an indwelling catheter is used it can be withdrawn on the first or second postoperative day when the patient is fully alert, hemodynamically stable, and the need to monitor urine output closely is no longer present. Even after proctectomy, the catheter can usually be removed earlier than after the same operation done for carcinoma because the pelvic dissection is carried out close to the wall of the rectum, and because prostatism is not a problem in the usual age group in which inflammatory bowel disease occurs. Because of the presence of perineal dressings and suction catheters, however, the logistics of voiding, particularly in females, can be trying, so that it is best to delay removal of the catheter until the perineal suction catheters are

FIG. 27-29. Intake and output flow sheet of patient who underwent subtotal colectomy and ileostomy for a severe and unrelenting relapse of chronic ulcerative colitis.

removed at about 5 days. In patients in whom the ability to void is questionable, it may be helpful to instill into the bladder 200 ml of sterile saline or an antibiotic solution before removing the urethral catheter, so that it can be determined immediately whether or not the patient is able to void without significant urinary residual.

A normally functioning, well-established ileostomy discharges 400 to 600 ml of fluid per day. In the early postoperative phase, however, losses of 800 to 1000 ml/24 hours are neither unusual nor a cause for alarm.[28] Losses in excess of 1000 ml suggest low-grade intestinal obstruction or may result from a proximally placed ileostomy. The losses are likely to be nearly isotonic with respect to body fluid, with the potassium content as high as 15 to 19 mEq/liter. If high output from an ileostomy is persistent, estimates of proper replacement therapy are greatly aided by analysis of a sample of ileostomy effluent for sodium, potassium, and chloride concentrations, determinations that can easily be done in any hospital clinical biochemistry laboratory. Bicarbonate losses can be estimated by calculation of the difference between the measured cations and anions. Patients with Crohn's disease having had long ileal resections, with or without ileostomy, may require some slowing of intestinal transit with codeine, deodorized tincture of opium, loperamide, or diphenoxylate-HCl, but this type of therapy is best deferred until normal intestinal function has returned unequivocally.

In the absence of demonstrated symptomatic abnormalities such as lactose intolerance or other malabsorption syndromes, special diets are not necessary for patients with inflammatory bowel disease. After either ileostomy or anastomosis, however, the patient is instructed to avoid excesses of food with undigestible residue such as corn, nuts, olives, raw fruit, and vegetables that might obstruct a relatively narrow segment of bowel such as the ileostomy or the site of the intestinal anastomosis.

Although in the absence of a proctectomy most patients are ambulatory on the first postoperative day, I continue prophylaxis for thromboembolic complications (such as "minidose" heparin) while the patient is in the hospital. This type of therapy is particularly indicated in patients after proctectomy who are confined to bed by the perineal suction catheters, one disadvantage of the method. Many surgeons for fear of disruption of the closed peritoneal floor restrict patients to bed for as long or longer than the 5-day-period that these tubes generally remain in place, however.

In patients with open perineal wounds, the drains should be removed about 7 days postoperatively, at which time irrigations of the perineal wound with saline should be begun. The wound should not be packed but, rather, a small amount of sterile gauze, changed several times a day, should be used to keep the edges separated to permit drainage. Later, it is mandatory for the surgeon to inspect these wounds weekly, or at least biweekly, to prevent premature bridging of superficial tissues and to promote healing by excising and cauterizing exuberant granulation tissue. At these times, hair at the edges of the wound should be shaved, instructions to the patient and family may be reiterated and reenforced, and minor changes in the method of dressing are made as necessary. The importance of such frequent inspection and care of the wound by the surgeon cannot be overemphasized, because persistent perineal sinus is more likely to occur when these tasks are relegated to those less knowledgeable of wound healing.

The management of the ileostomy has been simplified by a variety of new products that are helpful in implementing good ileostomy care. Chapter 28 is devoted to this subject. The essential principle is that the ileostomy effluent that is capable of digesting skin must never be allowed contact with the integument. Disposable Stomahesive* or karaya ring types of ileostomy appliances are extremely convenient for early postoperative care, and most patients can learn this technique with minimal difficulty. It is unusual at the present time for severe peristomal skin irritation to occur. When this does occur it usually reflects poor application technique or a local problem about the ileostomy such as a scar, a depression, an insufficiently protuberant ileostomy, or it represents a monilial infection. Peristomal skin irritation can be treated with a light dusting of karaya or nystatin powder followed by a skin sealant such as Skin Prep* and the application of "Stomahesive" type appliance with appropriate "build up" of depressions and the peristomal area with Stomahesive paste. Nonallergic adhesive tape placed around the periphery of the Stomahesive adds additional security.

Postoperative Complications

Chapter 30 is devoted to the diagnosis, prevention, and treatment of postoperative complications. It may be helpful, however, to comment upon two particularly troublesome ones in which my colleagues and I have had a special interest—the persistent perineal sinus and prestomal ileitis.

Persistent Perineal Sinus

The perineal wound closes and heals after proctectomy because the pelvic cavity is obliterated, not by granulation, but rather by a downward descent of the peritoneal floor and, to some extent, by the posterior movement of the urogenital structures anteriorly and by upward descent of the soft tissue of the perineum.[179] Our technique of primary closure of the perineal wound is based on these principles,[279] and it seems reasonable to believe that the descent of the peritoneum is aided and hastened by the suction catheters (Fig. 27-30). If primary closure is not employed, any factor such as packing or sepsis that delays descent and prolongs healing results in a thick-walled, rigid tract that cannot close because of its unyielding walls. The result is the development of a chronic sinus.[179] Analogous to the management of a thoracic empyema, in which healing occurs after adequate drainage by unroofing the rigid bony structures, marsupialization of a chronic perineal sinus may require excision of the coccyx and even the lower portion of the sacrum. Figure 27-31 depicts the

---

*E. R. Squibb Co.: Princeton, NJ 08540.

*United Surgical Co.: Largo, FL 33540.

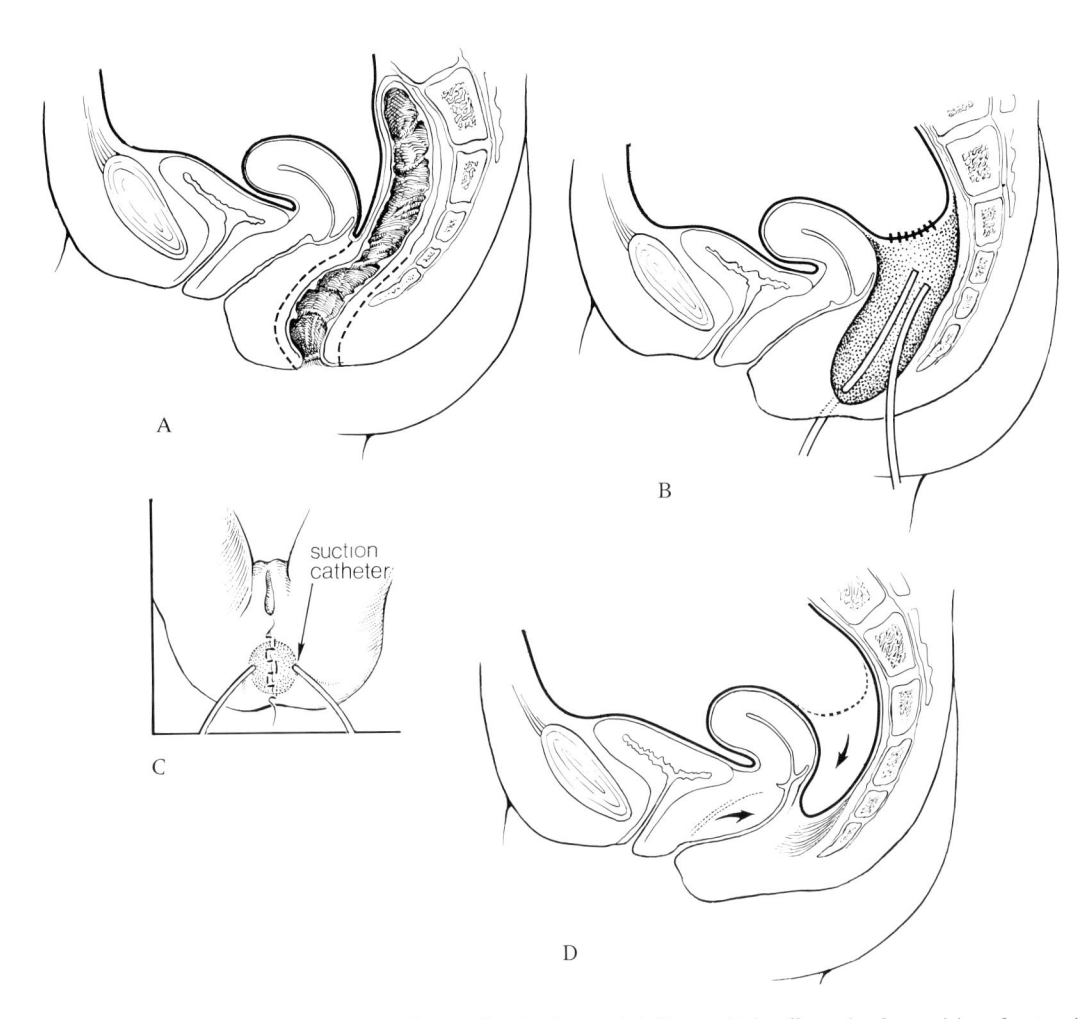

FIG. 27-30. Illustration of concept of primary closure of perineal wound. A: Space which will remain after excision of rectum is shown by dotted lines. B: Closure of pelvic peritoneum leaves a large space surrounded by totally unyielding bony walls posteriorly and laterally and by the relatively unyielding urogenital structures anteriorly. When primary closure is employed, the space is drained by large suction catheters (B,C). The space closes in large measure by descent of the pelvic peritoneum and to some extent by posterior displacement of the urogenital structures and upward movement of the perineum (D). (After Silen and Glotzer[179].)

steps in such an operation. A large defect results, but this remains clean, granulates beautifully, and heals usually within six months, a small price to pay for cure of such a devastating and persistent complication. Figure 27-32 shows a healed perineal wound after the unroofing operation. In our experience, failures of this technique are few, although some wounds require infinite patience on the part of the patient and the surgeon. Rarely, a large and chronic sinus or additional complicating factors may require the use of a more extensive procedure.[194] In these cases a definite place for obliterating the space (after debridement) exists, using well-oxgenated tissue in the form of muscular or myocutaneous flaps.[195-198]

Ileostomy Dysfunction and Prestomal Ileitis

A definitive exposition of ileostomy dysfunction and prestomal ileitis cannot be provided because of a lack of quantitative clinical studies done subsequent to the recognition of Crohn's disease of the colon. Prior to the 1950's, ileostomies were fashioned simply by bringing the ileum directly through the abdominal wall without primary suture of the intestine to the skin. The ileum was held in place by one means or another until the intestine became firmly adherent to the abdominal wall. The exposed serosa of the intestine developed granulation tissue on its surface, and over 4 to 6 weeks gradually

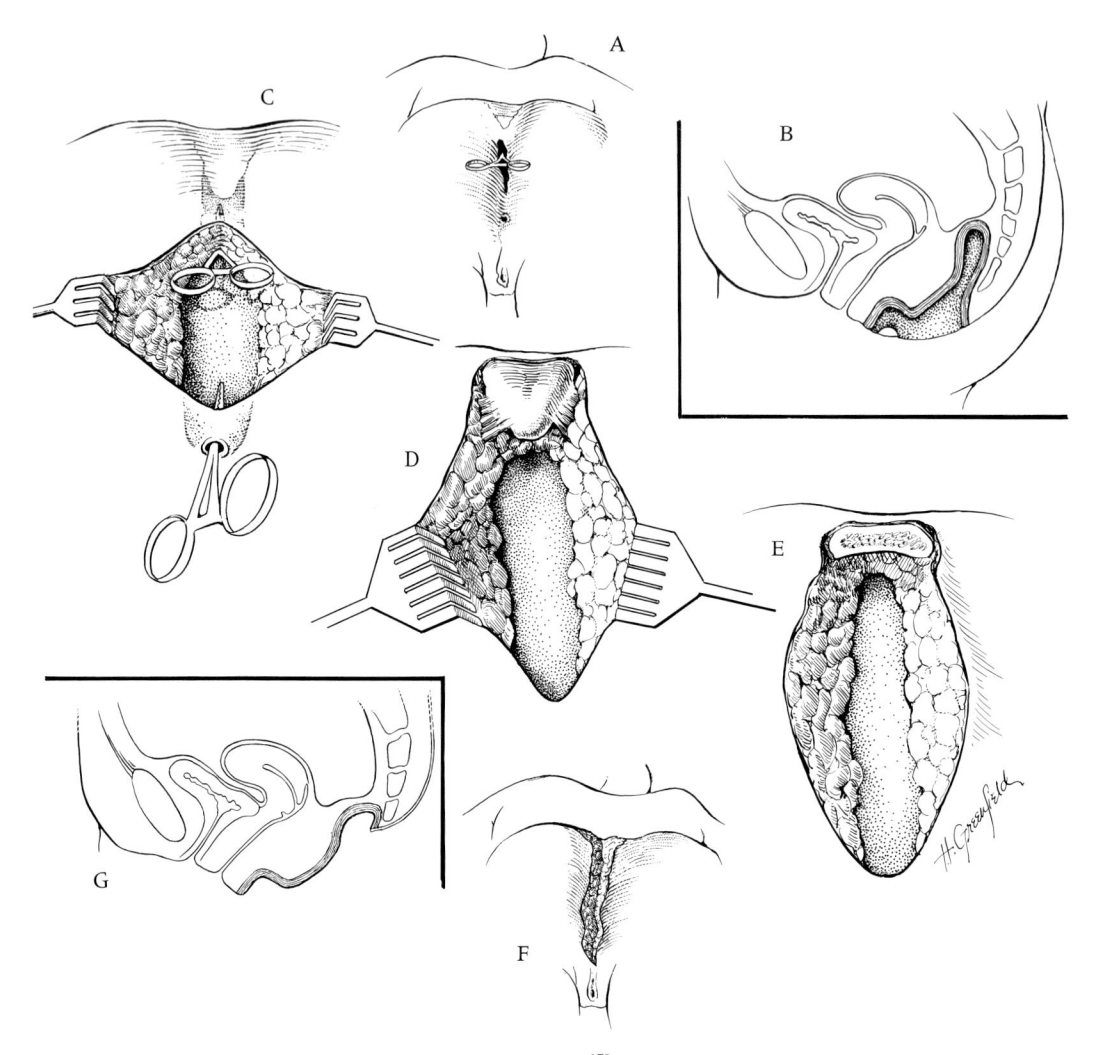

FIG. 27-31. Operation for persistent perineal sinus (Silen and Glotzer[179]). A: Hemostat placed in tract, which extends anterior to coccyx and sacrum. B: Tract in sagittal section showing the cephalad extent covered by unyielding coccyx and lower sacrum. C: Tract partially unroofed. D: Soft tissue portion of tract completely unroofed, but portion beneath coccyx and sacrum still covered. E: When coccyx and lower portion of sacrum are removed, the sinus is completely unroofed (F,G).

healed by approximation of the mucosa to the skin by eversion of the mucosa, a process termed "maturation" of the ileostomy.[24] It was also recognized that a protuberant, spout-like stoma was desirable and necessary to facilitate discharge of effluent from the ileostomy into an appliance, and to protect the peristomal skin. The skin-grafted ileostomy described by Dragstedt et al. represented an attempt to achieve the goal of a trouble-free ileostomy, but the grafted skin was no more resistant to digestion than the peristomal skin.[199] Warren and McKittrick described a syndrome of ileostomy dysfunction that occurred in more than 60% of their patients with nonmatured ileostomies.[200] These workers, along with Crile and Turnbull, Fleishner and Mandelstam, and others, elucidated the mechanism and sequelae of the established syndrome and its treatment and prevention.[24,201] The syndrome of ileostomy dysfunction is described briefly in the following. In the early postoperative period, patients often developed abdominal cramps and severe ileostomy diarrhea, which was often so copious (in excess of 5 liters/24 hours) that hypovolemic shock occurred if replacement of fluid and electrolytes was inadequate. The cramps and diarrhea could be alleviated by catheterization of the ileostomy. The mechanism therefore was thought to be a partial and functional obstruction secondary to a serositis of the exposed serosa of the ileum, with an inability of the muscu-

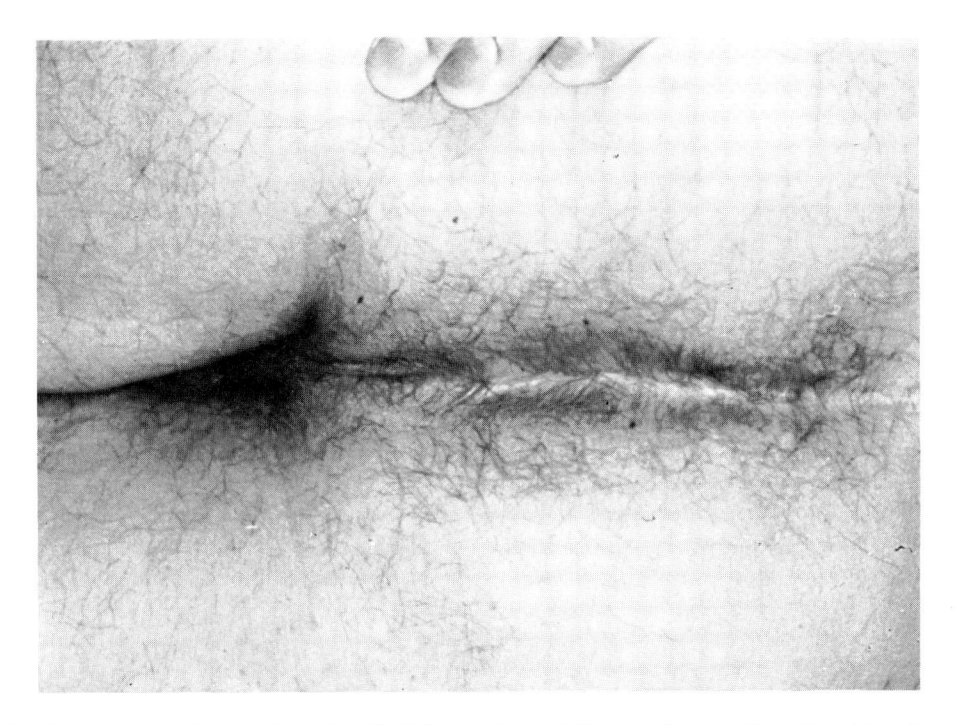

FIG. 27-32. Operation for persistent perineal sinus. Healed perineal wound after unroofing operation with excision of coccyx and portion of sacrum.

lar propulsive effort to the ileum to overcome the resistance of the narrowed stoma. Patients with established ileostomies were subject to periodic bouts of a similar type, thought to be produced by a decompensation of the balance between propulsive activity and obstruction secondary to a circumferential cicatricial stenosis, usually at the skin and subcutaneous level. Crile and Turnbull and Warren and McKittrick described the surgical relief of this syndrome by radial incision of the granulation tissue collar or by excision of the cicatricial band.[24, 200] Moreover, the classical contribution of Crile and Turnbull described the prevention of both the acute and the recurring syndrome by means of a primary surgical maturation of the ileostomy in which a segment of ileum, denuded of its serosa and muscularis, is turned back upon itself to produce a mucosa-covered ileostomy.[24] One year earlier, Brooke described his method of maturation of the ileostomy in which the full thickness of ileum is turned back upon itself and sutured to the skin.[25] It is not clear whether Brooke had in mind the prevention of the aforementioned morbid sequence, but his procedure has been universally accepted as the procedure of choice. In fact, the eponym, Brooke ileostomy, is generally used to denote conventional as opposed to continent ileostomy (Kock's pouch). Primary maturation of the ileostomy with per primam healing between the skin and ileum has obviated a great deal of morbidity after ileostomy, and, in the view of some, has eliminated entirely subsequent mechanical problems with the ileostomy.

It was recognized by numerous authors that some patients with ileostomy dysfunction developed ileitis in the prestomal ileum, about 8% in the experience of Warren and McKittrick.[200] This was of variable severity and longitudinal extent, and could lead to perforation, peritonitis, and even death. Various etiologies were suggested, including the possibility (which could not be substantiated) that prestomal ileitis was a continuation of "backwash" ileitis or an extension to the ileum of the underlying inflammatory process that had involved the colon. The concept gradually evolved, and was accepted, that this complication was secondary to ileostomy dysfunction. Certainly, the clearest clinical example supporting this point of view (and one in which there can be no implication of recurrence or persistence of an underlying inflammatory process) is the development of ileitis after colectomy for familial polyposis.[177,202,203] Obstructive colitis is probably another example of the same biologic phenomenon.[204,205]

The syndrome of ileostomy dysfunction and

dysfunctional ileitis was mainly described before the definitive and widespread recognition that Crohn's disease often involves the colon and can mimic, to a greater or lesser extent, ulcerative colitis. Nevertheless, as far back as Counsell's excellent publication,[177] it was recognized that some ileal inflammation after colectomy was granulomatous. Thayer and Spiro's paper on prestomal ileitis and that by Turnbull et al., both of which appeared before the heyday of Crohn's disease, left the etiology of most postcolectomy ileitis ambiguous.[206,207] It is now clear that many cases are instances of recurrent Crohn's disease in the ileum. The appearance of the ileum on x-ray study, at inspection at operation, or on gross pathologic examination can be absolutely typical of regional enteritis. Moreover, the microscopic finding of noncaseating granulomas or sinus tracts and, in most cases, the development of peristomal fistula are further evidence for recurrent Crohn's disease. With the acceptance of Crohn's disease of the colon as an entity and the advent of the matured ileostomy, however, it is now frequently assumed, either tacitly or expressly, that dysfunction of the ileostomy cannot occur, and that ileitis in the ileum after colectomy is, perforce, Crohn's disease. Knill-Jones, Morson, and Williams described two types of ileitis after colectomy for what was specifically diagnosed as ulcerative colitis however.[208] The first is an acute type that tends to occur early in the postoperative period and that requires operation because of a propensity for perforation. A second, latent type runs a more chronic course and may respond to steroids or limited resection. These authors felt that obstruction was not a pathogenetic factor (although dilatation of the ileum was common) and suggested that Crohn's disease was excluded by the pathologic findings both in the original colonic specimen and in the resected ileum. Adson et al. described a number of cases of ileitis after colectomy, the pathology of which reproduced that in the original colonic disease.[209] It was not made clear, however, whether all the ileostomies had been primarily sutured. Although Turnbull at first was vague on the subject of etiology,[207] he later felt that the acute type was of unknown etiology but that the latent type always resulted from Crohn's disease.[1] Menguy has even suggested that all postileostomy ileal inflammation is secondary to Crohn's disease and that if ileitis occurs, the original diagnosis of ulcerative colitis should be changed to Crohn's disease.[210] The following expresses this widely held point of view: (1) ulcerative colitis is always cured by operation, (2) primary maturation of the ileostomy prevents dysfunction of the ileostomy, and, (3) because recurrence is a more or less universal feature of Crohn's disease, any ileitis that develops after ileostomy establishes the diagnosis of Crohn's disease. This self-fulfilling prophesy cannot be disproved if the premises of the argument are accepted; however, we have encountered many instances of minimal or even extensive enteritis after colectomy for what clearly was ulcerative colitis by all recognized criteria. While most of these cases occurred before maturation of the ileostomy was practiced, others developed despite primary suture of the ileostomy. It is logical to surmise that the same morbid sequence must occur after colectomy for Crohn's disease. Thus, in many cases, the etiology of postcolectomy ileitis will remain extremely ambiguous. As a matter of fact, my long-term follow-up studies of Crohn's disease and ulcerative colitis showed that the incidence of ileostomy revision was not significantly higher in Crohn's disease when the diagnosis of the latter was made on the basis of combined clinical and histologic criteria.[95,96]

In light of the considerations just discussed, the following classification of prestomal ileitis must be recognized as being tentative.

Acute Prestomal Ileitis

The clinical picture includes abdominal cramps, distension, tenderness, fever, tachycardia, and copious malodorous ileostomy output. Digital examination of the ileostomy, x-ray study, and endoscopic examination may reveal ulceration. Because of the threat of perforation, prompt laparotomy, resection, and fashioning of a new ileostomy are required for proper treatment. This is a rare but devastating complication, and it may occur despite a primarily matured ileostomy.

Chronic (Nonspecific) Prestomal Ileitis

Knill-Jones et al. reported successful treatment with corticosteroids of some patients with latent ileitis.[208] I observed a patient who had undergone colectomy with matured ileostomy for clear-cut ulcerative colitis, and who, years later, developed diarrhea, cramps, and weight loss for which no cause could be found despite exhaustive work-up including negative endoscopic and radiographic studies. He was treated with a course of sulfasalazine and has remained free of symptoms and anatomic disease for 18 years.

Obstructive Dysfunctional Ileitis

The symptoms are those of ileostomy dysfunction with abdominal cramping pain, increased output by way of the ileostomy and consequent dehydration. Physical examination shows a tight stoma on digital examination, usually at the skin level. Radiographic study of the ileostomy shows dilatation, effacement, and edema of Kerckring's folds, and irregularity if inflammatory changes are present. Treatment consists of excision of the cicatricial stenosis (usually at skin level) and resuture of the ileal mucosa to the skin. With primary maturation of the ileostomy this complication is seen much less frequently now, but the following case history of a patient with Crohn's disease is instructive and intriguing with regard to this discussion.

An 18-year-old female had been treated for 6 years with sulfasalazine and corticosteroids for "ulcerative colitis" and was referred for colectomy because of failure to thrive, recurrent erythema nodosum, growth retardation, and lack of onset of menarche. One-stage panproctocolectomy was carried out. Examination of the specimen showed a long segment of ileal involvement. On microscopic study the inflammation was nonspecific, extending only to the muscularis propria. My colleagues and I would consider this a case of Crohn's ileocolitis by our combined criteria.[95,96]

The patient was well until 1 year postoperatively when she developed erythema nodosum and cramping abdominal pain, fever, diarrhea, and retraction of the ileostomy, which now appeared granular and inflamed. Ileostograms demonstrated extensive ileal ulceration, and inflammation and narrowing at the stoma. Laparotomy and resection of 30 cm of ileum resulted in complete resolution of all symptoms. The microscopic findings were nonspecific.

She was well for 16 months, at which time she returned with cramping abdominal pain, diarrhea, and erythema nodosum. The ileostomy had not retracted and its mucosa appeared to be normal. She had no fever. Ileostogram showed narrowing at the stoma and dilatation of the ileum proximal to the stoma, but no ulcerations. Simple revision of the ileostomy without resection of ileum but with widening at the skin and fascial levels resulted in complete and long-term resolution of the cramps, diarrhea, and erythema nodosum.

FRANK PRESTOMAL CROHN'S DISEASE

Recurrent Crohn's disease after ileostomy is usually found in the prestomal ileum and does not involve the external stoma for reasons that are unclear, mysterious, and intriguing. This phenomenon is reminiscent of the typical location of recurrent disease in the neoterminal ileum after restorative operation. In this regard it is interesting to note that biopsies of the external and prestomal mucosa of asymptomatic patients with ileostomy for colonic Crohn's disease regularly show the characteristic neuronal degeneration of Crohn's disease on electron microscopy, whereas similar biopsies from patients with ulcerative colitis do not.[156] The early symptoms of prestomal Crohn's disease are those of partial small bowel obstruction or ileostomy dysfunction with cramps, increased liquid content, and foul odor of the ileostomy effluent. Retraction or recession of the ileostomy stoma is frequent. Fever, abdominal pain, and peristomal tenderness may occur. Edema of the external stoma may occur, but actual involvement by the inflammatory process, as already noted, is rare. Peristomal abscess and peristomal fistula (after spontaneous or surgical drainage of an abscess) are not infrequent. The diagnosis is established by digital examination, radiographic study, and, occasionally, endoscopic examination with a pediatric proctoscope.

Should granulomatous prestomal ileitis be treated nonoperatively or by excision and revision of the ileostomy? I have seen patients who have done reasonably well for years with such a lesion with or without "specific" treatment by corticosteroids or sulfasalazine and have treated some patients in this manner. More recently I have taken a more aggressive approach, and now recommend for most patients the early surgical excision of the affected area with reconstruction of the ileostomy at the same site. This recommendation is based on two considerations: (1) a number of patients, while under observation and nonoperative treatment, have developed peristomal abscess and fistula that has added considerable morbidity and necessitated relocation of the ileostomy to a less desirable location, and (2) data on the long-term course of patients with Crohn's disease of the colon after ileostomy and colectomy indicate that one or more revisions of the ileostomy usually leads to restoration of health rather than to progressive proximal extension of disease.[95,96,211] Therefore, I recommend surgical revision in patients with prestomal Crohn's disease whose symptoms do not promptly abate with nonoperative management, or in the presence of any findings that suggest a developing peristomal abscess or fistula.

Results of Operation

Restorative Operation for Crohn's Disease

At the present time, elective restorative operation for Crohn's disease can be carried out with a mortality rate of under 3%. Mortality statistics reflect the stage of disease and condition of the patient at the time of referral, and also the time period during which the patient was treated. Even so, Banks et al., from my own institution, reported an operative mortality rate of 2.7% in a series of patients, some of whom were treated as early as 1929 (antedating Crohn's report), representing the efforts of diverse surgeons of varied experience.[212] More recently in my analysis of restorative operation for ileitis and ileocolitis at Beth Israel Hospital from 1942 through 1972, we found an operative mortality of 1.8% for initial operations and 3.6% for operations for recurrent disease.[55] I have never had a post operative fatality in a patient with classical Crohn's disease, whether the operation was a primary, secondary, or tertiary one, or whether the procedure was elective or emergent. This is not presented as braggadocio, but simply to emphasize the point that operation can be carried out with an acceptable mortality.

The immediate results of operation are generally excellent with respect to nutrition, freedom from disabling symptoms, cure of complications (including fistulas), and patient satisfaction.[213,214] Although the outcome with regard to the amount of diarrhea is unpredictable, it does depend to some extent upon the extent of disease and resection, and the amount of obstruction present preoperatively.[214] In most instances, however, diarrhea is not severe and it is difficult to predict whether it will be improved or exacerbated by operation.[214] In a general way, however, with longer resections the patient will have symptomatic diarrhea, but with shorter resections, especially in patients with prior significant obstructive symptoms, bowel function may be improved or at least not troublesome. The pathogenesis of postoperative diarrhea will differ from patient to patient and depend roughly upon the extent of resection. Hofmann has documented that, because of the loss of the specific site for the absorption of conjugated bile salts, bile salt catharsis is a significant cause of diarrhea in patients with resections of less than 100 cm.[215] The use of cholestyramine to bind bile salts and thereby ameliorate the cholerheic diarrhea in patients with more limited resections has proved to be a significant therapeutic advance, as documented by a double-blind crossover study.[216] In patients with resections of greater than 100 cm, steatorrhea is likely to be present and the cathartic action of fatty acids and hydroxylated fatty acids (by colonic flora) will be etiologic. Others have downplayed an important role for cholestyramine in the management of these patients and have relied instead upon antimotility agents and modest restriction of fat in the diet.[214] Patients with resections of this magnitude are also likely to have significant vitamin B_{12} malabsorption and require replacement by monthly B_{12} injections.[214]

Many physicians in evaluating the expected results of operation in ileal and ileocolonic Crohn's disease focus only on the high rate of recurrence, which we have found to be about 30% at 5 years, 50% at 10 years, 65% at 15 years, and 85% at 25 years.[55] Clearly the full picture of the expectations and benefits of surgical treatment is not reflected in the rate of recurrence. The early results have been enumerated in the previous paragraphs. In the long run, de Dombal, Burton, and Goligher found that unoperated patients with Crohn's disease were symptomatic during 4 out of every 5 years of living with disease whereas postoperative patients,[217] including those who may have developed recurrence or who had postoperative complications, spent 3 out of every 4 years in complete clinical remission. My associates and I found at the time of our review that the status of 78% of the patients having had an initial resection was excellent or good.[55]

Colectomy and Ileostomy for Ulcerative Colitis or Crohn's Disease of the Colon

Colectomy and ileostomy for colonic inflammatory bowel disease can be carried out with a mortality rate of less than 3%.[218] In my experience the single postoperative death was in an 81-year-old malnourished, psychotic man with fulminating colitis who died postoperatively of aspiration pneumonia (a complication that was present preoperatively) as a result of tube feedings that he required because he would not eat.

Clearly, operative mortality reflects to some extent the state of the patient referred for operation. Goligher et al. were disappointed to find, in collected statistics published from 1952 to 1967, an average mortality of 7.9% for colectomy and ileostomy without a pattern of continued improvement from earlier to later reports;[219] however, although their own average mortality was 9.2%, the mortality for elective operation was 2.9% and the mortality for urgent or emergency operation was 20.2%. Van Heerden et al. found a similar discrepancy between mortality for elective operation (1.3%) and that for emergency cases (25%).[218] The figures cited in Chapter 26, Table 26-3, show an 11% mortality rate for operation in nonperforated toxic megacolon, whereas in the presence of perforation, the mean mortality rate was 40%. Mortality rates in "elective" procedures also reflect the status of the patient at the time of referral for operation. A death after proctocolectomy in my hospital occurred in a young woman who was treated elsewhere for 3 months with massive doses of corticosteroids before she was referred for further treatment. At that time she had protein-calorie malnutrition with gross anasarca and fulminating staphylococcal pneumonia requiring immediate respirator treatment, with eventual development of lung abscess. The patient was unable to take nourishment and received intravenous and oral hyperalimentation. The proper timing of operation was difficult to determine and what was thought to be the optimal moment was chosen. Unfortunately, the patient died postoperatively of Clostridial peritonitis. This case illustrates in a tangible manner the problems in assessing postoperative mortality and emphasizes the points made in Chapter 26 about the proper timing of operation and the continuing of medical and surgical care in inflammatory bowel disease.

I would be remiss not to point out how well properly managed patients usually fare after such a major procedure as proctocolectomy. It is continually amazing and gratifying, particularly in the toxic patients, to observe the improvement in general appearance, mood, and vital signs, observations that are lost in a factual, cold recounting of morbidity and mortality statistics. Subsequently, the usual patient literally blooms with a dramatic weight gain and a feeling of well-being, and is rehabilitated socially and economically. Modern ileostomy construction and appliances have obviated many previously vexing problems.

The details of late morbidity are discussed in Chapters 30, 31, and 32. These include small intestinal obstruction, prestomal ileitis, recurrent carcinoma, or development of carcinoma in the rectal stump, renal lithiasis, psychiatric difficulties, and persistent perineal sinus. Recurrent Crohn's disease after colectomy and ileostomy is a problem that has been discussed already in several places. I sense that this issue is much less controversial than it has been in years past.[213,220] Patients with Crohn's disease of the colon can be expected to have somewhat more morbidity than those with ulcerative colitis after colectomy and ileostomy. Perhaps 10 to 20% can be expected to develop frank prestomal Crohn's disease at some point in their course, but this usually responds favorably to further ileal resection if necessary. Despite this potential for recurrent disease, in the patients we have followed eventual rehabilitation has been the norm after proctocolectomy both for ulcerative colitis and Crohn's disease of the colon. Steinberg et al. have described a susceptibility of patients with ileostomy for Crohn's disease to have periods of ileostomy diarrhea that they term "ileostomy flux," an omen in their experience of impending recurrent disease.[217] I have not observed "ileostomy flux" as a significant problem.

A number of older reports indicated a significant and cumulative late mortality after colectomy and ileostomy for ulcerative colitis, as high as 25% or more.[221-224] Parks found a yearly mortality of only 0.9%, however, of which more than 25% was caused by carcinoma.[225] Watts et al. found a late mortality of less than 3% after ileostomy and less than 0.7% annually.[226] Daly found that the mortality starting 2 years postoperatively approached that predicted in the absence of colitis, suggesting that if a patient survives proctocolectomy the subsequent life expectancy may become near normal.[29] Indeed, although exact actuarial data are needed on the risk of mortality subsequent to proctocolectomy and ileostomy, some insurance underwriters are aware of the favorable response of ulcerative colitis to operation and are willing to issue life and even disabiltiy insurance to these patients.

With regard to the quality of life with an ileostomy, a number of surveys have shown relatively little physical, social, or psychologic disability resulting from the ileostomy, and a high rate of rehabilitation.[29,226-234] Certainly in conducting surveys, as we have on the results of operation in Crohn's and ulcerative colitis,[95,96] and in following personal patients, one cannot fail to be impressed with the apparent state of well-being of ileostomates and with their positive attitudes toward life. Reports delving into the deeper feelings of patients with external stomas are sobering, however, and they clearly point out that the ileostomy is a trade-off of a definite psychologic handicap for physical well being.[235,236] Lenneberg and Rowbotham have also commented on a disparity between surface adjustment and problems at the internal psychologic level.[237] It remains to be seen whether the results of continent ileostomy or the ileoanal pull-through procedures will represent an overall improvement on the results of Brooke ileostomy. This statement is made with full awareness of a number of studies putatively showing that the satisfaction rates are better with these procedures, but the patients in these series are at least somewhat self-selected to be satisfied.

Sexual dysfunction in the male undergoing protocolectomy is a subject for concern in this generally young group of patients. Provided that the rectal dissection is carried out close to the rectum, the risk to sexual function should be minimal. Although patients should be warned of the possibility of altered function postoperatively, most studies have not found disability in the vast majority of male patients who have undergone operation for inflammatory bowel disease except in those who had a wide dissection for carcinoma.[29,227,229,238-244] The reports of Watts et al. and of May are less encouraging, however, but in common with the other studies cited, the difficulties seemed to increase with age, particularly in patients over 50.[226,245] Although the literature clearly indicates that the risk to totally intact sexual function is by no means nil, my experience leads me to believe, in common with Corman et al.,[242] that the incidence of sexual malfunction can be diminishingly small if careful, unhurried pelvic and perineal dissections are carried out.

A number of female patients after proctocolectomy and ileostomy at our institution have conceived and have delivered healthy children vaginally, and a number of reports detail similar experiences.[222,228,229,232,246-248] I have encountered three types of problems in pregnant patients with proctocolectomy and ileostomy. The simplest to deal with is enlargement of the ileal stoma that, together with the changed contour of the abdominal wall, makes it impossible for the patient to use her usual appliance, especially if it is one of the older types. I have advised an adhesive-backed temporary appliance with supplementary tape under these circumstances. A more troublesome and ominous problem is that of ileostomy prolapse that is contributed to by stomal enlargement and by softening and edema secondary to the gravid state. Use of an adhesive-backed appliance that is fixed to the skin by additional taping has helped this problem because it obviates the use of a tight belt that may increase the tendency to prolapse. The third problem I have encountered is that of intestinal obstruction, presumably resulting from changed relationships between intra-abdominal adhesions and the intestine because of the enlarging uterus. Retrograde intubation of the stoma has been helpful in some pregnant patients, as it may be in other patients with a similar problem. The physician is handicapped in diagnosis and management because of reluctance to use radiographic examination, particularly in the earlier stages of pregnancy. That this third mechanism is truly operative was demonstrated by a patient I treated who required induction of labor at near-term for particularly troublesome high-grade partial intestinal obstruction. Immediately after successful vaginal delivery the stoma began to function copiously on the delivery table, much to the chagrin of the staff. Scudamore et al. reported a similar experience.[246] My patient did not heed the advice to limit her family size and 1 1/2 years later an identical sequence occurred, happily with the same outcome.

It is not surprising that a number of surveys have indicated that the presence of a stoma and an appliance can be a psychologic impediment to normal sexual function in both males and females who are rehabilitated in other respects and who have no physical disability.[241,249,250] Clearly this is a major impetus for patients to seek continent ileostomies or sphincter-saving procedures, and to surgeons who advocate them. Objective studies are needed that will determine if the newer procedures accomplish the goal of rehabilitation in this respect better than a conventional ileostomy.

Operation is an effective modality of therapy in inflammatory bowel disease that is capable of restoring health with low mortality and morbidity.* Achieving these results requires knowledge of proper indications for and timing of operation, proper regard for the patient as a human being, and detailed attention to and correction of preoperative and postoperative biochemical and psychologic derangements. Proper selection of the type of procedure and attention to the technical details of operation are also important, even in the era of molecular medicine.

*Editors' note: see also, Voliulis, A. and Currie, D. J.: Surg. Gynecol. Obstet., *164*:27, 1987.

References

1. Goligher, J. C.: Surgery of the Anus, Rectum and Colon. 5th Ed. London, Baillière Tindall, 1984.
2. Crohn, B. B.: Regional Ileitis. New York, Grune and Stratton, 1949.
3. Marshak, R. H.: Granulomatous disease of the intestinal tract (Crohn's disease). Radiology, 114:3, 1975.
4. Colp, R., and Dreiling, D. A.: Persistent or recurrent proximal ileitis following surgery. Arch. Surg., 64:28, 1952.
5. Ginzburg, L.: The road to regional enteritis. Mt. Sinai J. Med., 41:272, 1974.
6. Hawkins, C.: Historical review. In Inflammatory Bowel Diseases. Edited by R. N. Allan, M. R. B. Keighley, J. Alexander-Williams, and C. Hawkins. London, Churchill Livingstone, 1983.
7. Glotzer, D. J.: The development of current surgical treatment of inflammatory bowel disease. In Recent Advances in Gastroenterology. Edited by A. Thomson, and L. R. DaCosta. New York, Plenum, 1986.
8. Makins, G. H.: Symposium on ulcerative colitis. Proc. R. Soc. Med., 2:75, 1909.
9. Klein, S. H., et al.: Emergency cecostomy in ulcerative colitis with acute toxic dilatation. Surgery, 47:399, 1960.
10. Turnbull, R. B., Jr., Hawk, W. A., and Weakley, F. L.: Surgical treatment of toxic megacolon: Ileostomy and colostomy to prepare patients for colectomy. Am. J. Surg., 122:325, 1971.
11. Corbett, R. S.: A review of surgical treatment of chronic ulcerative colitis. Proc. R. Soc. Med., 38:277, 1945.
12. Lockhart-Mummery, J. P., et al.: Discussion on the surgical treatment of idiopathic ulcerative colitis and its sequelae. Proc. R. Soc. Med., 3:637, 1940.
13. McIntyre, P. B., et al.: Therapeutic benefits from a poorly absorbed prednisolone enema in distal colitis. Gut, 26:822, 1985.
14. Friedman, G.: Tixocortal pivalate (JO 1016). Am. J. Gastroenterol., 78:529, 1983.
15. Peppercorn, M.: Sulfasalazine: Pharmacology, clinical use, toxicity, and related new drug development. Ann. Intern. Med., 377, 1984.
16. Brown, J. Y.: The value of complete physiological rest of the large bowel in the treatment of certain ulcerative and obstructive lesions of this organ: With descriptions of operative technique and report of cases. Surg. Gynecol. Obstet., 16:610, 1913.
17. Oberhelman, H. A., Jr., Kohatsu, S., Taylor, K. B., and Kivel, R. M.: Diverting ileostomy in the surgical management of Crohn's disease of the colon. Am. J. Surg., 115:231, 1968.
18. Truelove, S. C., Ellis, H., and Webster, C. U.: Place of a double-barreled ileostomy in ulcerative colitis and Crohn's disease of colon: A preliminary report. Br. Med. J., 1:150, 1965.
19. Miller, C. G., Gardner, C. McG., and Ripstein, C. B.: Primary resection of the colon in acute ulcerative colitis. Can. Med. Assoc. J., 60:584, 1949.
20. Ripstein, C. B.: Primary resection of the colon in acute ulcerative colitis. J. Am. Med. Assoc., 152:1093, 1953.
21. Counsell, P. B., and Goligher, J. C.: Surgical treatment of ulcerative colitis. Lancet, 2:1045, 1952.
22. Crile, G., Jr., and Thomas, C. Y., Jr.: The treatment of acute toxic ulcerative colitis by ileostomy and simultaneous colectomy. Gastroenterology, 19:58, 1951.
23. Ravitch, M. M.: Total colectomy and abdominoperineal resection (pancolectomy) in one stage. Ann. Surg., 144:758, 1956.
24. Crile, G., Jr., and Turnbull, R. B.: The mechanism and prevention of ileostomy dysfunction. Ann. Surg., 140:429, 1954.
25. Brooke, B. N.: Management of ileostomy including its complications. Lancet, 2:102, 1952.
26. Goligher, J. C.: Extraperitoneal colostomy and ileostomy. Br. J. Surg., 46:97, 1958.
27. Strauss, A. A., and Strauss, S. F.: Surgical treatment of ulcerative colitis. Surg. Clin. North Am., 24:211, 1944.
28. Hill, G. L.: Ileostomy. Surgery, Physiology, and Management. New York, Grune and Stratton, 1976.
29. Daly, D. W.: Outcome of surgery for ulcerative colitis. Ann. R. Coll. Surg. Engl., 42:38, 1968.
30. Devroede, G. J., et al.: Cancer risk and life expectancy of children with ulcerative colitis. N. Engl. J. Med., 285:17, 1971.
31. Kock, N. G.: Continent ileostomy. Prog. Surg., 12:180, 1973.
32. Taylor, B. M., et al.: The endorectal ileal pouch-anal anastomosis. Current clinical results. Dis. Colon. Rectum, 27:347, 1984.
33. Rothenberger, D. A., Buls, J. G., Nivatvongs, S., and Goldberg, S. M.: The Parks S ileal pouch and anal anastomosis after colectomy and mucosal proctectomy. Am. J. Surg., 149:390, 1985.
34. Schoetz, D. J., Jr., Coller, J. A., and Veidenheimer, M. C.: Ileoanal reservoir for ulcerative colitis and familial polyposis. Arch. Surg., 121:404, 1986.
35. Corbett, R. S.: Recent advances in the surgical treatment of chronic ulcerative colitis. Ann. R. Coll. Surg. Engl., 10:21, 1952.
36. Aylett, S.: Diffuse ulcerative colitis and its treatment by ileorectal anastomosis. Ann. R. Coll. Surg. Engl., 27:260, 1960.
37. Dennis, C., et al.: The response to vagotomy in idiopathic ulcerative colitis and regional enteritis. Ann. Surg., 128:479, 1948.
38. Schlitt, R. J., McNally, J. J., and Shafiroff, B. G.: Pelvic autonomic neurectomy for ulcerative colitis. Gastroenterology, 19:812, 1951.
39. Levy, R. W., et al.: Experiences with prefrontal lobotomy for intractable ulcerative colitis. J. Am. Med. Assoc., 160:1277, 1956.
40. Bucaille, M.: Selective frontal lobe operation for the treatment of some diseases of the gastrointestinal tract with special reference to ulcerative colitis. Surgery, 52:690, 1962.
41. Crohn, B. B., Ginzburg, L., and Oppenheimer, G. D.: Regional ileitis. A pathologic and clinical entity. J. Am. Med. Assoc., 191:825, 1932.
42. Garlock, J. H., Crohn, B. B., Klein, S. H., and Yarnis, H.: An appraisal of the long-term results of surgical treatment of regional enteritis. Gastroenterology, 19:414, 1951.
43. Hawker, P. C., Allan, R. N., Dykes, P. W., and Alexander-Williams, J.: Strictureplasty. A useful, effective surgical treatment in Crohn's disease. Gut, 24:A490, 1983.
44. Lee, E. C. G., and Papaioannou, N.: Minimal surgery for chronic obstruction with extensive or universal Crohn's disease. Ann. R. Coll. Surg. Engl., 64:229, 1982.
45. Lockhart-Mummery, H. E., and Morson, B. C.: Crohn's disease (regional enteritis) of the large intestine and its distinction from ulcerative colitis. Gut, 1:87, 1960.
46. Lockhart-Mummery, H. E., and Morson, B. C.: Crohn's disease of the large intestine. Gut, 5:493, 1964.
47. Lindner, A. E., et al.: Granulomatous colitis: A clinical study. N. Engl. J. Med., 269:379, 1963.
48. Jeejeebhoy, K. N., et al.: Total parenteral nutrition at home: Studies in patients surviving 4 months to 5 years. Gastroenterology, 71:943, 1976.

49. Fleming, C. R., et al.: Home parenteral nutrition for management of the severely malnourished adult patient. Gastroenterology, 79:11, 1980.
50. Wasser, R., Cohen, Z., and Langer, B.: Small intestinal transplantation. A closer reality. Dis. Colon Rectum, 28:908, 1985.
51. Ferguson, L. K.: Concepts in the surgical treatment of regional enteritis. N. Engl. J. Med., 264:748, 1961.
52. Garlock, J. H., and Crohn, B. B.: An appraisal of the results of surgery in treatment of regional enteritis. J. Am. Med. Assoc., 127:205, 1945.
53. Alexander-Williams, J., Fielding, J. F., and Cooke, W. T.: A comparison of results of excision and bypass for ileal Crohn's disease. Gut, 13:973, 1972.
54. Homan, W. P., and Dineen, P.: Comparison of the results of resection, bypass, and bypass with exclusion for ileocecal Crohn's disease. Ann. Surg., 187:530, 1978.
55. Trnka, Y. M., et al.: The long-term outcome of restorative operation in Crohn's disease. Influence of location, prognostic factors and surgical guidelines. Ann. Surg., 196:345, 1982.
56. Mekhjian, H. S. et al.: National Cooperative Crohn's Disease Study: Factors determining recurrence of Crohn's disease after surgery. Gastroenterology, 77:907, 1979.
57. Block, G. E., Enker, W. E., and Kirsner, J. B.: Significance and treatment of occult obstructive uropathy complicating Crohn's disease. Ann. Surg., 178:32, 1973.
58. Young, S., et al.: Results of surgery for Crohn's disease in the Glasgow region, 1961-1970. Br. J. Surg., 62:528, 1975.
59. Atwell, J. D., Duthie, H. L., and Goligher, J. C.: The outcome of Crohn's disease. Br. J. Surg., 52:966, 1965.
60. Alexander-Williams, J.: Progress report: The place of surgery in Crohn's disease. Gut, 12:739, 1971.
61. Heaton, L. D., et al.: President Eisenhower's operation for regional enteritis. A footnote to history. Ann. Surg., 159:661, 1965.
62. Mayo, C. W., Fly, O. A., and Connelly, M. E.: Fate of the remaining rectal segment after subtotal colectomy for ulcerative colitis. Ann. Surg., 144:753, 1956.
63. Moss, G. S., and Keddie, N.: Fate of rectal stump in ulcerative colitis. Arch. Surg., 91:967, 1965.
64. Binder, S. C., Miller, H. H., and Deterling, R. A., Jr.: Fate of the retained rectum after subtotal colectomy for inflammatory disease of the colon. Am. J. Surg., 131:201, 1976.
65. Korelitz, B. I., Dyck, W. P., and Klion, F. M.: Fate of the rectum and distal colon after subtotal colectomy for ulcerative colitis. Gut, 10:198, 1969.
66. Aylett, S. O.: Three hundred cases of diffuse ulcerative colitis treated by total colectomy and ileorectal anastomosis. Br. Med. J., 1:1001, 1966.
67. Baker, W. N. W., Glass, R. E., Ritchie, J. K., and Aylett, S. O.: Cancer of the rectum following colectomy and ileorectal anastomosis for ulcerative colitis. Br. J. Surg., 65:862, 1978.
68. Grundfest, S. F., et al.: The risk of cancer following colectomy and ileorectal anastomosis for extensive mucosal ulcerative colitis. Ann. Surg., 193:9, 1981.
69. Griffin, W. O., Jr., Lillehei, R. C., and Wangensteen, O. H.: Ileoproctostomy in ulcerative colitis: Long-term followup, extending in early cases to more than 20 years. Surgery, 53:705, 1963.
70. Jagelman, D. G., Lewis, C. B., and Rowe-Jones, D. C.: Ileorectal anastomosis: Appreciation by patients. Br. Med. J., 1:756, 1969.
71. Baker, W. N. W.: The results of ileorectal anastomosis at St. Mark's Hospital from 1953 to 1968. Gut, 11:235, 1970.
72. Adson, M. A., Cooperman, A. M., and Farrow, G. M.: Ileorectostomy for ulcerative disease of the colon. Arch. Surg., 104:424, 1972.
73. Tompkins, R. K., et al.: Reappraisal of rectum retaining operations for ulcerative and granulomatous colitis. Am. J. Surg., 125:159, 1973.
74. Watts, J. McK., and Hughes, E. S. R.: Ulcerative colitis and Crohn's disease: Results after colectomy and ileorectal anastomosis. Br. J. Surg., 64:77, 1977.
75. Jones, P. F., Munro, A., and Ewen, S. W. B.: Colectomy and ileorectal anastomosis for colitis: Report on a personal series with a critical review. Br. J. Surg., 64:615, 1977.
76. Khubchandani, I. T.: Ileorectal anastomosis for ulcerative and Crohn's colitis. Am. J. Surg., 135:751, 1978.
77. Farnell, M. B., van Heerden, J. A., Beart, R. W., Jr., and Weiland, L. H.: Rectal preservation in nonspecific inflammatory disease of the colon. Ann. Surg., 192:249, 1980.
78. Kock, N. G., Myrvold, H. E., and Nilsson, L. O.: Progress report on the continent ileostomy. World J. Surg., 4:143, 1980.
79. Cameron, A.: The continent ileostomy. Br. J. Surg., 60:785, 1983.
80. Goligher, J. C., and Lintott, D.: Experience with 26 reservoir ileostomies. Br. J. Surg., 62:893, 1975.
81. Thow, G. B., Manson, R. R., and Greenberg, E. M.: The Kock pouch continent ileostomy: Technique and results. Mod. Med., 43:71, 1975.
82. Gelernt, I. M., Bauer, J. J., and Kreel, I.: The reservoir ileostomy. Early experience with 54 patients. Ann. Surg., 185:179, 1977.
83. Goldman, S. L., and Rombeau, J. L.: The continent ileostomy. A collective review. Dis. Colon Rectum, 21:594, 1978.
84. Shrock, T. R.: Complications of continent ileostomy. Am. J. Surg., 138:162, 1979.
85. Dozois, R. R., Kelly, K. A., Beart, R. W., Jr., and Beahrs, O. H.: Improved results with continent ileostomy. Ann. Surg., 192:319, 1980.
86. Dozois, R. R., et al.: Factors affecting revision rate after continent ileostomy. Arch. Surg., 116:610, 1981.
87. Gerber, A., Apt, M. K., and Craig, P. H.: The Kock continent ileostomy. Surg. Gynecol. Obstet., 156:345, 1983.
88. Beahrs, O. H., Bess, M. A., Beart, R. W., Jr., and Pemberton, J. H.: Indwelling ileostomy valve device. Am. J. Surg., 141:111, 1981.
89. Ravitch, M. M., and Sabiston, D. C., Jr.: Anal ileostomy with preservation of the sphincter: A proposed operation in patients requiring total colectomy for benign lesions. Surg. Gynecol. Obstet., 84:1095, 1947.
90. Glotzer, D. J., and Pihl, B. G.: Preservation of continence after mucosal graft in the rectum and its feasibility in man. Am. J. Surg., 117:403, 1969.
91. Martin, L. W., LeCoultre, C., and Schubert, W. K.: Total colectomy and mucosal proctectomy with preservation of continence in ulcerative colitis. Ann. Surg., 186:470, 1977.
92. Parks, A. G., Nicholls, R. J., and Belliveau, P.: Proctocolectomy with ileal reservoir and anal anastomosis. Br. J. Surg., 67:533, 1980.
93. Utsonomiya, J., et al: Total colectomy, mucosal proctectomy and ileoanal anastomosis. Dis. Colon Rectum, 23:459, 1980.
94. Fonkalsrud, E. W.: Endorectal ileoanal anastomosis with isoperistaltic ileal reservoir after colectomy and mucosal proctectomy. Ann. Surg., 199:151, 1984.
95. Glotzer, D. J., et al.: Comparative features and course of ulcerative and granulomatous colitis. N. Engl. J. Med., 282:582, 1960.

96. Fawaz, K. A., et al: Ulcerative colitis and Crohn's disease of the colon: A comparison of the long-term postoperative courses. Gastroenterology, 71:372, 1976.
97. Burman, J. H., et al.: The effect of diversion of intestinal contents on the progress of Crohn's disease of the large bowel. Gut, 12:11, 1971.
98. Lockhart-Mummery, H. E.: Anal lesions of Crohn's disease. Clin. Gastroenterol., 1:377, 1972.
99. Ross, T. M., Fazio, V. W., and Farmer, R. G.: Long-term results of surgical treatment for Crohn's disease of the duodenum. Ann. Surg., 197:399, 1983.
100. Murray, J. J., et al.: Surgical management of Crohn's disease involving the duodenum. Am. J. Surg., 147:58, 1984.
101. Jones, T. W., et al.: A prime physiologic mechanism responsible for the failure of gastrojejunostomy in the treatment of peptic ulcer disease. Surgery, 43:781, 1958.
102. Sarr, M. G., Gladen, H. E., Beart, R. W., Jr., and van Heerden, J. A.: Role of gastroenterostomy in patients with unresectable carcinoma of the pancreas. Surg. Gynecol. Obstet., 152:597, 1981.
103. Herter, F. P., Cooperman, A. M., Ahlborn, T. N., and Antinori, C.: Surgical experience with pancreatic and periampullary cancer. Ann. Surg., 195:274, 1982.
104. Truelove, S. C.: Treatment of ulcerative colitis with local hydrocortisone hemisuccinate sodium: A report on a controlled therapeutic trial. Br. Med. J., 2:1072, 1958.
105. Truelove, S. C., and Witts, L. J.: Cortisone and corticotropin in ulcerative colitis. Br. Med. J., 1:387, 1959.
106. Truelove, S. C., and Witts, L. J.: Cortisone in ulcerative colitis: Final report on a therapeutic trial. Br. Med. J., 2:1041, 1955.
107. Summers, R. W., et al.: National Cooperative Crohn's Disease Study: Results of drug treatment. Gastroenterology, 77:847, 1979.
108. Howes, E. L., et al.: Retardation of wound healing by cortisone. Surgery, 28:177, 1950.
109. Pearce, C. W., et al.: The effect and interrelation of testosterone, cortisone, and protein nutrition on wound healing. Surg. Gynecol. Obstet., 111:274, 1960.
110. Schotte, O. E., and Smith, C. B.: Effects of ACTH and of cortisone upon amputational wound healing processes in mice digits. J. Zool., 146:209, 1961.
111. Hinshaw, D. B., Hughes, L. D., and Stafford, C. E.: Effects of cortisone on the healing of disrupted abdominal wounds. Am. J. Surg., 101:189, 1961.
112. Sandberg, N.: Time relationship between adminstration of cortisone and wound healing in rats. Acta Chir. Scand., 127:446, 1964.
113. Green, J. P.: Steroid therapy and wound healing in surgical patients. Br. J. Surg., 52:523, 1965.
114. McNamara, J. J., et al.: Effect of short-term pharmacologic doses of adrenocorticosteroid therapy on wound healing. Ann. Surg., 170:199, 1969.
115. Ehrlich, H. P., and Hunt, T. K.: The effects of cortisone and vitamin A on wound healing. Ann. Surg., 167:324, 1968.
116. Ehrlich, H. P., and Hunt, T. K.: The effects of cortisone and anabolic steroids on the tensile strength of healing wounds. Ann. Surg., 170:203, 1969.
117. Spark, R. F.: Hypothalamic-pituitary-adrenal axis in surgery. In Intensive Care. Edited by J. J. Skillman. Boston, Little Brown, 1975.
118. Jasani, M., et al.: Studies of the rise in plasma 11-hydroxycorticosteroids (11-OHC) in corticosteroid-treated patients with rheumatoid arthritis during surgery: Correlations with functional integrity of the hypothalamo-pituitary-adrenal axis. Q. J. Med., 37:407, 1968.
119. Graber, A. L., et al: Natural history of pituitary-adrenal recovery following long-term suppression with corticosteroids. J. Clin. Endocrinol. Metab., 25:11, 1965.
120. Danowski, T. S., et al: Probabilities of pituitary-adrenal responsiveness after steroid therapy. Ann. Intern. Med., 61:11, 1964.
121. Amatruda, T. T., Jr., Hurst, M. M., and D'Esopo, H. D.: Certain endocrine and metabolic facets of the steroid withdrawal syndrome. J. Clin. Endocrinol., 25:1207, 1965.
122. Bistrian, B. R., et al.: Protein status of general surgical patients. J. Am. Med. Assoc., 230:858, 1974.
123. Barot, L. R., et al.: Energy expenditure in patients with inflammatory bowel disease. Arch. Surg., 116:460, 1981.
124. Barot, L. R., Rombeau, J. L., Feurer, I. D., and Mullen, J. L.: Caloric requirements in patients with inflammatory bowel disease. Ann. Surg., 195:214, 1982.
125. Jeejeebhoy, K. N., et al.: Metabolic studies in total parenteral nutrition with lipid in man. Comparison with glucose. J. Clin. Invest., 57:125, 1976.
126. Dudrick, S. J., and Rubert, R. L.: Principles and practice of parenteral nutrition. Gastroenterology, 61:901, 1971.
127. Dickinson, R. J., et al.: Controlled trial of intravenous hyperalimentation and total bowel rest as an adjunct to the routine therapy of acute colitis. Gastroenterology, 79:1199, 1980.
128. Abel, R. M., et al: Malnutrition in cardiac surgical patients. Results of a prospective, randomized evaluation of early postoperative parenteral nutrition. Arch. Surg., 111:45, 1976.
129. Collins, J. P., Oxby, C. B., and Hill, G. L.: Intravenous aminoacids and intravenous hyperalimentation as protein-sparing therapy after major surgery. A controlled clinical trial. Lancet, 1:788, 1978.
130. Davis, G. R., Santa Ana, C. A., Morawski, S. G., and Fordtran, J. S.: Development of a lavage solution associated with minimal water and electrolyte absorption or secretion. Gastroenterology, 78:991, 1980.
131. Thomas, G., Brozinsky, S., and Isenberg, J. L.: Patient acceptance and effectiveness of a balanced lavage solution (Golytely) vs the standard preparation for colonoscopy. Gastroenterology, 82:435, 1982.
132. Glotzer, D. J., Boyle, P. L., and Silen, W.: Preoperative preparation of the colon with an elemental diet. Surgery, 75:535, 1974.
133. Washington, J. A., II, et al.: Effect of preoperative antibiotic regimen on development of infection after intestinal surgery. Prospective, randomized, double-blind study. Ann. Surg., 180:567, 1974.
134. Clarke, J. S., et al.: Preoperative oral antibiotics reduce septic complications of colon operations: Results of prospective, randomized, double-blind clinical study. Ann. Surg., 186:251, 1977.
135. Condon, R. E.: Bowel preparation for colorectal operations. Arch. Surg., 117:265, 1982.
136. Nichols, R. E., Condon, R. E., Gorbach, S. L., and Nyhus, L. M.: Efficacy of preoperative antimicrobial preparation of the bowel. Ann. Surg., 176:227, 1972.
137. Kakkar, V. V., and Corrigan, T. P.: Efficacy of low-dose heparin in preventing postoperative fatal pulmonary embolism: Results of an international multicentre trial. In Heparin: Chemistry and Clinical Usage. Edited by V. V. Kakkar, and D. P. Thomas. London, Academic Press, 1976.
138. The Multicenter Trial Committee: Dihydroergotamine-heparin prophylaxis of postoperative deep vein thrombosis. A multicenter trial. J. Am. Med. Assoc., 251:2960, 1984.
139. Heatley, R. V., et al.: Preoperative or postoperative deep-vein thrombosis? Lancet, 1:437, 1976.

140. Salzman, E. W., et al.: Intraoperative external pneumatic calf compression to afford long-term prophylaxis against deep vein thrombosis in urological patients. Surgery, 87:239, 1980.
141. Burke, J. F.: The effective period of preventive antibiotic action in experimental incision and dermal lesions. Surgery, 50:161, 1961.
142. Polk, H. C., Jr., and Lopez-Mayor, J. F.: Postoperative wound infection: A prospective study of determinant factors and prevention. Surgery, 66:97, 1969.
143. Glotzer, D. J., Goodman, W. S., and Geronimus, L. H.: Topical antibiotic prophylaxis in contaminated wounds.: Experimental evaluation. Arch. Surg., 100:589, 1970.
144. Kliman, A.: Red Cross blood and hepatitis (letter to editor). N. Engl. J. Med., 282:101, 1970.
145. Wilkins, J. L., et al.: Effects of neostigmine and atropine on motor activity of ileum, colon and rectum of anesthetized subjects. Br. Med. J., 1:793, 1970.
146. Goligher, J. C., et al.: A controlled clinical trial of three methods of closure of laparotomy wounds. Br. J. Surg., 62:828, 1975.
147. Malt, R. A.: Abdominal incision, sutures and sacrilege. N. Engl. J. Med., 297:722, 1977.
148. Stone, H. H., and Hester, T. R., Jr.: Incisional and peritoneal infection after emergency celiotomy. Ann. Surg., 177:669, 1973.
149. Engelholm, L., Mainguet, P., and Potliege, P.: Radiology in early Crohn's disease of small intestine. In The Management of Crohn's Disease. Edited by I. T. Weterman, A. S. Peña, and C. C. Booth. Amsterdam, Excerpta Medica, 1976.
150. Ferguson, R., Allan, R. N., and Cooke, W. T.: A study of the cellular infiltrate of the proximal jejunal mucosa in ulcerative colitis and Crohn's disease. Gut, 16:205, 1975.
151. Allan, R., et al.: Changes in the bidirectional sodium flux across the intestinal mucosa in Crohn's disease. Gut, 16:201, 1975.
152. Dunne, W. T., Cooke, W. T., and Allan, R. H.: Enzymatic and morphometric evidence for Crohn's disease as a diffuse lesion of the gastrointestinal tract. Gut, 18:290, 1977.
153. Salem, S. N., and Truelove, S. C.: Small intestinal and gastric abnormalities in ulcerative colitis. Br. J. Med., 1:827, 1965.
154. Dvorak, A. M., Connell, A. B., and Dickersin, G. R.: Crohn's disease: A scanning electron microscopic study. Hum. Pathol., 10:165, 1979.
155. Dvorak, A. M., Osage, J. E., Monahan, R. A., and Dickersin, G. R.: Crohn's disease: Transmission electron microscopic studies. III. Target tissues. Proliferation of and injury to smooth muscle and the autonomic nervous system. Hum. Pathol., 11:620, 1980.
156. Dvorak, A. M., and Silen, W.: Differentiation between Crohn's disease and other inflammatory conditions by electron microscopy. Ann. Surg., 201:53, 1985.
157. Rutgeerts, P.: National history of recurrent Crohn's disease at the ileocolonic anastomosis after curative surgery. Gut, 25:665, 1984.
158. Wenckert, A., Brahme, F., and Nilsson, R.: Operationsikndikationer vid Crohn's sjukom. Nord. Med., 83:334, 1970.
159. Colcock, B. P., and Braash, J. W.: Surgery of the Small Intestine in the Adult. Philadelphia, W. B. Saunders, 1968.
160. Van Patter, W. N., et al: Regional enteritis. Gastroenterology, 26:345, 1954.
161. Lee, E. C. G., and Papaioannou, N.: Recurrences following surgery for Crohn's disease. Clin. Gastroenterol., 9:419, 1980.
162. Pennington, L., Hamilton, S. R., Bayless, T. M., and Cameron, J. L.: Surgical management of Crohn's disease. Influence of disease at margin of resection. Ann. Surg., 192:211, 1980.
163. Heuman, R., Boeryd, B., Bolin, T., and Sjodahl, R.: The influence of disease at the margin of resection on the outcome of Crohn's disesase. Br. J. Surg., 70:519, 1983.
164. Hamilton, S. R., et al.: The role of resection margin frozen section in the surgical management of Crohn's disease. Surg. Gynecol. Obstet., 160:57, 1985.
165. Bergman, L., and Krause, U.: Crohn's disease: A long-term study of the clinical course in 186 patients. Scand. J. Gastroenterol., 12:937, 1977.
166. Karesen, R., Serch-Hanssen, A., Thoresan, B. O., and Hertzberg, J.: Crohn's disease: Long-term results of surgical treatment. Scand. J. Gastroenterol., 16:57, 1981.
167. Heen, L. O., Nygaard, K., and Bergan, A.: Crohn's disease. Results of excisional surgery in 133 patients. Scand J. Gastroenterol., 19:747, 1984.
168. Lindhagen, T., et al.: Recurrence rate after surgical treatment of Crohn's disease. Scand. J. Gastroenterol., 18:1037, 1983.
169. Lorenzo, G. A., Poticka, S. M., and Beal, J. M.: Mesenteric lymphatics in regional enteritis. Arch. Surg., 105:375, 1972.
170. Present, D. H., et al.: Obstructive hydronephrosis: A frequent but seldom recognizd complication of granulomatous disease of the bowel. N. Engl. J. Med., 280:523, 1969.
171. Nugent, W., Fromm, D., and Silen, W.: Pseudo-Crohn's disease. Am. J. Surg., 137:566, 1979.
172. Gerzof, S. G., et al.: Percutaneous catheter drainage of abdominal abscesses: A five-year experience. N. Engl. J. Med., 305:653, 1981.
173. Casola, G., and van Sonnenberg, E.: Percutaneous drainage of Crohn abscess: Results, uses, and problems. Radiology, 153:254, 1984.
174. Nasr, K., et al.: Free perforation of regional enteritis. Gut, 10:206, 1969.
175. Alexander-Williams, J.: Overview of surgical management and directions of future research. In Inflammatory Bowel Diseases. Edited by R. N. Allan, M. R. B. Keighley, and J. Alexander-Williams. New York, Churchill-Livingstone, 1983
176. Koudahl, G., and Aagaard, P.: The management of the rectal stump after subtotal colectomy for ulcerative colitis. Scand. J. Gastroenterol. (Suppl.), 9:127, 1971.
177. Counsell, P. B.: Lesions of the ileum associated with ulcerative colitis. Br. J. Surg., 44:276, 1956.
178. Goligher, J. C.: Extraperitoneal colostomy or ileostomy. Br. J. Surg., 46:276, 1956.
179. Silen, W., and Glotzer, D. J.: The prevention and treatment of persistent perineal sinus. Surgery, 75:535, 1974.
180. Risberg, B., Kock, N. G., and Myrvold, H.: Topography of the reconstructed pelvic peritoneum after proctectomy: Dis. Colon Rectum, 17:153, 1974.
181. Irvin, T. T., and Goligher, J. C.: A controlled clinical trial of three different methods of perineal wound management following excision of the rectum. Br. J. Surg., 62:287, 1975.
182. Warshaw, A. L., Ottinger, L. W., and Bartlett, M. K.: Primary perineal closure after proctocolectomy for inflammatory bowel disease. Am. J. Surg., 133:414, 1977.
183. Hubbard, T. B., Jr., et al.: The pathology of peritoneal repair: Its relation to the formation of adhesions. Ann. Surg., 165:908, 1967.

184. DeAlmeida, A. M., Dos Santos, N. M., Aldeia, F. J., and Gracias, J. W.: Primary pelviperineal closure without drainage, after abdominoperineal resection of the rectum—a comparative study. Acta Med. Port., 5:49, 1984.
185. Jones, J. H., Lennard-Jones, J. E., and Lockhart-Mummery, H. E.: Experience in the treatment of Crohn's disease of the large intestine. Gut, 7:448, 1966.
186. Lee, E.: Split ileostomy in the treatment of Crohn's disease of the colon. Ann. R. Coll. Surg. Engl., 56:94, 1975.
187. McIlrath, D. C.: Diverting ileostomy or colostomy in the management of Crohn's disease of the colon. Arch. Surg., 103:308, 1971.
188. Harper, P. H., et al.: Split ileostomy and ileocolostomy for Crohn's disease of the colon and ulcerative colitis. A 20 year survey. Gut, 24:106, 1983.
189. Glotzer, D. J., Glick, M. E., and Goldman, H.: Proctitis and colitis following diversion of the fecal stream. Gastroenterology, 80:438, 1981.
190. Korelitz, B. I., Cheskin, L. J., Sohn, N., and Sommers, S. C.: Proctitis after fecal diversion in Crohn's disease and its elimination with reanastomosis: Implications for surgical management. Report of four cases. Gastroenterology, 87:710, 1984.
191. Lusk, L. B., Reichen, J., and Levine, J. S.: Aphthous ulceration in diversion colitis. Clinical implications. Gastroenterology, 87:1171, 1984.
192. Binder, S. C., Patterson, J. F., and Glotzer, D. J.: Toxic megacolon in ulcerative colitis. Gastroenterology, 66:909, 1974.
193. Turnbull, R. B., Jr., et al.: Choice of operation for the toxic megacolon phase of nonspecific ulcerative colitis. Surg. Clin. North Am., 50:1151, 1970.
194. Brotschi, E., Noe, J. M., and Silen, W.: Perineal hernias after proctectomy. A new approach to repair. Am. J. Surg., 149:301, 1985.
195. Cohen, B. E., and Ryan, J. A.: Gracilis muscle flap for closure of the persistent perineal sinus. Surg. Gynecol. Obstet., 148:33, 1979.
196. Baek, S. M., Greenstein, A., McElhinney, A. J., and Aufses, A. H.: The gracilis myocutaneous flap for persistent perineal sinus after proctocolectomy. Surg. Gynecol. Obstet., 153:713, 1981.
197. Ryan, J. A., Jr.: Gracilis muscle flap for the persistent perineal sinus of inflammatory bowel disease. Am. J. Surg., 148:64, 1984.
198. Hurwitz, D. J., and Zwiebel, P. C.: Gluteal thigh flap repair of chronic perineal wounds. Am. J. Surg., 150:386, 1985.
199. Dragstedt, L. R., Dack, G. M., and Kirsner, J. B.: Chronic ulcerative colitis. A summary of evidence implicating bacterium necrophorum as the etiologic agent. Ann. Surg., 11:653, 1941.
200. Warren, R., and McKittrick, L. S.: Ileostomy for ulcerative colitis. Technique, complications and management. Surg. Gynecol. Obstet., 93:555, 1951.
201. Fleischner, F. G., and Mandelstam, P.: Roentgen observations of the ileostomy in patients with idiopathic ulcerative colitis. II. Ileostomy dysfunction. Radiology, 70:469, 1958.
202. Dennis, C., and Karlson, E.: Surgical measures as supplements to the management of idiopathic ulcerative colitis. Cancer, cirrhosis and arthritis as frequent complications. Surgery, 32:892, 1952.
203. Loygue, J., Florent, R., and Got, R.: Lesions de l'intestine grele et rectocolite ulcerohemorragique. Arch. Med. Appar. Dig., 48:308, 1959.
204. Glotzer, D. J., Roth, S. I., and Welch, C. E.: Colonic ulceration proximal to obstructing carcinoma. Surgery, 56:950, 1964.
205. Glotzer, D. J., and Pihl, B. G.: Experimental obstructive colitis. Arch. Surg., 92:1, 1966.
206. Thayer, W. R., and Spiro, H. M.: Ileitis after ileostomy: Prestomal ileitis Gastroenterology, 42:547, 1962.
207. Turnbull, R. B., Jr., Weakley, F. L., and Farmer, R. G.: Ileitis after colectomy and ileostomy for nonspecific ulcerative colitis. Dis. Colon Rectum, 7:427, 1964.
208. Knill-Jones, R. P., Morson, B. C., and Williams, R.: Perstomal ileitis; clinical and pathological findings in five cases. Q. J. Med., 39:287, 1970.
209. Adson, M. A., Benjamin, I., and Dockerty, M. B.: Postcolectomy ileitis and related disorders. Arch. Surg., 102:326, 1971.
210. Menguy, R. B.: Results of surgery and long-term complications. In Ulcerative and Granulomatous Colitis. Edited by Z. T. Berkovitz. Springfield, Charles C Thomas, 1973.
211. Goligher, J. C.: The long-term results of excisional surgery for primary and recurrent Crohn's disease of the large intestine. Dis. Colon Rectum, 28:51, 1985.
212. Banks, B. M., Zetzel, L., and Richter, H. S.: Morbidity and mortality in regional enteritis. Report of 168 cases. Am. J. Dig. Dis., 14:369, 1969.
213. Meyers, S., et al.: Quality of life after surgery for Crohn's disease. A psychosocial survey. Gastroenterology, 78:1, 1980.
214. Compston, J. E., and Creamer, B.: The consequences of small intestinal resection. Q. J. Med., 46:485, 1977.
215. Hofmann, A. F., and Poley, J. R.: Cholestyramine treatment of diarrhea associated with ileal resection. N. Engl. J. Med., 281:397, 1969.
216. Jacobsen, O., et al.: Effect of enterocoated cholestyramine on bowel habit after ileal resection: A double blind crossover study. Br. Med. J., 290:1315, 1985.
217. de Dombal, F. T., Burton, I., and Goligher, J. C.: The early and late results of surgical treatment of Crohn's disease. Br. J. Surg., 58:805, 1971.
218. Van Heerden, J. A., McIlrath, D. C., and Adson, M. A.: The surgical aspects of chronic mucosal inflammatory bowel disease (chronic ulcerative colitis). Ann. Surg., 187:536, 1978.
219. Goligher, J. C., et al.: Ulcerative Colitis. London, Baillière Tindall and Cassell, 1968.
220. Glotzer, D. J.: Recurrence in Crohn's colitis: The numbers game. World J. Surg., 4:173, 1980.
221. Steinberg, D. M., et al.: Sequelae of colectomy and ileostomy: Comparison between Crohn's colitis and ulcerative colitis. Gastroenterology, 68:33, 1975.
222. Rogers, A. G., Bargen, J. A., and Black, B. M.: Early and late experience of 124 patients with ileac stomas. Gastroenterology, 27:383, 1954.
223. Waugh, J. M., et al.: Surgical management of chronic ulcerative colitis. Arch. Surg., 88:556, 1964.
224. Rhodes, J. B., and Kirsner, J. B.: The early and late course of patients with ulcerative colitis after ileostomy and colectomy. Surg. Gynecol. Obstet., 121:1303, 1965.
225. Parks, A. G.: Prognosis of patients with an ileostomy. Proc. R. Soc. Med., 58:793, 1965.
226. Watts, J. McK., de Dombal, F. T., and Goligher, J. C.: The ultimate outcome of surgery for ulcerative colitis. Br. J. Surg., 53:1014, 1966.
227. Counsell, P. B., and Lockhart-Mummery, H. E.: Ileostomy: Assessment of disability and management. Lancet, 1:113, 1954.
228. Brooke, B. N.: Outcome of surgery for ulcerative colitis. Lancet, 2:532, 1956.

229. Bacon, H., Bralow, S. P., and Berkeley, J. L.: Rehabilitation and long-term survival after colectomy for ulcerative colitis. J. Am. Med. Assoc., 172:324, 1960.
230. Hughes, E. S. R., et al.: Ileostomy for ulcerative colitis. Aust. N. Z. J. Surg., 32:215, 1963.
231. Wilson, E.: The rehabilitation of patients with an ileostomy established for ulcerative colitis. Med. J. Aust, 1:842, 1964.
232. Roy, P. H., et al.: Experience with ileostomies. Evaluation of long-term rehabilitation in 497 patients. Am. J. Surg., 119:77, 1970.
233. Morowitz, D. A., and Kirsner, J. B.: Ileostomy in ulcerative colitis. A questionnaire study of 1,803 patients. Am. J. Surg., 141:370, 1981.
234. McLeod, R. S., et al.: Patient evaluation of the conventional ileostomy. Dis. Colon Rectum, 28:152, 1985.
235. Dyk, R. B., and Sutherland, A. M.: Adaptation of the spouse and other family members to the colostomy patient. Cancer, 9:123, 1956.
236. Dlin, B. M., Perlman, A., and Ringold, E.: Psychosexual response to ileostomy and colostomy. Am. J. Psychiatry, 126:374, 1969.
237. Lenneberg, E., and Rowbotham, J. L.: The Ileostomy Patient: A Descriptive Study of 1,425 Persons. Springfield, Charles C. Thomas, 1970.
238. Stahlgren, L. H., and Ferguson, L. K.: Influence on sexual function of abdominoperineal resection for ulcerative colitis. N. Engl. J. Med., 259:873, 1958.
239. Donovan, M. J., and O'Hara, E. T.: Sexual function following surgery for ulcerative colitis. N. Engl. J. Med., 262:719, 1960.
240. Davis, L. P., and Jelenko., C.: Sexual function after abdominoperineal resection. South. Med. J., 68:422, 1975.
241. Burnham, W. R., Lennard-Jones, J. E., and Brooke, B. N.: Sexual problems among married ileostomists. Survey conducted by The Ileostomy Association of Great Britain and Ireland. Gut, 18:673, 1977.
242. Corman, M. L., Veidenheimer, M. C., and Coller, J. A.: Impotence after proctectomy for inflammatory disease of the bowel. Dis. Colon Rectum, 21:418, 1978.
243. Yeager, E. S., and van Heerden, J. A.: Sexual dysfunction following proctocolectomy and abdominoperineal resection. Ann. Surg., 191:169, 1980.
244. Bauer, J. J., Gelernt, I. M., Salky, B., and Kreel, I.: Sexual dysfunction following proctocolectomy for benign disease of the colon and rectum. Ann. Surg., 197:363, 1983.
245. May, R. E.: Sexual dysfunction following rectal excision for ulcerative colitis. Br. J. Surg., 53:29, 1966.
246. Scudamore, H. H., et al.: Pregnancy after ileostomy for chronic ulcerative colitis. Gastroenterology, 32:295, 1957.
247. McEwan, H. P.: Pregnancy in patients with surgically treated ulcerative colitis. J. Obstet. Gynaecol. Br. Commonw., 72:450, 1965.
248. Hudson, C. H.: Ileostomy in pregnancy. Proc. R. Soc. Med., 65:281, 1972.
249. Gruner, O. P. N., Naas, R., Fretheim, B., and Gjone, E.: Marital status and sexual adjustment after colectomy. Results in 178 patients operated on for ulcerative colitis. Scand. J. Gastroenterol., 72:193, 1977.
250. Rolstad, B. S., Wilson, G., and Rothenberger, D. A.: Sexual concerns in the patient with an ileostomy. Dis. Colon Rectum, 26:170, 1983.

28 · The Conventional Ileostomy

DAVID G. JAGELMAN, M.S., F.R.C.S., F.A.C.S.

Surgical intervention in patients with ulcerative colitis or Crohn's colitis often involves the creation of an ileostomy. Over the years, patients' fear of such a burden has, in many instances, delayed the timing of appropriate surgical intervention when medical management had been exhausted. In addition, a distaste for the procedure on the part of the patient's physician has created some hesitancy in recommending it. Undoubtedly, an ileostomy following proctocolectomy can offer the patient good normal health, but at a price. Although improvements in surgical technique and the growth of enterostomal therapy have lessened the trauma of an ileostomy, an underlying abhorrence still exists among both patients and physicians that has generated a search for surgical alternatives for those with inflammatory bowel disease involving the large intestine. Nevertheless, proctocolectomy and conventional ileostomy remain mainstays in the methods of surgical treatment in such patients even though continent ileostomy, ileoanal anastomosis, or the ileoanal pouch procedures are becoming more attractive options in the treatment of ulcerative colitis (see Chap. 29).

Historical Perspective

In the early part of this century, the surgical management of "colitis" was primitive at best and was only used after all other means of therapy had failed. Needless to say, most patients who were operated on were almost in extremis and all were in a state of severe malnutrition. Appendicostomy was the procedure of choice at that time and it allowed the instillations of potassium permanganate, boric acid, and dilute bicarbonate solutions "to heal" the inflamed large bowel mucosa.[1] Later it was perceived that fecal diversion away from the ulcerated colonic mucosa was more important, so cecostomy was introduced.[2] It was soon realized that cecostomy produced only partial and inadequate fecal diversion, however, and in 1913 Brown recommended end-ileostomy and presented the results in ten patients subjected to the procedure.[3] The ileum was transected and exteriorized through the main incision, the distal end of the ileum being closed. A cecostomy was also fashioned for colonic irrigation with medications. This procedure remained the technique of choice for many years. As experience grew, a number of problems were encountered, and some alterations in the primary technique were recommended. In 1935, Cattell suggested exteriorizing both ends of the ileum following its transection.[4] Earlier he and Rankin had recognized that many of these patients developed severe dehydration because of excessive fluid and electrolyte loss from their ileostomies.[5] This complication became known as "ileostomy dysfunction" and created enormous problems in rehabilitation postoperatively. At that time it was thought to have been caused by bypassing the right colon and, therefore, not having its resorptive properties available. Further modifications of surgical technique by McKittrick and Miller described the importance of making a small, two-finger-size aperture in the abdominal wall to avoid parastomal hernia and prolapse.[6] In 1941, Dragstedt described the application of a skin graft around the base of the ileostomy to avoid skin ulceration.[7] It was later noted that skin-grafted stomas had less problems as far as ileostomy dysfunction was concerned. Unfortunately, they were also observed to become strictured because of constriction of the skin graft and, thus, required revision. From an analysis of 240 patients in 1951, Warren and McKittrick coined the term dysfunction in relationship to the excessive fluid loss from the ileostomy, and felt it was caused by partial obstruction at the ileostomy itself.[8] These patients were all treated with the Brown type of ileostomy, exteriorized by way of the main abdominal incision.[3] Apart from the problems associated with dehydration, most patients developed severe skin problems with leakage. Appropriate stomal equipment was not available and enterostomal therapy was nonexistent. In 1951, Lahey was the first surgeon to recommend placing the ileostomy through a separate stab incision rather than through the abdominal incision.[9] This was advocated to improve the fitting of the ileostomy appliance. Strauss and Strauss proselytized the use of an adherent appliance, a great step forward in stomal care, and indeed, the birth of enterostomal therapy as we know it today.[10]

The problem relating to ileostomy dysfunction was clarified by the work of Turnbull.[11] He showed that dysfunction was a result of partial obstruction at the ileostomy caused by the exteriorized peristomal surface of the ileum becoming infected. A form of local peritonitis created a lack of peristaltic activity, the lack of emptying led to small bowel dilatation, and the excess of small bowel contents resulted in dehydration. This dysfunction could be relieved by placing a catheter in the ileostomy. In those days, the exteriorized ileum took many weeks to "mature," that is, for the mucosa to reach skin level and prevent the external peritonitis. As a solution to this problem, in 1953, Turnbull recommended the use of the mucosal grafted ileostomy to shorten the maturation time.[11] He trimmed the ileostomy distally of half its muscular coat and then sutured it to the skin. This was a major advance that shortened the recovery time for many patients by avoiding ileostomy dysfunction. At about the same time, Brooke suggested eversion of the ileostomy through a separate stab wound, with primary suture to the skin.[12] This has become the routine technique for the construction of an ileostomy to this day.

In retrospect, surgeons were amiss in concentrating on the surgical aspects of ileostomy construction (even though important) while tending to ignore the more practical and day-to-day problems of ileostomy equipment and management. Fortunately, enterostomal therapy developed concurrently with surgical techniques through patient groups such as the Ostomy Association. The nursing profession also was somewhat late in getting involved in this difficult area of patient care, and Norma Bill, working with the encouragement of Dr. Rupert Turnbull at the Cleveland Clinic Foundation, was the first enterostomal therapist in the world. A stomal therapy school was established by them and has been the inspiration for many similar programs. New and innovative techniques have been established by close involvement with the patients and their problems, and by working with the manufacturers of stomal equipment. Today enterostomal therapy has developed into a highly specialized discipline and has improved the well-being of ileostomy patients both physically and psychologically.

Construction of the Conventional Ileostomy

As already emphasized, a patient requiring an ileostomy is fearful of the physical and emotional repercussions of accepting such a procedure. Even though he knows that an operation is necessary because of his poor health caused by colitis, the patient's fear is enormous. It is the duty of the surgeon and enterostomal therapist to provide emotional and educational support preoperatively, and it is then technically important to achieve a nonretracting, aesthetically acceptable ileostomy that will minimize the patient's physical and emotional turmoil. The ileostomy must be placed on the abdomen at a site where a leak-proof appliance can be worn, where it will not show through the clothes, and where bothersome parastomal hernias will not occur. Postoperatively, the patient will need daily care from an enterostomal therapist to prevent skin complications, to choose appropriate equipment to avoid leakage, and to learn the use of this equipment.

The site of stomal placement should be carefully chosen preoperatively. A point is selected on the right side of the abdomen that is flat and away from creases, previous incisions, and, indeed, the proposed new incision (see also Chapter 27). This point should be checked with the patient both lying down and sitting up. The stoma is best established through the rectus muscle rather than in a more lateral position, because the incidence of parastomal hernia and prolapse is lower (Fig. 28-1). Having selected such a site, a small pin-prick tattoo (using India ink) is made to mark the position with the use of marking rings that approximate to the size of the stomal equipment to be used subsequently. This marking is probably the most important aspect of creating an ileostomy, because without it it is impossible accurately to determine the correct site when the patient is on the operating table. Failure to take this time and effort may lead to difficulties in maintaining a suitably leak-proof appliance postoperatively, thus making the patient's life miserable because of persistent leakage.

At operation, following proctocolectomy the ileostomy is constructed through the right rectus muscle at the previously marked site (Fig. 28-1). The mesentery is trimmed to reduce its size and to allow its access through the abdominal wall, at the same time leaving a strip of mesentery 1.0 cm wide to the tip of the ileum to maintain its viability. The opening in the abdomen is kept small and should be a snug, "two-finger" sized aperture to reduce the incidence of hernia (Fig. 28-2), retraction, and prolapse. A small disc of skin approximately 2.0 cm wide is excised and all layers of the abdominal wall are divided longitudinally down to the rectus mus-

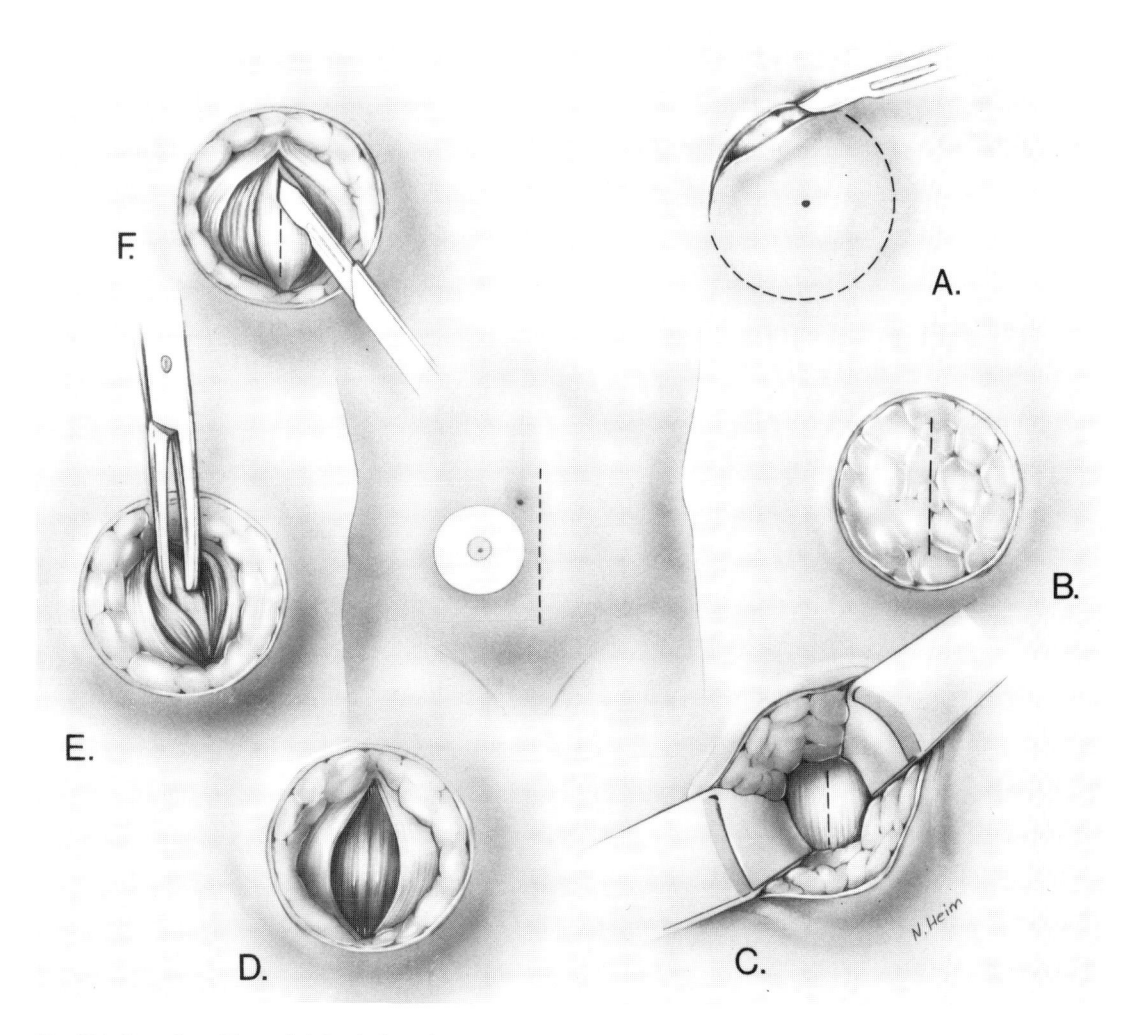

FIG. 28-1. Stomal marking and abdominal aperture.

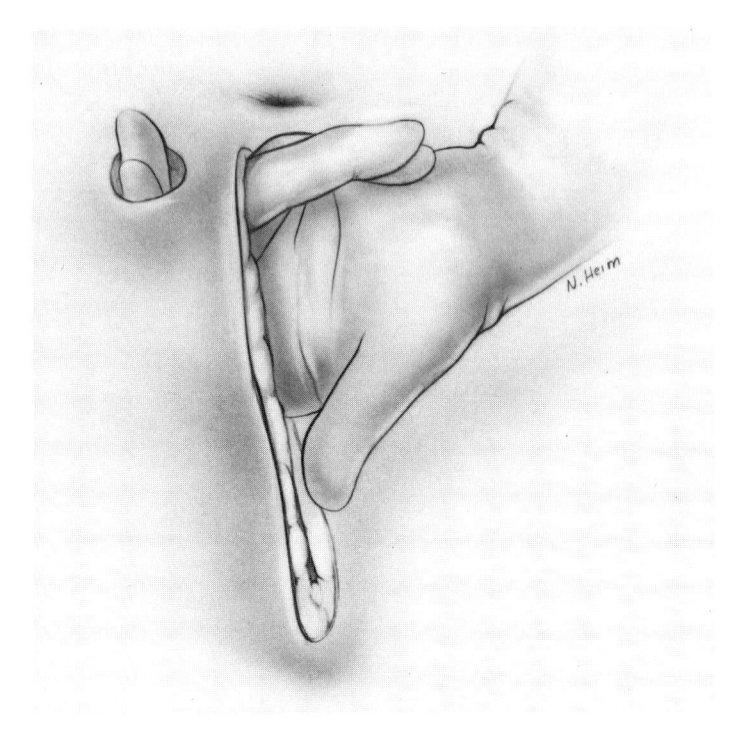

FIG. 28-2. Two finger sized opening.

cle. The rectus muscle fibers are separated longitudinally and the peritoneum divided (Fig. 28-1). Then the ileostomy is brought through without tension and checked for viability. Next, the cut edge of the small bowel mesentery is sutured to the anterior abdominal wall internally, using nonabsorbable suture material, in order to prevent volvulus around the fixed point of the ileostomy (Fig. 28-3). A slightly excessive length of ileum should be brought out to allow for trimming just prior to "maturation." Primary "maturation" is achieved following closure of the ab-

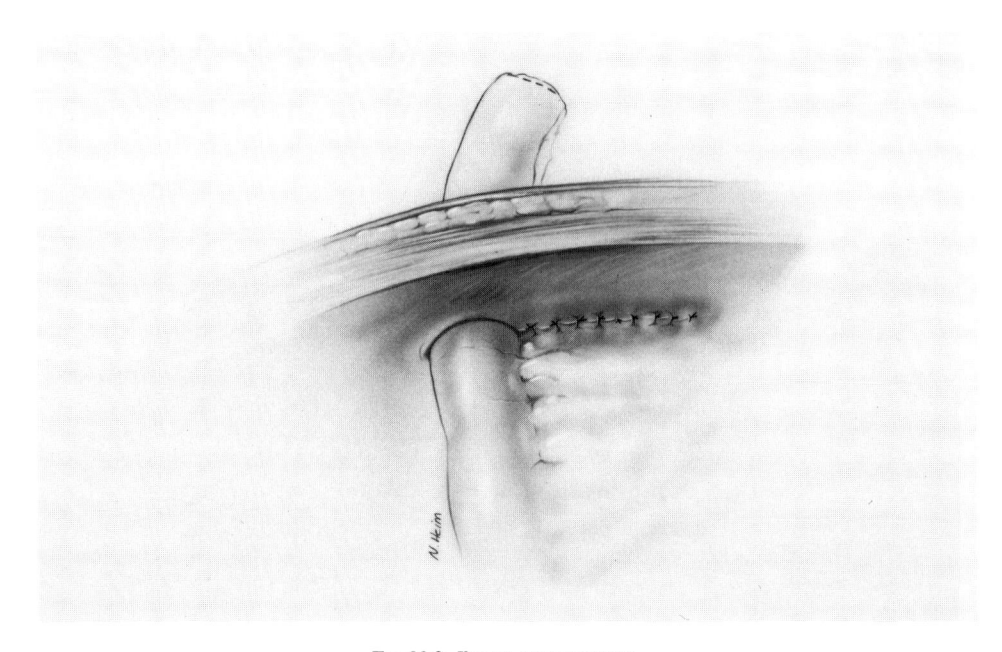

FIG. 28-3. Ileum: cut mesentery.

dominal incision to avoid contamination of the peritoneal cavity with intestinal contents. The staple closure of the ileum is trimmed at an appropriate point to allow for a 2.5 cm ileostomy. Viability of the stoma is reconfirmed but it is predictable if the mesentery has not been trimmed too much. Stabilizing sutures, of interrupted 3-0 catgut, are placed from Scarpa's fascia to the seromuscular layer beneath skin level, to help maintain stomal length and prevent a skin level ileostomy. All layers of the ileum are then sutured to the subcuticular layer circumferentially (Fig. 28-4). This suturing prevents the implantation of viable mucosa into the skin around the ileostomy. Meticulous attention to detail in surgical technique is essential to achieve a satisfactory ileostomy (see Chapter 27). Immediate use of a skin barrier such as karaya ring* or stomahesive† square prevents damage to the peristomal skin. Regular daily care by the enterostomal therapist postoperatively will maintain this situation and ensure a satisfactory result.

Complications of Ileostomy‡

Complications of an ileostomy may be early or late. Of the *early* complications the most urgent is that of *necrosis and retraction* (Fig. 28-5). Retraction may occur with or without ischemia and can be avoided through careful mesenteric trimming and the creation of an ileostomy without tension. On occasion, in obese patients with a short fat mesentery, a loop end or loop ileostomy may be necessary to avoid tension and to maintain the blood supply to the ileostomy. In the early postoperative period, *skin irritation* (Fig. 28-6) can be avoided by the use of skin barriers such as karaya and stomahesive (Fig. 28-7). These protect the skin, and an adhesive pouch is applied to the skin barrier rather than to the skin itself. *Parastomal abscesses* may occur in the first week or so following ileostomy construction and will require "unroofing" of the overlying skin as the latter tends to become necrotic because of the underlying infection (Fig. 28-8 A and B). An alteration in the stomal equipment then may be required until the skin that is "unroofed" heals by secondary intention.

Stomal fistulas occur occasionally, especially in Crohn's disease patients, either spontaneously or because of a seromuscular suture that is too deeply placed or too tightly tied. *Skin excoriation* results if the diameter of the stomal equipment is not reduced to compensate for the shrinkage of the ileostomy that occurs up to 6 weeks following its construction (Fig. 28-9). Patients may develop *allergic cutaneous reactions* to the skin barrier or to the adhesive tape used with the appliance, and appropriate alterations must be made (Fig. 28-10). *Fungal infection* is common if the peristomal skin becomes excoriated but can be treated by the application of nystatin (mycostatin powder).†

A *parastomal hernia* may become a problem over time (Fig. 28-11), and this can be resolved by relocating the stoma and by hernia repair. Such hernias usually can be obviated by placing the ileostomy in the rectus muscle at the original procedure, however, but if relocation becomes necessary it can be achieved without the need of a major laparotomy (Fig. 28-12). *Ileostomy prolapse*, another late complication, occurs when the opening in the abdominal wall is too large, and sometimes this develops in association with a paraileostomy hernia. *Retraction* of the ileostomy as a late complication may occur in Crohn's disease and is indicative of disease recrudescence. It may be associated with stomal ulceration, bleeding, cramping abdominal pain, and increased ileostomy output, all symptoms of such recrudescence. Lastly, injudicious eating of poorly digestible, high roughage foods (e.g., oranges, nuts, popcorn, or pizza) may promote leakage around an ileostomy and may be associated with symptoms suggestive of small bowel obstruction.

Most of these complications can be prevented by careful surgical technique, education, and good enterostomal therapy. Although an ileostomy can restore good health to a patient with severe unresponsive ulcerative colitis, a price must be paid. As previously indicated, ileostomy is not without its physical complications, let alone the psychologic ones that are difficult to measure and vary so much from patient to patient. In 1965, Rhodes and Kirsner reviewed 96 patients undergoing proctocolectomy and ileostomy for ulcerative colitis.[13] Thirty-four of them experienced food bolus obstruction, and only 55% had attained complete perineal wound healing at six months. Ileostomy problems occurred in two-thirds of the patients and additional surgical procedures were required in half the cases.

---

*Marlen Manufacturing and Development Company; Beford, OH 44146.

†E.R. Squibb Company; Princeton, NJ.

‡See also Chapters 30 and 31.

650   SEC. 6 THERAPY

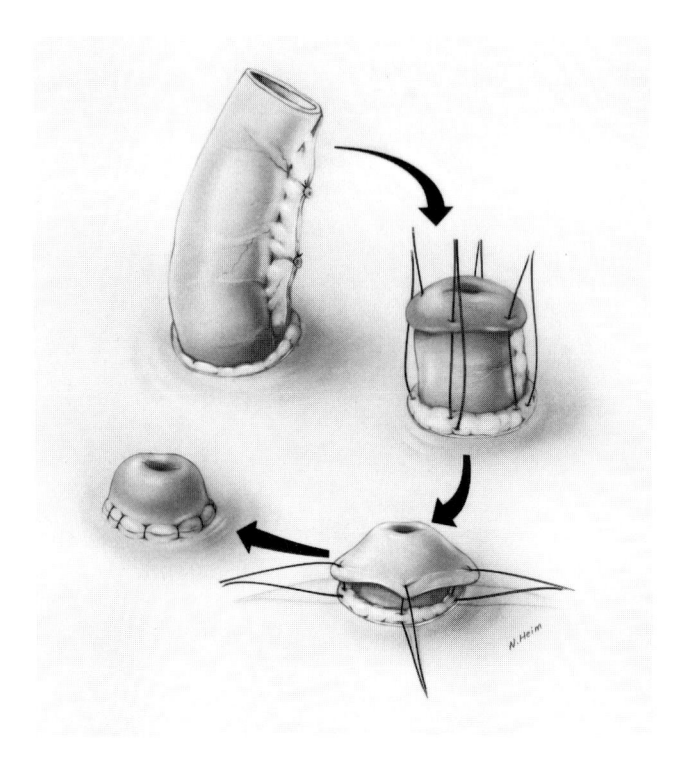

FIG. 28-4. Primary maturation, subcuticular suture.

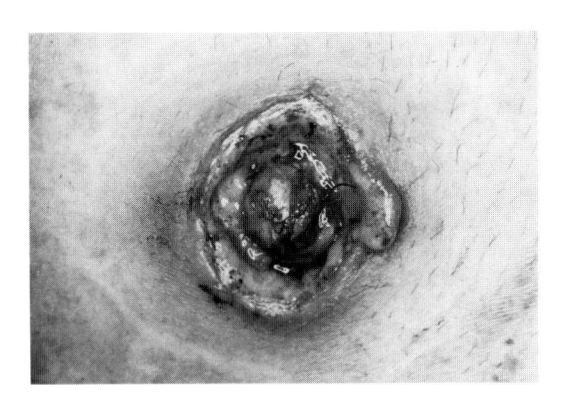

FIG. 28-5. Necrotic ileostomy occurring in early postoperative period.

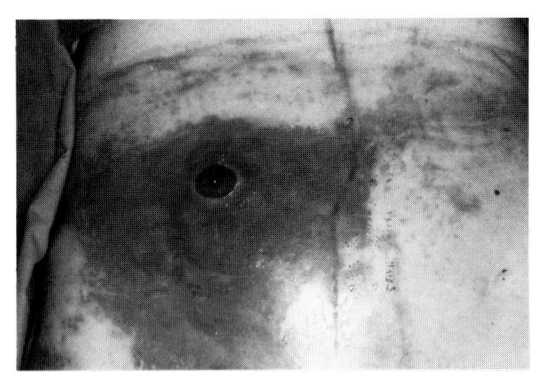

FIG. 28-6. Skin irritation caused by poor postoperative enterostomal care.

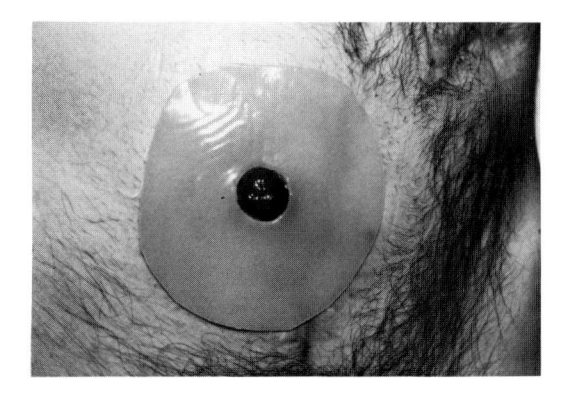

FIG. 28-7. Stomahesive skin barrier fitting ileostomy snugly.

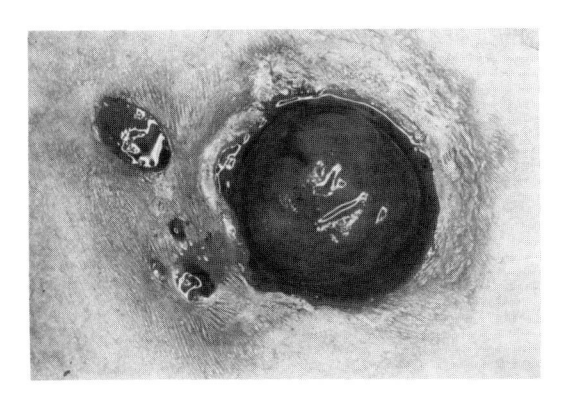

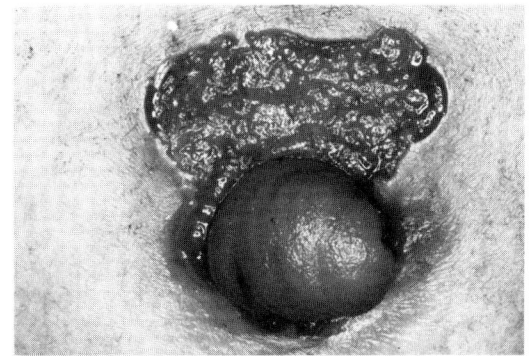

FIG. 28-8A. Parastomal abscess with skin breakdown. B. Debridement of parastomal abscess.

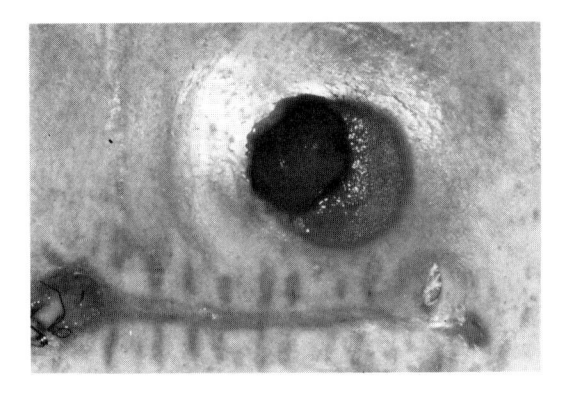

FIG. 28-9. Skin irritation caused by large aperture in the ileostomy appliance.

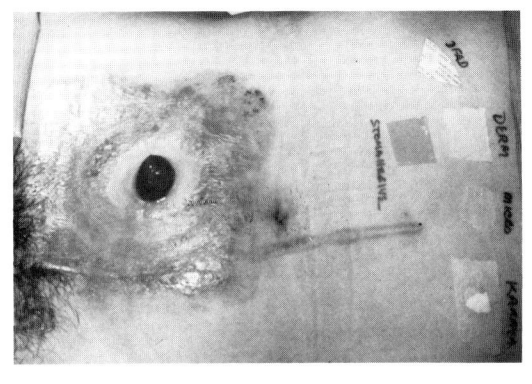

FIG. 28-10. Peri-ileostomy allergic reaction to skin barrier with test patches of equipment.

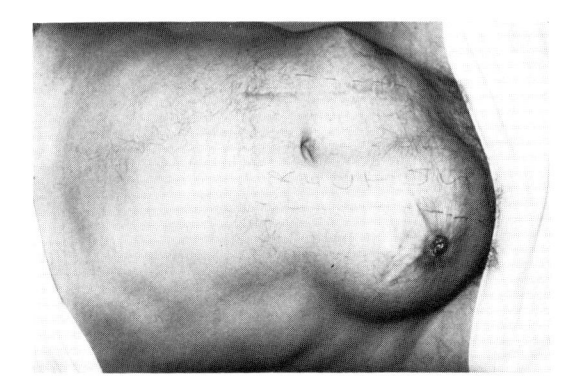

FIG. 28-11. Large paraileostomy hernia with stoma located lateral to rectus sheath.

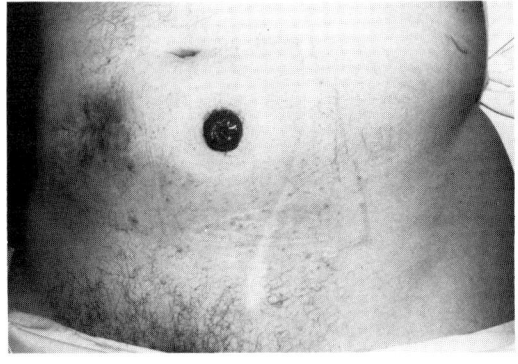

FIG. 28-12. Relocation of ileostomy and repair of parastomal hernia without laparotomy.

In 1966, Watts et al. reviewed 131 patients with conventional ileostomies and quoted reoperation rates of 13% the first year and 13% in the second year.[14] Skin excoriation occurred in 26% and recession or prolapse occurred in 21% of patients. Although these papers are approximately 20 years-old and surgical education and techniques have improved, problems associated with a conventional ileostomy still exist. An increasing awareness of this fact led to the search for surgical alternatives such as the ileoanal pouch or ileoanal anastomosis (see Chap. 29). Unfortunately, these procedures are not recommended for patients with Crohn's disease of the large intestine*. A "conventional" ileostomy therefore remains the only option for a considerable proportion of those with inflammatory bowel disease.

Biochemical Alterations

Following colectomy and ileostomy, the normal output in fluid volume will be from 1000 ml to 1500 ml in the early postoperative period, reducing to 500 ml to 600 ml by the time of discharge from the hospital. The sodium content of an ileostomy effluent in a well-balanced patient with a full length of small intestine will be from 50 to 100 mEq/L. This creates a chronic sodium deficit as well as a fluid loss. It has been found that the ileum compensates somewhat for this loss, but not completely. This chronic state of sodium and water deficit produces alterations in renal function that are manifest by a reduction in the renal excretion of water and sodium.[15,16] Patients with an ileostomy have an increased incidence of renal stones that would be expected with the aforementioned deficits (see also Chap. 31).[17] It is because of this chronic deficit that patients with an ileostomy are at risk of clinical dehydration if the output of the ileostomy increases. This can occur at the time of an unrelated viral illness or with an infectious diarrhea. Patients should always be encouraged to maintain a higher than normal water and sodium intake and to be particularly careful if diarrhea occurs. With a full length of small intestine all other absorptive functions seem to be maintained. If ileum has been resected, however, output is increased and vitamin B_{12} absorption may be compromised, and a disruption of bile salt absorption mechanisms may also occur and there is an increased incidence of gallstones in these patients (see Chap. 31).[18]

Proctocolectomy and "conventional" ileostomy remain mainstays of surgical management of colonic inflammatory bowel disease. In spite of newer procedures, commonly they are the most appropriate and may be requested to avoid some of the complications and uncertainties of the newer options. This is particularly true of older patients who wish to be rid of their "colitis" and who consider the adjustment to a "conventional" ileostomy to be an easier matter than may be the case in younger patients. An ideal operation for "colitis" does not exist; they all have advantages and disadvantages. However, there is no doubt that over the years refinements of surgical care and the growth of enterostomal therapy have made the rehabilitation of the ileostomate easier than before. Rehabilitation from a psychological point of view is more easily achieved if the physical problems of an ileostomy are minimized.*

General Management of the Ileostomy Patient (Editors' Comment)

We put no particular restrictions on the diets of ileostomy patients except for advising them to avoid eating large quantities of certain foods such as fresh fruit, vegetables, or nuts because, as mentioned above, their excessive intake may promote leakage around the ileostomy and provoke intestinal colic.

Because we encourage the patients to live as normal a life as possible, we advise no restrictions of any sort in their social lives, their employment, or their sporting activities, except the avoidance of diving during swimming. If patients wish to travel, we suggest only that they be feeling well and have no problems with the ileostomy. Because, effectively, all aircraft used for long-distance flying are pressurized, air travel should present no difficulties for the ileostomy. We do advise that, before traveling, patients ensure that they are self-sufficient for all their equipment needs for the care of the ileostomy during their trip.

The question of sexual activity is always of concern, and we stress heavily that patients should regard themselves as "normal" in this area of their lives. If young, married women with conventional ileostomies ask whether they can have a family, we raise no objections from the point of the ileostomy per se. Our emphasis throughout is to encourage ileostomy patients not to feel "different." This raises the question of "ileostomy clubs." We regard these as excellent if the patient needs such support in adapting to or living with the ileostomy; if not, we make no particular effort to persuade them to join. In either event, however, we ensure that they are followed up regularly by us or by their local physicians to be sure of their continuance in good health.

---

*Editors' note: see also, Bloom, A. J., et al.: Surg. Gynecol. Obstet., *162*:105, 1986. These authors concluded that continent ileostomy may be used in a few, highly selected patients with inactive Crohn's disease.

*Editors' note: see also, Meyers, S., et al.: Gastroenterology *78*:1, 1980, and Valiulus, A. and Currie, D. J.: Surg. Gynecol. Obstet., *164*:27, 1987.

References

1. Weir, R. F.: A new use for the useless appendix in surgical treatment of obstinate colitis. Med. Rec., *60*:101, 1902.
2. Allison, C. C.: Cecostomy. The operation of choice for temporary drainage of the colon. J. Am. Med. Assoc., *53*:1562, 1909.
3. Brown, J. Y.: Value of complete physiological rest of the large bowel in the treatment of certain ulcerative and obstructive lesions of this organ with description of operative technique and report of cases. Surg. Gynecol. Obstet., *16*:610, 1913.
4. Cattell, R. B.: The surgical treatment of ulcerative colitis. J. Am. Med. Assoc., *104*:104, 1935.
5. Rankin, F. W.: Total colectomy; its indications and technic. Ann. Surg., *94*:677, 1931.
6. McKittrick, L. S., and Miller, R. H.: Idiopathic ulcerative colitis: a review of 149 cases with particular reference to the value of and indications for surgical treatment. Ann. Surg., *102*:656, 1935.
7. Dragstedt, L. R., Dack, G. M., and Kirsner, J. B.: Chronic ulcerative colitis: a summary of evidence implicating Bacterium necrophorum as an etiologic agent. Ann. Surg., *114*:653, 1941.
8. Warren, R., and McKittrick, L. S.: Ileostomy for ulcerative colitis; technique, complications and management. Surg. Gynecol. Obstet., *93*:555, 1951.
9. Lahey, F. H.: Indications for surgical intervention in ulcerative colitis. Ann. Surg., *133*:726, 1951.
10. Strauss, A. A., and Strauss, S. F.: Surgical treatment of ulcerative colitis. Surg. Clin. North. Am., *24*:211, 1944.
11. Turnbull, R. B. Jr.: Symposium on ulcerative colitis: Management of the ileostomy. Am. J. Surg., *86*:617, 1953.
12. Brooke, B. N.: Management of ileostomy including its complications. Lancet, *2*:102, 1952.
13. Rhodes, J. B., and Kirsner, J. B.: The early and late course of patients with ulcerative colitis after ileostomy and colectomy. Surg. Gynecol. Obstet., *121*:1303, 1965.
14a. Watts, J. M., de Dombal, F. T., and Goligher, J. C.: Early results of surgery for ulcerative colitis. Br. J. Surg., *53*:1005, 1966.
14b. Watts, J. McK., de Dombal, F. T., and Goligher, J. C.: Long term complications and prognosis following major surgery for ulcerative colitis. Br. J. Surg., *53*:1014, 1966.
15. Gallagher, N. D., Harrison, D. D., and Skyring, A. P.: Fluid and electrolyte disturbances in patients with long established ileostomies. Gut, *3*:219, 1962.
16. Hill, G. L., Goligher, J. C., Smith, A. H., and Mair, W. S. J.: Long term changes in total body water, total exchangeable sodium and total body potassium before and after ileostomy. Br. J. Surg., *62*:524, 1975.
17. Maratka, Z., and Nedbal, J.: Urolithiasis as a complication of the surgical treatment of ulcerative colitis. Gut, *5*:214, 1964.
18. Hill, G. L., Mair, W. S. J., and Goligher, J. C.: Gallstones after ileostomy and ileal resection. Gut, *16*:932, 1975.

29 · Newer Operations for Ulcerative Colitis and Crohn's Disease

ROGER R. DOZOIS, M.D. AND KEITH A. KELLY, M.D.

Newer operations for ulcerative colitis and Crohn's disease are designed to replace older and imperfect procedures in an aim to be more ideal. To be ideal, an operation should be *safe*, that is, produce minimal morbidity and mortality, should be *effective* in preserving or restoring physiologic functions, and should improve the *quality of life* of patients. In the last decade or two, more progress has been made in approaching the ideal operation for ulcerative colitis than for Crohn's disease. This is probably not surprising. Because the inflammation is confined to the mucosa of the colon and rectum, ulcerative colitis can be cured by proctocolectomy, leaving the uninvolved small intestine for use in preserving and restoring physiologic function. In contrast, Crohn's disease is a nonspecific, inflammatory condition that can involve the whole of the gastrointestinal tract. Severely involved areas can be excised, but apparently uninvolved areas have not been used for reconstruction because of the risk of recurrence in them. Nonetheless, some progress has also been made in the surgical treatment of Crohn's disease. A review of the newer procedures for both diseases is the subject of this chapter.

Surgical Treatment for Ulcerative Colitis

Two newer procedures have emerged in the surgical treatment of ulcerative colitis—the ileal pouch-anal operation and the continent ileal reservoir (Kock pouch).

Ileal Pouch-Anal Anastomosis

The ileal pouch-anal anastomosis is designed to preserve fecal continence in patients with ulcerative colitis who require excision of their large intestine. In this operation, the cecum, the colon, and the proximal rectum are excised completely, but only the mucosa of the distal rectum is removed. Intestinal continuity is restored by the endorectal anastomosis of an ileal pouch to the anal canal at the dentate line. The operation preserves voluntary transanal defecation and maintains reasonable fecal continence. The operation, however, does impair fecal continence to some extent. An excellent review of the operation has been published.[1]

BACKGROUND

The combination of proctocolectomy and Brooke ileostomy has been the standard operation for ulcerative colitis. The procedure "cures" the disease, is safe, and improves the quality of an often previously miserable existence. The operation does not preserve fecal continence, however, an important physiologic function. Intestinal content and gas pass freely from the ileal stoma at any time. Consequently, an appliance must be worn continuously, day and night, to collect the discharge and prevent soiling. The psychologic and social disadvantages of having to wear a bag of ileal effluent attached to the anterior abdominal wall are a major handicap.

Moreover, about one-fourth of patients with a conventional ileostomy have significant problems that are directly or indirectly associated with the use of external appliances.[2] The ileal content, the appliance, or its adhesives may irritate the skin, causing weeping, itching, erythema, and edema. The appliances may be uncomfortable because of their weight and lack of porosity. The ever-present possibility of leakage and odor is an additional concern to patients. Appliances require upkeep and replacement, imposing a financial burden. Some patients also complain of the time required for daily care of their ileostomy.

To avoid an incontinent Brooke ileostomy, some surgeons, in the past and even today, have advocated colectomy and ileorectostomy rather than proctocolectomy and Brooke ileostomy. The ileorectostomy preserves the transanal path of defecation and anorectal continence, but it leaves behind a diseased rectum that causes symptoms and develops complications, including cancer. Thus, ileorectostomy does not fulfill the criteria for an ideal operation.

RATIONALE

The rationale for the ileal pouch-anal operation is that excision of the cecum, colon, proximal rectum, and distal rectal mucosa would remove all of the disease in patients with ulcerative colitis, and yet the ileal pouch-anal anastomosis would maintain an adequate fecal reservoir, preserve fecal continence and voluntary transanal defecation, and avoid ileostomy. In addition, because the distal rectal mucosa is removed endorectally, the chance of damage to the innervation of the bladder and genitalia during the operation would be minimized. Finally, because a complete proctectomy is not done, no perineal wound results, a wound which is sometimes difficult to heal.

THE OPERATION

The technique currently used at the Mayo Clinic in Rochester, Minnesota consists of excision of the cecum, colon, and proximal rectum, distal mucosal rectectomy, construction of a "J"-shaped ileal pouch, and ileal pouch-anal anastomosis.[3,4] A two-staged operative approach is used, protecting the pouch-anal anastomosis with a diverting loop ileostomy at the first operation and closing the loop ileostomy at a second operation about 2 months later.

The anesthetized patient is positioned on the operating table in the modified lithotomy position, giving access both to abdomen and perineum. A vertical midline incision is made. The abdomen is explored, and the presence of ulcerative colitis ascertained. The cecum and colon are mobilized, preserving the greater omentum. The rectum is freed down to the pelvic floor, keeping as close to the rectal wall as possible, thereby avoiding damage to the pelvic autonomic nerves.[5] The mobilized rectum is then divided about 7 cm proximal to the levator ani. A stapling device facilitates the division. The cecum, colon, and proximal rectum are removed and sent for pathologic examination to confirm the diagnosis.

Next, the ileal pouch is constructed from the distal 30 cm of ileum. Several types of ileal reservoirs are currently being employed, including the "J"-shaped,[6] "S"-shaped,[7] "W"-shaped,[8] and the lateral-lateral pouch.[9] Thus far, we have preferred the modified "J"-shaped reservoir of Utsunomiya that is simpler to construct, uses less intestine, and can be done more rapidly than other, more complex types of reservoirs, thus decreasing the chance of contamination and infection.[6] Moreover, the "J"-pouch gives clinical results comparable to those obtained with the other reservoirs. Also, from a physiologic point of view, the "J"-pouch will ultimately accommodate nearly 400 ml of content, preserve the anorectal angle by fitting the concavity of the sacrum, generate low but coordinated propulsive contractions, and, most importantly, can be emptied voluntarily.[10]

Pouch construction is begun by mobilizing the small intestinal mesentery from the retroperitoneum to allow the distal ileum to reach to the level of the dentate line. Dividing the visceral peritoneum along the right side of the superior mesenteric artery allows the mesentery to stretch and increases its length. If additional length is required, the ileocolic vessels or branches of the superior mesenteric vessels can be transected. When it is clear that the ileum will reach the dentate line, construction of the "J"-pouch is begun using the terminal 30 cm of ileum. The terminal ileum is folded into a "J"-shape. Continuous 2-0 chromic catgut or 2-0 polyglycolic acid sutures are used to approximate the seromuscular layers of the two 15 cm limbs (Figs. 29-1 and 29-2). The antimesenteric border of the limbs is incised and the mucosal surface

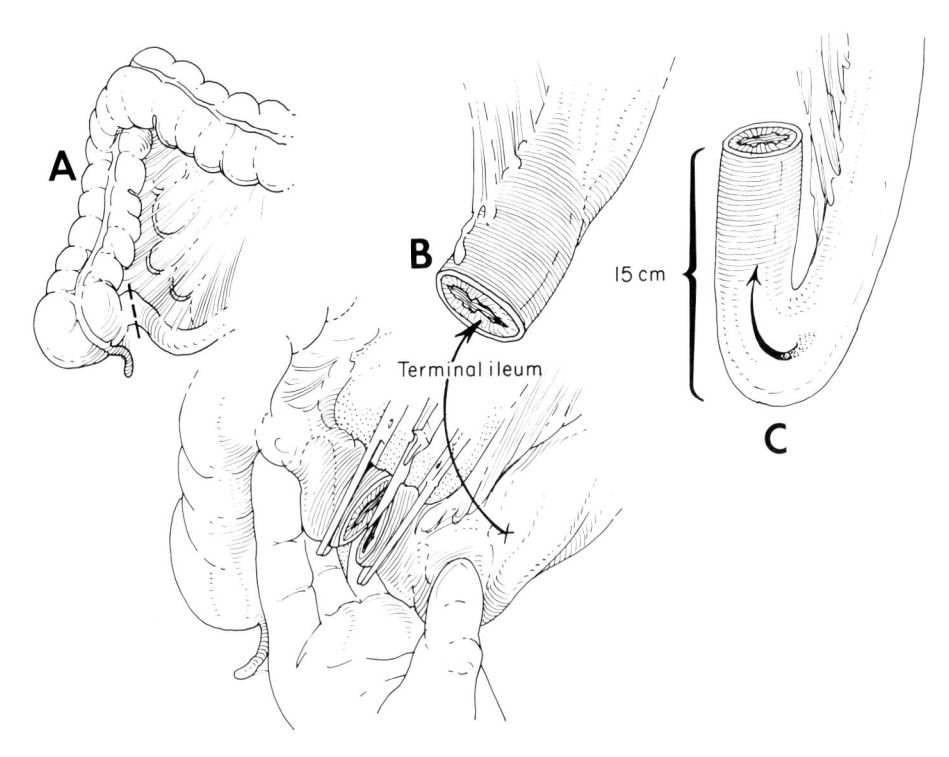

FIG. 29-1. Construction of a "J"-shaped ileal pouch. Initial steps. (Reprinted with permission from Kelly, K. A., and Dozois, R. R.: Chronic ulcerative colitis. *In* Surgical Treatment of Digestive Diseases. Edited by F. Moody. Chicago, Year Book Medical Publishers, 1985.)

of the newly-forming pouch exposed. A second row of sutures is used on the mucosal layer of the posterior wall. The anterior wall is then completed in the same two-layer fashion. Alternatively, the pouch may be constructed using a stapling device.

The surgeon then moves to the perineum to perform the removal of the distal rectal mucosa. The anus is effaced and dilated slightly by placing and opening two Gelpi self-retaining retractors at the anal verge. A dilute (1:100,000) solution of epinephrine is injected into the submucosa at the dentate line to aid separation of the mucosa from the underlying muscularis and to reduce bleeding. Dissection of the diseased rectal mucosa, using cautery or scissors, in the submucosal plane begins at the dentate line and extends proximally to a distance of 3 to 5 cm (Figs. 29-3 and 29-4). After the first 2 cm of mucosa are mobilized, the dissection is facilitated by everting the distal rectum onto the perineum. Using a tissue forceps passed per anum, the apex of the rectal stump is grasped and pulled inside-out (Fig. 29-5). Once 3 to 5 cm of distal rectal mucosa have been mobilized, the rectum is transected at this level and the more proximal rectum is excised (Fig. 29-6). The distal rectal muscular cuff is returned through the anus into the pelvis. An alternate technique is to excise the distal rectal mucosa without everting the rectum

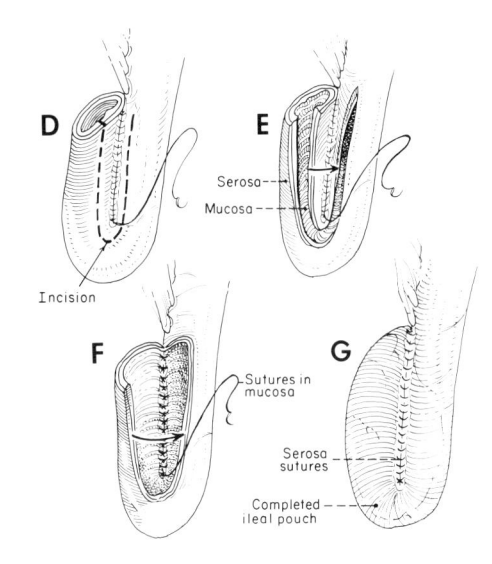

FIG. 29-2. Construction of a "J"-shaped ileal pouch. Final steps. (Reprinted with permission from Kelly, K. A., and Dozois, R. R.: Chronic ulcerative colitis. *In* Surgical Treatment of Digestive Diseases. Edited by F. Moody. Chicago, Year Book Medical Publishers, 1985.)

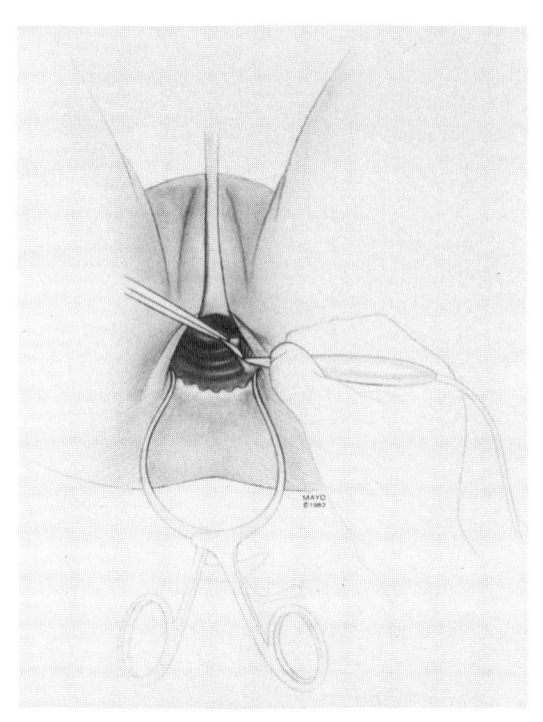

FIG. 29-3. Technique of rectal mucosectomy. Gelpi retractors are used to efface anus and expose dentate line.

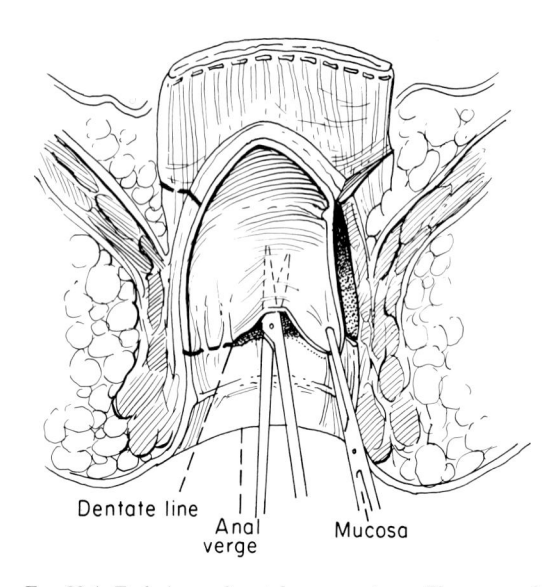

FIG. 29-4. Technique of rectal mucosectomy. The mucosal stripping begins at dentate line and extends to levator ani. (Reprinted with permission from Dozois, R. R.: Br. J. Surg. *(Suppl.)*, 72:S80, 1985.)

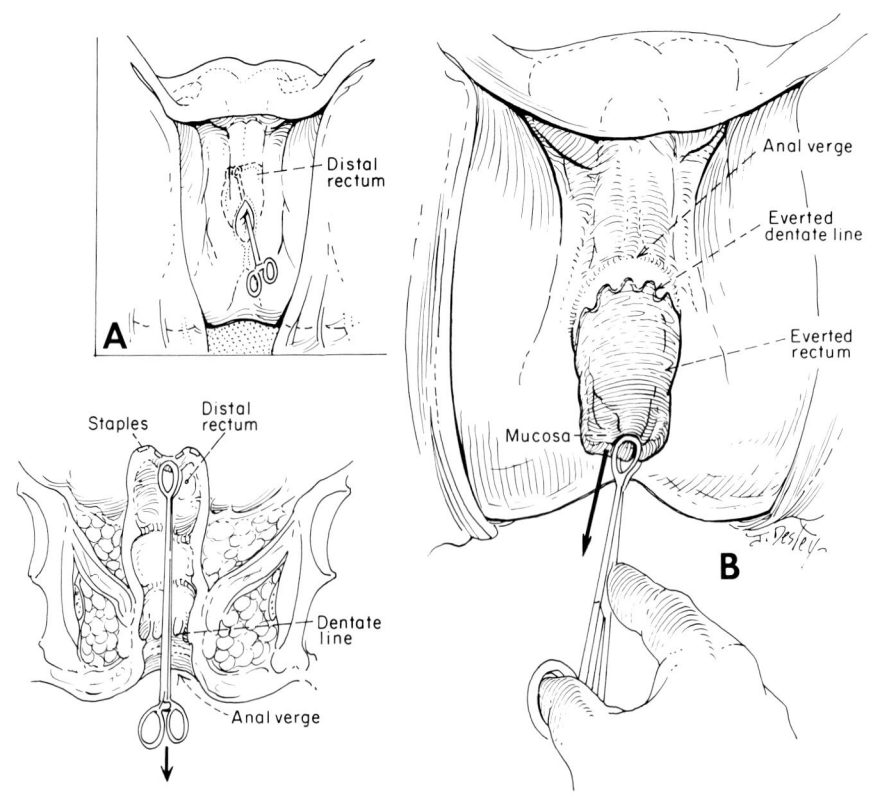

FIG. 29-5. Technique of rectal eversion to facilitate distal mucosal stripping. (Reprinted with permission from Kelly, K. A., and Dozois, R. R.: Chronic ulcerative colitis. *In* Surgical Treatment of Digestive Diseases. Edited by F. Moody. Chicago, Year Book Medical Publishers, 1985.)

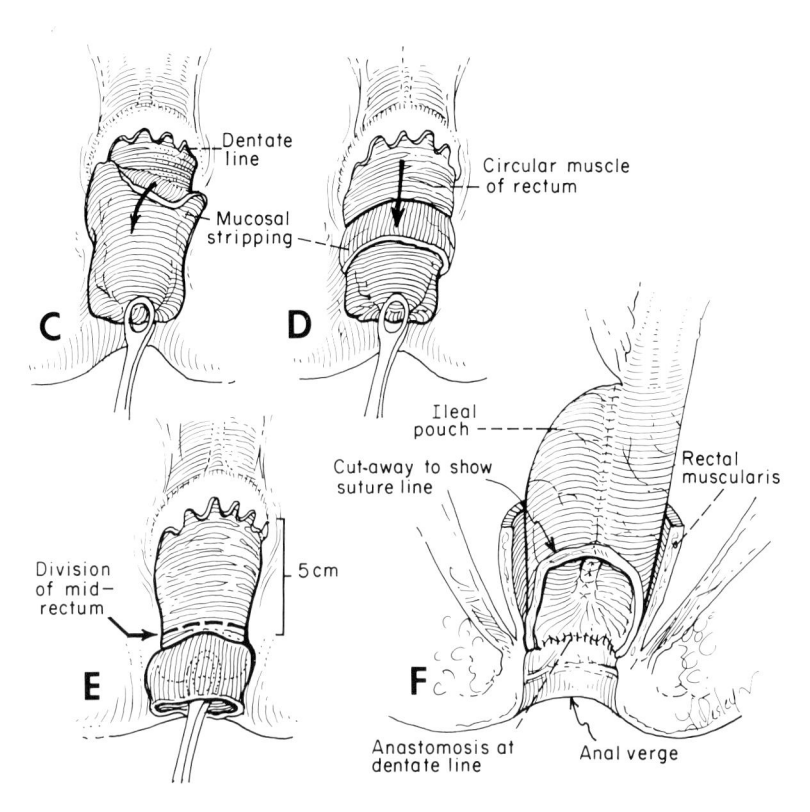

FIG. 29-6. Technique of distal mucosal rectectomy and ileal pouch-anal anastomosis. (Reprinted with permission from Kelly, K. A., and Dozois, R. R.: Chronic ulcerative colitis. *In* Surgical Treatment of Digestive Diseases. Edited by F. Moody. Chicago, Year Book Medical Publishers, 1985.)

by using anal dilatation and transanal dissection (Fig. 29-4). Currently, we favor the short 3 to 5 cm muscular cuff that reduces operating time, bleeding, and contamination, and thus the risk of pelvic sepsis, allows for better expansion of the neorectum and decreases the chance of leaving behind potentially premalignant mucosal cells.

The previously constructed ileal "J" pouch is then pulled endorectally through the muscular cuff, and its most distal portion is anastomosed to the anoderm at the dentate line, working intraluminally and using 3-0 absorbable sutures (Figs. 29-6 and 29-7). A soft, silastic drainage catheter, placed in the presacral space behind the pouch and brought out through a left abdominal wall stab wound, drains the space in the postoperative period. A loop ileostomy is then established through an opening made in the right lower abdominal wall.

The patient is allowed about 2 months to recover from the first operation, after which the second operation is performed. At this time, complete healing of the pouch and the anastomosis can usually be demonstrated radiographi-

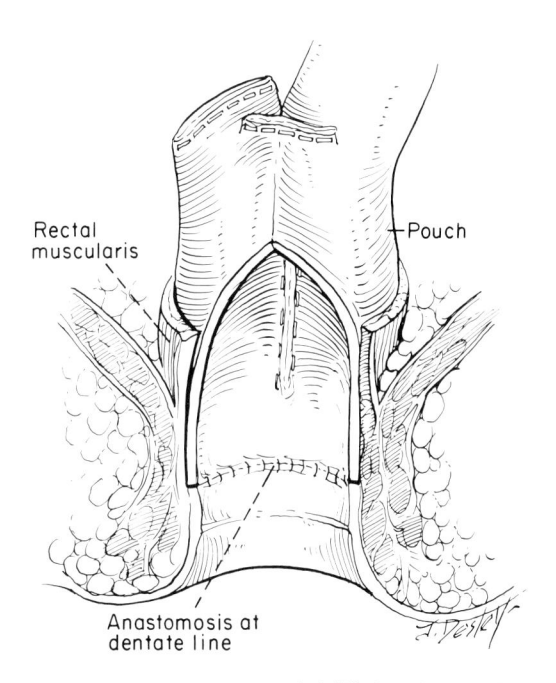

FIG. 29-7. Anastomosis of stapled "J"-shaped reservoir to dentate line. (Reprinted with permission from Dozois, R. R.: Br. J. Surg. *(Suppl.)*, 72:S80, 1985.)

cally, allowing enteric continuity to be restored. The loop ileostomy is mobilized through a small transverse, biconvex incision that encompasses the stoma. The defect in the bowel is closed using sutures. The repair is usually done without performing bowel transection or resection.

CLINICAL EVALUATION

THE PATIENTS. Between January, 1981 and August, 1987, about 650 adult patients have undergone the operation at the two hospitals affiliated with the Mayo Clinic. The operation was done for ulcerative colitis in approximately 93% of the patients and for familial polyposis coli in approximately 7% of the group. About equal numbers of men and women have undergone the operation. The mean age of the patients was 32 years; the ages ranged from 17 to 64 years. The mean hospital stay was 10 days after the first stage of the operation and 7 days after the second.

EARLY POSTOPERATIVE RESULTS. A detailed analysis of our initial 390 ulcerative colitis patients has been done. One of the patients died in the immediate postoperative period of pulmonary embolus. Pelvic sepsis developed in 21 patients (5%), and necessitated one or more abdominal operations in 12 patients, 5 of whom ultimately lost their reservoir. In the remaining 9 patients, local drainage and antibiotics sufficed to overcome the infection. Ileostomy closure was postponed for various periods of time in 15 patients because of asymptomatic delayed healing of the pouch-anal anastomosis. Other important complications included small bowel obstruction (21%), reservoir ileitis (14%), and anastomotic stricture requiring dilatation under anesthesia (5%). In all, 24 patients (6%) had their ileal reservoir excised and a permanent ileostomy established because of persistent sepsis despite surgical drainage, subsequent appearance of obvious Crohn's disease in the neorectum, or intractable diarrhea.

LATE POSTOPERATIVE RESULTS. All patients evacuated spontaneously; none had to use intubation to empty the pouch. At a follow-up of 1 to 6 years, 390 patients had a mean stool frequency (mean ± SD) of 6 ± 2 per day and 1 ± 1 at night.[11] A decrease in stool frequency occurred gradually during the 12 months following ileostomy closure,[11,12] and was associated with increasing capacity of the reservoir. Few patients had frank incontinence, but soiling and seepage did occur. Episodes of fecal soiling, defined as leakage serious enough to require the wearing of a protective pad, occurred in 2.5% of 157 patients during the day and 4.5% during sleep. Seepage, defined as minor staining or spotting of the underclothes, was more common, occurring more than twice a month in 25% of patients during waking hours and 47% at night (Table 29-1). Continence improved with time, following operation. Patients over 50 years of age had a greater stool frequency than younger patients.

QUALITY OF LIFE. Our group has compared performance status after performing Brooke ileostomy or ileoanal anastomosis.[13] Although the majority of patients (>90%) in each category were satisfied with their operation, a greater number of Brooke ileostomy patients stated they would consider a change (40% vs 6%, p < 0.001). Moreover, in each performance category, more ileoanal patients improved and fewer were restricted in pursuing daily activities than Brooke ileostomy patients (Table 29-2).

Most patients stated that their sexual function was unchanged or improved following operation. Thus, of the men, two percent developed impotence or failed to reach orgasm postoperatively, and 7 (4%) developed retrograde ejaculation.[11] In women, frequency of intercourse and ability to reach orgasm increased after operation, while dyspareunia decreased.[14] Six of 8 women who attempted to conceive succeeded and carried their pregnancy to term.[15] None of the 5 women who delivered vaginally demonstrated any perceptible alteration in subsequent continence.

TABLE 29-1. *Continence After Ileal Pouch-anal Anastomosis (157 patients).*

Factors Evaluated	Distribution by Degree of Continence (Percentage of Patients)		
	Perfect	Seepage*	Soilage*
Daytime	75	23	2
Nighttime	48	47	5
Daytime			
At 9 months	64	31	5
At 18 months	81	19	0
Disease treated			
Ulcerative colitis	72	25	3
Polyposis coli	90	10	0
Age			
<50 years	75	25	0
≥50 years	55	45	0

*See text for definitions.

TABLE 29-2. *Performance Status After Proctocolectomy.*

Type of Operation (Number of Patients)	Desire to Change (Percentage of Patients)	Activities (Percent Improved/Percent Restricted)		
		Sex	Social	Sports
Brooke (675)	40	15/29	28/21	15/43
Kock pouch (330)	11	31†/29	38†/17	26†/21†
Ileoanal (50)	6	34*/8**	56*/12**	40*/8**

* Ileoanal anastomosis > Brooke; p < 0.02
† Differs from Brooke, p < 0.05
** Ileoanal anastomosis < Brooke; p < 0.002

PHYSIOLOGIC RESULTS

Detailed physiologic studies have been performed on postoperative patients in order to define the alterations in fecal continence that occur as a result of the operation. Fecal continence depends upon a number of different factors. These include the anal sphincters, anorectal sensation, the puborectalis and the anorectal angle, the rectoanal inhibitory reflex, the distensibility and capacity of the rectum, rectal motility and "evacuability," the rapidity of transit through more proximal bowel, and the quality and quantity of the enteric content.

ANAL SPHINCTERS. Resting anal sphincteric tone is generally well-maintained after the operation, with only a slight decrease present compared to controls (Fig. 29-8). The mean maximum pressure ± SEM* among 10 patients was 71 cm H_2O ± 8 cm H_2O, compared to 87 cm H_2O ± 7 cm H_2O among healthy volunteers.[16] The decrease after operation may be a result of operative damage to the internal sphincter, to the external sphincter, or to the sphincteric innervation. Indeed, damage to the external sphincter or its innervation has been detected with electromyography in a few patients.[17] In those few patients in whom anal sphincteric resting tone was poor or absent after operation, gross fecal incontinence was more likely to be present. Thus, the maintenance of satisfactory resting sphincteric tone after operation is an essential factor in the maintenance of reasonable fecal incontinence in the postoperative period.

The anal squeeze mechanism is also usually intact after operation (Fig. 29-9). The pressure increases brought about by the squeeze after operation are largely unchanged from those found in healthy individuals. In a few patients, however, squeeze pressures were less than in controls, and in these patients a greater incidence of incontinence was found.

Overall, these findings suggest that the integrity of the anal sphincter and its extrinsic innervation is usually not greatly damaged by the operation. Also, the squeeze mechanism must not depend upon an intact proximal rectal muscular wall or upon intact rectal mucosa. After operation, as before operation, the squeeze mechanism likely acts to prevent leakage when propulsive forces from above stress the anal sphincter, but the squeeze mechanism is unlikely to maintain continence from hour to hour.

ANORECTAL SENSATION. The patients are able to detect the need for evacuation of the ileal pouch, and most can determine the nature of the content distending the neorectum.[18] Thus, the rectal mucosa must not be needed for anorectal sensation. Although the rectal mucosa was completely excised at the operation, sensory discrimination persisted. Sensation must arise, in part, in the anoderm of the anal canal, all of which has been preserved. A portion of the distal rectal tunica muscularis remains, however, and this could be responsible, in part, for the proprioceptive detection of distention of the underlying ileal pouch.

ANORECTAL ANGLE. The anorectal angle has not been studied extensively in ileoanal anastomosis patients to date (Fig. 29-10). The puborectalis muscle, however, is not usually disturbed by the distal mucosal rectectomy. Theoretically, the anorectal angle should be maintained after operation, because the apex of the pouch is pulled through the intact puborectalis loop. Tension at the anastomotic line, pelvic infection, and anastomotic dehiscence, however, may increase the angle and lead to gross fecal incontinence. Alternatively, if postoperative adhesions or kinks

* SEM = standard error of the mean.

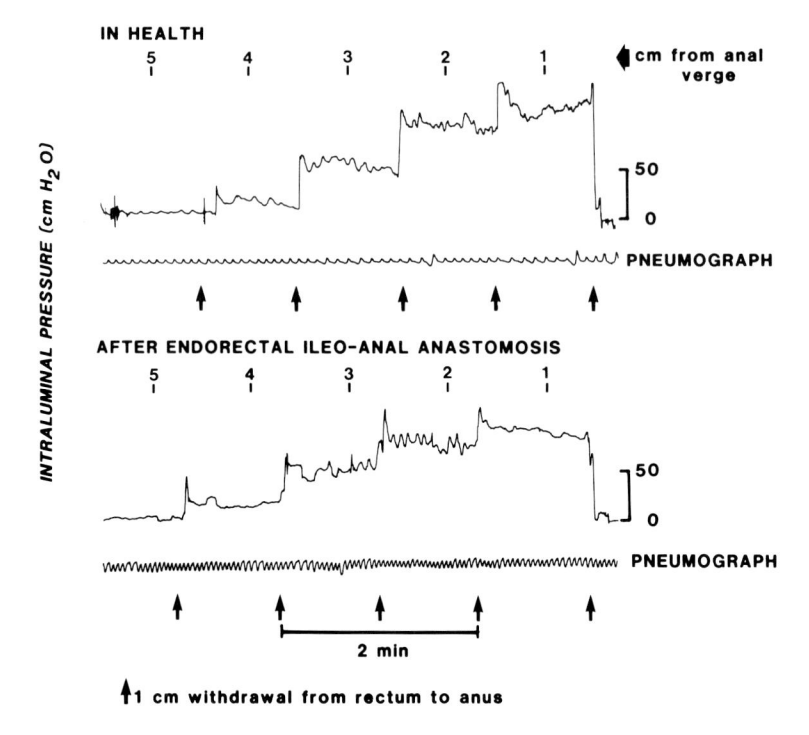

FIG. 29-8. Pull-through pressure profile of human anal sphincters in health and after ileoanal anastomosis. (Reprinted with permission from Kelly, K. A., and Pemberton, J. H.: Mechanisms of fecal continence: alterations with ileal pouch-anal anastomosis. *In* Cellular Physiology and Clinical Studies of Gastrointestinal Smooth Muscle. Edited by J. H. Szurszewski. Amsterdam, Elsevier/North-Holland Biomedical Press, 1987.)

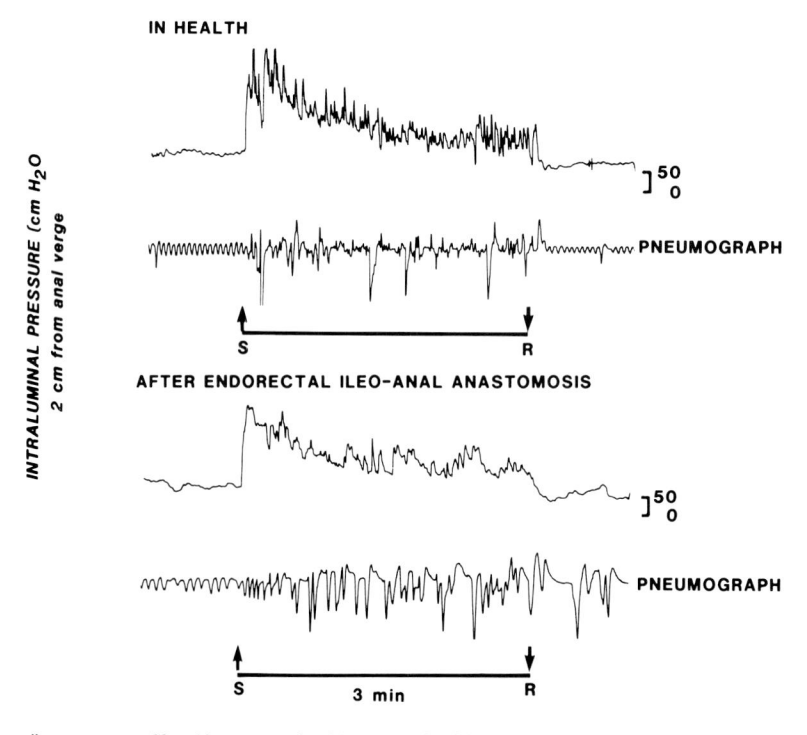

FIG. 29-9. "Squeeze" pressure profile of human anal sphincters in health and after ileoanal anastomosis. S = onset of squeeze, R = relaxation of squeeze. (Reprinted with permission from Kelly, K. A., and Pemberton, J. H.: Mechanisms of fecal continence: alterations with ileal pouch-anal anastomosis. *In* Cellular Physiology and Clinical Studies of Gastrointestinal Smooth Muscle. Edited by J. H. Szurszewski. Amsterdam, Elsevier/North-Holland, 1987.)

the anal canal. Distention of the pouch dilates the proximal canal. Thus, relaxation of the proximal part of the anal sphincter cannot be accurately measured by conventional intraluminal, pressure-sensitive devices.

The precise role of the rectal-anal inhibitory reflex is thrown into dispute by the finding that continence after ileoanal anastomosis is not hampered by the absence of the reflex. Patients in whom the reflex is lost may have perfect continence, and vice versa. The degree of continence does not correlate with the presence or absence of the rectal-anal inhibitory reflex.

NEORECTAL DISTENSIBILITY AND CAPACITY. The "J"-shaped ileal pouch we use has adequate distensibility and capacity. The distensibility of the "J"-pouch is similar to the distensibility of the healthy rectum (Fig. 29-12). The slope of the pressure-volume curve of the pouch patients during gradual pouch distention is nearly identical to the slope obtained from healthy subjects.[19] The capacity of the pouch (approximately 400 ml) is also similar to the capacity of the healthy rectum.

The satisfactory distensibility and capacity of the ileal pouch are reflected in the clinical results. The more distensible the pouch, the fewer the stools passed per day. Also, pouch distensibility prior to ileostomy closure correlates well with the postclosure stool frequency, the ability of the pouch to distend being reflected in a lower stool frequency.[20] Thus, the "J"-pouch provides a distensible, compliant, and capacious neorectum, a factor contributing to satisfactory postoperative fecal continence.

NEORECTAL MOTILITY. We studied the motility of the ileal pouch using open-tipped perfusion catheters and a flaccid, pressure-sensitive, distending bag placed in the pouch. It seemed possible that the differences in continence among patients were related to differences in the motility of the reservoirs. My colleagues and I, and other research groups, have found that large waves (mean ± SEM amplitude, 49 ± 2 cm H_2O) appeared in the pouches in response to distention (Figs. 29-12 and 29-13).[19-24] Pressures achieved in the pouch during the large waves sometimes even exceeded the resting anal sphincteric tone. When the large waves were present, our patients experienced the desire to evacuate. Voluntary squeeze contraction of the external anal sphincter was then required to maintain continence. Nonetheless, leakage of stool occasionally occurred. The frequency and

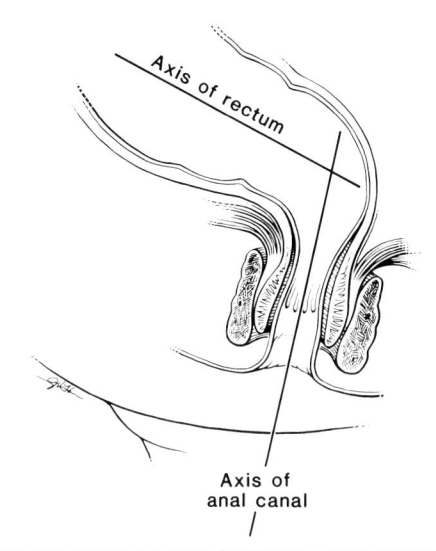

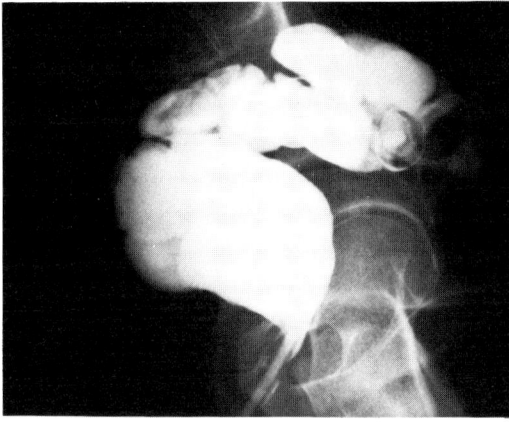

FIG. 29-10. Anorectal angle. A. in healthy man (diagram). B. after ileal "J"-pouch-anal anastomosis (lateral radiograph). (Reprinted with permission from Kelly, K. A., and Pemberton, J. H.: Mechanisms of fecal continence: alterations with ileal pouch-anal anastomosis. In Cellular Physiology and Clinical Studies of Gastrointestinal Smooth Muscle. Edited by J. H. Szurszewski. Amsterdam, Elsevier/North-Holland, 1987.)

accentuate the angle to 80° or less, content will not pass readily. Inefficient evacuation and overflow incontinence may then result.

RECTOANAL INHIBITORY REFLEX. The rectal-anal inhibitory reflex is usually lost after the operation (Fig. 29-11). In a few patients with a long rectal muscle cuff (8 to 12 cm), however, the rectoanal inhibitory reflex has been demonstrated postoperatively. The reflex, therefore, is likely to be initiated by proprioceptive receptors located in the muscular wall of the rectum. One problem in determining whether or not the reflex is present after the operation is that the distal point of the ileal pouch rests within the upper portion of

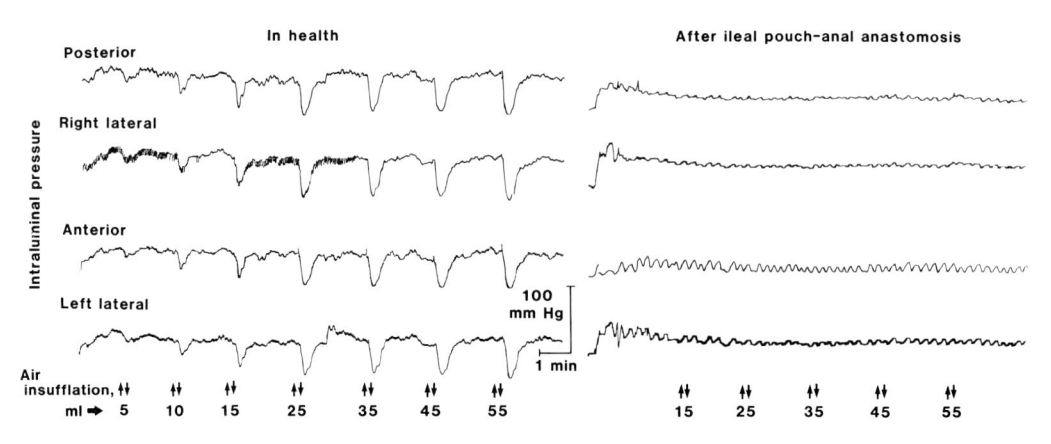

Fig. 29-11. Rectal-anal inhibitory reflex in response to increasingly large volumes of distal enteric distention before and after ileoanal anastomosis. The reflex is absent after operation. (Reprinted with permission from Stryker, S. J., et al.: Ann. Surg., 203:55, 1986.)

amplitude of the large waves were found to increase with time during fasting and following a meal, presumably as the pouch filled. With evacuation, the large waves promptly subsided.[24] It seemed, therefore, that the threshold volume at which the waves appear in the ileal pouch may be an important determinant of postoperative stool frequency.[19] As the threshold is a function of pouch capacity and distensibility, it would explain why both of these functions are also determinants of clinical outcome.

Clearly, the presence of large amplitude contractions in the ileal pouch with pouch distention contrasts with the absence of such contractions in the healthy rectum distended to the same degree. The large amplitude ileal pouch contractions are one factor that leads to less than perfect continence in the patients after operation.

EVACUATION OF NEORECTUM. Evacuation also occurred spontaneously and voluntarily after operation; none of our patients with a "J"-shaped pouch required intubation for evacuation. As in the healthy rectum, no obstruction to defecation

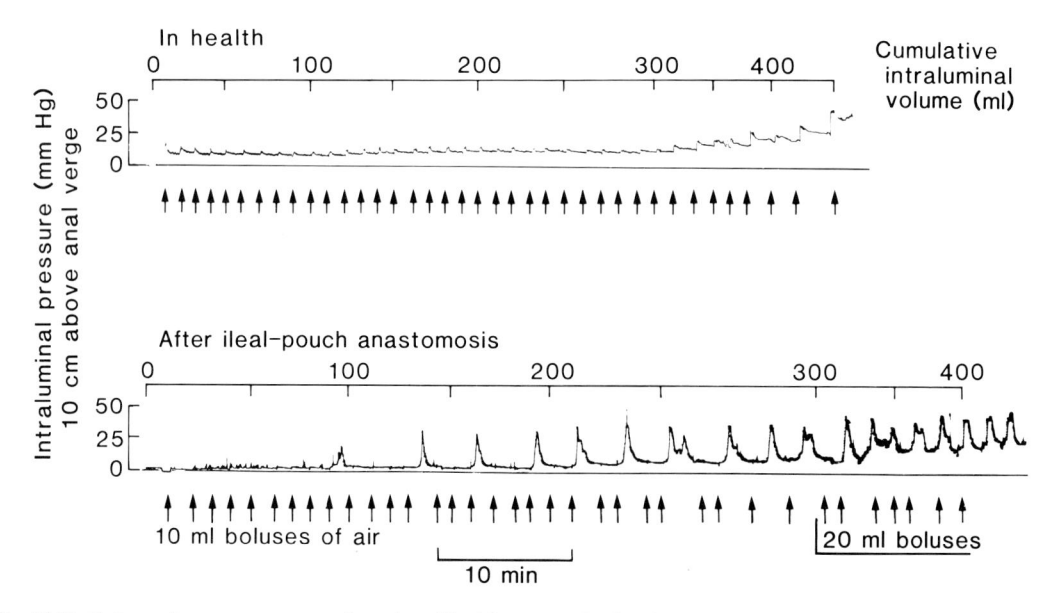

Fig. 29-12. Pattern of pressure waves on distention of healthy rectum (top) and neorectum (bottom) after ileoanal anastomosis. (Reprinted with permission from Kelly, K. A., and Pemberton, J. H.: Mechanisms of fecal continence: alterations with ileal pouch-anal anastomosis. In Cellular Physiology and Clinical Studies of Gastrointestinal Smooth Muscle. Edited by J. H. Szurszewski. Amsterdam, Elsevier/North-Holland, 1987.)

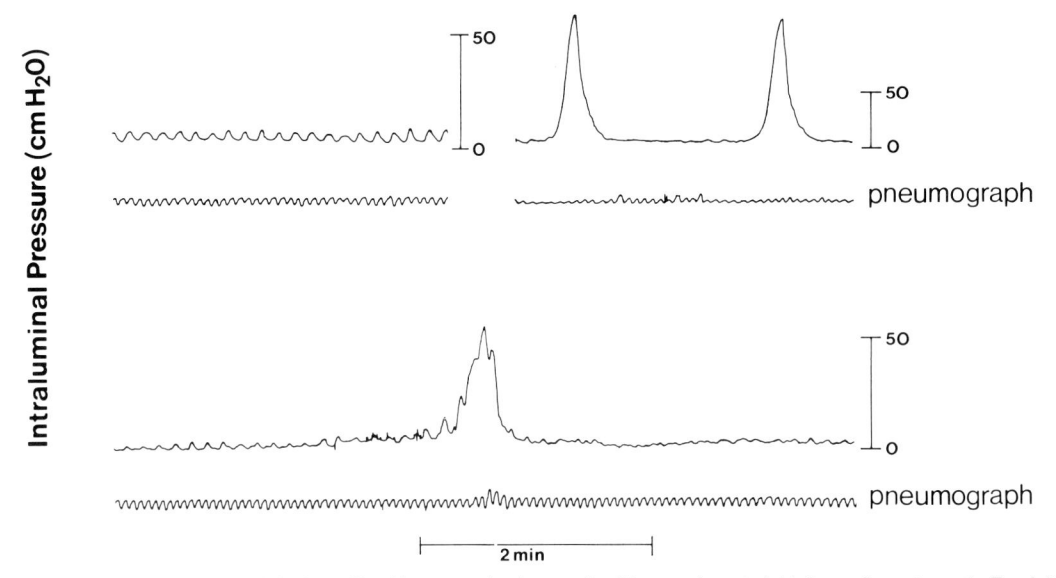

FIG. 29-13. Recordings of distal ileal motility 10 cm proximal to anal sphincter after straight ileoanal anastomosis. Top left: pressure waves of small amplitude and duration. Top right: waves of large amplitude and duration. Center: Waves of small and large amplitude. (Reprinted with permission from Heppell, J., Pemberton, J. H., Kelly, K. A., and Phillips, S. F.: Surg. Gastroenterol., 1:123, 1982.

by a segment of bowel distal to the reservoir was present. The pouch itself was anastomosed to the anal canal. The apex of the pouch lay partly within the pelvis and partly below the pelvic diaphragm within a short, 3 to 5 cm distal rectal muscular cuff.

Incomplete evacuation of other types of ileal pouches has been found to be a cause of poor postoperative results.[25] Therefore, it was of interest to study the completeness of pouch emptying in our "J"-pouch patients. Incomplete evacuation of any type of pouch would reduce the volume of stool required to distend the pouch again to its threshold volume, when large pressure waves and an urge to defecate would then appear. Using recovery of a semi-solid artificial stool instilled into the pouch to estimate efficiency of evacuation, we found that patients who emptied their pouch less completely had a greater daily stool frequency than those with more complete pouch emptying (Fig. 29-14).[22] Most patients studied could evacuate their pouches nearly as completely as could healthy persons, however. Patients evacuated 57% ± 3% of a semi-solid, artificial stool instilled per rectum compared to 73% ± 7% evacuated by healthy volunteers ($P > 0.05$).[26] Moreover, the voluntary onset of evacuation, the rate of fecal flow, and the use of Valsalva's maneuver to facilitate evacuation were, in general, similar to what was found in health. Thus, the fact that fecal evacuation is not greatly disturbed after ileal "J"-pouch-anal anastomosis probably contributes to the satisfactory fecal continence present after operation.

PROXIMAL ENTERIC MOTILITY. After operation, the migrating motor complexes characteristic of the healthy small bowel during fasting were still present in the jejunoileum (Fig. 29-15), and they were readily abolished by feeding. Large ileal pressure waves similar to those found in health were also present after ileal pouch-anal anastomosis, but they arose more proximally, perhaps because chyme is stored in the more proximal bowel after the operation. Unlike the large amplitude waves generated de novo in the ileal pouch, these more proximal waves did not result in a desire to defecate.[24] The abnormalities described by Summers et al. in mechanical small bowel obstruction were not seen in our studies.[27] Overall, the fasting and fed motor patterns in the proximal small bowel remained largely undisturbed after the operation.

Nonetheless, the pattern of ileal contractions after ileoanal anastomosis must differ from the pattern of contractions in the descending colon and sigmoid colon in health. The ileum may develop more propulsive waves when distended than does the distal colon. Such ileal propulsion could stress the mechanisms for continence more than would the colonic waves. This may be a factor leading to impaired continence after ileoanal anastomosis.

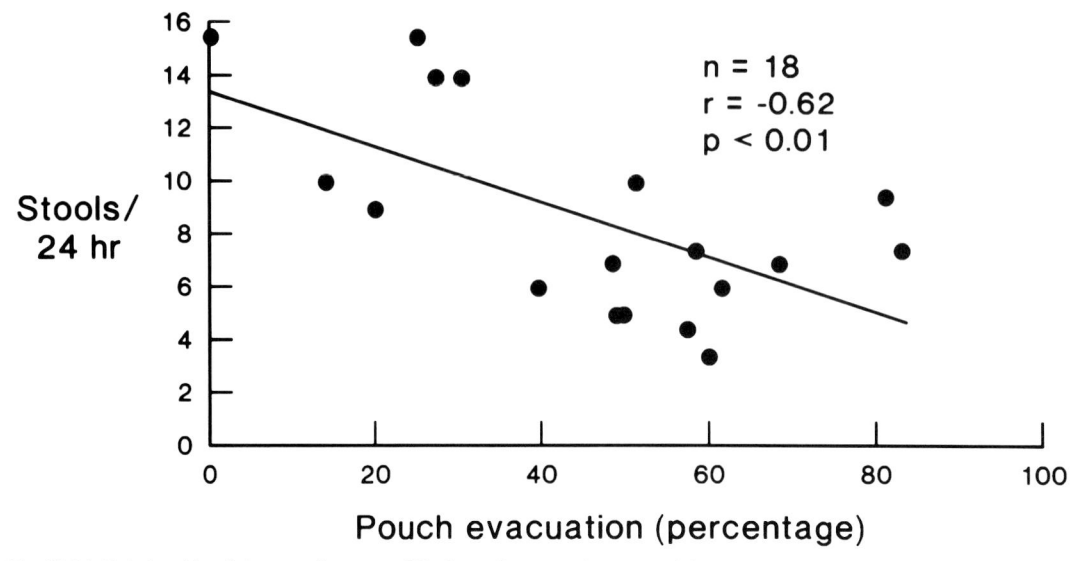

FIG. 29-14. Relationship of the completeness of ileal pouch evacuation to stool frequency after ileal pouch-anal anastomosis. (Reprinted with permission from Stryker, S. J., et al.: Ann. Surg., *203*:55, 1986.)

ENTERIC CONTENT. The output in our patients with ileoanal anastomosis was similar to that of ileostomy patients, about 650 ml of semi-solid stool per day. The stools were passed as five to seven 100-ml bowel movements per day. Dietary restriction and the use of bulk-forming agents had little effect on the volume excreted, but they did reduce urgency and perineal irritation by making the stool less liquid and possibly by binding the enteric bile salts. The use of agents to slow transit and improve absorption, such as loperamide hydrochloride, was also helpful in the initial weeks following ileostomy closure. The persistent passage of a large volume of semi-formed stool in the postoperative period, however, was a major factor in the frequent passage of stool, mild incontinence, and perineal irritation experienced by some patients after ileal pouch-anal anastomosis. The less the volume of stool passed, the better the result.

Other measures designed to slow small bowel transit, augment absorption, and reduce ileal output would be welcome. Possibilities under consideration at present are retrograde electrical pacing of the small bowel, which is effective in the canine short bowel syndrome model,[28] and the incorporation of an artificial valve in the ileum to slow enteric transit.[29]

DISCUSSION

As stated above, ileal "J"-pouch-anal anastomosis has been performed in about 650 adult patients at the Mayo Clinic since 1981. In all patients, the cecum, the colon, the rectal mucosa, and 70% of the rectal muscularis were excised. The anal sphincters, the puborectalis, the levator ani, 4 to 5 cm of distal rectal muscle, and all of the anoderm were retained. A neorectum was created and intestinal continuity restored with

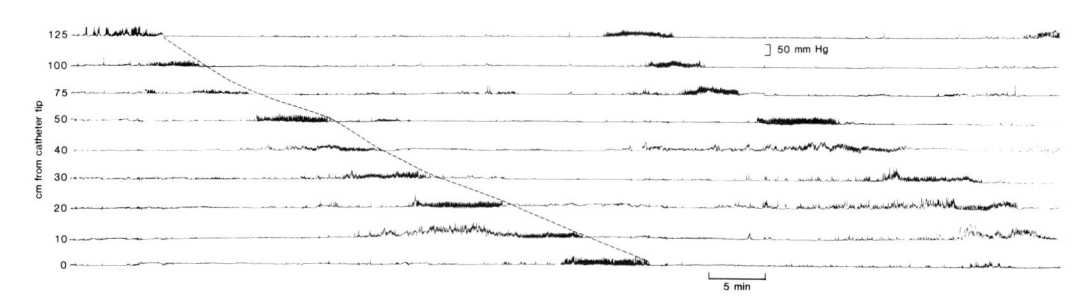

FIG. 29-15. Small intestinal migrating motor complexes during fasting in a patient after ileal pouch-anal anastomosis. Catheter tip is in distal ileum. Dotted line indicates distal propagation of complex. (Reprinted with permission from Stryker, S. J., et al.: Ann. Surg., *201*:351, 1985).

the ileal pouch-anal anastomosis. Use of the operation provided a unique opportunity for studying the relative importance of the recognized mechanisms of continence.

Satisfactory fecal continence was achieved after operation in over 90% of the patients. Some patients experienced intermittent leakage of intestinal content, particularly at night, but overall results were satisfactory in the majority. The maintenance of continence after operation depended primarily upon two factors: the preservation of a competent barricade to anorectal outflow and the creation of an adequate fecal reservoir. The operation almost always preserved the anal sphincters and probably the anorectal angle, and so a competent barricade to outflow was left undisturbed. The operation also created an adequate neorectal reservoir with the "J"-shaped ileal pouch. Such a pouch anastomosed directly to the anal canal was as distensible and capacious and as readily evacuated as is the rectum in health.

In those few patients in whom the anal sphincter had been damaged by the operation, incontinence usually resulted. Likewise, when the ileal pouch did not provide an adequate reservoir after the rectal excision, frequent passage of stool and poor fecal continence ensued.

Maintenance of anal sphincteric squeeze pressure, anorectal sensation, the anorectal angle, and a healthy pattern of proximal enteric motility after operation contributed to the satisfactory postoperative continence of our patients. Our findings further showed that fecal continence does not depend upon the presence of intact rectal mucosa, intact rectal tunica muscularis, or the rectoanal inhibitory reflex. The operation destroyed all three factors, and yet many patients still had excellent continence after operation.

Ileoanal patients, however, probably do not possess entirely "normal" patterns of fecal continence. With distal enteric distention, the frequent, large amplitude, propulsive contractions of the ileal pouch in patients stressed the anal sphincters more than the infrequent, small amplitude, nonpropulsive contractions of the healthy rectum. Moreover, our patients had to learn to recognize different signals of the impending need for evacuation. Large pressure waves occurring in the ileal pouch at threshold volume triggered the onset of evacuation after operation, although healthy persons may have evacuation initiated by a sensation of rectal fullness and the activation of the rectoanal inhibitory reflex.

The operation not only altered the anatomy, the reflex mechanisms, and the distal enteric contractions, but it also changed the consistency and the volume of enteric content. In healthy subjects, only about 150 ml of stool are passed per day, and the stool is formed. After the operation was performed, the volume usually increased to about 650 ml per day in our patients, and it assumed a semi-solid, mushy, or even liquid consistency. This placed greater strain on the anal sphincters in the patients. We found that the best results occurred in those with small outputs of stool ($\leq$500 ml/day), the consistency of which was semi-formed.

One broad definition of fecal continence states that continence depends on the ability to defer the act of defecation until a socially convenient time and place. If this definition is accepted, patients after ileoanal anastomosis are continent. The most important features of continence, a capacious reservoir and a well-functioning anal sphincter, are preserved by the operation. Other, more subtle, but probably no less important factors that work together to maintain continence are, however, changed. In the future, efforts directed toward achieving better continence in patients should focus upon decreasing the volume of stool excreted, increasing stool consistency, maximizing the threshold volume for ileal pouch contractions, ensuring complete pouch evacuation, and minimizing postoperative complications.

The ileal pouch-anal anastomosis can be performed safely in carefully selected patients, but the operation is associated with a significant risk of complications, even in the hands of surgeons experienced with the procedure. The procedure restores continence to a satisfactory, but not perfect, degree. Overall, the newest of the alternatives to the Brooke ileostomy provides a superior quality of life for most patients.

Continent Reservoir Ileostomy

The continent reservoir ileostomy (ileal pouch, Kock pouch) offers an alternative to a Brooke ileostomy for certain patients with ulcerative colitis requiring a proctocolectomy. The continent ileal reservoir is constructed entirely from the distal ileum and it consists of: (1) a pouch that collects and stores the ileal effluent, (2) a valve that makes the pouch continent for both gas and feces, and (3) a conduit leading to the stoma. Because the pouch is continent (except when drained by insertion of a catheter through the stoma), no external appliance need be worn.

BACKGROUND AND RATIONALE

In 1967, Kock reasoned that if an internal reservoir were constructed of terminal ileum, it would store fecal matter internally until emptied voluntarily by catheterization, obviating the need for an external appliance.[30] The pouch would need to hold about 500 ml so that it would not require emptying too often. Kock further suggested that incising the ileum along the antimesenteric border when making the pouch would help prevent ileal contractions, thereby keeping pressure low in the pouch as it filled.

Kock further recognized that an internal valve, also constructed from the terminal ileum, would be needed to separate the pouch from the stoma if continence were to be achieved. A catheter then could be passed through the stoma, through the valve, and into the pouch to drain the feces at appropriate intervals, convenient to the patient. Theoretically, between intubations, no stool should leak out of the reservoir, and therefore, the patient should not have to wear an external collecting device or bag.

Kock reported his first cases in 1969, with promising results.[30] A 30 cm segment of ileum was used to construct the pouch, which proved to be of adequate size. The valves that were constructed in the early operations were not always successful in providing continence, however. The use of an antiperistaltic limb of ileum between the pouch and the stoma, or the construction of an oblique course for the efferent ileal limb through a sling of rectus abdominis, did not always prevent leakage in Kock's patients,[31,32] nor did it do so when used by Beahrs et al. or Goligher and Lintott.[33,34]

Kock then devised a "nipple" valve made by "intussuscepting" the efferent ileal limb into the pouch for a distance of 3 to 5 cm, and anchoring the intussusceptum in place with nonabsorbable sutures. This valve proved to be more successful, and provided continence in 37 consecutive cases reported by Kock,[31] in 48 of 50 cases reported by Kelly and Beahrs,[35] and in 17 of 19 cases reported by Madigan.[36] The method of anchoring the intussusception has continued to evolve,[32] but to date the "nipple valve" remains the valve of choice.

We began constructing continent ileal reservoirs at the Mayo institutions in 1971. Currently, we still follow an operative plan similar to that used by Kock and Beahrs.

THE OPERATION

PREOPERATIVE PREPARATION. The patients are prepared for the operation with a thorough 48 hour cleansing of the gastrointestinal tract using laxatives and enemas. A clear liquid diet is given for the 24 hours preceding the operation. The patients also receive 1g neomycin and 0.5g erythromycin every 8 hours during the day before operation.

OPERATIVE TECHNIQUE. A vertical midline incision is made in the abdomen, skirting to the left of the umbilicus. The abdomen is thoroughly explored to establish the diagnosis of ulcerative colitis, the extent of disease, and especially to ascertain that the ileum is not involved. The terminal 3 cm of ileum, along with the cecum and colon, are then excised, and the rectum is stapled shut. The pelvic peritoneum is closed over the rectum but left lax enough to fall into the presacral space after the proctectomy is performed later in the operation.

The terminal 45 cm of ileum is used to form the pouch. Beginning 15 cm from the distal cut end of the ileum, a 30 cm segment of ileum is measured and fashioned into a "U"-shape. The antimesenteric borders of the two 15 cm limbs of the "U" are then approximated with continuous 2-0 chromic catgut. The antimesenteric borders of the limbs are then incised, exposing the mucosa. The incision on the afferent limb is made 4 to 5 cm longer than the incision on the efferent limb of the ileum, so that the afferent and efferent limbs of the pouch will separate as the pouch is constructed. A second row of chromic catgut sutures is used to control oozing from the cut edges of the bowel on what will become the posterior wall of the pouch (Fig. 29-16).

The valve is then fashioned from the terminal ileum. The serosal surface of the efferent limb of the ileum is scarified with the electrocautery beginning at the pouch and extending for a distance of 10 cm towards the distal cut end. The peritoneum is stripped off the mesentery adjacent to the 10 cm segment and the mesentery is "de-fatted." These maneuvers are designed to promote adherence of the ileum and its mesentery when the efferent limb is intussuscepted into the pouch to form the valve.

The efferent limb is intussuscepted into the pouch, forming a "nipple valve" about 5 cm in length. The intussusceptum is anchored in place

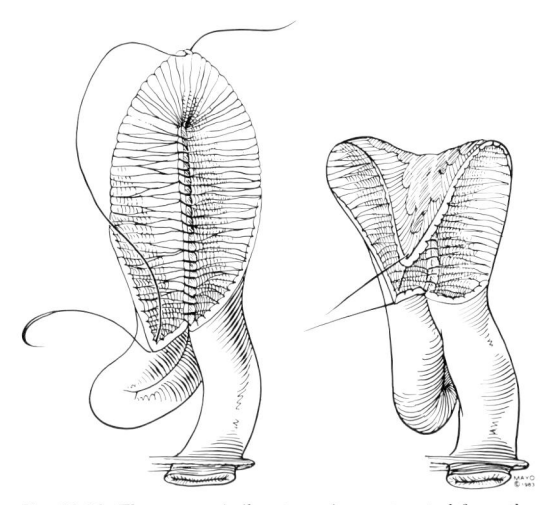

FIG. 29-16. The reservoir ileostomy is constructed from the distal 45 cm of ileum. The reservoir is made from two 15 cm limbs of ileum opened on the antimesenteric side, sutured together and folded over to form the anterior and posterior walls. (Reprinted with permission from Dozois, R. R., Kelly, K. A., Beart, R. W., and Beahrs, O. H.: Continent ileostomy: the Mayo Clinic experience. *In* Alternatives to Conventional Ileostomy. Edited by R. R. Dozois. Chicago, Year Book Medical Publishers, 1985.)

with interrupted 2-0 polyglycolic acid, through-and-through sutures and with 3 or 4 cartridges of stainless steel staples placed with the GIA autosuture apparatus (Figs. 29-17 and 29-18). Care is taken to avoid placing the sutures and staples through the vascular supply of the intussuscepted bowel. The placement of the sutures is facilitated by using a catheter (French scale, 28) as a stent in the lumen of the intussusceptum.

The bottom of the "U" is then folded over to form the anterior wall of the pouch. Closure is completed using two layers of continuous 2-0 chromic catgut. The efferent limb of the ileum is sutured to the pouch with interrupted 3-0 nonabsorbable sutures, just at the exit of the limb from the pouch, to further anchor the intussusceptum in place. In more recent cases, a piece of polyglycolic acid mesh has also been incorporated between the two layers of the intussuscepted ileum and sutured to the efferent limb at the site of exit.

Continence is now tested by clamping the afferent ileal limb of the pouch, passing a catheter

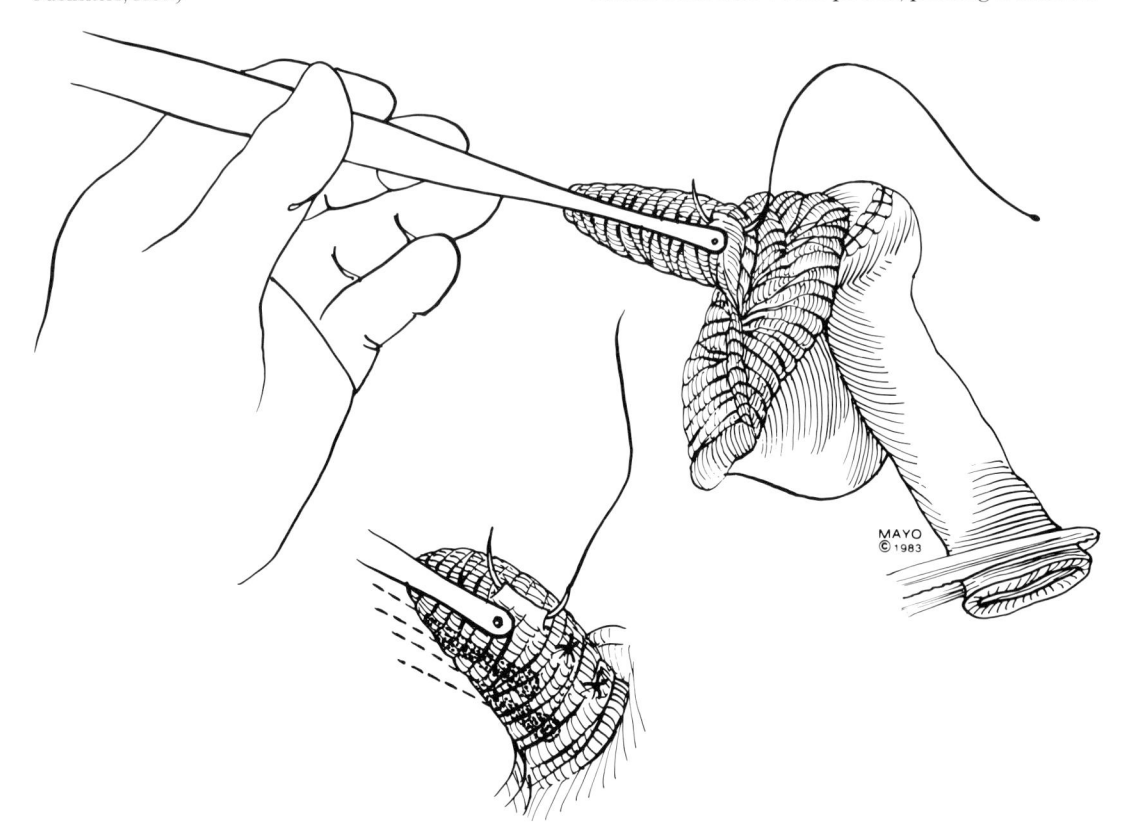

FIG. 29-17. A 10 cm segment of terminal ileum has been surgically intussuscepted to form the valve. (Reprinted with permission from Dozois, R. R., Kelly, K. A., Beart, R. W., and Beahrs, O. H.: Continent ileostomy: the Mayo Clinic experience. *In* Alternatives to Conventional Ileostomy. Edited by R. R. Dozois. Chicago, Year Book Medical Publishers, 1985.)

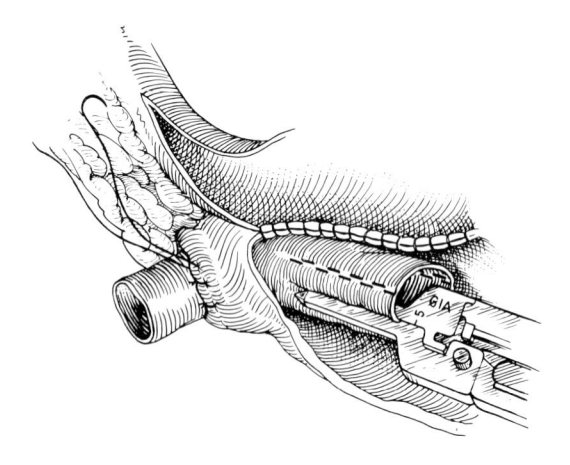

FIG. 29-18. Stainless staples and interrupted sutures of 2-0 polyglycolic acid between the base of reservoir and efferent ileal limb anchor the intussuscepted segment within the pouch and so form the valve. (Reprinted with permission from Dozois, R. R., Kelly, K. A., Beart, R. W., and Beahrs, O. H.: Continent ileostomy: the Mayo Clinic experience. *In* Alternatives to Conventional Ileostomy. Edited by R. R. Dozois. Chicago, Year Book Medical Publishers, 1985.)

through the valve into the pouch, and distending the pouch with air. When the catheter is removed, the distended pouch should hold the air without leakage through the nipple valve. The catheter is then reinserted, and the air is removed.

The site of the ileal stoma is located just above the pubic hairline in the right lower quadrant of the abdomen. After a circular defect has been created in the skin and another just below in the fascia, the terminal ileum leading from the pouch to the exterior is brought through the defects and cut off flush with the skin. The length of ileum between the pouch and the stoma is made as short as possible to prevent tortuosity and to facilitate later catheterization of the pouch. The pouch is sutured to the undersurface of the anterior abdominal wall just at the exit of the terminal ileum from the abdomen to prevent the pouch from retracting into the abdominal cavity postoperatively. These stitches also insure that the "nipple valve" will be directly posterior to the stoma (Fig. 29-19). The distal cut end of the ileum is then sewn to the edges of the surrounding skin using interrupted 4-0 chromic catgut.

A catheter (French scale, 28) is passed through the stoma and valve, and its tip is positioned within the lumen of the pouch just before the abdominal incision is closed. A suture is tied around the catheter at the level of the stoma, so that the exact position of the catheter can easily be ascertained in the postoperative period. The abdomen is irrigated with 154 mM NaCl, after which the abdominal incision is closed without intraperitoneal drainage.

The patient is then placed in the lithotomy position, and the rectum and anus are excised. Two silastic catheters (Jackson-Pratt, 6.3) are placed in the presacral space and brought to the surface through separate perineal stab wounds. These catheters are used for continuous irrigation and suction of the perineal wound in the postoperative period.[37] The perineal wound is closed primarily.

POSTOPERATIVE CARE. The patient is given intravenous feeding, nasogastric suction, and nothing by mouth for the first 3 to 5 days postoperatively, after which a liquid diet and then a general diet is given.

The pouch is intubated continuously and kept on gravity drainage for the first 4 weeks after the operation. The catheter draining the pouch is irrigated every 4 to 6 hours with 25 ml of sterile 154 mM NaCl to assure patency. After the fourth week, the catheter is removed and intermittent intubation is begun. The pouch is intubated every 2 hours during the day and twice at night during the fifth postoperative week. The interval between intubations is then gradually increased by 1 hour each week, until the patient is intubating 2 to 4 times per day, but not at night. Antibiotics are not used in the postoperative period unless specific infections develop.

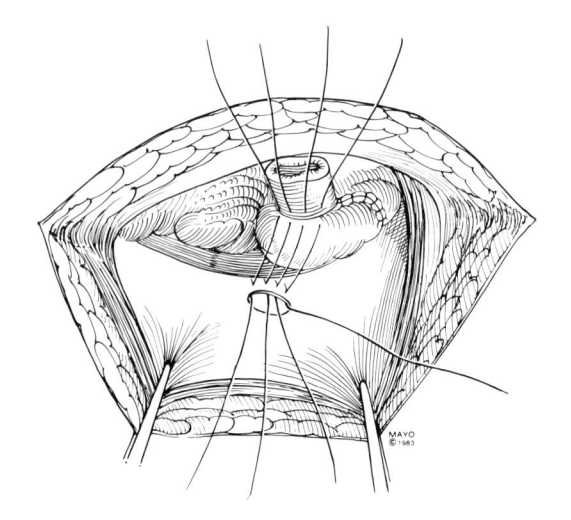

FIG. 29-19. The reservoir is anchored to undersurface of abdominal wall immediately underneath stoma. (Reprinted with permission from Dozois, R. R., Kelly, K. A., Beart, R. W., and Beahrs, O. H.: Continent ileostomy: the Mayo Clinic experience. *In* Alternatives to Conventional Ileostomy. Edited by R. R. Dozois. Chicago, Year Book Medical Publishers, 1985.)

POST-HOSPITALIZATION CARE. On leaving the hospital, patients are given a catheter designed specifically for use in draining the pouch (either an Ileostomy Catheter, M8730, Atlantic Surgical Co., Inc., Marrick, NY; or an Ileal Pouch Catheter, Dow-Corning Co., Midland, MI). The Atlantic Ileostomy Catheter has a diameter of about 9 mm (French scale, 28) and a length of 30 cm, and the Dow-Corning Ileal Pouch Catheter has a diameter of about 1 cm (French scale, 30) and a length of about 64 cm. Some patients prefer the shorter and some the longer catheter. Each catheter has a thin wall and large holes at the insertion end just proximal to its blunt tip (Fig. 29-20). The patient keeps the catheter in a small plastic case, which is carried at all times.

Patients report a sensation of fullness when the pouch needs to be emptied. To empty the pouch, the patient passes the catheter through the stoma into the pouch, usually when in the sitting position. The ileal contents are allowed to drain spontaneously (by gravity) through the catheter into the toilet or another suitable receptacle (Fig. 29-21). The Valsalva's maneuver and direct manual compression of the abdomen over the pouch are sometimes used to facilitate drainage, but irrigations are not required. The catheter is then removed from the pouch, rinsed clean, and placed in its case for later use. A soft gauze pad with a waterproof surface is taped over the stoma to absorb any mucus secreted by the stoma. Patients rapidly become expert at this procedure, which requires about 5 to 10 minutes to complete. None of our patients has ever perforated the pouch with the catheter.

Some patients have found that partially digestible substances, such as seeds, apple skins, celery, and mushrooms, may plug the catheter, and so have avoided these foods. Others have found that all foods can be eaten, however, provided they are thoroughly chewed before being swallowed. Bezoars have not developed in the pouches.

No restrictions are placed on physical activities when the patient has fully recovered at about 4 to 6 weeks after the operation. Pregnancy is not contraindicated. Many of our patients have become pregnant. Several have delivered healthy babies by caesarean section. Others have had normal vaginal deliveries.

CLINICAL EVALUATION

INDICATIONS AND CONTRAINDICATIONS. Although the ileoanal anastomosis is now preferred by most patients requiring proctocolectomy, the continent ileostomy remains a viable alternative to the Brooke ileostomy for certain patients in the following groups:

1. Those who already have a conventional Brooke ileostomy, who have lost their anal sphincter, and who wish to improve their quality of life
2. Those who need a proctocolectomy to preserve continence, but are not candidates for an ileoanal anastomosis, usually because of poor anal sphincter function
3. Those who prefer a continent ileostomy to an ileoanal anastomosis (usually patients who are away from toilet facilities for prolonged periods of time because of their jobs)
4. Those who had a failed ileoanal anastomosis and still prefer a continence-preserving procedure to the wearing of an external appliance

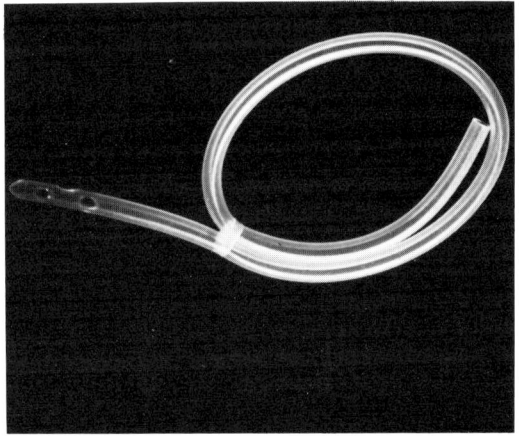

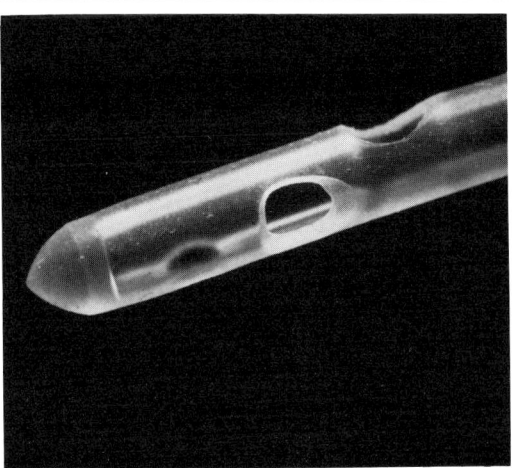

FIG. 29-20. The catheter used to drain the ileal pouch has a length of about 64 cm and a diameter of about 1 cm (A). Large holes are present in its thin wall just proximal to its "bullet tip" (B).

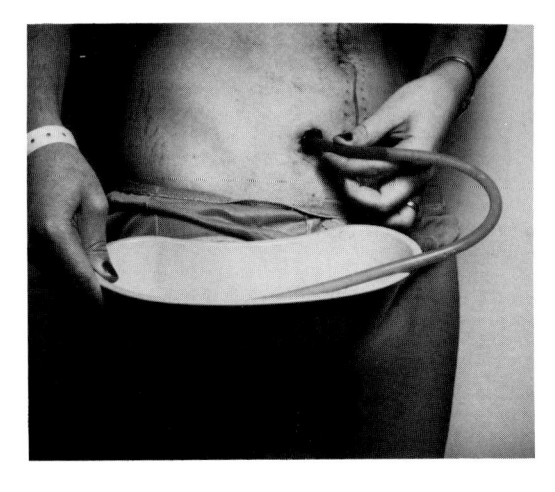

FIGURE 29-21. The patient passes the catheter through the stoma into the pouch. Ileal contents drain spontaneously through the catheter into a suitable receptacle (or directly into the toilet).

The operation should be *discouraged* in:

1. Older patients, who may be more prone to postoperative complications, including valve dysfunction, and may not tolerate a reoperation
2. Patients with Crohn's disease*
3. Obese patients
4. Critically ill patients, such as those plagued by toxic megacolon, in whom a staged procedure may be safer
5. The psychologically unfit patient, because of the inability to intubate properly or to tolerate reoperation if necessary

MAYO CLINIC PATIENT POPULATION. Continent ileal reservoirs were constructed in 460 patients at the two Mayo-affiliated hospitals during the years between November 1, 1971 and January 1, 1982. Nearly equal numbers of men and women were in the series, their ages ranging from 16 years to 67 years; the mean age was 32 years.

Most of the 460 patients had chronic ulcerative colitis (92%), as did those in Kock's series.[31,32] The remainder had familial polyposis coli (7%) or Crohn's disease of the large intestine (<1%) (Table 29-3). None of the patients with Crohn's disease had involvement of the esopha-

---

*Editors' comment: However, see also Bloom, R. J., et al.: Surg. Gynecol. Obstet., *162*: 105, 1986. In this study it was concluded that the Kock continent ileostomy may be used in a few, highly selected patients with the disease inactive for in excess of 5 years.

TABLE 29-3. *Diseases Treated (460 Patients).*

Disease	Number of Patients (Percentage)
Chronic ulcerative colitis	420 (92)
Familial polyposis	35 (7)
Crohn's disease	5 (1)

gus, stomach, or small intestine at the time the pouch was made. About two-thirds of our patients had the pouch constructed in conjunction with proctocolectomy, and chose a continent ileostomy to avoid a conventional ileostomy (Table 29-4). Three-tenths were dissatisfied with their incontinent Brooke ileostomy and sought change to an ileal pouch. Sixteen patients had had a continent ileostomy constructed elsewhere and came to the Mayo Clinic for revision of a poorly functioning pouch.

Patients in a debilitated condition, those with severe "backwash ileitis," and those undergoing acute, emergent operations were not considered candidates for the procedure, nor were grossly obese patients. Many patients were chronically ill, however, and many were taking corticosteroids at the time their pouch was constructed. The benefits and risks of the continent ileostomy relative to those of a conventional ileostomy were thoroughly discussed with the patients prior to operation.

SAFETY. No pouch-related deaths occurred intraoperatively or postoperatively, and patients generally convalesced satisfactorily. The mean postoperative stay in the hospital was about 10 days. Compared to patients with conventional ileostomy, the patients with ileal reservoirs experienced more abdominal cramps and distention in the postoperative period and returned to a general diet more slowly, a reflection of the intestinal obstruction produced by the pouch and its valve. These symptoms gradually disappeared as the pouch dilated in the postoperative period (Fig. 29-22).

TABLE 29-4. *Operative Procedures (460 Patients).*

Operation	Number of Patients (Percentage)
Proctocolectomy, pouch	306 (66)
Conversion of conventional ileostomy to pouch	138 (30)
Revision of a pouch originally constructed elsewhere	16 (3)

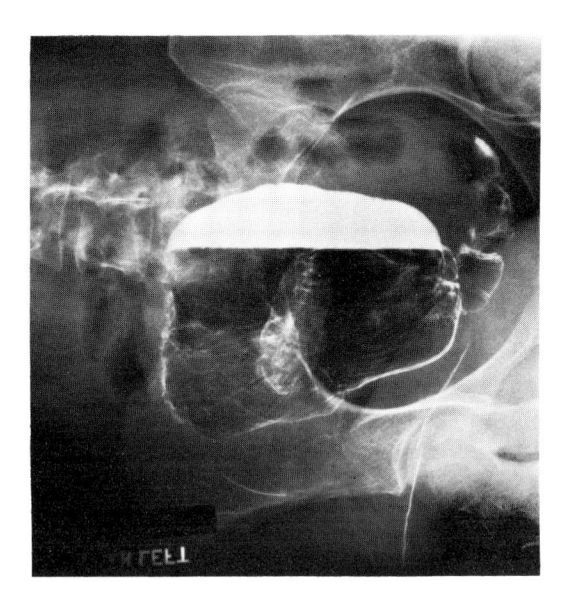

FIG. 29-22. Barium-contrast roentgenogram of continent ileal reservoir one year after its construction. The reservoir occupies the right lower quadrant of the abdomen and the pelvis. The nipple valve protrudes about 5 cm into the lumen of the pouch.

With increasing experience, the need for excision of the reservoir has been reduced from about 10% in our early patients to about 3% more recently.[38-40] This was accomplished by avoiding its use in those with Crohn's colitis and by favoring revision over excision when serious complications took place. Occasionally, the establishment of a temporary diverting loop-ileostomy is being used both by us and by Kock.[32]

EFFECTIVENESS. Long-term follow-up (up to 16 years) has shown excellent results in the series. Most of the pouches have remained continent, with almost no peristomal irritation of the skin or unpleasant odors from the stoma. Moreover, social, sexual and psychologic disability have apparently been absent or minimal. In general, the patients have gained weight, returned to good health, and taken up their former employment or occupation.

Malfunction of the Nipple valve. Incontinence and difficult intubation of the pouch caused by malfunction of the nipple valve have been the major difficulties in our overall series, requiring reoperation in about 20% of our patients, as in Kock's series. The malfunction has appeared between 1 and 39 months after construction of the pouch; however, all but four instances occurred within the first year (Fig. 29-23). The risk of malfunction, necessitating revision or excision of the pouch, decreases with time.

The reason for malfunction of the nipple valve appears to be as follows. The intestine, in an effort to relieve the complete intestinal ob-

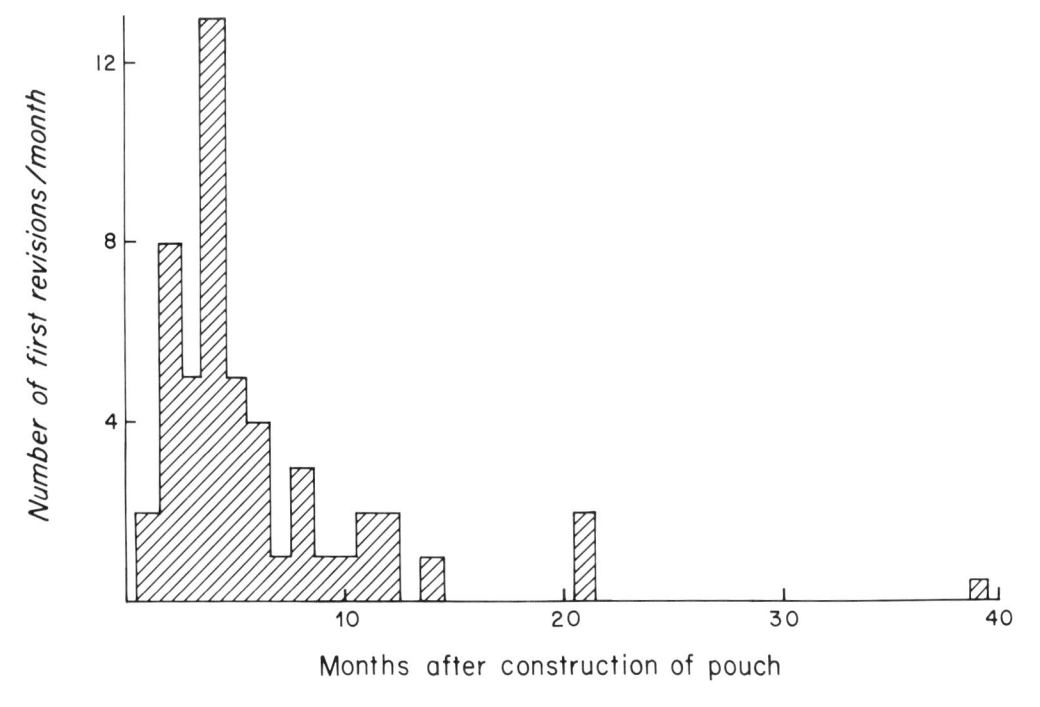

FIG. 29-23. The number of patients requiring revision of the nipple valve is greatest 2 to 6 months after construction of the pouch. Only four patients in a series of 129 patients required revision after one year.

struction created by the valve, spontaneously extrudes the valve out along its mesenteric attachment, rendering the pouch partially incontinent. The pouch leaks, yet it is difficult to intubate. The efferent limb leading from the pouch to the exterior becomes longer and more tortuous with the valve extruded. The catheter used for draining the pouch gets entrapped in the folds of the efferent limb and cannot be advanced into the lumen of the pouch (Fig. 29-24). Persistent efforts usually are successful. Occasionally, it has been necessary to intubate the pouch with a proctoscope first, and then to pass the catheter through the instrument into the pouch.

Reoperation is required when malfunction of the valve occurs. The pouch and ileostomy are taken down from the anterior abdominal wall. An incision is made through the anterior wall of the pouch. The nipple valve is pulled back into the pouch and reanchored with stainless steel staples. The incision in the anterior wall of the pouch is then closed, and the pouch and stoma are fixed again in the right lower quadrant of the abdomen, as described previously. Nipple valve revision has been successful, in that ultimately 95% of patients again have a continent valve and never have to wear an appliance.

Several factors would appear to influence the risk of valve revision.[38-40] Younger patients (<40 years) required fewer revisions than older patients (≥40 years), and the older the patient, the greater the probability of revision (Fig. 29-25). Also, fewer revisions were required in women than men, in patients who had their continent reservoir constructed at the same time as the colectomy compared to those who had a previously constructed Brooke ileostomy converted to a continent ileostomy, and in nonobese compared to obese patients (Table 29-5). With the technical modifications described, we have considerably reduced this problem, but about 20% of patients still need revisional surgical treatment of the valve at some point in their postoperative course.

Diarrhea. About 5% of our patients have developed episodes of watery diarrhea in the late postoperative period. Staphylococcus aureus, Campylobacter, or other pathogens have been cultured from the ileal content in some instances, and the diarrhea subsided when appropriate antibiotic therapy was given. Other patients have had diarrhea secondary to a mechanical obstruction of the small intestine. Lysis of adhesions resolved the diarrhea. Still others had reddened, friable, edematous mucosa in the pouch without evidence of abnormal fecal flora or mechanical obstruction of the small intestine proximal to the nipple valve. These patients usually respond to metronidazole per os, suggesting that the overgrowth of anaerobic bacteria in the pouch or in the jejunoileum proximal to the pouch might be responsible for the syndrome.[41,42]

QUALITY OF LIFE. The crucial consideration in assessing the value of the continent ileostomy is whether it is continent enough so that patients do not need to wear an external appliance. At

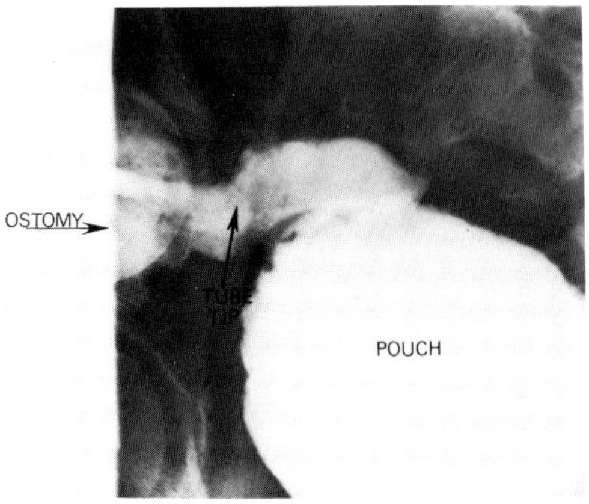

FIG. 29-24. Barium-contrast roentgenogram of an ileal reservoir with a reduced nipple valve. The tip of the catheter used for intubation becomes entrapped in the redundant efferent ileal limb and cannot be advanced into the lumen of the pouch.

TABLE 29-5. *Factors Influencing Valve Revision in Continent Ileostomies.*

Factors	Revision, %	P*
Age		
<40 years	20	
≥40 years	35	<0.05
Sex		
Women	17	
Men	28	<0.05
Operation		
Colectomy and pouch	16	
Conversion of ileostomy	30	<0.05
Obesity**		
Yes	75	
No	23	

*Estimates of cumulative probability were based on multivariate analysis.
**Derived from Schrock, T. R.: Am J. Surg., *138*:162, 1979.

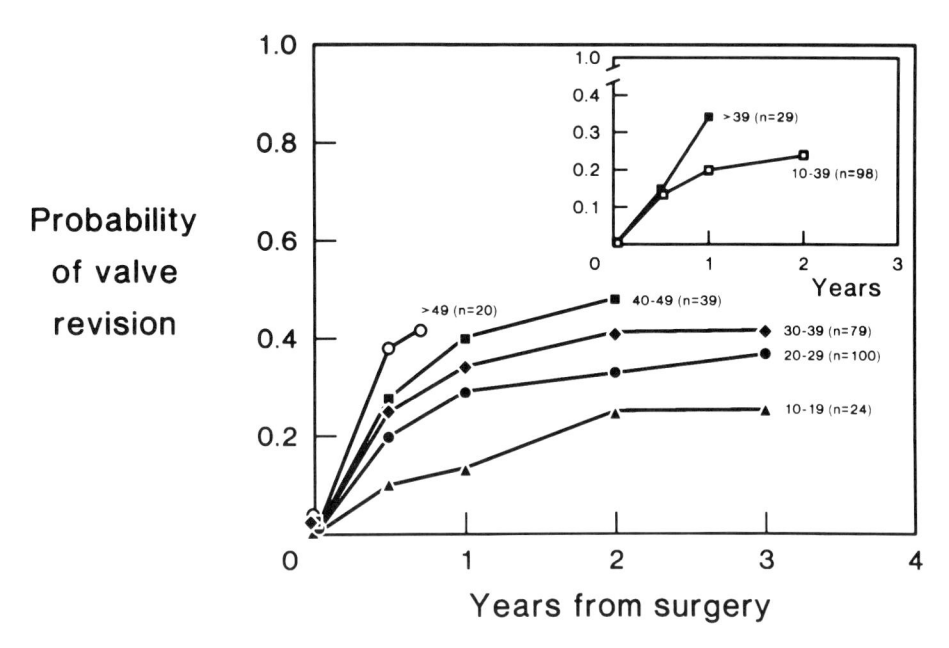

FIG. 29-25. The risk of revision of the nipple valve increases with increasing age.

the time of follow-up, 75% of our patients stated they had always been continent for gas and stool, and ultimately 95% of the entire group never have to wear an appliance.[40] When the quality of life after continent ileostomy was compared to that after Brooke ileostomy, our group found that absolute satisfaction was greater and the desire for change less in Kock pouch patients than in Brooke ileostomy patients (Table 29-2).[43] Also, in each performance category, more patients with continent ileostomy improved in their daily activities than did patients with a Brooke ileostomy.

ANATOMIC AND PHYSIOLOGIC RESULTS

Numerous questions are raised when a new surgical procedure is first undertaken, especially when the new technique replaces one of proven value. These questions can have considerable theoretic interest as well as obvious practical importance. Surgical construction of a "stagnant loop" of ileum raises certain questions. For example, what are the absorptive capabilities of an ileal pouch? Does retention of fecal material in the pouch change the constituent flora, and, if so, are mucosal function and structure altered? What influence does a pouch have on functions of the proximal intestine? Clearly, this list of uncertainties could be easily expanded; however, some of the answers, at least in the short-term, are known, and the available information is summarized in Table 29-6.

VOLUME OF THE POUCH. Although the length of ileum used to construct the reservoir is standardized, considerable variation has been noted in the measured capacity of different patients' pouches. Moreover, the adaptability of pouches to distention will vary between patients over time. Our measurements were made by inflating a flaccid balloon in the pouch, thereby preventing reflux into the ileum. In different individuals, 150 to 800 ml could be instilled before a sensation of fullness and discomfort was noted. Inflation to the point of discomfort was associated with increases in baseline pressure within the balloon of 10 to 20 cm of H_2O.[44] In most patients studied, the pouch adapted acutely to distention showing no increase in intraluminal pressure above 10 to 20 cm H_2O, despite increased distention (Fig. 29-26). Cameron studied the capacity of the pouch by introducing radiopaque fluid.[45] He reported pressures of 40 cm H_2O, after which fluoroscopic reflux into the afferent limb of ileum was noted.

PATTERN OF MOTILITY. Surgical experience has focused increasingly on careful construction of the nipple valve, as its proper function appears crucial for continence. Not surprisingly, therefore, measurements of pressure in a continent pouch show that the nipple valve constitutes a high-pressure barrier, with higher resting pressures in the nipple segment than in the pouch.[46,47]

TABLE 29-6. *Anatomical and Functional Results of Continent Ileostomy in Man.*

Characteristic Studied		Reference
Volume of Pouch	400-600 ml	30
	150-250 ml; pouch pressure when distended, 30-40 cm H$_2$O with reflux into ileum	44
	200-800 ml; pouch pressure when distended, 20-20 cm H$_2$O	45
Pattern of motility	High pressure valve at nipple	46
	Continuous low pressure basal contractions (8/min) and intermittent high pressure contractions	48
Mucosal morphology	Shortened-clubbed villi, shortened microvilli	49,50
	"resembled colonic mucosa"	44
	Variable pattern of villi and colonic features	52
Bacteriology	10^4 and 10^9 organisms per ml of effluent anaerobes > aerobes	49,54
Absorption from pouch	Water and electrolytes absorbed quantitatively and quantitatively similar to normal ileum	44
	Vitamin B$_{12}$ absorption is "active"	44,55
	Bile acids absorbed	52
	Absorption of d-xylose, phenylalanine unchanged during follow-up of 1 year	49
	Mucosal electrical potential similar to normal ileum	44
Absorption from entire bowel	Stomal outputs of volume and fat Similar to conventional ileostomies	56,57
	Schilling test usually normal	44,55
	Bile acid metabolism similar to conventional ileostomies	44

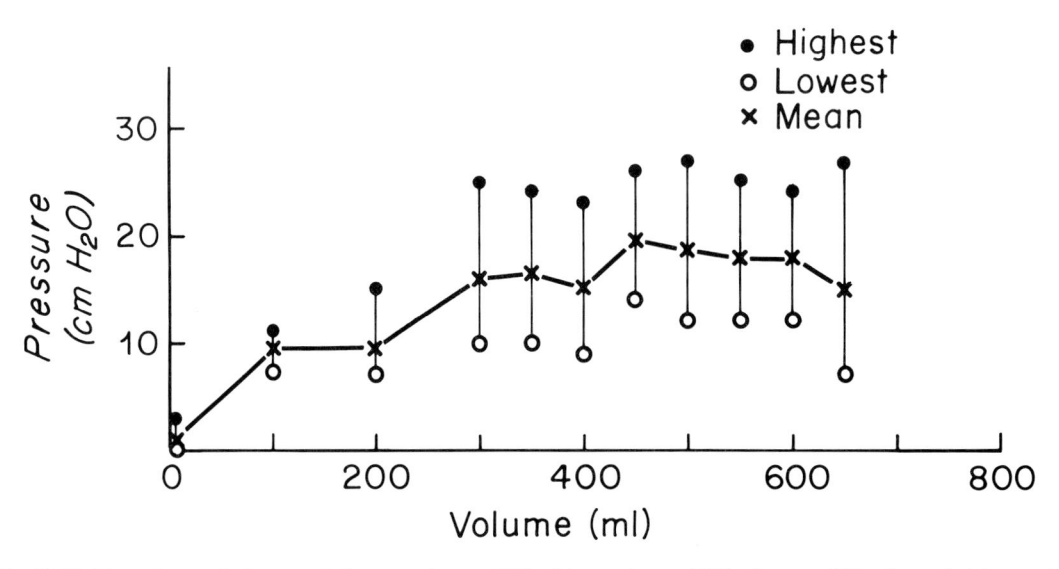

FIG. 29-26. Distending an ileal reservoir from a volume of 300 ml to a volume of 650 ml causes little change in intrapouch pressure. The ileal reservoir accommodates to distention.

Our measurements of pressure in the pouch showed a basal motor pattern in which the contractions were of low pressure (2.5 cm H_2O), regular (8/minute), and brief (5.5 seconds).[48] This resembled the "Type I" activity recorded from normal ileum. This basal pattern was seen in empty pouches and during distention. Although the pouch was thought to be constructed to negate contractile forces, studies showed that wave patterns corresponding to basal ileal activity were still clearly present. Additional high pressure "phasic" contractions (mean amplitude, 26 cm H_2O; duration, 80 seconds; and frequency, 1 per 3 minutes) were seen during distention. The threshold volume for these waves, which appear to correspond to "Type IV" waves of normal ileum and colon, was 50 to 800 ml. Most were accompanied by reported sensations of fullness and spasmodic discomfort.

MUCOSAL MORPHOLOGY. Kock's group found that the villi seen in mucosal biopsy specimens of human reservoirs were shorter, more clubbed, more leaf-like, and more variable than those of the normal ileum.[49] On electron microscopy, however, a normal brush border and microvillous pattern were seen. Kock's group also constructed experimental pouches in dogs and cats so that morphometry and mitotic indexes could be determined.[50,51] The shorter villi were associated with increased turnover of cells. Cameron described a "coloniform" appearance in human mucosal biopsy specimens, but gave no further details.[45]

Our findings in humans, using scanning electron microscopy, were of an extremely variable mucosa.[52] Among different patients, and even on biopsy specimens from the same patient, a villous architecture comparable to normal ileum or a mucosal appearance similar to that of normal colon were observed (Fig. 29-27). The significance of these morphologic alterations is uncertain; however, the long-term effects of increased cellular turnover and a change to-

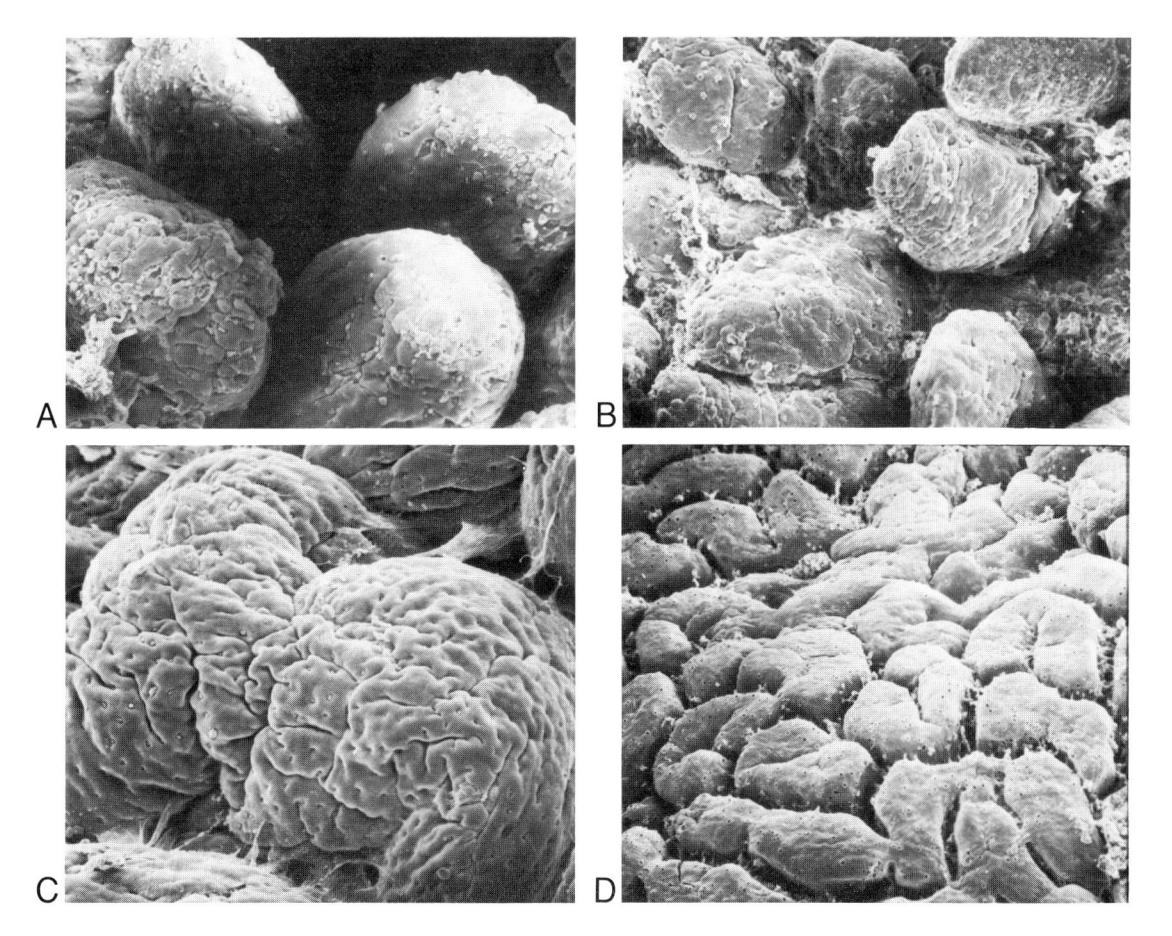

FIG. 29-27. Compared to villi from normal ileum (A), villi from an ileal reservoir may show little change (B), may be fused (C), or may be absent, so that a "coloniform" pattern is present (D). Scanning electron micrographs (×100-200).

wards a colonic pattern must be of concern in relation to premalignant potential. To date, no increased incidence of malignancy has appeared.

BACTERIOLOGY. The ileal flora in patients who have undergone conventional ileostomies is known to differ from that of the normal ileum and that of normal stools. The total organisms present and the ratio of anaerobes to aerobes fall between these two patterns.[53] By analogy, and not surprisingly, the flora of ileal pouches falls between that of conventional ileostomies and that of normal stools.[42,49,54] In some patients with diarrhea, an increase in jejunal anaerobic flora also occurs.[42]

ABSORPTION FROM THE POUCH. We studied absorption from the ileal pouch in eight patients who had satisfactory pouches present for at least 6 months.[44] Nasointestinal intubation was done to a point in the ileum just proximal to the pouch. Using marker infusion and aspiration, we were able to obviate problems caused by contamination of the pouch from above. Test solutions were introduced into and aspirated from the pouch before and after a study period of 1 hour (Fig. 29-28).

We compared functions of the pouch to those known for normal ileum, specifically: (1) active absorption of sodium ions against steep electrochemical gradients, (2) absorption of chloride ions against large gradients of concentration, (3) secretion of bicarbonate ions, (4) low resting negative mucosal potential differences that are augmented by intraluminal glucose, and (5) active absorption of vitamin B_{12}. In our experiments, the mucosa of the pouch retained the first four of these established and characteristic functions of ileal mucosa. We also compared the amount of absorption from the pouch with that reported in the literature for normal ileum. Because studies of normal ileum have involved techniques different from those we used to study the pouch (usually constant perfusion of the ileum), comparison between normal ileum and pouch was difficult. The absorption of sodium chloride was quantitatively similar in pouches and in normal ileum, however (Fig. 29-29).

Vitamin B_{12} absorption was also studied. Addition of intrinsic factor was shown to increase absorption of the vitamin, suggesting that "active" absorption persists in the pouch.[44] This confirmed and extended the findings of Kock's group who demonstrated the absorption of vitamin B_{12} when combined with intrinsic factor.[55] In other studies, they also showed that absorption of sugar (d-xylose) and amino acid (l-phenylalanine) was constant over a 1-year period of

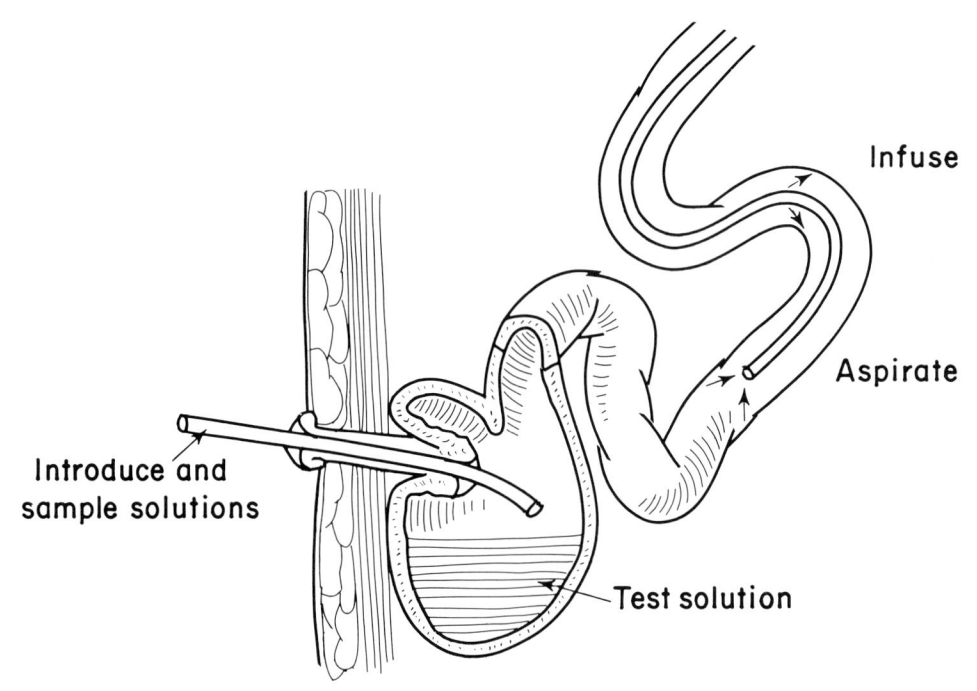

FIG. 29-28. Test solutions were instilled through the stoma into an ileal reservoir, while contamination from proximal ileal content was assessed by a marker infusion-aspiration technique using a nasointestinal tube.

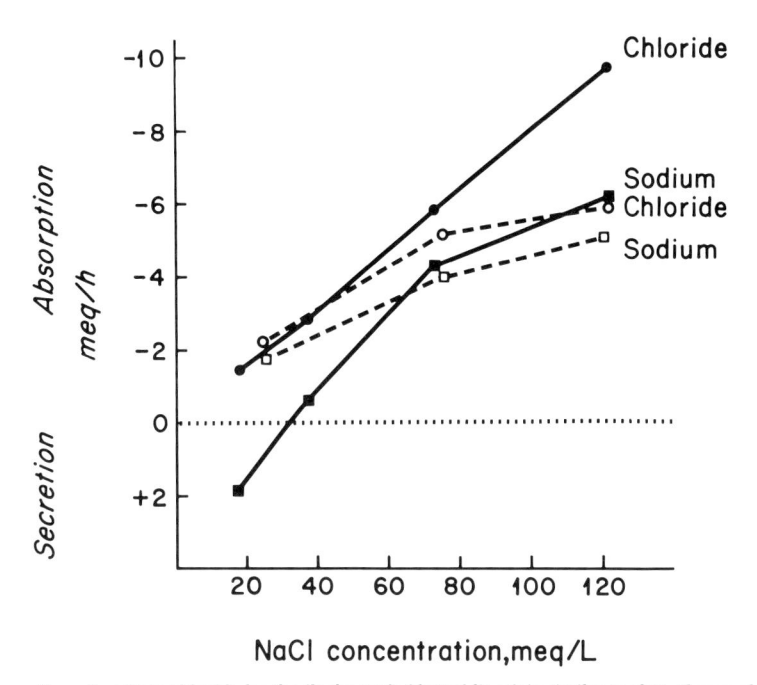

FIG. 29-29. The absorption of sodium chloride by the ileal pouch (dotted lines) is similar to that of normal ileum (solid lines) when solutions of both high and low concentrations of sodium chloride are tested. (Data of normal ileum are from Fordtran, J. S., et al., J. Clin. Invest., 47:884, 1968.)

follow-up.[49] Long-term follow-up showed few adverse metabolic consequences.[56]

We had planned to establish the presence or absence of active bile acid transport. Unfortunately, precision was required that was beyond the limits of our methodology, primarily because minute contamination of the pouch with bile from small intestinal fluids created excessive artifact. We were able to show that glycine conjugates of the common bile acids were absorbed at least as well as unconjugated bile acids, however. The most rational explanation for our findings is that glycine deconjugation preceded absorption of the conjugate.

ABSORPTION FROM THE ENTIRE BOWEL. Kock's group has shown that outputs from the stoma (mean output, 642g/24 hours; mean total fat, 8.3g/24 hours) were similar to those from conventional stomas.[57] Absorption of d-xylose and l-phenylalanine, following oral loads, was also similar in patients with pouches and in those with conventional stomas.

The results of standard Schilling tests usually were normal.[44,55] Kock's series included 34 patients studied 1 to 6 years after surgical treatment. Normal absorption of vitamin B_{12} was found in 29 patients; 4 were borderline, and only 1 was clearly abnormal. Associated resection of terminal ileum was present in some patients with abnormal tests, so that the effect of the pouch per se cannot be evaluated.

We assessed the metabolism of bile acids by examining the composition of duodenal samples of bile.[44] After colectomy and conventional ileostomy, the bile acid pool has a lesser exposure to bacterial biotransformation, and secondary bile acids are strikingly absent.[58] This phenomenon was also seen in patients with the pouch (Fig. 29-30), implying that stagnation in the pouch did not recreate the conditions of bacterial metabolism of bile acids that occur with an intact colon.

Concerns that ileal stasis might lead to bacterial overgrowth in the small bowel and development of "blind loop syndrome" were increased by the report of patients with pouches showing evidence of steatorrhea and malabsorption of vitamin B_{12}.[41] In our series, approximately one-third of 50 patients studied by using metabolic balance had excessive outputs of volume,[59] electrolytes, and fat. Some of these patients had, in addition, evidence of superficial inflammation of the pouch mucosa. The role of an altered fecal flora and the effect of treatment with antibiotics remains to be evaluated thoroughly.

Thus, ileal pouches can possess many of the functions of normal ileum. Moreover, they do not alter intestinal function in ways that differ

Normal
25–40%

Brooke ileostomy
0–10%; Mean 2·5; n=11

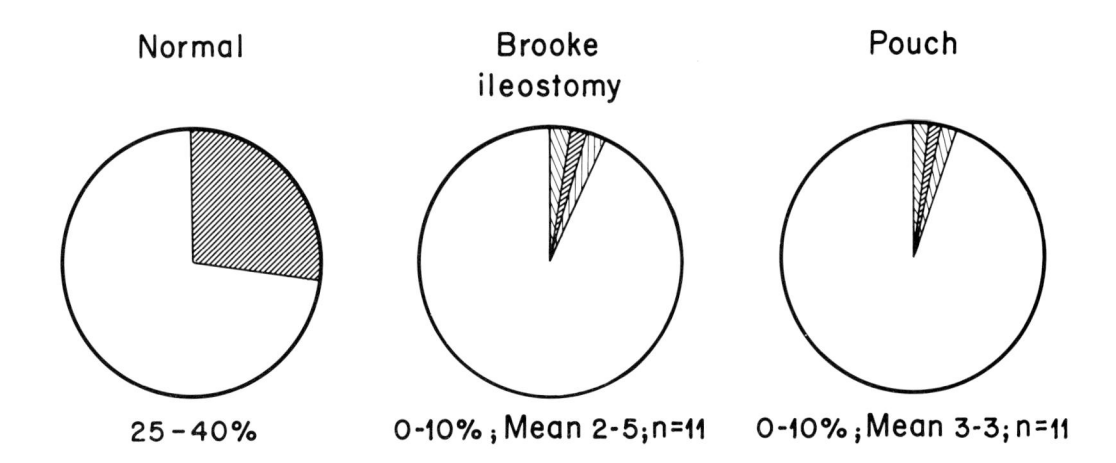

Pouch
0–10%; Mean 3·3; n=11

Morris, Scand. J. Gastro. (1972)

FIG. 29-30. Secondary bile acids (hatched areas) constitute 25 to 40% of the bile acids found in the bile of normal persons with an intact colon, but their percentage is much reduced in patients with an ileal pouch, just as in patients with a conventional Brooke ileostomy. Dark hatching = mean percentage; light hatching = standard error. (Data from Morris, J. S., et al., Scand. J. Gastroenterol., 8:425, 1973.)

greatly from those following colectomy and conventional ileostomy. Some concerns should be expressed that the presence of an iatrogenic blind loop could have deleterious effects on the distal bowel, however, and other variables of potential significance remain to be explored. For example, the frequency of evacuation or the completeness of emptying may influence the resident flora, thereby creating a functional blind loop.

DISCUSSION

In general, then, our experience with the continent ileostomy confirms that reported by Kock and encourages continued use of the operation.[30-32] The current operative approach offers a high probability of complete continence, and the patients are pleased, even enthusiastic, with the pouch. Ileostomy with construction of an internal reservoir is a more complex operation than a conventional ileostomy, however, requiring a longer convalescence. In addition, the patient faces a one-in-five chance of having to undergo a second operation to maintain continence. To date, nearly all of our patients have opted for a revision; few have wanted to lose the pouch.

The operation continues to be most attractive to young people, especially unmarried individuals, who are concerned about the social, psychologic, and sexual disadvantages of an incontinent ileostomy. Such younger patients are also more suitable candidates than elderly individuals, because they are better able to withstand additional operations should these become necessary. We have not performed this operation on any children, although we believe responsible children who could be taught to intubate and care for the pouch would be suitable candidates.

We continue to believe that patients with Crohn's disease should *not* receive a pouch. In our series, the disease recurred in the pouch and excision was required in 4 of 17 cases at risk. We decided that it would be unwise to construct a second pouch in any patient whose initial pouch had been excised for recurrent Crohn's disease or for other reasons. The possibility of the loss of an additional 45 cm of ileum should the second pouch become diseased or not function properly was an important factor in this decision.

The major technical problem has been maintaining competence of the nipple valve and continence of the pouch. Improvements in the design and construction of the valve are being considered. For example, a mechanical or magnetic appliance could be implanted that would intermittently occlude the efferent limb of the pouch, but we are concerned about infection. Consequently, a valve of living tissue remains preferable.

Metabolic, nutritional, hepatic, renal, or oncologic complications have not appeared in our patients yet, but the long-term consequences of chronic ileal stasis are unknown.

Until the technical challenges and the long-term consequences of the continent ileostomy are understood more thoroughly, the continent ileostomy should be done mainly in centers where the operation will be performed in sufficient numbers to enable the surgical team to become proficient and where careful follow-up will be available.

In summary, a clinically satisfactory, continent ileal pouch can be constructed in patients with chronic ulcerative colitis and familial polyposis of the large intestine with little or no mortality. Acceptance by the patients has been excellent, but about one-fifth have required reoperation on the valve of the pouch to maintain continence. Nutritional, hepatic, renal, or oncologic complications have not appeared to date, but the long-term consequences of chronic ileal stasis are unknown. Continued careful evaluation in selected medical centers is required.

Surgical Treatment for Crohn's Enterocolitis

Currently available surgical treatment for Crohn's enterocolitis still mainly employs resection or bypass of diseased segments (see Chap. 27). Nonetheless, a newer operation called stricture-plasty has emerged that can relieve the obstruction caused by Crohn's disease, and yet preserve bowel.

Stricture-plasty

RATIONALE

Chronic obstruction, which is one of the most common indications for surgical treatment in Crohn's disease, results from fibrous strictures caused by maturation of granulation tissue. A longitudinal incision across the narrowed segment followed by transverse suturing should relieve the obstruction and yet preserve bowel.

THE OPERATION

The longitudinal incision in the strictured segment is made with the scalpel, extending into normal or near-normal, nonstenosed bowel on either side of the stricture. The longitudinal opening is closed transversely using one layer of interrupted 3-0 vicryl inverting sutures (Fig. 29-31 A and B). Conceivably, several such stricture-plasties can be done in an individual patient.

CLINICAL EVALUATION

Few reports on the use of this approach can be found in the current literature. Alexander-Williams, who has proposed the procedure, performed 31 such stricture-plasties in 16 patients.[60] None of the patients died postoperatively, and none developed serious complications, with the exception of one patient who developed an enterocutaneous fistula that resolved spontaneously. Four other patients exhibited minor symptoms that suggested local peritonitis soon after the operation, but these resolved spontaneously. In a 2-year follow-up, none of the patients showed recrudescence of their disease at the stricture-plasty site.

Lee and co-workers also used this technique in 13 patients without leakage and with excellent results over a 4-year follow-up period.[61] At the Mayo Clinic, stricture-plasty has been done in only 4 patients with obvious localized sites of chronic obstruction. No mortality or morbidity has occurred because of the procedure (unpublished observations).

In conclusion, few new operations have been designed for the management of Crohn's dis-

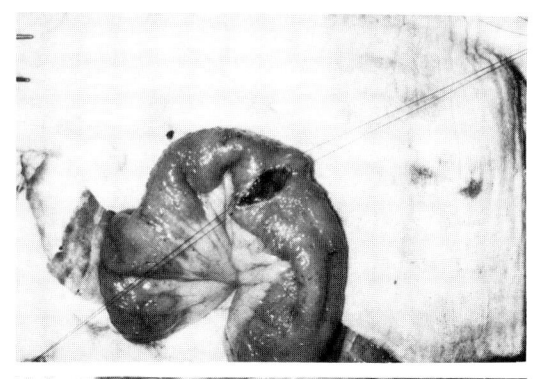

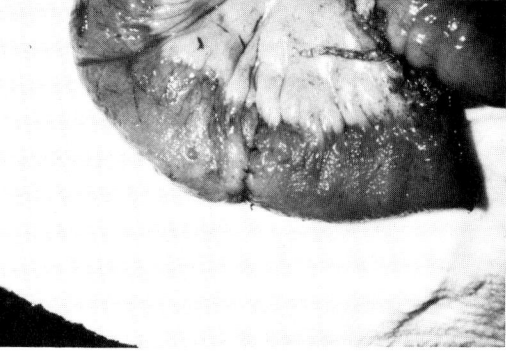

FIG. 29-31. Diagram of stricture-plasty for a short segment of Crohn's disease. A. The longitudinal incision through the stricture is stretched transversely. B. The incision has been closed.

ease. In cases of diffuse disease and areas of localized obstruction, one or more stricture-plasty of the narrowed areas may have a role in avoiding extensive, resective surgical treatment. The procedure is safe and effective in relieving the obstruction. It improves the patient's clinical status, at least over the short-term. What is needed now is a prospective study comparing stricture-plasty to conventional excisional surgery in the management of obstructive Crohn's disease.

References

1. Williams, N. S., and Johnston, D.: The current status of mucosal proctectomy and ileo-anal anastomosis in the surgical treatment of ulcerative colitis and adenomatous polyposis. Br. J. Surg., 72: 159, 1985.
2. Roy, P. H., Sauer, W. G., Beahrs, O. H., and Farrow, G. M.: Experience with ileostomies. Evaluation of long-term rehabilitation in 497 patients. Am. J. Surg., 119:77, 1970.
3. Kelly, K. A.: Ileal pouch-anal anastomosis after proctocolectomy. Surg. Rounds, 8:48, 1985.
4. Dozois, R. R.: Ileal "J" pouch-anal anastomosis. Br. J. Surg., 72(Suppl.):S80, 1985.
5. Lee, J. F., Maurer, V. M., and Block, G. E.: Anatomic relations of pelvic autonomic nerves to pelvic operations Arch. Surg., 107:324, 1973.
6. Utsunomiya, J., et al.: Total colectomy, mucosal proctectomy and ileoanal anastomosis. Dis. Colon Rectum, 23:459, 1980.
7. Parks, A. G., Nicholls, R. J., and Belliveau, P.: Proctocolectomy with ileal reservoir and anal anastomosis. Br. J. Surg., 67:533, 1980.
8. Nicholls, R. J., and Pezim, M. E.: Restorative proctocolectomy with ileal reservoir for ulcerative colitis and familial adenomatous polyposis: A comparison of three reservoir designs. Br. J. Surg., 72:470, 1985.
9. Fonkalsrud, E. W.: Total colectomy and endorectal ileal pull-through with internal ileal reservoir for ulcerative colitis. Surg. Gynecol. Obstet., 150:1, 1980.
10. Kelly, K. A., and Pemberton, J. H.: Mechanisms of fecal continence: Alterations after ileal pouch-anal anastomosis. In Cellular Physiology and Clinical Studies of Gastrointestinal Smooth Muscle. Edited by J. H. Szurszewski. Amsterdam, Elsevier-North Holland, 1987.
11. Pemberton, J. H., et al.: Ileal pouch-anal anastomosis for chronic ulcerative colitis: long-term results. Ann. Surg. 206:504, 1987.
12. Taylor, B. M., et al.: The endorectal ileal pouch-anal anastomosis: current clinical results. Dis. Colon Rectum, 27:347, 1984.
13. Pemberton, J. H., Phillips, S. F., Ready, R. L., and Zinsmeister, A. R.: Comparing performance status after Brooke ileostomy and ileal pouch-anal anastomosis. Gastroenterology, 88:1535, 1985.
14. Metcalf, A. M., Dozois, R. R., and Kelly, K. A.: Sexual function in women after proctocolectomy. Ann. Surg. 204:624, 1986.
15. Metcalf, A. M., et al.: Pregnancy following J pouch-anal anastomosis. Gastroenterology, 88:1501, 1985.
16. Heppell, J., et al.: Physiologic aspects of continence after colectomy, mucosal proctectomy, and endorectal ileoanal anastomosis. Ann. Surg., 195:435, 1982.
17. Stryker, S. J., et al.: Anal sphincter electromyography after colectomy, mucosal rectectomy, and ileoanal anastomosis. Arch. Surg., 201:713, 1985.
18. Beart, R. W., Dozois, R. R., Wolff, B. G., and Pemberton, J. H.: Mechanisms of rectal continence: lessons from the ileoanal procedure. Am J. Surg., 149:31, 1985.
19. O'Connell, P. R., Pemberton, J. H., and Kelly, K. A.: Motor correlates of defecation after ileal pouch-anal anastomosis. Dig. Dis. Sci., 30:785, 1985.
20. Heppell, J., et al.: Predicting outcome after endorectal ileoanal anastomosis. Can. J. Surg., 26:132, 1983.
21. Taylor, B. M., et al.: A clinico-physiological comparison of ileal pouch-anal and straight ileoanal anastomosis. Ann. Surg., 198: 462, 1983.
22. Stryker, S. J., et al.: Anal and neorectal function after ileal pouch-anal anastomosis. Ann. Surg., 203:55, 1986.
23. Rabau, M. Y., Percy, J. P., and Parks, A. G.: Ileal pelvic reservoir: a correlation between motor patterns and clinical behaviour. Br. J. Surg., 69:391, 1982.
24. Stryker, S. J., et al.: Motility of the small intestine after proctocolectomy and ileal pouch-anal anastomosis. Ann. Surg., 201:351, 1985.
25. Parks, A. G., Nicholls, R. J., and Belliveau, P.: Proctocolectomy with ileal reservoir and anal anastomosis. Br. J. Surg., 67:533, 1980.
26. O'Connell, P. R., Pemberton, J. H., Brown, M. L., and Kelly, K. A.: Neorectal emptying after ileal "J" pouch-anal anastomosis. Br. J. Surg., 72:1026, 1985.
27. Summers, R. W., Anuras, S., and Green, J.: Jejunal manometry patterns in health, partial intestinal obstruction, and pseudo-obstruction. Gastroenterology, 85:1290, 1983.
28. Gladen, H. E., and Kelly, K. A.: Enhancing absorption in the canine short bowel syndrome by intestinal pacing. Surgery, 88:281, 1980.
29. Williams, N. S., and King, R. F. G. J.: The effect of reversed ileal segment and artificial valve vs intestinal transit and absorption following colectomy and low ileorectal anastomosis in the dog. Br. J. Surg., 72:169, 1985.
30. Kock, N. G.: Intra-abdominal "reservoir" in patients with permanent ileostomy. Preliminary observations on a procedure resulting in fecal continence in five ileostomy patients. Arch. Surg., 99:223, 1969.
31. Kock, N. G.: Continent ileostomy. Prog. Surg., 12:180, 1973.
32. Kock, N. G.: A new look at ileostomy. Surg. Annu., 8:241, 1976.
33. Beahrs, O. H.: Use of ileal reservoir following proctocolectomy. Surg. Gynecol. Obstet., 141:363, 1975.
34. Goligher, J. C., and Lintott, D.: Experience with 26 reservoir ileostomies. Br. J. Surg., 62:893, 1975.
35. Kelly, K. A., and Beahrs, O. H.: A clinical assessment of the continent ileal pouch. In, Syllabus for Postgraduate Course, American Gastroenterological Association, Miami Beach, Florida, 1976.
36. Madigan, M. R.: The continent ileostomy and the isolated ileal bladder. Ann. R. Coll. Surg. Engl., 58:62, 1976.
37. Waits, J. O., Dozois, R. R., and Kelly, K. A.: Primary closure and continuous irrigation of the perineal wound after proctectomy. Proc. Mayo Clin., 57:185, 1982.
38. Dozois, R. R., Kelly, K. A., Beart, R. W., and Beahrs, O. H.: Improved results with continent ileostomy. Ann Surg., 192:319, 1980.
39. Dozois, R. R., et al.: Factors affecting revision rate after continent ileostomy. Arch. Surg., 116:610, 1981.
40. Dozois, R. R., Kelly, K. A., Beart, R. W., and Beahrs, O. H.: Continent ileostomy: the Mayo Clinic experience. In, Alternatives to Conventional Ileostomy. Edited by R. R. Dozois. Chicago, Year Book Medical Publishers, 1985.

41. Schjønsby, H., Halvorsen, J. F., Hofstad, T., and Hovdenak, N.: Stagnant loop syndrome in patients with continent ileostomy (intra-abdominal ileal reservoir). Gut, *18*:795, 1977.
42. Kelly, D. G., et al.: Dysfunction of the continent ileostomy: clinical features and bacteriology. Gut, *24*:193, 1983.
43. Pemberton, J. H., et al.: Quality of life in ileostomy patients. *In*, Alternatives to Conventional Ileostomy. Edited by R. R. Dozois. Chicago, Year Book Medical Publishers, 1985.
44. Gadacz, T. R., Kelly, K. A., and Phillips, S. F.: The continent ileal pouch: absorptive and motor features. Gastroenterology, *72*:1287, 1977.
45. Cameron, A.: The continent ileostomy. Br. J. Surg., *60*:785, 1973.
46. Hahnloser, P., et al.: Kontinente ileostomy—indikation und moglichkeiten. Schweiz. Med. Wochenschr., *105*:800, 1975.
47. Berglund, B., Kock, N. G., and Myrvold, H. E.: Volume capacity and pressure characteristics of the continent-ileostomy reservoir. Scand. J. Gastroenterol., *19*:683, 1984.
48. Akwari, O. E., Kelly, K. A., and Phillips, S. F.: Myoelectric and motor patterns of continent pouch and conventional ileostomy. Surg. Gynecol. Obstet., *150*:363, 1980.
49. Philipson, B., et al.: Mucosal morphology, bacteriology and absorption in intra-abdominal ileostomy reservoir. Scand. J. Gastroenterol., *10*:145, 1975.
50. Philipson, B., et al.: Function and structure of the mucosa of continent ileostomy reservoirs in dogs. Gut, *16*:132, 1975.
51. Philipson, B.: Morphology in the cat ileal mucosa following construction of an ileal reservoir or transposition of patches to different locations. Scand. J. Gastroenterol., *10*:369, 1975.
52. Gadacz, T. R., Kelly, K. A., and Phillips, S. F.: unpublished observations.
53. Gorbach, S. L., et al.: Studies of intestinal microflora. IV. The microflora of ileostomy effluent: a unique microbial ecology. Gastroenterology, *53*:874, 1967.
54. Brandberg, A., Kock, N. G., and Philipson, B.: Bacterial flora in intraabdominal ileostomy reservoir: a study of 23 patients provided with "continent ileostomy." Gastroenterology, *63*:413, 1972.
55. Jagenburg, R., Kock, N. G., and Philipson, B.: Vitamin B_{12} absorption in patients with continent ileostomy. Scand. J. Gastroenterol., *10*:141, 1975.
56. Nilsson, L. O., et al.: Absorption studies in patients six to ten years after construction of ileostomy reservoirs. Gut, *20*:499, 1979.
57. Jagenburg, R., et al.: Absorption studies in patients with "intraabdominal ileostomy reservoirs" and in patients with conventional ileostomies. Gut, *12*:437, 1971.
58. Morris, J. S., Low-Beer, T. S., and Heaton, K. W.: Bile salt metabolism and the colon. Scand. J. Gastroenterol., *8*:425, 1973.
59. Branon, M. E., Phillips, S. F., Smith, L. H., and Kelly, K. A.: Excessive stomal outputs from continent ileostomies. Gastroenterology, *74*:1151, 1978.
60. Alexander-Williams, J.: New directions for future research: surgical/clinical. *In* Inflammatory Bowel Diseases. Vol. III. Edited by D. Rachmilewitz. London, Martinus Nijhoff, 1982.
61. Lee, E. C. G., and Papaionnou, N.: Minimal surgery for chronic obstruction in patients with extensive or universal Crohn's disease. Ann. R. Coll. Surg. Engl., *64*:229, 1982.

30 · Complications of the Surgical Treatment of Ulcerative Colitis and Crohn's Disease

GEORGE E. BLOCK, M.D., F.A.C.S. AND WOLFGANG H. SCHRAUT, M.D., PH.D., F.A.C.S.

The decision to perform an operation for the treatment of the patient suffering from idiopathic inflammatory bowel disease is essentially a value judgement made by the physician and the surgeon in concert with the informed patient (see Chapters 26 and 27). The decision-making process essentially compares the benefits of a particular clinical circumstance against the risks of complications or death. The decision, then, becomes almost a mathematical balance between the desired result and the known hazards.

An awareness of the possible complications in a given operative procedure, the ability to avoid them, or to recognize and successfully treat them becomes the sine qua non if the patient is to receive the greatest benefit while exposed to the least risk.

Operations on the diseased bowel are attended by special complications in addition to those hazards associated with any major abdominal operation. The problems inherent in surgical treatment for inflammatory bowel disease are generally those of sepsis and inanition. In addition, specific organ abnormalities may be encountered in the operative and postoperative period in these patients.

This chapter is not intended to be a compendium of the hazards and complications of general surgical treatment. Rather, it is a presentation of the special, serious problems associated with operations on the patient suffering from inflammatory disease of the gut. These special problems are presented so that they may be anticipated, avoided, or, if present, properly treated.

Wound

Incision

The placement of the abdominal incision should be made to afford ready access to the organs to be manipulated, yet must resist dehiscence, evisceration, and hernia. Operations upon the diseased bowel may carry the surgeon from the duodenum to the splenic flexure and the deep pelvis. The most popular incision for colonic operations is some modification of the longitudinal incision.[1] Although the longitudinal midline incision allows fast and easy access to the abdominal and pelvic cavity, it is prone to herniation, and, if infected, leads to difficult ventral hernias.[2] We prefer a horizontal or transverse infraumbilical incision usually extending from one anterior axillary line to the other (Fig. 30-1).[3]

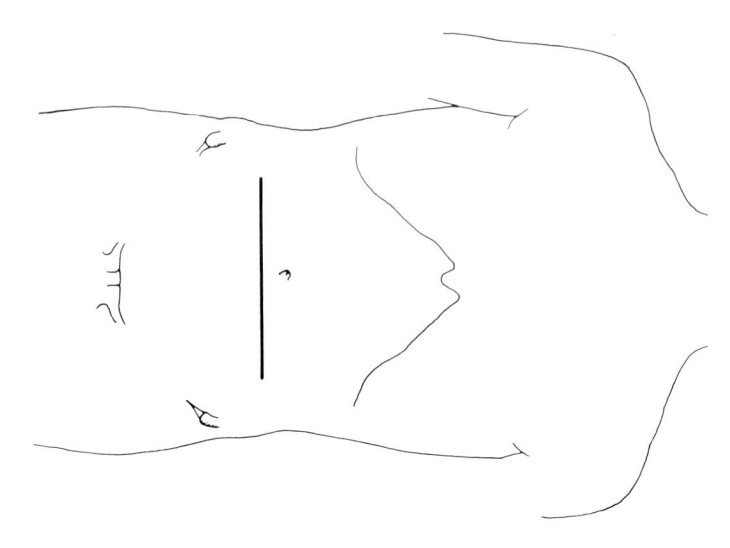

Fig. 30–1. Our choice of abdominal incision for operations for inflammatory bowel disease.

Infection

Reliable reports of the frequency of wound infection following operations for inflammatory bowel disease give conflicting data. Ritchie states that abdominal wound complications are uncommon,[4] but Barker reports a wound infection rate as high as 38%.[5] Cole and Bernard indicate that 14% of wounds through which the intestine is opened become infected.[6] At the University of Chicago Medical Center, we encountered a 7% wound infection rate in 149 consecutive resections for Crohn's ileocolitis. Delayed closure or nonclosure was elected in 82 patients (35% of 231 patients) who presented with either peritonitis, large abscesses, or extensive fistulous disease, or who were operated on under emergency conditions. Less than 4% of patients specifically operated for inflammatory bowel disease required rehospitalization for wound complications.[7]

The rate of wound infection is influenced by such factors as age, severity of disease, and preoperative nutritional state of the patient. The most important predisposing factors to wound infection are the presence of intra-abdominal septic foci, operative technique, preoperative bowel preparation, avoidance of obvious contamination, and methods of closure.[8]

The most common site of wound infection is in the subcutaneous tissue. The frequency of such sources of contamination as fistulas, intra-abdominal abscesses, as well as the inevitable contamination associated with transection of the bowel, would seem to make wound infections inevitable. Contamination cannot be eliminated, however, but the contaminated wound may be prevented from developing a frank abscess by a number of means.[9] Careful technique and the avoidance of "dead space" are paramount. Although adjuvant measures, such as local wound irrigation with antibiotic solutions and routine subcutaneous drainage of the wound,[10] are advocated by some surgeons, they do not replace meticulous operative technique nor completely obviate the possibility of wound sepsis. A uniformly accepted ("standard") and effective adjuvant to sound operative technique is available in the administration of prophylactic perioperative antibiotics. If a wound becomes contaminated, delayed- or nonclosure should be elected.

If frankly contaminated regions are in juxtaposition to the wound, or if the wound has gross fecal contamination, the prudent surgeon will elect a delayed- or nonclosure of the superficial wound and subcutaneous tissue.[11] The use of this technique will prevent almost all true wound infections, decrease postoperative hospitalization, and result in an acceptable cosmetic result.

The organisms most frequently encountered in the infected wound are those of colonic origin. Usually more than one organism is involved. Bacteroides, E. coli, streptococci, and staphylococci are the most common offenders. If a wound abscess is suspected, the wound should be widely opened, the exudate cultured, the wound copiously irrigated, and then lightly packed with fine mesh gauze. Frequent changes of packing and irrigation will result in healthy granulations within 4 to 5 days; at this time the surgeon can elect either secondary closure at the bedside, or closure by secondary intention. The patient may be discharged from the hospital with a healthy granulating wound that is not completely healed.

Systemic antibiotics are not required for the usual superficial wound infection. Tetanus, necrotizing fasciitis, and gas gangrene are extremely rare complications. If, however, systemic manifestation of sepsis is obvious, or if other conditions such as cardiac valvular lesions exist, then appropriate antibiotics are warranted. Their selection should be determined by the culture identification of the offending organisms and their sensitivity to antibiotics as determined in vitro.[12]

Although it is impossible to sterilize the contents of the bowel completely, most surgeons attempt to decrease the population of the colonic bacteria by some preoperative antibiotic preparation in combination with mechanical cleansing.[13] Such preparation will decrease the likelihood of postoperative infections, but its injudicious use may result in the proliferation of resistant strains and increase the likelihood of catastrophic septic complications and the development of pseudomembranous enterocolitis.[14] Both systemic and enteral prophylaxis reduce septic complications, but no clear superiority of either method has been proved. Lewis et al. compared systemic cephaloridine with intraluminal neomycin and erythromycin, and found no significant difference between the incidences of infectious complications in the two groups.[15] Although Dion found no difference between oral and parenteral use of metronidazole as prophylaxis in surgical treatment of the colon,[16] Keighley et al. demonstrated a superiority of systemic versus oral preparation using metronidazole and kanamycin.[17] Stone and Polk have shown the efficacy of parenteral prophylactic antibiotic administration in situations in which the likelihood of infection is great and the consequence of such infection is catastrophic.[18,19] In "clean-contaminated" (most operations upon gut) and frankly contaminated cases, Stone has decreased the incidence of postoperative infections from a control rate of 16% to only 6% in those patients receiving parenteral cefazolin prior to operation, during operation, and in the early postoperative period. Stone stresses that for such a regimen to be successful, the antibiotic chosen must be appropriate to the organism encountered, have adequate circulating blood levels, and be present in the local tissues at the time of the expected contamination. We strongly advocate such a program for patients suffering from inflammatory bowel disease whose gut is to be transected.

The frankly obstructed or grossly diseased colon cannot be cleansed nor adequately prepared. In these situations, resections may be done with safety, but primary anastomosis should be avoided. Here the prudent surgeon will consider the wound to be contaminated and leave it open to heal by secondary intention.

Wound Separation

Improper closure and inadequate healing of the abdominal wound may result in postoperative complications ranging from minor separations to complete dehiscence and evisceration. These latter catastrophes are associated with an eventual mortality rate up to 35%.[19]

Causal factors for wound separation include infection, faulty technique, obesity, and increased abdominal tension and stress. Corticosteroid administration has often been indicted in the genesis of separation, but persuasive data are lacking.[20]

Most major wound separations are associated with the use of some variety of longitudinal incision inadequately supported by retention sutures.[21] The use of the transverse incision is, perhaps, the single most important factor in the prevention of these complications. Singleton and Blocker report no disruptions in 470 transverse abdominal incisions and eventual herniation in 5% of patients.[2] Our experience is similar. In a consecutive series of 231 patients operated on for Crohn's ileocolitis through a transverse incision, we have encountered no wound disruptions nor incisional hernias. The transverse incision divides the transversalis fascia in the direction of its fibers, parallel to the vectors of stress. Further, the denervation and devascularization of the abdominal wall musculature are minimal.

Wound disruption may only be heralded by the subjective sensation of "something giving way" at the wound site. However, more commonly, a serosanguinous discharge from the wound of a febrile distended patient announces the disruption. Such a discharge occurs in approximately one-half of the patients suffering disruption.[22] When a discharge is observed or a dehiscence is suspected, the wound should be examined under sterile conditions; a few sutures may be removed to search for hematoma, pus, or a concealed loop of bowel. When separation has occurred, any exposed bowel should be covered with moist, sterile dressings, the abdomen supported, and the patient should be operated on immediately for definitive closure.

Debridement of the wound is then accomplished, any occult abscesses drained, and the abdominal cavity heavily irrigated with 0.85% saline solution. Some surgeons advocate the use of antibiotic irrigants, but these offer no advantage to saline in the prevention of postoperative sepsis.[23] Aminoglycosides in the anesthetized patient may prolong and potentiate the actions of muscle relaxants, leading to respiratory insufficiency.[24] Solutions containing sulfonamides are notorious for causing a chemically adhesive peritonitis.[25] We prefer the traditional saline irrigation, supplemented with appropriate systemic antibiotics, for the patient suffering evisceration after bowel resection.

Reclosure is effected with stout nonabsorbable sutures. In longitudinal wounds, a through and through suture well back from the wound is necessary. Although the necrotic effect of these retention sutures on the skin and abdominal wall can be reduced, partial necrosis almost invariably occurs and compounds local sepsis (Fig. 30-2). To avoid this we employ a one layer closure using number 4 monofilament wire that encompasses the entire fibrotic, indurated wound margins with the exception of the skin and subcutaneous tissue. Once all sutures have been placed, the wound edges are approximated by tightening the wire ends. The skin and subcutaneous tissue are left open. Tension can be relieved, if necessary, by lateral relaxing incisions in the flank (Fig. 30-2).

On occasion, the extent of separation may be too great to permit reapproximation of the edges. In these situations, it may be judicious to employ a Marlex mesh to fill the defect.[26] Aggressive measures to prevent further peritonitis are undertaken, including intestinal decompression, diversion of the fecal stream when appropriate, and massive antibiotic administration. Total parenteral nutrition (TPN) is useful to restore these patients to the anabolic state.*

Incisional Hernia

A late wound complication may be the development of an incisional or ventral hernia. The incidence following operation for inflammatory bowel disease is from 0.5 to 3.9%.[4,27] This is no higher than the expected incidence in laparotomies in general.[28] The choice of the incision and

*Editors' note: see also: Parenteral nutrition in the surgical patient (Review). Br. J. Surg., 74: 172, 1987.

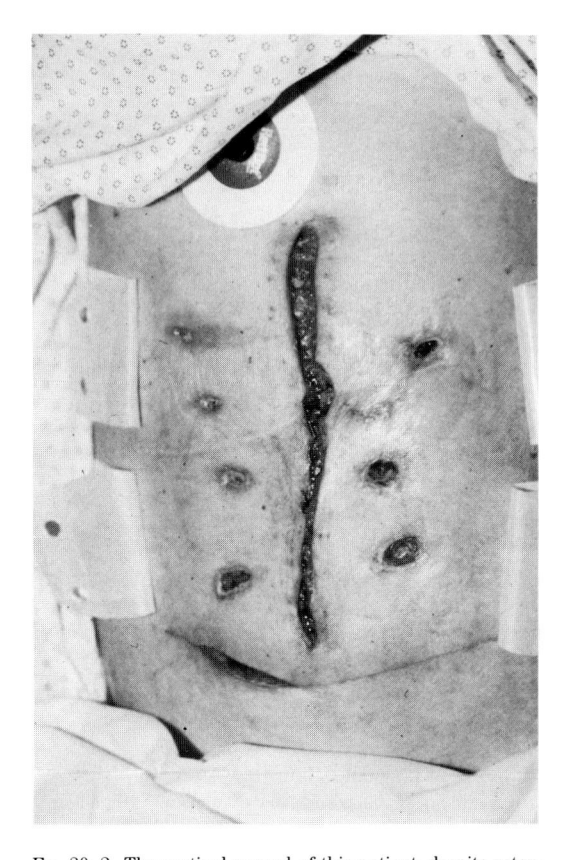

FIG. 30–2. The vertical wound of this patient, despite retention sutures, dehisced. Successful closure with #4 wire is shown which closes the fascia, but not the skin and subcutaneous tissue. Note the abdominal wall necrosis caused by the previous retention sutures and the ready healing of the subsequent transverse incision.

the presence of drains or infections influence the rate of occurrence of this complication. Wound infection is noted in about 25% of patients who eventually develop an incisional hernia.

Most incisional hernias present as painless swellings at the site of the old scar, usually within 60 days of operation. Of course, these hernias are subject to the same complication of intestinal obstruction as are other hernias.

Incisional hernias are best repaired by excision of the sac and a precise anatomic repair of the abdominal wall. Incisional hernias occurring through longitudinal incisions are, in general, more difficult to repair than those occurring through transverse incisions.[29] Large defects in the abdominal wall may require closure by employment of fascial graft or Marlex prosthesis. The use of prosthetic material may be avoided by the employment of bilateral or unilateral relaxing incisions through the oblique muscles down to the transversalis layer at the flanks. This allows a tension-free closure of a wide midline incisional hernia. The lateral skin incisions can always be closed over the muscle incisions because tension at the skin level rarely occurs.

Sepsis

The most dreaded postoperative complication of surgical therapy of the colon is peritonitis. A certain amount of contamination occurs during every operation, but gross contamination by fecal spillage, inadvertent rupture of an inflamed viscus, or failure of an anastomosis present overwhelming challenges to the peritoneal cavity with resultant, and often fatal, bacterial peritonitis.

In 1971, Ritchie reported 81 postoperative deaths in 453 patients undergoing operation for inflammatory bowel disease.[7] Peritonitis and "systemic infection" accounted for 24 of these fatalities. de Dombal indicted peritonitis in 17 of 24 postoperative deaths occurring in patients with Crohn's disease.[27]

Acute peritonitis may be diffuse or localized, and from an etiologic view may be conveniently classified as *primary*, *secondary*, or *postoperative*. For the purposes of this section, we shall consider only *secondary* and *postoperative* peritonitis, whether localized or diffuse. Secondary peritonitis may be the terminal event of perforation of an inflamed bowel, and postoperative peritonitis is a relatively common sequel to abdominal operations involving the opening or transection of a hollow viscus.[30]

Thirty years ago, the mortality rate of *secondary* peritonitis was 30%; today it is less than 10%.[31] *Postoperative* peritonitis, especially that associated with anastomotic failures, ends in death in almost one-half of the patients.[32]

Aird has stated that the peritoneum is well adapted to combat;[8] however, if continued soiling of the peritoneum occurs it is unable to withstand the bacterial attack. Peritonitis secondary to fecal contamination involved 16 species of aerobic microorganisms and 18 species of anaerobes in 100 patients studied by Altemeier.[33,34] The biologic relationships of bacteria are of great significance in the production of peritonitis. The action between aerobes and anaerobes is synergistic, and so-called nonpathogenic bacteria may exist in synergy during fecal peritonitis.[35] In general, the greater the number of bacterial species present in the peritoneal exudate, the more virulent and clinically severe the peritonitis.

The common bacterial flora of secondary or postoperative peritonitis include such common aerobic bacteria as Escherichia coli, Aerobacter aerogenes, various streptococci, Klebsiella, Pseudomonas, Proteus, Staphylococcus aureus, yeasts, and diphtheroids. Anaerobic bacteria are represented by Bacteroides fragilis, Clostridia, and several species of streptococci and staphylococci.[35] Bacteroides fragilis is the most prevalent organism.

The peritoneal lining of the abdominal cavity represents a large surface that approximates the total body surface area. Any trauma to this membrane, either planned or accidental, results in hyperemia and edema. Contaminating bacteria are usually dealt with adequately, but clinical peritonitis will result when the bacterial inoculum is large or virulent, or if the host's local defenses are compromised because of chronic illness, the presence of intraperitoneal foreign bodies or blood, or drugs that interfere with the inflammatory response. The exudative potential of the peritoneum is responsible for the sequestration of tremendous volumes of fluid during peritonitis. These third space losses may range from 4 to 12 liters during a 24-hour period.[30] This fluid is not usable by the patient for circulatory support and must be parenterally replaced. The impaired and inflamed peritoneum will allow the absorption of toxic materials from the peritoneal cavity, particularly bacterial toxins and metabolites.[30,36]

The metabolic and circulatory responses to peritonitis have been studied by a number of investigators.[37,38] Although effects of peritonitis are pansystemic, circulatory and respiratory failure and the derangement of metabolic homeostasis are clinically prominent. Cardiac output is generally insufficient to meet the increased circulatory demands.[37] Striking alveolar-arterial oxygen differences are commonly encountered, probably representing phenomena of intrapulmonary shunting.[38] Metabolic acidosis is common as an expression of circulatory deficiencies coupled with end-product absorption from the altered peritoneal surfaces.

Totally, the terminal stage of peritonitis is metabolic degeneration from combined fluid volume changes, circulatory insufficiency, disturbed oxygen transfer, and metabolic acidosis.

Postoperative sepsis may appear as either localized or generalized peritonitis. Although the diagnosis may be difficult, a surgical infection must be distinguished from a nonsurgical infection. Awareness by the surgeon of the possibility of a technical error leading to a localized abscess or, more unfortunately, anastomotic disruption resulting in generalized peritonitis, is the key to early diagnosis. An unexplained fever, a tachycardia inappropriate to the clinical situation, the diminution of bowel sounds, and, finally, the appearance of frank ileus or the accumulation of intraperitoneal gas on roentgenograms of the abdomen, point to peritoneal sepsis. In our experience, the classical findings of leukocytosis or abdominal pain are not of great value, and their absence, particularly in patients receiving corticosteroids, can be misleading. Abdominal wall rigidity is, however, a reliable indication of peritoneal irritation under these circumstances.

The search for intra-abdominal abscesses or generalized peritonitis has been tremendously enhanced by the use of computerized axial tomography of the abdomen (CT scan). The CT scan is the initial diagnostic procedure of choice; sonography is less useful because collections may be camouflaged by overlying air or fat and fluid-filled or air-filled viscera. Opacification of the gut with contrast material is essential for proper use of the CT scan.[39]

Once the diagnosis of peritoneal sepsis is established, the surgeon must then differentiate between localized and general peritonitis and provide an appropriate operative attack, adequate chemotherapy, and metabolic support.

Treatment of Generalized Peritonitis

ANTIMICROBIAL TREATMENT. The rational use of antibacterial drugs should be based upon two principles. The first is to establish a bacteriologic diagnosis and the second is to make an accurate estimate of the antimicrobial agent(s) that will be effective in vivo. From a practical standpoint, these objectives may not be attainable in each patient prior to the institution of treatment. Positive blood, wound, or peritoneal cultures may be lacking at the crescendo of the patient's illness. Further, imperfect collection and culture techniques may fail to reveal anaerobic organisms that are abundantly present. Given the clinical picture of peritonitis, the clinician may assume that the offending agents are enteric, both aerobic and anaerobic, and that a mixed, or polymicrobial, infection exists.[35]

Antibiotic therapy should begin as soon as peritonitis is diagnosed, even before samples of the peritoneal fluid have been cultured. We prefer a combination of antimicrobials in the presence of suspected or proven peritonitis. These drugs must be given via a parenteral route in high concentrations. Therapy can be modified by subsequent knowledge of the exact identification of the organism(s) and its drug sensitivities.

Most clinically important anaerobes are susceptible to penicillin with the exception of the most common organism in the colon, Bacteroides fragilis.[40] Chloramphenicol, clindamycin, metronidazole, and the newer cephalosporins are effective against Bacteroides fragilis and most other anaerobic species.[41,42]

Chloramphenicol is effective both against gram-negative and gram-positive aerobic and anaerobic pathogens (including enterococci and Bacteroides fragilis) and does not require dose adjustment in patients with renal failure. Chloramphenicol may be inactivated by some anaerobes, but is usually effective in fecal peritonitis. It has been associated with numerous blood dyscrasias; however, a mild, dose-related anemia is common but the severe hypersensitivity reaction responsible for pancytopenia and death is extremely rare.[43] The metabolism of chloramphenicol is not affected by the presence of renal insufficiency.[44]

A number of antibiotics, particularly clindamycin, have been associated with the diarrhea and pseudomembranous colitis caused by toxins produced by Clostridium difficile.[45] If diarrhea occurs with treatment, colitis may be prevented by cessation of therapy. Vancomycin is the drug of choice for the treatment of antibiotic-associated colitis caused by C. difficile.

Considering the potential problems with both chloramphenicol and clindamycin, metronidazole appears to be the preferred drug for anaerobic coverage.

Second and third generation cephalosporins, such as moxalactam, cefotaxime, and cefaperazone, are effective against gram-negative organisms and Bacteroides fragilis, but they have not been shown to be superior to a combination of an aminoglycoside and clindamycin or metronidazole.

Altemeier suggests the use of systemic penicillin because of its effectiveness against gram-positive cocci and bacilli commonly associated with peritonitis.[35] Large doses of penicillin inhibit the growth of virulent gram-positive bacteria, particularly of the anaerobes, lessening the number of organisms at growth and their known synergistic effect.[46]

The aminoglycosides are weakly effective against anaerobes, but represent a wise choice for the aerobic and coliform species present.[41] They are effective against most strains of E. coli, Klebsiella, Enterobacter, and Proteus. Pseudomonas is rarely an initial problem in peritonitis. For the aminoglycosides gentamicin and tobramycin, appropriate peak and trough blood levels are sought; peak blood levels should not be below 6 μg/ml or above 12 μg/ml; trough levels should always be below 2 μg/ml. These concentrations supply appropriate therapeutic levels and limit toxicity. In patients with impaired renal function the dosage should be appropriately reduced. In all instances, aminoglycoside blood levels should be monitored and "rules of thumb" or therapeutic recipes should not be substituted for actual blood level determinations.[42,47]

In fecal peritonitis, enterococci are usually part of the polymicrobial flora causing the sepsis. These organisms are best treated by ampicillin. Thus, a triple antibiotic program relying on a combination of penicillin, an aminoglycoside, and an agent effective against anaerobes is recommended.[48]

If clostridial organisms are identified, or if the clinical situation suggests the possibility of tetanus infection, both active and passive immunity are supplied to the patient.[49]

OPERATIVE TREATMENT OF ACUTE PERITONITIS. Although antibiotics are essential in the treatment of peritonitis, the decision to treat peritonitis by operation is usually determined by identification of the source of the contamination. Spreading peritonitis in the postoperative period indicates an intra-abdominal catastrophe that will require operative correction. Primary repair of the contaminating intestinal leak is usually inadvisable; the surgeon should rely on the principle of "diversion of the fecal stream." These operative maneuvers are, of course, supplemented both by antimicrobial and supportive measures.

Occasionally, the source of peritoneal contamination is a sequel to the original disease state and operation, and not a direct consequence of the technical aspects of the operation. Such instances include free perforation of a peptic ulcer, strangulation-obstruction of the small bowel or ischemic necrosis of a hollow viscus. In these circumstances, the complication is treated on its own merits by closure or resection.

However, certain catastrophes occur during the postoperative period in the patient who has undergone operation for inflammatory disease of the bowel that require specific operative correction by an experienced surgeon.

A common cause of peritonitis is the retained rectal or sigmoid stump. For a number of reasons, the prudent surgeon may wish to perform total colectomy by way of a two-stage procedure, or to preserve the rectosigmoid for possible future anastomosis with the small bowel. The inexperienced surgeon may attempt closure of an overtly or occultly diseased segment of rectosigmoid and replace it into the peritoneal cavity. This is fraught with dangers; the closure may disrupt, leading to generalized peritonitis, or a minor leakage may occur with ensuing pelvic abscess and bowel obstruction. Should one be faced with this problem, it can be handled by a variety of means. The safest and most reliable approach is reoperation to exteriorize the peritoneal portion of the rectosigmoid as a mucous fistula. If the segment is too short or too "bound-down" by the inflammatory response, the surgeon may elect intubation of the proximal lumen and attachment to the parietal peritoneum. This will result in a controlled fistula. Occasionally, in minor peritoneal soiling, the rectum may be resected and reclosed beneath the peritoneal reflection.

To avoid this sequence, it is best to establish a mucous fistula from the retained distal segment at the cutaneous level. A slight modification of this technique is to close the distal stump and to exteriorize the closed end at the fascial level. If closure is successful, the patient is not bothered by the mucous stoma. If closure is unsuccessful, leakage will occur to the exterior. A third, but less reliable option, is to resect the rectum beneath the peritoneal reflection to afford an extraperitoneal closure.

Disruption of an enterocolic anastomosis is a catastrophe that demands prompt recognition. The first step in its recognition is to accept the definite diagnostic possibility. Too often the surgeon will not admit such a possibility to himself, and needlessly procrastinates. If the enterocolic anastomosis is readily accessible within the free peritoneal cavity, the area of the anastomosis may be exteriorized. Such an exteriorization is best accomplished through a separate incision, although the original incision is used to obtain access to the peritoneal cavity. The surgeon may elect to resect or take down the previous anastomosis and convert it into a temporary enterostomy (usually ileostomy) and distal mucous fistula. This is the safest and most effective approach. In these instances, the ileostomy is fashioned with the same care and attention as during a primary operative procedure.

If an ileoproctostomy has been performed

previously, making exteriorization difficult or impossible, a proximal loop ileostomy supplemented by copious irrigation of the peritoneal cavity is performed. This is a simple procedure that can be performed expeditiously and may be life saving. After healing, the ileostomy can be simply repaired and intestinal continuity reestablished. This time interval is usually from 6 to 8 weeks.

Irrigation with a sterile saline solution is useful for diluting and washing out contaminating bacteria and debris. After fibrin forms, however, such irrigation is of limited value. Irrigation with antimicrobial solutions is not universally accepted.[35,50] Postoperative peritoneal irrigation through indwelling intra-abdominal catheters is favored by some authors,[51] but its advantages are not clear-cut and the danger exists of erosion of the edematous, boggy bowel by the indwelling catheters.

We have successfully used peritoneal debridement in severe peritonitis to remove peritoneal debris, pseudomembranes, and exudates. Although time consuming, peritoneal debridement can diminish postperitonitis abscess formation and result in increased survival, if carefully done. Debridement is accomplished by removal of membranes from all visceral and parietal surfaces throughout the abdomen, supplemented by copious irrigation.[52]

Localized Peritoneal Sepsis

Intraperitoneal abscesses occurring in the postoperative period represent areas of localized infection subsequent to secondary or postoperative peritonitis.[32] Such an abscess is a continuing site of sepsis that has been isolated by the inflammatory response. The pathogenesis of these abscesses is usually by one of two means: (1) loculation in anatomically dependent areas following a diffuse peritonitis, or (2) infection contiguous to an active disease process. The bacterial flora of these abscesses are identical to those listed in the discussion of generalized peritonitis.

The diagnosis of an abscess is made by a number of circumstantial factors including spiking fever, partial bowel obstruction, profound neutrophilic leukocytosis, pleural effusion, and air-fluid levels visible on roentgenograms. The CT scan is an especially helpful diagnostic tool in these patients.

Although the postoperative patient may develop abscesses in any recess of the peritoneal cavity, certain common sites of predilection exist.[35,53]

Pelvic Abscess

The differentiation of a pelvic abscess from a pelvic inflammatory mass, or phlegmon, may require a trial of therapy. The latter will often improve by simple antimicrobial therapy; the former will not. Depending upon the extent of the operative dissection, a postoperative pelvic abscess may be drained by a number of routes. The surgeon may wish to approach a large pelvic abscess transabdominally, but extraperitoneally. After locating the site of the abscess, appropriate dependent and/or sump drainage is established. Although pelvic abscesses may be drained through the vagina in the parous patient, vaginal drainage in immature females is inadequate and dangerous. If the rectum is in place, the pelvic abscess may be drained through the rectum, but this procedure should be avoided in patients with inflammatory bowel disease for fear of causing damage to an entrapped loop of small bowel, with a resulting enterorectal fistula. If the rectum has been removed, or the supralevator space has been dissected, the pelvic abscess may be drained through the perineum. This drainage is usually accomplished in the presacral space and extends above the remnants of the levator sling. Appropriate antibiotics supplement the care of patients before, during, and after manipulation of the abscess. Such abscesses can occur at any time postoperatively. Most will make their clinical appearance within 30 days of operation; however, we have encountered such abscesses 5 years after the original operative procedure. Abscesses appearing after this period in patients suffering from Crohn's disease may indicate a recrudescence of the disease rather than a postoperative complication.

Subphrenic and Subhepatic Abscesses

These collections of pus may be described by their relation to the falciform ligament and the liver. They are often insidious and difficult to diagnose. Most make their appearance within two weeks of peritoneal soiling; 30- to 90-day intervals are not uncommon. A high index of suspicion, plus several diagnostic radiographic studies, are aids to diagnosis. Pleural effusions, displacement of the gastric outline, and air-fluid levels within the abscess may all indicate such an abscess on flat or upright chest and abdominal roentgenograms. Subphrenic abscesses are best drained extraperitoneally. Computerized tomography (CT scan) has replaced the transmission-emission scan and is the radiographic maneuver of choice to diagnose and localize any intra-abdominal abscesses. A single, well localized abscess may be drained percutaneously using stereotaxic localization. In our experience, however, this maneuver often fails to completely eradicate a postoperative abscess of enteric origin because of loculation of the abscess or the high viscosity of its contents. Failure of percutaneous drainage, as manifested by the continued septic state, requires open drainage. For anterior abscesses a Clairmont subcostal incision is advocated, and the posterior approach of Ochsner through the bed of the 12th rib is ideal for posterior presentations.[54] Adjuvant antimicrobial therapy is, of course, used.

Retroperitoneal Abscesses

Altemeier and Alexander have described the anatomic boundaries of the retroperitoneal space.[55] Most retroperitoneal abscesses associated with inflammatory bowel disease occupy the anterior retroperitoneal space. Only rarely does enteric disease result in a posterior retroperitoneal infection. The majority of these abscesses are present preoperatively, and their appearance in the postoperative period implies that they were overlooked or inadequately drained at the time of operation. Complete evacuation, thorough debridement, and adequate drainage, combined with appropriate antimicrobial therapy, are essential for proper treatment.

Intermesenteric Abscesses

Occasionally, loculations of pus will occur between leafs of mesentery or loops of small bowel. These lesions are notoriously difficult to diagnose, but an awareness of the possibility of their existence and the use of abdominal CT scans will disclose the abscesses. Because extraperitoneal drainage is often impossible with intermesenteric abscesses, their treatment may require transperitoneal drainage or bowel resection.

Hepatic Abscesses

Hepatic abscess is an extremely rare occurrence in the patient with inflammatory bowel disease who has not had a septic complication of the disease. In our experience we have encountered only three patients with hepatic abscesses who did not have evidence of another septic complication, such as perforation, intra-abdominal abscess, or an anastomotic leak. Treatment must be individualized and includes percutaneous drainage, open drainage, a combination of the two approaches, and, occasionally, partial hepatic resection.

Supportive Therapy

Some manifestations of postoperative infection require only proper antimicrobial therapy and supportive measures without operative intervention. Gram-negative sepsis is essentially treated by elimination of the offending organism, plus the rapid and efficient support of the circulatory and ventilatory requirements of the patient.[38,56] This requires monitoring and managing the patient in an intensive care unit.

Supportive treatment of the septic patient requires attention to the circulatory and ventilatory requirements. The needs of the patient are best determined by careful and frequent bedside observations, supplemented by appropriate laboratory studies of bodily fluids and monitoring of fluid dynamics and oxygen tension. Swan-Ganz catheterization, determination of cardiac indices, rhythms, and output are essential to the proper management of the seriously ill individual.

Adequate fluid replacement, including water for urinary and insensible loss, a "balanced" saline solution to counteract third space fluid shifts, and blood administration are all necessary to compensate for the tremendous fluid volume redistribution accompanying peritonitis.

Respiratory toilet and support with a ventilator by way of an endotracheal tube or tracheostomy are often lifesaving, because many of these patients have both mechanical and physiologic respiratory inadequacies that become manifest by lowered peripheral oxygen tension (adult respiratory distress syndrome).

A nasogastric tube should be in place to decompress the paralyzed foregut. Corticosteroids must be continued in the stressful postoperative situation for those patients whose endogenous adrenocortical mechanism has atrophied because of chronic medication by exogenous corticosteroids.

Patients who are epidemiologically at risk for thromboembolism because of inflammatory bowel disease, treatment with corticosteroids, immobilization, or obesity may be treated with prophylactic, low-dose herapin. 5,000 units of herapin is given subcutaneously every 12 hours, and in certain disease entities other than inflammatory bowel disease, this regimen has been shown to decrease the incidence of deep venous thrombosis and fatal pulmonary emboli, without fear of undue bleeding.[57] The presence of deep venous thrombosis or the suspicion or documentation of a pulmonary embolus mandates more vigorous therapy. Systemic heparinization is called for in these patients. Certain individuals, however, are at great risk for hemorrhage, because the unresected diseased bowel may bleed with systemic heparinization. Heparinization is contraindicated in the early postoperative period following proctocolectomy or other large dissections because the raw retroperitoneal surfaces resulting from the dissection may bleed. For these patients, prophylactic or therapeutic caval clipping or interruption by an indwelling filter is indicated.[58,59,60] We have frequently employed these procedures without incident, and none of our patients had a subsequent clinically evident pulmonary embolus.

For the chronically ill patient, long-term TPN may be lifesaving (see also Chap. 24).[61] In the presence of acute sepsis, however, the use of TPN is often accompanied by ketoacidosis, requiring parenteral insulin and potassium supplementation. It is not uncommon for these patients to require 300 mg of potassium per day. The stressed patient attempting to heal wounds is best supplemented with 1000 mg of ascorbic acid per day.[62]

Persistent Perineal Wound or Sinus

The persistent perineal wound or residual sinus is merely a failure of healing of the posterior wound. An open or infected wound or sinus remaining after 6 months is usually considered to fulfill the definition of persistence. We have treated wounds that had persisted for up to 22 years.

Although many of the persistent wounds are minor cutaneous sinuses and are merely a nuisance to the patient, others are huge, purulent cavities with unhealthy granulations that interfere with the patient's health, rehabilitation and social acceptance. The incidence of the unhealed perineal wound following total proctocolectomy is quoted as from 10 to over 40%.[27,63] Of more practical importance is that prolonged hospitalization is often necessary for the closure of these wounds, and multiple operative procedures may be entailed.[7]

Corticosteroids apparently do not play a role in the persistence of the open wound.[64] Crohn's colitis is more often associated with nonhealing than is ulcerative colitis. Only one-fourth of de Dombal's patients with ulcerative colitis suffered wound failure,[65] but one-half of his patients with granulomatous colitis developed this complication.

This late complication is more common in women, particularly when the perineal wound is packed.[65] This suggests that lack of pelvic support plays an etiologic role. An occasional wound failure, when investigated, will reveal the explanation for persistence, such as retained mucosa, fistula to bladder or gut, or neoplasia. When these uncommon situations exist, the removal of the cause and re-excision of the walls of the wound will suffice for cure.

Jalan and Myers et al. agree that the avoidance of pelvic sepsis, combined with primary closure of the perineum and the early removal of small, effective drainage, is the best prevention of this complication.[63,66]

These additional observations will aid in the prevention of persistent perineal wounds. First, precise hemostasis must be achieved in the pelvis and perineum and the introduction of foreign bodies, such as packing, should be avoided. We use only a small posterior suction drain in the presacral space for 24 to 48 hours after operation. Secondly, the perineal wound should be closed in layers, the levator ani, the subcutaneous tissue, and the skin, without the formation of a "dead space."

If the surgeon is confronted by a large, infected persistent perineal wound, he must first verify that no fistula, foreign body, or unrecognized abscess is to blame. If these are present, they are treated appropriately. Usually, however, the surgeon will be faced with a chronic, thick-walled, fibrous cavity bearing pale, infected granulations. Under anesthesia, the entire thick fibrous wall of this cavity must be excised. Adequate excision may include the coccyx and portions of the sacrum. Curettage is inadequate treatment because it fails to remove the thick fibrous wall. During this procedure the surgeon must be careful to avoid injury to the bladder and urethra anteriorly, and must also realize that the small bowel may be in close proximity to the superior portion of the cavity. Preoperative visualization by contrast roentgenograms is often useful in delineating sites of possible hazard. An indwelling urethral catheter should always be used so that the course of the urethra is easily discernable.

The wound then is left open and will heal spontaneously within a few weeks in the majority of instances. Continuing attention by the surgeon, however, is required to insure proper healing. Hair must be shaved from the area to prevent pilonidal sinus formation, and superficial infection of the granulation tissue may require topical or systemic antimicrobial and antimonilial agents. Daily irrigation of the cavity is mandatory.

In certain individuals, re-excision alone of the perineal abscess cavity either will not suffice or it will require an unrealistically long time for healing. Patients who have harbored a persistent perineal wound for many months or years, those who have deep or voluminous cavities, and female patients in whom there are sinus tracts to the posterior vaginal wall are candidates for myocutaneous flaps. Although some authors advocate the use of such flaps at the time of cavity excision, we prefer a two-staged approach that allows for subsidence of the local infection. One or two gracilis muscles are transposed into the cavity, depending on its size. The configuration of the perineal wound will dictate a simple muscle flap or a myocutaneous flap. If the perineal destruction is large, a myocutaneous flap is used to afford skin closure of the perineum. In other individuals, the cavity is obliterated by the muscle transposition and the perineal skin closed primarily.[67]

In some unfortunate patients, tremendous perineal sepsis is present with multiple abscesses and sinus tracts originating from the persistent perineal wound. In these situations, the defect is often not deep and the superior portion will close by excision of the cavity, coccyx, and appropriate portions of the sacrum. The defect that remains is a two-dimensional defect, in the female often running from the introitus to the coccyx and to the medial aspect of each thigh. In such instances, a posterior thigh flap consisting of skin, subcutaneous tissue, and fascia without muscle is transferred to the now clean perineum, with excellent results. In female patients whose posterior vaginal wall has been completely or partially destroyed, the transposition of a gracilis myocutaneous flap is advocated, with the cutaneous portion being used for reconstruction of the posterior vagina.

The use of these techniques will uniformly result in the closure of these persistent and bothersome wounds (Fig. 30-3).

Complications Associated with Ileostomy*

The problems associated with a permanent ileostomy are important when considering proctocolectomy for inflammatory bowel disease. Jacob, Pace, and Thomford reported that 14% of their patients required revision of the stoma

*See also Chapters 28, 29.

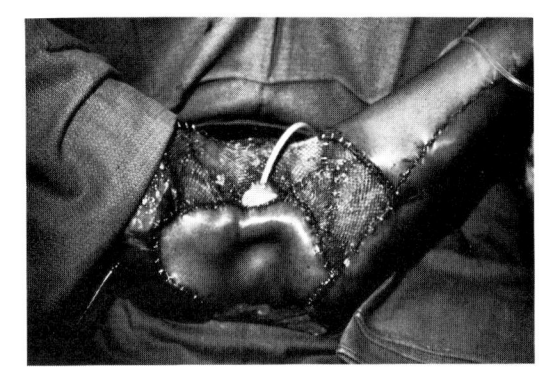

FIG. 30–3. The perineum of this patient was involved with extensive necrosis and suppuration resulting from a persistent perineal wound open for 20 years after proctectomy. Following excision of the fibrotic cavity, vaginal hysterectomy, and extensive perineal, inguinal and buttocks debridement, closure was obtained utilizing a posterior-thigh fasciocutaneous flap and meshed split-skin grafts.

within 10 years.[68] In a study of the late causes of mortality after proctocolectomy, Ritchie cited complications related to the ileostomy as a major cause of death.[7]

Ileostomy Dysfunction

In 1951, Warren and McKittrick defined ileostomy dysfunction as partial obstruction of the stoma resulting in cramps and increased stomal output.[69] This was seen in 61.9% of their 210 patients and resulted in 7 deaths, being second only to peritonitis as the leading cause of postoperative death. This stomal obstruction was thought to be caused by local serositis and a cutaneous cicatrix about the terminal ileum. The advent of the Brooke ileostomy in 1952 substantially eliminated this entity, so that Brooke was able to report its occurrence in only 1 of 71 patients.[70,71] Nevertheless, partial obstruction of the ileostomy is still seen today as a result of improper ileostomy construction. The leading cause of stomal dysfunction today is construction of a short conventional ileostomy.[72,73] Converted to a continent ileostomy, the complication rate decreased from 18 to 5%. Continence was achieved in 90 to 95% of the patients.[86–91]

Operative Mortality of the Continent Ileostomy

The first experiences with the continent ileostomy resulted in a mortality rate of from 4 to 9%,[92,93] but several recent series of patients were operated upon without deaths.[93-96] The continent-ileostomy procedure now can be considered a safe operation when performed by experienced surgeons.

Early Postoperative Complications of the Continent Ileostomy

The immediate postoperative complications of the continent ileostomy are predictable from the nature of the procedure. The reports by Kock et al. and Goldman et al. give comprehensive reviews of the spectrum of these complications.[90,97] Intestinal obstruction, anastomotic leak, intra-abdominal bleeding, wound complications, ileostomy dysfunction, fistula, complications of the nipple valve (necrosis, fistula, prolapse, sliding, or obstruction), and reservoir dysfunction ("pouchitis") are the major postoperative problems.

Mechanical obstruction of the small intestine occurs in 2 to 6%.[94,97] It must be differentiated from obstruction at the nipple-valve either because of obturation (fecal plug) or kinking, slippage, or eversion of the nipple valve. The clinical presentation of these two problems usually allows a clear differentiation. Sudden difficulties with intubation of the stoma point towards valve dysfunction, and the absence of fecal material and flatus from the reservoir indicates a mechanical obstruction of the small bowel proximal to the reservoir. Abdominal radiographs allow a clear distinction and further corroborate the clinical impression by demonstrating absence of the familiar reservoir bubble or the presence of air-fluid levels in the proximal small bowel.

Anastomotic leakage with localized or diffuse peritonitis is the most serious complication and can be expected occasionally because of the lengthy suture lines. Specifically, the area between the anterior suture line of the pouch and the intussuscepting valve, a zone where the blood supply may be compromised, constitutes a site of predilection for leak. The reported incidence of leakage ranges from 3 to 8.8%.[90,97] Once the clinical diagnosis is made, prompt surgical intervention is necessary, usually requiring the removal of the reservoir and the establishment of a conventional ileostomy. A localized perforation with abscess may be approached by open or percutaneous drainage of the abscess and does not necessarily require reservoir. The enterocutaneous fistula that will probably develop may close after prolonged catheter drainage of the reservoir aided by "bowel rest" and TPN.

Intra-abdominal bleeding requiring reoperation, wound infection, or intra-abdominal abscess are complications that may occur after any intestinal operation; their treatments follow established principles modified by the individual circumstances. Not unexpectedly, reoperations required for nipple valve dysfunction have a high incidence of these problems.[94]

Necrosis of the nipple valve has been reported with greater frequency as maneuvers are employed to achieve a stronger lasting bonding between the two sleeves of the intussuscepting bowel. Methods currently in use to achieve the adherence include mesenteric stripping with stapling or through and through sutures of the nipple valve, the mesenteric rotation procedure, and stapling of the valve with placement of Marlex mesh or a fascial sling between the two serosal surfaces. Although these techniques achieve a secure valve, they may compromise the blood supply to the nipple, and cause total or partial sloughing or fistulas.[90,94,95] The degree of necrosis dictates the extent and timing of the operative intervention. If the necrosis is confined to the nipple within the reservoir, an expectant attitude may be taken and reconstruction of the fibrosed, stenotic, and now incontinent ileostomy may be undertaken at a later date.

Late Postoperative Complications of Continent Ileostomy

Two major problems may occur at varied times following the operative procedure: nipple valve dysfunction, leading to incontinence, and reservoir dysfunction ("pouchitis").

Spontaneous reduction (prolapse, sliding) of the nipple valve has been the most common late complication reported from all centers. Usually this occurs during the first year after construction of the valve. Patients troubled by a malfunctioning valve complain of increasing difficulties with intubation of the stoma that can lead to acute fecal retention, or complete or intermittent incontinence. Reduction of the prolapse and prolonged intubation may be successful in some instances but, most often, operative reconstruction is required. The incidence of nipple valve dysfunction ranges from 2.8 to 22%, and it varies with the techniques used to construct the valve.[88-90] Overall, a continence rate of 80 to 95% is reported.[98] Although various surgeons advocate their particular method of nipple valve construction, long-term evaluation of any of the methods is still lacking. A standard technique to achieve a strong union between the two serosal surfaces of the nipple valve and, thus, prevent eversion without complications has not yet evolved to the satisfaction of all clinicians.

Patients with a malfunctioning nipple valve should be examined by retrograde contrast radiography of the stoma. This will usually disclose a tortuous outflow tract with leakage of the contrast material to the outside. If decompression of the reservoir proves unsuccessful, repair of the existing malfunctioning valve is necessary. Frequently the valve must be excised, the pouch rotated, and a new valve constructed from the inflow tract, as suggested by Goligher.[95]

Late fistulas result from unsuspected Crohn's disease or erosion, caused either by the Marlex sling, the through and through sutures, or the staples of the nipple valve. Radiographs and endoscopic examination will verify the suspected fistula. In these circumstances, revisional surgical treatment, which amounts to construction of a new nipple valve, is required.

Ileostomy stricture at the skin level is uncommon if a disk of skin is excised and care is taken to make the stoma flush with the skin rather than beneath the skin level. Stenosis of the stoma is easily corrected by local revision at the skin level.

The patient with a continent ileostomy is heir to several potential complications caused by altered intestinal physiology (see also Chapter 31). These complications are not the result of faulty operative technique, but rather are changes inherent in the continent ileostomy and reservoir. Normal intestinal physiology in a patient with a continent ileostomy is altered. The colon is absent so that the patient is exposed to all of the complications of fluid and mineral loss of any colectomized patient. In addition, the ileal reservoir harbors large volumes of fecal material; a state of fecal stasis exists that results in increased bacterial colonization in the ileal reservoir.[99,100] Several studies report bacterial counts in the pouch effluent similar to those normally found in the stool.[101,102] This "colonic" flora is constantly in contact with the ileal mucosa of the pouch and may produce morphologic mucosal abnormalities such as villous blunting, reversion to a colonic pattern, and increased cell turnover.

Ileostomy diarrhea and malabsorption have been reported in 30% of the patients studied at the Mayo Clinic.[103] Kock et al. report a 17% incidence of single or repeated episodes of nonspecific ileitis responsive to antimicrobial therapy.[90] It is accepted that "pouchitis" is an almost inescapable episodic complication of the continent ileostomy. Because the patient with the continent ileostomy has an almost normal life expectancy, the occurrence of these episodes can not be ignored, although their long-term significance is still uncertain. Investigating the underlying cause of ileostomy diarrhea and malabsorption, Kelly et al. noted that malabsorption was more common in patients with stomal outputs in excess of 1000g /24 hours than in patients with less effluent.[104] Again, increased fecal output and malabsorption may be the result of an increased number of bacteria in these patients' intestinal effluent. Although Kelly et al. found no difference in the quantitative cultures of effluents between patients with well-functioning continent ileostomies and those who had inflammation and diarrhea,[102] others noted a significant difference.[101,105,106] The bacterial cause of this complication is further supported by the fact that reservoir inflammation and its clinical sequelae of ileostomy diarrhea and abdominal pain are almost always corrected by a course of antimicrobial therapy.

These physiologic alterations have clinical implications. When the function of an ileal pouch is abnormal, evidence of mechanical failure of the nipple valve should be sought by endoscopic and radiographic studies. A mechanical complication will require operative correction. Most often, however, signs of mucosal inflammation are found only by endoscopy: mucosal erythema, contact bleeding, pinpoint erosions, and occasionally ulcerations. Although histology is not a reliable guide to the origin of inflammation, biopsy material should be obtained to rule out Crohn's disease. Taking a fecal culture is advisable to exclude specific pathogens, but the identification of a specific fecal pathogen is unlikely. Empiric treatment with antimicrobials is then advocated.

If one antibiotic should fail, another may succeed, and some patients will require repeated courses of antibiotics. The use of metronidazole has been most successful in these instances.

From the accumulated experience of many surgeons, particularly Kock,[90] it is now evident that the incidence of both the early and late complications associated with the continent ileostomy can be decreased to an acceptable level. Because of the complexity of the procedure and the demanding postoperative management, however, the continent ileostomy operation should be performed only by surgeons familiar with the procedure. Because of the long-term changes within the continent reservoir and the uncertainty as to their eventual physiologic effects, the patient with a continent ileostomy and his surgeon must accept the necessity for indefinite observation.

Ileostomy Prolapse

Today, this is a rare complication of conventional ileostomy. Warren has, however, reported prolapse occurring in 13% of his patients.[69] Prolapse may be uniformly prevented by the secure anchoring of the mesentery of the bowel to the transverse layer of the abdominal wall by nonabsorbable suture material adjacent to the internal abdominal wall defect. Sutures that include the serosal surface of the bowel should be avoided, because these do not prevent the sliding hernia and may cause fistulas. Construction of an ileostomy without anchoring the small bowel mesentery will often result in evisceration of the ileostomy in the immediate postoperative period.

Incarcerated prolapse is an indication for urgent operation, release or resection of the prolapsed portion of bowel, and reconstruction of a proper ileostomy.

Paraileostomy Hernia

A prolapsed ileostomy may present as an interstitial hernia with protrusion of ileal tissue into the subcutaneous layers of the abdominal wall. A paraileostomy hernia is diagnosed by the presence of obstructive symptoms and palpation of the defect and sac through the stoma. Revision of the ileostomy with excision of the sliding sac and lateral repair of the abdominal defect is usually the treatment of choice. Other options exist, however, depending on the size of the hernia, the condition of the abdominal wall and the presence of contamination accompanying ileal fistulas. Goligher recommends relocation of the ileostomy to the opposite abdominal site, with closure of the original defect.[74] Sugarbaker advocates repair of the fascial defect in large parastomal hernias, using Marlex mesh.[75] This prosthetic repair is best used in noncontaminated situations.[75] Internal hernias in the lateral space following ileostomy will usually be manifested by intestinal obstruction.

Ileostomy Fistulas

Ileocutaneous fistulas are a relatively common problem that may necessitate ileostomy revision and/or relocation. Fistulas are caused by: (1) damage to the ileum at the time of operation; (2) an ill-fitting appliance and mechanical irritation of the ileum; (3) self-manipulation of the stoma; (4) chronic and continued compromise of the ileostomy by such entities as a tight fascial ring; and (5) the occurrence of stomal or prestomal ileal inflammatory disease.

If the ileostomy fistula occurs above the level of the skin, the output will be diverted from the orifice without causing serious local sepsis. If, however, the fistula is at skin level or below, abscess and wound infection invariably will result. This will necessitate drainage of the abscess and fistula and revision of the ileostomy. If the right lower abdominal wall is massively involved by an inflammatory process, relocation of the ileostomy to another site will become necessary. When possible, however, relocation should be avoided, because left-sided ileostomies can be troublesome because of inadequate length and the inability to close the lateral space.

Prestomal or Stomal Ileitis

Ileitis appearing at or near the stoma may occur because of a number of factors: (1) persistence or recrudescence of Crohn's disease in the small bowel;[76] (2) the rare prestomal ileitis that mimics histologically the pre-existing colon lesion, but is separate from it both geographically and temporally;[77] (3) the so-called backwash ileitis reported by Warren[69] and others.[77-79]

Although granulomatous disease of the colon is only associated infrequently with recrudescence of the disease in the small bowel, this does occur, and its presence in the patient with a stoma may require resection on its own merits. This may entail revision of the ileostomy.

Adson, et al. reported a form of prestomal ileitis mimicking the histopathology of the resected colon.[77] In several of his cases it was impossible to rule out simple obstruction as the cause of the nonspecific ileitis. In these instances, revision with resection was adequate for cure.

Although "backwash" ileitis is frequently mentioned as a cause of stomal ileitis, in our experience it is a rare or nonexistent lesion. The so-called backwash ileitis is usually nonspecific in nature and is most likely an inflammation associated in ulcerative colitis with the propinquity of the small bowel to the involved colon. It is usually a radiographic and not a clinical or specific histologic diagnosis. The fear of this lesion should not lead the surgeon routinely to resect the last few inches of ileum. Empiric resections of this type rob the patient of valuable reabsorptive water surface and may result in a copious ileostomy output.

Dermatitis*

Selection of the site of the ileostomy, proper protection of the skin, and the fitting of an appropriate appliance will routinely protect the patient from paraileostomy dermatitis. For detailed accounts of methods of mechanical skin protection by adherents or protective devices, see the numerous medical articles on the subject,[80-83] as well as bulletins and manuals of the United Ostomy Association.[84] It is sufficient to state that once established, most paraileostomy dermatitis can be corrected by protection of the skin with a Karaya gum or similar substance, the use of a liquid latex adherent and a properly fitting appliance. Consultation with ileostomy clubs and the cooperation of an enterostomal therapist is invaluable in the treatment of this and many other bothersome problems associated with ileostomy.

The Future for the Patient with an Ileostomy

Generally, the outlook for the patient after a proctocolectomy and ileostomy is excellent and the surgeon can be optimistic. Patients with an ileostomy can engage in all types of physical activity and professions, with no restriction on sexual activity or child bearing. The ileostomy patient may look forward to a life expectancy the same as an individual without colitis of the same age and sex, although metabolic and mechanical complications can and do occur (see also Chap. 31).[85]

Complications of the Ileoanal Anastomosis Procedures†

The operative procedure, commonly referred to as ileoanal anastomosis or restorative proctocoletomy, involves an abdominal colectomy, endorectal mucosal excision, and endorectal pull-through of the ileal reservoir or ileum with ileoanal anastomosis. This technique has evolved as a curative operation and a valid alternative to the conventional ileostomy for nearly all patients with chronic ulcerative colitis and familial polyposis, excluding those with malignant involvement of the rectum and with sphincteric destruction. Patients with perineal sepsis and those requiring an emergency colectomy can undergo an abdominal colectomy with creation of a Hartmann's closure or mucous fistula and end-ileostomy and still be eligible for an ileoanal anastomosis at a later time.

The major premise of the ileoanal anastomosis procedure is to "cure" the underlying mucosal disease, which it does, and to maintain anorectal continence. The latter does not occur instantly, but is attained eventually in most patients. The eventual outcome in terms of defecatory frequency, continence, and ability to evacuate spontaneously is influenced by whether a reservoir is used, by the type of reservoir employed, and by its proximity to the anal anastomosis. Mucosal proctectomy with preservation of the sphincter and direct (without reservoir) ileoanal anastomosis results in removal of all diseased tissue, but function is often unsatisfactory. The mean frequency of defecation has been reported to be approximately 7 to 8 times every 24 hours, including night evacuation in almost all patients without a reservoir.[107,108] The addition of an ileal reservoir has alleviated defecatory frequency; comparison of patients with proctocolectomy and ileoanal anastomosis with or without a reservoir have demonstrated the superiority of the reservoir.[109] The necessity to employ a proximal ileal reservoir, however, has not been universally accepted. For the pediatric or adolescent patient, a complementary ileal reservoir may not be required because the terminal ileum of the young patient (thought to possess a higher compliance rate than in adults) may dilate within several months and allow eventually for reservoir-like continence.[110] Although the need for a reservoir has been generally accepted for the adult patient, the type of the reservoir and its size are still a matter of laboratory and clinical evaluation.

Two types of ileal pouch configuration have achieved clinical popularity. The "S"-shaped reservoir, first used by Parks et al., is constructed by side-to-side anastomosis of a triple loop of distal ileum in which an outflow tract remains for ileoanal anastomosis.[111] This reservoir is peristaltically inert,[112] and, if combined with a lengthy ileal outflow conduit, may lead to difficulty in spontaneous evacuation that then necessitates transanal catheterization.[113,114] This impairment of reservoir evacuation can be avoided or minimized by constructing a smaller reservoir than that suggested by Parks,[111] and by shortening the outflow tract.[115] A side-to-side anastomosis of two loops of terminal ileum forms the basic design for the "J"-pouch described by Utsonomiya,[116] and the lateral side-

---

*Editors' note: see also, Wilkins, T. D.: Gastroenterology, 93: 389, 1987.

†See also Chapter 29.

to-side pouches proposed by Fonkalsrud in 1981 and Schraut and Block in 1982.[117,118] The side-to-side reservoirs are less prone to fecal stasis, excessive reservoir dilatation, and fecal retention than the "S"-shaped reservoir.[119,120]

Irrespective of the type of reservoir used and despite the various methods to achieve the mucosal proctectomy, major differences in the overall rate of operative complications have not been experienced. The ileoanal anastomosis operation is a technically difficult and often lengthy procedure that requires expertise and knowledge of anorectal physiology and anatomy. Complications have become less frequent and continence has improved as experience with the ileoanal anastomosis procedure has increased.

Mortality

In experienced hands, total colectomy and ileoanal anastomosis is a safe operative procedure. A reported operative mortality of less than 1% compares favorably with other major abdominal operations. Nicholls reported on over 400 procedures with only 1 operative death.[121]

Morbidity

Morbidity after the ileoanal anastomosis procedure has been significant and is undoubtedly an expression of the extent and intricacy of this procedure. Septic complications, usually within the pelvis (0 to 27%), bowel obstruction (9 to 18%), recurrent episodes of pouchitis (6 to 27%), and complete failure requiring take-down of the ileoanal anastomosis with construction of an end-ileostomy (0 to 9%) are the most frequently reported postoperative problems.[115,121-126]

Like the continent ileostomy procedure, septic complications occurring usually in the pelvis and often associated with anastomotic leaks have been common (11 to 60%).[115] Spillage of rectal contents if a rent develops in the friable mucosal sleeve during the mucosal proctectomy, and the inevitable contamination that occurs during the lengthy construction of the reservoir may in part be the responsible factors. Careful dissection combined with meticulous hemostasis, shorter operative time, and copious irrigation of the pelvis and rectal muscular sleeve will decrease the incidence of septic complications, but are unlikely to prevent them completely. Lengthy anastomotic suture lines contribute to the sepsis rate by anastomotic leakage that has been encountered in up to 18% of reported cases.[127-129] Major pelvic sepsis and spreading peritonitis are readily recognized and require prompt surgical intervention with removal of the ileoanal anastomosis and construction of an end-ileostomy.

A complication peculiar to the ileoanal anastomosis procedure is the development of a cuff abscess, that is, an abscess developing between the rectal muscular cuff and the ileum or ileal reservoir (Fig. 30-4). Copious irrigation before the pull-through and placement of a soft drain between the mucosal sleeve and the ileal reservoir are recommended to reduce the incidence of this problem. If a pelvic abscess occurs, it may be treated by simple drainage either transanally or presacrally for low lying abscesses or transabdominally for higher or more extensive collections. Because every patient with an ileoanal anastomosis procedure has a proximal diverting ileostomy, a low-output fecal fistula can be expected. Although the septic focus can be cleared in some of these patients without resorting to takedown of the ileoanal anastomosis and construction of an end-ileostomy, failure of local drainage will require the more aggressive approach.

Anastomotic strictures at the anal anastomosis develop frequently. According to the Mayo Clinic, they occur in 13.6% of patients.[130] If accompanied by induration and perirectal tenderness, closure of the loop ileostomy should be postponed until the inflammation has subsided and fibrosis is complete. Repeated dilatation of the web-like stricture will almost invariably alleviate the problem. Impairment of continence has not been a reported sequel to anastomotic strictures.

Small-bowel obstruction after ileoanal anastomosis is the second most common complication, with an incidence reportedly as high as 18%.[115] The extensive mesenteric mobilization, often combined with transverse incision of the mesenteric peritoneum to gain adequate mesenteric length for a tension-free pull-through, is a likely cause for this complication. A trial of suction and intravenous fluid replacement will often be successful in the early postoperative period. Enterolysis is necessary for complete or unremitting obstructions. Partial obstruction associated with stomal edema will usually resolve spontaneously.

Impairment of genitourinary function is a rare occurrence after the ileoanal anastomosis procedure. Impotence in the male has not been reported, although temporary retrograde ejaculation has been encountered in 9% of the patients.[130]

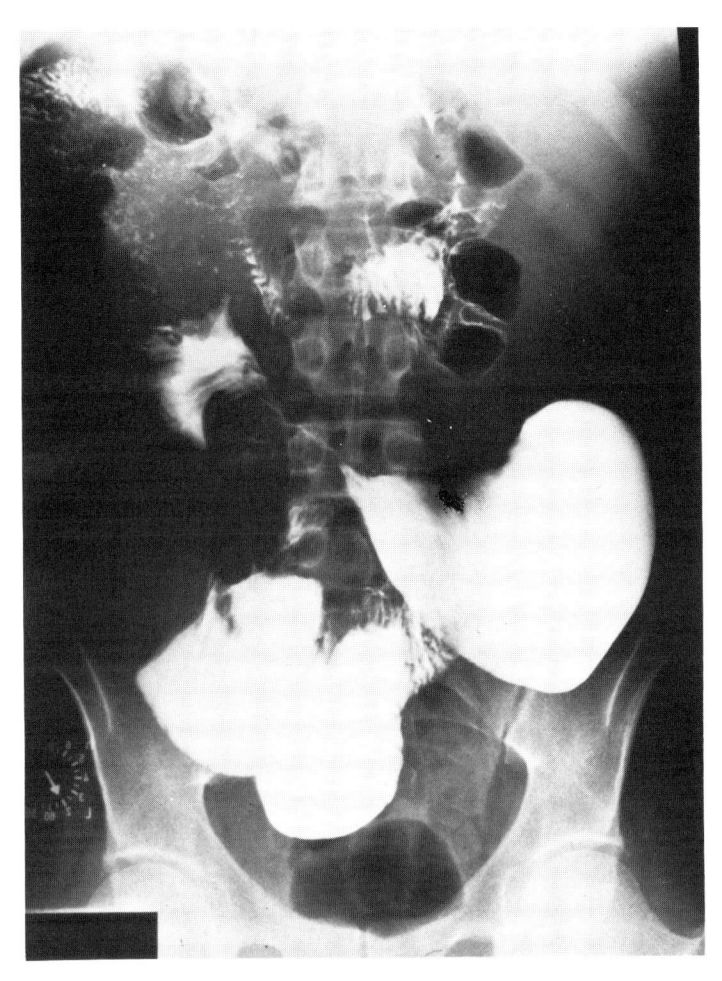

FIG. 30-4. The "chain-of-lakes" deformity demonstrated in this patient with multiple strictures from jejunal-ileal Crohn's disease resulted in symptoms of cramping and obstruction. A combination of bypass and open dilatation of strictures was successful in obtaining complete relief of symptoms.

Clinical Results

The long-term results achieved with the ileoanal anastomosis (with or without complementary reservoir) depend on physiologic (ileal or reservoir compliance and peristaltic patterns) and anatomic (reservoir design and anal proximity) factors. A successful outcome can be expected if a compliant ileum or ileal reservoir, which is capable of generating propulsive peristalsis on complete distention, is placed directly or in close proximity to the anus. It must be understood that an ileoanal anastomosis can only approximate the normal physiology and function of the anorectum. Nevertheless, this procedure provides eventual anal continence in over 90% of the patients treated.[115] The period of adaptation, which may range from weeks to months, appears to be shorter in children and adolescents, who regain total continence, particularly nighttime continence, sooner than adults.

Prolonged, and sometimes persistent, diarrhea and defecatory frequency are noted in patients with direct ileoanal anastomoses.[107,108,110] With time, however, defecatory frequency appears to abate. The physiologic basis underlying this improvement is thought to be in the development of a neoampulla, i.e., progressive ileal dilatation. The time and extent to which this develops vary from patient to patient.[131] Intermittent transanal balloon dilatation promotes the development of a neoampulla.[132]

The "S"-shaped reservoir alleviates diarrhea and frequency after the operative procedure rather rapidly. The further course, however, may be complicated by inability to evacuate spontaneously, thereby requiring transanal intubation and evacuation. Although these sequelae have been alleviated by shortening the outflow tract and constructing a smaller size reservoir, only long-term evaluation will determine if this problem has been corrected or is an inevitable sequel inherent to the "S"-shaped reservoir. The "J"-type and double-barreled reservoirs are free from this problem.[112] Within several months, the majority of the patients (98%) with these reservoirs attain normal daytime bowel habits and, somewhat later, nighttime continence as the reservoir enlarges.[130] With the passage of time, the need to administer antidiarrheal agents decreases.

Reservoir inflammation ("pouchitis") is similar in its reported frequency (6 to 27%), and in its presumed cause and treatment, to that encountered with the continent ileostomy.[112] The episodes of pouchitis (sudden onset of diarrhea with or without lower abdominal crampy pain) are easily controlled by antimicrobials, particularly metronidazole, indicating that bacterial (anaerobic) overgrowth is a major cause of the inflammation.

Intestinal Obstruction

Any abdominal operation may be complicated by intestinal obstruction. The risk is increased after operations for inflammatory bowel disease, especially after proctocolectomy and ileostomy. Complete small bowel obstruction occurred in 7.7% of the patients undergoing operation at St. Mark's Hospital (London, U.K.) between 1960 and 1964.[4] Obstruction as a cause of late death was second only to carcinoma in the series reported by Ritchie.[133]

The mechanical nature of the various operations for inflammatory bowel disease may predispose to adhesion formation and potentially creates spaces for internal herniae. Ellis contends that serosal defects closed under tension become ischemic, promote adhesion formation, and finally, bowel obstruction.[134] This phenomenon, coupled with the large peritoneal defects associated with excision of the rectum and construction of an ileostomy or colostomy, make the patient with inflammatory bowel disease a prime candidate for postoperative bowel obstruction.

Bowel obstruction in the postoperative period may be conveniently classified as follows:

1. Incomplete—early
   a. neurologic
   b. mechanical
2. Incomplete—late
   a. mechanical on the basis of adhesions
   b. mechanical-anastomotic recurrence of disease
3. Complete

In the immediate postoperative period some degree of paralytic ileus is always present. Overzealous attempts at feeding may result in a prolonged or recurrent ileus. These episodes are readily treated by gastric decompression and cessation of oral feedings. Similarly, incomplete mechanical obstruction appearing in the immediate postoperative period usually will resolve with continued intestinal decompression. Persistent high-grade partial mechanical obstruction requires operative intervention with lysis of adhesions and/or resection.

The bowel obstruction associated with recrudescence of Crohn's disease at or near a site of enterocolic anastomosis is usually partial and remitting, but progressive. This is a classic complication of the disease process and is an indication for reoperation. de Dombal comprehensively studied the results of surgical treatment of Crohn's disease and concluded that operations short of colectomy were subject to reoperation of some type in over one-third of patients.[27] Obstruction was the second most common complication necessitating reoperation in his series.

Complete mechanical small bowel obstruction in the postoperative patient is an urgent indication for operation. Ellison observed an improved survival and a lower rate of complications after prolonged intestinal intubation was abandoned in favor of resuscitation and early operation.[135] By following this program, the incidence of intestinal gangrene was only 10% and the overall mortality rate was 4%.

Mechanical obstruction in the patient with inflammatory bowel disease is usually caused by adhesions. Three potential hazards, however, are also particularly prominent in these patients: (1) lateral space hernias with incarceration at the site of the ileostomy or colostomy; (2) adhesions to the pelvic floor; and (3) herniation through the pelvic floor with entrapment. The treatment of these situations is facilitated by their early recognition followed by appropriate operation. The prevention of these serious complications may be aided by the secure closure of the lateral space. The parietal peritoneum is secured to the cut edge of the mesentery rather than to the serosa of a potentially diseased viscus.

The pelvic floor may be secured by a number of methods. To prevent postoperative adhesions, a closure under tension should be avoided. A tense closure is also prone to dehiscence and entrapment of bowel. If the pelvic peritoneum remaining at the termination of the procedure is inadequate for easy reapproximation, which is rare in operations for inflammatory bowel disease, the surgeon should leave the pelvis widely open and close the pelvic floor securely. If the perineal wound is also inadequate for closure, support can be achieved by packing the perineum and pelvis over a protecting sheet of Owens surgical material.* The Owens material is nonreactive, and satisfactory regrowth of the peritoneum can be anticipated in 1 week.

Multiple and/or Recurrent Strictures†

Multiple strictures of the small bowel, manifested by symptoms of partial obstruction and weight loss, are usually associated with the jejunoileal variety of Crohn's disease, but are occasionally encountered in patients whose disease is recrudescent after an ileocolic resection (Fig. 30-5). Resection is usually contraindicated for these patients because the strictures are often multiple and resection would result in a short gut. Bypass is rarely applicable to all of the strictured areas. We have adopted the suggestion made by Alexander-Williams and have successfully dilated these strictures in a number of patients, with gratifying results.[136] We have used strictureplasty as advocated by Alexander-Williams occasionally for short strictures in patients with relatively quiescent disease.[136] Alexander-Williams and Haynes reported a clinical leak in 7% of patients following strictureplasty, "painful episodes" in 9.3%, and wound infections in another 9.3%.[137] Our approach is to explore the entire small bowel and determine the extent and location of the strictures. The multiple strictures will often give a "chain of lakes" configuration to the bowel that is amenable to a combination of bypass, strictureplasty, and dilatation. For those areas to be dilated, we perform an enterotomy in "normal" bowel adjacent to the stricture and serially pass Hager dilators through the lumen of the strictured bowel, "fracturing" the fibrosis, until the lumen corresponds to that of the nonstrictured gut. The enterotomy is then closed in a standard fashion. We have had no complications from these maneuvers and the obstructive symptoms have abated for months and even years. Our series is too small for statistical analysis. Nevertheless, this maneuver appears to be at least an excellent palliative approach for a vexing surgical problem.

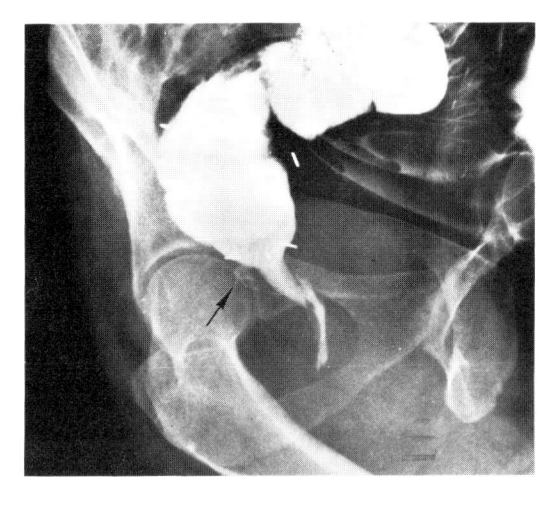

FIG. 30–5. Barium study of an ileoanal anastomosis with a J-type reservoir. The arrow indicates a small blind sinus tract extending from the anus into the rectal muscular cuff. The sinus tract cleared without an additional surgical intervention. The anastomotic stricture could be easily dilated. The patient is continent following closure of the loop ileostomy 5 months after the initial operation.

Malabsorption–Short Bowel Syndrome‡

Serial, massive, or injudicious resections of the small bowel for patients suffering from Crohn's disease may result in the complexities of intestinal malabsorption known as the "short bowel syndrome." The following are important factors influencing post resection absorption:

1. The extent and site of the small bowel resected
2. The presence of the ileocecal valve
3. The condition of the remaining bowel and related digestive organs
4. The adaptation of the remaining small bowel and stomach

The loss of adequate small bowel function results in protracted diarrhea and the malabsorption of essential nutrient substances.

Resections of up to one-half of the small bowel may be performed with safety, and, if the

---

*Davis & Geck, American Cyanamid Company, Pearl River, NY 10965.
†See also Chapter 27.
‡See also Chapter 31.

remaining small bowel is normal, little diarrhea and malabsorption will ensue. Survival is rare, however, if less than 2 feet of jejunum and ileum remains, although several patients have survived with only 6 to 18 inches of jejunum and an intact duodenum.[138] The average length in vivo of the human intestine is approximately 20 feet. Resection of from one-third to one-half of this may represent the upper limit of safety. When resections exceed this, particularly in the absence of the colon, absorption is markedly altered and poses significant management problems. In addition, the loss of a specialized function of the ileum can lead to vexing diarrhea and specific malabsorption even after seemingly "conservative" resections.

Although many substances are absorbed throughout the length of the small intestine, certain nutrients seem to be absorbed in one region more than others. Regional resection may result in malabsorption of these substances unless the remaining bowel can adapt. The proximal small intestine is the major site of absorption of iron, calcium, water soluble vitamins (except B_{12}), and fat (monoglycerides and fatty acids). Sugars are absorbed both in the jejunum and ileum. The major absorption of amino acids appears to occur in the jejunum, and the distal ileum is the site for absorption of bile salts and vitamin B_{12}. The colon is important for the absorption of water and electrolytes. Patients who have a colectomy superimposed on an extensive small bowel resection are difficult to manage.

Inadequate absorptive area and short transit time leads to incomplete digestion of carbohydrates, fats, and proteins, and efficient segmental absorption cannot occur. Loss of ileal function leads directly to malabsorption of bile salts and vitamin B_{12}. Subsequent diminution of the enterohepatic circulation of bile acids gives rise to inadequate micellar formation and contributes to malabsorption in the remaining jejunum. Consequently, severe steatorrhea is more prominent after ileal resection than jejunal loss.[139] The presence of fatty acids and bile acids in the colon seem to interfere with salt and water absorption, further promoting diarrhea.[140] This so-called "bile salt enteropathy" is often successfully treatable by oral cholestyramine, 8 to 12 g per day. This preparation binds unabsorbed bile acids to prevent their effect upon the colon. Loss of vitamin B_{12} will result in a megaloblastic anemia and combined system diseases. Steatorrhea and fat malabsorption cause loss of the fat soluble vitamins A, C, and K. Deficiencies in vitamin D and increased excretion of calcium and magnesium with fecal fat can lead to severe deficits in these minerals and serious neurologic and metabolic abnormalities.[141]

Therapy for patients with short bowel is directed at the replacement of fluid and electrolytes, adequate caloric intake, and supplementation of inadequately absorbed nutrients, vitamins, and minerals. Some degree of eventual intestinal adaptation can be expected, and malabsorption should improve. The capacity of the ileum to adapt is greater than that of the jejunum.[142]

Initially, we rely on total parenteral nutrition (TPN) during the immediate postoperative period until oral feedings can be resumed (see also Chap. 24). TPN can reverse the catabolic effects of operation and nutritionally support the patient while intestinal anastomoses are healing and the bowel is starting to adapt. Wilmore, Dudrick, and associates have demonstrated the beneficial effects of TPN on small intestinal adaption after massive resection.[143]

With the resolution of postoperative ileus, the remaining bowel's absorptive capacity can be more accurately assessed and oral intake resumed. At this point, treatment is based on overcoming specific absorptive defects so the patient may be weaned from TPN. Intestinal adaptation takes place over a variable period of time and may require months. The transition to oral feedings must be gradual. At first, feedings must be small and frequent. We use an elemental diet similar to that reported by Voidk et al.[144] Such diets demand no digestive effort by the compromised gut and need a minimal absorptive surface. Proteins are given as hydrolysates or amino acids, and fats are delivered as medium-chain triglycerides that are easily absorbed directly into the portal circulation and contribute minimally to steatorrhea. We limit the intake of these triglycerides to about 20 g per day. The major drawback of these diets is their unpalatability. Usually, they are delivered by way of a soft nasogastric feeding tube. In addition, these formulas are uniformly hyperosmolar. They must be diluted and the serum osmolarity must be monitored frequently. Attempts to control diarrhea with diphenoxylate or loperamide often fail, and usually paregoric or codeine are required, although the disadvantages of their use are obvious.

As the patient's condition improves, solid foods are given, slowly and in small quantities at first, while continuing the elemental diet. Feedings are frequent, aimed at supplying 20 to 25 kilocalories per pound of ideal body weight. Total caloric intake has to be greater, however, because many of the calories will be lost in the stool. Protein intake should supply at least 50 g per day and total fat intake should be kept as low as the patient will tolerate. Medium-chain triglycerides should continue to be given as a supplement. Fat soluble vitamins will continue to be lost with steatorrhea and must be supplemented along with calcium and magnesium. Malabsorption of water-soluble vitamins is usually not a problem, except of course for vitamin B_{12}, after ileal resection. This should be administered parenterally. Milk products should be avoided because these patients frequently cannot tolerate lactose and the diarrhea is worsened.[145]

Patients who survive and adjust to oral feedings strike a delicate balance between their disability and the rigorous treatment necessary to maintain life. They must be carefully followed and specific nutritional and metabolic derangements corrected as they occur. Recurrence of inflammatory bowel disease or unrelated illnesses may worsen already marginal bowel function. At the first sign of deterioration, the patient should be rehospitalized, and an elemental diet or parenteral alimentation resumed.

Many patients are now maintained at home for prolonged periods of time with TPN with either total or supplemental parenteral nutrition.[146] This mode of support is no longer experimental and affords a reasonable life and prolonged survival for patients with complete excision of the gut. The use of the Silastic, "long-term," cuffed catheters has replaced the PVC catheter for the chronic patient. The Silastic catheters are associated with a lower incidence of thrombosis than the PVC catheters and "catheter sepsis" is reduced. The use of the double-or triple-lumen catheter implying the manipulation of the catheter for purposes other than alimentation results in increased incidence of sepsis as compared to the single-lumen catheter. Thrombosis of the axillary veins or superior cava in patients requiring long-term TPN is a vexing problem. Transsternal atrial catheterization may be used. Recanalization of one or both axillary veins may allow for eventual reuse of these sites.[147,148] Lower extremity access has not been universally accepted, but has come into some use recently. It is fraught with all of the thrombotic and septic complications that are seen with the preferred subclavian approach.[148]

Urogenital Complications

Problems affecting the urogenital system in the postoperative period are either a direct result of operative trauma or of residual inflammatory disease, or are indirect sequelae of metabolic derangements coincident to ileostomy dysfunction.

By far, urinary and sexual problems occur most frequently after resection of the rectum.[149] One or both ureters may be injured, perineal-urinary fistulas may develop, urinary retention may occur, and the male patient may become impotent. Basically, all of these complications are associated with operative trauma or manipulation.

If ureteral injury has been sustained, diagnosis will usually be accomplished by excretory or retrograde pyelography. The level and the type of injury dictate the appropriate therapy. Most ureteral injuries occur at the upper level of the rectum immediately beneath the peritoneal reflection. In most instances, ureteroneocystostomy can eventually be established after adequate drainage or diversion of the urinary stream has allowed inflammation to subside. Occasionally, nephroureterectomy is necessary.

Bladder or urethral fistulas to the perineal wound will usually close spontaneously with long-term ureteral catheter drainage.[150] Occasionally, secondary closure supplemented by cystostomy may be warranted.

Persistent right-sided hydroureter occurring in Crohn's disease has been reported.[151] Ureterolysis of the involved ureter and appropriate drainage of the associated retroperitonitis uniformly leads to recovery.

Postoperative Urinary Bladder Dysfunction

Difficulty in bladder emptying has been reported following total proctocolectomy in up to 16% of patients, and male or female patients may suffer this complication.[149,150] If prolonged urethral drainage fails to result in spontaneous voiding, the patient should be investigated by excretory pyelography and cystometrogram.[150] Partial or complete motor-neuron paralysis is the usual cause of the dysfunction. In these patients, the pelvic autonomic nerves have probably been damaged at the sacral promontory or lateral and anterior to the rectum in the retrovesical and retrouterine spaces. To avoid this problem, dissection should be carried out close to the rectum and anterior to the endopelvic fascia. Decompensated or atonic bladders in either sex are often rehabilitated by a program of cholinergic stimulation. Therapy is administered by 7.5 to 10.0 mg Urecholine* every 4 hours subcutaneously for 24 hours. When the residual urine is less than 30 ml on each of 3 consecutive days, the urecholine may be tapered gradually to an oral dose of urecholine or mycholine chloride† every 4 to 6 hours, depending upon the state of micturition.

If endoscopy reveals vesical-neck contracture or obstructing prostatic hypertrophy, correction of these lesions is best performed several weeks after coloproctectomy. Transurethral resection of the obstruction is the procedure of choice. This condition is usually seen in male patients, but occasionally females are similarly affected by urethral stricture.[150]

Sexual Dysfunction

Although sexual dysfunction following adequate abdominoperineal resection for cancer may be considered to be a "necessary" consequence of an adequate cancer operation, it is distressing and unnecessary to render the young male with inflammatory bowel disease impotent.

Watts reported 11 of 41 males with some impairment of sexual function following proctectomy.[152] This was related to age. Only 5 of 33 men younger than 50 reported any postoperative sexual dysfunction. Of these, two experienced permanent failure of ejaculation, two suffered temporary impotence, and one patient was permanently impotent.

In Watts' series, only an occasional female patient suffered sexual dysfunction. Here the dysfunction was associated with other conditions, including perineal fistula, vaginal stenosis, and emotional instability.

Bauer et al. reported on 291 patients undergoing proctectomy.[153] Of 135 males, four (3%) had a permanent deficit in sexual function. Only 2 of 156 females complained of any physical sexual dysfunction. Both of these patients suffered temporary dyspareunia. Bauer and colleagues also discuss the anatomy and physiology of the pelvic autonomic nervous system, and detail the technical features that avoid injury to these structures during proctectomy.[153]

Sexual function in the male is under the control of the autonomic pelvic plexus, and avoidance of injury to these delicate structures is the only preventative for postoperative sexual dysfunction. The second, third, and fourth sacral nerves give rise to the nervi erigenti, course through the inferior hypogastric plexus, and fan out to the pelvic viscera. Sympathetic fibers reach the inferior hypogastric plexus by way of the presacral nerves and travel with parasympathetic fibers to their end organs. Damage to these structures usually occurs at the superior hypogastric plexus. This plexus is of variable size and is separated from the great vessels of the pelvis by the strong endopelvic fascia. The pelvic viscera lie medially, separated from the plexus by loose areolar tissue. These nerves can be avoided by dividing the mesentery as close to the bowel as possible at the sigmoid colon and rectum, and by preserving a generous portion of pelvic peritoneum.[154–156]

If impotency in the young male is persistent after 3 months, the operative insertion of various devices will afford erection.[157] This allows him to engage in intercourse but will, of course, not enable him to ejaculate. Occasionally, dissection in the region of the seminal vesicles will result in retrograde ejaculation, and no specific therapy is available for this condition.

Ureteronephrolithiasis

Deren has studied stone disease in 271 patients suffering from inflammatory bowel disease.[158] Of these, 2.1% had stone disease. From 7 to 13% of patients with ileostomies eventually develop urinary stones. Deren found calcium stones, uric acid stones, as well as "unclassified" varieties. Previous steroid therapy, urinary tract infection, hyperuricemia, hypokalemic alkalosis, and consistently acidic urine have been implicated in the genesis of these stones.[158]

Excessive ileostomy loss with concomitant, decreased urinary volume appears to be an attractive thesis for the genesis of such stones.[159] Also implicated in an occasional patient is excessive bile salt loss and the associated derangement of calcium metabolism. In spite of this long list of causative factors, the most conspicuous alteration is the relative oliguria and persistently acidic urine in stone-forming patients. The diminished urine output is prominent in the formation of all other stones, but the persistently acidic reaction of the urine appears to account for the high incidence of uric acid stones.

Maintenance of an adequate urinary output, correction of electrolyte depletion, alkaliniza-

---

*Bethanechol Chloride, Merck, Sharp and Dohme, West Point, PA.

†Bethanechol Chloride, Glenwood Laboratories, Tenafly, NJ.

tion of urine, treatment of infection, and the use of xanthine inhibitors in patients with hyperuricemia are the appropriate measures for the prevention of recurrent stone disease.

Neurologic Complications

The central nervous system complications associated with the administration of steroids, with septicemia, or shock may occasionally be observed in the patient suffering inflammatory bowel disease. These complications are, however, not specific to inflammatory bowel disease. Postoperative seizures are sometimes seen, particularly in young patients suffering from inflammatory bowel disease, and steroid administration, fluid retention, and arterial hypertension are common to these patients.[160]

Peripheral neuropathies involving the branches of the sciatic nerve are commonly observed, in varying severity, in those individuals who have undergone total proctocolectomy in the lithotomy position. These neuropathies are a direct result of pressure trauma to the peripheral nerves coincident to the position of the patient.[161]

Some modification of the lithotomy position is used in most procedures in which there is a perineal dissection of the rectum. Those positions that use support or tension at the knee are prone to injure the common peroneal (external popliteal) nerve as it courses laterally to the head of the fibula. The injuries are usually transient and may involve either the superficial (musculocutaneous) or deep peroneal (anterior tibial) components of the nerve.[29] Although transient, peroneal nerve injuries may persist for up to 6 months after injury. Prevention of these injuries is achieved by scrupulous attention to positioning and padding of the patient. We use at least two thicknesses of a bath towel and blanket between the head of the fibula and any possible pressure area.

Those positions that involve extension of the leg may inadvertently cause stretching injuries to the tibial and/or peroneal nerves by hyperextension and pressure on the tibial plateau. At least 10 to 15 degrees of flexion should be maintained at the patient's knees at all times to avoid these complications.

We have encountered three patients with partial or complete femoral nerve palsy following resection of ileum from which a sinus tract had penetrated the substance of the right psoas muscle with a resultant chronic psoas abscess. Whether the inflammatory process itself or the manipulation of the muscle mass coincident to resection and evacuation of the chronic abscess cavity was the cause of the palsy is unclear. In all of the patients, the weakness was temporary and all had full return of function.

Hepatitis*

The colitic patient is at risk both for clinical hepatitis and for infection of his attendant personnel because of his increased exposure to transfusion of blood and blood products. Multiple blood transfusions for the colitic patient are more the rule than the exception and these patients must be considered at risk for hepatitis. Long-term corticosteroid administration may contribute to incubation of a viral hepatitis without clinical demonstration of the disease.[162]

Post-surgical Recurrence, Morbidity, and Mortality

After listing the depressing litany of the minor complications and major catastrophes to which the inflammatory bowel disease patient is heir after operation, it is appropriate to summarize the general postoperative fate of the colitic patient (see Table 30-1).

Prohaska concluded that approximately one-half of those undergoing operation for inflammatory bowel disease have ulcerative colitis, 7% harbor granulomatous colitis, and the remainder display variable sites of Crohn's enterocolitis.[163] Approximately one-quarter of the colitic population will require colectomy in any given year. To assess the efficacy and limitations of operative therapy, the colitic population can be evaluated as a whole, according to the histologic character of the disease, or by the operative therapy applied.[164]

Ritchie studied 453 patients who underwent excisional therapy for either ulcerative and Crohn's colitis in one geographic area of England between the years 1955 and 1966.[7] She concluded that various factors are operative in the mortality rate. Advancing age adversely affected the mortality rate: for those patients under 50 years of age, the mortality rate was 11%; operations in patients over 50 years of age were associated with a mortality rate of 25%. The severity of the disease and the preoperative clinical state of the patient were also factors in the outcome. The necessity for emergency operation and the existence of conditions such as toxic megacolon

*See also Chapter 27.

that dictated urgent operation adversely affected mortality. She reported, however, that with each passing year the mortality rate improved so that the rate fell from 17.2% at the beginning of the series to 10.8% at its termination. Over half of the patients suffered complications of some degree of severity, and 34.5% of the patients at risk required readmission to the hospital.

Ulcerative Colitis

In a subsequent publication, Ritchie reported on a 15-year experience with ulcerative colitis treated by operation at St. Mark's Hospital.[4] Of 117 cases, 21 experienced major complications and 37 were recorded as experiencing minor complications. In this group of patients, age, urgency of operation, and clinical status were predictably operative in a successful or nonsuccessful outcome. Of special interest is Ritchie's observation, when combining several reported series of patients with ulcerative colitis, that the life expectancy of the patients, in the absence of malignant change, is normal after 1 year has elapsed following colectomy.

Survival after total proctocolectomy for colorectal carcinoma in ulcerative colitis[165] was reported to be as low as 6% by Dennis,[166] but only 3 of Prohaska's 7 patients survived 5 years. Of Bargen's 101 patients, 32% survived.[167]

Ileorectal anastomosis for chronic ulcerative colitis has been advocated by Aylett who reported 183 successes in 213 attempts.[168] Prohaska reported eventual failure of the procedure in all of his patients, however.[171] Although 17 of Adson's carefully selected 24 patients had a satisfactory result with ileorectal anastomosis,[169] Adson cautions that the younger patients are, however, usually candidates for proctectomy.

The popularity and widespread use of the various sphincter-saving operations for ulcerative colitis have added a new dimension to the analysis of quality of life for the colitic patient following operation (see also Chap. 29). Oakley et al. reported on 145 patients from the Cleveland Clinic with an ileorectal anastomosis;[170] this group represented 26% of the patients operated upon for ulcerative colitis. Oakley and colleagues concluded that the operation is safe and that the functional results are good for a majority of the patients; however, they noted that a cancer risk still exists and that regular surveillance is mandatory. Sexual dysfunction is avoided by this procedure and it still allows for some other type of continence-preserving operation at a later date.

At the Mayo Clinic in Rochester, Minnesota, Stryker et al. studied 20 patients with ileal pouch-anal anastomoses and compared them to 12 healthy volunteers.[171] They concluded that 85 to 90% of their patients had a satisfactory outcome up to 35 months after endorectal ileoanal anastomoses.

Crohn's Disease

Any assessment of operative therapy for Crohn's disease must be made with the realization that the geographic extent of the disease in the large bowel will dictate the operative procedure (see also Chap. 27), the dangers encountered, and, ultimately, the recurrence rate. de Dombal, Burton, and Goligher reported on 295 patients undergoing 415 operative procedures for Crohn's disease.[27] The operative mortality rate was 4.1% for primary operation, 8.2% for reoperation, and 5.2% overall. The overall late mortality rate was 13%; 7% were directly related to Crohn's disease. The reoperation rate varied considerably after different primary operations; the lowest rate was for proctocolectomy and the highest followed bypass operations and ileorectal anastomoses.

Patients whose disease is primarily restricted to the large bowel have a slightly higher mortality rate than those whose disease is confined to the foregut.

The increased risk of carcinoma of the colon in Crohn's disease has been established (see also Chap. 15).[172] Greenstein and coworkers noted that such cancers in patients with Crohn's disease are prone to occur in segments of bowel that have been bypassed or defunctionalized.[173] Whether this is a reflection of the bypass per se or chronicity is not clear. The prognosis for patients with "Crohn's carcinoma" is poor, probably because the malignant lesions are discovered late in their course.[173]

The surgeon who elects a bypass operation for Crohn's disease must also accept the fact that partial diversion of the fecal stream does not cure Crohn's disease and the bypassed segments of bowel may become the sites of enteric fistulas, perforations, hemorrhage[174] or carcinoma.

Korelitz et al.[175] have reported that 46% of their patients with Crohn's disease of the colon treated by proctocolectomy and ileostomy subsequently developed evidence of recrudescent regional enteritis.[175] This is in contrast to a report from the Beth Israel Hospital of Boston indicating that gross disease occurring in the small bowel after proctocolectomy for granulomatous colitis is rare.[176] Our experience has paralleled de Dombal's;[177] recurrences in such situations are seen, but are infrequent, occurring in only 5 to 10% of the operated population. Crohn's disease of the small bowel observed at the time of colectomy is frequently associated with recurrence in the neoileum.[178]

As a general statement, the prognosis in terms of recurrence in Crohn's colitis can be directly correlated with the length of the bowel segments involved and the existence of rectal fistulas.

Baker states that ileorectal anastomoses for Crohn's disease has a lower operative mortality than the same operation performed for ulcerative colitis.[179] The long-term prognosis is worse, however, because of recrudescent disease and serious inflammatory anal lesions. Burman, Cooke, and Williams reported that 32% of their patients with ileorectal anastomoses developed nonfatal anastomotic leaks.[180] Their overall recurrence rate was 60%. This was not influenced by age, duration of the disease or steroid therapy. Recrudescence was directly related to the presence of concurrent small-bowel disease and by residual rectal disease at the site of anastomosis.

TABLE 30-1. *Incidences of Major Complications of Surgical Treatment; Data Derived From Representative Series of Patients with Inflammatory Bowel Disease.*

Nature of the Complication	Ritchie[4] (1972)	Ritchie[7] (1971)	Watts, et al.[65] (1966)	de Dombal, et al.[27] (1971)
Abdominal wound				
Infection	2.2%	3.8%		
Disruption			4.6%	3.4%
Hernia	0.4%	1.3%		
Peritonitis and postoperative sepsis	7 deaths per 226 patients	17 deaths per 453 patients	33.3% resulting in 6 deaths per 151 patients	3.9%
Persistent perineal wound	7.1%	40.0%	24.7%	42.6%
Ileostomy				All types—30% (usually dermatitis)
Dysfunction			2.0%	
Prolapse		1.6%	2.5%	
Paraileostomy hernia		0.8%	2.5%	
Fistulas		0.5%	0.8%	
Dermatitis	0.9%	3.1%	25.0%	
Required reconstruction for any reason	3.5%	10.8%	11.6%	
Intestinal obstruction				
Complete	8.9%	7.8%	Total 8.4%	Total 8.4%
Incomplete	6.2%	7.0%		
Urogenital				
Sexual dysfunction			1.7% of males	
Stones	2.7%			1.7%

Block and Schraut 1972–1982

Infection	6%
Disruption	0
Hernia	1.3%
Anastomotic leak	2.2%
Abscess	4%
Obstruction	9%
Death	0.4%

*231 patients undergoing ileocolectomy for Crohn's ileocolitis

Operations for inflammatory bowel disease are attended by numerous complications; some of which may be serious or fatal. The patient suffering inflammatory bowel disease is often far from an ideal candidate for operation. In general, the operations are not truly elective—most are either urgent or emergent. A knowledge of the hazards involved in the operative treatment of these patients will, it is hoped, contribute to a lessening of the complications and deaths, and improve the ability of the surgeon to safely treat his patient.

References

1. Griffen, W. O., Jr., and Jewell, W. R.: The colon. *In* Operative Surgery: Principles and Techniques. Edited by P. F. Nora. Philadelphia, Lea & Febiger, 1972.
2. Singleton, A. O., and Blocker, T. G.: The problem of disruption of abdominal wounds and postoperative hernia. J. Am. Med. Assoc., *112*:122, 1939.
3. Rees, V. L., and Coller, F. A.: Anatomic and clinical study of the transverse abdominal incision. Arch. Surg., *47*:136, 1943.
4. Ritchie, J. K.: Ulcerative colitis treated by ileostomy and excisional surgery: Fifteen years' experience at St. Mark's Hospital. Br. J. Surg., *59*:345, 1972.
5. Barker, K., et al.: The relative significance of preoperative oral antibiotics, mechanical bowel preparation and preoperative peritoneal contamination in the avoidance of sepsis after radical surgery for ulcerative colitis and Crohn's disease of the large bowel. Br. J. Surg., *58*:270, 1971.
6. Cole, W. R., and Bernard, H. R.: Origin of abdominal wound contaminants. J. Int. Coll. Surg., *40*:1, 1963.
7. Ritchie, J. K.: Ileostomy and excisional surgery for chronic inflammatory disease of the colon: A survey of one hospital region. Gut, *12*:528, 1971.
8. Maingot, R.: Abdominal Operations. 5th Ed. New York, Appleton Century Crofts, 1969.
9. Polk, H. C., and Lopez-Mayor, J. F.: Postoperative wound infection: A prospective study of determinant factors and prevention. Surgery, *66*:97, 1969.
10. Moylan, J. A., and Brockenbrough, E. C.: Antibiotic wound irrigation in the prevention of surgical wound infection. Surg. Forum, *19*:66, 1968.
11. Coller, F. A., and Valk, W. L.: The delayed closure of contaminated wounds. Ann. Surg., *112*:256, 1940.
12. Todd, J. C.: Wound infection: Etiology, prevention and management. Surg. Clin. North Am., *48*:787, 1968.
13. Nichols, R. L., and Condon, R. E.: Preoperative preparation of the colon. Surg. Gynecol. Obstet., *132*:323, 1971.
14. Altemeier, W. A., Hummel, R. P., and Hill, E. O.: Staphylococcal enterocolitis following antibiotic therapy. Ann. Surg., *157*:847, 1963.
15. Lewis, R. T., et al.: Antibiotics in surgery of the colon. Can. J. Surg., *21*:339, 1978.
16. Dion, Y. M., et al.: The influence of oral versus parenteral preoperative metronidazole on sepsis following colon surgery. Ann. Surg., *192*:221, 1980.
17. Keighley, M. R. B., et al.: Comparison between systemic and oral antimicrobial prophylaxis in colorectal surgery. Lancet, *1*:894, 1979.
18. Stone, J. H., et al.: Antibiotic prophylaxis in gastric, biliary and colonic surgery. Ann. Surg., *184*:443, 1976.
19. Polk, H. C., and Lopez-Mayor, J. F.: Postoperative wound infection: A prospective study of determinant factors and prevention. Surgery, *66*:97, 1969.
20. Alexander, H. C., and Prudden, J. F.: The causes of abdominal wound disruption. Surg. Gynecol. Obstet., *122*:1223, 1966.
21. Eisenstat, M. S., and Hoerr, S. O.: Courses and management of surgical wound dehiscence. Cleve. Clin. Q., *39*:33, 1972.
22. Mayo, C. W., and Lee, M. J.: Separations of abdominal wounds. Arch. Surg., *62*:883, 1951.
23. Rambo, W. M.: Irrigation of the peritoneal cavity with cephalothin. Am. J. Surg., *123*:192, 1972.
24. Foldes, F. F., Lunn, J. N., and Benz, H. G.: Prolonged respiratory depression caused by drug combinations: Muscle relaxant and intraperitoneal antibiotics as etiologic agents. J. Am. Med. Assoc., *183*:672, 1963.
25. Crutcher, R. R., Daniel, R. A., and Billins, F. T.: The effects of sulfanilamide, sulfathiazole and sulfadiazine on the peritoneum. Ann. Surg., *117*:677, 1943.
26. Markgraf, W. H.: Abdominal wound dehiscence: A technique for repair with marlex mesh. Arch. Surg., *105*:728, 1972.
27. de Dombal, F. T., Burton, I., and Goligher, J. C.: The early and late results of surgical treatment for Crohn's disease. Br. J. Surg., *58*:805, 1971.
28. Akman, P. C.: A study of five hundred incisional hernias. J. Int. Coll. Surg., *37*:125, 1962.
29. Anson, B. J., and McVay, C. B.: Surgical Anatomy. 5th Ed. Vol. I. Philadelphia, W. B. Saunders, 1971.
30. Davis, J. H.: Current concepts of peritonitis. Am. Surg., *33*:673, 1967.
31. Dawson, J. L.: A study of some factors affecting the mortality rate in diffuse peritonitis. Gut, *4*:368, 1963.
32. Debas, H. T., and Thomson, F. B.: A critical review of colectomy with anastomosis. Surg. Gynecol. Obstet., *135*:747, 1972.
33. Altemeier, W. A.: Bacterial flora of acute perforated appendicitis with peritonitis: Bacteriologic study based upon 100 cases. Ann. Surg., *107*:517, 1938.
34. Altemeier, W. A.: The pathogenicity of the bacteria of appendicitis peritonitis. Ann. Surg., *114*:158, 1941.
35. Altemeier, W. A., Culbertson, W. R., and Fuller, W. D.: Intra-abdominal sepsis. *In* Advances in Surgery. Edited by C. E. Welch, and J. D. Hardy. Chicago, Year Book Medical Publishers, 1971.
36. Welch, C. E., and Hedberg, S. E.: Complications in surgery of the colon and rectum. *In* Complications in Surgery and Their Management. 2nd Ed. Edited by C. P. Artz, and J. D. Hardy. Philadelphia, W. B. Saunders, 1967.
37. Clowes, G. H., Vucinic, M., and Weidner, M. G.: Circulatory and metabolic alterations associated with survival or death in peritonitis: Clinical analysis of 25 cases. Ann. Surg., *163*:866, 1966.
38. Skillman, J. J., Bushnell, L. S., and Hedley-Whyte, J.: Peritonitis and respiratory failure after abdominal operations. Ann. Surg., *170*:122, 1969.
39. Rubenstein, W. A., Yong, H. A., and Kazam, E.: Computed tomography of the abdomen. Adv. Surg., *17*:171, 1984.
40. Kislak, J. W.: The susceptibility of Bacteroides fragilis to 24 antibiotics. J. Infect. Dis., *125*:295, 1972.
41. Lorber, B., and Swenson, R.: The bacteriology of abdominal infections. Surg. Clin. North Am., *55*:1349, 1975.
42. Sanford, J. P., et al.: Panel discussion of the treatment of serious gram negative infections. Postgrad. Med. J., *47*:25, 1971.
43. Meyler, L., et al.: Blood dyscrasias attributed to chloramphenicol. Postgrad. Med. J. *50*:123, 1974.

44. Goodman, L. S., and Gilman, A.: The Pharmacological Basis of Therapeutics. 4th Ed. New York, Macmillan, 1970.
45. Tedesco, F. J., Barton, R. W., and Alpers, D. H.: Clindamycin associated colitis—A prospective study. Ann. Intern. Med., 81:429, 1974.
46. Finegold, S. M., Bartlett, J. G., and Chow, A. W.: Management of anaerobic infections. Ann. Intern. Med., 83:375, 1975.
47. Noone, P., Pattison, J. R., and Davies, D. G.: The effective use of gentamycin in life threatening sepsis. Postgrad. Med. J. (Suppl.), 50:9, 1974.
48. Simmons, R. L., and Ahrenholz, D. H.: Therapeutic principles in peritonitis. Topics in intra-abdominal surgical infection. Edited by R. L. Simmons, New York, Appleton Century Croft, 1982.
49. Furste, W., and Wheeler, W. L.: Tetanus: A team disease. Curr. Probl. Surg., 3, 1972.
50. Burnett, W. E., et al.: The treatment of peritonitis using peritoneal lavage. Ann. Surg., 145:675, 1957.
51. DiVincenti, F. C., and Cohn, I.: Prolonged administration of intraperitoneal kanamycin in the treatment of peritonitis. Am. Surg., 37:177, 1971.
52. Hudspeth, A. S.: Radical surgical debridement in the treatment of advanced generalized bacterial peritonitis. Arch. Surg., 110:1233, 1975.
53. Autio, V.: The spread of intraperitoneal infection: Studies with contrast medium. Acta Chir. Scand. 321, 1964.
54. Ariel, I. M., and Kazarian, K. K.: Classification, diagnosis and treatment of subphrenic abscesses. Rev. Surg., 28:1, 1971.
55. Altemeier, W. A., and Alexander, J. W.: Retroperitoneal abscess. Arch. Surg., 83:512, 1961.
56. Hechtman, H. B., Utsunomiya, T., Krausz, M. M., and Shepro, D.: The management of cardiorespiratory failure in surgical patients. In Advances in Surgery. Edited by L. D. MacLean. Chicago, Year Book Medical Publishers, 1981.
57. Verstraete, M.: The prevention of postoperative deep vein thrombosis and pulmonary embolism with low dose subcutaneous heparin and dextran. Surg. Gynecol. Obstet., 143:981, 1976.
58. Bergan, J. J., Kaupp, H. A., and Trippel, O. H.: Critical evaluation of vena cava plication in prevention of pulmonary embolism. Arch. Surg., 88:1016, 1964.
59. DeWeese, M. S., and Hunter, D. C.: A vena cava filter for the prevention of pulmonary embolism: A five-year clinical experience. Arch. Surg., 86:852, 1963.
60. Greenfield, L. J., et al.: Clinical experience with the Kim-Ray Greenfield vena cava filter. Ann. Surg., 185:692, 1977.
61. Dudrick, S. J., et al.: Intravenous hyperalimentation. Med. Clin. North Am., 54:577, 1970.
62. Doolas, A.: Planning intravenous alimentation in surgical patients. Surg. Clin. North Am., 50:103, 1970.
63. Jalan, K. N., et al.: Perineal wound healing in ulcerative colitis. Br. J. Surg., 56:749, 1969.
64. Jalan, K. N., et al.: Influence of corticosteroids on the results of surgical treatment for ulcerative colitis. N. Engl. J. Med., 282:588, 1970.
65. Watts, J. McK., de Dombal, F. T., and Goligher, J. C.: Long-term complications and prognosis following major surgery for ulcerative colitis. Br. J. Surg., 53:1014, 1966.
66. Myers, R. T., and Hightower, F.: Critical follow-up of surgically treated ulcerative colitis. Ann. Surg., 167:920, 1968.
67. Cohen, B. E., and Ryan, J. A.: Gracilis muscle flap for closure of persistent perineal sinus. Surg. Gynecol. Obstet., 148:33, 1979.
68. Jacob, R. A., Pace, W. G., and Thomford, N. R.: The hazards of a permanent ileostomy. Arch. Surg., 99:549, 1969.
69. Warren, R., and McKittrick, L. S.: Ileostomy for ulcerative colitis: Technique, complications, and management. Surg. Gynecol. Obstet., 93:555, 1951.
70. Brooke, B. N.: The management of an ileostomy including its complications. Lancet, 2:102, 1952.
71. Brooke, B. N.: Discussion of ileostomy. Proc. R. Soc. Med., 49:949, 1956.
72. Wright, H. K., and Tilson, M. D.: A method for testing the functional significance of tight ileostomy stomas. Am. J. Surg., 123:417, 1972.
73. Irving, M.: Ileostomy. Clin. Gastroenterol., 11:237, 1982.
74. Goligher, J. C.: Surgery of the Anus, Rectum and Colon. 3rd Ed. London, Baillière Tindall, 1975.
75. Sugarbaker, P. H.: Peritoneal approach to prosthetic mesh repair of paraostomy hernias. Ann. Surg., 201:344, 1985.
76. Goligher, J. C.: Ileal recurrence after ileostomy and excision of the large bowel for Crohn's disease. Br. J. Surg., 59:253, 1972.
77. Adson, M. A., Benjamin, I., and Dockerty, M. B.: Postcolectomy ileitis and related disorders. Arch. Surg., 102:326, 1971.
78. Knill-Jones, R. P., Morson, B., and Williams, R.: Prestomal ileitis: Clinical and pathological findings in five cases. Q. J. Med., 154:287, 1970.
79. Thayer, W. R., and Spiro, H. M.: Ileitis after ileostomy: Pre-stomal ileitis. Gastroenterology, 42:547, 1962.
80. Lyons, A. S., and Brockmeier, M. J.: Mechanical management of the ileostomy stoma. Surg. Clin. North Am., 52:979, 1972.
81. Turnbull, R. B.: Management of the ileostomy. Am. J. Surg., 86:617, 1953.
82. Sachs, D., and Barker, W.: Immediate postoperative management of the ileostomy. Surgery, 59:373, 1966.
83. Honesty, H.: Essentials of Abdominal Ostomy Care. New York, Springer Publishing Company, 1972.
84. Lyons, A. S.: An ileostomy club. J. Am. Med. Assoc., 150:812, 1952.
85. Hill, G. L.: Ileostomy. Part 3. Metabolic complications of ileostomy. Clin. Gastroenterol., 11:260, 1982.
86. Kock, N. G.: Continent ileostomy. Prog. Surg., 12:180, 1973.
87. Kock, N. G., et al.: The quality of life after proctocolectomy and ileostomy: A study of patients with conventional ileostomies converted to continent ileostomies. Dis. Colon Rectum, 17:287, 1974.
88. Dozois, R. R., et al.: Improved results with continent ileostomy. Ann. Surg., 192:319, 1980.
89. Gerber, A., Apt, M. K., and Craig, P. H.: The Kock continent ileostomy. Surg. Gynecol. Obstet., 156:345, 1983.
90. Kock, N. G., et al.: Continent ileostomy: The Swedish experience. In Alternatives to Conventional Ileostomy. Edited by R. R. Dozois. Chicago, Year Book Medical Publishers, 1985.
91. Dozois, R. R., Kelly, K. A., Beart, R. W., and Beahrs, O. H.: Continent ileostomy: The Mayo Clinic experience. In Alternatives to Conventional Ileostomy. Edited by R. R. Dozois. Chicago, Year Book Medical Publishers, 1985.
92. Halvorsen, J. F., Hoel, R., and Nygaard, K.: The continent reservoir ileostomy: Review of a collective series of 36 patients from three surgical departments. Br. J. Surg., 62:65, 1975.
93. Kock, N. G., and Myrvold, H. E.: Progress report on the continent ileostomy. World J. Surg., 4:143, 1980.
94. Schrock, T. R.: Complications of continent ileostomy. Am. J. Surg., 138:162, 1979.

95. Goligher, J. C.: The quest for continence in the surgical treatment of ulcerative colitis. *In* Advances in Surgery. Edited by G. L. Jordon. Chicago, Year Book Medical Publishers, 1980.
96. Fazio, V. W.: Comments on the continent ileostomy: The Swedish experience. *In* Alternatives to Conventional Ileostomy. Edited by R. R. Dozois. Chicago, Year Book Medical Publishers, 1985.
97. Goldman, S. L., and Rombeau, J. L.: The continent ileostomy: A collective review. Dis. Colon Rectum, 21:594, 1978.
98. Gunby, P.: Results of continent reservoir ileostomy procedure improving. J. Am. Med. Assoc., 244:1763, 1980.
99. Gorbach, S. L., Nahas, L., and Weinstein, L.: Studies of intestinal microflora: The microflora of ileostomy effluent. A unique microbial etiology. Gastroenterology, 53:874, 1967.
100. Philipson, B., et al.: Mucosal morphology, bacteriology and absorption in intra-abdominal ileostomy reservoir. Scand. J. Gastroenterol., 10:1, 1975.
101. Schjonsby, H., et al.: Stagnant loop syndrome in patients with continent ileostomy (intra-abdominal ileal reservoir). Gut, 18:795, 1977.
102. Kelly, D. G., et al.: Dysfunction of the continent ileostomy: Clinical features and bacteriology. Gut, 24:193, 1983.
103. Phillips, S. F.: Altered physiology. *In* Alternatives to Conventional Ileostomy. Edited by R. R. Dozois. Chicago, Year Book Medical Publishers, 1985.
104. Kelly, D. G., et al.: Diarrhea after continent ileostomy. Gut, 21:711, 1980.
105. Gelernt, I. M.: Continent ileostomy forum. Ostomy Q., 16:56, 1979.
106. Loeschke, K., et al.: Bacterial overgrowth in ileal reservoirs (Kock pouch): Extended functional studies. Hepatogastroenterology, 27:310, 1980.
107. Martin, L. W., LeCoultre, C., and Schubert, W. K.: Total colectomy and mucosal proctectomy with preservation of continence in ulcerative colitis. Ann. Surg., 186:477, 1977.
108. Telander, R. L., and Perrault, J.: Colectomy with rectal mucosectomy and ileoanal anastomosis in young patients. Arch. Surg., 116:623, 1981.
109. Taylor, B. M., et al.: A clinico-physiological comparison of ileal pouch-anal and straight ileoanal anastomosis. Ann. Surg., 198:462, 1983.
110. Coran, A. G., et al.: The endorectal pull-through for the management of ulcerative colitis in children and adults. Surgery, 197:99, 1983.
111. Parks, A. G., and Nicholls, R. J.: Proctocolectomy without ileostomy for ulcerative colitis. Br. Med. J., 2:85, 1978.
112. Schraut, W. H., Rosemurgy, A. S., Wang, C. H., and Block, G. E.: Determinants of optimal results after ileoanal anastomosis: Anal proximity and motility patterns of the ileal reservoir. World J. Surg., 7:400, 1983.
113. Parks, A. G., Nicholls, R. J., and Belliveau, P.: Proctocolectomy with ileal reservoir and anal anastomosis. Br. J. Surg., 67:533, 1980.
114. Rothenberger, D. A., et al.: Restorative proctocolectomy with ileal reservoir and ileoanal anastomosis. Am. J. Surg., 145:82, 1983.
115. Wong, W. D., Rothenberger, D. A., and Goldberg, S. M.: Ileoanal pouch procedures. Curr. Probl. Surg., 22:3, 1985.
116. Utsunomiya, J., et al.: Total colectomy, mucosal proctectomy and ileoanal anastomosis. Dis. Colon Rectum, 23:459, 1980.
117. Fonkalsrud, E. W.: Endorectal ileal pull-through with lateral ileal reservoir for benign colorectal disease. Ann. Surg., 194:761, 1981.
118. Schraut, W. H., and Block, G. E.: Ileoanal anastomosis with proximal ileal reservoir: An experimental study. Surgery, 91:275, 1982.
119. Kojima, Y., Sanada, Y., and Fonkalsrud, E. W.: Comparison of endorectal ileal pull-through following colectomy with and without ileal reservoir. J. Pediatr. Surg., 17:653, 1982.
120. Rosemurgy, A. S., Schraut, W. H., and Block, G. E.: The physiologic effects of ileal reservoirs and efferent conduits complementing ileo-anal anastomosis: An experimental study. Surgery, 94:697, 1983.
121. Nicholls, R. J., and Pezim, M. E.: Restorative proctocolectomy with ileal reservoir—a comparison between the 3-loop and 2-loop reservoir. Read before the Annual Meeting of the American Society of Colon and Rectal Surgeons, New Orleans, May 6-11, 1984.
122. Handelsman, J. C., et al.: Endorectal pull-through operation in adults after colectomy and excision of rectal mucosa. Surgery, 93:247, 1983.
123. Martin, L. W., and Fischer, J. E.: Preservation of anorectal continence following total colectomy. Ann. Surg., 196:700, 1982.
124. Taylor, B. M., et al.: The endorectal ileal pouch-anal anastomosis: Current clinical results. Dis. Colon Rectum, 27:347, 1984.
125. Peck, B. A.: Rectal mucosal replacement. Ann. Surg., 191:294, 1980.
126. Fonkalsrud, E. W.: Endorectal ileoanal anastomosis with isoperistaltic ileal reservoir after colectomy and mucosal proctectomy. Ann. Surg., 199:151, 1984.
127. Nicholls, R. J., Moskowitz, R. L., and Shepherd, N. A.: Restorative proctocolectomy with ileal reservoir. Br. J. Surg., 72:S76, 1985.
128. Rothenberger, D. A., et al.: Restorative proctocolectomy with ileal reservoir and ileoanal anastomosis for ulcerative colitis and familial polyposis. Dig. Surg., 1:19, 1984.
129. Metcalf, A., et al.: Ileal pouch-anal anastomosis. The procedure of choice? Presented at the American Society of Colon and Rectal Surgeons, New Orleans, May, 1984.
130. Beart, R. W., Metcalf, A. M., Dozois, R. R., and Kelly, K. A.: The J-ileal pouch-anal anastomosis: The Mayo Clinic experience. *In* Alternatives to Conventional Ileostomy. Edited by R. R. Dozois. Chicago, Year Book Medical Publishers, 1985.
131. Heppell, J., et al.: Physiologic aspects of continence after colectomy, mucosal proctectomy, and endorectal ileoanal anastomosis. Ann. Surg., 195:435, 1982.
132. Telander, R. L., Perrault, J., and Hoffman, A. D.: Early development of the neorectum by balloon dilatation after ileoanal anastomosis. J. Pediatr. Surg., 16:911, 1981.
133. Ritchie, J. K.: The causes of late mortality in ileostomists. Proc. R. Soc. Med., 65:73, 1972.
134. Ellis, H.: The cause and prevention of postoperative intraperitoneal adhesions. Surg. Gynecol. Obstet., 133:497, 1971.
135. Ellison, E. H.: Gastric suction and early operation for small bowel obstruction. *In* Current Surgical Management III. Edited by J. H. Mulholland, E. H. Ellison, and S. R. Freisen. Philadelphia, W. B. Saunders, 1960.
136. Alexander-Williams, J.: Overview of surgical management and direction of future research. *In* Inflammatory Bowel Disease. Edited by R. N. Allan, M. R. B. Keighly, J. Alexander-Williams, and C. Hawkins. Edinburgh, Churchill Livingstone, 1983.

137. Alexander-Williams, J., and Haynes, I. G.: Conservative operations for Crohn's disease of the small bowel. World J. Surg., 9:945, 1985.
138. Winawer, S. J., and Zamcheck, N.: Pathophysiology of small intestinal resection in man. In Progress in Gastroenterology. Vol. I. Edited by G. B. J. Glass. New York, Grune and Stratton, 1968.
139. Wester, E.: The management of patients after small bowel resection. Gastroenterology, 71:146, 1976.
140. Ammon, H. V., and Phillips, S. F.: Inhibition of colonic water absorption by fatty acids in man. Gastroenterology, 65:744, 1973.
141. Swenson, S. A., Lewis, J. W., and Sebby, K. R.: Magnesium metabolism in man with special reference to jejuno-ileal bypass for obesity. Am. J. Surg., 127:250, 1974.
142. Dowling, R. H.: Intestinal adaptation. N. Engl. J. Med., 288:520, 1973.
143. Wilmore, D. W., et al.: The role of nutrition in the adaptation of the small intestine after massive resection. Surg. Gynecol. Obstet., 132:673, 1971.
144. Voitk, A. J., et al.: Use of elemental diet during the adaptive stage of short gut syndrome. Gastroenterology, 65:419, 1973.
145. Richards, A. J., Concon, J. R., and Mallison, C. M.: Lactose intolerance after extensive small bowel resection. Br. J. Surg., 58:493, 1971.
146. Jeejeebhoy, K. N., et al.: Total parenteral nutrition at home for 23 months without complication and good rehabilitation. Gastroenterology, 65:811, 1973.
147. Brennan, M. F., and Horowitz, G. D.: Total parenteral nutrition in surgical patient. Adv. Surg., 17:1, 1984.
148. Pollack, P. F., et al.: 100 Patient years' experience with the Broviac Silastic catheter for central venous nutrition. JPEN, 5:32, 1981.
149. Baumrucker, G. O., and Shaw, J. W.: Urological complications following abdominoperineal resection of the rectum. Arch. Surg., 67:502, 1953.
150. Tank, E. S., et al.: Urinary tract complications of anorectal surgery. Am. J. Surg., 123:118, 1972.
151. Enker, W. E., and Block, G. E.: Occult uropathy complicating Crohn's disease. Arch. Surg., 101:319, 1970.
152. Watts, J. McK., de Dombal, F. T., and Goligher, J. C.: Early results of surgery for ulcerative colitis. Br. J. Surg., 53:1005, 1966.
153. Bauer, J. L., Gelernt, I. M., Salky, B. and Kreel, I.: Sexual dysfunction following proctocolectomy for benign disease of the colon and rectum. Ann. Surg., 197:363, 1983.
154. Lee, J. B., Maurer, V. M., and Block, G. E.: The anatomic relations of the pelvic autonomic nerves. Arch. Surg., 107:324, 1973.
155. Strahlgren, L. H., and Ferguson, L. K.: Influence on sexual function of abdominoperineal resection for ulcerative colitis. N. Engl. J. Med., 259:873, 1958.
156. Harris, J. W.: Sexual dysfunction and tardiness in wound healing after proctocolectomy for ulcerative colitis. J. Int. Coll. Surg., 35:379, 1961.
157. Pearman, R. O.: Insertion of a Silastic penile prosthesis for the treatment of organic sexual impotence. J. Urol., 107:802, 1972.
158. Deren, J. J., et al.: Nephrolithiasis as a complication of ulcerative colitis and regional enteritis. Ann. Intern. Med., 56:845, 1962.
159. Maratka, Z., and Nedbal, J.: Urolithiasis as a complication of the surgical treatment of ulcerative colitis. Gut, 5:214, 1964.
160. Levine, A. M., Pickett, L. K., and Touloukian, R. J.: Steroids hypertension and fluid retention in the genesis of postoperative seizures with inflammatory bowel disease in childhood. J. Pediatr. Surg., 9:715, 1974.
161. Kline, D. G.: Operative management of major nerve lesions of the lower extremity. Surg. Clin. North Am., 52:1247, 1972.
162. Torisu, M., et al.: Immunosuppression, liver injury and hepatitis in renal, hepatic, and cardiac homograft recipients: With particular reference to the Australia antigen. Ann. Surg., 174:620, 1971.
163. Van Prohaska, J.: The inflammatory diseases of the large and small bowel. Curr. Probl. Surg., 3, 1969.
164. Rhodes, J. B., and Kirsner, J. B.: The early and late course of patients with ulcerative colitis after ileostomy and colectomy. Surg. Gynecol. Obstet., 121:1303, 1965.
165. Goldgraber, M. B., and Kirsner, J. B.: Carcinoma of colon complicating ulcerative colitis: report of 10 cases. Dis. Colon Rectum, 7:336, 1964.
166. Dennis, C., and Karlson, K. E.: Cancer risk in ulcerative colitis: formidability per patient-year of late disease. Surgery, 50:568, 1961.
167. Bargen, J. A., and Gage, R. P.: Carcinoma and ulcerative colitis: prognosis. Gastroenterology, 39:385, 1960.
168. Aylett, S.: Ulcerative colitis treated by total colectomy and ileorectal anastomosis: A ten-year review. Proc. R. Soc. Med., 56:183, 1963.
169. Adson, M. A., Cooper, A. M., and Farrow, G. M.: Ileorectostomy for ulcerative disease of the colon. Arch. Surg., 104:424, 1972.
170. Oakley, J. R., et al.: Complication and quality of life after ileorectal anastomoses for ulcerative colitis. Am. J. Surg., 148:230, 1985.
171. Stryker, S. J., et al.: Anal and neorectal function after ileal pouch-anal anastomosis. Ann. Surg., 203:55, 1986.
172. Weedon, D. D., et al.: Crohn's disease and cancer. N. Engl. J. Med., 289:1099, 1973.
173. Greenstein, A. J., et al.: Cancer in Crohn's disease after diversionary surgery. A report of seven carcinomas occurring after excluded bowel. Ann. Surg., 135:86, 1978.
174. Pollock, A. V.: Crohn's disease. Br. J. Surg., 46:193, 1958.
175. Korelitz, B. I., et al.: Recurrent ileitis after ileostomy and colectomy for granulomatous colitis. N. Engl. J. Med., 287:110, 1972.
176. Glotzer, D. J., et al.: Comparative features and course of ulcerative colitis and granulomatous colitis. N. Engl. J. Med., 282:582, 1970.
177. de Dombal, F. T., Burton, I., and Goligher, J. C.: Recurrence of Crohn's disease after primary excisional surgery. Gut, 12:519, 1971.
178. Karim, A. F., et al.: Ulcerative colitis and Crohn's disease of the colon—A comparison of the long term postoperative courses. Gastroenterology, 71:372, 1976.
179. Baker, W. N. W.: Ileo-rectal anastomosis for Crohn's disease of the colon. Gut, 12:427, 1971.
180. Burman, J. H., Cooke, W. T., and Williams, J. A.: The fate of ileorectal anastomosis in Crohn's disease. Gut, 12:432, 1971.

31 · Physiologic Consequences of Surgical Treatment For Inflammatory Bowel Disease

D. L. EARNEST, M.D.

Surgical removal of a diseased segment of the intestinal tract can result in significant improvement in selected patients with inflammatory bowel disease. Such treatment may also produce new problems that result from loss or impairment of normal intestinal function, however. Resection of a short segment of intestine, such as 25 to 50 centimeters, is usually well tolerated. In contrast, a more extensive resection can lead to a spectrum of clinical problems, varying from a mere change in stool frequency and consistency to a deficiency of specific nutrients or even to life-threatening malabsorption. The current understanding of intestinal physiology and the effects of intestinal resection should enable the physician to predict consequences of bowel resection and to develop a plan for postoperative management.

The stomach and small intestine are tasked with accepting, chemically simplifying, and absorbing a wide variety of nutrients presented in diverse forms and volumes. The colon functions mainly to absorb water and sodium and to provide a reservoir allowing discharge of its contents at a convenient time. The obvious effect of removal of an intestinal segment is a reduction in the surface area available to absorb water, electrolytes, and nutrients. The intraluminal phase of digestion, the solubility of lipophilic substances in aqueous intestinal contents, the transit time through the intestine, and the resulting contact time with remaining mucosa may all be diminished and cause malabsorption. As shown in Table 31-1, the clinical picture following surgical resection of part of the small or large intestine depends on a number of factors including the specific segment removed, the length of the resection, the preservation or absence of the ileocecal valve and colon, the function of remaining small intestine and colon, the ability of remaining intestine to undergo adaptation, and also the status of other digestive organs, especially the stomach, liver, and pancreas. This chapter reviews how each of these important factors may affect clinical outcome.

Specific Factors Affecting Intestinal Absorption After Bowel Resection

Extent and Area of Intestinal Resection

The average length of the small intestine at autopsy is 657 centimeters.[1] In contrast, measurements made in vivo, where there is maintenance of normal muscular tone, demonstrates the length to be somewhat less, in the range of 421 to 643 cm.[2,3] The large absorptive surface of the small intestine, estimated to be approximately 100 square meters, results not only from the length of the bowel but also from the villous configuration of the mucosa. Mucosal villi are larger in the jejunum than the ileum, and thus the proportion of total small bowel surface area

TABLE 31-1. *Important Factors Affecting Intestinal Absorption Following Extensive Bowel Resection.*

Specific segment removed
Length of resection
Preservation of the ileocecal valve and colon
Function of remaining small intestine and colon
Adaptive change in remaining small intestine and colon
Functional status of stomach, pancreas and liver

present in the jejunum is greater than that in the ileum.[4] Accordingly, resection of jejunum will remove more surface area than is apparent from measurement of the length of the resected specimen.

Most nutrients in a standard meal are absorbed across mucosa in the proximal 100 centimeters of the small intestine.[5] The remaining surface area in the ileum provides a functional reserve to absorb intermittent large feedings as well as sites for absorption of certain specific nutrients and substances such as vitamin B_{12} and bile salts. Resection of an extensive segment of small intestine can cause malabsorption by deleting a specific absorptive site (Table 31-2), by accelerating passage of nutrients across the remaining mucosal surface without adequate time for absorption, by facilitating colonization of proximal intestine by colon bacteria, by interrupting the normal enterohepatic circulation of bile salts, or by a combination of these factors. In addition, resection of the proximal small intestine conceivably could impair the important contributions of the pancreas and liver to intraluminal digestion. The duodenal and proximal jejunal mucosa release peptide hormones such as secretin, pancreazymine, and cholecystokinin in response to intraluminal hydrogen ions and amino acids and fat in the meal. These hormones stimulate secretion of bicarbonate and enzymes by the pancreas, and flow of bile from the biliary tree.[6] Enterokinase, which activates pancreatic trypsinogen to trypsin, is secreted by mucosa of the duodenum and proximal jejunum.[7] Impaired release of these intestinal hormones and enzymes is thought to contribute to maldigestion and malabsorption occurring with primary intestinal mucosal diseases such as sprue,[8,9] and also to discoordinate mixing of intestinal contents and pancreaticobiliary secretions that can occur following gastric drainage procedures.[10,11] Thus, resection of an extensive amount of proximal small intestine can cause a degree of functional pancreatic and biliary insufficiency that contributes to nutrient malabsorption.

Effect of Small Intestine Resection on Absorption of Specific Nutrients

Digestion and absorption of carbohydrate, protein, fat, and most minerals, as well as water soluble vitamins, except B_{12}, occur in the duodenum and jejunum. After intestinal resection, adaptive changes occur that may eventually produce almost normal absorption of many nutrients by the remaining intestine. These adaptive changes will be discussed after a consideration of the clinical picture and potential for ultimate development of a deficiency state for each major nutrient.

CARBOHYDRATE, PROTEIN, AND FAT

The major carbohydrate in most North American diets is starch. This is followed in amount by the disaccharides sucrose and lactose, the monosaccharides fructose and glucose, and, finally, a variety of poorly or nonabsorbed carbohydrates. In total, carbohydrates provide more than half of our daily caloric needs. Most absorbable dietary carbohydrates consist of a complex of two or more monosaccharides linked by glycosidic bonds that must be split before the individual monosaccharides can be absorbed. Starch, a polymer of glucose, is split in the intestinal lumen by salivary and pancreatic amylases to maltose and isomaltose. These disaccharides, as well as sucrose and lactose, require further hydrolysis by specific enzymes in the intestinal mucosa before the monosaccharide products glucose, galactose, and fructose can be absorbed. Normal absorption of carbohydrate thus depends upon adequate intraluminal hydrolysis of starch, adequate exposure of the epithelial cell brush border to the carbohydrate, adequate

TABLE 31-2. *Mechanisms Causing Malabsorption After Resection of the Small Intestine.*

Loss of surface area and specific absorptive sites
Rapid transit time of luminal nutrients causing inadequate mucosal contact
Overgrowth of colon bacteria in proximal intestine
Functional pancreatic insufficiency
Interruption of bile salt enterohepatic circulation
Hypersecretion of gastric acid

mucosal content and activity of the specific disaccharidase enzymes, and, finally, normal transport of the released monosaccharides into the cell.

Intestinal resection impairs carbohydrate absorption mainly by decreasing the amount of available mucosal disaccharidase enzymes. Other factors that may play a role include inadequate intraluminal hydrolysis of starch and reduced exposure time of the carbohydrate to mucosa because of rapid transit. The mucosal content of most intestinal disaccharidase enzymes, except lactase, is greatest in the duodenum and jejunum. Lactase activity peaks more distally in the mid-small bowel and its hydrolysis is slower than the other disaccharides.[12] Residual lactase activity is usually most decreased after small bowel resection.[13,14] Thus, the milk sugar should be excluded from the diet as part of early management of any postoperative diarrhea. Ingestion of large amounts of sucrose can also cause diarrhea after extensive resection of the small bowel. This, presumably, results not only from a decrease in sucrase but also from malabsorption of the component monosaccharide fructose.[15] Fructose is absorbed more slowly than glucose or galactose, and its absorption occurs along the entire length of the small intestine by facilitated diffusion.[16,17] Normal persons may develop diarrhea after ingestion of large amounts of fructose, caused by its incomplete absorption. The problem of sucrose malabsorption is magnified in patients with a reduced small bowel surface area.[18]

Malabsorbed carbohydrates are fermented by colonic bacteria to osmotically active substances such as short chain organic acids, which are partly absorbed and used for energy by the colonic mucosa.[19-21] Those metabolites that are not absorbed increase the osmotic activity and lower the pH in fecal contents and thereby inhibit colonic absorption of electrolytes and water.[22] Bacterial metabolism of malabsorbed carbohydrate also produces gas, especially hydrogen and carbon dioxide.[23] Therefore, symptomatic carbohydrate malabsorption after small bowel resection is generally manifested by watery diarrhea and increased flatus. If malabsorption is severe, weight loss from caloric deprivation will also occur.

Protein digestion and absorption normally occurs in the stomach and proximal intestine. Polypeptides released by peptic digestion in the stomach are hydrolyzed in the intestinal lumen by pancreatic peptidases to amino acids and dipeptides and tripeptides.[24] Amino acids are normally absorbed by active transport, mainly in the jejunum.[25] In contrast, the dipeptides and tripeptides are both hydrolyzed and absorbed in the more distal jejunum and proximal ileum.[26,27] Extensive resection of the proximal intestine can impair protein digestion and absorption by causing functional pancreatic insufficiency, as mentioned previously, and by reducing the surface area for small intestinal hydrolysis and absorption of amino acids and peptides. Adaptive changes do occur with time that result in an increase in enterokinase and peptide hydrolase activity in the residual mucosa, however.[28] The degree of nitrogen malabsorption that finally results is roughly parallel to the degree of steatorrhea.[29] Significant malabsorption of protein causes negative nitrogen balance and eventually leads to impaired hepatic protein synthesis, hypoalbuminemia, decreased immune function, impaired growth, and response to injury.

The absorption of dietary fat, particularly triglyceride, occurs mainly across the mucosa of the jejunum after emulsification in the stomach, hydrolysis by pancreatic lipase, dispersion of the released fatty acids and monoglyceride into bile salt micelles, and diffusion of the mixed micelle across an unstirred layer of water adjacent to the microvillus membrane.[5,30] Diffusion of lipophilic substances through this unstirred water layer is more of a hindrance to mucosal absorption than is actual penetration of the microvillous membrane.[30] One implication of this aqueous diffusion barrier is that bile acid micelles are necessary for normal fat absorption. In the absence of bile, significant malabsorption of long-chain fatty acids occurs. Moreover, nonpolar compounds such as cholesterol, fat soluble vitamins, and hydrocarbons are essentially not absorbed unless micelles are present. In contrast, medium-chain fatty acids (C8-C12) are more soluble in water and thus can be absorbed in the absence of bile.[31,32] Because normal fat absorption requires interaction between almost all digestive organs, measurement of steatorrhea gives a good estimate of the residual digestive and absorptive function after small bowel resection.

Surgical resection of ileum has a more significant effect on fat absorption than does resection of a similar segment of jejunum. The reasons for this are two-fold. First, adaptive changes in the mucosa, which enhance absorption, are greater in the ileum following resection of the jejunum than vice versa.[31,33] Secondly, the ileum is necessary for maintenance of normal enterohepatic circulation of bile salts.[34] Bile salts are absorbed in the ileum by an active transport process. This absorption mechanism is not present in the jejunum and does not develop, or appear, after ileal resection.[33,35] Normally, more than 90% of bile salts secreted into the small intestine are conserved by ileal absorption and returned to the liver, forming the enterohepatic circulation. Excessive loss of bile acid into stool is replaced by new synthesis in liver, but this compensatory mechanism is limited. Thus, a pool of bile acids (2 to 4 g in size) is secreted by the liver, stored in the gallbladder and under the influence of cholecystokinin delivered into the upper intestine during a meal. The bile acid pool cycles 2 to 4 times with each meal and functions in the digestion process to solubilize dietary lipids in the aqueous phase of intestinal contents and to transport them in mixed micelles across the unstirred water layer adjacent to the mucosa. The purpose of this conservation and recycling of bile salts appears to be at least two-fold. The enterohepatic circulation maintains a quantity of bile salts in the upper intestine that is above the critical micellar concentration (CMC) necessary for formation of micelles. Secondly, it prevents flow of excess bile acid into the colon that can cause diarrhea, as discussed in the following. Resection of the ileum interrupts bile salt homeostasis by breaking the enterohepatic cycle. If the length of ileal resection is great enough, more bile salt is lost into stool than can be replaced by hepatic synthesis. As a consequence, the concentration of bile salts in the duodenum and jejunum decreases.[34] When it falls below the critical micellar concentration, intraluminal solubilization of lipid is impaired and fat malabsorption results. As a rule of thumb, patients with an ileal resection of less than 100 centimeters usually excrete less than 15 to 20 grams of fat in stool daily during a normal diet. More extensive ileal resection usually causes more severe malabsorption of fat.[36]

It should be remembered that steatorrhea occurring after resection of the small intestine can be of diverse origin and its severity may depend as much on the functional status of other digestive organs as it does on the length and location of intestine removed. For example, any previous gastroduodenal ulcer surgical treatment, especially with antrectomy, can impair emulsification of fat and magnify the effect of bowel resection. Functional pancreatic insufficiency can result from malnutrition as well as impaired release of mucosal secretagogues. Gastric acid hypersecretion, discussed in more detail in the following, can contribute to steatorrhea by at least two mechanisms: (1) the intraluminal pH may be reduced by excess acid below the optimum for lipase activity; and (2) at an acid pH dihydroxy bile salts precipitate from solution, a situation that impairs micelle formation.[37] Following removal of the ileocecal valve, colonization of proximal intestine by colonic bacteria may lead to deconjugation and absorption of bile acids in the proximal intestine, a situation that short-circuits the enterohepatic bile salt circulation.[38,39] Extensive ileal resection obviously impairs bile salt reabsorption and can deplete the bile acid pool. All of these situations lead to maldigestion and malabsorption of fat.

Malabsorption of other nonpolar or lipophilic substances may result from the retention of malabsorbed fat in the intestinal lumen. For example, in cases of pancreatic insufficiency or lipase inactivation, a large amount of unhydrolyzed triglyceride often remains in the intestinal lumen. This can be recognized clinically by passage of an orange oil in stool. Other fat soluble substances in diet, such as vitamins and drugs, may partition into this intraluminal fat phase and be carried through the small intestine into the colon, also escaping absorption. If pancreatic hydrolysis is adequate but formation of bile salt micelles is impaired or mucosal absorption is interrupted, the malabsorbed fatty acids may precipitate from solution as calcium soaps, or partition into an intraluminal bulk oil phase and be passed in stool.

MINERALS

Absorption of minerals occurs throughout the entire small intestine. Although the rate of absorption for iron and calcium is greatest in the duodenum, these minerals can be absorbed along most of the upper small intestinal surface.[40,41] Intestinal absorption of calcium is complex and influenced by intraluminal solubility of the ion, by mucosal uptake, and largely by the circulatory levels of $1,25(OH)_2$ vitamin D_3. With vitamin D deficiency, intestinal mucosal transport of calcium is minimal or absent.[40] Following intestinal resection, malabsorption of calcium is likely to be more related to a reduced dietary intake, to coprecipitation with malabsorbed fatty acids, and to a deficiency of vitamin D than it is to a reduction in the available absorptive surface. Hypocalcemia may result from impaired intestinal absorption of calcium, but it may also reflect hypoalbuminemia or, in some cases, hypoparathyroidism caused by magnesium deficiency.[42] Magnesium is necessary both for normal release of parathyroid hormone from the parathyroid gland and for its actions on peripheral tissues, such as calcium mobilization.[43] Magnesium replacement in deficient patients with hypocalcemia often will result in complete "normalization" of the serum calcium.[44]

Diminished iron absorption is usually a manifestation of a mucosal disease of the duodenum, such as sprue or Crohn's disease, and not of surgical intervention because resection of the duodenum is rare for any cause. Iron malabsorption may occur with gastroduodenal surgical treatment for peptic ulcer disease as a consequence of reduced gastric acid secretion, impaired gastric protein digestion, and bypass of, or rapid transit through, the duodenum of intraluminal contents. Iron deficiency developing after a small bowel resection should raise the possibilities of occult blood loss and unrecognized small intestinal mucosal disease.

Magnesium is absorbed throughout the small intestine. Although the rate of magnesium absorption is greatest in the proximal intestine,[45] the bulk of magnesium absorption probably occurs in the ileum because of the slower transit time of luminal contents through the distal small intestine. Extensive resection of the jejunum may significantly impair magnesium absorption early after the operation, before adaptive changes in ileum have occurred. The hypomagnesemia is often of short duration, however. Resections of the distal ileum sufficient to cause steatorrhea can lead to a serious and persisting magnesium deficiency both from a decrease in absorptive surface and from impaired magnesium solubility resulting from coprecipitation of magnesium with malabsorbed fatty acids. Of note, the magnesium salts that are formed with short or medium-chain fatty acids are more soluble in aqueous intestinal contents than are magnesium salts of long-chain fatty acids.[46] Thus, substitution of medium chain triglyceride for normal long-chain fat in the diet may be a useful method for reducing magnesium malabsorption in patients with extensive small bowel resections and severe steatorrhea. It already was noted that magnesium deficiency could lead to hypocalcemia and it should also be recognized that magnesium deficiency may be related to refractory potassium deficiency.[47,48]

Zinc is an important cofactor in the enzyme systems necessary for protein synthesis. Chronic deficiency of zinc can lead to impaired growth and sexual maturation, and a reduced appetite and sense of taste. Acute zinc deficiency has been described in patients with malabsorption caused by Crohn's disease, that developed when they were maintained on intravenous alimentation.[49] The quartet of observed symptoms included acrodermatitis, alopecia, diarrhea, and mental changes with disturbances in mood, irritability, and depression. Zinc is usually complexed in food with protein and carbohydrate. Thus, normal digestion is required for release of zinc into solution for intestinal absorption. Although mucosal absorption of zinc occurs at all levels of the small intestine,[50] in vivo radioisotopic absorption studies in man showed that peak levels occur in blood approximately 3 hours after oral ingestion of the radioisotope.[51] This suggests that the bulk of normal zinc absorption occurs primarily in the duodenum and proximal jejunum. Large resections of the proximal intestine impair zinc absorption. Diseases or resection of the ileum that cause steatorrhea can also lead to zinc deficiency resulting from binding of zinc with malabsorbed fatty acids.[52] A low molecular weight ligand has been described in exocrine pancreatic secretions that stimulates intestinal absorption of zinc.[53] Thus, functional pancreatic exocrine insufficiency resulting from malnutrition, or due to reduced secretion of cholecystokinin/pancreazymin after extensive proximal intestinal resection, conceivably could contribute to impaired zinc absorption.

Copper is normally absorbed in the upper small intestine.[54] Malabsorption of copper may result after intestinal resection, because of removal of absorptive sites or from its precipitation with malabsorbed fatty acids. The prevalence and clinical significance of copper deficiency from malabsorption remains uncertain because copper deficiency is rare in Americans. A deficiency of copper has been associated with development of kinky hair and also with a hypochromic microcytic anemia similar to that seen in iron deficiency. After massive small bowel resection, copper deficiency has been recognized mainly when it was not included in intravenous solutions used for total parenteral nutrition.[55,56] Malabsorption of copper with lowered copper levels in blood has also been reported after intestinal bypass surgical procedures for obesity.[57]

Deficiency of two other trace elements may be of concern in patients, especially children, with extensive bowel resection who are maintained for long periods (probably more than 6 months) on total parenteral nutrition. Selenium and chromium are essential trace elements in various animal species. A deficiency of selenium may result in hepatic necrosis and noninflammatory degeneration of cardiac and skeletal muscle associated with an increase in serum SGOT and low blood and tissue levels of glutathione peroxidase.[58,59] Symptomatic selenium deficiency has been reported in humans maintained on prolonged parenteral nutrition.[60-62] Chromium is necessary for normal metabolism of glucose; it appears to act as a cofactor in the peripheral action of insulin.[63,64] Chromium administration has been shown to improve IV glucose tolerance in malnourished children.[65] Chromium deficiency should be considered in patients receiving long-term parenteral nutrition for bowel resection or disease who are found to develop glucose intolerance.[66]

WATER SOLUBLE VITAMINS

Water soluble vitamins, except for B_{12}, are absorbed primarily in the proximal small intestine. The large amounts of vitamin C in diets in the U.S.A. are absorbed by passive diffusion. Of interest, an active sodium-dependent transport site for vitamin C is also found in the ileum.[67] Deficiency of ascorbic acid caused by resection or disease of only the ileum has not been observed, however. Deficiency of ascorbic acid is usually a consequence of inadequate dietary intake, even after intestinal resection. Vitamin C deficiency is manifest clinically by malaise and weakness, bone pain, perifollicular hemorrhages, hyperkeratotic hair follicles, and coiled hairs. In the late stages of vitamin C deficiency, or scurvy, petechiae on the skin and enlarged, bleeding gums are seen. Deficiency of vitamin C is rare after intestinal resection, but can be assessed by measuring levels of ascorbate in leukocytes.

Thiamine (vitamin B_1) deficiency also usually occurs as a consequence of inadequate dietary intake. Physiologic amounts of thiamine in the diet are absorbed by an active transport process that is greatest in the duodenal mucosa and progressively less active in the distal small intestine.[68] In contrast, pharmacologic doses of thiamine are absorbed by passive diffusion. The effect of a marginal dietary intake of thiamine can be magnified by extensive small intestinal disease or resection, and lead to clinical deficiency.[69] Severe thiamine depletion results in beriberi and the Wernicke-Korsakov syndrome. Less severe manifestations include anorexia, nausea, paresthesias, personality disturbances, hypotension, and reduced gastrointestinal motility. The presence of thiamine deficiency should always be considered in patients with extensive small bowel resection or bypass who are not on replacement therapy. A deficiency can be assessed clinically by measuring erythrocyte transketolase activity and its response to thiamine replacement.[70]

Pyridoxyl phosphate (vitamin B_6) absorption occurs in the proximal intestine by passive diffusion and is not usually affected by distal ileal or short proximal intestinal resections.[71] Thus, a clinical deficiency of vitamin B_6 because of primary intestinal diseases or malabsorption after bowel resection is rare, if it exists. Of note, vitamin B_6 deficiency can be seen in individuals who are taking drugs that block intestinal absorption of the vitamin, such as isoniazide. Accordingly, supplements of vitamin B_6 should be prescribed for patients with intestinal resection who are given isoniazide. Deficiency of vitamin B_6 may cause sideroblastic anemia, glossitis, cheilosis, angular stomatitis, seborrheic dermatitis, and irritability or depression. Evidence for a deficiency of vitamin B_6 can be assessed by measuring urinary excretion of xanthenuric acid before and after a tryptophan load. Excretion of xanthenuric acid is increased in vitamin B_6 deficiency.[72]

Niacin is absorbed largely in the jejunum by a sodium-dependent carrier mechanism.[73] Except for massive intestinal resection, clinical deficiency causing pellagra or nicotinamide encephalopathy usually arises from poor dietary intake of niacin or of tryptophan from which approximately 50% of niacin requirements are normally derived. The deficiency state progresses through dermatitis, diarrhea, dementia, and, unless corrected, death. Early symptoms include glossitis, stomatitis, insomnia, anorexia, irritability, abdominal pain, burning paresthesias, forgetfulness, and unexplained fears. An erythematous rash develops that becomes hyperpigmented and desquamates. Diarrhea is seen in almost half of cases and may be accompanied by steatorrhea. The potential for niacin deficiency should be considered in patients with extensive small bowel resection, and niacin replacement should be provided.

Riboflavin is rapidly absorbed in the proximal intestine and its uptake facilitated by the presence of bile acids.[74] Body stores of riboflavin are large and its synthesis by colonic bacteria with subsequent absorption by colonic mucosa tends to make a deficiency state uncommon.[75] A poor diet, however, plus severe malabsorption, can lead to a symptomatic deficiency that is manifested by sore burning lips, mouth, and tongue, angular stomatitis, glossitis (magenta tongue), photophobia, and burning itchy eyes. A burning foot syndrome has also been attributed to riboflavin deficiency, but it is not always corrected by replacement of the vitamin.[76]

No information is available about the mechanism of biotin absorption in man. In the hamster, absorption appears to be in the proximal intestine by an active sodium-dependent mechanism.[77] Biotin is synthesized by intestinal bacteria, and 3 to 6 times more biotin is excreted in urine than is ingested.[78] Thus, a true clinical biotin deficiency from reduced dietary intake or absorption is not recognized. Biotin deficiency can be induced, however, by eating large amounts of raw egg white, which contain avidin, a substance that binds biotin and prevents its absorption. The deficiency state in an experimental situation is characterized by pallor, lassitude, anorexia, insomnia, scaling dermatitis, anemia, and muscular and chest pains. Although biotin deficiency would not necessarily be expected after intestinal resection, a deficiency state has been reported in humans who chronically consumed raw eggs.[79,80]

Folates are absorbed primarily in the duodenum and proximal jejunum, although some absorption can occur in the ileum.[81] Pteroylpolyglutamates in the diet are deconjugated by intestinal epithelial brush border enzymes to the monoglutamate derivative, which is absorbed into portal blood. The exact location for the deconjugating enzyme (folate deconjugase) is unclear but appears to be in or near the brush border of the epithelial cells.[82] Hydrolysis of folate seems to be rate-limiting for subsequent absorption and becomes a clinical problem only when the intestinal mucosa is diseased or shortened by surgical treatment. The proportion of natural folates in the diet that is absorbed depends partly on the length of the polyglutamate chain. For example, only 50 to 80% of polyglutamates are absorbed, but almost all of the monoglutamate is absorbed. When used in therapeutic doses, folic (pteroylglutamic) acid is almost completely absorbed unchanged from the proximal intestine because it is a poor substitute for the reducing enzyme dihydrofolate reductase. Folate undergoes an enterohepatic circulation that may be important for conservation of the vitamin in deficiency states.[83] Whether this is disturbed sufficiently by ileal resection to cause a clinical deficiency remains unclear, but it appears not to be the case. Of note, intestinal bacteria synthesize folates.

When bacterial overgrowth of the proximal intestine occurs, the bacterially-synthesized folate is absorbed and can lead to high folate levels in blood.

A deficiency of folate caused by malabsorption occurs mainly with diseases of the proximal intestinal mucosa such as sprue, but can occur with inflammatory bowel disease or after extensive jejunal resection. Chronic use of certain drugs such as sulfasalazine, methotrexate, isoniazide, phenytoxin, oral contraceptives, and, possibly, cholestyramine can also result in folate malabsorption. This effect of drug therapy could add to the tendency of intestinal resection to impair overall folate absorption and its enterohepatic circulation. Folic acid deficiency is characterized by macrocytic anemia, megaloblastosis of bone marrow, diarrhea, and glossitis. Weight loss also may occur. The development of megaloblastic anemia in patients with intestinal resection should not be attributed to folate deficiency without assuring normal absorption of vitamin B_{12}. Replacement doses of folic acid correct the megaloblastic anemia seen with vitamin B_{12} deficiency, but they will not correct the neurologic impairment caused by vitamin B_{12} deficiency.

Vitamin B_{12} is absorbed by an active transport process in the distal small intestine that is dependent on recognition of the B_{12}-intrinsic factor complex.[84] Vitamin B_{12} in the diet is tightly bound to proteins and is released either by the process of cooking or by peptic digestion in the stomach. When released into gastric contents, vitamin B_{12} is rapidly bound to intrinsic factor, a glycoprotein that is secreted in excess by gastric parietal cells. Some vitamin B_{12} ($\pm 30\%$) may also be bound in the stomach to a low molecular weight protein known as R-protein.[85] In the duodenum, R-protein is removed by hydrolysis by pancreatic enzymes. The liberated B_{12} then binds with free intrinsic factor.[86] The main function of R-protein appears to be in binding nonphysiologic analogues of vitamin B_{12} to make them unavailable for absorption. The B_{12}-intrinsic factor complex passes down the intestine to interact with specific receptors present in epithelial cells from the mid small bowel to the ileocecal valve.[87] Significant malabsorption leading to clinical deficiency of vitamin B_{12} usually results when the last 100 centimeters of terminal ileum are removed.[88]

A deficiency of vitamin B_{12} does not lead to a compensatory increase in vitamin B_{12} absorption. To the contrary, megaloblastic changes occur in the intestinal epithelium with vitamin

B_{12} deficiency just as in the bone marrow, and the resulting abnormal ileal surface cells may have impaired vitamin B_{12} absorption. Measurable impairment of intestinal absorption of vitamin B_{12} occurs only after more than 50 to 55 centimeters of terminal ileum are resected.[88,89] As part of the adaptive change in ileum that occurs following resection of proximal intestine, increased absorption of vitamin B_{12} per unit length of remaining ileal mucosa may occur.[90] In contrast, no adaptive development of receptors exists for the intrinsic factor-B_{12} complex in proximal intestine following ileal resection.[33]

Malabsorption of vitamin B_{12} can occur from a variety of causes in patients with gastrointestinal disease, and should be considered as potentially contributing to a deficiency of vitamin B_{12} in patients with intestinal resection. These include gastric causes (e.g., intrinsic factor deficiency resulting from extensive resection of stomach, and also pernicious anemia), intestinal causes (e.g., primary mucosal disease such as sprue, stasis with bacterial overgrowth, infestation with fish tapeworm, radiation damage, and competitive effects of drugs such as methformin), and possibly a pancreatic cause (inadequate enzyme secretion resulting in impaired hydrolysis of the R-protein-vitamin B_{12} complex). Hepatic stores of vitamin B_{12} are usually sufficient to last for 3 to 5 years. Therefore, symptomatic vitamin B_{12} deficiency develops late after intestinal resection and may not be discovered until a significant clinical problem develops. It is advisable to quantitate intestinal absorption of vitamin B_{12} in all patients soon after ileal resection in order to determine if an adequate absorptive surface remains. Replacement should be started as soon as vitamin B_{12} malabsorption is found and before any signs of a deficiency state develop.

FAT SOLUBLE VITAMINS

The fat soluble vitamins A, D, E, and K are absorbed both in the jejunum and the ileum. Although their absorption can be impaired by extensive reduction in small intestinal mucosal surface by surgical intervention, the usual reason for deficiency of fat soluble vitamins after intestinal resection is diminished absorption consequent to reduced solubility in the aqueous intestinal contents. Fat soluble vitamins are fairly nonpolar molecules and are taken up into bile salt micelles for transport to the mucosal epithelium where they partition into the microvillous membranes. In the presence of steatorrhea, fat soluble vitamins can partition either into bile salt micelles or into the intraluminal bulk phase of malabsorbed fat. A clinically significant deficiency of fat soluble vitamins usually develops only when severe steatorrhea is prolonged, such as occurs with pancreatic insufficiency, extensive small bowel disease, or resection, and with inadequate luminal bile salt concentration consequent to extensive ileal resection, small intestinal bacterial overgrowth, chronic obstructive liver disease, or intestinal fistulas. Clinical symptoms of fat soluble vitamin deficiency may readily develop for vitamins A, D, and K.

Vitamin A occurs in diet mainly as retinyl esters, beta carotene, or other carotinoids (0.3 μg retinol = 6 μg beta carotene = 12 μg dietary carotinoids in vitamin A activity). For normal absorption to occur, retinyl esters are first hydrolyzed by pancreatic and mucosal retinyl hydrolase. Beta carotene is cleaved by pancreatic dioxygenase and yields two molecules of retinol. Retinyl esters, retinol, and beta carotene are dispersed in bile salt micelles in intestinal contents to permit their movement to the brush border where absorption occurs, probably by diffusion into the lipid membrane. Within the cell, retinol is re-esterified to retinyl ester and incorporated into chylomicrons for subsequent transport to the liver.[91] Thus, a deficiency of vitamin A could result from a number of factors after intestinal resection including inadequate dietary intake, reduced pancreatic enzyme secretion, impaired intestinal micellar solubilization, inadequate mucosal surface for absorption, and reduced re-esterification and incorporation into chylomicrons. Deficiency of vitamin A most commonly occurs from inadequate dietary intake; however, it may also develop with malabsorption and present early with impaired dark adaptation of the retina causing symptomatic night blindness. More severe deficiency causes significant eye changes with xerophthalmia and white spots (Bitot's spots) on the conjunctiva. Keratomalacia and, ultimately, blindness are late sequelae. Vitamin A also has an important role in maintenance of fertility and of epithelial surfaces. Symptomatic deficiency is manifested early by dryness and thickening of the skin. Vitamin A deficiency can be detected by measuring the level of carotene in blood or by the more specific and sensitive method of measuring dark adaptation by the retina.

Approximately 90% of circulating vitamin D_3 (25-hydroxy-cholecalciferol) is produced endogenously by the effect of ultraviolet radiation in sunlight on 7-dihydroxy-cholecalciferol in skin. In winter, or during times of prolonged reduced skin exposure to sunlight, intestinal absorption of vitamin D becomes more important. Impaired intestinal absorption of vitamin D thus increases the risk of significant vitamin D deficiency. Vitamin D is absorbed mainly in the duodenum and jejunum and undergoes an enterohepatic circulation.[92,93] This may be interrupted by surgical reduction in mucosal surface, by cholestasis or by bacterial overgrowth in the small intestine.[92,94] Absorption of vitamin D is enhanced by adequate bile salts and by normal mucosal absorption of fatty acids and monoglycerides. Absorbed vitamin D is converted in the liver to 25-hydroxy vitamin D_3 that is further hydroxylated in the kidney to the active metabolites 1,25-dihydroxy-cholecalciferol (1,25-DHCC) or 24,25-dihydroxy-cholecalciferol. Both active and passive intestinal absorption of calcium are stimulated by 1,25-DHCC. Hypocalcemia would develop more frequently in vitamin D deficiency were it not for the compensatory increase in secretion of parathyroid hormone that causes mobilization of calcium from bone. Thus, chronic malabsorption and deficiency of vitamin D can lead to secondary hyperparathyroidism. As already discussed in the mineral malabsorption section, a coexisting deficiency of magnesium may impair this parathyroid hormone response and promote development of symptomatic hypocalcemia.[94]

Two different types of gastrointestinal surgical therapy place patients at increased risk for developing vitamin D and calcium deficiency. First, partial or total gastric resection may lead to reduced dietary intake of vitamin D, to rapid gastric emptying with diminished mucosal contact time in the proximal intestine, and to poor intestinal mixing and fat malabsorption. Osteomalacia, secondary hyperparathyroidism, and osteoporosis have been reported in up to 30% of such patients.[94-96] Bacterial overgrowth in the proximal bowel after gastric surgical treatment may also play a contributory role by interrupting the enterohepatic circulation of vitamin D metabolites. Administration of antibiotics to such patients can correct a postgastrectomy deficiency of vitamin D.[97] Secondly, patients with intestinal resection or with bypass for obesity may develop low serum levels of calcium, phosphate, and vitamin D from the induced intestinal malabsorption. In this latter group, malabsorption of magnesium may play a critical role in whether hypocalcemia develops.

Vitamin E is present in diet as tocopherols and tocotrienols. These compounds undergo intraluminal hydrolysis by pancreatic enzymes, are solubilized by bile salt micelles, and are absorbed mainly in the proximal small intestine, probably by passive diffusion. Body stores of vitamin E are large, and the development of a deficiency state after intestinal resection may require years to occur. Low serum levels of vitamin E are found more commonly with severe exocrine pancreatic insufficiency, prolonged cholestasis, intestinal lymphangiectasia, and with untreated sprue than they are with extensive small bowel resection, possibly because vitamin E replacement is often included with nutritional rehabilitation following surgical treatment. Vitamin E functions as a biologic antioxidant and may also play a role in neurologic function. Severe vitamin E deficiency is usually manifest by development of a peroxide-sensitive hemolytic anemia and accumulation of brown lipofuscin pigment in tissues. Fertility may also be impaired. More severe deficiency, such as occurs with abetalipoproteinemia and long-standing cholestasis, is occasionally manifested by a neurologic syndrome consisting of areflexia, cerebellar ataxia, and loss of positional sense. Administration of vitamin E can improve or reverse these neurologic abnormalities.[98] Such severe symptomatic vitamin E deficiency, however, has not been described after small intestinal resection.

Vitamin K_1 (phylloquinone) is a normal constituent of many plant foods, vitamin K_2 (menaquinone) is synthesized by colon bacteria, and vitamin K_3 (menadione) is a synthetic molecule that is not found in the diet. Intestinal absorption of both vitamin K_1 and K_2 occurs in the distal small intestine and requires adequate micellar solubilization of the vitamin. In contrast, vitamin K_3 is much more water soluble and can be absorbed in the proximal intestine. Vitamin K_2 is important in maintaining vitamin K balance in rodents but plays an unclear role as a physiologic source of vitamin K in man. Malabsorption of vitamin K occurs with any chronic disease or situation that interrupts bile acid micelle formation, such as extensive ileal resection, chronic cholestasis, bacterial overgrowth in the proximal intestine, or treatment with high doses of cholestyramine. A decrease in intestinal surface area by disease or by surgical resection, and also obstruction of lymphatics by tumor or fibrosis, may impair vitamin K absorption and lead to symptomatic vitamin K deficiency.

Vitamin K is required for post-translational

carboxylation of gamma-glutamic acid residues in a variety of proteins, especially those in coagulation factors II, VII, IX, and X that are synthesized in liver.[99,100] The carboxylation reaction is necessary for final synthesis of the active protein. Impaired carboxylation leads to formation of nonfunctional proteins. A lack of vitamin K is thus reflected clinically by prolongation of the prothrombin-time and reduced levels in blood of active Factors II, VII, IX, and X.[101] A number of situations can cause an absolute or functional vitamin K deficiency, in addition to malabsorption with intestinal resection or disease. These include treatment with antibiotics that sterilize the gut, advanced liver disease with a defective carboxylase enzyme reaction, anticoagulation therapy with coumarin drugs, and also large doses of vitamin E which potentiate the effects of marginal vitamin K deficiency and of coumarin drugs.[102-104]

Preservation of the Ileocecal Valve

The transit time of intraluminal contents through the ileum is slower than that through the jejunum. Although this results in part from a slower intrinsic myoelectric activity of the distal small intestine,[105] the presence of an intact ileocecal valve itself has been demonstrated experimentally to reduce transit of intraluminal contents through the distal small intestine. Thus, removal of the ileocecal valve leads to more rapid movement of luminal contents through the small bowel, and thereby reduces mucosal contact time.[106] In patients with intestinal resection, loss of the ileocecal valve is often associated with more severe diarrhea and malabsorption.

The ileocecal valve functions as a mechanical barrier, preventing reflux of colonic contents into the more proximal small intestine. Absence of this barrier increases colonization of the proximal small intestine by colonic bacteria.[39] The consequences of this can be dramatic and are much the same as those that occur with small intestinal overgrowth from stasis with a blind loop or impaired motility. For example, colonic bacteria in the small intestine may bind and metabolize vitamin B_{12}, preventing its absorption by any remaining ileum.[89] The bacteria also deconjugate bile salts and thereby shortcircuit the enterohepatic bile salt circulation, causing more severe steatorrhea.[34] Carbohydrates may be abnormally fermented, with production of excessive organic acids and gas. A significant amount of ingested protein may be deaminated and further metabolized to urea and ammonia by the luminal bacteria.[107] Enzymes produced by the bacteria also can worsen absorption of carbohydrates and proteins by damaging the epithelial cell brush border and causing a decrease in activity of disaccharidases and peptidases.[108] Excessive degradation and loss of protein in the gut may impair hepatic protein synthesis and lead to hypoalbuminemia and reduced immune function. Bacterial metabolism of cholic acid increases luminal concentrations of deoxycholic acid, and metabolism of malabsorbed fatty acids produces hydroxylated fatty acids, such as hydroxysteric acid. These bile and fatty acids stimulate secretion of water and electrolytes by remaining in the small intestine and colon.[109-111] Thus, removal of the ileocecal valve can significantly worsen malabsorption and also cause diarrhea. It follows that every attempt possible should be made to preserve this important part of intestinal anatomy.

When the ileocecal valve is resected, variable amounts of proximal colon usually are also removed. Often, not enough consideration is given at the time of surgical treatment to the large absorptive capacity of the colon, especially the ascending colon. The normal colon can absorb up to 5,700 milliliters of water, 816 milliequivalents of sodium, and 44 milliequivalents of potassium daily.[112] Even in the setting of abnormal delivery of malabsorbed nutrients to the colon, significant absorption of water and short-chain fatty acids can occur before osmotic diarrhea develops.[18] Thus, every attempt should be made at the time of surgical treatment to leave as much colon intact as possible, because following small bowel resection, the stool volume and frequency depend more on the length of colon that remains than on the length of small bowel removed.[106,113] Also, patients who have removal of the ileocecal valve and part of the ascending colon at the time of ileal resection, have greater malabsorption of nutrients and water than do those with a similar extent of small bowel resected but with an intact ileocecal valve and colon.[114]

Intestinal Adaptation

Improvements in surgical technique and in postoperative parenteral nutritional support allow most patients today to survive for at least the first few weeks after extensive resection of the intestine for inflammatory bowel disease or other causes. Subsequent attempts to use the gastrointestinal tract for its normal absorptive and excretory functions are usually complicated early by malabsorption of nutrients, electrolytes, and water. A key element in determining the ultimate outcome of the surgical procedure is the adaptive response in the remaining intestinal tract. Considerable evidence shows that permanent alterations occur in mucosal structure and function that can be considered true compensatory changes. In patients who have had resection of 50 to 80% of the small bowel, oral biopsy of the remaining intestine shows an increase in number (hyperplasia) of cells on the intestinal villi.[115] The absorption of carbohydrates, fat, and nitrogen gradually improves, and diarrhea lessens over a period of weeks to months following surgical therapy.[116,117] In vivo intestinal perfusion studies have demonstrated corresponding slight but significant increases in segmental absorption of glucose.[118] Absorption of water and electrolytes is also enhanced.[119] Most control studies of intestinal adaptation following extensive bowel resection have been done in experimental animal models, especially in the rat and the dog. Accordingly, the information presented in the following section must be viewed from this perspective, although no significant differences in the adaptive response of the intestine have been noted between the various animal species studied to date.

Changes in Intestinal Morphology

Following small bowel resection, the remaining intestine becomes dilated and may elongate slightly (Figure 31-1). Mucosal crypt depth and villous height also increase. These changes are generally proportional in magnitude to the length of bowel resected, that is, they are most prominent with very extensive resections.[120] The changes in morphology are also influenced by which segment of intestine was removed. For example, the adaptive response in remaining ileum following jejunal resection is significant, whereas changes in the remaining jejunum after ileal resection are more modest.[121] Adaptive growth of intestine is accompanied by increased segmental weight and thickening of the entire wall, especially the mucosa. Figure 31-2 shows an example of the hyperplasia that occurred in the ileal mucosae of rats 1 month after jejunal resection.

The adaptive changes occur on both sides of the surgical anastomosis but are always greatest in the more distal intestine.[121] It is clear that adaptive growth also occurs in the cecum and proximal colon after resection of the ileum.[122,123] Although some hyperplasia of colonic mucosa occurs following jejunal resection, the early response usually diminishes with time.[124] Thus, adaptive changes in the intestine following resection of the small intestine develop in both the remaining small and large bowel.

The morphologic response in the crypts of the small intestine to the adaptive stimulus is slightly different from that which occurs in the villi.[125] Cells on the villi arise from progenitor stem cells in the crypts. Several crypts may contribute cells to a single villus. An equilibrium normally exists between cell formation in the crypts and cell loss into the lumen from the villus tip. By this process of cell migration up the crypts and villi, the surface epithelium is replaced every 2 to 6 days in rodents and in man.[33] Epithelial cell renewal probably occurs from a pluripotential crypt stem cell that gives rise to an amplification cell compartment that, in turn, may undergo several divisions as the cells move up the crypt and villus.[125] Studies using tritiated thymidine to measure mitosis in sham and bowel-resected rats show that the average time a cell spends in the proliferative compartment is approximately 11 hours. After partial small bowel resection, the number of stem cells in crypts both proximal and distal to the resection is increased. The cell cycle time is also reduced, mainly by a decrease in the "S" phase. The net

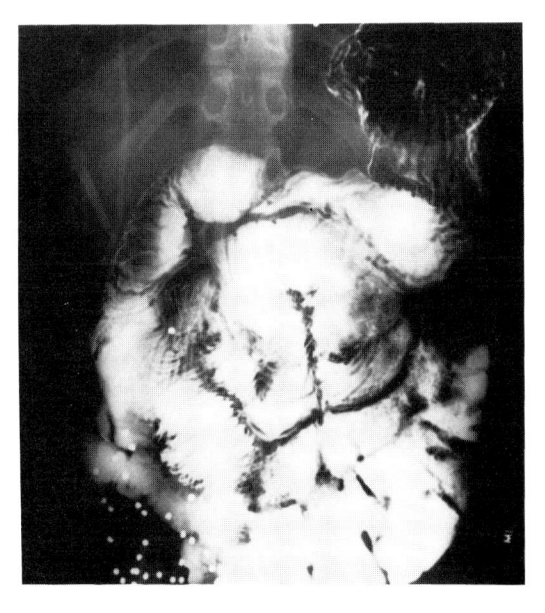

FIG. 31-1. X-ray showing dilatation and elongation of the jejunum in a 30-year-old man two years after resection of all but eight inches of proximal small intestine. (Courtesy of George F. Sheldon, M. D.)

result is more crypt cells that have an increased rate of cycling.[126] The increase in size of the proliferative cell compartment is proportional to the extent of bowel resection, tends to maintain an unchanged total growth fraction of mucosal epithelial cells, and appears to be permanent.[120] Figure 31-3 shows that the adaptive increase in number of crypt stem cells begins within a few days after intestinal resection and is complete by the end of 12 days. The hyperplastic response in each crypt appears to be independent of its position in the intestine. Also, the total number of residual crypts in each intestinal segment does not increase after bowel resection.[125]

Although no gross morphologic difference exists between crypts in the jejunum and those in ileum, the morphology of the villi in each of the two segments is considerably different. The villi in the duodenum and jejunum are tall and slender, but those in the ileum are much shorter. Also, more cells are found per villus in the jejunum than in the ileum. For example, the number of epithelial cells per villus decreases from 85 in rat jejunum to 40 in lower ileum.[127] Thus, a proximal to distal gradient is found in villous height, cell count, and functional absorptive surface in the small intestine. Resection of the proximal intestine in rats causes a rapid increase in cellularity (Fig. 31-3) and eventually height (Fig. 31-2) of the more distal ileal villi.[125] Within one week after a 30 to 50% proximal intestinal resection, the RNA and DNA content of remaining ileal mucosa reaches a peak that is approximately 175% of control values.[124] This postoperative villous hyperplasia persists for at least 6 months and possibly indefinitely.[128]

The speed of the adaptive change probably varies from species to species. Although it begins in the rat within 1 to 2 days after resection, reaches a maximum by 1 to 2 weeks, and is fully developed by one month,[121] it appears to take considerably longer in the dog.[129] No similar quantitative studies have been done in man, but clinical observations suggest that up to 1 year may be required for the adaptive change with improvement in intestinal function to be complete.[116]

Adaptation of the colon after small bowel resection is important because the remaining colon seems to have a great influence on clinical consequences of extensive small bowel resection. Similar to the small intestine, the adaptive response of colon mucosa has been mainly studied in rats. Following ileal resection, hyperplasia of colonic crypt cells is similar to that seen in the distal ileum after jejunal resection.[122,123] Some

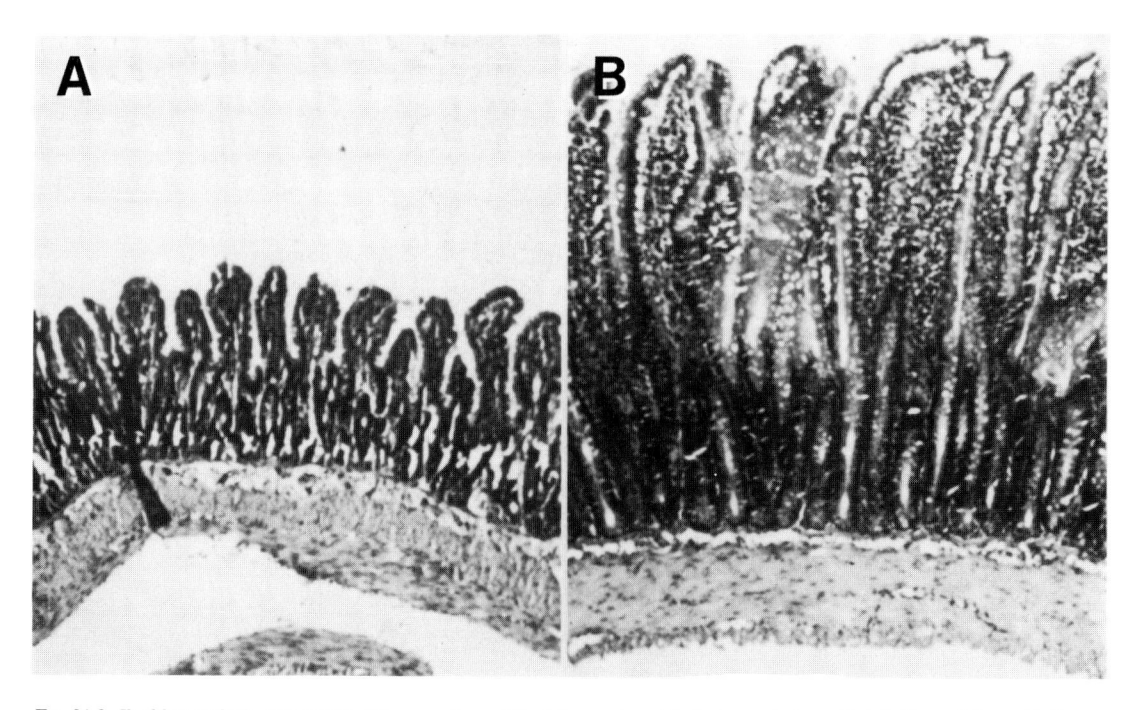

FIG. 31-2. Ileal hyperplasia one month after resection of the jejunum in rat fed a normal chow diet. A. Normal ileum. B. Ileum from resected rat. Formalin fixed, hematoxylin and eosin-stained tissue. Original magnifications × 1000. (Reproduced with permission of Elliot Weser, M. D., from: Viewpoints on Digestive Diseases. Vol. 10, March 1978.)

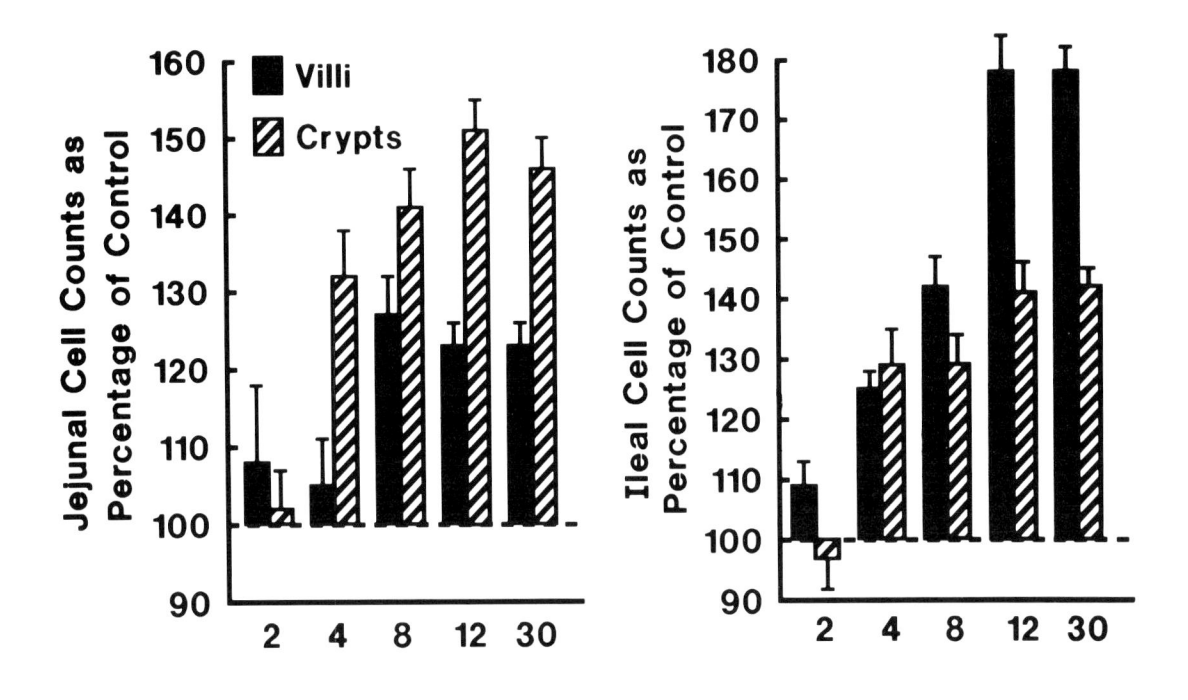

FIG. 31-3. These graphs show results of counts of epithelial cells in the villi and crypts of remaining small intestine measured at increasing times after a 70% small bowel resection. The results are expressed as a percentage of the initial or control cell count (100%) quantitated at the time of surgical transection. Note that the adaptive increase in number of both crypt and villous cells begins a few days after the intestinal resection and reaches a maximum by 12 days. In resected jejunum, the increase in the number of crypt cells exceeded the increase in villous epithelial cells. In contrast, the increase in villous cell count significantly exceeded the increase in crypt cell count in the ileum. Morphologically, this is reflected by a noticeable increase in the length of villi in ileal mucosa. (Adapted from Hanson, W. R. and Osborne, J. W.: Gastroenterology, 60:1087, 1971.)

hyperplasia also occurs in colonic crypts after resection of the jejunum, but the response decreases as any remaining ileum adapts.[124] Of interest, subtotal colectomy causes compensatory hyperplasia both in the ileum and the distal rectum.[130-132] Possibly, this adaptive change in the ileum after partial colectomy compensates for the loss of colonic function because cecectomy causes little effect on the remaining colon unless the terminal ileum is also resected.[133]

In humans, adaptive changes have been shown to occur after resection or exclusion of the colon. Within the first few weeks after colectomy, the height of the villi in terminal ileum is increased, the absorption by ileal mucosa is increased, and ileostomy fluid output is reduced.[134] Exclusion of the distal colon from the fecal stream by a colostomy causes hypoplasia of distal colonic mucosa. Subsequent closure of the colostomy induces a burst of the cell proliferative activity in crypts of the previously excluded mucosa.[135] Ultimately, the mucosa returns to normal. Thus, the diarrhea that often occurs in such patients after reanastomosis of colonic segments probably reflects impaired mucosal absorptive function in the distal segment induced by exclusion of the epithelium from normal colonic contents. The diarrhea is usually temporary, and it is assumed that the gradual improvement reflects an adaptive response after reanastomosis.[136]

Mechanisms Causing the Adaptive Change

A number of experiments suggest that complex mechanisms control the adaptive changes in epithelial morphology after resection. When a segment of distal ileum with intact nerve and blood supply is surgically inserted into the proximal jejunum, the villi increase in size to resemble those of the adjacent jejunum.[121] If the ampulla of Vater with intact biliary and pancreatic secretions is transposed into the distal ileum, the ileal villi are then transformed to resemble jejunal villi.[4] These results suggest a role in the adaptive response for substances in the intestinal lumen that reach the upper intestinal mucosa first, such as the diet and salivary, gastric, pancreatic, and biliary secretions. If a segment of jejunum or ileum is entirely removed from contact with these luminal contents and formed into a Thiry-Vella fistula, the mucosal villi undergo atrophy.[124,137] This supports an important role for the mere presence of luminal contents in maintaining normal villous morphology. In contrast, if extensive resection of the intestine remaining in continuity is performed in the animals with a Thiry-Vella fistula, the villi in the excluded intestine undergo a normal adaptive response, increase in size and develop a morphology similar to that of the remaining functionally intact intestine.[138,139] This observation suggests that some systemic or humoral factor also plays an important role in small bowel adaptation. A consideration of the mechanisms postulated to be responsible for causing the adaptive response is thus conveniently divided into evidence supporting roles for luminal nutrition, for pancreatic and/or biliary secretions, for hormonal factors, and for other possible contributors such as blood flow and innervation.

Role of Luminal Nutrients

Epithelia of the duodenum and jejunum normally are exposed to high concentrations of luminal nutrients following a meal. Thus, it should not be surprising that withdrawal of this nutrient exposure has an adverse effect on mucosal structure and function. Restriction of food intake orally, or maintenance of total nutrition by only a parenteral route rapidly reduces both the number and migration of proliferating enterocytes.[140,141] The mucosa becomes hypoplastic and the individual epithelial cells become hypermature.[142] As mentioned previously, surgical bypass of a segment of jejunum stimulates growth of villi in the ileum that then receives nutrients first. The jejunal mucosa, which is no longer exposed to luminal nutrients, becomes hypoplastic with shorter villi, diminished absorption, and reduced mucosal enzyme activity per length of intestine as compared to normal.[143] Thus, when oral delivery of nutrients to the proximal intestine is stopped or bypassed, the jejunal mucosa is affected the most, and the hypoplastic changes that follow result in loss of the normal jejunoileal gradient of villous height and absorptive surface. The process can be reversed by refeeding or by reestablishing intestinal continuity.[144]

Experimentally, if nutrients are infused directly into bypassed proximal intestine, postoperative hypoplasia can be prevented. Much study has been directed at determining precisely which nutrient or combination of nutrients is responsible for mucosal growth and prevention of hypoplasia. Infusion of glucose, galactose, and various amino acids, which are actively transported and possibly metabolized by the mucosa, all are effective in preventing hypoplasia in self-emptying loops.[145,146] A similar effect can be shown by infusion of specific nutrients into the ileum of animals with jejunal resection that are maintained on total parenteral nutrition.[147] The effect of these nutrients on the adaptive response does not seem to result from mucosal metabolism of the infused substance, because both galactose and 3-0 methyl-glucose, which are actively absorbed but not metabolized in the mucosa, also stimulate mucosal hyperplasia.[147] Even substances that are not actively absorbed but cross the epithelium by facilitated transport or move with bulk water flow, such as mannose and mannitol, also stimulate mucosal growth. Thus, it is not clear whether active mucosal transport, mucosal metabolism, or some other parameter related to the absorption of individual nutrients plays a role in the adaptive hyperplasia. Of all the individual nutrients that have been studied, long-chain fatty acids seem to have the greatest stimulating effect on the mucosal adaptive response. For example, in jejunectomized rats, when only 20% of the total caloric requirement was provided intragastrically as long-chain triglyceride, the structure and function of remaining small intestine was maintained intact and similar to that seen in normal rats fed a whole diet.[148] Thus, the exact mechanism by which luminal nutrition affects mucosal growth and adaptation in the small intestine is unknown, appears to vary with the specific nutrients and may even be different in the jejunum versus the ileum.

Exclusion of luminal nutrition also causes hypoplasia in the colonic mucosa, with associated prolongation of the crypt cell cycle.[135,140] Reapplication of luminal nutrients as well as of simple mechanical distention of the colon by intestinal bulk reverses the changes induced by withdrawal of luminal nutrition.[121,149]

In contrast to the mucosal hypoplasia caused by nutrient exclusion, hyperphagia induces hyperplasia of intestinal villi. Hyperphagia is associated with increased growth of the intestine in a number of experimental conditions including hyperthyroidism, hypothermia, diabetes mellitus, and lactation.[33] The mechanism for this response appears to be complex and may involve humoral factors as well as increased luminal nutrition.

As a group, the aforementioned observations support the concept that some factor related to intraluminal nutrition affects mucosal growth. Also, the normal morphologic differences between jejunal and ileal mucosa seem to result in part from the fact that nutrients normally reach the proximal intestine first, and in higher concentrations. Thus, in order for adaptive development to occur after small bowel resection, nutrition must be provided to the remaining intestine by a luminal route. Total parenteral nutrition alone abolishes post-resectional mucosal hyperplasia.[150,151] In contrast, similar nutritional support administered as a liquid elemental diet taken by mouth induces normal small bowel adaptive change.[152] Such chemically defined oral feedings, however, may not protect the colonic mucosa from undergoing hypoplasia because there is generally complete absorption of the elemental nutrients in the small bowel and also lack of intraluminal bulk.[153,154] Thus, after resection of the small intestine for inflammatory bowel disease or another cause, it is important to begin oral nutrition as soon as possible to maximize early adaptive changes in the remaining intestinal mucosa.

Role of Pancreaticobiliary Secretions

The possible importance of pancreatic or biliary secretions in stimulating mucosal growth and adaptive change was first suggested by experiments in which the site of entry of these secretions into the lumen was changed by transposing the ampulla of Vater to self-emptying loops of ileum.[155] This resulted in growth of the ileal villi to resemble those in the jejunum normally adjacent to the ampullary orifice. Also, introduction of preharvested pancreatic secretions into the ileal loops had the same effect on villous growth as did endogenous stimulation of pancreatic secretion by a meal. The consequences of deprivation of proximal intestinal mucosa from pancreatic secretions is not settled, however, because both hypoplasia and some hyperplasia have been reported.[156,157]

The initial observation that pancreaticobiliary secretions caused growth of ileal mucosa led to a variety of experiments that confirmed the phenomenon and showed that these secretions also potentiate the adaptive response in ileum after jejunal resection. A number of studies have attempted to determine which, if either, of the two secretions is the important factor. The results showed that both pancreatic juice and bile are independently trophic to ileal mucosa.[156,158,159] One problem with most of these studies has been the fact that the high protein content, especially in pancreatic secretions, may itself serve as a source of luminal nutrition. The effect of pancreaticobiliary secretions in stimulating hyperplasia also does not appear to occur by way of improved digestion, because similar results were obtained when oral nutrition was provided as whole food or as a chemically defined elemental diet.[158] Thus, the exact mechanism for potentiation of mucosal growth by pancreaticobiliary secretions still remains unclear. Nevertheless, these secretions appear to play an important contributory role to the adaptive response.

Hormones and Polyamines as Factors in Intestinal Adaptation

Both exogenous and endogenous hormones and peptides have been extensively examined as candidates for a role as an enterotropin. Gastrin, cholecystokinin, secretin, pancreatic glucagon and enteroglucagon, growth hormone, prolactin, thyroid hormone, and corticosteroids are only a few that have been studied in detail.[160] Much attention was initially focused on gastrin because it is known to have a trophic effect on the stomach, duodenum, and colon. Gastrin levels in blood initially were reported as being increased following small bowel resection.[161] Subsequent reports, however, did not confirm this and also cast doubt on the existence of any significant role for gastrin.[162] For example, several studies failed to find any evidence for a trophic effect of exogenously administered gastrin on jejunal or ileal mucosa of fed animals.[154,163] Induced alterations in endogenous secretion of gastrin also had no effect on causing mucosal growth.[164] Moreover, hyperplasia of mucosa in the jejunum and ileum is not seen as part of the Zollinger-Ellison syndrome, which shows an excess of gastrin and a trophic response of gastric mucosa. Thus, the bulk of current information does not support a primary role for gastrin in causing adaptive intestinal hyperplasia after small bowel resection.

Secretin that inhibits the trophic effects of gastrin on the stomach appears to have no significant effect on the growth of intestinal mucosa.[165] Exogenous cholecystokinin alone also does not produce a trophic effect, at least on the duodenal mucosa.[161] Administration of both secretin and cholecystokinin, however, prevents intestinal mucosal hypoplasia associated with total parenteral nutrition.[166] Hypoplasia of the pancreas also occurs with prolonged total parenteral nutrition, and both cholecystokinin and secretin stimulate pancreatic growth.[129] It is of interest that partially administered cholecystokinin octapeptide stimulates pancreatic growth but has little effect on the morphology of intestinal mucosa.[167] Thus, it is conceivable that secretin and cholecystokinin play an indirect role in maintaining small bowel mucosal structure and function by promoting normal pancreatic growth and by stimulating secretion of pancreatic enzymes, protein, and, possibly, growth factors.

The hypoplasia of small intestinal mucosa that follows hypophysectomy can be prevented in part by replacing the individual hormones removed, for example, growth hormone, ACTH, TSH, and prolactin.[168] The response to the first three appears to be primarily related to the fact that these hormones stimulate food intake and not to a specific effect of the hormone itself on the mucosa, however. Prolactin has a trophic effect on a variety of tissues; however, studies in rats showed no evidence that prolactin causes hyperplasia of intestinal mucosa in normal rats or that the hormone plays any role in intestinal adaptation after small bowel resection.[169]

Oral glucocorticoids, such as prednisolone, have little effect on intestinal morphology or cell kinetics in normal or resected intestine.[170] Corticosteroids do enhance the maximum absorptive capacity of the mucosa, however. This effect occurred mainly by an increase in carrier-mediated transport without a change in number of the epithelial cell population. Treatment with prednisolone led to an increase in synthesis of brush border proteins and to enhanced glycoprotein content of the microvillous membrane. Following jejunal resection, short-term treatment with prednisolone enhanced the effects of adaptive hyperplasia on intestinal absorption by maximizing the functional capacity of the remaining epithelial cells.[171] Whether this effect is significant enough to justify corticosteroid administration to humans after intestinal resection has not been sufficiently studied.

Enteroglucagon is the strongest current candidate for a hormone that plays a major role in causing mucosal adaptation and hyperplasia after intestinal resection. The recent focus on enteroglucagon resulted from studies in a patient with an enteroglucagon-secreting tumor of the right kidney who was found to have dilatation of the small intestine, villous hyperplasia, and high blood levels of enteroglucagon. All of these abnormalities normalized when the tumor was removed.[172] Subsequent analysis of the tumor tissue showed it to contain gut-derived rather than pancreatic-derived glucagon.[173] The highest concentrations of enteroglucagon are normally found in mucosa of the terminal ileum. Significant but somewhat smaller concentrations of enteroglucagon are also present in the colonic mucosa.[174] Enteroglucagon is released from the mucosae of the small and large intestine by the presence of fat and carbohydrate.[175] Accordingly, malabsorption consequent to proximal intestinal resection or mucosal disease would allow these nutrients to reach ileal and colonic mucosa in higher than normal concentrations. Indeed, increased concentrations of enteroglucagon in blood have been reported in patients with intestinal bypass for obesity, proximal intestinal resection, and also active sprue, all of whom had hyperplasia of more distal small intestinal mucosa.[176] This association does not necessarily prove a cause and effect relationship between elevated blood enteroglucagon and intestinal mucosal hyperplasia. A number of observations do create compelling evidence to suggest that this indeed may be the case, however. First, a strong correlation exists between crypt cell production rate and the basal level of immunoreactive enteroglucagon in blood.[177] Also, manipulation of the level of enteroglucagon in blood by administering regulatory peptides that influence enteroglucagon release causes proportional changes in crypt cell production rate.[178] Somatostatin inhibits and bombesin stimulates release of enteroglucagon. In rats with a 75% proximal intestinal resection, somatostatin depressed plasma enteroglucagon levels and also diminished crypt cell proliferation. In contrast, administration of bombesin increased the plasma enteroglucagon concentration and was associated with a significant increase in crypt cell production.[178] Lastly, enteroglucagon cell hyperfunction has been demonstrated in the rat ileum after resection of the proximal small intestine.[179] Although the results of these studies suggest that a change in enteroglucagon level may influence intestinal adaptation, a prime effect of the regulating hormone on cell replication itself has not yet been excluded. Nevertheless, partially purified enteroglucagon has been reported to stimulate DNA synthesis in cultured jejunal mucosa.[180] Thus, enteroglucagon is currently the best candidate for a hormonal stimulator of the adaptive hyperplasia and mucosal growth that follows small bowel resection. It remains to be seen if exogenous administration of enteroglucagon can itself, in the absence of bowel resection, exert a hyperplastic effect on the intestinal mucosa.

Recently, interest has turned to the possibility that enteroglucagon or other trophic substances may have their final and common effect through modification of enzymes that regulate polyamine synthesis in intestinal mucosa. For years, it has been recognized that polyamines influence tissue growth.[181] Measurement of polyamines in the mucosa of small intestine shows a proximal to distal gradient, with polyamine concentration being greatest in the duodenum and least in the ileum.[182] The rate-limiting factor for synthesis of putracine, an important polyamine, is the enzyme ornithine decarboxylase (ODC). Although ODC is present in all tissues, almost 90% of the body stores are in the villi of the small intestine.[183] These facts suggest that ODC and polyamines may somehow play a role in the normal regulation of crypt cell and villous growth, and also in the adaptive response to intestinal resection. Indeed, changes in intestinal activity of ODC occur during the process of intestinal maturation and also during repair following mucosal injury.[184] Transient increases in ODC activity have been associated with the onset of adaptive mucosal hyperplasia.[185,186] It is conceivable that the aforementioned factors that appear to regulate mucosal adaptive response could operate by affecting ODC activity. For example, some peptide hormones that affect adaptive hyperplasia are known to increase the activity of ODC.[186] Also, following proximal intestinal resection or diversion of pancreaticobiliary secretions to the distal ileum, the polyamine content in ileal mucosa significantly increases.[182] When DMFO, a specific blocker of ODC activity, was given to a group of rats with pancreaticobiliary diversion to the ileum, the adaptive changes were inhibited.[182] In summary, preliminary data suggest that regulation of polyamine synthesis may be of primary importance in causing adaptive hyperplasia in the intestine. Factors that modify the adaptive response, such as luminal nutrients, pancreaticobiliary secretions and hormones may actually exert their trophic effects through modulation of polyamine synthesis. More information needs to be developed about this intriguing possibility.

Neurovascular Effects on the Adaptive Response

After adaptation has occurred, visual inspection of the hyperplastic segment of intestine clearly demonstrates that blood flow increases. The question of whether the increased blood flow occurred first or was consequent to the adaptive response has not been clearly answered, although preliminary reports suggest it may precede the increase in tissue mass.[187] Therefore, the ability to increase tissue blood flow could be an important factor limiting recovery of those individuals who undergo intestinal resection for ischemic disease.

Neural factors may also play a role in the adaptive response. Epinephrine inhibits mucosal mitosis, and beta-adrenergic blocking drugs can reverse this phenomenon.[188] Sympathectomy also inhibits cell proliferation and cholinergic drugs reportedly stimulate cell division.[189] Abdominal vagotomy leads to intestinal hypoplasia but with stimulated cell turnover.[190] Transection of the afferent fibers of the vagus nerve was shown in pigs to blunt the adaptive response of remaining intestine after partial small bowel resection.[191] Whether this reflects a primary neural response or one manifested by a change in other factors modified by vagotomy is unclear. For example, vagotomy blunts the postprandial rise in cholecystokinin and subsequent contraction of the gallbladder.[192]

It should be apparent from the previous discussion that intestinal adaptation is a complex situation, and that a variety of mechanisms have been invoked to explain the changes in intestinal morphology and function that occur following intestinal resection. It is hoped that a specific endogenous factor or factors will be identified that can be used to supplement or improve spontaneous adaptive changes. To date, however, none have emerged that can be tested in clinical situations. At the current time, early institution of oral nutrition, with chemically defined diets as a supplement to total parenteral nutrition, remains the best way to stimulate endogenous adaptive mechanisms in patients with extensive small bowel resection.

Functional Status of the Remaining Intestine and Other Digestive Organs

The functional status of the remaining intestine, as well as that of other digestive organs can be critically important in determining the course and overall outcome of extensive small bowel resection. Persisting foci of inflammatory bowel disease, the presence of other intestinal disorders such as sprue, radiation enteritis, or idiopathic pseudo-obstruction can significantly impair the absorptive function in the remaining intestine. Unfortunately, the presence of intestinal disease may be first suspected during clinical evaluation of an unexplained absorptive defect: for example, iron malabsorption in a patient with resection of only the distal ileum. The best example is probably preexisting disaccharidase deficiency, especially lactase deficiency. This can significantly magnify clinical problems with diarrhea and excess flatus from carbohydrate malabsorption induced by resection of the mid small intestine.

Diseases of the stomach that complicate small bowel resection are generally related to gastric acid hypersecretion and the consequences of vagotomy with intestinal drainage for peptic ulcer. Excess acid secretion may develop during the early days after extensive small bowel resection. This is discussed later in more detail. Acute peptic ulcer disease, hypovolemia alkalosis, and hypokalemia can result, unless the excess gastric secretion is controlled by administering histamine-2 receptor blocking drugs such as ranitidine and cimetidine. With the availability of these drugs to control gastric secretion, acute peptic ulcer disease following small intestinal resection is now much less a problem than in the past.

Gastric surgical intervention for peptic ulcer disease should be avoided if possible in patients with extensive intestinal resection because intestinal absorption and nutritional status may be impaired. Gastric resection and vagotomy may worsen steatorrhea by decreasing gastric emulsification of fat and by promoting rapid passage of luminal contents through the intestine without adequate mixing with digestive enzymes or contact time with intestinal mucosa. A similar admonition holds for removal of the gallbladder in patients with extensive small bowel resection. As discussed below, the frequency of cholesterol gallstones is increased in patients with Crohn's disease and ileal resection. In these individuals, the normal enterohepatic circulation of bile acid is sufficiently interrupted to cause a reduction in size of the bile acid pool. Obviously, gallstones are only one consequence of a reduced bile acid pool. Impaired reabsorption of bile salts in the ileum leads to a progressive decrease in the amount of bile salts delivered into the upper intestine after each meal. Late in the day, the concentration of bile salt in the duodenum may fall below the critical micellar concentration, and fat malabsorption results.[193] Patients with this situation are best able to absorb fat in meals consumed early in the day because the gallbladder forms an important reservoir for storage of bile acids synthesized overnight. Simply rearranging nutrient intake so that breakfast is the major meal of the day helps maximize intestinal absorption and often leads to weight gain. When cholecystectomy is performed, the patient loses the overnight bile salt reservoir. Absorption of dietary lipids is impaired because bile salts secreted overnight are directly emptied into the intestine, passing into the distal intestine before arrival of the ingested meal. It is not uncommon for patients with ileal resection or disease to lose weight after cholecystectomy because of this change in fat absorption. Consequently, the gallbladder should not be removed unless acute cholecystitis or recurrent severe biliary colic is present.

Functional pancreatic insufficiency can occur in patients with short bowel syndrome because of either protein malnutrition associated with malabsorption, diminished mucosal release of cholecystokinin-pancreazymin consequent to resection of the proximal intestine, or, possibly, interruption of the enteropancreatic circulation of pancreatic enzymes thought to play a regulatory role in maintaining adequacy of enzyme secretion.[194,195] Accordingly, patients with preexisting pancreatic insufficiency would be expected to have their nutritional problems or malabsorption symptoms magnified by an extensive intestinal resection. A similar deleterious effect of coexisting chronic liver disease might also be predicted. Significant malabsorption of peptides and amino acids can further impair hepatic protein synthesis. Malabsorption of other nutrients, such as the fat soluble vitamins, may magnify defects in hepatic synthesis, such as the effect of vitamin K malabsorption on hepatic synthesis of coagulation factors. Disease of the colonic mucosa can impair its important role in absorption of water and electrolytes, as discussed in the section on preservation of the ileocecal valve and colon. Problems with diarrhea and water balance are magnified in those patients with small bowel resection who, for various reasons, later undergo a colostomy. Clearly, preservation of as much intact and functioning colon as possible should be a surgical goal in any patient undergoing resection of the small intestine.

Specific Syndromes Associated with Intestinal Resection

Gastric Hypersecretion

Gastric hypersecretion has been reported in approximately half the patients with extensive small bowel resection and usually begins within 24 hours after surgical treatment.[196,197] Both fasting and meal-stimulated levels of gastrin in blood may be elevated in the post-operative period. Although the increased level of circulating gastrin and gastric acid secretion is usually of short duration, the abnormality can persist for months or even years.[198] The degree of gastric hypersecretion roughly correlates with the length of small intestine resected. No real factor has been identified that is related to resolution or persistence of the abnormality.

Gastric hypersecretion after intestinal resection has been produced in a variety of experimental animal models. Morphologically, a hyperplastic response occurs in the gastric mucosa, characterized by an increase in the number of parietal, chief, and mucous cells.[199] The increase in chief and mucous cells suggest that the hyperplastic response may result from factors other than only gastrin. Based on the obtained data, several explanations for the phenomenon have been advanced; however, all involve a mechanism leading to increased levels of gastrin. First, the small intestine normally removes a significant amount of gastrin from the circulation.[200,201] As a consequence of bowel resection, intestinal catabolism of gastrin is diminished and gastrin levels in blood rise. An alternative possibility is that intestinal resection leads to loss of an inhibitor of gastrin release. This is supported in part by the observation that gastric acid output is reduced if antrectomy precedes the bowel resection. Unfortunately, little is known about changes after intestinal resection in the plasma levels of inhibitory substances, such as somatostatin and gastric inhibitory polypeptide (GIP). Both of these hormones suppress gastric acid secretion and a reduction in their levels following surgical treatment of the bowel could explain acid hypersecretion. Of note, just the opposite was found in one study, where a 50% small bowel resection in the rhesus monkey was followed by an elevation of blood levels of GIP.[202]

It is important to be aware that gastric acid hypersecretion is a potential consequence of extensive small bowel resection in order to avoid serious consequences. When hypersecretion occurs, the large volume of hydrogen ions and water entering the upper intestine may cause acute peptic ulceration of the duodenum and also facilitate breakdown of the small bowel anastomosis with formation of fistulas. Routine postoperative nasogastric suction will demonstrate the excessive fluid volume. Unless gastric secretion is controlled by intravenous administration of histamine-2 receptor blocking drugs (cimetidine or ranitidine) and careful fluid and electrolyte balance is maintained, the patient may also rapidly develop hypovolemia, alkalosis, and hypokalemia.

The effects of excess gastric acid on intraluminal digestion and, consequently, on nutrition are similar to those seen with the Zollinger-Ellison syndrome. The excess hydrogen ion causes damage to the intestinal epithelium, precipitation of bile salts in the proximal bowel, and inactivation of pancreatic lipase.[37] The resultant malabsorption may be severe, especially in patients with ileal resection who have an additional cause for bile acid depletion. A number of reports have shown that the control of gastric acid secretion by histamine-2 receptor blocking drugs leads to increased solubility of bile acids in the intestinal lumen, improved fat absorption and consequently, reduced steatorrhea.[203,204] Thus, patients with severe steatorrhea following extensive bowel resection should be evaluated for gastric acid hypersecretion, even if many months have elapsed since the operation.

D-lactic Acidosis

A few patients with short bowel syndrome have been described who developed a sudden onset of an acute neurologic syndrome characterized by ataxia, dysarthria, and confusion. This illness is accompanied by a hyperchloremic metabolic acidosis, an excessive anion gap in the blood, and increased concentrations of D-lactate in the blood and urine.[205,206] This syndrome has also been observed in patients following a jejunoileal bypass for obesity.[207] The disorder results from an accumulation of D-lactate that is an isomer of the ubiquitous L-lactate, a normal product of anaerobic metabolism. The mechanism for D-lactic acidosis appears to be the production of large amounts of D-lactate by colonic bacteria from malabsorbed carbohydrate.[208] Colonic bacteria metabolize simple sugars to pyruvate by the anaerobic glycolytic pathway and both isomers of lactic acid are produced. The resulting decrease in fecal pH inhibits the growth of the normal flora and favors emergence of acid-resistant bacteria that produce D-lactate. These include Bifidobacterium, Lactobacillus, and Eubacterium. Stools from patients with D-lactic acidosis and short bowel syndrome have been shown to have an increased content of these bacteria.[205,207] Absorbed L-lactate is rapidly metabolized by L-lactate dehydrogenase. The D-lactate cannot be metabolized and contributes to development of the acidosis.

Several pitfalls may make diagnosis of the condition difficult. Conventional laboratory tests for lactate may measure only the L-isomer. Thus, patients with this disorder may have normal blood and urine levels of L-lactate. Therefore, a specific test for total lactate or for the D-isomer must be used. Secondly, the hyperchloremia that is often present may give rise to a lower anion gap in serum than would be predicted from the concentrations of D-lactate in blood.[208] Thus, a high degree of clinical suspicion for the disorder is probably the most helpful factor in leading to an early diagnosis. The exact cause for the encephalopathy with D-lactic acidosis is unclear, but it may be related to an abnormality or deficiency in brain metabolism of pyruvate.[208]

Treatment should be instituted by attempting to decrease production of D-lactate by the colonic bacteria. Reportedly this can be achieved both by reducing the carbohydrate intake in the diet, and by administering a broad spectrum antibiotic for 10 to 14 days to change the intestinal bacterial flora.[205] One should also make sure the intake of vitamins, trace elements, and, especially, thiamine is adequate. The latter is possibly of practical importance because the encephalopathy is similar to that seen with other acquired disorders of pyruvate metabolism, including primary thiamine deficiency, or that secondary to severe alcoholism.[208]

Interruption of Bile Salt Enterohepatic Circulation

Interruption of the bile salt enterohepatic circulation by ileal resection can produce a variety of clinical syndromes. These result either from the effects of excess, malabsorbed bile acid on the colon, or from an inadequate amount of bile salts in the enterohepatic circulation. The clinical consequences that result are diarrhea, impaired absorption of dietary lipid, and enhanced formation of gallbladder and kidney stones. Effective treatment is available for each and is based on our current understanding of alterations in intestinal physiology induced by ileal resection or disease.

Cholerrheic and Steatorrheic Diarrhea

Resection of the distal ileum causes diarrhea by at least two mechanisms. They should be differentiated clinically because control of symptoms requires separate forms of therapy. Bile salts that are not reabsorbed into the enterohepatic circulation cause water secretion by the colonic mucosa.[109] This fluid, along with secreted mucus, contributes to normal stool consistency and facilitates passage by the colon. Reduced entry of bile acids into the colon as occurs in chronic cholestasis is often associated with constipation. In the opposite circumstance in which excessive amounts of bile salt enter the colon, diarrhea can result.[36] The dihydroxy bile acids, deoxycholic, and chenodeoxycholic (chenic) acids increase the permeability of the colonic mucosa, thereby impairing net absorption of ions and water.[209] When these bile acids are present in the aqueous phase of colon contents in concentrations above approximately 3mM, they also stimulate net secretion of chloride by the epithelium, an effect that may be mediated by increased mucosal content of cyclic AMP.[210] Accompanying net ion secretion is a net movement of water into the bowel lumen. If the luminal flux of ions and water is sufficiently large, the absorptive capacity of the mucosa is overwhelmed and diarrhea results.

Conjugated bile salts are normally absorbed by an active transport mechanism in the distal ileum. Following resection of the ileum, this function is not replaced by an adaptive change in the more proximal jejunum,[33,129] and the extent of the resection directly correlates with the degree of interruption of the bile salt enterohepatic circulation. Two consequences of this are an increased delivery of bile salts into the colon and a decreased return of bile salt to the liver. Each of these plays an important role in determining the clinical response to ileal resection. Short ileal resections, such as 25 cm or less, may cause no symptoms, because most bile salts are reabsorbed and the effects on colonic mucosa of those that are malabsorbed are not sufficient to overwhelm normal colon absorptive function. When a larger amount of ileum is removed, however, increased amounts of bile salts are malabsorbed and enter the colon. Malabsorbed cholate and chenodeoxycholate are normally deconjugated and dehydroxylated by colonic bacteria to form deoxycholic and lithocholic acids respectively. These secondary bile acids, especially lithocholic acid, precipitate from solution at the alkaline pH of colon contents. When the amount of bile acids entering the colon becomes excessive, however, bacterial dehydroxylation of chenodeoxycholic acid may be incomplete, and excessive amounts of this dihydroxy primary bile acid remain in fecal water.[36] Moreover, the pH of colonic contents may also become more acidic, secondary to malabsorbed carbohydrate and fatty acids. In this situation, the reduced pH favors increased solubility both of chenodeoxycholic and deoxycholic acids.[211] The net result is enhanced bile acid interaction with the colonic mucosa and, accordingly, increased mucosal secretion and diarrhea, as already discussed. This condition has been called cholerrheic enteropathy.[212] Because it results from the increased presence of bile acid in fecal water, it often can be effectively managed by oral administration of anion exchange resins such as cholestyramine and colestipol that bind bile acids and decrease their activity in fecal water below a point where the effect on mucosal permeability and secretion is no longer significant.[36] Although these resins often produce spectacular control of diarrhea in patients with short ileal resections, a number of potential clinical problems may develop. Too much or prolonged administration of the resin can result in constipation. Thus, the dose should be titrated and also periodically reduced or discontinued as daily treatment is often not necessary. Secondly, the concentration of bile acids in the proximal intestine will be reduced by large amounts of the resin. If the concentration of bile salts in the upper intestine is already low because of the ileal malabsorption, the additional sequestration of bile salts by the resin may significantly worsen fat absorption. Lastly, the resins exchange chloride for bile acid and most of the chloride is absorbed. If renal failure is present, hyperchloremic acidosis may develop.[213,214]

The second mechanism causing diarrhea occurs in patients with an extensive resection of the ileum, usually 100 cm or greater, and is caused by malabsorption of fat. The bile acid pool normally cycles through the enterohepatic circulation two or three times with each meal. When there has been extensive resection of the terminal ileum, a large fraction of the bile salt pool is malabsorbed with each cycle. This leads to progressive depletion of the pool throughout the day. As already discussed, after an overnight fast the concentration of bile salts in the duodenum and the jejunum may facilitate normal fat absorption, because the liver has had almost 12 hours after the last meal to synthesize and secrete bile acid for storage in the gallbladder. With subsequent meals, however, the bile salt pool is depleted by malabsorption and the concentration of bile salts in the proximal intestine may fall below the critical micellar concentration, causing significant steatorrhea. In this circumstance, one might be tempted to use orally administered bile salts to improve fat absorption. Such oral supplementation could briefly increase the concentration of bile salts in the upper intestine; however, the quantity of bile salts entering the colon would also be increased and the effect would be significant diarrhea. Thus, oral bile salt supplements should not be used in such patients. If the patient has an ileostomy, however, the effect of bile acids on the colon would not be of concern. At least one patient with extensive ileal resection, an ileostomy, and severe malabsorption has been reported in whom oral bile salt supplements improved steatorrhea without a significant increase in ileostomy fluid output.[215]

In the absence of adequate intraluminal bile salts, hydrolysis of dietary fat by pancreatic enzymes proceeds normally, but the products of lipolysis cannot be transported normally in aqueous intestinal contents to the mucosa for absorption. The result is severe fat malabsorption. Patients with extensive ileal resection generally excrete more than 15 to 20 grams of fat daily in the stool. The concentration of bile acids in fecal water is low, because of both depletion of the bile salt pool and precipitation of bile acid from fecal water.[211] In this circumstance, diarrhea is caused by either malabsorbed osmotically active substances, such as carbohydrates, or more likely by fatty acids and their hydroxylated metabolites formed by colonic bacteria.[111] Similar to the effect of dihydroxy bile salts on colonic mucosa but more potent in effect, hydroxy fatty acids cause increased permeability of colonic mucosa and stimulate net electrolyte secretion and water movement into the lumen.[216,217] Thus, the mechanism for diarrhea occurring after resection of greater than 100 cm of ileum relates to malabsorption of fat and not bile acids.[36,212] Accordingly, treatment of such patients with cholestyramine would not be anticipated to be of benefit. Instead, treatment should proceed by reducing both the amount of malabsorbed, osmotically active carbohydrate, and by strict adherence to a low fat diet (20 to 40 g/day). If restriction of dietary fat is not sufficient to control the steatorrheic diarrhea or if weight loss ensues, one can substitute medium-chain triglyceride for a portion of normal long-chain triglyceride in the diet.[36,218,219] Medium-chain triglycerides do not require bile salt micelles for absorption in the proximal intestine. Their use in the diet will decrease steatorrhea and thereby the amount of hydroxy fatty acids in the colon. Diarrhea is usually improved. Other beneficial effects include improved absorption of calories, of fat soluble vitamins, and of cations such as magnesium, calcium, and zinc.

Cholesterol Gallstones

Patients with ileal disease or resection have an increased prevalence of gallstones.[220,221] The pathogenesis of gallstone disease is complex and has been extensively reviewed elsewhere.[222] The cause for increased gallstone formation in patients with ileal resection or disease appears to be primarily a reduction in size of the bile salt pool consequent to excessive bile acid loss into stool.[223] Reduction in size of the bile-salt pool can lead to diminished hepatic bile salt secretion. Because cholesterol secretion into bile is not commensurately reduced, hepatic bile becomes supersaturated with cholesterol, or "lithogenic".[224] As a consequence, cholesterol crystals form, nucleate, and grow to form cholesterol gallstones.

Two concerns should be mentioned regarding the treatment of gallstones in this specific group of patients. First, one should strongly consider not recommending elective cholecystectomy merely for the presence of stones, because removal of the gallbladder may cause significant worsening of malabsorption and of the patient's nutritional status. The mechanism for this has already been discussed.

Secondly, it is now possible to dissolve cholesterol gallstones in some patients by oral administration of chenodeoxycholic or ursodeoxycholic acid. Administration of large amounts of chenodeoxycholic acid to patients with ileal resection would be unwise, as previously discussed, because it would cause significant diarrhea. In contrast, ursodeoxycholic acid does not stimulate water secretion by the colonic mucosa or enhance its permeability to the same degree as chenodeoxycholic acid.[209] Although oral administration of ursodeoxycholic acid conceptually might be useful in dissolving cholesterol gallstones in some patients with a short ileal resection, no clinical experience or evidence of its efficacy in this specific situation has been reported.

Enhanced Formation of Kidney Stones

For more than 20 years, it has been recognized that up to 10% of patients with inflammatory bowel disease develop renal stones.[225] This incidence is in dramatic contrast to the 0.1% incidence found for the general population.[226] Moreover, those patients who have had their inflammatory bowel disease treated surgically have the highest incidence of nephrolithiasis.[225] Two different types of renal stones predominate, and each tends to occur in a clinical setting with different contributing factors. Medical management for each, especially to prevent recurrence, is based on correcting underlying abnormalities in intestinal absorption and in urine composition that promote abnormal crystal formation and growth. When the activity of various ions in urine exceeds their formation product for crystallization, insoluble salt crystals may develop. Various substances, such as magnesium and citrate, stabilize urine and prevent crystal formation and precipitation. Thus, whether or not renal stone formation occurs depends on a number of factors including the degree of saturation of urine by individual ions and the presence of substances that promote or inhibit crystal formation, growth, and macroaggregation. These factors have been reviewed in detail elsewhere.[227] Patients with ulcerative colitis, chronic diarrhea, and especially those with an ileostomy, have a tendency to form uric acid stones. In contrast, patients with regional enteritis, especially after extensive resection of the distal ileum sufficient to cause steatorrhea, may form calcium oxalate renal stones. Because the pathophysiology causing formation of the two stone types is different, they will be discussed separately.

URIC ACID STONES

The incidence of uric acid kidney stones is increased in patients with ulcerative colitis as well as in those with any type of chronic diarrhea. Three factors that predispose to the formation of uric acid renal stones are the increased excretion of uric acid in urine, an increased concentration of the urine, and a persistently low urinary pH. Patients who have chronic ulcerative colitis, an ileostomy, or an extensive small intestinal resection or bypass do not necessarily excrete increased amounts of uric acid in the urine. The loss of water, sodium, and bicarbonate in the stool is increased, however, especially in the ileostomy patients. As a consequence, the urinary pH is almost always low (5 to 5.5), the volume is reduced and the concentration of uric acid is increased. Because the pKa of uric acid is 5.42, much of the urinary urate will be present as the protonated, poorly soluble acid form rather than the salt. The solubility of uric acid in urine is almost 12 times less at pH 5 than it is at pH 7. Thus, the concentrated, acid urine often produced by these patients predisposes to crystallization and formation of uric acid stones. The coexistence of a chronic urinary tract infection, a structural abnormality causing stasis, or an increase in urine calcium or urate itself further enhances the tendency to stone formation.

Treatment of patients with intestinal disease and uric acid renal stones has been discussed in detail elsewhere.[228] Briefly, any recovered stone should be analyzed precisely to determine its composition. If it is mostly uric acid, initial therapy in patients with chronic diarrhea should be directed towards correcting the abnormality in urine volume and acidity while excluding chronic urinary tract infection and obstruction. Oral hydration should be increased to produce a urine volume of 1500 to 2000ml/day. A persistently acid urine pH can be corrected by oral administration of a potassium/sodium citrate mixture such as Polycitra.* Urine pH should be increased to at least 6 or greater in order to maximize uric acid solubility. Sodium bicarbonate can also be used and certainly will alkalinize the urine. The excess sodium, however, along with increased alkalinity, may enhance the risk of forming calcium stones.[229] If the 24-hour urinary excretion of uric acid is increased, allopurinol should be added to the treatment program.

Some evidence exists that the formation of uric acid crystals may be an important factor in enhancing nucleation and growth of oxalate crystals in the early stages of calcium oxalate stone formation.[230] Thus, in the subsequent discussion regarding hyperoxaluria and calcium oxalate nephrolithiasis, it should be kept in mind that the urinary concentration of uric acid and also the urinary pH may require specific evaluation and treatment as well as factors specifically related to oxalate.

CALCIUM OXALATE STONES

The most common type of kidney stone found in the United States is composed mainly of calcium

* Willen Drug Co., Baltimore, MD 21202.

oxalate; however, most persons who form calcium oxalate stones have no abnormality in oxalate metabolism and do not excrete increased amounts of oxalate in urine. Thus, the pathogenesis of oxalate renal stones is usually related to an abnormality of oxalate solubility in urine. In contrast, two patient groups with abnormal gastrointestinal function have increased formation of calcium oxalate renal stones caused by increased intestinal absorption and renal excretion of oxalate. They are patients with extensive ileal disease or resection, particularly from regional enteritis, and patients with jejunoileal bypass for obesity. The cause for increased nephrolithiasis appears to be hyperoxaluria combined with fluid and electrolyte depletion.[231] Other patients with various digestive diseases have increased intestinal absorption of oxalate and hyperoxaluria but do not appear excessively to form oxalate renal stones. They include persons with pancreatic insufficiency, with small bowel bacterial overgrowth, with sprue, or with hepatic cirrhosis. The common factor in all these conditions is fat malabsorption. The source of the excess urinary oxalate is preformed oxalate in the diet, although some evidence suggests that certain substances in food may be converted to oxalate in the intestine.[232]

Our current understanding of the mechanism responsible for excessive intestinal absorption of oxalate in the presence of malabsorption of other nutrients has evolved over the past 10 to 15 years. Two separate abnormalities contribute to the enhanced oxalate absorption. The first involves a change in oxalate solubility in intestinal water. Oxalic acid is a strong acid with a pKa_2 of 1.23 and pKa_2 of 4.14. Thus, at the pH of intestinal fluid and urine, oxalate is present mainly as a salt. Oxalic acid is only moderately soluble in water (8.7g/100ml at 20°C). It readily forms salts with a number of alkaline metal ions (Ca^{++}, K^+, Na^+ and Li^+) and also ferrous salts. The calcium salt, which is the one most commonly formed in the intestine, is almost insoluble in water (0.58mg/100ml at 18°C). At the pH of intestinal contents, the affinity of the carboxyl groups of oxalic acid is greater for calcium than other metal ions normally present. Accordingly, most dietary oxalate, liberated from its form in food by digestion, rapidly complexes with luminal calcium, precipitates from solution as calcium oxalate, and thus is unavailable for mucosal absorption. Normal persons absorb and excrete in urine about 6% or less of oxalate in the diet.[233] In contrast, patients with enteric hyperoxaluria absorb 30 to 40% or more, and this is excreted in urine.

The two most important factors that promote enhanced solubility of oxalate in the intestinal lumen are excessive amounts of malabsorbed fatty acids and a decrease in calcium ion activity. Like oxalic acid, fatty acids combine with calcium to form insoluble complexes; however, the affinity of calcium for fatty acids is greater than that for oxalic acid.[234] Therefore, when fatty acid malabsorption is large, formation of calcium soaps is excessive and it significantly reduces both calcium activity in intestinal water and the formation of calcium oxalate. More soluble salts of oxalate are formed, remain in solution and are absorbed by intestinal mucosa.

Normal intestinal absorption of dietary oxalate is thought to occur in the small intestine by a passive mechanism.[235] In contrast, studies both in rats and in humans have shown that the absorption of excessive oxalate in enteric hyperoxaluria occurs in the colon.[236,237] Recent investigations have demonstrated the presence of active, possibly chloride-like transport of oxalate across the colonic mucosa.[238] The magnitude of this active transport process, however, is probably small or insignificant in patients with enteric hyperoxaluria in comparison to the passive flux of soluble oxalate across colonic mucosa.

The second mechanism for enhanced intestinal absorption of food oxalate is an increase in the permeability of the colonic mucosa.[239] In vitro studies in rat and rabbit colonic mucosa, as well as in vivo studies in monkeys and in man, have convincingly demonstrated that dihydroxy bile salts (deoxycholate and chenodeoxycholate) and also hydroxy fatty acids (such as ricinoleic acid) increase the permeability of the colonic mucosa.[209] As a result, the flux of oxalate is increased across the mucosa down a concentration gradient from bowel lumen to blood. Obviously, the effects of increased colonic permeability on enhancing oxalate absorption becomes significant only when oxalate solubility in the colonic contents is increased by excess fatty acid and decreased calcium activity. This is reflected clinically by the fact that hyperoxaluria almost never occurs in patients with malabsorption unless the steatorrhea exceeds 12 to 15g/day.

Successful outpatient treatment and control of enteric hyperoxaluria is difficult. Foods that are high in oxalate should be excluded from the diet. Most reviews on treatment of enteric hyperoxaluria and standard food texts list the oxalate content of food;[228] however, the oxalate content of some common foods is not precisely known. This makes dietary restriction alone an inadequate way to achieve satisfactory control of urine oxalate excretion. The most important aspect of treatment is to control the severity of fat malabsorption. This can be achieved by prescribing a low-fat diet, by substituting medium-chain triglycerides for long-chain fat in the diet, and by providing pancreatic enzymes if pancreatic insufficiency is present. A combination of all three approaches is often necessary. The reduction in steatorrhea will decrease the effect of malabsorbed fatty acids on colon permeability. Reduced steatorrhea also presumably increases calcium activity in fecal water, and consequently decreases the solubility of oxalate, as already discussed. Thus, control of fat malabsorption itself may be all that is needed to "normalize" urine oxalate excretion. If urine oxalate excretion is not "normalized," cholestyramine resin may be added.[240] The beneficial effect of this resin may result both from its binding oxalate in the intestinal lumen and from its complexing with bile acids and fatty acids to prevent their effects on colonic permeability. One can also supplement the diet with large amounts of calcium (1-3g/day, elemental calcium) as the gluconate or lactate salt.[241] This increases calcium ion activity in fecal water and reduces oxalate solubility; however, the consequences of this approach to treatment must be closely monitored. Urinary calcium excretion often is low in patients with enteric hyperoxaluria, reflecting the diminished intestinal absorption of dietary calcium. Large supplements of calcium may be sufficiently absorbed to increase the amount of calcium excreted in the urine. Unless urinary oxalate excretion is "normalized" by the calcium treatment, the rise in the increase in urinary calcium may increase the risk of renal stone formation.[242] It is reasonable to recommend a diet containing up to 1000 mg of calcium daily for these patients. Supplementation of the diet with higher doses of calcium should be done with caution, however, and only after other methods of controlling urine oxalate have failed. During calcium treatment, urinary calcium and oxalate excretion should be monitored closely. Finally, the solubility of oxalate in urine is enhanced by the presence both of magnesium and citrate. Patients with malabsorption and steatorrhea have diminished intestinal absorption of citrate and increased renal tubular reabsorption of this organic acid.[243] Both situations contribute to low concentrations of citrate in urine. Urinary excretion of citrate may not be "normalized" completely even by dietary supplementations until any coexisting magnesium deficiency has been corrected.

In summary, patients with a variety of gastrointestinal diseases are at increased risk for development of renal stones. It is important to consider this possibility in routine evaluation and management. Such patients should have appropriate screening for the risk factors discussed, and when such are found, preventative treatment is indicated.

References

1. Underhill, B. M. L.: Intestinal length in man. Br. Med. J., 2:1243, 1955.
2. Backman, L., and Hollenberg, D.: Small intestinal length. An intraoperative study in obesity. Acta Chir. Scand. 140:57, 1974.
3. Cook, G. C., and Carruthers, R. H.: Reaction of human small intestine to an intraluminal tube and its importance in jejunal perfusion studies. Gut, 15:545, 1974.
4. Altmann, G. G., and Leblond, C. P.: Factors influencing villus size in the small intestine of adult rats as revealed by transposition of intestinal segments. Am. J. Anat., 127:15, 1970.
5. Borgstrom, B., Dahlquist, A., Lundh, G., and Sjovall, J.: Studies of intestinal digestion and absorption in the human. J. Clin. Invest., 36:1521, 1957.
6. MacGregor, I. L., Parent, J. A., and Meyer, J. H.: Gastric emptying of liquid meals and pancreatic and biliary secretion after subtotal gastrectomy or truncal vagotomy and pyloroplasty in man. Gastroenterology, 72:195, 1977.
7. Brunne, H., et al.: Gastric emptying and secretion of bile acids, cholesterol and pancreatic enzymes during digestion. Mayo Clin. Proc., 49:251, 1974.
8. DiMagno, E. P., Go, V. L. W., and Summerskill, W. H. J.: Impaired cholecystokinin-pancreozymin secretion, intraluminal dilution and maldigestion of fat in sprue. Gastroenterology, 63:25, 1972.
9. Rhodes, R. A., Tai, H. H., and Chey, W. Y.: Impairment of secretin release in celiac sprue. Am. J. Dig. Dis., 23:833, 1978.
10. Allan, J. G., Gerskowitch, V. P., and Russell, R. I.: The role of bile acids in the pathogenesis of post vagotomy diarrhoea. Br. J. Surg., 61:516, 1974.
11. Mayer, E. A., et al.: Gastric emptying and sieving of solid food and pancreatic and biliary secretion after solid meals in patients with truncal vagotomy plus antrectomy. Gastroenterology, 83:184, 1982.
12. Gray, G. M., and Santiago, N. A.: Disaccharide absorption in normal and diseased intestine. Gastroenterology, 51:489, 1969.
13. Richards, A. J., Concon, J. R., and Mallison, C. M.: Lactose intolerance following extensive intestinal resection. Br. J. Surg., 58:493, 1971.
14. Cockenek, W. J., Narczewska, B., and Gizegieluch, M.: Effect of massive proximal small bowel resection on intestinal sucrase and lactase activity in the rat. Digestion, 9:224, 1973.
15. Ravich, W. J., Bayless, T. M., and Thomas, M.: Fructose: Incomplete intestinal absorption in humans. Gastroenterology, 84:26, 1983.
16. Gray, G. M., and Ingelfinger, F. J.: Intestinal absorption of sucrose in man: interrelation of hydrolysis and monosaccharide product absorption. J. Clin. Invest., 45:388, 1966.
17. Kimmich, G. A.: Intestinal absorption of sugar. In Physiology of the Gastrointestinal Tract. Edited by L. R. Johnson. New York, Raven Press, 1981.
18. Bond, J. H., Currier, B. E., Buchwald, H., and Levitt, M. D.: Colonic conservation of malabsorbed carbohydrate. Gastroenterology, 78:444, 1980.
19. Stevens, C. E.: Physiological implications of microbial digestion in the large intestine of mammals: relation to dietary factors. Am. J. Clin. Nutr., 31:5161, 1978.
20. Arzenzio, R. A., Southworth, M., and Stevens, C. E.: Sites of organic acid production and absorption in the equine gastrointestinal tract. Am. J. Physiol., 226:1043, 1974.
21. Roediger, W. E. W.: Nutrition of the colonic mucosa. In Topics in Gastroenterology. Edited by S. C. Truelove, and C. P. Willoughby. London, Blackwell Scientific Publications, 1979.
22. Christopher, N. L., and Bayless, T. M.: Role of the small bowel and colon in lactose-induced diarrhea. Gastroenterology, 60:845, 1971.
23. Levitt, M. D., Lasser, R. B., Schwartz, J. S., and Bond, J. H.: Studies of a flatulent patient. N. Engl. J. Med., 295:260, 1976.
24. Adibi, S. A.: Intestinal phase of protein assimilation in man. Am. J. Clin. Nutr., 29:205, 1976.
25. Adibi, S. A.: The influence of molecular structure of neutral amino acids on their absorptive kinetics in the jejunum and ileum of human intestine in vivo. Gastroenterology, 56:903, 1969.
26. Matthews, D. M., and Adibi, S. A.: Peptide absorption. Gastroenterology, 71:151, 1976.
27. Silk, D. B. A., et al.: Functional differentiation of human jejunum and ileum: a comparison of the handling of glucose, peptide and amino acids. Gut, 15:444, 1974.
28. McCarthy, D. M., and Kim, Y. S.: Changes in sucrase, enterokinase and peptide hydrolase after intestinal resection. J. Clin. Invest., 52:942, 1973.
29. Earnest, D. L., and Hammerman, K.: Nitrogen balance during elemental diet treatment of patients with inflammatory bowel disease and steatorrhea. Gastroenterology, 74:1121, 1978.
30. Westergaard, H., and Dietschy, J. M.: The mechanism whereby bile acid micelles increase the rate of fatty acid and cholesterol uptake into the intestinal mucosal cell. J. Clin. Invest., 58:97, 1976.
31. Thompson, A. B. R., and Dietschy, J. M.: Intestinal lipid absorption: Major extracellular and intracellular events. In Physiology of the Gastrointestinal Tract. Edited by L. R. Johnson. New York, Raven Press, 1981.
32. Bach, A. C., and Babayan, V. K.: Medium chain triglycerides: An update. Am. J. Clin. Nutr., 36:950, 1982.
33. Williams, R. C. N.: Intestinal adaptation: structural, functional and cytokinetic changes. N. Engl. J. Med., 298:1393, 1978.
34. VanDeest, B. W., Fordtran, J. S., Morawski, S. G., and Wilson, J. D.: Bile salt and micellar fat concentration in proximal small bowel contents of ileectomy patients. J. Clin. Invest., 47:1314, 1968.
35. Krag, E., and Phillips, S. F.: Active and passive bile acid absorption in man. Perfusion studies of the ileum and jejunum. J. Clin. Invest., 53:1686, 1974.
36. Hofmann, A. F., and Poley, J. R.: Role of bile acid malabsorption in pathogenesis of diarrhea and steatorrhea in patients with ileal resection. Gastroenterology, 62:918, 1972.

37. Go, V. L. W., Poley, J. R., Hofmann, A. F., and Summerskill, D. M.: Disturbances in fat digestion induced by acidic jejunal pH due to gastric hypersecretion in man. Gastroenterology, 58:638, 1970.
38. Kim, Y. S., et al.: The role of altered bile acid metabolism in the steatorrhea of experimental blind loop. J. Clin. Invest., 45:956, 1966.
39. Issacs, P. E. T., and Kim, Y. S.: The contaminated small bowel syndrome. Am. J. Med., 67:1049, 1969.
40. Kenny, A. D.: Intestinal Calcium Absorption and its Regulation. Boca Raton, CRC Press, 1981.
41. Powell, L. W., and Halliday, J. W.: Iron absorption and overload. Clin. Gastroenterol., 10:707, 1981.
42. Fuh, S. M., Tasjian, A. A., and Matuso, N.: Pathogenesis of hypocalcemia in primary hypomagnesemia. J. Clin. Invest., 52:153, 1973.
43. Rude, R. K., Oldham, S. B., and Singer, F. R.: Functional hypoparathyroidism and parathyroid hormone end-organ resistance in human magnesium deficiency. Clin. Endocrinol., 5:209, 1976.
44. Muldowney, F. P., et al.: Parathormone-like effect of magnesium replenishment in steatorrhea. N. Engl. J. Med., 281:61, 1970.
45. Graham, L. A., Caesar, J. J., and Burger, A. S. V.: Gastrointestinal absorption and excretion of Mg_{28} in man. Metabolism, 9:646, 1960.
46. Tantibhedhyangkul, P., and Hashim, S. A.: Medium chain triglyceride feeding in premature infants: Effects on calcium and magnesium absorption. Pediatrics, 61:537, 1978.
47. Whang, R., et al: Magnesium depletion as a cause for refractory potassium repletion. Arch. Intern. Med., 145:1686, 1985.
48. Shils, M. E.: Experimental human magnesium deficiency. Medicine, 43:61, 1969.
49. Tasman-Jones, C.: Zinc deficiency states. In Advances in Internal Medicine. Edited by G. H. Stollerman. Chicago, Year Book Medical Publishers, 1980.
50. Kowarski, S., Blair-Stuneck, C. S., and Schacter, D.: Active transport of zinc and identification of zinc-binding protein in rat jejunal mucosa. Am. J. Physiol., 226:401, 1974.
51. Andersson, K. E., Brutt, L., Denker, H., and Lanner, E.: Some aspects of the intestinal absorption of zinc in man. Eur. J. Clin. Pharmacol., 9:423, 1976.
52. Ladefoged, K., Nicolaidou, P., and Jarnum, S.: Calcium, phosphorous, magnesium, zinc and nitrogen balance in patients with severe short bowel syndrome. Am. J. Clin. Nutr., 33:2137, 1980.
53. Evans, C. W., Grace, C. I., and Votara, H. J.: A proposed mechanism for zinc absorption in the rat. Am. J. Physiol., 228:501, 1975.
54. Sternlieb, I.: Gastrointestinal copper absorption in man. Gastroenterology, 52:1038, 1967.
55. Fleming, C. R., Hodges, R. E., and Hurley, L. S.: A prospective study of serum copper and zinc levels in patients receiving total parenteral nutrition. Am. J. Clin. Nutr., 29:70, 1976.
56. Karpel, J. T., and Peden, V. H.: Copper deficiency in long-term parenteral nutrition. J. Pediatr., 80:32, 1972.
57. Atkinson, R. L., et al.: Plasma zinc and copper in obesity and after intestinal bypass. Ann. Intern. Med., 89:491, 1978.
58. Ganther, H. E., et al.: Selenium and glutathione peroxidase in health and disease—a review. In Trace Elements in Human Health and Disease. Vol. II. Edited by A. S. Prasad, and D. Oberleas. New York, Academic Press, 1976.
59. Fleming, C. R., et al.: Selenium deficiency and fatal cardiomyopathy in a patient on home parenteral nutrition. Gastroenterology, 83:689, 1982.
60. van Rij, A. M., Thompson, C. D., McKenzie, J. M., and Robinson, M. F.: Selenium deficiency in total parenteral nutrition. Am. J. Clin. Nutr., 32:2076, 1979.
61. Johnson, R. A., et al.: An occidental case of cardiomyopathy and selenium deficiency. N. Engl. J. Med., 304:1210, 1981.
62. Kien, C. L., and Ganther, H. E.: Manifestations of selenium deficiency in a child receiving total parenteral nutrition. Am. J. Clin. Nutr., 37:319, 1983.
63. Mertz, W.: Chromium occurrence and function in biological systems. Physiol. Rev., 49:163, 1969.
64. Hambridge, K. M.: Chromium nutrition in man. Am. J. Clin. Nutr., 27:505, 1974.
65. Levander, O. A.: Selenium and chromium in human nutrition. J. Am. Diet. Assoc., 66:338, 1975.
66. Jeejeebhoy, K. N., et al.: Chromium deficiency, glucose intolerance and neuropathy reversed by chromium supplementation in a patient receiving long-term total parenteral nutrition. Am. J. Clin. Nutr., 30:531, 1977.
67. Mellors, A., Nagrwold, D. C., and Rose, R. C.: Ascorbic acid fluxes across mucosal border of guinea pig and human ileum. Am. J. Physiol., 233:E2172, 1977.
68. Hoyumpa, A. M., Middleton III, H. M., Wilson, F. A., and Schenker, S.: Thiamine transport across the rat intestine. Gastroenterology, 68:1218, 1975.
69. Thomson, A. D.: The absorption of radioactive sulfur-labelled thiamine hydrochloride in control subjects and in patients with intestinal malabsorption. Clin. Sci., 31:167, 1966.
70. Dreyfus, P. M.: Clinical application of blood transketolase determinations. N. Engl. J. Med., 276:596, 1962.
71. Brain, M., and Booth, C. C.: The absorption of tritium-labelled pyridoxine HCl in control subjects and in patients with intestinal malabsorption. Gut, 5:241, 1964.
72. Baker, E. M., et al.: Vitamin B_6 requirement for adult men. Am. J. Clin. Nutr., 15:59, 1964.
73. Rose, R. C.: Absorption of water soluble vitamins. In Physiology of the Gastrointestinal Tract. Vol. II. Edited by L. R. Johnson. New York, Raven Press, 1981.
74. Morrison, A. B., and Campbell, J. A.: Vitamin absorption studies: I Factors involving the excretion of oral test doses of thiamine and riboflavin by human subjects. J. Nutr., 72:435, 1960.
75. Levy, G., and Jusko, W.: Factors affecting the absorption of riboflavin in man. J. Pharmacol. Sci., 55:285, 1966.
76. Pallis, C. A., and Lewis, P. D.: Other vitamin deficiencies. In The Neurology of Gastrointestinal Disease. Edited by C. A. Pallis, and P. D. Lewis. London, W. B. Saunders, 1974.
77. Berger, E., Long, E., and Semenza, G.: The sodium activation of biotin absorption in hamster small intestine in vitro. Biochim. Biophys. Acta (Amsterdam), 225:873, 1972.
78. Appel, T. W.: Studies of biotin metabolism in man. J. Med. Sci., 204:856, 1942.
79. Baugh, C. M., Malone, J. M., and Butterworth, C. E.: Human biotin deficiency. A case history of biotin deficiency induced by raw egg consumption in a cirrhotic patient. Am. J. Clin. Nutr., 21:173, 1968.
80. Scott, D.: Clinical biotin deficiency (egg white injury). Acta Med. Scand., 169:69, 1958.
81. Rosenberg, I. H.: Absorption and malabsorption of folates. Clin. Hematol., 5:589, 1976.
82. Halsted, C. H.: The intestinal absorption of folates. Am. J. Clin. Nutr., 32:846, 1979.

83. Pratt, R. F., and Copper, B. A.: Folates in plasma and bile of man after feeding folic acid-^{3}H and 5-formyltetrahydrofolate (folinic acid). J. Clin. Invest., *50*:455, 1971.
84. Ellenbogen, L.: Uptake and transport of cobolamines. *In* Biochemistry of Nutrition. Vol. 27. Edited by A. Neuberger, and T. H. Jukes. International Review of Biochemistry. Baltimore, University Park Press, 1979.
85. Allen, R. H.: Human vitamin B_{12} transport proteins. Prog. Hematol., *9*:57, 1975.
86. Allen, R. H., Seetharam, B., Podell, E., and Alpers, D. H.: Effect of proteolytic enzymes on the binding of cobolamin to R protein and intrinsic factor. J. Clin. Invest., *61*:47, 1978.
87. Hagedorn, C. H., and Alpers, D. H.: Distribution of intrinsic factor-vitamin B_{12} receptors in human intestine. Gastroenterology, *73*:1019, 1977.
88. Filipsson, S., Hulten, L., and Lindstedt, G.: Malabsorption of fat and vitamin B_{12} before and after intestinal resection for Crohn's disease. Scand. J. Gastroenterol., *13*:529, 1978.
89. Lindenbaum, J.: Aspects of vitamin B_{12} and folate metabolism in malabsorption syndromes. Am. J. Med., *67*:1037, 1979.
90. MacKinnon, A. M., Short, M. D., Elias, E., and Dowling, R. H.: Adaptive changes in vitamin B_{12} absorption in celiac disease and after proximal small bowel resection in man. Am. J. Dig. Dis., *20*:835, 1975.
91. Goodman, D. S.: Overview of current knowledge of metabolism of vitamin A and carotenoids. J. Natl. Cancer Inst. *73*:1375, 1984.
92. Goldsmith, R. S.: Enterohepatic cycling of vitamin D and its metabolites. Miner. Electrolyte Metab., *8*:289, 1982.
93. Weisner, R. H., Kumar, R., Seeman, E., and Go, V. L. W.: Enterohepatic physiology of 1,25 dihydroxy vitamin D_3 metabolites in normal man. J. Lab. Clin. Med., *96*:1094, 1980.
94. Meridith, S. C., and Rosenberg, I. H.: Gastrointestinal hepatic disorders and osteomalacia. Clin. Endocrinol. Metab., *9*:131, 1980.
95. Eddy, R. L.: Metabolic bone disease after gastrectomy. Am. J. Med., *50*:442, 1971.
96. Duncombe, V. M., and Reeve, J.: Calcium homeostasis in digestive disorders. Clin. Gastroenterol., *10*:653, 1981.
97. Stamp, T. C. B.: Intestinal absorption of 25-hydroxycholecalciferol. Lancet, *2*:121, 1974.
98. Muller, D. P. R., Lloyd, J. K., and Wolff, O.: Vitamin E and neurological function. Lancet, *1*:225, 1983.
99. Stenflo, J.: Vitamin K-dependent formation of γ-carboxyglutamic acid. Ann. Rev. Biochem., *46*:157, 1977.
100. Gallop, P. M., Lian, J. B., and Hauschka, P. V.: Carboxylated calcium-binding proteins and vitamin K. N. Engl. J. Med., *302*:1460, 1980.
101. Jackson, C. M., and Suttie, J. W.: Recent developments in understanding the mechanism of vitamin K and vitamin K antagonist drug action and the consequences of vitamin K action in blood coagulation. Prog. Hematol., *10*:333, 1977.
102. Blanchard, R. A., et al.: Acquired vitamin K dependent carboxylation deficiency in liver disease. N. Engl. J. Med., *305*:242, 1981.
103. Corrigan, J. J., Jeter, M., and Earnest, D. L.: Prothrombin antigen and coagulant activity in patients with liver disease. J. Am. Med. Assoc., *248*:1736, 1982.
104. Corrigan, J. J., Jr.: Coagulation problems relating to vitamin E. Am. J. Pediatr. Hematol. Oncol., *1*:169, 1979.
105. Weisbrodt, N. W.: Motility of the small intestine. *In* Physiology of the Gastrointestinal Tract. Vol. I. Edited by L. Johnson. New York, Raven Press, 1981.
106. Cummings, J. H., James, W. P. T., and Wiggins, H.: Role of the colon in ileal-resection diarrhea. Lancet, *1*:344, 1973.
107. Jones, E. A., et al.: Protein metabolism in the intestinal stagnant loop syndrome. Gut, *9*:466, 1968.
108. Jonas, R., Flanagan, P. R., and Forstner, G. C.: Pathogenesis of mucosal injury in the blind loop syndrome. Brush border enzyme activity and glyco-protein degradation. J. Clin. Invest., *60*:1321, 1977.
109. Mekhjian, H. S., Phillips, S. F., and Hofmann, A. F.: Colonic secretion of water and electrolytes induced by bile acids. Perfusion studies in man. J. Clin. Invest., *50*:1569, 1971.
110. Gaginella, T. S., et al.: Perfusion of rabbit colon with ricinoleic acid: dose-related mucosal injury, fluid secretion, and increased permeability. Gastroenterology, *73*:95, 1977.
111. Ammon, H. V., Thomas, P. J., and Phillips, S. F.: Effects of oleic and ricinoleic acid on net jejunal water and electrolyte movement: Perfusion studies in man. J. Clin. Invest., *53*:374, 1974.
112. Debongnie, J. C., and Phillips, S. F.: Capacity of the human colon to absorb fluid. Gastroenterology, *74*:698, 1978.
113. Mitchell, J. E., et al.: The colon influences ileal resection diarrhea. Dig. Dis. Sci., *25*:33, 1980.
114. Cosnes, J., Gendre, J. P., and LeQuintree, Y.: Role of the ileocecal valve and site of intestinal resection in malabsorption after extensive small bowel resection. Digestion, *18*:329, 1978.
115. Porus, R. L.: Epithelial hyperplasia following massive small bowel resection in man. Gastroenterology, *48*:753, 1965.
116. Winawar, S. J., et al.: Successful management of massive small bowel resection based on assessment of absorption defects and nutritional needs. N. Engl. J. Med., *274*:72, 1966.
117. Scheflan, M., Galli, S. J., Perrotto, J., and Fischer, J. J.: Intestinal adaptation after extensive resection of the intestine and prolonged administration of parenteral nutrition. Surg. Gynecol. Obstet., *143*:757, 1976.
118. Dowling, R. H., and Booth, C. C.: Functional compensation after small bowel resection in man. Lancet, *2*:146, 1966.
119. Weinstein, L. D., Shoemaker, C. P., Hersh, T., and Wright, H. K.: Enhanced intestinal absorption after small bowel resection in man. Arch. Surg., *99*:560, 1969.
120. Hanson, W. R., Osborn, J. W., and Sharp, J. G.: Compensation by the residual intestine after intestinal resection in the rat. I. Influence of amount of tissue removed. Gastroenterology, *73*:692, 1977.
121. Dowling, R. H., and Booth, C. C.: Structural and functional changes following small intestinal resection in the rat. Clin. Sci., *32*:139, 1967.
122. Nundy, S., et al.: Onset of cell proliferation in the shortened gut. Colonic hyperplasia after ileal resection. Gastroenterology, *72*:263, 1977.
123. Williamson, R. C. N., Lyndon, P. J., and Tudway, A. J. C.: Effects of anticoagulation and ileal resection on the development and spread of experimental intestinal carcinomas. Br. J. Cancer, *42*:85, 1980.
124. Williamson, R. C. N., Bauer, R. L. R., Ross, J. S., and Malt, R. A.: Proximal enterectomy stimulates distal hyperplasia with bypass or pancreaticobiliary diversion. Gastroenterology, *74*:16, 1978.
125. Hanson, W. R.: Proliferative and morphological adaptation of the intestine to experimental resection. Scand. J. Gastroenterol. (Suppl.), *17*:11, 1982.
126. Hanson, W. R. and Osborne, J. W.: Epithelial cell kinetics

in the small intestine of the rat 60 days after resection of 70 percent of the ileum and jejunum. Gastroenterology, 60:1087, 1971.
127. Hanson, W. R., Osborne, J. W., and Sharpe, J. G.: Compensation by the residual intestine after intestinal resection in the rat. Gastroenterology, 72:701, 1977.
128. Weser, E., and Tawil, T.: Epithelial cell loss in remaining intestine after small bowel resection in the rat. Gastroenterology, 71:412, 1976.
129. Dowling, R. H.: Small bowel adaptation and its regulation. Scand. J. Gastroenterol. (Suppl.), 17:53, 1982.
130. Masesa, P. C., and Forrester, J. M.: Consequences of partial and subtotal colectomy in the rat. Gut, 18:37, 1977.
131. Buckholtz, T. W., Malamud, D., Ross, J. S., and Malt, R. A.: Onset of cell proliferation in the shortened gut: Growth after subtotal colectomy. Surgery, 80:601, 1976.
132. Owen, R. J., and Lyttle, J. A.: Rectal adaptation to colectomy and ileorectal anastomosis in the rat. Gut, 20:444, 1979.
133. Scarpello, J. H. B., Cary, B. A., and Sladen, G. E.: Effects of ileal and coecal resection on the colon of the rat. Clin. Sci. Mol. Med., 54:241, 1978.
134. Wright, H. K., Cleveland, J. C., Tilson, M. D., and Herskovic, T.: Morphology and absorptive capacity of the ileum after ileostomy in man. Am. J. Surg., 117:242, 1969.
135. Terpstra, O. T., et al.: Colostomy closure promotes cell proliferation and dimethylhydrazine induced carcinogenesis in rat distal colon. Gastroenterology, 81:475, 1981.
136. Tilson, M. D., Fellner, B. J., and Wright, H. K.: A possible explanation for postoperative diarrhea after colostomy closure. Am. J. Surg., 131:94, 1976.
137. Garrido, A. B., Jr., Freeman, H. J., and Kim, Y. S.: Amino acid and peptide absorption in bypassed jejunum following jejunoileal bypass in rats. Dig. Dis. Sci., 26:107, 1981.
138. Tilson, M. D., and Wright, H. K.: Adaptation of functioning and bypassed segments of ileum during compensatory hypertrophy in the gut. Surgery, 67:687, 1970.
139. Williamson, R. C. N., Buckholtz, T. W., and Malt, R. A.: Humoral stimulation of cell proliferation in small bowel after transection and resection in rats. Gastroenterology, 75:249, 1978.
140. Hageman, R. F., and Stragand, J. J.: Fasting and refeeding: Cell kinetic response of jejunum, ileum and colon. Cell Tissue Kinetics, 10:3, 1977.
141. Koga, A., and Kimura, S.: Influence of restricted diet on the cell renewal of the mouse small intestine. J. Nutr. Sci. Vitaminol. (Tokyo), 25:265, 1979.
142. Dowling, R. H.: Compensatory changes in intestinal absorption. Br. Med. Bull., 23:275, 1967.
143. Gleeson, M. H., Cullen, J. and Dowling, R. H.: Intestinal structure and function after small bowel bypass in the rat. Clin. Sci., 43:731, 1972.
144. Altman, G. G.: Influence of starvation and refeeding on mucosal size and epithelial renewal in the rat small intestine. Am. J. Anat., 133:391, 1972.
145. Menge, H., Werner, H., Lorenz-Meyer, H., and Riecken, E. O.: The nutritive effect of glucose on the structure and function of jejunal self-emptying blind loops in the rat. Gut, 16:462, 1975.
146. Clark, R. M.: "Luminal nutrition" versus "functional work-load" as controllers of mucosal morphology and epithelial replacement in the rat small intestine. Digestion, 15:411, 1977.
147. Weser, E., Vandeventer, A., and Tawil, T.: Nonhormonal regulation of intestinal adaptation. Scand. J. Gastroenterol. (Suppl.), 17:105, 1982.

148. Morin, C. L., Grey, V. L., and Carofalo, C.: Influence of lipids on intestinal adaptation after resection. In Mechanisms of Intestinal Adaptation. Edited by J. W. L. Robinson, H. R. Dowling, and E. O. Riecken. Lancaster, MTP Press, 1982.
149. Stragand, J. J., and Hagemann, R. F.: Effect of lumenal contents on colonic cell replacement. Am. J. Physiol., 233:E208, 1977.
150. Levine, G. M., Deren, J. J., and Yezdimir, E.: Small bowel resection: oral intake is the stimulus for hyperplasia. Am. J. Dig. Dis., 21:542, 1976.
151. Morin, C. L., Ling, V., and Van Caillie, M.: Role of oral intake on intestinal adaptation after small bowel resection in growing rats. Pediatr. Res., 12:268, 1978.
152. Fenijo, G., and Hallbert, D.: The influence of a chemical diet on the intestinal mucosa after jejuno-ileal bypass in the rat. Acta Chir. Scand., 142:270, 1976.
153. Ryan, G. F., Dudrick, S. J., Copeland, E. M., and Johnson, L. R.: Effects of various diets on colonic growth in rats. Gastroenterology, 77:658, 1979.
154. Morin, C. L., and Ling, V.: Effect of pentagastrin on the rat small intestine after resection. Gastroenterology, 75:224, 1978.
155. Altman, G. C.: Influence of bile and pancreatic secretions on the size of the intestinal villi in the rat. Am. J. Anat., 132:167, 1971.
156. Gelinas, M. D., and Morin, C. L.: Effects of bile and pancreatic secretions on intestinal mucosa after proximal small bowel resection in rats. Can. J. Physiol. Pharmacol., 58:1117, 1980.
157. Miazza, B., Levan, H., Vaja, S., and Dowling, R. H.: Pancreaticobiliary diversion (PBD) by duodenal transposition: a new model for stimulating jejunal and pancreatic adaptation. Gut, 21:A917, 1980.
158. Weser, E., Heller, R., and Tawil, T.: Stimulation of mucosal growth in the rat ileum by bile and pancreatic secretions after jejunal resection. Gastroenterology, 73:524, 1977.
159. Williamson, R. C. N., Bauer, F. L. R., Ross, J. S., and Malt, R. A.: Contributions of bile and pancreatic juice to cell proliferation in ileal mucosa. Surgery, 83:570, 1978.
160. Williamson, R. C. N.: Intestinal adaptation. Mechanism of control. N. Engl. J. Med., 298:1444, 1978.
161. Johnson, L. R.: The trophic effect of gastrointestinal hormones. Gastroenterology, 70:278, 1976.
162. Mayston, P. D., Barrowman, J. A., and Dowling, R. H.: Effect of pentagastrin on small bowel structure and function on the rat. Digestion, 12:78, 1975.
163. Mak, K. M., and Chang, W. W. L.: Pentagastrin stimulates epithelial cell proliferation in duodenal and colonic crypts in fasted rats. Gastroenterology, 71:1117, 1976.
164. Oscarson, J. E. A., et al.: Compensatory post-resectional hyperplasia and starvation atrophy in small bowel: dissociation from endogenous gastrin levels. Gastroenterology, 72:890, 1977.
165. Johnson, L. R., and Guthrie, P. D.: Secretin inhibition of gastrin-stimulated deoxyribonucleic acid synthesis. Gastroenterology, 67:601, 1974.
166. Hughes, C. A., and Dowling, R. H.: Speed of onset of adaptive mucosal hypoplasia and hypofunction in the intestine of parenterally fed rats. Clin. Sci., 59:317, 1980.
167. Hughes, C. A., et al.: The effect of cholecystokinin and secretin on intestinal and pancreatic structure and function. In Mechanisms of Intestinal Adaptation. Edited by J. W. L. Robinson, R. H. Dowling, and E.O. Riecken. Lancaster, MTP Press, 1982.
168. Riecken, E. O., at al.: Effect of pair feeding on intestinal adaptation after hypophysectomy. In Intestinal Adaptation. Edited by R. H. Dowling, and E. O. Riecken. Stuttgart-New York, Schattauer Verlag Publishers, 1974.

169. Muller, E., and Dowling, R. H.: Prolactin and the small intestine. Gut, *22*:558, 1981.
170. Batt, R. M., and Scott, J.: Response of the small intestinal mucosa to oral glucocorticoids. Scand. J. Gastroenterol. (Suppl.), *17*:75, 1982.
171. Scott, J.: Physiological, pharmacological and pathological actions of glucocorticoids on the digestive system. Clin. Gastroenterol., *10*:627, 1981.
172. Gleeson, M. H., et al: Endocrine tumor of kidney affecting small bowel structure, motility, and absorptive function. Gut, *12*:773, 1971.
173. Bloom, S. R.: An enteroglucagon tumor. Gut, *13*:520, 1972.
174. Sagor, G. R., et al: The effect of altered luminal nutrition on cellular proliferation and plasma concentrations of enteroglucagon and gastrin after small bowel resection in the rat. Br. J. Surg., *69*:14, 1982.
175. Jian, R., et al: Colonic inhibition of gastric secretion in man. Dig. Dis. Sci., *26*:195, 1981.
176. Bloom, S. R., et al: Gut hormone profile following resection of large and small bowel. Gastroenterology, *76*:1101, 1979.
177. Bloom, S. R., and Polak, J. M.: The hormonal pattern of intestinal adaptation. A major role for enteroglucagon. Scand. J. Gastroenterol. (Suppl.), *17*:93, 1982.
178. Sagor, G. R., et al: Evidence for a hormonal mechanism after small bowel resection: exclusion of gastrin but not enteroglucagon. Gastroenterology, *84*:902, 1983.
179. Buchan, A. M. J., Griffiths, C. J., Morris, J. F., and Polak, J. M.: Enteroglucagon cell hyperfunction in rat small intestine after gut resection. Gastroenterology, *88*:8, 1985.
180. Uttenthal, L. O., Batt, R. M., Carter, M. W., and Bloom, S. R.: Stimulation of DNA synthesis in cultured small intestine by partially purified enteroglucagon. Regul. Pept., *3*:84, 1982.
181. Boynton, A. L., Whitfield, J. F., and Walker, P. R.: The possible roles of polyamines in prereplicative development and DNA synthesis: a critical assessment of the evidence. *In* Polyamines in Biochemical Research. Edited by J. M. Gaugas. London, John Wiley and Sons, 1980.
182. Dowling, R. H., et al: Hormones and polyamines in intestinal and pancreatic adaptation. Scand. J. Gastroenterol. (Suppl.), *20*:84, 1985.
183. Baylin, S. B., Stevens, S. A., and Shakir, K. M. M.: Association of diamine oxidase and ornithine decarboxylase with maturing cells in rapidly proliferating epithelium. Biochim. Biophys. Acta (Amsterdam), *541*:415, 1978.
184. Luk, G. D., Marton, L. J., and Baylin, S. B.: Ornithine decarboxylase is important in intestinal mucosal maturation and recovery from injury in rats. Science, *210*:195, 1980.
185. Luk, G. D., and Baylin, S. B.: Polyamines and intestinal growth—increased polyamine biosynthesis after jejunectomy. Am. J. Physiol., *245*:G656, 1983.
186. Luk, G. D., and Baylin, S. B.: Ornithine decarboxylase in intestinal maturation, recovery and adaptation. *In* Mechanisms of Intestinal Adaptation. Edited by J. W. L. Robinson, R. H. Dowling, and E. O. Riecken. Lancaster, MTP Press, 1982.
187. Touloukian, R. J., Aghajanian, G. K., and Roth, R. H.: Adrenergic denervation of the hypertrophied gut remnant. Ann. Surg., *176*:633, 1972.
188. Tutton, P. M. J., and Helme, R. D.: The influence of adenoceptor activity on crypt cell proliferation in the rat jejunum. Cell Tissue Kinet., *7*:125, 1974.
189. Tutton, P. J. M.: Neural and endocrine control systems acting on the population kinetics of the intestinal epithelium. Med. Biol., *55*:201, 1977.
190. Liavog, I., and Vaage, S.: The effect of vagotomy and pyloroplasty on the gastrointestinal mucosa in the rat. Scand. J. Gastroenterol., *7*:23, 1972.
191. Laplace, J. P.: Effects of afferent sensory vagotomy on intestinal adaptation in the pig. *In* Mechanisms of Intestinal Adaptation. Edited by J. W. L. Robinson, R. H. Dowling, and E. O. Riecken. Lancaster, MTP Press, 1982.
192. Maton, P. N., Selden, A. C., and Chadwick, V. S.: Measurement of plasma cholecystokinins using high pressure liquid chromatography and radioimmunoassay: Response to oral fat and effect of atropine. Regul. Pept., *3*:76, 1982.
193. Krone, C. L., Theodor, E., Sleisenger, M. H., and Jeffries, G.: Studies on the pathogenesis of malabsorption. Medicine, *47*:89, 1968.
194. Liebow, C., and Rothman, S. S.: Enterohepatic circulation of digestive enzymes. Science, *189*:472, 1975.
195. Diamond, J. M.: Reabsorption of digestive enzymes: playing with poison. Nature, *271*:111, 1978.
196. Aber, G. M., Ashton, F., Carmalt, M. H. B., and Whitehead, T. P.: Gastric hypersecretion following massive small bowel resection in man. Am. J. Dig. Dis., *12*:785, 1967.
197. Windsor, C. W. O., et al: Gastric secretion after massive small bowel resection. Gut, *10*:779, 1969.
198. Strauss, E., Gerson, C. D., and Yallow, R. S.: Hypersecretion of gastrin associated with short bowel syndrome. Gastroenterology, *66*:175, 1974.
199. Seelig, L. L., Winborn, W. B., and Weser, E.: Effect of small bowel resection on the gastric mucosa in the rat. Gastroenterology, *74*:421, 1977.
200. Becker, H. D., Reeder, D. D., and Thompson, J. C.: Extraction of circulating endogenous gastrin by the small bowel. Gastroenterology, *65*:903, 1973.
201. Temperly, J. M., Stagg, B. H., and Wylie, J. H.: Disappearance of gastrin and pentagastrin in the portal circulation. Gut, *12*:372, 1971.
202. Moosa, A. R., Hall, A. W., Skinner, D. B., and Winans, C. S.: Effect of fifty percent small bowel resection on gastric secretory function in rhesus monkeys. Surgery, *80*:208, 1976.
203. Fitzpatrick, W. J. F., Zentler-Munro, P. L., and Northfield, T. C.: Ileal resection: effect of cimetidine and taurine on intrajejunal bile acid precipitation and lipid solubilization. Gut, *27*:66, 1986.
204. Cortot, A., Fleming, C. R., and Malagelada, J. R.: Improved nutrient absorption after cimetidine in short bowel syndrome with gastric hypersecretion. N. Engl. J. Med., *300*:79, 1979.
205. Stalbert, L., et al: D-lactic acidosis due to abnormal gut flora: diagnosis and treatment of two cases. N. Engl. J. Med., *306*:1344, 1982.
206. Scoorel, E. P., Giesberts, M. A. H., Blom, W., and Van Geldren, H. H.: D-lactic acidosis in a boy with short bowel syndrome. Arch. Dis. Child., *55*:810, 1980.
207. Dahlquist, N. R., Perrault, J., Callaway, C. W., and Jones, J. D.: D-lactic acidosis and encephalopathy after jejunoileostomy: response to overfeeding and fasting in humans. Mayo Clin. Proc., *59*:141, 1984.
208. Cross, S. A., and Callaway, C. W.: D-lactic acidosis and selected cerebellar ataxis. Mayo Clin. Proc., *59*:202, 1984.
209. Chadwick, V. S., et al: Effect of molecular structure on bile acid-induced alteration in absorptive function, permeability, and morphology in perfused rabbit colon. J. Lab. Clin. Med., *94*:661, 1979.
210. Saunders, D. R., et al: Morphological and functional effects of bile salts on rat colon. Gastroenterology, *68*:1236, 1975.
211. McJunkin, B., Fromm, H., Sarva, R. P., and Amin, P.: Factors in the mechanism of diarrhea in bile acid malab-

sorption: fecal pH a key determinant. Gastroenterology, 80:1454, 1980.
212. Hofmann, A. F.: The syndrome of ileal disease and the broken enterohepatic circulation: cholerheic enteropathy. Gastroenterology, 52:752, 1967.
213. Eaves, E. R., and Korman, M. G.: Cholestyramine induced hyperchloremic metabolic acidosis. Aust. N. Z. J. Med., 14:670, 1984.
214. Hartline, J. V.: Hyperchloremia, metabolic acidosis, and cholestyramine. J. Pediatr., 89:155, 1976.
215. Fordtran, J. S., Bunch, F., and Davis, G. R.: Ox bile treatment of severe steatorrhea. An ileectomy-ileostomy patient. Gastroenterology, 82:564, 1982.
216. Bright-Asare, P., and Binder, H. J.: Stimulation of colonic secretion of water and electrolytes by hydroxy fatty acids. Gastroenterology, 64:81, 1973.
217. Ammon, H. V., and Phillips, S. F.: Inhibition of colonic water and electrolyte absorption by fatty acids in man. Gastroenterology, 65:744, 1973.
218. Bochenek, W., Rodgers, J., and Balint, J. A.: Effects of changes in dietary lipids on intestinal fluid loss in the short bowel syndrome. Ann. Intern. Med., 72:205, 1970.
219. Greengerger, N. J., and Skillman, T. G.: Medium chain triglycerides. Physiologic considerations and clinical implications. N. Engl. J. Med., 280:1045, 1969.
220. Cohen, S., Kaplan, M., Gottleib, L., and Patterson, J.: Liver disease and gallstone disease in regional enteritis. Gastroenterology, 60:237, 1971.
221. Heaton, K. W., and Read, A. G.: Gallstones in patients with disorders of the terminal ileum and disturbed bile salt metabolism. Br. Med. J., 3:494, 1969.
222. Holzbach, R. T.: Pathogenesis and medical treatment of gallstones. In Gastrointestinal Disease. 3rd Ed. Edited by M. H. Sleisenger, and J. S. Fordtran. Philadelphia, W. B. Saunders Co., 1983.
223. Aburre, R., Gordon, S. G., Mann, J. G., and Kern, F., Jr.: Fasting bile salt pool size and composition after ileal resection. Gastroenterology, 57:679, 1969.
224. Dowling, R. H., Bell, G. D., and White, J.: Lithogenic bile in patients with ileal dysfunction. Gut, 13:415, 1972.
225. Gelzayd, E. A., Breuer, R. I., and Kirsner, J. B.: Nephrolithiasis in inflammatory bowel disease. Am. J. Dig. Dis., 13:1027, 1968.
226. Boyce, W. H., Garvey, F. K., and Strawcutter, H. E.: Incidence of urinary calculi among patients in general hospitals, 1948-1952. J. Am. Med. Assoc., 161:1437, 1956.
227. Nancollas, G. H.: Urine supersaturation: the nucleation, growth and dissolution of stones. In Urolithiasis and Related Clinical Research. Edited by P. O. Schwille, L. H. Smith, W. G. Robertson, and W. Vahlensieck. New York, Plenum Press, 1985.
228. Earnest, D. L.: Hyperoxaluria and renal stones complicating intestinal disease. In Current Therapy in Gastroenterology and Liver Disease 1984-1985. Edited by T. M. Bayless. Philadelphia, B. C. Decker, 1984.
229. Pak, C. Y. C., et al.: Mechanism of calcium urolithiasis among patients with hyperuricosuria. J. Clin. Invest., 59:426, 1977.

230. Coe, F. L., Strauss, A. L., Tembe, V., and Dunn, M. S. L.: Uric acid saturation in calcium nephrolithiasis. Kidney Int., 17:662, 1980.
231. Dobbins, J. W.: Nephrolithiasis associated with intestinal disease. In Urolithiasis and Related Clinical Research. Edited by P. O. Schwille, L. H. Smith, W. G. Robertson, and W. Vohlensieck. New York, Plenum Press, 1985.
232. Hofmann, A. F., et al.: Complex pathogenesis of hyperoxaluria after jejunoileal bypass surgery: oxalogenic substances in diet contribute to urinary oxalate. Gastroenterology, 84:293, 1983.
233. Earnest, D. L., Johnson, G., Williams, H. E., and Admirand, W. H.: Hyperoxaluria in patients with ileal resection: an abnormality in dietary oxalate absorption. Gastroenterology, 66:1114, 1974.
234. Earnest, D. L., Williams, H. E., and Admirand, W. H.: A physicochemical basis for treatment of enteric hyperoxaluria. Trans. Assoc. Am. Physicians, 88:224, 1975.
235. Binder, H. J.: Intestinal oxalate absorption. Gastroenterology, 67:441, 1974.
236. Saunders, D. R., Sillery, J., and McDonald, G. B.: Regional differences in oxalate absorption in the rat intestine: evidence for excessive absorption by the colon in steatorrhea. Gut, 16:543, 1975.
237. Dobbins, J. W., and Binder, H. J.: Importance of the colon in enteric hyperoxaluria. N. Engl. J. Med., 296:298, 1977.
238. Hatch, M., Freel, R. W., Goldner, A. M., and Earnest, D. L.: Oxalate and chloride absorption by the rabbit colon: sensitivity to metabolic and anion transport inhibitors. Gut, 25:232, 1984.
239. Fairclouth, P. D., Feest, T. G., Chadwick, V. S., and Clark, M. L.: Effect of sodium chenodeoxycholate on oxalate absorption from the excluded human colon—a mechanism for "enteric" hyperoxaluria. Gut, 18:240, 1977.
240. Stauffer, J. Q., Humphreys, M. H., and Weir, G. J.: Acquired hyperoxaluria with regional enteritis after ileal resection: role of dietary oxalate. Ann. Intern. Med., 79:383, 1973.
241. Stauffer, J. Q.: Hyperoxaluria and calcium oxalate nephrolithiasis after jejunoileal bypass. Am. J. Clin. Nutr., 30:64, 1977.
242. Barilla, D. E., Notz, C., Kennedy, D., and Pak, C. Y. C.: Renal oxalate excretion following oral oxalate loads in patients with ileal disease and with renal and absorptive hypercalciurias. Effect of calcium and magnesium. Am. J. Med., 64:579, 1978.
243. Rudman, D., et al.: Hypocitraluria in patients with gastrointestinal malabsorption. N. Engl. J. Med., 303:657, 1980.
244. Weser, E.: Intestinal adaptation after small bowel resection. Viewpoints on Digestive Diseases. Vol. 10, March, 1978.

Section 7 · *Prognosis*

32 · Prognosis of Idiopathic Inflammatory Bowel Disease

THEODORE M. BAYLESS, M.D.

The Clinical Variability of Inflammatory Bowel Disease in Relation to Prognosis—Problems of Assessment

The word prognosis, coming from the Greek phrase for "a knowing beforehand," is derived from "pro" plus "gignoskeia," [to know], and is defined as the forecast of the course of a disease. Prognostication in inflammatory bowel disease (IBD) is especially difficult because of the varied individual situations and complications, and because of the many unresolved aspects of IBD. Certain predictions can be made confidently. For example, today the chance of surviving ulcerative colitis without a colectomy exceeds 75% and the possibility of living a reasonably normal life span has improved to more than 95% in the last 30 years. However, the patient with severe bloody diarrhea, anemia, fever, and abdominal pain during a first attack of ulcerative colitis is at increased risk of perforation, surgery, and death although these risks, with steadily improving medical support, have decreased substantially. The patient with severe mucosal dysplasia in several areas of the colon, especially when associated with a "mass," is at a high risk of developing colon cancer within the next 6 years, and has a 50% chance of already having a colonic malignancy.

In Crohn's disease, the increasing use of nutritional supports will further lower the mortality rate from surgical treatment in Crohn's disease, just as earlier surgical intervention for fulminant colitis and megacolon dramatically lowered the surgical fatality rate for first attacks of ulcerative colitis. Other situations in patients either with ulcerative colitis or with Crohn's disease are more difficult to predict. For example, are patients with ulcerative colitis with ileal pouches, Kock pouches, or ileoanal anastomoses more susceptible to neoplasia because of the associated bacterial and bile salt stasis? Will the long term use of immunosuppressives, such as 6-mercaptopurine and azathioprine, or of metronidazole increase the risk of neoplasia in patients with idiopathic inflammatory bowel disease? Are those patients with Crohn's disease of the colon who are able to avoid colectomy because of improved medical treatment at greatly increased risk for the development of colonic carcinoma? Will knowledge of the mediators of inflammatory responses permit the development of "cocktails" of therapeutic agents directed at multiple stages in the biochemical cascade characterizing the inflammatory reaction, thereby lessening the inflammatory response and thus improving the ultimate course? Will effective anti-inflammatory therapy diminish the fibrosis and reduce the frequency of strictures and intestinal obstruction characteristic of "late" Crohn's disease of the small intestine? Unlikely; despite the fact that symptoms in patients with small bowel Crohn's disease may be controlled for years by alternate day prednisone therapy and sulfasalazine or antibiotics,[1] years later they may develop obstruction and require surgical treatment.[2]

Ideally, as in all other illnesses, accurate prognosis in IBD, would be helpful; identifying those who would respond to medical therapy; those who would not relapse after suppressive medications are slowly discontinued; those who would require surgical intervention for Crohn's colitis; and those who would not have a recrudescence of small bowel disease after ileocolonic resection. Even ulcerative proctitis, the presumably mildest form of idiopathic inflammatory bowel disease, occasionally will progress despite medical therapy, and require surgical resection. Other patients with a seemingly limited proctitis at the outset, will develop pancolitis within the first year of the onset of disease.[4] The individual variability in the course of ulcerative colitis and of Crohn's disease make it impossible initially to predict the precise outcome in each patient. Because at least one-fifth of the patients with mild to moderately active Crohn's disease in the National Cooperative Study in the United States experienced prolonged remission on placebo,[3] occasional patients will do well with almost no therapy; others, despite all therapeutic efforts, experience a progressive and relentless course. In view of these considerations, predictions in IBD should be conservative.

Some of the observations on the clinical course and complications in this chapter will overlap with data given elsewhere in this book. It is necessary to consider prognosis in relation to subsets of patients, such as those with ulcerative (idiopathic) proctitis as distinct from ulcerative colitis. Also, grouping patients with Crohn's disease into subgroups by anatomic distribution, such as jejunoileitis, terminal ileitis, ileocolitis, and colitis, has proven helpful in recognizing differences in clinical course.[5] Patients who have had two or three resections for Crohn's disease have a prognosis different from those who have never required surgical treatment. Patients with "aggressive" Crohn's disease initially, may experience a similarly severe course when the disease recrudesces after resective therapy.[6] Children and adolescents may have a more difficult course with severe colitis or with severe Crohn's disease than adult patients, many requiring colectomy within 1 to 2 years[7]. Elderly patients with severe colitis are increasingly vulnerable to a poor outcome, in part because of cardiovascular, pulmonary, or renal concomitants.

Earlier statements on prognosis usually were based on retrospective reviews from large referral centers.[8] Data from such centers, both then and now, generally include the more complicated and more severely ill patients, thus presenting a skewed view of overall prognosis. Studies of large geographic catchment areas (e. g., Copenhagen County, Denmark) include a broader clinical spectrum ranging from mild ambulatory patients to severely ill, hospitalized individuals, and show a more representative and generally more favorable prognosis.[9,10] A study from Rochester, Minnesota involving 138 patients between 1960 and 1979 reached similar conclusions; mainly that "the clinical severity of chronic ulcerative colitis in communities is less than is commonly thought; most have mild disease and the risk of cancer, though increased, is perhaps less than suggested by data from referral centers.[11] In addition, previous studies often were inadequately defined in terms of patient selection, diagnostic criteria, duration of disease, and length of follow-up. The use of simple mortality and complication percentages now has been replaced by more accurate actuarial methods, including life-table analysis.[12] Ideally, a homogeneous population at risk of a particular complication or outcome is determined, and the rate of that complication can be precisely related to disease duration and completeness of follow-up ascertainment.

In general, the survival of those with ulcerative colitis or with Crohn's disease has improved substantially in the past 50 years, in part reflecting advances in general medical, nutritional, and surgical care, and also the inclusion of more representative series of patients in the studies.

Chronic Ulcerative Colitis

Chronic ulcerative colitis involves the rectum and colon in a continuous, relatively diffuse inflammatory process. In idiopathic proctitis the inflammation and mucosal damage may be grossly and histologically limited to the rectum, however, and whether this is a separate illness or a stage in the development of ulcerative colitis is not settled. In about 20 to 25% of patients with proctitis, the disease progresses to involve the rectosigmoid and descending colon. A smaller proportion, with time, develop generalized ulcerative colitis. Occasional patients, years later, are found to have Crohn's disease rather than ulcerative proctitis.

"Left-sided" colitis is the term used when gross inflammation and ulceration apparently extend from the rectum to the splenic flexure or mid-transverse colon. In many such cases, double contrast barium enemas and colonoscopy with multiple biopsies show that the disease is more diffuse than suggested by the single contrast barium enema. Histologic evidence of active colitis or of prior mucosal inflammation with crypt distortion and destruction commonly is found in areas appearing normal to the endoscopist, and the patient previously classified as having "left-sided" colitis may have histologic evidence of disease extending to the hepatic flexure or into the ascending colon. If so, is the cancer risk now the same as in the patient with gross evidence of pancolitis? Probably yes. On the basis of this newer information, earlier prognostic assessments of some patients diagnosed as having "left-sided" colitis require revision to the category of extensive colitis or pancolitis.[13]

In addition to variations in the extent of colitis, the clinical severity of the disease varies from mild to moderate to severe. Most patients with severe ulcerative colitis have pancolitis, but patients with "left-sided" colitis may be extremely ill, and at increased risk of complications.

The severity of the initial attack may determine whether the patient requires an emergency or semielective colectomy early in the course of the illness. Most patients (approximately 60%) proceed into remission after the initial attack, however, only to relapse within a year or so, the *acute intermittent* type. Twenty percent of those with CUC do not achieve a complete remission and disease activity continues, a *chronic unremitting* form of colitis. A *fulminant* course can occur de novo or complicate either of these two types of CUC.

Survival

Mortality rates as high as 55% were reported in the mid-1950's,[14] but by the mid-1960's the mortality rate had decreased to less than 10%;[15,16] reports in the 1970's documented further declines in mortality. Studies using life table methods reported in the 1970's (Fig. 32-1) that survival was lower than in the general population over the entire period of follow-up; however,[17] importantly, almost all of the increased mortality occurred in the first and second years of ul-

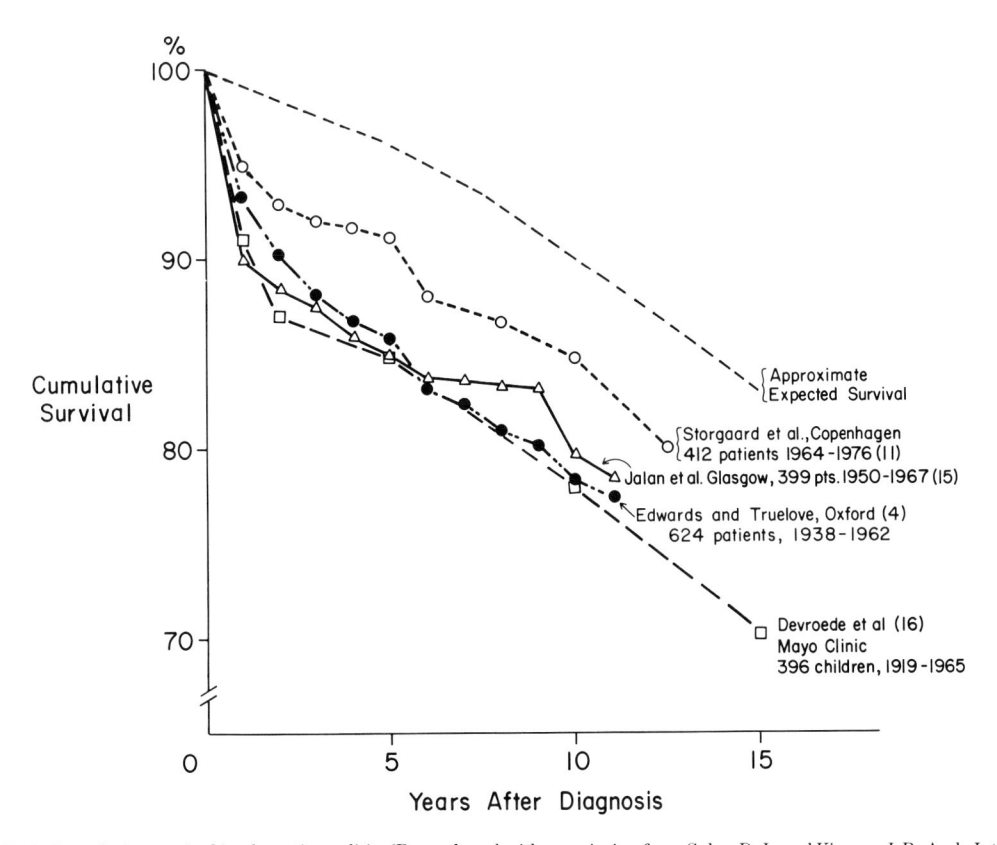

FIG. 32-1. Cumulative survival in ulcerative colitis. (Reproduced with permission from Sales, D. J., and Kirsner, J. B.: Arch. Intern. Med., *143*:294, 1983.)

cerative colitis.[18-21] Subsequently the slope of the survival curves was similar to that for the general population, indicating little, if any, excess mortality.

In Copenhagen County, a study of 783 patients with ulcerative colitis diagnosed between 1960 and 1978 indicated that an excellent survival outlook exists when an entire catchment population is considered.[10] The period of observation averaged 8 years, with 100% follow-up. At the time of diagnosis, 16% had pancolitis, 41% had disease above the rectum, and 41% had proctitis, as determined radiographically, presumably by single contrast barium enema. For the 441 women in the group the survival rate did not differ from that in the background population. A slight excess mortality of 2.1% existed among the 341 men during the first year of diagnosed illness, and the excess mortality was 1.5% in the second year. Subsequently, the survival rate did not differ from that in the general population. Interestingly, the excess mortality in the first 2 years was only statistically significant for the men who were over 40 years of age at the time of diagnosis (Fig 32-2). The excellent prognosis found in this study was influenced in part by the inclusion of ambulatory cases of CUC and the high proportion of proctitis patients.

The early mortality in ulcerative colitis usually is caused by severe or fulminant disease with its increased risk of potentially fatal complications including massive bleeding, toxic megacolon, or perforation, requiring emergency or semiurgent surgical treatment. The mortality rate may be as high as 2% for elective total colectomy but escalates to 20% or more if colonic perforation has occurred. In the past decade, the hazard of the initial severe attack of ulcerative colitis has diminished appreciably as a direct result of improved general, nutritional, and anti-inflammatory supportive measures.

Death in ulcerative colitis can be attributed to the illness itself in about one-third of patients, to colitis-related problems in another third, and to other causes in the remainder. In a Copenhagen study, 35% or 17 deaths in patients with CUC between 1960 and 1971 were directly attributable to the ulcerative colitis.[19] Similar findings had been reported earlier from the University of Chicago covering a period from 1930 to 1966.[22] Thirty-four percent of the 137 Chicago fatalities were caused by the colitis per se, including fulminant disease and operative and postoperative problems. An additional 30% were classified as colitis-related, including carcinoma of the colon (16 patients), suicide (6 patients), chronic liver disease (5 patients), thrombophlebitis (3 patients), and therapeutic complications (14 patients).

The improvement in survival rates for ulcerative colitis over the past 30 years, including the substantially decreased mortality rate for total proctocolectomy, can be attributed both to medical and surgical advances. The trend toward early surgical intervention (within 24 to 72 hours) for fulminant colitis, with or without "toxic dilation" of the colon, has been an important factor. Since the introduction of adrenal corticosteroids in the 1950's, the mortality rate for severe colitis has decreased by 50%. Improved antibiotic coverage and nutritional support systems also have ameliorated severe disease and decreased the need for emergency high-risk surgical treatment (Figs. 32-3 and 32-4). The prolonged survival of patients with extensive colitis not requiring a colectomy theoretically increases the pool of individuals at risk for developing problems such as sclerosing cholangitis, however. Thus, by sparing more people from colectomy through more effective medical therapy, and by confirming the absence of epithelial dysplasia by way of colonoscopic surveillance, more patients may become eligible for other late, colitis-related complications.

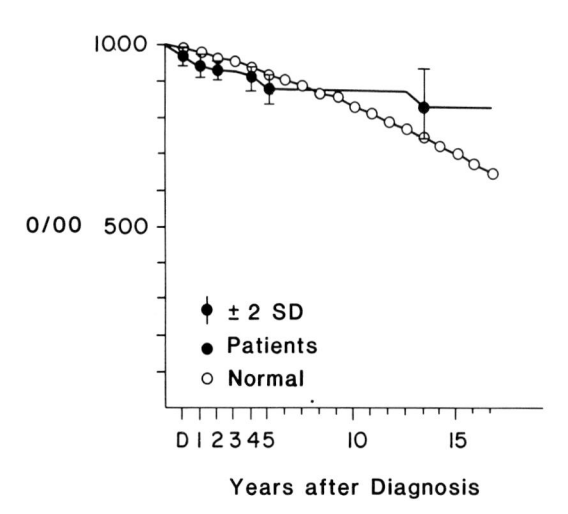

FIG. 32-2. Survival of men with ulcerative colitis compared with an age and sex-matched population. (Reproduced with permission from Hendriksen, et al.: Gut, 26:158, 1985.)

Prognostic Factors

Prognostic factors directly correlating with a high mortality rate include the following: (1) the severity of initial attack; (2) a requirement for surgical intervention during the initial at-

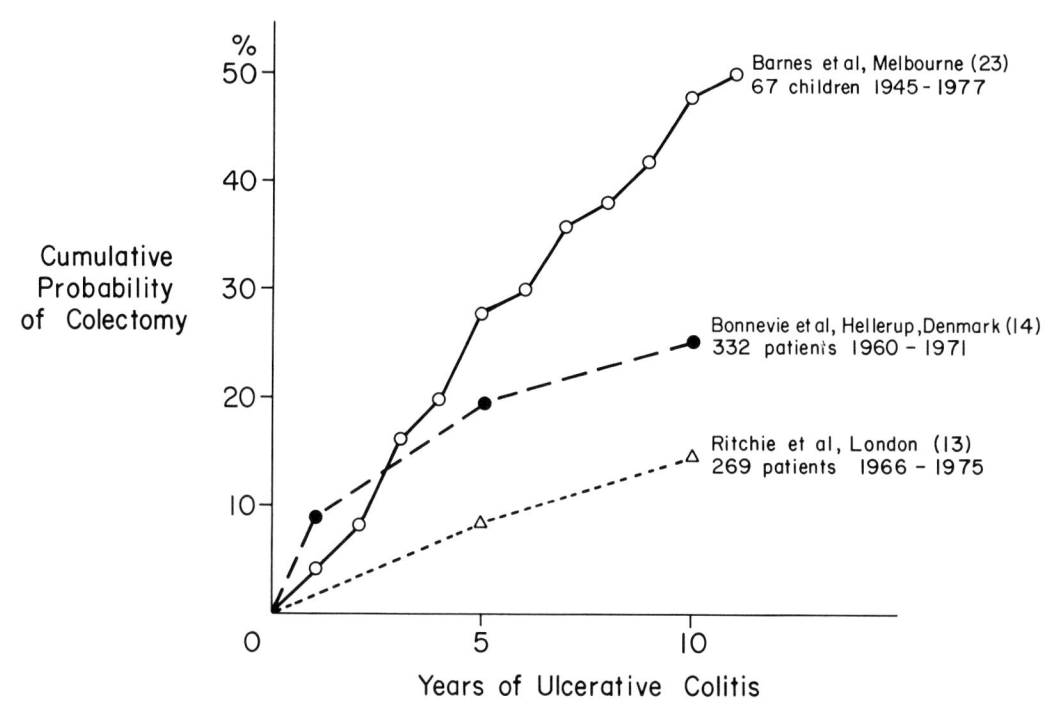

FIG. 32-3. Probability of colectomy in ulcerative colitis. (Reproduced with permission from Sales, D. J. and Kirsner, J. B.: Arch. Intern. Med., *143*:294, 1983.)

tack;[18,19,23] (3) a short duration prior to diagnosis;[19] (4) extensive colitis, which also influences cancer risk;[19,23-25] and (5) an onset during childhood and adolescence or when over 50 years of age.[18,19,24,26]

Prognosis is directly related to the extent of colitis because most of the colitis-related deaths are in patients with pancolitis. Individuals with proctitis are *not* at significantly increased risk either of death, developing cancer, or colectomy. As a practical matter, it would seem reasonable for insurance companies to consider those patients with histologic evidence of inflammation and mucosal injury limited to the lower 20 to 30 cm of the large intestine for 5 years as a separate group, with approximately normal mortality risk. Patients with "left-sided" colitis are in an intermediate mortality risk category in terms of cancer development and a need for colectomy.

Sex distribution has not been a consistent prognostic factor. Ulcerative colitis affects males and females approximately equally. Also, despite divergent results,[10,19,21,23,26] the short- and long-term survival rates appear to be similar for both sexes.[18,24]

As in most chronic illnesses that may require surgery, age is a factor in prognosis. Individuals with an onset of CUC after age 50 have a worse prognosis than patients with a disease onset between ages of 20 and 50.[10,18,21,24,26,27] In fact, as already mentioned, the Copenhagen report disclosed an increased mortality in ulcerative colitis only in men over 40, chiefly because of the increased mortality during the initial attack of

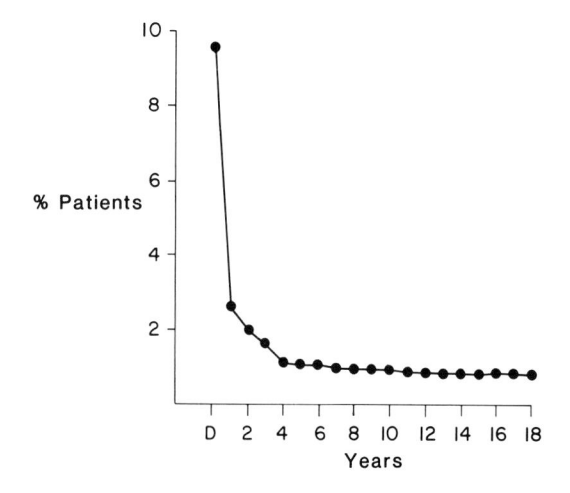

FIG. 32-4. Colectomy rates in the years after the diagnosis of ulcerative colitis. (Reproduced with permission from Hendriksen, C., et al.: Gut, *26*:158, 1985.

colitis.[10] For patients over the age of 50, surgical mortality rates are higher and drug side-effects and colitis-related morbidity may be more pronounced. This older population also is susceptible to the non-colitis-related degenerative problems that affect an aged-matched population. Ischemic enteritis or colitis may be difficult to distinguish from idiopathic inflammatory bowel disease. In fact, ischemia may be the sole cause of the bowel disease in some patients, especially in elderly individuals with ileocolitis of short duration. In others, ischemic injury may be superimposed upon an underlying colitis.

In children developing ulcerative colitis, a larger proportion have extensive colitis and a smaller proportion have proctitis. The initial attacks tend to be more severe and require colectomy more commonly than among adults. After an initial clustering of colitis-related deaths, however, the overall mortality for childhood-onset ulcerative colitis is similar to that of adult-onset disease. Nevertheless, because most children, adolescent and young adult patients subsequently have a longer duration of colitis, problems such as dysplasia, cancer, sclerosing cholangitis, and the need for colectomy tend to be more prevalent than in adults with a shorter duration of illness.

Colectomy

In contrast to Crohn's disease, ulcerative colitis is "cured" by the surgical removal of the colon and rectum.* Most newly diagnosed patients with ulcerative colitis view colectomy and ileotomy as the major threat of the illness, however. Although the improvement in surgical ileostomy techniques,† in appliances, and in support services including stomal therapy and ostomy associations, has made ileostomy more acceptable, alternatives to ileostomy continue to be sought.

In the past decade, the development of such procedures as the Kock pouch and ileal pouch-anal anastomoses, and the availability of mechanical ostomy caps has made it easier for patients to view colectomy as a socially acceptable procedure. Physicians also are less reluctant now to consider colectomy for patients with severe colitis. Even before the availability of alternatives to conventional ileostomy, the probability of colectomy varied considerably among medical centers in the United States and abroad. Colectomy for fulminant colitis before perforation is credited with much of the improved survival of patients with severe initial attacks or with severe relapses. Many colectomies are done during the first few years after diagnosis,[20,24,27,28] but the need for colectomy continues at a more modest rate for at least 10 or 20 years after the onset (Figs. 32-3, 32-4). In the Copenhagen series, which included proctitis patients, 10% of the CUC patients had an operation in the initial year and 3% in the second year. From the 4th to the 18th year, about 1% of the at-risk population underwent colectomy yearly. By 18 years, the cumulative operated rate was up to 31% of the total ulcerative colitis-proctitis population. This trend of a persistent, albeit small, need for colectomy will continue because of the "ileostomy-alternative" operations and because surveillance programs probably will identify dysplasia in 1 to 3% of the at-risk population each year.[29]*

The extent of colitis and the severity of disease are two factors clearly related to the need for colectomy. Most people undergoing colectomy have either pancolitis or involvement from the rectum at least to the hepatic flexure.[8,24,26] Severe disease, especially in the initial attack, also correlates with the need for colectomy, but because most patients with severe disease have extensive colitis, both factors are interrelated.[24]

Although cumulative colectomy rates of 35 to 50% are not unusual in pediatric series,[28,30] comparable adult rates are 20 to 25%.[8,19,20] At the Boston Children's Hospital, half of the children with severe colitis, either ulcerative colitis or Crohn's colitis, underwent colectomy during that hospitalization, and another one-fourth required surgical treatment in the next 2 years.[7] This series was accumulated before the use of hyperalimentation or immunosuppressive medications for Crohn's colitis. In the past, growth retardation in prepubescent adolescents has been another indication for colectomy, but awareness of the substantial nutritional requirements and their correction, including by parenteral nutrition, has greatly decreased this need (see also Chap. 24).

Ileostomy revisions and reoperations for intestinal obstruction are necessary in about 10% of patients who undergo proctocolectomy and ileostomy (see Chap. 30). Some of these problems result because the primary illness was Crohn's disease and not ulcerative colitis. Because 10 to 20% of patients with colitis without small bowel involvement may be diagnosed as "indeterminant colitis" despite radiologic, endo-

---

*See also Chapter 27.
†See also Chapter 29.

*See also Chapter 15.

scopic, and histologic examinations, the problem of unrecognized Crohn's disease will continue until more precise "biologic markers" are identified. The reoperation rate with Kock pouches is at least 20%, probably closer to 30%. It is not yet clear how often ileoanal anastomoses will require repair or conversion to a Kock pouch or Brooke ileostomy. Preliminary unpublished observations suggest that this conversion rate is increasing. Ileorectal anastomoses may be followed by recurrence in the rectum or by the development of cancer. In one series of ileorectal anastomoses, more than 20% of the patients developed rectal cancer after 20 years of ulcerative colitis.[31]

Neoplasia

As improving medical therapy has enhanced the response rate in initial and severe attacks of ulcerative colitis, the population at risk for development of carcinoma has enlarged. In the United States and the United Kingdom, it is generally accepted that the risk of colorectal cancer is increased in patients with CUC, but whether such an increased risk exists in other parts of the world is unknown. The identifiable risk factors include the duration of the colitis, the extent of colonic involvement, and the presence of mucosal dysplasia. In contrast to earlier beliefs that the risk was greater in those with the onset of CUC in childhood, apparently the risk is increased greatly and the lag period is shorter for the development of colorectal cancer in patients whose CUC symptoms develop at a later age.[32] An intriguing, as yet unclarified factor in the cancer risk of CUC may be environmental influences, including the eating habits (e.g., eating foods such as animal fat) that characterize countries with high incidences of colorectal cancer, such as the United States and Great Britain.

Cancers have been detected during the eighth year of pancolitis or extensive CUC. By 10 years, the incidence is at least 2%. Another 10 to 15% of patients develop colon cancer during the second decade of pancolitis. After 30 years, 30 to 40% of patients apparently will develop carcinoma of the colon (Fig. 32-5).

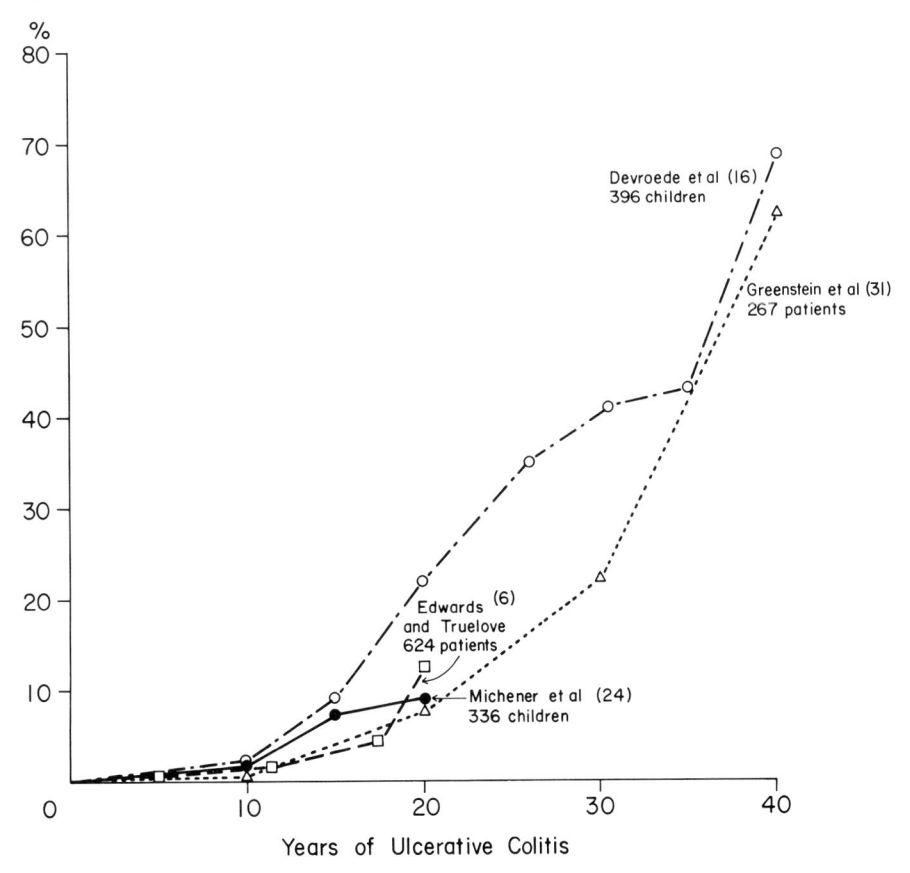

FIG. 32-5. Cumulative risk of developing colorectal cancer in ulcerative colitis. (Reproduced with permission from Sales, D. J. and Kirsner, J. B.: Arch. Intern. Med., 143:294, 1983.)

The onset of cancer may be somewhat delayed in those with "left-sided" colitis (defined by single contrast barium enema) to periods of 15 to 20 years after the onset of colitis.[13] As pointed out earlier, histologic recognition of universal colitis (as at colonoscopy) moves a patient with macroscopic "left-sided" colitis into a higher risk group. Chronic ulcerative colitis patients with ileorectal anastomoses are still at increased risk of developing cancer, in contrast to patients with proctitis, who probably are not at increased risk. Cancers have been found in individuals with proctitis, but only in their 7th decade at which time non-colitis-related colorectal cancers can be expected, as in the general population.

The aforementioned statistics may overestimate cancer risk because they derive from several studies of patients in tertiary referral centers; commonly, such have diseases of longer duration and increased severity than those in "catchment" areas. A study of 258 unselected patients with ulcerative colitis from a single practice yielded cancer risks of 6.6% at 26 years duration and 11.4% at 32 years.[33] This study probably underestimated cancer risk by including patients with Crohn's colitis who were possibly "nursing" right-sided cancer.[34] The recent Rochester, Minnesota community-wide study reinforces the belief that cancer risk data will be lower if proctitis and proctosigmoiditis patients are included, because they comprise almost half of such population study groups.[11] Although CUC patients should not become unduly alarmed by the threat of cancer, neither should they be complacent. The degree of activity of ulcerative colitis does not always correlate directly with cancer risk. Patients asymptomatic for 10 to 15 years may develop colon cancer. Patients with chronic continuously active disease have the highest incidence of colon cancer,[8,18] but in recent years more of such individuals are being treated earlier by colectomy because of the continued clinical activity. Patients with single attacks or with mild intermittent disease probably now comprise the "greatest risk" group.[35,36]

Dysplasia, an epithelial change identifiable in the colonic mucosa in over 95% of patients with ulcerative colitis and colon cancer, is a definite risk factor for subsequent cancer development. Dysplastic changes were highlighted as a possible marker for cancer risk by Morson and Pang after finding them in patients with over 10 years of ulcerative colitis.[37] In a series of colectomy specimens, Kewenter et al. have demonstrated a linearly increasing frequency of dysplasia with the duration of ulcerative colitis.[38] Dysplasia without cancer was found after 4 years of ulcerative colitis. By 30 years, 70% cumulative incidence of dysplasia was found in the small number of subjects still at risk.

The lag time between the discovery of dysplasia and the development of invasive carcinoma is not known precisely. Kewenter's data suggested a 7 year difference between the curve for cumulative frequency of dysplasia and the cumulative frequency of cancer in another series of ulcerative colitis patients. Our data also suggest that 7 or 8 years is an approximate interval. For example, patients with ulcerative colitis and colon cancer had an average duration of colitis of 20 years, whereas those only with dysplasia had colitis for an average duration of 13 years.[36]

The presence of an adenomatous colonic polyp in a patient with ulcerative colitis without dysplasia elsewhere in the colon may be a chance association. If dysplasia is found on the stalk of the polyp or in the tissue surrounding the base, however, or if other adenomatous polyps are present, colectomy appears to be a reasonable recommendation.

The prognosis for patients with colon cancer and ulcerative colitis is the same as the outlook for patients with non-colitis-related colon cancer, when similar Dukes's stages are compared.[39] Unfortunately, before the advent of surveillance colonoscopy programs, most cancers in ulcerative colitis were discovered after the patients become symptomatic and were already at an incurable stage. In a group of 18 patients with colon cancer and ulcerative colitis seen in our institution between 1958 and 1968, none survived over 16 months after cancer diagnosis. The prognosis now is improved because most of the cancers discovered by surveillance programs are Dukes's A or B; however, some asymptomatic patients found to have dysplasia at their first colonoscopy already have developed metastases to lymph nodes.[40]

It is hoped that cancer-related premature deaths in the ulcerative colitis population will continue to decrease as surveillance programs for dysplasia are more widely applied. If this approach can be supplemented by biologically more "specific" histochemical stains, the prognosis of chronic ulcerative colitis should improve further.

Quality of Life

Most individuals who develop ulcerative colitis have a relatively benign course. Except for the first few years, about 90% of those in the 1984 Copenhagen survey were fully capable of work.[10] Less than 5% received any disability pensions and most of these were not for ulcerative colitis. Their work capacity and disability rates were similar to those of the general Danish population aged 1 to 66 years. The 1963 report from Oxford, England of the follow-up of 501 surviving patients seen from 1938 to 1962 concluded that 69% led an entirely normal life and an additional 19% were essentially "normal" except for the need of medical supervision. Six percent continued in their former occupation but with some interruptions. Five percent were fully active but had changed occupations. None were chronic invalids.[8] A different type of assessment was made of 308 patients first seen at the Cleveland Clinic as children or adolescents.[35] Only 25% considered themselves to be in good health, and 72% chose a rating of "fair" to describe their quality of life. Seven percent said their life was "poor." These differences in quality of life may be caused by, in part, the more severe nature of colitis in children. Only 10% of the population had a single attack, 20% had intermittent symptoms, 50% had chronic but not incapacitating problems, and 20% were chronically involved. Among the 92 colitis-related deaths reported from the University of Chicago for the 36 year period ending in 1966, 6 younger patients committed suicide, possibly related to the fact that teenagers are more troubled by alterations in health, appearance, diet, and activity capacity.

Studies of "social prognosis" suggest that most ulcerative colitis patients are similar to age- and sex-matched control populations in terms of marital status, frequency of severe family or sexual problems, leisure activities, physical and earning capaciy, the incidence of mental disorders, and the intake of alcohol and other psychopharmacologic drugs.

In summary, small but significant numbers of patients with ulcerative colitis are at increased risk for colectomy, colon cancer, and/or early mortality, but the great majority are able, with a supervised therapeutic approach, to lead a "relatively acceptable" lifestyle. Unfortunately, the term "relatively acceptable" is like beauty, it is defined only by the eye of the beholder.

Ulcerative Proctitis

Definition and Activity of Disease

Proctitis is defined as a chronic inflammatory process limited to the rectum. It can be subdivided into: (1) those whose disease never extends above 20 cm (even by rectosigmoid biopsy) and are the clinically mildest and most predictable group, and (2) those whose inflammatory process extends, even if only histologically, into the descending colon, who are less likely to respond to topical steroids and sulfasalazine. As emphasized earlier, in some epidemiologic studies, as in Copenhagen and Rochester, Minnesota, proctitis patients were included in the overall ulcerative colitis population,[10,11] but in others, especially those based on hospital populations, proctitis patients were not included because they are seldom admitted to a hospital. In 80% of proctitis patients the inflammatory process remained localized to the rectum; approximately 10 to 20% developed ulcerative colitis. However, much of this "follow-up" was based on earlier studies using single contrast barium enemas. The availability of flexible sigmoidoscopy and colonoscopy has now provided important histologic evidence of the presence of ulcerative proctitis/colitis even when the disease is in clinical remission.

No initial clinical features predict the therapeutic response in proctitis. The response may be rapid and virtually complete but, not infrequently, seemingly mild proctitis may be resistant to usual therapy (sulfasalazine, steroid enemas). Approximately 70 to 80% of these patients may respond to retention enemas with 5-aminosalicylic acid, but the tendency to recurrence is ever present. Prolonged use of 5-aminosalicylate enemas may lessen the number of proctosigmoiditis patients who are affected by chronic unremitting symptoms.

Progression of proctitis into generalized or left-sided ulcerative colitis usually occurs in the first year or two of illness. No specific prognostic features separate these patients from those with persistently limited proctitis. Approximately 5% of patients thought to have proctitis for several years are later found to have Crohn's disease of the colon, but the early use of biopsy in persistent proctitis and an increased awareness of the subtle histologic features of Crohn's disease, such as focal inflammation or scattered granulomas, should keep such diagnostic errors to a minimum.

Surgical Treatment

Although it is rare for a patient with ulcerative proctitis to require proctocolectomy, occasionally the tissue reaction may be so severe as to destroy the entire rectal mucosa. Prior to colectomy in such patients, histologic evidence of colitis involving at least half of the colon usually is found. Severe, unremitting ulcerative proctitis with intense inflammatory changes usually will require a total colectomy, despite the relatively limited anatomic extent of disease.

Cancer Risk

In proctitis the risk of large bowel cancer is not increased over that of the general population, matched for age. When rectal cancers do occur, usually these are in patients in their 60s or 70s, as in the general population.

Survival

As a group, survival in proctitis is equivalent to that of the general population controlled for age. If the inflammation extends into the colon, the patient then assumes the characteristics and the prognosis of the ulcerative colitis patient, considered earlier in this chapter.

Crohn's Disease

Crohn's disease affects patients of all ages, all parts of the alimentary system (mouth, esophagus, stomach, small intestine, colon, and rectum) and "metastatic lesions" may be found. The clinical course varies from individual to individual. Potential complications are numerous and may affect all bodily systems but occur in only a small proportion of patients. Surgical treatment is required in at least 50%, involving multiple operations in some. Useful estimates of prognosis, therefore, require evaluations of groups of patients with approximately similar clinical features.

In general, the gross lesions of Crohn's disease are distributed as follows: approximately 50% of patients have ileocolitis, 20% have predominantly ileitis, 20% have "pure" colitis, and 10% have oral, esophageal, gastric, or duodenal involvement. Perianal disease is present in about 30% of patients; however, the widespread but focal distribution of microscopically detectable areas of inflammation and the asymptomatic aphthous ulcers noted at meticulous endoscopic scrutiny of the host show that the disease is much more extensive than is obvious by conventional roentgen studies. This quality of Crohn's disease explains the so-called "recurrent" nature of the illness, and handicaps the validity of frozen sections of the bowel at the time of surgical treatment.[41]

It is important to separate patients with *active inflammation* (diarrhea, fever, intestinal complications, extraintestinal manifestations) from those with "*late*" and "*inactive*" stages of the disease, characterized by fibrosis and severe narrowing of the bowel lumen. Active Crohn's disease often responds to medical therapy, especially if it is limited to the distal ileum and/or the cecum. Fistulas that occur early in the course of the illness may not require resection initially and can be left intact as the active inflammation is treated and, hopefully, suppressed.[42] In contrast, the late or fibrotic phase of Crohn's disease in the small bowel will not resolve completely with medical therapy, and, when advanced to the point of recurrent obstruction, often is an indication for surgical resection[2] or perhaps for the new procedure of stricturoplasty. Experience with balloon dilatation of narrowed bowel in Crohn's disease is too limited to assess at present.

The natural history of "pure" Crohn's disease of the colon is less predictable. Some patients with extensive, apparently severe disease experience a prolonged remission on "simple" medical therapy. Others require more intense treatment with steroids, metronidazole, immunosuppressives, and parenteral hyperalimentation. A relatively small proportion do not respond to any available medical treatment and require bowel resection.

Survival

The excess mortality rates for Crohn's disease increase throughout the course of the illness. Nevertheless, most patients are able to lead a reasonably normal life despite occasional recurrences. Mortality is greatest during the initial 5 years after the illness becomes clinically recognizable, but a slightly shortened survival continues through the next 25 years of the disease. This sort of survival was reported in 1980 by the Birmingham, England group, based upon a 20 year follow-up. The mortality rate in 174 patients was 1.5 times that expected in the general population.[43]

Survival in Crohn's disease has improved during the past 30 years (Fig. 32-6). The survival rate approximated 90% after 20 years of illness in 240 patients seen at the Mayo Clinic during the 1953

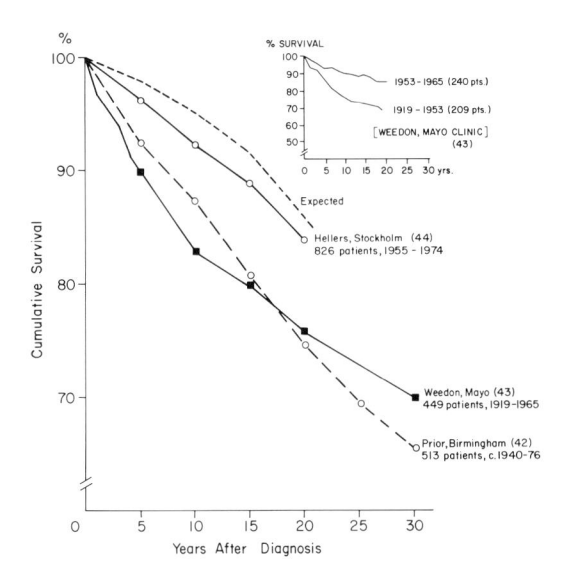

FIG. 32-6. Cumulative survival in Crohn's disease. (Reproduced with permission from Sales, D. J. and Kirsner, J. B.: Arch. Intern. Med., 143:294, 1983.)

to 1965 period, compared to a 70% survival rate in 209 seen between 1919 and 1953.[44] Although steroid therapy was considered a major factor in this improved course, other therapeutic advances including improved nutritional and medical support and more opportune and increasingly skillful surgical intervention also contributed. A contrasting opinion has implicated steroids and their concomitant side effects in an increased mortality from Crohn's disease.[45]

Unfortunately, the mortality rate is regrettably higher than expected in younger patients. In a 1981 series of 513 patients from Birmingham, England, the mortality for the entire study population was twice that expected, but the mortality of patients aged 5 to 29 was 4.4 times the expected rate, the rates being similar in males and females.[45] This trend toward a higher mortality rate in young patients was not observed in studies in Copenhagen and in Uppsala, however.[46,47]

Causes of Death

Approximately half the deaths of patients with Crohn's disease can be related directly to the disease or its complications. Of these disease-related deaths, one-half to two-thirds are attributable to postoperative complications. For example, Sales and Kirsner reviewed series from Oxford,[48] Birmingham, England,[8,43,45] Stockholm,[9] and Boston,[49] which reported 229 deaths among 1728 patients. Fifty-five percent were directly disease related,[125] and 64% of these deaths were associated with postoperative problems.[17] In a Swedish series 34 of 70 deaths (among 826 patients followed from 1955 to 1974) were attributable to Crohn's disease.[46] The 22 postsurgery deaths resulted from anastomotic leaks, abscesses, fistula formation, invasion of the bloodstream by fungi, or from the effects of the short-bowel syndrome.

Suicide and narcotic overdosage are among the causes of death indirectly related to Crohn's disease, and four suicides and one heroin overdosage were recorded among 36 non-Crohn's disease related deaths in the 1979 Stockholm series.[9] Three of 100 deaths, all three in women, were caused by suicide, according to a report from Birmingham, England; this represented a statistically significantly increased rate over that in an age and sex matched control population.[44,46] Amyloidosis accounted for three of six deaths in 214 patients reported from Oslo.[50]

The extent of Crohn's disease seems to be a more consistent prognostic factor than its site. Patients with extensive small bowel or colonic disease experience greater morbidity and mortality. In various series of childhood Crohn's disease, those with colonic disease had a slightly worse prognosis,[30,51] but in an adult series, the mortality rate was highest with ileocolitis,[52] perhaps in part because of the high "recurrence" rates after ileocolonic resection.

Complications

Complications obviously influence the clinical course of Crohn's disease, and their nature relates to the area of involvement. In a Cleveland Clinic series intestinal obstruction occurred in 44% of patients with ileocolonic disease.[5] Thirty-eight percent had perianal and rectal fistulas and 34% had internal or cutaneous fistulas. Among those with predominantly colonic disease, 46% had rectal bleeding, 36% had perianal fistulas, 11% had toxic megacolon, and 16% had arthritis. The lowest morbidity was associated with small bowel disease; 35% of these patients experienced intestinal obstruction. A similar relationship between clinical pattern and morbidity has been found among children at Yale,[51] in adults in Stockholm,[9] and in the United States National Cooperative Crohn's Disease study.[53]

Surgical Treatment

The majority of patients with small bowel Crohn's disease require at least one bowel resection. The clinical pattern of Crohn's disease is a

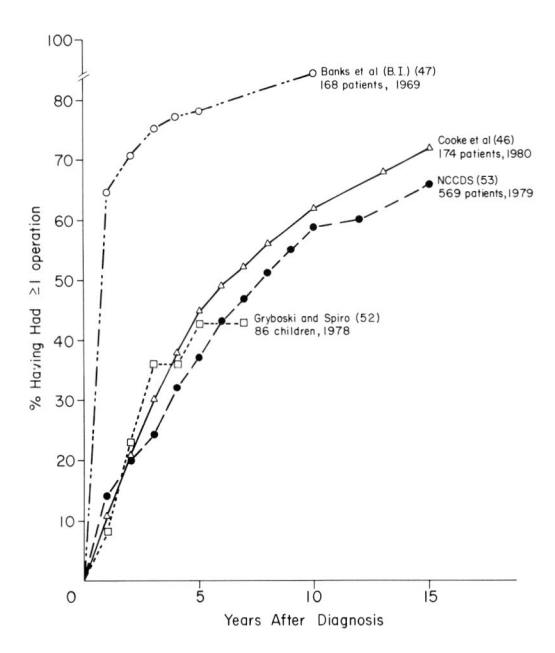

FIG. 32-7. Chance of requiring surgery in Crohn's disease. (Reproduced with permission from Sales, D. J. and Kirsner, J. B.: Arch. Intern. Med., *143*:294, 1983.)

predictor of the chance of requiring surgical treatment.[52] A second variable is the therapeutic "philosophy" of the particular medical center. Surgical rates at many reporting institutions are highest for the first attack.[45,53,57] At others the cumulative risk is steady at approximately 40% at 5 years for the entire Crohn's disease population, rising to 60% at 10 years, and to 70% 15 years after diagnosis (Fig. 32-7).[43,46,51,53,54] Even after 15 years without surgical intervention, the risk continues at approximately 6% per year.[43] Computer-aided systems may allow an accurate prediction of the need for surgical treatment in some patients.[55]

Patients with ileocolonic Crohn's disease are more likely to require an operation during the initial attack, and cumulatively during their course, than those with colonic or small bowel disease, but the differences are small. de Dombal and his colleagues in England reported a "short-term" surgical treatment rate for first attacks of 65% for ileocolonic disease, 58% for ileal disease, and 47% for colonic disease in a series of 332 patients.[54] In a similar short-term (3.6 years) study at the Cleveland Clinic, 73% of those with ileocolonic disease underwent surgical procedure compared to 50% of those with either "pure" ileal or colonic disease.[52] At St. Mark's Hospital in London, 20 of 57 patients (39%) with colonic Crohn's disease required surgical treatment within 10 years of its onset, most having their operation during the first five years. Ten had an operation for an acute attack, and 10 for chronic symptoms. At the end of the follow-up period, 11 of 14 surviving patients treated surgically had a permanent abdominal stoma. Among the 28 who were treated only medically, all were well, 17 on no medications, 8 on sulfasalazine (plus steroids in 1 case), and 3 on steroids (plus azathioprine in 1). This experience suggested that about half of all patients with colonic Crohn's disease can be treated medically without abdominal surgical treatment, and that the need for treatment with drugs tends to decrease with time.[56] Groups using immunosuppressive agents, at times combined with parenteral alimentation, apparently are requiring fewer colonic resections.[57]

RECRUDESCENCES

"Recurrence" of active inflammation after bowel resection is so common in Crohn's disease treated by intestinal resection and reanastomosis that surgical treatment is palliative rather than curative (Table 32-1; Figs. 32-8 and 32-9). The risk of reoperation is greatest in the first five postoperative years, ranging from 20 to 40%. By 15 years after the first resection, 40

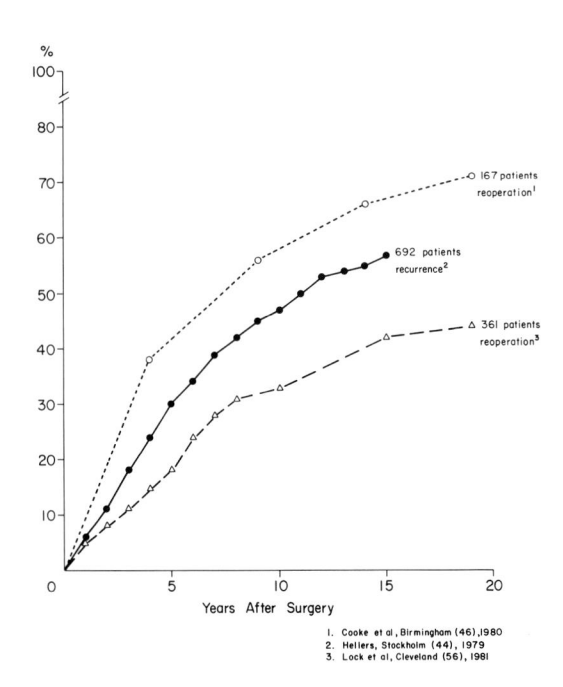

FIG. 32-8. Recrudescence rates after surgery for Crohn's disease. (Reproduced with permission from Sales, D. J. and Kirsner, J. B.: Arch. Intern. Med., *143*:294, 1983.)

TABLE 32-1. *Factors Reported to be Associated with Recrudescence of Crohn's Disease after Resection*

Factors Inherent to Crohn's Disease	Factors Influenced by Surgical Technique
Clinical Factors	
Young age at onset	Staged operation
Young age at resection	Ileorectal anastomosis
Male sex	in patients with
Female sex	Crohn's colitis
Long duration of disease	
Short duration of disease	
Previous resection	
Intractability	
Pathologic Factors	
Site of involvement	Gross disease at resection
Ileocolitis > colitis	margin
Ileitis > colitis	Histopathologic disease at
Long length of involved bowel	resection margin
Paucity of granulomas	Short margin length
Pyloric metaplasia	No resection of regional lymph nodes

(Reference 63)

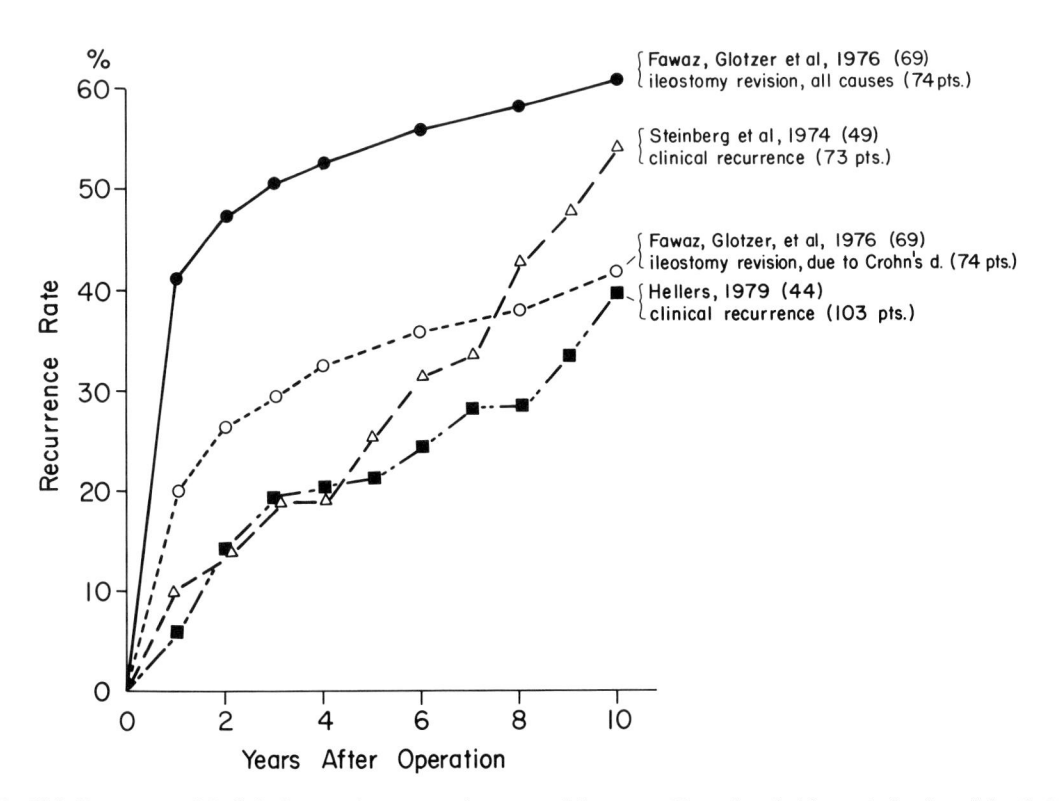

FIG. 32-9. Recurrence of Crohn's disease after proctocolectomy and ileostomy. (Reproduced with permission from Sales, D. J. and Kirsner, J. B.: Arch. Intern. Med., *143*:294, 1983.)

to 70% will have required another operation.[17,52,58,59]

Risk factors for recurrence include the site and pattern of the gross disease. The risk of recrudescence is greatest for those with ileocolonic disease and least for those with colonic Crohn's disease.[59] For example, among 26 patients with colonic disease treated by total colectomy and ileostomy and followed for an average of 9.8 years, only 1 had a recurrence, and 21 were well.[47] The ages at onset and at the time of resection also influence the rate of recurrence. Patients under age 25 have a higher rate than those over age 40.[9,59,60] The extent of the initial resection of the small bowel also correlates directly with recurrence rate.[61] Fistulas recur more commonly and earlier if fistulas are present initially. Extensive perianal disease tends to recur if bowel continuity is maintained or reestablished even after a lengthy period of bowel rest.[61]

The presence or absence of granulomas in the resected bowel or the margins of resection does not seem to influence the rate of recrudescence. The status of the resection margins in terms of the presence or absence of microscopic inflammation also does not influence the recurrence rate.[9,45,61-63] The incidences of immediate postoperative complications, late recurrences, or need for reoperation were the same whether the resection margins were normal or inflamed.[62] Similarly, the use of frozen sections to monitor the extent of bowel resection was not helpful.[41] Because neither the short-term nor the long-term outcome was improved by histologic examination of the anastomotic margin, this suggested that bowel resection should be limited to gross disease and viable bowel should not be sacrificed to achieve histopathologically uninvolved anastomotic margins.[62] It was shown in one study that radical bowel resection with 10 cm margins, analogous to a cancer operation as advocated by some surgeons,[18] did not decrease the frequency of "late" recurrences.[47] One long-term study of 186 patients in Uppsala, Sweden yielded a different conclusion, however.[47] After a mean follow up of 18 years, 31% of patients undergoing "radical" resection at their first operation had recurrent disease. This outcome contrasted with an 83% recurrence rate after "non-radical" resection. Unfortunately, it is not clear how patients were selected for the initial "radical" or "non-radical" approach. Thus, those with a long area of disease and a higher chance of recurrence might have been spared a radical resection by the surgeon. Currently, it would appear that a conservative approach is reasonable when resecting bowel involved by Crohn's disease.

Crohn's Colitis

The course of Crohn's disease limited to the colon is variable. Occasional patients develop fulminant disease and require surgical treatment in the first 1 or 2 years of illness, especially among children and teenagers. Others follow a more benign course. In general, as mentioned earlier, the prognosis for Crohn's colitis is the most favorable of all of the disease patterns in Crohn's disease.[9,51,52,54,56]

The recurrence rate or need for ileostomy revision after total colectomy and ileostomy ranges from 20 to 30% at 5 years and 35 to 50% at 10 years.[9,64,65] This is clearly a group with a favorable prognosis especially if the ileum is grossly uninvolved at the time of colectomy.[65]

Recurrence rates after partial colonic resection with reanastomosis are substantially higher, especially with ileorectal anastomoses, being as great as 75%.[9,59,66-68] In the Uppsala series, 15 of 25 patients with ileorectal anastomoses had recurrent disease;[47] however, in the Johns Hopkins series only 3 of 13 patients with subtotal colectomy, with or without immediate ileorectal anastomoses experienced recurrence. Segmental resections are acceptable, especially if a long segment of uninvolved left colon can be retained.[69]

Cancer

In patients with Crohn's colitis the risk of colorectal cancer is increased four- to twenty-fold[44,70-72] compared to the general population. The risk factors, as with ulcerative colitis, include a long duration of illness and presumably the extent of disease. In the small bowel and in the colon, obstructed or bypassed loops of bowel are particularly high risk areas. Most of the cancers arise in areas grossly involved by Crohn's disease,[73] but cancer may develop at apparently uninvolved sites.[74]

Dysplasia was found contiguous with the resected carcinomas in all 10 patients reviewed by Hamilton.[70] Although the finding of dysplasia would support surveillance programs for patients with colorectal Crohn's disease or with a bypassed segment of bowel, the variations in clinical course make this a complicated situation. Although 8 of the 10 patients reported by Hamilton had a 24-year average duration of disease, 2 patients presented with colorectal carcinoma initially and only later were found to have undiagnosed Crohn's disease. In 1 patient the cancer developed 4 years before the initial diagnosis of Crohn's disease. Two of the cancers were in bypassed and strictured rectums.

The outlook for Crohn's disease-associated cancers may be poorer than for noncolitis related cancers and even that for ulcerative colitis-associated tumors, because of the difficulties of examining the small bowel, bypassed loops of bowel, or strictured areas of colon, and the resulting long delay before clinical or surgical recognition of the lesion.

Quality of Life

Even though Crohn's disease may be a serious chronic illness with significant morbidity, a high likelihood of requiring surgical treatment, a continuing possibility of recurrence, risk of intestinal cancer, and increased mortality, most patients with the disease report a surprisingly good quality of life.[75] Obviously exceptions exist because of individual problems, such as multiple operations, short bowel syndrome, extraintestinal manifestations, and because of the apparently increased suicide rate. A major factor in assessing the quality of life is the personality of the patient; it is axiomatic that cheerful, optimistic individuals are more likely to evaluate their course more positively than those who are discouraged or depressed.

Out of 121 patients followed for over 20 years in Birmingham, England, 119 reported that they were leading a normal life, free of medical restrictions.[43] In a New York series of 53 patients who had undergone elective surgical treatment, however, a less than satisfactory quality of life was found when they were surveyed 5 to 10 years later.[75] Those with recrudescent disease had the greatest impairment of activity. Despite their medical/surgical problems, 92% of the patients said they were "satisfied" with the surgical outcome, which seems somewhat contradictory. In a Swedish study, 89% of 152 patients followed for more than 14 years reported a "good" quality of life, 8.6% had moderate symptoms, and 2.6% had pronounced symptoms.[47] In contrast, a pessimistic report from the Cleveland clinic in 1979 found that two-thirds of 552 patients with a childhood or adolescent onset of Crohn's disease considered their state of health to be suboptimal when surveyed an average of 8 years later, although only 6% of the patients thought they had a "poor" quality of life. In this study, the quality was least satisfactory in those with colonic disease.[30]

In a 1984 report from Copenhagen, the working capacity was normal in about 75% of patients for all years except the year of diagnosis.[46] Although symptoms persisted in some despite medical treatment and surgical intervention, most were capable of work and were leading a relatively "normal" life.

Current medical therapy suppresses disease activity in many patients, especially those with ileal disease. The results of medical therapy for more extensive small bowel disease and for colonic disease are less predictable. Repeated or massive intestinal resections may result in serious and at times incapacitating abnormalities in intestinal function. Fortunately, now fewer patients develop "short bowel" syndromes because of the increased efforts to preserve as much bowel as possible. The adaptation of patients to Crohn's disease is greatly aided by adequate information and peer support, such as that provided by the patient's informed and understanding physician, his or her family, and by The National Foundation for Ileitis and Colitis. Nevertheless, it must be accepted that a significant proportion of patients with Crohn's disease are unhappy with their situation, despite protestations that their quality of life is "satisfactory."

References

1. Whittington, P. F., Barnes, H. V., and Bayless, T. M.: Medical management of Crohn's disease in adolescence. Gastroenterology, 72:1338, 1977.
2. Schwartz, J. B., Bayless, T. M., and Hamilton, S. R.: Crohn's disease: is there a predictable pattern of late ileal complications? Gastroenterology, 90:1623, 1986.
3. Summers, R. W., et al.: National Cooperative Crohn's disease study: results of drug treatment. Gastroenterology, 77:847, 1979.
4. Farmer, R. G.: Long-term prognosis for patients with ulcerative proctosigmoiditis. J. Clin. Gastroenterol., 1:47, 1979.
5. Farmer, R. G., Whelan, G., and Fazio, V. W.: Long-term follow-up of patients with Crohn's disease. Relationship between the clinical pattern and prognosis. Gastroenterology, 88:1818, 1985.
6. Greenstein, A. J., et al.: Concordance of surgical indications from initial to subsequent operations for Crohn's disease. Gastroenterology, 90:1438, 1986.
7. Kelts, D. G., and Grand, R. J.: Inflammatory bowel disease in children and adolescents. Curr. Probl. Pediatr., 10:1, 1980.
8. Edwards, F. C., and Truelove, S. C.: The course and prognosis of ulcerative colitis (Parts 1-4). Gut, 4:1, 299, 1963.
9. Hellers, G.: Crohn's disease in Stockholm County, 1955-1974. Acta Chir. Scand. (Suppl.), 490:1, 1979.

10. Hendriksen, C., Kreiner, S., and Binder, V.: Long term prognosis in ulcerative colitis—based on results from a regional patient group from the county of Copenhagen. Gut, 26:158, 1985.
11. Stonnington, C. M., Phillips, S. F., Melton, L. J., Zinsmeister, A. R., and Phillips, S. F.: Chronic ulcerative colitis: Incidence and prevalence in a community. Gut, 28:402, 1987.
12. Devroede, G., and Taylor, W. F.: On calculating cancer risk and survival of ulcerative colitis patients with the life table method. Gastroenterology, 71:505, 1976.
13. Greenstein, A. J., et al.: Cancer in universal and left-sided ulcerative colitis: factors determining risk. Gastroenterology, 77:290, 1979.
14. Wheelock, F. C., Jr., and Warren, R.: Ulcerative colitis: follow-up studies. N. Engl. J. Med., 252:421, 1955.
15. Spencer, J. A., et al.: Immediate and prolonged therapeutic effects of corticotropin and adrenal steroids in ulcerative colitis. Gastroenterology, 42:113, 1962.
16. Korelitz, B. I., and Lindner, A. E.: The influence of corticotropin and adrenal steroids on the course of ulcerative colitis: a comparison with the presteroid era. Gastroenterology, 46:671, 1964.
17. Sales, D. J., and Kirsner, J. B.: The prognosis of inflammatory bowel disease. Arch. Intern. Med., 143:294, 1983.
18. Jalan, K. N., et al.: An experience of ulcerative colitis, III Long-term outcome. Gastroenterology, 59:598, 1970.
19. Bonnevie, O., Binder, V., Anthonisen, P., and Riis, P.: The prognosis of ulcerative colitis. Scand. J. Gastroenterol., 9:81, 1974.
20. Ritchie, J. K., Powell-Tuck, J., and Lennard-Jones, J. E.: Clinical outcome of the first ten years of ulcerative colitis and proctitis. Lancet, 1:1140, 1978.
21. Storgaard, L., et al.: Survival rate in Crohn's disease and ulcerative colitis. Scand. J. Gastroenterol., 14:225, 1979.
22. Morowitz, D. A., and Kirsner, J. B.: Mortality in ulcerative colitis: 1930 to 1966. Gastroenterology, 57:481, 1969.
23. Devroede, G. J., et al.: Cancer risk and life expectancy of children with ulcerative colitis. N. Engl. J. Med., 285:17, 1971.
24. Lanfranchi, G. A., et al.: Clinical course of ulcerative colitis in Italy. Digestion, 20:106, 1980.
25. de Dombal, F. T.: Ulcerative colitis: epidemiology and aetiology, course and prognosis. Br. Med. J., 1:649, 1971.
26. Gilat, T., et al.: Risk factors in ulcerative colitis. Digestion, 14:400, 1976.
27. Jalan, K. N., et al.: An experience of ulcerative colitis, II Short-term outcome. Gastroenterology, 59:589, 1970.
28. Binder, V., et al.: Ulcerative colitis in children: treatment, course and prognosis. Scand. J. Gastroenterol., 8:161, 1973.
29. Nugent, F. W., and Haggitt, R. C.: Results of a long-term prospective surveillance program for dysplasia in ulcerative colitis. Gastroenterology, 86:1197, 1984.
30. Farmer, R. G., and Michener, W. M.: Prognosis of Crohn's disease with onset in childhood or adolescence. Dig. Dis. Sci., 24:752, 1979.
31. Aylett, S.: Cancer and ulcerative colitis. Br. Med. J., 2:203, 1971.
32. Lashner, B. A., Silverstein, M. D., Evans, A. A., and Hanauer, S. B.: Hazard rates for dysplasia and cancer in an ulcerative colitis surveillance program. Gastroenterology, 90:1513, 1986.
33. Katzka, I., Brody, R., Morris, E., and Katz, S.: Assessment of colorectal cancer risk in patients with ulcerative colitis: experience from a private practice. Gastroenterology, 85:22, 1983.
34. Yardley, J. H., Ransohoff, D., Riddell, R., and Goldman, H.: Cancer in inflammatory bowel disease: how serious is the problem and what should be done about it? Gastroenterology, 85:197, 1983.
35. Michener, W. M., Farmer, R. G., and Mortimer, E. A.: Long-term prognosis of ulcerative colitis with onset in childhood or adolescence. J. Clin. Gastroenterol., 1:301, 1969.
36. Yardley, J. H., Bayless, T. M., and Diamond, M. P.: Cancer in ulcerative colitis. Gastroenterology, 76:221, 1979.
37. Morson, B. C., and Pang, L. S. C.: Rectal biopsy as an aid to cancer control in ulcerative colitis. Gut, 8:423, 1967.
38. Kewenter, J., Ahlman, H., and Holten, L.: Cancer risk in extensive ulcerative colitis. Ann. Surg., 188:824, 1978.
39. Hughes, R. G., et al.: The prognosis of carcinoma of the colon and rectum complicating ulcerative colitis. Surg. Gynecol. Obstet., 146:46, 1978.
40. Nugent, F. W., et al.: Malignant potential of chronic ulcerative colitis: preliminary report. Gastroenterology, 76:1, 1979.
41. Hamilton, S. R., et al.: The surgical management of Crohn's disease: an appraisal of frozen section examination of resection margins for selecting an anastomotic site. Surg. Gynecol. Obstet., 160:57, 1985.
42. Broe, P. J., Bayless, T. M., and Cameron, J. L.: Crohn's disease: are enteroenteral fistulas an indication for surgery? Surgery, 91:249, 1982.
43. Cooke, W. T., Mallas, E., Prior, P., and Allan, R. N.: Crohn's disease: course, treatment and long-term prognosis. Q. J. Med., 49:363, 1980.
44. Weedon, D. D., et al.: Crohn's disease and cancer. N. Engl. J. Med., 289:1099, 1973.
45. Prior, P., et al.: Mortality in Crohn's disease. Gastroenterology, 80:307, 1981.
46. Binder, V., Hendriksen, C., and Kreiner, S.: Prognosis in Crohn's disease-based on results from a regional patient group from the county of Copenhagen. Gut, 26:146, 1985.
47. Krause, U., Ejerblad, S., and Bergman, L.: Crohn's disease. A long-term study of the clinical course in 186 patients. Scand. J. Gastroenterol., 20:516, 1985.
48. Truelove, S. C., and Peña, A. S.: Course and prognosis of Crohn's disease. Gut, 17:192, 1976.
49. Banks, B. M., Zetzel, L., and Richter, H. S.: Morbidity and mortality in regional enteritis. Am. J. Dig. Dis., 14:369, 1969.
50. Lind, E., Fausa, O., Gjone, E., and Mogensen, S. B.: Crohn's disease. Treatment and outcome. Scand. J. Gastroenterol., 20:1014, 1985.
51. Gryboski, J. D., and Spiro, H. M.: Prognosis in children with Crohn's disease. Gastroenterology, 74:807, 1978.
52. Farmer, R. G., Hawk, W. A., and Turnbull, R. B.: Clinical patterns in Crohn's disease. Gastroenterology, 68:627, 1975.
53. Mekhjian, H. S., et al.: National cooperative Crohn's disease study: factors determining recurrence of Crohn's disease after surgery. Gastroenterology, 77:907, 1979.
54. de Dombal, F. T., Burton, I. L., Clamp, S. E., and Goligher, J. C.: Short-term course and prognosis of Crohn's disease. Gut, 15:435, 1974.
55. de Dombal, F. T., et al.: Production of individual patient prognosis. Value of computer-aided systems. Decision Making, 6:18, 1986.
56. Elliott, P. R., Ritchie, J. K., and Lennard-Jones, J. E.: Prognosis of colonic Crohn's disease. Br. Med. J., 291:178, 1985.
57. Present, D. H., et al.: Treatment of Crohn's disease with 6-mercaptopurine: a long-term randomized double blind study. N. Engl. J. Med., 302:981, 1980.

58. McDermott, F. T., et al.: An Australian experience of Crohn's disease. Aust. N. Z. J. Surg., 50:470, 1980.
59. de Dombal, F. I., Burton, I., and Goligher, J. C.: Recurrence of Crohn's disease after primary excisional surgery. Gut, 12:519, 1971.
60. Greenstein, A. F., Sachar, D. B., Pasternak, B. S., and Janowitz, H. D.: Reoperation and recurrence in Crohn's colitis and ileocolitis: crude and cumulative rates. N. Engl. J. Med., 293:685, 1975.
61. Gump, F. E., Sakellariadis, P., Wolff, M., and Broell, J. R.: Clinical-pathological investigation of regional enteritis as a guide to prognosis. Ann. Surg., 176:233, 1972.
62. Pennington, L., Hamilton, S. R., Bayless, T. M., and Cameron, J. L.: Surgical management of Crohn's disease: influence of disease at margin of resection. Ann. Surg., 192:311, 1980.
63. Hamilton, S. R.: Pathologic features of Crohn's disease associated with recrudescence after resection. In Pathology Annual. Edited by S. C. Somers, and P. P. Rosen. Norwalk, CT, Appleton-Century Crofts, 1983.
64. Steinberg, D. M., et al.: Excisional surgery with ileostomy for Crohn's colitis with particular reference to factors affecting recurrence. Gut, 15:845, 1974.
65. Fawaz, K. A., et al.: Ulcerative colitis and Crohn's disease of the colon—a comparison of the long-term postoperative courses. Gastroenterology, 71:372, 1976.
66. Weterman, I. T., and Peña, A. S.: The long-term prognosis of ileorectal anastomosis and proctocolectomy in Crohn's disease. Scand. J. Gastroenterol., 11:185, 1976.
67. Steinberg, D. M., Allan, R. N., Cooke, W. T., and Williams, J. A.: The place of ileorectal anastomosis in Crohn's disease. Aust. N. Z. J. Surg., 46:49, 1976.
68. Himal, H. S., and Belliveau, P.: Prognosis after surgical treatment of granulomatous enteritis and colitis. Am. J. Surg., 142:347, 1981.
69. Sanfey, H., Cameron, J. L., and Bayless, T. M.: Crohn's disease of the colon. Is there a role for limited resection? Am. J. Surg., 147:38, 1984.
70. Hamilton, S. R.: Colorectal carcinoma in patients with Crohn's disease. Gastroenterology, 89:398, 1985.
71. Riddell, R. H., et al.: Dysplasia in inflammatory bowel disease: standardized classification with provisional clinical applications. Hum. Pathol., 14:931, 1983.
72. Kirsner, J. B., and Shorter, R. G.: Recent developments in "nonspecific" inflammatory bowel disease. N. Engl. J. Med., 306:775, 1982.
73. Traube, J., et al.: Crohn's disease and adenocarcinoma of the bowel. Dig. Dis. Sci., 25:939, 1980.
74. Greenstein, A. J., et al.: Patterns of neoplasia in Crohn's disease and ulcerative colitis. Cancer, 46:403, 1980.
75. Meyers, S., et al.: Quality of life after surgery for Crohn's disease: a psychosocial survey. Gastroenterology, 78:1, 1980.

33 · The Fallibility of Activity Indices in Crohn's Disease (CD)

ROY G. SHORTER, M.D.

Since this book reached "proof stage" in its preparation, a special report on the use of activity indices in CD has appeared in the literature.[1] The study was carried out by the International Organization for the Study of Inflammatory Bowel Disease (IOIBD); 15 members (with some colleagues) independently reviewed a series of "real life cases," each observer ascribing indices of activity to each of the patients, using eight different methods for their estimation. Those taking part included physicians from the United States, Canada, the United Kingdom, Scandinavia, France, the Netherlands, and West Germany.

As is well known, a Crohn's disease activity index (CDAI) was first developed by the National Cooperative Crohn's disease study group in the United States[2] to provide a "standard" method for quantifying disease activity before and after the introduction of various medical treatments in clinical trials, and perhaps for the management of individual patients. As a result of criticisms of the index because of bias introduced by certain highly subjective variables in its calculation, subsequently not only was it modified by its developers,[3] but also by others.[4,5] Various different methods for deriving indices of activity have been proposed for general use,[6,7] serving as a further illustration, if one were needed, of "tot homines quot sententiae." Unfortunately, as de Dombal and Softley pointed out, no group published any results of testing the various methods, and without a high degree of reproducibility the merit of any such index to clinical use is highly suspect. Accordingly, the IOIBD decided to evaluate the CDAI,[2,3] Harvey and Bradshaw's CDAI,[4] an IOIBD method, the Leeds CDAI,[1] the European AI,[1] a Dutch AI,[6] an Oxford scoring,[7] and a South African index (unpublished).

The study consisted of four parts. In the first, 5 consultant gastroenterologists and surgeons and 2 research assistants were asked individually to calculate the 8 activity indices for each of 10 patients with Crohn's disease, using case histories as the sources of information. In the second part, from case data, 15 physicians each calculated the 8 indices for a single patient. Then, after some discussion about discrepancies, the first part of the study was repeated as part 3. Part 4 involved interviewing 6 patients with Crohn's disease by a panel of 6 gastroenterologists with considerable experience in IBD. The case histories also were made available. Each physician in the study was provided with the methods for calculating the various indices.

Analysis of the information obtained used simple nonparametric analyses wherever possible, which inevitably involved some bias to the particular index under evaluation.[1] The analytic methods were discussed fully in an appendix to the report.[1]

The findings were, to put it mildly, "most unfortunate." In part one, the scatter of values for each patient was startling, and part two did nothing to encourage the hope of achieving consistency between observers. While part three produced some improvement, part four showed wide variations in each of the indices tested, the least being with the Dutch AI.[6]

After discussing some of the possible limitations of the study, de Dombal and Softley sounded a solemn note. First, they emphasized that the study had gone to great lengths to co-opt a group of physicians who might be expected to use such activity indices in their daily practice. Secondly, based on the considerable experience of Crohn's disease possessed by most of the medical participants, it was anticipated that the groups would be able to score each of the indices reproducibly. The fact that obviously they could not raises considerable doubt as to the validity of results obtained by studies that have used the various indices.[1] However, the report ended by suggesting that the use of ranking methods may be a remedial approach to the difficulties encountered by the IOIBD study and for future evaluations of Crohn's disease activity.

The significance of these findings to new therapeutic trials and to individual patient management is sufficient to justify this brief finale to the book. The data also serve as a caveat when reviewing the background to some of the modalities in current use in IBD. The IOIBD report was timely, indeed.

References

1. de Dombal, F. T., and Softley, A.: IOIBD Report No. 1: Observer variation in calculating indices of severity and activity in Crohn's disease. Special Report. Gut, *28*:474, 1987.
2. Best, W. R., Becktel, J. M., Singleton, J. W., and Kern, F. J., Jr.: Development of a Crohn's disease activity index. National Cooperative Crohn's Disease Study. Gastroenterology, *70*:439, 1976.
3. Best, W. R., and Becktel, J. M.: The Crohn's disease activity index as a clinical instrument. *In* Recent Advances in Crohn's Disease. Edited by A. S. Peña, I. T. Weterman, C. C. Booth, and W. Strober. Boston, Martinus Nijhoff Publishers, 1981.
4. Harvey, R. F., and Bradshaw, J. M.: A simple index of Crohn's disease activity. Lancet, *1*:514, 1980.
5. Myren, J., et al.: The OMGE multinational inflammatory bowel disease survey 1976-1982. A further report on 2657 cases. Scand J Gastroenterol, *19* (Suppl. 95):1, 1982.
6. van Hees, P.A.M., van Elteren, Ph., van Lier, H. J. J., and van Tongeren, J. H. M.: An index of inflammatory activity in patients with Crohn's disease. Gut, *21*:279, 1980.
7. Data from a 1981 meeting (in Oxford, U.K.) of a study group forming the IOIBD; cited by Myren J., et al. in reference 5.
8. Geobell, H., Jeskinsky, J. H., Weinbeck, M., and Schomerus, H.: European Co-operative Crohn's Disease Study (ECECS): An index of severity and activity in Crohn's disease (SAI). In press, 1987; cited by de Dombal, F. T. and Softley, A., in reference 1.

Index

Page numbers in *italics* indicate figures; page numbers followed by "t" indicate tables.

Abdominal pain, 247–250, *248, 249*
   clinical approaches to, 249–250
   in Crohn's disease, 176
      in children, 228
Abscess, cuff, 700, *701*
   in Crohn's disease, as indication for surgery, 541–543, 556–557, 576
   in ulcerative colitis, as indication for surgery, 570
   intra-abdominal, 264–265, 265t
      undernutrition and, 244
   intraperitoneal, 692
   modification of ileocolectomy imposed by, 602–603
   parastomal, with ileostomy, 649, *651*
   perianal. *See* Perianal abscess.
   perirectal, as indication for surgery, 576
   postoperative, hepatic, 693
      intermesenteric, 693
      pelvic, 692
      retroperitoneal, 693
      subphrenic and subhepatic, 692–693
Acetic acid, production of intestinal inflammation in animals by, 38
ACTH therapy, 530
   in ulcerative colitis, 450–455
      adverse effects of, 454–455, 455t
      clinical trials and, 451–452
      mechanism of action and, 450–451
ADCC. *See* Antibody dependent cellular cytotoxicity.
Adenomatous polyps, 753
   colonoscopy and, 356
Age, course of ulcerative colitis and, 171, 172–173
   epidemiology of inflammatory bowel disease and, 13–14, 14t–16t, 16
Agglutination pattern, of sera, 110
Alexithymia, 216
Allergic colitis, 130, 235
Allergic cutaneous reactions, with ileostomy, 649, *651*
Allergic proctitis, differential diagnosis of, 193
Allergy, 130
   gastrointestinal, 70–71
   to sulfasalazine, management of, 446t, 446–447
Amebiasis, differential diagnosis of, 198, *199–200*, 200
   endoscopy and, 361
   pathology of, 54
Aminocaproic acid, in ulcerative colitis, 457
Aminoglycosides, in peritonitis, 690–691
5-Aminosalicylic acid, 447–448. *See also* Sulfasalazine.
   azo-bond pro-drugs of, 449–450
   in Crohn's disease, 481–482, 483–484, *484*
      clinical studies and, 484
   in ulcerative colitis, 441
   oral non-linked, 450
Amyloid, 306

Anal anastomosis. *See* Anastomosis, anal; Ileal pouch-anal anastomosis.
Anal canal lesions, 259–260
Anal fistulae, treatment of, 261
Anal lesions, as indication for surgery, 576
   in Crohn's disease, 340
   in ulcerative colitis, 336
Anal sphincters, ileal pouch-anal anastomosis and, 661, *662*
Anal stenosis, 259
   treatment of, 261
Analgesics, in ulcerative colitis, 437–438
Anaphylatoxins, 112, 114
Anastomosis, anal, individual operations for, 600–604
   recurrence and, 596–598
   surgical strategy and principles of, 598–600
   ileal pouch-anal. *See* Ileal pouch-anal anastomosis.
   ileoanal, 368, *426*, 426–427, *427*, 699–702
   ileorectal, 589, 708, 709
   in Crohn's disease, 573–574
   leakage of, following ileostomy, 696
   technique of, 596, *597*
Anastomotic strictures, 700
Anemia, 308
   iron deficiency, in children, 509
   megaloblastic, sulfasalazine and, 444
Anergy, systemic cellular immunity and, 138
Anesthesia, 595–596
Angiography, 425
   mesenteric, massive hemorrhage and, 263, *263*
Animal models, intestinal inflammation in, 37–43
   animal transmission studies and, 41t, 41–43, 42t
   by immunologic methods, 40–41
   by indirect manipulation, 37–38
   by topical application of irritant chemicals, 38–40
   psychosocial factors and, symptom onset and exacerbation and, 211–212
   spontaneous, 43–45
      idiopathic disorders and, 44–45, 45t
      infections and, 43, 44t
Ankylosing spondylitis, *304*, 304–305, *305*
   association with inflammatory bowel disease, 20, 22, 23, 92–93
Anorectal angle, ileal pouch-anal anastomosis and, 661, 663, *663*
Anorectal complications, 257–262, 258t
   in Crohn's disease, as indication for surgery, 545
   of anal canal, 259–260
   of skin, 258–259, *259*
   treatment of, 261–262
Anorectal sensation, ileal pouch-anal anastomosis and, 661
Anorexia, 239–241, *241, 242*
   clinical approaches to, 240–241

Anthropomorphic measurements, nutritional assessment and, 516, 516t
Antibiotic therapy, in Crohn's disease, 488–490, 494
　anti-tuberculous, 489
　broad-spectrum, 488–489
　in pseudomembranous enterocolitis, 205
　in severe colitis, 461–462
　in toxic megacolon, 566
　preoperative, 594
　wound infection and, 687
Antibiotic-associated colitis, endoscopy and, 361–362
Antibodies, against microbial pathogens, 56–57
　against normal flora bacteria, 56
　autoantibodies, 110–111
　response to immunizations and, 111–112
　systemic humoral immunity and, 108–112
　to bacteria, 109–110
　to food antigens, 109
　to viruses, Mycoplasma, and Chlamydia, 108–109
Antibody dependent cellular cytotoxicity (ADCC), 72, 136
　anti-colon antibodies and, 143–144
　circulating cells and, 106
　cytotoxicity of, 144
Anticholinergic drugs, in ulcerative colitis, 436
Anti-colon antibodies, as etiologic theory, 142t, 142–144
Antidepressants, in ulcerative colitis, 437
Antidiarrheal drugs, in ulcerative colitis, 436–437
　pregnancy and, 324–325
Antigen(s), epithelial cell-associated, 143, 145
　HLA, 20, 97–99, 100t–101t, 102–103
　as genetic markers, 20, 92
　major histocompatibility complex, 97–98
　regulation of intestinal response to, 125
Antigen-presenting cells (APC), 129
Antigen-sensitive cells. See Lymphocytes.
Antilymphocyte globulin, in ulcerative colitis, 456
Antimicrobial therapy. See also Antibiotic therapy.
　in peritonitis, 690–691
　in ulcerative colitis, 457
Antipsychotic drugs, in ulcerative colitis, 437
Antispasmodic drugs, in children, 504
　in ulcerative colitis, 436
APC (antigen-presenting cells), 129
Aphthous ulcers. See Ulcer(s), aphthous.
Apical membranes, of M cells, 78
Appendectomy, in Crohn's disease, 550–551
Appendicitis, in Crohn's disease, 550–551
　perforated, 407, 407
Appendicostomy, 585–586, 645
Arabinomannan, 56
Arachidonic acid, intestinal cellular immunity and, 139
　metabolism of, redirection of, in ulcerative colitis, 442
Arachidonic acid cascade, 245
　in ulcerative colitis, 441–442
Arteritis, 308
Arthritis, 118, 302
　colitic, 303–304
　in children, 230
Arthus reaction, 116–117
5-ASA. See 5-Aminosalicylic acid.
Ascorbic acid, absorption of, impairment by resection, 720
　requirements for, 524
Atrophic changes, in ulcerative colitis, lack of, 336–337
　specificity of, 336
　of crypts, 361

Autoantibodies, 110–111
Autoimmunity, as etiologic theory, 142–145, 144t
Aylett operation, 626–627
　in ulcerative colitis, 589
Azathioprine, 455–456
　adverse effects of, 313
　circulating cells and, 106
　in Crohn's disease, in children, 506
　pregnancy and, 321–322
Azo-bond preparations, 449–450
Azodisalicylate (Olsalazine; Dipentum), 449
Azulfidine. See Sulfasalazine.

B cells, 105
　mucosal immune system and, 122, 123
Bacillary dysentery. See Shigellosis.
Bacille Calmette Guerin (BCG) vaccine, in Crohn's disease, 491
Backwash ileitis, 251, 698
　in ulcerative colitis, 335
Bacteria. See also Flora; Mycobacteria.
　antibodies to, 56, 109–110
　continent reservoir ileostomy and, 678
　extraintestinal manifestations and, 313
　in Crohn's disease, 55–56
　intra-abdominal abscess and, 264
　mucosal relationships of, 52
　transport by M cells, 80–81
Bacterial endotoxin, 109
Bacterial overgrowth syndrome, 252, 253
Bacteroides necrophorum, 52–53
Bacteroides vulgatus, experimental colitis and, 57
Balantidium coli, endoscopy and, 362
Barbiturates, in ulcerative colitis, 437
Barium studies, in children, 234
　in Crohn's colitis, 189, 190–192, 191
　in Crohn's disease, cancer and, 290
　in gonorrheal proctitis, 196
　in ischemic disease, 203
　in pseudomembranous enterocolitis, 205
　in radiation colitis, 202
　in toxic megacolon, 271
　in ulcerative colitis, cancer and, 284
BCG (Bacille Calmette Guerin) vaccine, in Crohn's disease, 491
"Bear claw" ulcers, 358
Behavioral interventions, 222–223
Bile acid(s), as intestinal defense, 67
　ileostomy and, 251
　metabolism of, with continent pouch ileostomy, 679
"Bile acid diarrhea," 246
Bile salt enterohepatic circulation, postoperative interruption of, 734–739
　cholerrheic and steatorrheic diarrhea and, 734–736
　cholesterol gallstones and, 736
　kidney stones and, 736–739
Biliary tract cancer, 291–292
Biochemical markers, 21
Biopsies, colonoscopic, detection of dysplasia and, 369–370, 371t
　differential diagnosis and, 359–360
　for cancer surveillance, frequency of, 370, 372
　in Crohn's disease, 342–344
　　multiple, from same level, 344
　　multiple, from variety of levels, 344
　　single, 342–344
　rectal, detection of dysplasia and, 369

Biotin, absorption of, 721
  requirement for, 524
Bladder dysfunction, postoperative, 705–706
Bleeding. *See also* Hemorrhage.
  rectal, 250
Blood chemistry, nutritional assessment and, 516–517
Blood film, nutritional assessment and, 516
Blood groups, as genetic markers, 91–92
Bone loss, steroid therapy and, 454
Bowel. *See* Colon; Duodenum; Ileum; Intestine; Small intestine.
Bowel rest, 513
  in Crohn's disease, 526
Breast milk, as intestinal defense, 67–68
  epidemiology of inflammatory bowel disease and, 25–26
  in Crohn's disease, 483
Bronchopulmonary manifestations, 309
Bypass surgery, 587–588
  cancer and, 289
  exclusion, modification of ileocolectomy imposed by, *603*, 603–604
  in Crohn's disease, 708

Calcium, absorption of, impairment by resection, 718
  nutritional assessment and, 517
  requirement for, 525
  urinary excretion of, 738
Calcium deficiency, 514, 718
Calcium oxalate stones, postoperative enhanced formation of, 737–739
Campylobacter fetus subspecies jejuni, differential diagnosis of, 195
  endoscopy and, 362
Cancer. *See also* Dysplasia; Malignancy; Neoplasia.
  etiology of, 292
  extraintestinal, 291–292
  in Crohn's disease. *See* Crohn's disease, cancer in.
  in ulcerative colitis, 281–287
    as indication for surgery, 567–570, 568t
    bile duct carcinoma, 291
    diagnosis of, 283–284
    extent of risk for, 281–283
    pathologic features of, 283, *283*
    surveillance for, 285–287, *286*, *287*
    treatment and prognosis for, 284–285, *285*
  in ulcerative proctitis, prognosis of, 756
  inflammatory polyps and, 336
  intestinal, 291
  of biliary tract, 291–292
Carbohydrates, malabsorption of, 242–243
  small intestine resection and, 716–718
Carcinoid, differentiation of Crohn's disease from, 416, *417*, *418*
  intestinal, 291
Carcinoma. *See also* Cancer; Dysplasia; Malignancy; Neoplasia.
  as indication for surgery, 534–535
  colonoscopy and, 355
  in children, 229
  in Crohn's disease, 708
    as indication for surgery, 421, 545–546, 558–559, 575
  in ulcerative colitis, radiography and, 384, *393–395*
  squamous, intestinal, 291
  weighing risk factors for, 535
Carrageenan, experimental colitis and, 57
  production of intestinal inflammation in animals by, 39

Case-control study, 6
Catabolism, of complement, 114
Catheter, postoperative, 628–629
CDAI (Crohn's Disease Activity Index), 179, 179t
Cecostomy, 645
Cell membranes, direct penetration of, 66
Cellular effector system, 103
Cell-wall defective bacteria, 58–59
Central nervous system, alterations in immune function and, 213–214
  postoperative complications and
Chemokinesis, 119
Chemotaxis, 119–120
Children, 227t, 227–236
  cholelithiasis in, 230
  clinical presentation in, 228t, 228–229, 229t
  complications in, 229–232
    extraintestinal, 230
    growth failure as, 230–232, 231t
    intestinal, 229–230
  Crohn's disease in. *See* Crohn's disease, in children.
  differential diagnosis in, 235–236, 236t
  epidemiology of inflammatory bowel disease in, 6, 228, 228t
  evaluation of, 232–235, 233t
    history in, 232
    ^{111}-indium-labeled leukocyte scan in, 234
    laboratory studies in, 232–233, 233t
    pathology and, 235
    physical examination in, 232
    radiology in, 233–234, 234t
    sigmoidoscopy and colonoscopy in, 234–235, 235t
    ultrasonography and computed tomography in, 234
  medical management in, 503–510
    approach to patient and, 503–504
    sulfasalazine therapy and, 447
  ulcerative colitis in, 752
    medical management of, 504–505
    surgical intervention in, 505
Chlamydia, antibodies to, 108–109
Chloramphenicol, in peritonitis, 690
Chloride deficiency, 514
Cholangiocarcinoma, 312
Cholangitis, sclerosing, *311*, 311–312
  radiology and, *424*, 424–425, *425*
Cholelithiasis, 312
  in children, 230
Chromium, absorption of, impairment by resection, 719–720
  requirements for, 522
Circulating cells, effect of treatment on, 106–107
  systemic humoral immunity and, 104–107
Cirrhosis, 310–311
Clonidine, in ulcerative colitis, 437, 457
Clostridium difficile, 57–58
  in Crohn's colitis, 189
Clubbing, 305
Coagulopathy, 308
Cobblestoning, differential diagnosis and, 358, 359
  in Crohn's colitis, 191
  in Crohn's disease, 339, *339*
Colectomy, completion as proctocolectomy, *609–613*, 610–612
  conduct of, *605*, 605–626, *606–609*
  in children, 505
  in toxic megacolon, 628
  in ulcerative colitis, 173, 589

Colectomy, in ulcerative colitis, *(Continued)*
  prognosis of, 752–753
  prophylactic, 569–570
  results of, 636–638
  subtotal, *605*, 608–610
    in ulcerative colitis, 589
    risk of cancer and, 372
  toxic megacolon and, 335
Colitic arthritis, 303–304
Colitis, acute self-limited, differential diagnosis of, 346, *347*
  allergic, 130, 235
  amebic. *See* Amebiasis.
  antibiotic-associated, endoscopy and, 361–362
  collagenous, differential diagnosis of, 193, 347–348
  Crohn's. *See* Crohn's colitis.
  diarrhea in, pathophysiology of, 244–245, 245t, 246t
  diversion, differential diagnosis of, 348–349
  drug-induced, differential diagnosis of, 348
  fulminant. *See* Fulminant colitis.
  granulomatous. *See* Crohn's disease.
  "indeterminate," 344–345
  infectious, differential diagnosis of, 193–194, *194*
  ischemic, endoscopy and, 365
  pseudomembranous, in children, 236
    radiologic appearance of, 387, 392
  radiation, differential diagnosis of, 201–202
    endoscopy and, 366
  toxic, acute, in Crohn's disease, 408–409
Collagenous colitis, differential diagnosis of, 193, 347–348
"Collar button" ulcerations, in Crohn's colitis, 191
Colon, common infections of, endoscopy and, 361–364, 362t
  contrast examination methods for, 378
  dilatation of, in toxic megacolon, 462
  diverticular disease of, 364–365
  free perforation of, 268
  in Crohn's disease, distensibility of, 397, *401–404*
    distinction from other diseases and, 406–408, *406–409*
    fistulae and. *See* Fistulae, in Crohn's disease.
    radiology in. *See* Radiology, in Crohn's disease.
    segmental involvement of, 397, *399–401*
  infections of, differential diagnosis of, 194–205
  lymphoma of, 408, *409*
  massive hemorrhage of, 262–263
  normal flora of, 51
Colonoscopy, 353–373, 354t
  cancer detection and, 284, 286, 569
    frequency of, 370, 372
  colonic infections and, 361–364, 362t
  complications of, 372
  differential diagnosis of inflammatory bowel disease and, 356–361, 358t, 359t
  dysplasia and, 369–370, 370t, 371t, 372, 568
  ileostomy and, 366–368
  in children, 235, 235t
  in Crohn's disease, 189, 189t
  in evaluation of unexplained diarrhea, 368
  in ulcerative colitis, 170, 171t, 434
    cancer and, 284, 286
  in upper gastrointestinal involvement by Crohn's disease, 372–373
  inflammatory conditions of colon and, 364–366
  massive hemorrhage and, 264
  postoperative, in Crohn's disease, 366
  preparation for, diarrhea and, 368

screening for premalignant and malignant features with, 368–369
strictures and mass lesions and, 355–356
to evaluate extent of inflammatory bowel disease, 354–355
Colorectum, adenocarcinoma of, 288–289
Colostomy, in Crohn's disease, 560
  left-sided or rectal, 574
Complement, levels in inflammatory bowel disease, 114
  metabolism and activation of, 114–115
  systemic humoral immunity and, 112, *113*, 114–115
Complement fixation test, in Lymphogranuloma venereum, 197
Computerized tomography, *423*, 423–424, *424*
  in evaluation of pediatric patients, 234
Conflict, 215
Conjunctivitis, 308
Contraceptives, oral, epidemiology of inflammatory bowel disease and, 27
Contrast examination. *See also* Barium studies; Radiology.
  methods of, 377–378
Control mechanisms, microflora and, 52
Copper, absorption of, impairment by resection, 719
  requirements for, 522
Corticosteroids, circulating cells and, 106
  growth failure and, 231
  in acute colitis, 460, 461
  in children, 504, 505, 506
  in Crohn's disease, 484–488
    adverse effects and, 487–488
    clinical studies and, 484, 485t, 486
    in children, 506
    mechanism of action and, 487
    pharmacology and, 487
    pregnancy and, 488
  in sepsis, 693
  in toxic megacolon, 273–274
  in ulcerative colitis, 459
  intestinal absorption and, 730
  length of therapy with, 539
  leukotrienes and, 139
  neutrophil function and, 121
  postoperative, 628, 693
  pregnancy and, 322
  surgery and, 591–593, 592t
Crohn's colitis, differential diagnosis of, 187–188
  prognosis for, 760
  signs and symptoms of, 186–187
Crohn's disease. *See also* Inflammatory bowel disease.
  active, pathology of, 339
  anastomotic procedures for, 596–604
    individual operations for, 600–604
    recurrence and, 596–598
    surgical strategy and principles in, 598–600
  aphthous ulcer in, 126, *342*, 342–343
  bacterial flora in, 55–56
  biopsy diagnosis of, 342–344
    with multiple biopsies from same level, 344
    with multiple biopsies from variety of levels, 344
    with single biopsy, 342–344
  cancer in, 287–291
    diagnosis of, 290
    extent of risk of, 287–289
    pathologic features of, 290
    prognosis for, 290, 760–761
    surveillance for, 290–291

treatment of, 290
clinical patterns and disease locations in, 177t, 177–178, 178t
cobblestone mucosa and linear ulceration in, development and resolution of, 339, *339*
coexistent with ulcerative colitis, 345–346
differential diagnosis of, *186–188*, 186–191, 188t, 346–349
  endoscopy and, 189, 189t
  laboratory findings and, 189
  pathology and, 191
  radiography and, 189, *190–192*, 191
disease activity indices in, 179t, 179–180, 180t
duodenal, 177–178
  choice of operations in, 590–591
  indications for surgery in, 546, 551–553
  radiology and, 416–418, *419–421*
erythema nodosum in, 301
fissures and fistulae in, 340, *340*
free perforation in, 268–269
gastric, choice of operation in, 590–591
  indications for surgery in, 546, 551–553
granulomas in, 340–341
histologic features of, resected bowel and, 341
  traps in diagnosis and, 341–342
HLA antigens in, 98–99, 100t, 102–103
ileal or ileocolonic, ileocolic resection for, 600, *601*
immunologic features of, compared with ulcerative colitis, 147
in children, 505–510
  medical treatment of, 505–507
  nutritional intervention in, 507–510
  surgical intervention in, 510
in pregnancy, 323
in remission, approach to, 494
"indeterminate colitis" and, 344–345
indications for surgery in, 535–546, 535t–539t, 549–562, 571–576
involving foregut and midgut, 549–562
involving substantial portions of colon, choice of operation in, 590
laboratory features of, 178–179
medical therapy of, 477–494
  antibiotics and, 488–490
  approach to patient and, 492, 494
  corticosteroids and. See Corticosteroids, in Crohn's disease.
  diet and nutrition and, 477–479
  failure of, as indication for surgery, 536, 539–540, 553–554
  for upper gastrointestinal disease, 492
  immunosuppressive therapy and, 490–491
  in children, 505–507
  placebo and, 492, 493t
  psychotherapy and, 479
  sulfasalazine and. See Sulfasalazine, in Crohn's disease.
  sulfasalazine-related drugs and, 483–484, *484*
metastatic, 302, *303*
mild, approach to, 492, 494
moderate, approach to, 492, 494
pathology of, 338–342
postoperative endoscopy in, 366
prestomal, 635–636
prognosis of, 181–182, 756–761
  cancer and, 760–761
  causes of death and, 757
  complications and, 757
  Crohn's colitis and, 760
  quality of life and, 761
  surgical treatment and, 757–760, *758*
  survival and, 756–757, *757*
quality of life and, 182, 761
radiography in. See Radiology, in Crohn's disease.
recrudescent, ileostomy in, 352
rectal bleeding in, 250
segmental operations in, 626
severe, approach to, 494
small intestinal, indications for surgery in, 553t, 553–562
strictures in, 277–278
  colonic, 277
  of small intestine, 278
surgical treatment for, 681–682
  choice of operation and, 587–588
  in children, 510
  indications for, 180t, 180–182, 181t, 535–546, 535t–539t, 549–562
  prognosis for, 757–760, *758*
  recurrences following, 180–181, 551, 708–710
  results of, 636
symptoms and signs of, 175–177
total parenteral nutrition as primary therapy for, 526
toxic megacolon in, 269
transmural inflammation in, 340
upper gastrointestinal involvement by, endoscopy in, 372–373
Crohn's Disease Activity Index (CDAI), 179, 179t
Crohn's Ileocolitis, 410–416, *410–416*
Crypt(s), architecture of, 361
  atrophy of, 361
  following bowel resection, 725–726
  in quiescent ulcerative colitis, 332–333, *333*
Cuff abscess, 700, *701*
Cultural factors, 212
Cutaneous hypersensitivity, nutritional assessment and, 517
Cyclosporine, in ulcerative colitis, 456
Cytomegalovirus, endoscopy and, 362
Cytomegalovirus occlusion disease, differential diagnosis of, 198
Cytotoxic cells, as etiologic theory, 144t, 144–145
  intestinal cellular immunity and, 140–141
  systemic cellular immunity and, 136–137

DALM (dysplasia associated mucosal masses), 534, 569
Deep vein thrombosis, 308
Dehydration, with ileostomy, 652
Demographic characteristics, 13–19
Depression, 218
Dermatitis, ileostomy and, 699
DFMO (difluoromethyl ornithine), production of intestinal inflammation in animals by, 38
Diagnosis-related groups, case ascertainment and, 5
Diarrhea, "bile acid," 246
  changes in microflora and, 53–54
  cholerrheic and steatorrheic, postoperative, 734–736
  clinical approaches to, 247, *247*
  continent reservoir ileostomy and, 674
  following ileostomy, 697
  in collagenous colitis, 193
  in Crohn's disease, in children, 228–229
  in ileostomy patients, 251–252
  in salmonellosis, 194
  in ulcerative colitis, 168
  pathophysiology of, 244–247

Diarrhea, pathophysiology of, *(Continued)*
  in colitis, 244–245, 245t, 246t
    in disease of small intestine, 245–247
  sulfasalazine and, 445
  unexplained, endoscopy in evaluation of, 368
Diet. *See also* Nutrition.
  defined formula, enteral feeding of, 517–518, 519t
  elemental, in Crohn's disease, 478–479
  epidemiology of inflammatory bowel disease and, 25–26
  for children, 504, 508
  in Crohn's disease, 477–479
  in ulcerative colitis, 436, 460
  postoperative, 630
Dietary supplements, in children, 508
Difluoromethyl ornithine (DFMO), production of intestinal inflammation in animals by, 38
Dilatation, in ulcerative colitis, 334–335, *335*
Dinitrochlorobenzene (DNCB), production of intestinal inflammation in animals by, 40
  response to, 137
Dipentum (azodisalicylate), 449
Diphenoxylate, in ulcerative colitis, 437
Diphtheria toxoid, response to, 111–112
Disease activity indices, in children, 507
  in Crohn's disease, 179t, 179–180, 180t
Disodium cromoglycate, in Crohn's disease, 491
Distensibility, of colon, in Crohn's disease, 397, *401–404*
Diversion colitis, differential diagnosis of, 348–349
Diversion proctitis, differential diagnosis of, 193
Diverticulae, intramural, tiny, 408, *409*
Diverticular disease, 364–365
  differential diagnosis of, 191–193
  endoscopy and, 364–365
  perforated, 406–407, *407*
DNCB (dinitrochlorobenzene), response to, 137
Drug effects. *See also specific drugs and drug types.*
  on course of pregnancy, 321–322
  on digestion and absorption, 244, 245t
  pathogenetic, 240
Drug-induced colitis, differential diagnosis of, 348
Duodenum, contrast examination methods for, 378
  endoscopy and, 372–373
  in Crohn's disease. *See* Crohn's disease, duodenal.
Dysplasia. *See also* Cancer; Malignancy; Neoplasia.
  colonoscopy and, 568
  detection of, colonoscopic biopsies and, 369–370, 371t
    frequency of, 370, 372
    rectal biopsies and, 369
    retained rectal segment and, 372
  in ulcerative colitis, radiography and, 384–385, *395, 396*
  prognosis and, 753, 760–761
Dysplasia associated mucosal masses (DALM), 534, 569

ECA (enterobacterial common antigen), 71–72
  neonatal sensitization to, 71–72, *72*
ECAC (epithelial cell-associated components), 143, 145
Education, incidence of inflammatory bowel disease related to, 18, 19
Eh (oxidation-reduced potential), low, 51–52
Electrolytes, abnormalities of, in ulcerative colitis, 435
  deficiencies of, 514
  nutritional assessment and, 516–517
  replacement of, postoperative, 628
  requirements for, 524–525

Elemental diet, in Crohn's disease, 478–479
End-jejunostomy syndrome, as indication for total parenteral nutrition, 520–521
Endocrine manifestations, 309
  growth failure and, 231
Endocytosis, nonselective, 65–66, *66, 67*
  receptor-mediated, 65
Endoscopy. *See* Colonoscopy.
Energy, expenditures of, 241
  requirements for, 522
Enteral feeding. *See also* Total parenteral nutrition.
  of defined formula diets, 517–518, 519t
Enteric content, ileal pouch-anal anastomosis and, 666
Enteric infections, in Crohn's disease, in children, 507
Enteric motility, proximal, ileal pouch-anal anastomosis and, 665, *666*
Enteritis, acute, choice of operation in, 588
  mucosal, 252
  proximal, in Crohn's disease, as indication for surgery, 560
  regional. *See* Crohn's disease.
Enterobacterial common antigen (ECA), 71–72
  neonatal sensitization to, 71–72, *72*
Enterocolitis, pseudomembranous, differential diagnosis of, 203, *204*, 205
Enterocutaneous fistulae. *See* Fistulae, enterocutaneous.
Enteroenteral fistulae, 266–267, *267*
  as indication for surgery, 555
Enteroglucagon, intestinal absorption and, 730–731
Enterovesical fistulae, 265–266, *266*
  as indication for surgery, 556
Environmental factors, genetic factors separated from, 6–7
  heredity and, 93–94, 94t
Eosinophils, 331–332
Epidemiology, psychosocial factors and, symptom onset and exacerbation and, 212–213
Episcleritis, *307*, 307–308
Epithelial cell(s), colonic, cells cytotoxic for, 144t, 144–145
  membranous. *See* Membranous epithelial cells.
Epithelial cell-associated components (ECAC), 143, 145
Erythema nodosum, *301*, 301–302
Erythrocyte sedimentation rate (ESR), in ulcerative colitis, 433
Escherichia coli, production of intestinal inflammation in animals by, 40
Esophagus, radiology and, 378, 416–418, *421, 422*
ESR (erythrocyte sedimentation rate), in ulcerative colitis, 433
Ethnicity, epidemiology of inflammatory bowel disease and, 17t, 17–18
Exclusion bypass, modification of ileocolectomy imposed by, *603*, 603–604
Extraintestinal manifestations, 299–314
  bronchopulmonary, 309
  cancer, 291–292
  hematologic and vascular, 308–309
  hepatobiliary, 309–312
  in children, 229, 230
  in Crohn's disease, as indication for surgery, 576
    in children, 229
  in patients without inflammatory bowel disease, 313
  in ulcerative colitis, 169, 173t, 173–174, 463–465
    as indication for surgery, 571

metabolic and endocrine, 309
musculoskeletal, 302–305
ocular, 307–308
of skin and mucous membranes, 299–302
pathogenesis of, 313–314
renal and genitourinary, 305–306
therapy related, 312–313

Familial aggregation, 19–20, 20t
Family, approach to, 465–466
　distribution of inflammatory bowel disease cases within, 87t, 87–91, 88t
　　impact of ulcerative colitis on, 435
　　involving in treatment, 222
　　positive history of inflammatory bowel disease in, 89–91, 89t–91t
Fat, malabsorption of, diarrhea and, 735–736
　hyperoxaluria and, 738
　small intestine resection and, 717–718
Fat distribution, steroid therapy and, 454
Fatty acids, requirements for, 522
Fatty liver, 309–310
Fecal continence, with ileal pouch-anal anastomosis, 667
Femoral nerve palsy, postoperative, 707
Fertility, in men, 320, 320t
　in women, 319–320
　medical management of inflammatory bowel disease in regard to, 324–325, 325t
　sulfasalazine and, 444–445
Fiber, epidemiology of inflammatory bowel disease and, 25
Fissure in ano, 259
Fissures. *See* Anal lesions.
Fistula in ano, 260–261
Fistulae, anal, treatment of, 261
　as indication for total parenteral nutrition, 521
　enterocutaneous, 266
　　as indication for surgery, 555–556, 576
　　surgery and, 602
　enteroenteral, 266–267, *267*
　　as indication for surgery, 555
　enterovesical, 265–266, *266*
　　as indication for surgery, 556
　following ileostomy, 697
　ileo right colic, in Crohn's disease, 555
　ileocecal, in Crohn's disease, 555
　ileocutaneous, following ileostomy, 698
　ileosigmoidal, in Crohn's disease, 555
　ileostomy, 698
　ileovesical, surgery and, 602
　in Crohn's colitis, 191
　in Crohn's disease, 340, *340*, 399, *405*, *406*
　　anastomotic procedures and, 599
　　as indication for surgery, 541–543, 555–556, 576
　　immunosuppressive therapy for, 267–268
　　perianal, 559
　in ulcerative colitis, as indication for surgery, 570
　modification of ileocolectomy imposed by, 601–602
　of urinary tract, 265–266, *266*
　perianal. *See* Perianal fistulae.
　rectovaginal, 265
　　as indication for surgery, 542–543
　stomal, with ileostomy, 649
Flora. *See also* Bacteria; Microflora.
　postoperative peritonitis and, 689
Fluid replacement, in sepsis, 693
　postoperative, 628, 693
Fluid requirements, 524

Folic acid, requirements for, 523–524
Follicle-associated epithelial cells. *See* Membranous epithelial cells.
Food antigens, antibodies to, 109
Frei test, in lymphogranuloma venereum, 197
Friability, differential diagnosis and, 358, 358t, 359t
Fulminant colitis, as indication for surgery, 532–533, 564, 566–567
　in Crohn's disease, 576
　rectal sparing and irregular transition to active disease in, 338
　surgical treatment of, 627–628
　V-shaped ulcers in, 341–342
Fungal infection, with ileostomy, 649, *651*

Gallbladder, small bowel resection and, 732
Gallstones, 312
　cholesterol, postoperative, 253–254, 736
GALT (gut-associated lymphoid tissue), 121–125, *122*
　sensitization to antigens, 71
Gastric acid, control of microorganisms by, 52
Gastric Crohn's disease. *See* Crohn's disease, gastric.
Gastric emptying, delayed, in Crohn's disease, 240
Gastric hypersecretion, ileostomy and, 252
　postoperative, 733
Gastroduodenum, involvement of, 240
Gastrointestinal complications, 257–278, 258t. *See also specific complications.*
　anorectal, 257–262, 258t
　　treatment of, 261–262
　hemorrhagic, 262–264
　　colonic, 262–263
　　in upper gut, 263
　　treatment of, *263*, 263–264
　steroid therapy and, 454–455
Gastrojejunostomy, posterior, in Crohn's disease, 591
Gay bowel syndrome, differential diagnosis of, 200–201
　endoscopy and, 364
Genetic factors, 20–21, 87–94
　distribution of inflammatory bowel disease cases within families and, 87t, 87–91, 88t
　environment and, 6–7, 93–94, 94t
　genetic markers and, 91–93
Genetic markers, 91–93
　associations with other disorders and, 92–93
Genetic susceptibility, 93
Genitourinary manifestations, 305–306
　after ileoanal anastomosis, 700
Goblet cells, in quiescent ulcerative colitis, 333
Gonadotropins, sexual maturation and, 510
Gonorrheal proctitis, differential diagnosis of, 196–197
Graft-versus-host disease, production of intestinal inflammation in animals and, 41
Granularity, differential diagnosis and, 357, 358, 358t, 359t
Granuloma(s), in children, 236
　in Crohn's disease, 340–341, 342
　　biopsy diagnosis and, 342
　　noncaseating, 302, *303*
　　solitary, significance of, 341
　in "indeterminate colitis," 345
　in ulcerative colitis, 337–338
　transfer of, 59–60
Granulomatous colitis. *See* Crohn's disease.
Growth failure, 230–232, 231t
　as indication for total parenteral nutrition, 521
　in Crohn's disease, 229, 507–508, 508t
　　as indication for surgery, 544, 561

Growth failure, *(Continued)*
  in ulcerative colitis, 564
  undernutrition and, 244
Growth-promoting hormones, in Crohn's disease, 509–510
Gut-associated lymphoid tissue (GALT), 121–125, *122*
  sensitization to antigens, 71
Gut irrigation, in Crohn's disease, 491

Health care costs, 219, 219t
Hematologic manifestations, 308
Hematologic studies, in Crohn's disease, in children, 232–233
Hematopoietic system, sulfasalazine and, 444
Hemoglobin, nutritional assessment and, 516
Hemorrhage, as indication for surgery, 534
  in Crohn's disease, 543–544, 576
    in ulcerative colitis, 567
    following ileostomy, 696
  massive, 262–264
    colonic, 262–263
    of upper gut, 263
    treatment of, *263*, 263–264
  of bowel, in ulcerative colitis, 435
Hemorrhoids, 258–259
Heparin, in sepsis, 693–694
  preoperative, 594, 693–694
Hepatic abscess, abscess, 693
Hepatic dysfunction, in children, 230
Hepatic factors, affecting macromolecular transport, 68–69, *69*, *70*
Hepatic reactions, to sulfasalazine, 444
Hepatitis, chronic active, 310
  granulomatous, 311
  postoperative, 707
Hepatobiliary manifestations, 309–312
Hermansky-Pudlak syndrome, association of inflammatory bowel disease with, 92
Hernia, incisional, 688–689
  paraileostomy, 698
  parastomal, with ileostomy, 649, *651*
Histoplasmosis, differential diagnosis of, 197
  endoscopy and, 362
History, in evaluation of pediatric patients, 232
Histrionic personality, 218
HLA antigens, 20, 97–99, 100t–101t, 102–103
  as genetic markers, 20, 92
HLA typing, in diagnosis of ankylosing spondylitis/sacroiliitis, 305
Homosexuality. *See* Gay bowel syndrome.
Hormones, intestinal adaptation and, 729–731
Humoral effector system, 103
Humoral immunity, intestinal. *See* Immunology, intestinal humoral immunity and.
  systemic. *See* Immunology, systemic humoral immunity and.
Hydronephrosis, obstructive, in Crohn's disease, 306
Hydrophilic mucilloids, in ulcerative colitis, 437
Hyperalimentation, complications of, 313
Hyperoxaluria, 738
Hyperplasia, lymphoid, nodular, differential diagnosis of, 358
Hypersensitivity reactions, to sulfasalazine, 443–444
Hypertrophic osteoarthropathy, 305
Hypoalbuminemia, 243
Hypocalcemia, 514, 718
Hypochondriasis, 218
Hypogammaglobulinemia, 108, 146–147

Hypomagnesemia, 514–515, 517, 718–719
Hypophosphatemia, 515

IBD. *See* Inflammatory bowel disease.
IEL (intraepithelial lymphocytes), mucosal immune system and, 124
IgA, in inflammatory bowel disease, 129–130
  secretory, mucosal immune system and, 124–125
  transport of, 69
IgE, 130
Ileal pouch, *425*, 425–426, *426*
Ileal pouch-anal anastomosis, 253
  in ulcerative colitis, 655–667, 708
    background of, 655–656
    clinical evaluation of, 660
    physiologic results of, 661, 663–666
    rationale for, 656
    technique for, 656–657, *657–659*, 659–660
Ileal resection, diarrhea and, 245–246
Ileitis, acute, 549–551
  backwash, 251, 698
    in ulcerative colitis, 335
  dysfunctional, obstructive, 635–636
  prestomal, 251, 633–635, 698
    acute, 634
    chronic, 634–635
  stomal, 698
  terminal, in Crohn's disease, biopsy diagnosis and, 343, *343*
Ileo right colic fistulae, in Crohn's disease, 555
Ileoanal anastomosis, 368, *426*, 426–427, *427*
  complications of, 699–702
Ileoanal pull-through procedures, 627
Ileocecal fistulae, in Crohn's disease, 555
Ileocecal valve, control of microorganisms by, 52
  preservation of, nutrient absorption and, 724
  regulation of microflora by, 55
Ileocolectomy, modification of, imposed by complications, 601–603
Ileocolic resection, for ileal or ileocolic Crohn's disease, 600, *601*
Ileocolitis, choice of operation in, 587–588, 590
  Crohn's, 410–416, *410–416*
  indications for surgery in, 572–573
Ileocutaneous fistulae, following ileostomy, 698
Ileoproctostomy, in Crohn's disease, 590
  resection and, 626–627
Ileorectal anastomosis, in Crohn's disease, 709
  in ulcerative colitis, 589, 708
Ileorectostomy, 656
Ileoscopy, 360
Ileosigmoidal fistulae, in Crohn's disease, 555
Ileostomy, 250–253, 562–563, 586
  alternatives to, 562–563
  anal, in ulcerative colitis, 589
  Brooke, 620, 655–656
  complications of, 251, 695–699
  construction of, 616–621
    Brooke ileostomy and, 620
    extraperitoneal, 616–620, *626–620*
    maturation and, 620–621, *622*, *623*
    reperitonealization and closure of abdomen and, 621
  continent, 252–253, 367, 425–427
    early postoperative complications of, 696
    ileal pouch and, *425*, 425–426, *426*
    ileoanal anastomosis and, *426*, 426–427, *427*
    late postoperative complications of, 696–698

operative mortality of, 695–696
continent reservoir, 667–681
  anatomic and physiologic results of, 675, *676*, 676t, 677–680
  background and rationale for, 668
  clinical evaluation of, 671–675
  post-hospitalization care and, 671, *671*, *672*
  postoperative care and, 670
  technique for, 668–670, *669*, *670*
conventional, 252, 645–652
  biochemical alterations and, 652
  complications of, 649, *650*, *651*, 651–652
  construction of, 646–649, *647*, *648*, *650*
  general patient management and, 652
  historical perspective on, 645–646
  in ulcerative colitis, 589
dermatitis and, 699
diarrhea and, 251–252
discharges from, 629
diversionary, in Crohn's disease, 574, 627
dysfunction of, 631–634
early use of, 585–586
endoscopy and, 366–368
fistulae and, 698
functional sequelae of, 251
future for patient with, 699
in ulcerative colitis, 588–589
ligation of blood supply and preparation of ileum for, 612–615, *613–616*
management of perineal wound and, 623–626, *624*, *625*
outputs from, 250–251
paraileostomy hernia and, 698
prestomal or stomal ileitis and, 698
previously established, effects of pregnancy on, 324
prolapse of, 649, 698
quality of life with, 637–638
results of, 636–638
site of, 605, *605*
"Ileostomy clubs," 652
Ileostomy dysfunction, 645–646, 695
Ileovesical fistulae, surgery and, 602
Ileum, in tuberculosis, 196
  local, obstructive lesions of, 240
  terminal, in Crohn's disease, 410–411, *410–416*, 413, 415–416
    in ulcerative colitis, radiography and, 385–386, *388*, *389*, *396*
Illness behaviors, 217–218
Immune complex, extraintestinal manifestations and, 313
  production of intestinal inflammation in animals and, 40–41
  systemic humoral immunity and, 115–118
Immune complex disease, localized, 115–117
  systemic, 117–118
  systemic humoral immunity and, 115–118
Immune mechanisms, neonatal sensitization to microbial/mammalian cross-reacting antigen and, 71–72, *72*
Immunizations, response to, 111–112
Immunodeficiency, as etiologic theory, 142
Immunoglobulins. *See also* IgA; IgE.
  deficiency of, 108
  synthesis of, 146–147
  systemic humoral immunity and, 107–108
  turnover of, 107–108

Immunology, 97–147
  immunogenetics and, 97–99, 100t–102t, 102–103
  intestinal humoral immunity and, 121–147
    comparison of immunologic features of ulcerative colitis and Crohn's disease and, 147
    etiologic theories and, 141–147
    intestinal cellular immunity and, 138–141
    mucosal immune system and, 121–132, *122*
    systemic cellular immunity and, 132–138, *133*
  macromolecular transport and, 67–68, *68*
  systemic humoral immunity and, 103–121, *104*
    circulating cells and, 104–107
    complement and, 112–115
    immune complex disease and, 115–118
    neutrophils and, 118–121
    serum antibodies and, 108–112
    serum immunoglobulins and, 107–108
Immunomodulation, in ulcerative colitis, 455–456
  drugs and, 455–456
  immunostimulation and, 456
Immunoregulation, abnormal, 145–147
Immunostimulants, in Crohn's disease, 491
Immunosuppressive therapy, anorectal lesions and, 262
  for fistulae, in Crohn's disease, 267–268
  in Crohn's disease, 490–491
  pregnancy and, 325
  side effects of, 313
Incision, anastomotic procedures in Crohn's disease and, 598
  closure of, 596
  complications of, 685, *686*
Incisional hernia, 688–689
"Indeterminate colitis," 344–345
Index of Crohn's Disease Activity, simple, 179, 179t
[111]-Indium-labeled leukocyte scan, in evaluation of pediatric patients, 234
Infantilism, in Crohn's disease, as indication for surgery, 561
Infection, differential diagnosis of, 194–205, 346, *347*
  differentiation of ulcerative colitis from, 387, 392
  enteric, in Crohn's disease, in children, 507
  fungal, with ileostomy, 649, *651*
  of wound, 686–687
  superimposed, acute exacerbation of ulcerative colitis by, 337
Infectious agents, 23–24
Infectious colitis, differential diagnosis of, 193–194, *194*
Inflammation, continuity of, in ulcerative colitis, radiography and, 381–382, *388–389*
  "disproportionate," biopsy diagnosis and, 343
  in Crohn's disease, 360
  transmural, in Crohn's disease, 340
Inflammatory bowel disease (IBD). *See also* Crohn's disease; Ulcerative colitis.
  association with other diseases, 21–22, *23*
  Clostridium difficile and, 57–58
  differential diagnosis of, endoscopy and, 356–361, 358t, 359t
  effect on patient, 218–219
  epidemiology of, 3–29
  experimental, 37–45
    production of intestinal inflammation in animals and, 37–43
    spontaneous animal models of ileitis and colitis and, 43–45
  general findings on, 28t
  problems in approaches to, 3–7

Inflammatory bowel disease (IBD), problems in approaches to, *(Continued)*
  demographic characteristics and, 13–19
  genetic and environmental hypotheses and, 19–27
  morbidity and mortality and, 7–13
  prognosis of, 747–761
    clinical variability in relation to, 747–748
Inflammatory infiltrates, 331, 334
Inflammatory mass, in Crohn's disease, as indication for surgery, 556–557, 576
Inflammatory mediators, intestinal cellular immunity and, 138–139
Inflammatory polyps, in Crohn's disease, 397, 399, *401, 402, 404, 405*
  in ulcerative colitis, 335–336
    radiography and, 382–383, *386–388, 390, 391*
Informed consent, obtaining, 591
Inheritance. *See also* Genetic factors.
  risk of, 320–321
Intercellular junctions, passage through, 66
Interferon, in Crohn's disease, 491
Intermesenteric abscess, 693
International Classification of Disease codes, 5
International Organization for the Study of Inflammatory Bowel Disease (IOIBD), 176
Interpersonal relationships, 215–216
Intestinal absorption. *See also* Malabsorption.
  after resection, 715–724
    extent and area of resection and, 715–716, 716t
    preservation of ileocecal valve and, 724
    specific nutrients and, 716–724
Intestinal adaptation, postoperative, 725–731
  changes in intestinal morphology and, 725–727, *725–727*
  hormones and polyamines and, 729–731
  luminal nutrients and, 728–729
  mechanisms causing, 727–728
  neurovascular effects on, 731
  pancreatobiliary secretions and, 729
Intestinal defenses, 65–72
  immune mechanisms as, 71–72
  macromolecular transport mechanisms as, 65–66
    factors affecting, 66–69, 67t
    pathologic, clinical conditions associated with, 70, 70–71
Intestine. *See also* Colon; Duodenum; Ileum; Small intestine.
  cancers of, 291
  postsurgical functional status of, 731–732
  resected, histologic features in, 341
  surgically bypassed, cancer in, 289
Intra-abdominal abscesses, 264–265, 265t
  undernutrition and, 244
Intraepithelial lymphocytes (IEL), mucosal immune system and, 124
Intraperitoneal abscess, 692
Iodine, requirements for, 523
IOIBD (International Organization for the Study of Inflammatory Bowel Disease), 176
Iritis, 307
Iron, absorption of, impairment by resection, 719
Iron deficiency anemia, in children, 509
Iron supplements, in ulcerative colitis, 436
Ischemia, differential diagnosis of, 202–203, *203*, 346–349
  segmental, 406, *406, 407*
Ischemic colitis, endoscopy and, 365

J-chain, 124
Jejunoileitis, choice of operation in, 588
  in Crohn's disease, as indication for surgery, 560, 574
Jews, incidence of inflammatory bowel disease among, 17t, 17–18
J-pouch, 656–667

Kidney stones. *See* Renal calculi.
Kock pouch. *See* Ileostomy, conventional.
Kveim antigen, response to, 137–138

Laboratory studies. *See also specific studies.*
  for medical therapy in ulcerative colitis, 433
  in colitic arthritis, 303
  in Crohn's disease, 178–179
  in evaluation of pediatric patients, 232–233, 233t
  in toxic megacolon, 272
  in ulcerative colitis, 169t, 170
  intra-abdominal abscess and, 264
Lactation, sulfasalazine and, in Crohn's disease, 483
  sulfasalazine therapy and, 447
D-Lactic acidosis, postoperative, 733–734
Lactose, malabsorption of, 242
Lactose intolerance, in children, 504
LAK (lymphokine-activated killer) cell, 141
Lamina propria, intestinal cellular immunity and, 138
  isolated cells of, 131t, 131–132
  lymphocytes of, mucosal immune system and, 123–124
  plasma cells in, immunohistochemistry of, 127–128
Lectins, mitogenic, 133
  production of intestinal inflammation in animals by, 39
Leprosy, relation of Crohn's disease to, 59
Leukemia, acute, 292
Levamisole, in Crohn's disease, 491
  in ulcerative colitis, 456
L-forms, 58–59
Lidamidine, in ulcerative colitis, 437
Linear ulceration, in Crohn's disease, 339, *339*
Lipid A, 109
Lipopolysaccharide, 109
Liver, fatty, 309–310
Liver disease. *See also* Hepatitis.
  associated with inflammatory bowel disease, 571
Loperamide, in ulcerative colitis, 437
Lymph nodes, anastomotic procedures in Crohn's disease and, 598
  regional, immunopathology of, 127
Lymphatic obstruction, production of intestinal inflammation in animals by, 37–38
Lymphocyte(s), antibodies to, 110–111
  intraepithelial, mucosal immune system and, 124
  of lamina propria, mucosal immune system and, 123–124
  proliferation of, intestinal cellular immunity and, 138
  regulation of, 146
  systemic cellular immunity and, 133–134
Lymphocyte subsets, systemic humoral immunity and, 104–105
Lymphoepithelial cells. *See* Membranous epithelial cells.
Lymphogranuloma venereum, differential diagnosis of, 197, *198*
Lymphoid tissue, in "indeterminate colitis," 345
Lymphokine(s), intestinal cellular immunity and, 138–139
  systemic cellular immunity and, 134–135

Lymphokine-activated killer (LAK) cell, 141
Lymphoma, differentiation of Crohn's disease from, 416
  intestinal, 291
  of colon, 408, 409

M cells. See Membranous epithelial cells.
Macromolecular transport, by M cells, 78–79, 79t
  factors affecting, 66–69, 67t
  mechanisms of, 65–66
  pathologic, clinical conditions associated with, 70, 70–71
Macrophages, intestinal cellular immunity and, 139–140
  systemic cellular immunity and, 135
Magnesium, absorption of, impairment by resection, 718–719
  nutritional assessment and, 517
  requirement for, 525
Magnesium deficiency, 514–515, 517, 718–719
Major histocompatibility complex (MHC) antigens, 97–98
Malabsorption. See also Intestinal absorption.
  following ileostomy, 697
  growth failure and, 232
  in short bowel syndrome, postsurgical, 703–705
  of lactose, 242
  of starch, 242–243
Malignancy. See also Cancer; Neoplasia.
  immunosuppressive drugs and, 456
  screening for, endoscopy and, 368–369
Malnutrition, 513–518. See also Undernutrition.
  as indication for total parenteral nutrition, 520
  etiology of, 513–514, 514t
  growth failure and, 231–232
  in Crohn's disease, in children, 229
  physiologic effects of, 515–517
  prevention and treatment of, 517–518. See also Nutritional support.
  specific deficiencies in, 514–515
Manganese, requirements for, 523
Marital status, epidemiology of inflammatory bowel disease and, 18
Mass lesions, endoscopy and, 355–356
  in Crohn's disease, as indication for surgery, 556–557, 576
Mast cell(s), 131
Mast cell stabilizers, in ulcerative colitis, 456
Medical management, drugs in, 121
  for strictures, 276–277
  in Crohn's disease. See Crohn's disease, medical therapy of.
  in regard to pregnancy and fertility, 324–325, 325t
  in toxic megacolon, 273t, 273–274
  in ulcerative colitis. See Ulcerative colitis, medical therapy in.
  of pediatric patient, 503–510
    approach to patient and, 503–504
Megaloblastic anemia, sulfasalazine and, 444
Membranous epithelial (M) cells, 75–82
  apical membranes of, 78
  distribution and renewal on Peyer's patch domes, 81–82
  function of, 78–81, 79t, 80
  importance of, 82
  morphology of, 76, 77, 78
  origin of, 81

Men, fertility in, 320, 320t
  proctocolectomy in, 638
6-Mercaptopurine, 455–456
  in Crohn's disease, 490
    in children, 506
  pregnancy and, 321–322
  side effects of, 268, 313, 490
Metabolic complications, of total parenteral nutrition, 525t, 525–526
Metabolic management, intraoperative, 594–595
Metabolic manifestations, 309
  in ulcerative colitis, 435
Metabolism, of complement, 114
Metal deficiencies, 514–515
Metaplasia, pyloric, in Crohn's disease, biopsy diagnosis and, 343–344
Metastatic Crohn's disease, 302, 303
Metronidazole, anorectal lesions and, 261–262
  in Crohn's disease, 489–490, 492, 545
    in children, 506
  microflora and, 55
  pregnancy and, 321, 325
  side effects of, 262
MHC (major histocompatibility complex) antigens, 97–98
MICC (mitogen-induced cellular cytotoxicity), 140
Microbial pathogens, antibodies against, 56–57
Microflora, intestinal, 51–61. See also Bacteria; Flora.
  antibodies against, 56
    chronic ulcerative colitis and bacillary dysentery and, 54–55
    Clostridium difficile and inflammatory bowel disease and, 57–58
    experimental colitis and, 57
  in Crohn's disease, 55–56
  mycobacterial, 59–61
  normal, 51–54
  novel, 58–59
  pathogenic, antibodies against, 56–57
Mineral(s), absorption of, small intestine resection and, 718–720
Mineral imbalance, in children, 509
Minnesota Multiphasic Personality Inventory (MMPI), 217
Mitogen-induced cellular cytotoxicity (MICC), 140
Mixed lymphocyte reaction (MLR) assay, 134
MMPI (Minnesota Multiphasic Personality Inventory), 217
Molybdenum, requirements for, 523
Monocytes, systemic cellular immunity and, 135–136
Morbidity, 7–10, 8t–10t
  postoperative, 707–710
Mortality, 12t, 12–13
  of inflammatory bowel disease, 12t, 12–13
  postoperative, 707–710
Motility, control of microorganisms by, 52
  ileal pouch-anal anastomosis and, 665, 666
Mucin depletion, 331
Mucosa, 302, 302
  bacterial relationships of, 52
  cobblestone, 191, 339, 339, 358, 359
  in ulcerative colitis, 170, 171t
  lacking regenerative changes, active ulcerative colitis superimposed on, 337
  morphology of, continent reservoir ileostomy and, 677, 677–678
Mucosal bridges, differential diagnosis and, 359

Mucosal disease, focal, in Crohn's disease, biopsy diagnosis and, 343
Mucosal enteritis, 252
Mucosal immune system, 121–132, *122*
 in inflammatory bowel disease, 125–132
 intraepithelial lymphocytes and, 124
 lamina proprial lymphocytes and, 123–124
 Peyer's patches and, 121–123, *122*
 regulation of response to antigen in intestine and, 125
 secretory IgA and, 124–125
Muscle function, nutritional assessment and, 517
Muscle mass, steroid therapy and, 454
Muscularis mucosae, hypertrophy of, 333
Musculoskeletal manifestations, 302–305
Mycobacteria, 59–61
 antibodies to, 110
 culture isolation studies of, 60–61
 early studies of, 59–60
 in Crohn's disease, 60–61
Mycoplasma, antibodies to, 108

Natural killer (NK) cell, 103, 136–137
 cytotoxicity of, 140–141, 144
Nausea, 239–241, *241*, *242*
 clinical approaches to, 240–241
NBT (nitroblue tetrazolium) dye reduction test, 120
Necrosis, of nipple valve, 696
 with ileostomy, 649, *650*
Necrotizing enterocolitis (NEC), 70
Neonate, sensitization to microbial/mammalian cross-reacting antigen, 71–72, *72*
Neoplasia. See also Cancer; Dysplasia; Malignancy.
 in ulcerative colitis, prognosis of, *753*, 753–754
Neorectal distensibility and capacity, ileal pouch-anal anastomosis and, 663, *664*
Neorectal evacuation, ileal pouch-anal anastomosis and, 664–665, *666*
Neorectal mobility, ileal pouch-anal anastomosis and, 663–664, *664*, *665*
Nephrolithiasis, 305–306
Neuritis, retrobulbar, 308
Neurogenic manipulation, production of intestinal inflammation in animals by, 38
Neurologic complications, postoperative, 707
Neuronal proliferation, in "indeterminate colitis," 345
Neurovascular effects, intestinal adaptation and, 731
Neutrophil(s), drug therapy and, 121
 migration of, 119
 systemic humoral immunity and, 118–121
Neutrophil enzyme markers, 120–121
Niacin, absorption of, impairment by resection, 720
Niacinamide, requirements for, 523
Nipple valve, dysfunction of, 696–697
 necrosis of, 696
Nitroblue tetrazolium (NBT) dye reduction test, 120
NK (natural killer) cell, 103, 136–137
 cytotoxicity of, 140–141, 144
Nodular lymphoid hyperplasia, differential diagnosis of, 358
Nonwhites, incidence of inflammatory bowel disease among, 16–17
Nutrients, requirements for, in children, 232
Nutrition. See also Diet; Intestinal absorption; Malnutrition; Total parenteral nutrition; Undernutrition.
 in Crohn's disease, 477–479
 in ulcerative colitis, 435, 436

Nutritional assessment, 515–516
Nutritional intervention, in Crohn's disease, in children, 507–510
Nutritional support, 518–526
 anorectal lesions and, 262
 selection of patients for, 518, 520

Obstruction, as surgical complication, 702–703
 in Crohn's disease, 249
  as indication for surgery, 540–541, 554–555
  modification of ileocolectomy imposed by, 601
 of small bowel, after ileoanal anastomosis, 700
  following ileostomy, 696
 ileostomy and, 252
Obstructive dysfunctional ileitis, 635–636
Obstructive hydronephrosis, in Crohn's disease, 306
Obstructive uropathy, anastomotic procedures and, 600
 in Crohn's disease, as indication for surgery, 558
Occupation, incidence of inflammatory bowel disease related to, 18–19
Ocular manifestations, 307–308
ODC (ornithine decarboxylase), intestinal absorption and, 731
Olsalazine (azodisalicylate), 449
OMGE (World Organization of Gastroenterology), 176
Oral contraceptives, epidemiology of inflammatory bowel disease and, 27
Oral mucosal manifestations, 302, *302*
Ornithine decarboxylase (ODC), intestinal absorption and, 731
Orosomucoids, in Crohn's disease, 179
Osteoarthropathy, hypertrophic, 305
Osteomyelitis, pelvic, 305
Osteonecrosis, steroid therapy and, 454
Osteoporosis, steroid therapy and, 454
Oxidation-reduced potential (Eh), low, 51–52

Pancreatic insufficiency, small bowel resection and, 732
Pancreatobiliary secretions, intestinal adaptation and, 729
Paneth cells, in quiescent ulcerative colitis, 333
Panproctocolectomy, 586
 in Crohn's disease, 590
 in toxic megacolon, 628
Pantothenic acid, requirements for, 523
Paraileostomy hernia, 698
Parastomal abscesses, with ileostomy, 649, *651*
Parastomal hernia, with ileostomy, 649, *651*
Pathogens. See also *specific pathogens*.
 antibodies against, 56–57
 novel, 58–59
Patient, approach to, 220–223, 465–466
 in Crohn's disease, 492, 494
 educating, 222
 effect of inflammatory bowel disease on, 218–219, 435
 postoperative care of, 628–630, 629t
 preoperative preparation of, 593–594
 psychologic preparation of, for surgery, 591
Patient evaluation, for medical therapy in ulcerative colitis, 431–434
 chronicity and, 434, *434*
 clinical features and, 432–433, 433t
 general principles of, 431, 432t
 histology and, 434
 laboratory studies and, 433

new cases and, 431–432, *432*
radiography and, 434, 434t
Patient selection, for nutritional support, 518, 520
Pelvic abscess, postoperative, 692
Pelvic osteomyelitis, 305
Penicillin, in peritonitis, 690
Pepsin inhibitors, production of intestinal inflammation in animals by, 38
Peptides, 213
immune function and, 214–215
production of intestinal inflammation in animals by, 40
Perforation, as indication for surgery, 534
free, 268–269
colonic, 268
in Crohn's disease, as indication for surgery, 557–558
modification of ileocolectomy imposed by, 601
of small intestine, 268–269
in Crohn's disease, as indication for surgery, 544–545, 556–558, 576
in ulcerative colitis, as indication for surgery, 564, 566–567
Perianal abscess, 259–260, *260*
in Crohn's disease, 559
as indication for surgery, 576
treatment of, 261
Perianal disease, in Crohn's disease, in children, 230
Perianal fistulae, in Crohn's disease, 559
in ulcerative colitis, as indication for surgery, 570
treatment of, 261
Perianal lesions, in Crohn's disease, 177
"Pericholangitis," 310, *310*
Perineal complications, in Crohn's disease, as indication for surgery, 545, 559–560
Perineal sinus, persistent, 694–695
as surgical complication, 630–631, *631–633*
Perineal wound, persistent, 694–695, *695*
Peripheral neuropathies, postoperative, 707
Perirectal abscess, in Crohn's disease, as indication for surgery, 576
Peritonitis, in Crohn's disease, as indication for surgery, 557–558
localized, postoperative, 692
treatment of, 690–692
antimicrobial, 690–691
operative, 691–692
Personality, characteristic, in inflammatory bowel disease patients, 215–216
Peyer's patches, 75–76
distribution and renewal of M cells on domes of, 81–82
mucosal immune system and, 121–123, *122*
Phenobarbital, in ulcerative colitis, 437
Phosphate deficiency, 515
Phosphorus, requirement for, 525
Physical examination, in evaluation of pediatric patients, 232
Physicians, opinions regarding psychosocial factors, 210–211
Plaques, in pseudomembranous enterocolitis, 203, *204*, 205
Plasma albumin, nutritional assessment and, 517
Plasma cells, in deeper layers of bowel wall, immunohistochemistry of, 128
in lamina propria, immunohistochemistry of, 127–128
Plasma chemistry, nutritional assessment and, 516–517
Plasmaphoresis, in Crohn's disease, 491

Pleuropericarditis, 309
Polyamines, intestinal adaptation and, 729–731
Polyarteritis nodosa, cutaneous, 302
Polymorphonuclear leukocytes, sulfasalazine and, 443
Polyps, adenomatous, 753
colonoscopy and, 356
inflammatory, in Crohn's disease, 397, 399, *401*, *402*, *404*, *405*
in ulcerative colitis, 335–336, 382–383, *386–388*, *390*, 391
post-inflammatory, in ulcerative colitis, 464
Potassium, nutritional assessment and, 516
requirement for, 525
Potassium deficiency, 514
Pouchitis, 252, 253, 367, 702
differential diagnosis of, 348–349
Precancer, in ulcerative colitis, as indication for surgery, 567–570, 568t
Pregnancy, corticosteroids and, 488
effects on previously established ileostomy, 324
influence of drug therapy on course of, 321–322
influence of inflammatory bowel disease on outcome of, 322–323, 323t
influence on course of inflammatory bowel disease, 323t, 323–324, 324t
during postpartum period, 324
medical management of inflammatory bowel disease in regard to, 324–325, 325t
proctocolectomy and, 638
sulfasalazine therapy and, 447, 483
Prestomal ileitis. *See* Ileitis, prestomal.
Proctectomy, secondary, 626
Proctitis, allergic, differential diagnosis of, 193
diversion, differential diagnosis of, 193
drug-induced, differential diagnosis of, 348
gonorrheal, differential diagnosis of, 196–197
ulcerative, 167–168
approach to, 458–459
prognosis of, 755–756
Proctocolectomy, *609–613*, 610–612, 655–656. *See also* Colectomy; Ileoanal anastomosis.
in Crohn's disease, 590, 708–709
in ulcerative colitis, 588–589, 708
male sexual dysfunction and, 638
management of perineal wound and, 623–626, *624*, *625*
massive hemorrhage and, 264
perineal phase of, 621, 623, *624*, *625*
pregnancy and, 638
Proctocolitis, 201, 407, *408*
Proctoscopy, in salmonellosis, 194
Proctosigmoiditis, 244–245
Prostaglandins, diarrhea and, 245
in ulcerative colitis, 442
intestinal cellular immunity and, 139
Prostanoids, 245
Protein, absorption of, impairment by resection, 716–717
small intestine resection and, 717–718
requirements for, 521
for children, 508–509, 509t
Pseudomembranous colitis, in children, 236
radiologic appearance of, 387, 392
Pseudomembranous enterocolitis, differential diagnosis of, 203, *204*, 205
Pseudopolyposis, 275–276, *276*
"Pseudopolyps," 335–336
Psychologic preparation, for surgery, 591

Psychosocial factors, 24, 209–224
　in diagnosis and treatment, 219–223
　　approach to patient and, 220–223
　　case analysis and, 223–224
　　need for integrated model and, 219–220
　in ileostomy, 652
　in ulcerative colitis, 435
　literature review and, 210–219, 211t
　　characteristic personality features and, 215–216
　　doctors' opinions and, 210–211
　　impact of disorder and, 217–219
　　mediating mechanisms and, 213–215, *215*
　　psychiatric diagnoses and, 216–217
　　symptom onset and exacerbation and, 211–213
Psychotherapy, 223, 479
Puberty, delayed, 244, 507–508
Pulmonary manifestations, 309
Pyloric metaplasia, in Crohn's disease, biopsy diagnosis and, 343–344
Pyoderma gangrenosum, *300*, 300–301, *301*
Pyostomatitis vegetans, 301
Pyridoxyl phosphate, absorption of, impairment by resection, 720
Pyroxidine, requirements for, 523

Quality of life, continent reservoir ileostomy and, 674–675
　ileal pouch-anal anastomosis and, 660, 661t
　ileostomy and, 637–638
　in Crohn's disease, 182, 761
　in ulcerative colitis, 755

Race, epidemiology of inflammatory bowel disease and, 16t, 16–17
Radiation colitis, differential diagnosis of, 201–202
　endoscopy and, 366
Radiology, 377–427. *See also* Angiography; Computerized tomography; Ultrasound.
　in amebiasis, 200
　in Crohn's disease, 189, *190–192*, 191, 392, 397–420
　　carcinoma and, 421
　　colon and, 397–409, *399–406*
　　esophagus, stomach, and duodenum and, 416–418, *419–422*
　　small intestine and, 409–416, *410–418*
　in evaluation of pediatric patients, 233–234, 234t
　in radiation colitis, 201–202
　in toxic megacolon, 271–272, *272*
　in ulcerative colitis, 169t, 170, 378–392, *379–388*
　　carcinoma and, 384, *393–395*
　　continuity of inflammatory process and, 381–382, *388–389*
　　distinction from other diseases of colon and, 387, 392, *396–398*
　　dysplasia and, 384–385, *395*, *396*
　　inflammatory polyps and, 382–383, *386–388*, *390*, *391*
　　medical therapy and, 434, 434t
　　strictures and, 383–384, *391–393*
　　terminal ileum and, 385–386, *388*, *389*, *396*
　methods of contrast examination and, 377–378
　strictures and, 276
Rectal bleeding, 250
Rectal gonorrhea, 196–197
Rectal sparing, differential diagnosis and, 358–359
　in fulminant colitis, 338
　in "indeterminate colitis," 345
Rectoanal inhibitory response, ileal pouch-anal anastomosis and, 663, *664*

Rectovaginal fistulae, 265
　as indication for surgery, 542–543
Refined sugars, epidemiology of inflammatory bowel disease and, 25
Regenerative changes, in ulcerative colitis, lack of, 336–337
　specificity of, 336
Regional enteritis. *See* Crohn's disease.
Renal calculi, 253, 306
　enhanced formation of, 736–739
　in children, 230
　postoperative, 253–254
Renal manifestations, 305–306
Reoviruses, transport by M cells, 79–80, *80*
Resection, 586
　ileal, diarrhea and, 245–246
　ileocolic, 600, *601*
　ileoproctostomy and, 626–627
　in Crohn's disease, 590
　intestinal absorption after. *See* Intestinal absorption, after resection.
　syndromes associated with, 733–734
Resection margins, anastomotic procedures in Crohn's disease and, 598–599, *599*
Reservoir inflammation. *See* Pouchitis.
Respiratory toilet, in postoperative sepsis, 693
Retraction, of ileostomy, 649
Retrobulbar neuritis, 308
Retroperitoneal abscess, 693
Riboflavin, absorption of, impairment by resection, 720–721
　requirements for, 523
Rural distribution, epidemiology of inflammatory bowel disease and, 18

Sacroiliitis, *304*, 304–305, *305*
Salazopyrin. *See* Sulfasalazine.
Salicylazosulfapyridine. *See* Sulfasalazine.
Salmonellosis, differential diagnosis of, 194–195
　endoscopy and, 363
SASP. *See* Sulfasalazine.
Schistosomiasis, endoscopy and, 363
Sclerosing cholangitis, *311*, 311–312
　radiology and, *424*, 424–425, *425*
Sedatives, in ulcerative colitis, 437
Segmental operations, in Crohn's disease involving colon, 626
Selenium, absorption of, impairment by resection, 719–720
　requirements for, 522–523
Sepsis. *See also* Peritonitis.
　bacterial flora and, 689
　following ileostomy, 700
　postoperative, 689–694
　　localized, 692
　　supportive therapy in, 693–694
Serologic tests, in amebiasis, 200
　in histoplasmosis, 197
Sex, epidemiology of inflammatory bowel disease and, 13, 13t
Sexual development, delayed, 244
Sexual dysfunction, male, proctocolectomy and, 638
　postoperative, 706
Sexual function, with ileal pouch-anal anastomosis, 660
Shigellosis, differential diagnosis of, 195
　endoscopy and, 363
　ulcerative colitis and, 54–55

Short bowel syndrome, as indication for total parenteral nutrition, 520
  as surgical complication, 703–705
Sick role, 217–218, 221
Sigmoidoscopy, in amebiasis, 200
  in evaluation of pediatric patients, 234–235
  in ischemic disease, 203
  in pseudomembranous enterocolitis, *204*, 205
  in radiation colitis, 201
  in ulcerative colitis, in children, 234–235
Sinus, perineal, persistent, 694–695
Skin involvement, 299–302
  allergic, nutritional assessments and, 517
    with ileostomy, 649, *651*
  excoriation of, with ileostomy, 649, *651*
  irritation of, with ileostomy, 649, *650*
  lesions of, anorectal, 258–259, *259*
  reactions of, to sulfasalazine, 444
Skin tags, edematous, 258
Skin test responses, systemic cellular immunity and, 137–138
Skip lesions, proximal, modification of ileocolectomy imposed by, 603
Small intestine. *See also* Ileum, terminal.
  adenocarcinoma of, in Crohn's disease, 288
  contrast examination methods for, 378
  disease of, pathophysiology of diarrhea in, 245–247
  free perforation of, 268–269
  in Crohn's disease, radiology and, 409–416, *410–418*
  obstruction of, after ileoanal anastomosis, 700
    as indication for total parenteral nutrition, 521
    following ileostomy, 696
  resection of, effect on absorption of nutrients. *See* Intestinal resection, resorption after.
Smoking, epidemiology of inflammatory bowel disease and, 26t, 26–27
Socioeconomic factors, epidemiology of inflammatory bowel disease and, 18–19
Sodium, requirement for, 524–525
Sodium deficiency, 514
  with ileostomy, 652
Solitary rectal ulcer syndrome, differential diagnosis of, 347, *348*
  endoscopy and, 365–366
Somatomedins, growth and, in children, 509
Spermatozoa, sulfasalazine and, 444–445
S-pouch, 701–702
Spouses, inflammatory bowel disease cases among, 89
Squamous carcinoma, intestinal, 291
Stagnant-loop syndrome, 55–56
  as indication for surgery, 561
Starch, malabsorption of, 242–243
Steatorrhea, 243
  resection and, 718
Steroids. *See also* Corticosteroids.
  in acute colitis, 460
  in Crohn's disease, 494
  in ulcerative colitis, 450–455
    adverse effects and, 454–455, 455t
    clinical trials and, 451–452
    local, 453–454
    maintenance therapy and, 453
    mechanism of action and, 450–451
  in ulcerative proctitis, 458
  pregnancy and, 325
  side effects of, 312–313, 454–455, 455t
Stomach, contrast examination methods for, 378
  diseases of, complicating small bowel resection, 732
  endoscopy and, 372
  in Crohn's disease, radiology and, 416–418, *419*, *420*
Stomal fistulae, with ileostomy, 649
Stomal ileitis, 698
Stool, bloody, in ulcerative colitis, 168
Stool examination, in Crohn's disease, in children, 233
  in salmonellosis, 194
Stress, immune function and, 214–215
  ulcerative colitis and, 437
Stricture(s), 276–278
  anastomotic, 700
  benign, in ulcerative colitis, 335
  endoscopy and, 355–356
  following ileostomy, 697
  in Crohn's disease, 277–278
    as indication for surgery, 560, 575
    colonic, 277, *277*
    of small intestine, 278
  in lymphogranuloma venereum, 197, *198*
  in ulcerative colitis, 276–277
    as indication for surgery, 560, 570, 575
    radiography and, 383–384, *391–393*
  multiple or recurrent, as surgical complication, 703, *703*
Strictureplasty, in Crohn's disease, *681*, 681–682
  modification of ileocolectomy imposed by, 604, *604*
Subhepatic abscess, 692–693
Submucosal inflammation, disproportionate, in Crohn's disease, biopsy diagnosis and, 343
Subphrenic abscess, 692–693
Sucralfate, in ulcerative colitis, 457
Sugars, epidemiology of inflammatory bowel disease and, 25
Sulfapyridine. *See* Sulfasalazine.
Sulfasalazine, circulating cells and, 106
  in acute colitis, 460
  in children, 504, 505, 506
  in Crohn's disease, 479–483, 492, 539
    adverse effects and desensitization and, 482–483
    clinical studies and, 479, 480t, 481
    drug interactions and, 483
    in children, 506
    pharmacology and, 481–482, *482*
    pregnancy and nursing and, 483
  in severe colitis, 462
  in ulcerative colitis, *438*, 438–447, 459, 464
    adverse reactions and, 443–445
    clinical experience with, 438–439
    intolerance and allergy and, 446t, 446–447
    maintenance therapy with, 439, *439*
    mechanism of action and, 441–443, *442*
    pharmacology and, 439–441, *440*
    pregnancy, lactation, and children and, 447
  in ulcerative proctitis, 458
  leukotrienes and, 139
  neutrophil function and, 121
  pregnancy and, 321, 324–325, 447, 483
  side effects of, 240, 312, 443–445, 482–483
Sulfonamides, microflora and, 55
Sulphasalazine. *See* Sulfasalazine.
Superoxide dismutase, in Crohn's disease, 491–492
Supportive therapy, in postoperative sepsis, 693–694
  in ulcerative colitis, 436
Suppositories, 5-ASA, 448
Surgery, 585–638. *See also specific procedures.*
  anorectal lesions and, 262
  choice of operation and, 586–591, 587t
  complications of, 685–710. *See also specific complications and surgical procedures.*

Surgery, complications of, *(Continued)*
    neurologic, 707
    septic, 689–694
    urogenital, 705–707
    wound and, 685–689
  diversion proctitis and, 193
  historic perspective on, 585–586
  in Crohn's disease. *See* Crohn's disease, surgical treatment for.
  in peritonitis, 691–692
  in pyoderma gangrenosum, 301
  in toxic megacolon, 274–275, 463
  in ulcerative colitis. *See* Ulcerative colitis, surgical treatment for.
  in ulcerative proctitis, prognosis of, 756
  indications for, 529–546, 549–576
    in colonic inflammatory disease, 562t, 562–576
    in Crohn's disease, 535–546, 535t–539t, 549–562
    in ulcerative colitis, 529–535
  intraoperative physiologic and metabolic management and, 594–596, *595*
  management of corticosteroids and, 591–593, 592t
  physiologic consequences of, 715–739, 716t
    factors affecting intestinal absorption and, 715–724
    functional status of remaining intestine and digestive organs and, 731–732
    interruption of bile salt enterohepatic circulation and, 734–739
    intestinal adaptation and, 724–731
    syndrome associated with intestinal resection and, 733–734
  postoperative care and, 628–630, 629t
  postoperative complications and, 250–254, 630–636
  pregnancy and, 323
  preoperative preparation of patient and, 593–594
  psychologic preparation and informed consent and, 591
  results of operation and, 636–638
  specific techniques in, 596–628
  total parenteral nutrition prior to, 520
Susceptibility, genetic, 93
Systemic complications, in Crohn's disease, as indication for surgery, 561–562
Systemic immunity, sulfasalazine and, 443

T cell(s), cytotoxic, 132, 136, 140
  immunology and, 104–105
  in intestinal lesions, immunohistochemistry of, 129
  mucosal immune system and, 122–123, 124
  regulatory function of, 146
  suppressor, 125
T cell subsets, systemic humoral immunity and, 105–106
Terminal ileitis, in Crohn's disease, biopsy diagnosis and, 343, *343*
Terminal ileum. *See* Ileum, terminal.
Tetanus toxoid, response to, 111–112
Tetracycline, pregnancy and, 322
Therapeutic relationship, establishing, 221–222
Therapy related manifestations, 312–313
Thiamine, absorption of, impairment by resection, 720
  requirements for, 523
Thrombosis, deep vein, 308
"Thyrogastric complex," 111
TNB (trinitrobenzenosulfonic acid), production of intestinal inflammation in animals by, 38

Total parenteral nutrition (TPN), 520–526
  administration routes for, 521
  adverse effects of, 313
  complications of, 525t, 525–526
  in children, 508
  in Crohn's disease, 478, 545
    in children, 508
  in malabsorption-short bowel syndrome, 704
  in postoperative sepsis, 694
  in severe colitis, 461
  in toxic megacolon, 273
  in ulcerative colitis, 457–458
  indications for, 520–521
  nutritional requirements and, 521–525
  pregnancy and, 322
Toxic colitis, acute, in Crohn's disease, 408–409
Toxic megacolon, 334–335, *335*
  acute, 269–275
    diagnostic features of, 271–272
    pathophysiology of, 269–270
    risk factors for, 270t, 270–271
    treatment of, 273–275
  approach to, 462–463
  as indication for surgery, 566
    in Crohn's disease, 575–576
    in fulminant colitis, 532–533
    in ulcerative colitis, 564, 565t, 566–567
  in ulcerative colitis, 334–335, *335*
    as indication for surgery, 564, 565t, 566–567
    in children, 229
  surgical treatment of, *627*, 627–628
Trace elements, deficiency of, 239–240
  requirements for, 522–523
Tranexamic acid, in ulcerative colitis, 457
Transcobalamins, 120–121
Transfer factor, in Crohn's disease, 491
Transmural inflammation, in Crohn's disease, 340
Trinitrobenzenosulfonic acid (TNB), production of intestinal inflammation in animals by, 38
Tuberculin responses, 137
Tuberculosis, differential diagnosis of, 195–196
  differentiation of Crohn's disease from, 416, *418*
  endoscopy and, 363
  in children, 236
Turnbull's multiple "ostomy" procedure, 628
Turner's syndrome, association of inflammatory bowel disease with, 92, 93
Twin studies, 21, 22t, 88–89

Ulcer(s), aphthous, differential diagnosis and, 358
  in Crohn's disease, 126, *342*, 342–343
  "bear claw," 358
  "collar button," in Crohn's colitis, 191
  differential diagnosis and, 358
  fissuring, in "indeterminate colitis," 345
  linear, in Crohn's disease, 339, *339*
  metastatic, 258
  rectal, solitary, differential diagnosis of, 347, *348*
    endoscopy and, 365–366
  V-shaped, in fulminant colitis, 341–342
Ulcerative colitis. *See also* Inflammatory bowel disease.
  acute, approach to, 460
    pathology of, *330*, 330–332
  acute exacerbation by superimposed infection, 337
  anal lesions in, pathology of, 336
  bacillary dysentery and, 54–55
  backwash ileitis in, pathology of, 335

Ulcerative colitis, (Continued)
 benign strictures in, pathology of, 335
 cancer in. See Cancer, in ulcerative colitis.
 chronically active, pathology of, 333
 coexistent with Crohn's disease, 345–346
 course of, 170–172
  following first attack, 172t, 172–174
 degrees of severity of, 185–186
 differential diagnosis of, 185–186, 187–188
 distal, 185, 186
 endogenous microflora in, 52–54
 experimental, 57
 granulomas in, 337–338
 HLA antigens in, 98–99, 101t, 102–103
 immunologic features of, compared with features of Crohn's disease, 147
 in children, 752
  medical management of, 504–505
  severity of, 504–505
  surgical intervention in, 505
 in pregnancy, 323–324
 inflammatory polyps in, pathology of, 335–336
 initial attack of, 168–170, 169, 169t
 left-sided, 748–749
  approach to, 459–460
 medical therapy in, 431–466
  approach to patient and family and, 465–466
  approaches to clinical situations and, 458–460
  complications of, 435
  corticosteroids in, 459
  diet and nutritional factors and, 436
  extensive disease and, 460–463
  extraintestinal complications and, 464–465
  failure of, as indication for surgery, 529–532, 530t–532t
  intestinal complications and, 464
  maintenance, 464
  medical management and, 435
  patient evaluation and, 431–434
  psychosocial factors and, 435
  refractory disease and, 463–464
  sulfasalazine in. See Sulfasalazine, in ulcerative colitis.
  therapeutic agents and, 436–457
  total parenteral nutrition and, 457–458
 mild, in children, 504
 moderate, approach to, 460–461
  in children, 504
 pathology of, 329–336
  distribution of disease and, 330
  histologic findings and, 330
 postsurgical recurrence, morbidity and mortality in, 708
 preclinical, pathology of, 338
 prognosis of, 748–755
  colectomy and, 752–753
  neoplasia and, 753, 753–754
  prognostic factors and, 750–752
  quality of life and, 755
  survival and, 749–750, 749–751
 quiescent, pathology of, 332, 332–333, 333
 radiology in. See Radiology, in ulcerative colitis.
 refractory, approach to, 463–464
 resolving, pathology of, 332
 severe, approach to, 460–462
  in children, 504–505
  pathology of, 333–334, 334
 strictures in, 276–277

 surgical treatment for, 172, 173, 173, 655–681
  cancer and, 284–285
  choice of operation and, 588–590
  in children, 505
  indications for, 529–535, 563–571
 symptoms of, 168
 toxic dilatation and perforation in, pathology of, 334–335, 335
 toxic megacolon in, 269
 unusual biopsy appearances in, 336–338
Ulcerative proctitis, 167–168
 approach to, 458–459
 incidence of, 7–8
 prognosis of, 755–756
  cancer risk and, 756
  definition and activity of disease and, 755
  surgical treatment and, 756
  survival and, 756
Ultrasound, 422, 422–423
 in evaluation of pediatric patients, 234
Undernutrition, 241–244, 243, 245t
Upper gut, massive hemorrhage of, 263
Urban distribution, epidemiology of inflammatory bowel disease and, 18
Ureteronephrolithiasis, postoperative, 706–707
Urinary stones, 306
 uric acid, postoperative enhanced formation of, 736–737
Urinary tract fistulae, 265–266, 266
Urogenital complications, postoperative, 705–707, 736–737
Uropathy, obstructive, anastomotic procedures and, 600
Uveitis, 307, 307
 in children, 230

Vagotomy, in Crohn's disease, 591
Vascular changes, production of intestinal inflammation in animals by, 38
Vascular manifestations, 308–309
Vasculitis, 302, 308–309
Vasopressin, massive hemorrhage and, 263–264
Vennimun, in Crohn's disease, 491
Viruses, antibodies to, 108
Vitamin deficiencies, 515
Vitamins, absorption of, small intestine resection and, 720–724
 requirements for, 523–524
Vomiting, 239–241, 241, 242
 clinical approaches to, 240–241

Water, deficit of, with ileostomy, 652
 requirement for, 524
Weight loss, in Crohn's disease, 176
Women, fertility in, 319–320
World Organization of Gastroenterology (OMGE), 176
Wound, perineal, persistent, 694–695, 695
Wound infection, 686–687
Wound separation, 687–688, 688

Yersinia, endoscopy and, 363
 in acute enteritis, 550

Zinc, absorption of, impairment by resection, 719
 requirements for, 522
Zinc deficiency, 239–240, 719
 in children, 509